CONNECTING MEDICAL INFORMATICS AND BIO-INFORMATICS

Studies in Health Technology and Informatics

This book series was started in 1990 to promote research conducted under the auspices of the EC programmes' Advanced Informatics in Medicine (AIM) and Biomedical and Health Research (BHR) bioengineering branch. A driving aspect of international health informatics is that telecommunication technology, rehabilitative technology, intelligent home technology and many other components are moving together and form one integrated world of information and communication media. The complete series has been accepted in Medline. Volumes from 2005 onwards are available online.

Series Editors:
Dr. J.P. Christensen, Prof. G. de Moor, Dr. A. Famili, Prof. A. Hasman, Prof. L. Hunter, Dr. I. Iakovidis, Dr. Z. Kolitsi, Dr. O. Le Dour, Dr. A. Lymberis, Dr. P. Niederer, Prof. A. Pedotti, Prof. O. Rienhoff, Prof. F.H. Roger France, Dr. N. Rossing, Prof. N. Saranummi, Dr. E.R. Siegel and Dr. P. Wilson

Volume 116

Recently published in this series

ISSN 0926-9630

Connecting Medical Informatics and Bio-Informatics

Proceedings of MIE2005

The XIXth International Congress of the European Federation for Medical Informatics

Edited by

Rolf Engelbrecht

*Institute for Medical Informatics, GSF National Research Centre
for Environment and Health, Munich-Neuherberg, Germany*

Antoine Geissbuhler

Service of Medical Informatics, University Hospitals of Geneva, Switzerland

Christian Lovis

Service of Medical Informatics, University Hospitals of Geneva, Switzerland

and

George Mihalas

*Department of Biophysics and Medical Informatics, "Victor Babes"
University of Medicine and Pharmacy, Timisoara, Romania*

IOS
Press

Amsterdam • Berlin • Oxford • Tokyo • Washington, DC

ISBN 1-58603-549-5
Library of Congress Control Number: 2005930831

Publisher
IOS Press
Nieuwe Hemweg 6B
1013 BG Amsterdam
Netherlands
fax: +31 20 620 3419
e-mail: order@iospress.nl

Distributor in the UK and Ireland
IOS Press/Lavis Marketing
73 Lime Walk
Headington
Oxford OX3 7AD
England
fax: +44 1865 750079

Distributor in the USA and Canada
IOS Press, Inc.
4502 Rachael Manor Drive
Fairfax, VA 22032
USA
fax: +1 703 323 3668
e-mail: iosbooks@iospress.com

Connecting Medical Informatics and Bio-Informatics
R. Engelbrecht et al. (Eds.)
IOS Press, 2005

v

Preface

After a successful MEDINFO in 1992, the Swiss Society for Medical Informatics hosts again a major event in medical informatics – the 19th Medical Informatics Europe Conference, under the generic name of MIE2005. The host city, Geneva, is well known for its commitment in international healthcare, being the residence of several international organisations, including WHO. Geneva is also synonym with other major medical informatics achievements: the DIOGENE hospital information system and Natural Language Processing, both strongly connected to Geneva and its University Hospital.

The motto of the conference, "Connecting Medical Informatics and Bio-Informatics" emphasizes the convergence of these disciplines, illustrated by the Swiss Institute of Bioinformatics, also founded in Geneva, and home of the SwissProt database. It also reflects the growing role of the co-operation of different disciplines in healthcare, co-operation which tends to become integration.

The major challenge of this decade is to develop and extend the use of information technology for the improvement of patient oriented health care. It has to integrate results from other areas and scientific disciplines, and interoperability will be the key problem to be solved. All these trends were already reflected in MIE2005 submissions and addressed a large palette of topics, including classical topics as standards, terminology, coding, imaging etc.

The selection process was a difficult task for the Scientific Program Committee. We kept the scientific quality as the major determinant criterion for selection. There were over 300 submitted papers to be presented orally or as poster. A score was given by 2 and more reviewers selected from a panel of more than 160 experts. The reviews were accompanied by suggestions and advice about possible improvements of the submitted paper. The type of presentation was sometimes modified from oral presentation to a short oral presentation combined with a poster or just a poster for detailed presentation and deep discussion. In a second step, when creating the scientific programme, there were a few modifications of the presentation type, mainly due to the limited time slots available for oral presentations.

The result of SPC activity is reflected by the Conference programme and the Proceedings. The printed version has limited pages and therefore limited numbers of papers of all types of presentations (oral and poster presentations) which are most qualified. It will be cited in Medline. The full content was proposed for the CD version of the proceedings; it is an EFMI publication and contains all accepted papers in the revised version and also the workshops. This way of publishing enables searching keywords, the title and the full content.

Workshops were offered to the participants like in previous MIEs, organised or supported by EFMI working groups. A clearer distinction between presentations in workshops and presentations in scientific sessions was aimed: while a pure scientific paper presents results in a classical manner, a workshop paper would rather present and comment unfulfillments or raise questions. The workshop procedure comprises a brief introduction (usually invited), followed by several short statements or presentations. The major output is expected from discussions. The results which might be achieved will be published after MIE2005 separately. All documents, (material from the workshops) available at publishing time will be included on the CD proceedings. We plan to make it also available on the EFMI web site by the moment of this material publication.

We shall also mention that the call for tutorials resulted in a set of high ranked contributions, included in the "scientific workflow" of each MIE conference. They will provide basics and deep insight into certain disciplines and topics related to medical informatics. It may help to develop a better understanding of some presentations and workshops during MIE2005. In this context tutorials are a substantial part and the material developed should be available to a broader community.

The proceedings are an integrated part of MIE2005. We would like to thank all those who have made the printed volume and the CD possible, the authors, the scientific programme committee, the reviewers, and the teams in Geneva and Munich, Robert Baud, Jérôme Billet, Henning Müller, Claudia Hildebrand, Ruslan David, Jutta Balint, Alfred Breier, Silvia Weinzierl and some more.

Rolf Engelbrecht
Antoine Geissbuhler
Christian Lovis
Gheorghe Mihalas

Reviewers for MIE2005

The following reviewers, listed in alphabetical order, contributed to the selection process of the papers.

Abidi, Raza
Afrin, Lawrence
Åhleldt, Hans
Albuisson, Eliane
Ammenwerth, Elske
Pitsillides, Andreas
Angelidis, Pantelis
Aronsky, Dominik
Arredondo, María Teresa
Bainbridge, Mike
Barber, Barry
Barton, Amy
Baud, Robert
Bellazzi, Riccardo
Betts, Helen
Beuscart, Régis
Beuscart-Zéphir, Marie-Catherine
Blobel, Bernd
Bodenreider, Olivier
Boire, Jean-Yves
Brender, Jytte
Brigl, Birgit
Bruins Slot, Harm
Brunetaud, Jean Marc
Bruun-Rasmussen, Morten
Bryden, John S.
Bürkle, Thomas
Ceinos, Carmen
Charlet, Jean
Christian, Lovis
Chute, Christopher
Cimino, James
Cinquin, Philippe
Cornet, Ronald
Darmoni, Stefan
David, Ruslan
de Keizer, Nicolette
de Lusignan, Simon
Demichelis, Francesca

Demiris, Thanos
Dudeck, Joachim
Dumitru, Roxana Corina
Effken, Judith
Eich, Hans-Peter
Eils, Roland
Engelmann, Uwe
Frankewitsch, Thomas
Fruman, Amir
García-Rojo, Marcial
Garde, Sebastian
Geissbuhler, Antoine
Gell, Guenther
Gibaud, Bernard
Goetz, Christoph
Goh, Hsien Ming
Grimson, Jane
Grimson, William
Hasman, Arie
Heinzl, Harald
Hildebrand, Claudia
Hippe, Zdzislaw
Hirose, Yasuyuki
Hoelzer, Simon
Horsch, Alexander
Hovenga, Evelyn
Huet, Bernard
Isaacs, Sedick
Jao, Chiang
Jaulent, Marie-Christine
Jávor, András
Jenders, Robert
Joubert, Michel
Juhola, Martti
Jung, Benjamin
Kern, Josipa
Kindler, Hauke
Knaup, Petra
Kokol, Peter

Kondo Oestreicher, Mitsuko
Krauthammer, Michael
Kuma, Hisao
Kverneland, Arne
Kwak, Yun Sik
Laforest, Frederique
Lampe, Kristian
Landais, Paul
Le Beux, Pierre
Le Duff, Franck
Legrand, Louis
Lehmann, Thomas
Lehmann, Christoph
Leiner, Florian
Li, Jack
Liaskos, Joseph
Lippert, Soren
Lorenzi, Nancy
Lungeanu, Diana
Maglaveras, Nicos
Makikawa, Masaaki
Marsh, Andy
Martin-Sanchez, Fernando
Mast, Oliver
Mazzoleni, M.Cristina
Meinzer, Hans-Peter
Mihalas, George
Minato, Kotaro
Moehr, Jochen
Moisil, Ioana
Nishibori, Masahiro
Nordberg, Ragnar
Olivieri, Nora
Oswald, Helmut
Øyri, Karl
Petrovecki, Mladen
Pharow, Peter
Popper, Mikulas

Power, Michael
Punys, Vytenis
Rajkovic, Vladislav
Reichert, Assa
Renard, Jean-Marie
Rigby, Michael
Roberts, Jean
Roger France, Francis
Rossing, Niels
Ruotsalainen, Pekka
Sadan, Batami
Saranummi, Niilo
Sboner, Andrea
Serio, Angelo
Seroussi, Brigitte
Shahsavar, Nosrat
Shifrin, Michael
Simon, Pál
Skiba, Diane
Sousa Pereira, Antonio
Stoicu-Tivadar, Lacramioara
Stroetmann, Karl A.
Surján, György
Suselj, Marjan
Takabayashi, Katsuhiko
Talmon, Jan
Trpisovsky, Tomas
Tschopp, Mathias
van Bemmel, Jan H.
Vellidou, Eleftheria
Vimarlund, Vivian
Vovc, Victor
Wathelet, Bernard
Weber, Patrick
Weltner, János
Yuasa, Tetsuya
Zvárová, Jana

Contents

Section 4. Educational Technologies and Methodologies

Section 5. Handheld and Wireless Computing

Section 6. Healthcare Networks

Section 7. Imaging Informatics

Section 8. Implementation & Evaluation of Clinical Systems

Section 9. Terminologies, Ontologies, Standards and Knowledge Engineering

Section 10. Natural Language, Text Mining and Information Retrieval

Section 11. Online Health Information & Patient Empowerment

Section 12. Organization Change, Information Needs

Section 13. Public Health Informatics, Clinical Trials

Section 1

Bioinformatics and Medical Genomics

Connecting Medical Informatics and Bio-Informatics
R. Engelbrecht et al. (Eds.)
IOS Press, 2005

3

Immunogenetics Sequence Annotation: the Strategy of IMGT based on IMGT-ONTOLOGY

Véronique Giudicelli[a], Denys Chaume[a], Joumana Jabado-Michaloud[a], Marie-Paule Lefranc[a, b]

[a]*Laboratoire d'ImmunoGénétique Moléculaire, LIGM, Université Montpellier II, Institut de Génétique Humaine, Montpellier, France*
[b]*Institut Universitaire de France, 103 Boulevard Saint Michel, 75005 Paris, France*

Abstract

> *IMGT, the international ImMunoGeneTics information system® (http://imgt.cines.fr) created in 1989, by the Laboratoire d'ImmunoGénétique Moléculaire (LIGM), Université Montpellier II and CNRS, Montpellier, France, is a high quality integrated information system, specialized in immunoglobulins (IG), T cell receptors (TR), major histocompatibility complex of human and other vertebrates and related proteins of the immune system that belong to the IgSF and Mhc superfamilies. IMGT/LIGM-DB, the first and the largest IMGT database, manages more than 92,000 IG and TR nucleotide sequences from human and 150 other vertebrate species in May 2005. IMGT/LIGM-DB provides expertly annotated sequences and standardized knowledge based on IMGT-ONTOLOGY, the first ontology for immunogenetics and immunoinformatics. The strategy developed by IMGT, for the IG and TR nucleotide sequence annotation, involves two different approaches that depend on the nature of the sequences, genomic DNA (gDNA) or complementary DNA (cDNA).*

Keywords:
Immunogenetics; IMGT; Immunoinformatics; Sequence annotation; Database; Immunoglobulin; T cell receptor; Antibody

1. Introduction

IMGT, the international ImMunoGeneTics information system® (http://imgt.cines.fr) [1], created in 1989, by the Laboratoire d'ImmunoGénétique Moléculaire (LIGM), at the Université Montpellier II and CNRS, Montpellier, France, is a high quality integrated information system, specialized in immunoglobulins (IG), T cell receptors (TR), major histocompatibility complex of human and other vertebrates and related proteins of the immune system that belong to the IgSF and MhcSF superfamilies. IMGT® is the international reference in immunogenetics and immunoinformatics and consists of several sequence, genome and structure databases, of Web resources and of interactive tools [2]. IMGT/LIGM-DB is the first and the largest IMGT database in which are managed, analysed and annotated more than 92,000 IG and TR nucleotide sequences (in May 2005) from human and 150 other vertebrate species. The expert annotation of these sequences and the added standardized knowledge are based on IMGT-ONTOLOGY [3], the first ontology developed in the field of immunogenetics and immunoinformatics. IMGT genome annotation has allowed the IG and TR genes to be entered in the genome database, LocusLink and Entrez Gene at NCBI [4,5]. This has been a crucial IMGT contribution as these genes were not identified in the large sequencing project, owing to their unusual structure (non classical exon/intron structure). In contrast to other loci, where genome annotation means gene identification usually obtained with automatic procedures, genome annotation of IG and TR loci can only be performed manually by experts. The IMGT strategy for the sequence annotation takes into account the complexity of the IG and TR synthesis and genetics [4, 5] and the need of an automatic procedure due to the acceleration of the sequencing rate of expressed repertoires.

This strategy involves two different approaches that depend on the nature of the sequences, genomic DNA (gDNA) or complementary DNA (cDNA): (i) the annotation of gDNA (germline or rearranged sequences) includes the search of specific IG and TR motifs and requires a high quality manual curation, by an expert, for the characterization and the classification of new genes in large sequences. The gene and allele related knowledge, based on the IMGT-ONTOLOGY CLASSIFICATION concept, is managed, for the human and mouse, in IMGT/GENE-DB [6], the IMGT gene database, and for the other vertebrates, in IMGT Repertoire, the IMGT Web resources [7]; (ii) the annotation of cDNA (rearranged sequences), despite the complexity of the IG and TR synthesis, has been automatised. This has been possible as the necessary rules for the automatic annotation include the identification of the sequences, the description of the constitutive motifs and the codon and amino acid numbering. These rules, described in the IMGT Scientific chart, correspond to the IMGT-ONTOLOGY IDENTIFICATION, DESCRIPTION and NUMEROTATION concepts [3], respectively. They have been encoded in IMGT/Automat [8], a Java program developed by IMGT, which automatically annotates the IG and TR cDNA sequences. IMGT/Automat implements the IMGT/V-QUEST tool [9] for the gene and allele identification and classification, and the amino acid numbering, and the IMGT/JunctionAnalysis tool [10] for the detailed analysis of the V-J or V-D-J junction. More than 9,000 human and mouse cDNA have already been successfully automatically annotated.

The two different approaches of the IMGT sequence annotation strategy for gDNA and cDNA, respectively, guarantee, by their complementarity, the validity, the accuracy and the coherence of the annotations of the nucleotide sequences in IMGT/LIGM-DB. Annotation accuracy and reliability are the determining factors for the exploitation of the immunogenetic sequences in sectors as exacting as fundamental research, therapeutical approaches and medical research, veterinary research and antibody engineering.

2. Material and methods

IMGT/LIGM-DB entries

IMGT/LIGM-DB manages all IG and TR sequences published in the generalist EMBL/DDBJ/GenBank [11-13]. These sequences mostly belong to the 'HUM', 'MUS', 'ROD', 'MAM' and 'VRT' divisions. IG and TR sequences include germline (not rearranged) gDNA sequences, rearranged gDNA sequences that result from V-J or V-D-J gene recombination in B or T cells, and rearranged cDNA sequences. A prototype of the molecular organization of the 3 types of IG or TR sequences, with the main IMGT feature labels, is shown in Figure 1 [4, 5].

Annotation of the gDNA sequences

The annotation of the gDNA sequences consists in the localization of genes, the prediction of exons, the determination of regulation signals such as promoters and splicing sites, and the similarity evaluation with other known genes. The programs that usually accomplish these tasks,

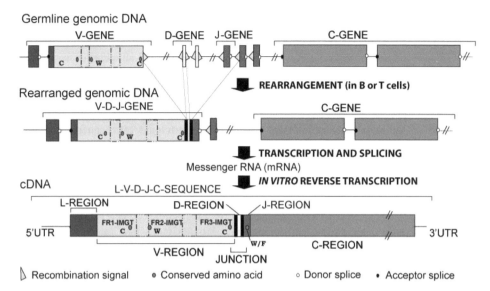

Figure 1-Prototypes of IG or TR germline genomic DNA (gDNA), rearranged gDNA and cDNA [4,5]. The IMGT labels (in capital letters) are according to the DESCRIPTION concept of IMGT-ONTOLOGY [3]. Messenger RNA (mRNA) and cDNA have the same structure and share the same labels. Note that sequences qualified as mRNA in the databases are actually cDNA.

are inefficient to find IG and TR genes owing to the particular structure of these genes: as an example, Figure 1 shows that the second exon of a variable gene in germline configuration (V-GENE) does not end with a stop codon in 3', but instead ends with a characteristic IG or TR recombination signal which is involved in the V-J or V-D-J DNA rearrangement. The diversity genes (D-GENE) and junction genes (J-GENE) do not begin with an initiation codon in 5' [4, 5]. Moreover their coding regions are very short (less than 20 amino acids) and the classical tools are not able to predict them correctly. IMGT has therefore developed a program to search for specific IG and TR motifs, LIGMotif, based on the recognition of the recombination signals, splicing sites and the IMGT standardized numbering of the codons which allows, in particular, to localize the conserved amino acids (Figure 1). IMGT has defined a reference sequence for each gene and allele. The sets of these reference sequences constitute the IMGT reference directory. The coding regions of the new identified genes are then compared, by BLAST, FASTA and IMGT/V-QUEST, to the sequences of the IMGT reference directory. The manual curation by an expert is essential and crucial for the gene identification and classification, the characterization of its alleles, the definition of its structure and of its functionality. These annotations are based on the IMGT-ONTOLOGY concepts [3] and on the rules of the IMGT Scientific chart [2, 7].

Annotation of the cDNA sequences

The cDNA represent more than one half of IMGT/LIGM-DB and most of these sequences are from human and mouse. The IG and TR genomic loci of these species have been studied in IMGT extensively, and all known genes and alleles from human and mouse [4-6] have been characterized. The corresponding coding sequences are in the IMGT reference directory [2]. Since the human and mouse cDNA sequences result from the rearrangement of known IMGT genes and alleles, these sequences can successfully be analysed by the IMGT sequence analysis tools, and then automatically annotated by IMGT/Automat [8].

IMGT/Automat, a Java program, analyses a cDNA sequence and produces a totally automatic and complete annotation. IMGT/Automat relies on the main concepts of IMGT-ONTOLOGY [3]. The four main tasks of IMGT/Automat are shown in Figure 2. IMGT/Automat implements the previously developed software IMGT/V-QUEST [9] that compares and aligns the cDNA sequences with the IMGT reference directory sequences of the same species and of the same type. IMGT/Automat deduces the IDENTIFICATION of the chain type, the CLASSIFICATION of the V, D, and J genes and alleles and the numbering of the codons and amino acids according to the NUMEROTATION concept. Then IMGT/Automat performs the DESCRIPTION of the IG and TR specific constitutive motifs. It delimits the framework regions (FR-IMGT) and complementarity determining regions (CDR-IMGT) according to the biological rules described elsewhere [4,5].

The description of the junction between the V-D-J or or V-J genes is performed by the IMGT/JunctionAnalysis tool [10]. Java methods, based on motif comparison, allow the delimitation of the signal peptide (location of the initiation codon), of the constant region (location of the stop codon), of the untranslated sequences in 5' and in 3', and of the composed coding regions (for example: L-V-D-J-C-REGION or L-V-J-C-REGION). In a third step, the functionality of the sequence is defined according to the biological rules of the IMGT Scientific chart [2,4,5]. The biological origin and the methodology used (part of the OBTENTION concept), when indicated by the authors, are integrated in the annotation. Finally, the complete annotation is integrated in IMGT/LIGM-DB. At each step, IMGT/Automat checks the meaning and the coherence of the results. The annotation is validated, at the end of the first step, if the alignment score of the V-GENE performed by IMGT/V-QUEST is higher than a fixed value.

This score is reliable since the alignment is always performed on sequences of about 330 nucleotides. Our background in the analysis of IMGT/V-QUEST alignments led us to set this value to 1000. Under this value, the automatic annotation is stopped. The annotation is validated, at the end of the second step (description), if the delimitation of the motifs is in agreement with the prototype of the cDNA (Figure 1). Coherence of the third step verifies the functionality of the cDNA, and validates the annotation of sequences that are defined as «productive». The other sequences, defined as «unproductive», are set apart as they need an additional manual expertise.

3. Results

The annotation of IG and TR gDNA sequences, based on the search of specific motifs and manual expertise, represents the essential and indispensable step to identify, to characterize and to classify all the germline genes and alleles, for a given species and a given chain type. That expertise has completely been realized by IMGT, for the genes and alleles from human and mouse, and data are available in IMGT/GENE-DB [6]. The nomenclature elaborated by IMGT for the human IG and TR [4,5] was accepted in 1999 by the HUGO Nomenclature Committee (HGNC) [14] and has become the international reference. Thus, reciprocal direct links have been set up between IMGT/GENE-DB and LocusLink and Entrez Gene at NCBI, GDB, GENATLAS and GeneCards.

The annotation of cDNA sequences by IMGT/Automat allows to deal with a high number of sequences which represent more than 50% of IMGT/LIGM-DB. Currently IMGT/Automat is used to annotate human and mouse cDNA. IMGT/LIGM-DB includes more than 18,000 fully annotated cDNA, 9,000 of them were treated and validated by IMGT/Automat. We estimate to 4,000 the number of rejected sequences by IMGT/Automat because of incoherency or need of

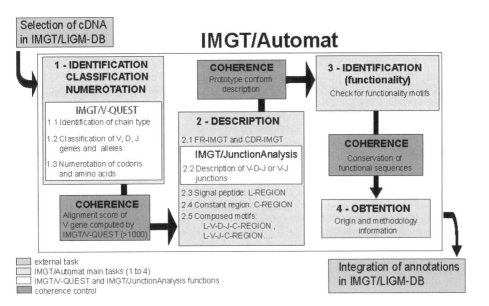

Figure 2-IMGT/Automat main tasks

additional manual expertise. IMGT/Automat allows also the verification and the update of already annotated cDNA sequences when a new gene or a new allele is integrated in IMGT.

4. Conclusion

IMGT has adopted, for the annotation of IMGT/LIGM-DB nucleotide sequences, a strategy that comprises two approaches based on IMGT-ONTOLOGY. That strategy takes into account the specific requirements linked to the complexity of the IG and TR synthesis and genetics, and to the increasing need of automation. The annotation of gDNA sequences is based on an important manual expertise. Indeed, the robustness and the accuracy of this manual annotation are required for the development, in a second time, of the automatic annotation by IMGT/Automat, of the cDNA sequences of the same species and of the same chain type. In a remarkable way, the quality of the cDNA automatic annotation is equivalent to the quality of the annotation achieved by a human expert. This is due to the high score value set up in IMGT/Automat that works in such a way that the tool either provides a result which is necessarily correct or gives no result at all.

This automation will be applied to the annotation of rearranged genomic sequences, through an improvement of the method. Annotations provided by IMGT, the international reference in immunogenetics and immunoinformatic, are particularly used in medical research [15] for the study of IG and TR repertoires in normal and pathological situations (immune and infectious diseases, AIDS, leukemias, lymphomas, myelomas), in biotechnology and antibody engineering (combinatorial libraries, phage displays) and for the therapeutical approaches (grafts, immunotherapy). The IMGT strategy that combines manual expertise and automatism is currently the only way, in the field of immunogenetics, to guarantee the annotation quality and the management of an always increasing number of nucleotide sequences.

6. Acknowledgments

We thank A. Andreou, C. Belessi, K. Stamatopoulos, F. Davi, O. Clément and G. Lefranc for the helpful discussion. IMGT is funded by the Centre National de la Recherche Scientifique (CNRS), the Ministère de l'Education Nationale, de l'Enseignement Supérieur et de la Recherche (MENESR) (Université Montpellier II Plan Pluri-Formation, BIOSTIC-LR2004 Région Languedoc-Roussillon and ACI-IMPBIO IMP82-2004). Subventions have been received from the Association pour la Recherche sur le Cancer (ARC) and the Région Languedoc-Roussillon.

7. References

[1]   Lefranc M-P, Giudicelli V, Kaas Q, Duprat E, Jabado-Michaloud J, Scaviner D, Ginestoux C, Clément O, Chaume D, Lefranc G. IMGT, the international ImMunoGeneTics information system®. *Nucleic Acids Res* 2005: 33: D593-D597.

[2]   Lefranc M-P, Clement O., Kaas Q., Duprat E., Chastellan P., Coelho I., Combres K., Ginestoux C., Giudicelli V., Chaume D. and Lefranc G. IMGT-Choreography for Immunogenetics and Immunoinformatics. In *Silico Biol.* 2005: 5: 0006 http://www.bioinfo.de/isb/2004/05/0006/

[3]   Giudicelli V. and Lefranc M-P. Ontology for Immunogenetics: the IMGT-ONTOLOGY. *Bioinformatics* 1999: 12: 1047–1054.

[4]   Lefranc M-P and Lefranc G. *The Immunoglobulin FactsBook*. Academic Press, London, UK, 458 pages, 2001.

[5]   Lefranc M-P and Lefranc G. *The T cell receptor FactsBook*. Academic Press, London, UK, 398 pages, 2001.

[6]   Giudicelli V, Chaume D, Lefranc M-P. IMGT/GENE-DB: a comprehensive database for human and mouse immunoglobulin and T cell receptor genes. *Nucleic Acids Res* 2005: 33: D256-D261.

[7]   Lefranc M-P, Giudicelli V, Ginestoux C, Bosc N, Folch G, Guiraudou D, Jabado-Michaloud J, Magris S, Scaviner D, Thouvenin V, Combres K, Girod D, Jeanjean S, Protat C, Yousfi Monod M, Duprat E, Kaas Q, Pommié C, Chaume D and Lefranc G. IMGT-ONTOLOGY for Immunogenetics and Immunoinformatics. *In Silico Biol*, 2004: 4: 17–29.

[8]   Giudicelli V, Protat C and Lefranc M-P. The IMGT strategy for the Automatic annotation of IG and TR cDNA sequences: IMGT/Automat. *ECCB'2003, EuropeanConference on Computational Biology*. Ed DISC/Spid DKB-31, 2003; pp103–104.

[9]   Giudicelli V, Chaume D and Lefranc M-P. IMGT/V-QUEST, an integrated software program for immunoglobulin and T cell receptor V-J and V-D-J rearrangement analysis. *Nucleic Acids Res*. 2004: 32: W435–W440.

[10] Yousfi Monod M, Giudicelli V, Chaume D and Lefranc M-P. IMGT/JunctionAnalysis: the first tool for the analysis of the immunoglobulin and T cell receptor complex V-J and V-D-J JUNCTIONs. *Bioinformatics* 2004: 20: I379–I385.

[11] Kanz C, et al. The EMBL Nucleotide Sequence Database. *Nucleic Acids Res*. 2005: 33: D29-D33.

[12] Tateno Y, Saitou N, Okubo K, Sugawara H and Gojobori T. DDBJ in collaboration with mass-sequencing teams on annotation. *Nucleic Acids Res*. 2005: 33: D25-D28.

[13] Benson DA, Karsch-Mizrachi I, Lipman DJ, Ostell J and Wheeler DL. GenBank. *Nucleic Acids Res.*, 2005: 33: D34-D38

[14] Wain HM, Bruford EA, Lovering RC, Lush MJ, Wright MW and Povey S. Guidelines for human gene nomenclature. *Genomics*, 2002: 79: 464–470.

[15] Lefranc M-P. IMGT® databases, web resources and tools for immunoglobulin and T cell receptor sequence analysis, http://imgt.cines.fr. *Leukemia*, 2003: 17: 260–266.

Address for correspondence

Marie-Paule Lefranc,
Laboratoire d'ImmunoGénétique Moléculaire LIGM, UPR CNRS 1142 , Institut de Génétique Humaine IGH 141 rue de la Cardonille , 34396 Montpellier Cedex 5, France ,
Tel: +33 4 99 61 99 65 , Fax: +33 4 99 61 99 01
Email: lefranc@ligm.igh.cnrs.fr, URL : http://imgt.cines.fr

Connecting Medical Informatics and Bio-Informatics
R. Engelbrecht et al. (Eds.)
IOS Press, 2005

9

An Integrated Data-Warehouse-Concept for Clinical and Biological Information

Dominik Brammen[a], Christian Katzer[a], Rainer Röhrig[a], Katja Weismüller[a], Michael Maier[b], Hamid Hossain[c], Thilo Menges[a], Gunter Hempelmann[a], Trinad Chakraborty[c,d]

[a]Department of Anaesthesiology, Intensive Care Medicine and Pain Therapy, University Hospital Giessen, Germany
[b]Department of Medical and Administrative Data Processing, University Hospital Giessen, Germany
[c]Department of Medical Microbiology, University Hospital Giessen, Germany
[d]Network Infection and Inflammation, NGFN-2

Abstract

The development of medical research networks within the framework of translational research has fostered interest in the integration of clinical and biological research data in a common database. The building of one single database integrating clinical data and biological research data requires a concept which enables scientists to retrieve information and to connect known facts to new findings.
Clinical parameters are collected by a Patient Data Management System and viewed in a database which also includes genomic data. This database is designed as an Entity Attribute Value model, which implicates the development of a data warehouse concept.
For the realization of this project, various requirements have to be taken into account which has to be fulfilled sufficiently in order to align with international standards.
Data security and protection of data privacy are most important parts of the data warehouse concept. It has to be clear how patient pseudonymization has to be carried out in order to be within the scope of data security law.
To be able to evaluate the data stored in a database consisting of clinical data collected by a Patient Data Management System and genomic research data easily, a data warehouse concept based on an Entity Attribute Value datamodel has been developed.

Keywords:
Data warehouse; Clinical data; Genomic data; Pseudonymization

1. Introduction

The development of medical research networks within the framework of translational research has fostered interest in the integration of clinical and biological data in a common database [1, 2]. Clinical data are required to analyse the relevance and importance of the biological systems investigated. Within the scope of the German "Nationales Genom Forschungsnetzwerk 2 (NGFN-2)", the University Hospital Giessen is engaged in a project dealing with molecular biology of infection and inflammation in different clinical pictures. Its goal is the generation of prognostic scores concerning sepsis out of genomic and clinical data. Clinical data on intensive care units are collected automatically by a Patient Data Management System (PDMS) [3]. The aim of this project is the formulation of requirements on a data warehouse concept dealing with data collected from the PDMS combined with data resulting from genomic research.

2. Materials and Methods

2.1. Genomic Data

Blood samples are taken from patients attending intensive care units of the University Hospital Giessen, presenting with a disease which may lead to a severe sepsis or already suffering from it. Sepsis is a complex clinical picture showing parallel tracks of inflammation and antiinflammation resulting in a severe disease with mortality up to 60% [4]. The RNA of the patients who have volunteered for the study is isolated from these blood samples and examined using microarrays. After processing the raw data from these microarrays, it is possible to state whether the expression of certain genes is significantly high or low.

2.2. Patient Data Management System (PDMS)

In 1999, the PDMS ICUData (IMESO GmbH, Hüttenberg) was installed at the Operative Intensive Care Unit (Operative ICU) of the University Hospital Giessen [3]. Actually, the system is used in two other departments which are participating in the project.

The PDMS is a message based four-tier system. For communication between the applications of the PDMS and between the different tiers (applications, application servers, distribution layer, data storage) the TCP/IP and the HL7 protocol are used.

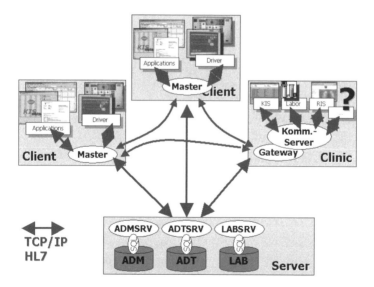

Figure 1-The architecture of the PDMS

Data are stored in logically and physically distributed instances of the database: The instance for the administrative data supplies the PDMS with information for the graphical user interface (GUI) and user authorisation. This instance also contains a medical data dictionary (MDD) to define parameters and their contents. Another instance stores the data of patient administration, whereas the third instance contains the clinical data (including results from routine laboratory tests, values from standard physiologic monitoring devices and settings of standard treatment devices such as ventilators). The design of these database instances varies from a stringent relational design in the administrative sections (system administration, patient administration) to a semantic network in the medical data dictionary and an entity attribute value (EAV) model for storing medical data items [5].

The dynamic GUI is designed for the various and changing demands of the clinical documentation (Figure 2). Since medical data have to be interpreted in time context, every information owns a timestamp for storage and presentation.

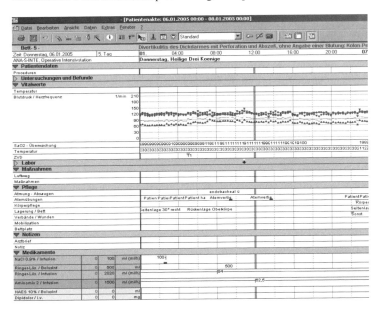

Figure 2- A screenshot of the GUI of the PDMS

2.3. Scientific requirements

First aim of this project is the formulation of requirements on a data warehouse concept. The data warehouse should include information from clinical medicine as well as information from genomic research to allow combined analysis. Since a non-hypothetical approach to scientific problems was chosen, the progress of the project will continuously create new questions, scientific problems and new assessment of the data. Therefore, it is a vital requirement to provide the possibility of expanding the database.

2.4. Data security and protection of data privacy

The handling of clinical data from patients and their genomic data demands a very sensible proceeding of these data. Data security and protection of data privacy has to be provided in accordance with valid laws for data security. Also, the patient has the right to gain insight into data concerning herself or himself, especially in case the patient might have a benefit towards the disease he or she is suffering from.

3. Results

In order to comply with the requirements, a design concept for a data warehouse model integrating clinical and genomic research data was chosen following the principles of incremental architected data marts [6]. The first development step was focused on the data mart for clinical data.

The data collected by the PDMS are stored routinely in an Oracle™ database. A daily updated image of the clinical data database is provided on a different computer for clinical research using Oracle™ distributed computing techniques. The mirroring was necessary for performance issues of the production database. Based on the mirrored database, the data are transformed into the data warehouse structure for structural and semantic standardization. This level of the data warehouse is meant only for administrative issues with no user accessibility. In a next step, patients are pseudonymisized and personal data as well as anything referring to personal data are extinguished. On this pseudonymization level, user access is granted to domain specialists. A study flag assigned in an exclusive sector of the PDMS by the research physician recruits the patients to the study. For recruited patients, clinical data according to the study definition are selected by domain specialists to populate the study data mart. On the data mart level, access is granted to researchers for data queries and data extraction.

Data derived from microarray experiments are stored in a proprietary database. The data sets are labelled with a pseudonym right from the beginning of genomic examination. Genomic data are connected with the clinical data by the trusted research physician, who is linking both pseudonyms.

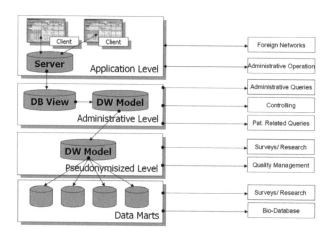

Figure 3-Organisation of the clinical data warehouse

On the administrative level, a trustee administers the pseudonyms and is the only one who is able to re-identify a patient. Scientists using the data warehouse will not be able to re-identify patients. They will have a view on the database adapted to their individual scientific problem, this means that they will not have access to all the data stored in the database concerning one patient or a group of patients, but only have access to previously defined parameters necessary for their scientific project.

The pseudonymisation procedure in use actually will be replaced by the upcoming data security concept of the "Telematikplattform für Medizinische Forschungsnetze e.v." (TMF – national medical IT board) [7] as soon as the concept is launched.

4. Discussion

As we chose a non-hypothetical approach to scientific problems, the progress of the project will continuously create new scientific questions and problems; new technologies could contribute as well to the scientific work in the laboratories and to the data-management. Therefore, it is a vital requirement to provide the possibility of expanding the database on a basic level. To support this dynamic process, we chose the EAV model which is defined by a flat structure of organization. Thus, it is much more easily expandable than a data model consisting of a more rigid structure, e.g. a strictly relational database. The PDMS is presently already stored in a data model based on HL-7. In earlier work, existing clinical scores were successfully calculated on data from the PDMS and procedures for the score generation were validated [8].

The development of the data warehouse presented in this paper was led by the objectives performance, transparency and security. These goals were realized by the concept of a level organized data warehouse. Mirroring of the production database on the administrative level reduces the workload for the database of the PDMS and guarantees a complete data basis on which necessary standardizations are possible. Pseudonymization on the next level provides data security and data privacy. Selection of patients and data according to the study definition on the data mart level provides an efficient and comprehensive view for the researcher and allows for the linkage between clinical and genomic data.

Besides projects for quality improvement and outcome studies [9], there are no known projects utilising routine clinical data from PDMSs for data warehouses. The integration of clinical data from PDMSs and genomic data for biological research broadens the data basis for research, although its usage obtains some obstacles. The semantic standardization at the administrative level needs ongoing refinements and should conform to semantic standards like Logical Observation Identifiers Names and Codes (LOINC), which are not implemented at the actual version.

In case relevant diagnostic findings are revealed in course of the study, a pseudonymization of the patients is more preferable than an anonymization in order to re-identify the patient. The information gained from the genomic examination could possibly influence the patient's therapy and thus eventually affect the course of his or her disease. If this situation should occur, it could be considered non-ethical to withhold this information from the patient. Actually, the pseudonymization follows a locally developed algorithm which will be replaced by the upcoming pseudonymization algorithm from the TMF. This algorithm will support the linkage between clinical and genomic data without need for the trusted research physician to link both pseudonyms.

The data marts defined by the domain specialists, containing the study protocol, defined clinical data for included patients provide the researcher with the needed clinical data. At the actual implementation of the concept, data are extracted into flat files from the data mart as well as from the proprietary database for microarray research data. With these flat files, analysis tools are populated.

Several tools exist for microarray viewing and analysis, featuring interfaces to process data formatted according to established standards like MAGE-ML [9]. For clinical data, the Clinical Data Interchange Standards Consortium (CDISC) and the Health Level 7 group (HL7) are designing data standards to enable system interoperability. Assuming the use of analysis tools operating with standardised data, the implementation of interfaces to exchange data in a standardised format is scheduled. These interfaces will also enable data exchange with external data sources.

5. Conclusion

The data warehouse presented in this paper provides an efficient, transparent and secure access to the clinical data collected by the PDMS. The working basis of the data warehouse concept is data security and protection of data privacy according to valid data security laws. The level organised data processing as well as the flexibility of an EAV model database based on the HL-7 RIM allows for an integration of all resulting data, clinical data and genomic data. Since score generation and computation with clinical data from the PDMS using pre-assigned views and procedures has already been successfully realized, these concepts can now be extended to the integration of the genomic research data.

6. Acknowledgements

The authors would like to thank NGFN-2 and all colleagues who in many ways supported this work.

7. References

[1] Altman RB, Klein TE. Challenges for Biomedical Informatics and Pharmacogenomics. *Annu Rev Pharmacol Toxicol* 2002;42:113-33.

[2] Yue L, Reisdorf WC. Pathway and ontology analysis: emerging approaches connecting transcriptome data and clinical endpoints. *Bioinformatics* 2005; 5(1):11-21.

[3] Michel A, Benson M, Junger A, Sciuk G, Hempelmann G, Dudeck J, Marquardt K. Design principles of a clinical information system for intensive care units (ICU Data). *Stud Health Technol Inform* 2000; 77: 921-4.

[4] Brun-Buisson C, Doyon F, Carlet J, Dellamonica P, Gouin F, Lepout Mercier JC, Offenstadt G, Regnier B. Incidence, risk factors, and outcome of severe sepsis and septic shock in adults. A multicenter prospective study in intensive care units. French ICU group for severe sepsis. *JAMA* 1995; 274(12):968-74.

[5] Huff SM, Haug PJ, Stevens LE, Dupont RC, Pryor TA. HELP the next generation : a new client server architecture. *Proc Annu Symp Comput Appl Med Care* 1994;15:271-5.

[6] Hackney D. Architectures and Approaches for Succesful Data Warehouses. *Oracle White Papers* 2002.

[7] Pommerening K, Reng M. Secondary use of the Electronic Health Record via pseudonymisation. *In: Bos L, Laxminarayan S, Marsh A (eds.): Medical Care Compunetics 1. Amsterdam: IOS Press* 2004:441-446.

[8] Junger A, Böttger S, Engel J, Benson M, Michel A, Röhrig R, Jost A, Hempelmann G. Automatic calculation of a modified APACHE II score using a patient data management system (PDMS). *Int J Med Inform* 2002;65:145-57.

[9] Tjandra D, Wong S, Shen W, Pulliam B, Yu E, Esserman L. An XML message broker framework for exchange and integration of microarray data. *Bioinformatics.* 2003;19(14):1844-5.

8. Address for correspondence

Dr. med. Christian Katzer
Department of Anaesthesiology, Intensive Care Medicine and Pain Therapy
University Hospital Giessen
Rudolf-Buchheim-Str.7
35392 Giessen

Connecting Medical Informatics and Bio-Informatics
R. Engelbrecht et al. (Eds.)
IOS Press, 2005

Time Series Models on Analysing Mortality Rates and Acute Childhood Lymphoid Leukaemia

Maria Kis

University of Debrecen, Debrecen, Hungary

Abstract

In this paper we demonstrate applying time series models on medical research. The Hungarian mortality rates were analysed by autoregressive integrated moving average models and seasonal time series models examined the data of acute childhood lymphoid leukaemia.
The mortality data may be analysed by time series methods such as autoregressive integrated moving average (ARIMA) modelling. This method is demonstrated by two examples: analysis of the mortality rates of ischemic heart diseases and analysis of the mortality rates of cancer of digestive system. Mathematical expressions are given for the results of analysis. The relationships between time series of mortality rates were studied with ARIMA models. Calculations of confidence intervals for autoregressive parameters by tree methods: standard normal distribution as estimation and estimation of the White's theory and the continuous time case estimation. Analysing the confidence intervals of the first order autoregressive parameters we may conclude that the confidence intervals were much smaller than other estimations by applying the continuous time estimation model.
We present a new approach to analysing the occurrence of acute childhood lymphoid leukaemia. We decompose time series into components. The periodicity of acute childhood lymphoid leukaemia in Hungary was examined using seasonal decomposition time series method. The cyclic trend of the dates of diagnosis revealed that a higher percent of the peaks fell within the winter months than in the other seasons. This proves the seasonal occurrence of the childhood leukaemia in Hungary.

Keywords:
Time series analysis; Autoregressive integrated moving average models; Mortality rates; Seasonal decomposition time series method; Acute childhood lymphoid leukaemia

1. Introduction

Time series analysis is a well-known method for many years. Box and Jenkins provided a method for constructing time series models in practice [1], [2]. Their method often referred to as the Box-Jenkins approach and the autoregressive integrated moving average models (ARIMA). This method has been applied in the beginning such fields as industry and economics later in medical research as well as [3], [4], [5], [6].

The method of seasonal time series analysis can be used in various fields of the medicine. With such time series one can detect the periodic trend of the occurrence of a certain disease [7], [8], [9]. Among other diseases, the seasonal periodicity of the childhood lymphoid leukaemia was also analysed using statistical methods [10], [11]. The pathogenesis of the childhood lymphoid leukaemia is still uncertain, but certain environmental effects may provoke the manifestation of latent genes during viral infections, epidemics or pregnancy.

The date of the diagnosis of patients were statistically analysed to determine the role, which the accumulating viral infections and other environmental effects may play during the conception and fatal period on the manifestation of the disease. Because the available data is rather limited and controversial, it seemed logical to make an in-depth analysis of the date of diagnosis of the acute lymphoid leukaemia in Hungarian children.

2. Methods

Autoregressive moving average models

The mortality data often change in the form of 'time series'. Data of frequencies of mortality rates are usually collected in fixed intervals for several age groups and sexes of the population. Let the value of the mortality rates z_t, z_{t-1}, z_{t-2}, … in the years t, t-1, t-2, … . For simplicity we assume that the mean value of z_t is zero, otherwise the z_t may be considered as deviations from their mean. Denote a_t, a_{t-1}, a_{t-2}, … a sequence of identically distributed uncorrelated random variables with mean 0 and variance σ_a^2. The a_t are called white noise.

The autoregressive moving average model of order p, q (ARMA(p, q)) can be represent with the following expression [1], [12]: $z_t = \phi_1 z_{t-1} + … + \phi_p z_{t-p} + a_t + \theta_1 a_{t-1} + … + \theta_q a_{t-q}$. Where ϕ_1, ϕ_2, … , ϕ_p and θ_1, θ_2, … , θ_q are parameters, p means the p order of autoregressive process and q denotes the q order of moving average process.

There are special cases of the ARMA(p,q) models: the autoregressive model of order p (AR(p) model) and the moving average model of order q (MA(q) model). The AR(p) [1], [12]: zt=ϕ1zt-1+…+ϕpzt-p+at. The MA(q) [1], [12]: zt=at+θ1at-1+…+θqat-q. The special case of AR(p); when p=1; zt=ϕ1zt-1+at. zt is linearly dependent on the previous observation zt-1 and the random shock at. The special case of MA(q); when q=1; zt=at+θ1at-1. In this case zt is linear expression of the present and previous random shock.

The time series that has a constant mean, variance, and covariance structure, which depends only on the difference between two time points, is called stationary. Many time series are not stationary. It has been found that the series of first differences is often stationary. Let wt the series of first differences, zt the original time series, than wt=zt-zt-1=∇zt. The Box-Jenkins modelling may be used for stationary time series [1], [12].

The dependence structure of a stationary time series zt is described by the autocorrelation function: ρk=correlation(zt;zt+k); k is called the time lag. This function determines the correlation between zt and zt+k.

To identify an ARIMA model Box and Jenkins have suggested an iterative procedure [1]:

- for provisional model may be chosen by looking at the autocorrelation function and partial autocorrelation function
- parameters of the model are estimated
- the fitted model is checked
- if the model does not fit the data adequately one goes back to the start and chooses an improved model.

Among different models, which represent the data equally well, one chooses the simplest one, the model with fewest parameters [1], [12].

The relation between two time series zt and yt can be give by the cross correlation function (ρzy(k)); ρzy(k)=correlation(zt;yt+k); where k=0, ±1, ±2, … . The cross correlation function determines the correlation between the time series as a function of the time lag k [1].

Estimations for confidence intervals

For estimation the parameter of first order autoregressive model two methods are well known: apply the standard normal distribution as estimation and the White method [13]. These methods cannot be applied in non-stationary case. Little known for estimation of the parameter of first order autoregressive parameter is the application of estimation for continuous time case processes [13], [14]. This method can be applied properly in each case.

Seasonal time series

The time series usually consist of three components: the trend, the periodicity and the random effects. The trend is a long-term movement representing the main direction of changes. The periodicity marks cyclic fluctuations within the time series. The irregularity of the peaks and drops form a more-or-less constant pattern around the trend line. Due to this stability the length and the amplitude of the seasonal changes is constant or changes very slowly. If the periodic fluctuation pattern is stable, it is called a constant periodic fluctuation. When the pattern changes slowly and regularly over the time, we speak of a changing periodicity. The third component of the time series is the random error causing irregular, unpredictable, non-systematic fluctuations in the data independent from the trend line.

An important part of the time series analysis is the identification and isolation of the time series components. One might ask how these components come together and how we can define the connection between the time series and its components with a mathematical formula. The relationship between the components of a time series can be described either with an additive or a multiplicative model.

Let $y_{i,j}$ (i=1, ... , n; j=1, ... , m) mark the observed value of the time series. The index i stands for the time interval (i.e. a year), the j stands for a particular period in the time interval (i.e. a month of the year). By breaking down the time series based on the time intervals and the periods we get a matrix-like table. The rows of the matrix show the values from the various periods of the same time interval; while in the columns show the values from the same periods over various time intervals.

$y_{1,1}; y_{1,2}; ...; y_{1,m};$

$y_{2,1}; y_{2,2}; ...; y_{2,m};$

$y_{3,1}; y_{3,2}; ...; y_{3,m};$

...

$y_{n,1}; y_{n,2}; ...; y_{n,m}.$

Let $d_{i,j}$ (i=1,2, ... , n; j=1,2, ... , m) mark the trend of the time series, $s_{i,j}$ (i=1,2, ... , n; j=1,2, ... , m), the periodic fluctuation and $\varepsilon_{i,j}$ (i=1,2, ... , n; j=1,2, ... , m), the random error. Using these denotations the additive seasonal model can be defined as $y_{i,j}=d_{i,j}+s_{i,j}+\varepsilon_{i,j}$, (i=1,2, ... , n; j=1,2, ... , m), the multiplicative model as $y_{i,j}=d_{i,j}*s_{i,j}*\varepsilon_{i,j}$; (i=1,2, ... , n; j=1,2, ... , m).

The trend of a time series can easily be computed with moving averages or analytic trend calculation. Moving averaging generates the trend as the dynamic average of the time series. Analytic trend calculation approximates the long-term movement in the time series with a simple curve (linear, parabolic or exponential curve) and estimates its parameters.

The indices of the periodic fluctuation are called seasonal differences (in the additive model) or seasonal ratios (in the multiplicative model). These indices represent the absolute difference from the average of the time interval using the additive model or the percentile difference using the multiplicative model. Seasonal adjustment is done by subtracting the j seasonal difference from the j data value of each i season (additive model) or by dividing the j data value of each i season by the j seasonal ratio (multiplicative model). The seasonally adjusted data reflect only the effect of the trend and the random error.

3. Results

Analysing the mortality rates

The SPSS program-package was used for analysing. ARIMA models were identified for some mortality rates. The results demonstrate two cases from Hungarian mortality rates. The mortality rates of cancer of the digestive system over age 65 for male and female were examined. The autocorrelation functions decay for both data series.

The partial autocorrelation functions have a significance value at $k=1$ lag. The first order autoregressive model can be acceptable on the basis of autocorrelation and partial autocorrelation functions. So the stochastic equation over age 65 years of male: $zt=0,742zt-1+\varepsilon t$. The model over age 65 of female is the following: $zt=0,756zt-1+\varepsilon t$. When the fitted model is adequate then the autocorrelation of residuals have $\chi 2$ distribution with (K-p-q) degree of freedom [1]. On the basis of test the selected models were adequate because $\chi 2male=8,475$; $\chi 2female=5,794$; $\chi 20,05;5=11,07$.

The cross correlation function before fitting model and after fitting model was examined. The function has more significance values before fitting model. The cross correlation function for the residuals has not significance values after fitting model. From behaviour of residuals we may be conclude that between examined time series isn't "synchronisation" [4].

The changes in the mortality rates of ischemic heart diseases for age class 0-64 years between male and female were examined as well. The stochastic equation for the mortality rates of male: $zt=0,884zt-1+\varepsilon t$; data of female: $zt=0,72zt-1+\varepsilon t$. On the basis of the $\chi 2$ test the selected models were adequate; because $\chi 2male=10,795$; $\chi 2female=6,56$; $\chi 20,05=11,07$ [4].

The cross correlation function for residuals has significance value at $k=0$ lag on 95% significance level. It may be concluded that there is a "synchronisation" between time series. In those years when the mortality rates for male increased the mortality rates for female increased as well.

The confidence intervals were carried out by the three mentioned methods. For the calculations of the confidence limits we used the tables of the known exact distribution of the maximum-likelihood estimator of the damping parameter of an autoregressive process [13], [14]. The confidence intervals for different significance levels for the first order autoregressive parameter of stochastic equation for males of ischemic heart diseases can be seen in Table 1.

Table 1 - Confidence intervals for different significance levels for the first order autoregressive parameter of stochastic equation for male of ischemic heart diseases

$\phi \approx 0,884$ (male)	p=0,1	p=0,05	p=0,01
Normal distribution	(0,7338;1,0342)	(0,7005;1,0675)	(0,6402;1,1278)
White method	(0,7364;1,0316)	(0,706;1,0619)	(0,6444;1,1236)
Continuous time process	(0,8095;0,9864)	(0,7828;0,9579)	(0,7332;0,9725)

Analysing the periodicity of acute childhood lymphoid leukaemia

The databank of the Hungarian Paediatric Oncology Workgroup contains the data of all the patients with lymphoid leukaemia diagnosed between 1988 and 2000. In this time interval a total of 814 children were registered (of which 467 were boys). The patients were 0-18 years old, with a mean age of 6.4 years and a median of 5.4 years.

The components of the time series can be identified and isolated using statistical program packages. The analysis of the seasonal periodicity of the acute childhood lymphoid leukaemia was done with the SPSS 9.0 statistical program package.

The analysis of the periodicity of acute childhood lymphoid leukaemia was performed on the basis of the date of the diagnosis (year + month) of the disease. We analysed three data series. The first data series contained the number of all the patients diagnosed monthly, the second contained the number of those patients younger than the value of the median, the third series contained the number those older than the value of the median.

The seasonal components of all patients revealed 9 peaks (peak=values of seasonal components greater than 6). 6 of these peaks fell within the winter months (November-February), 1 in the autumn period (September-October), 1 in the summer months (June-August) and 1 in the spring months (March-May).

The seasonal components of the younger age group showed 7 peaks (peak=values of seasonal components greater than 3) in the winter, 1 in the spring and 1 in the summer months.

The seasonal components of the older age group showed 7 peaks (peak=values of seasonal components greater than 3) in the winter, 1 in the spring, 1 in the autumn and 4 in the summer months.

4. Discussions

The Box-Jenkins models may be useful for analysing epidemiological time series. The method described the relationships between time series of mortality rates. It reveals strong synchronised behaviour of ischemic heart diseases between the sexes. For time series of mortality data for cancer of digestive system over age 65 years no such synchronisation is found between subgroups.

From the analysis of the first order autoregressive parameters it may be seen that by applying the normal distribution as estimation and White method the confidence intervals are near equal. For the upper estimations of confidence limits we can get larger than one applying these methods. Applying the continuous time process for the estimation of the confidence intervals they are much smaller and it can be used in each case [13].

Analysis of the seasonality of childhood lymphoid leukaemia in Hungary was performed both on the total number of patients and on the data series divided at the median. This way the characteristics can be observed more easily.

A certain periodicity was found in the dates of the diagnosis in patients with leukaemia. Although there was some difference in the patterns of the seasonal components peaks of the three time series, the majority of the peaks fell within the winter months in all three-time series. This was more significant in the group of all the patients and in the younger age group. The results of the analyses proved the seasonal occurrence of the childhood lymphoid leukaemia. Some studies reported similar seasonality [15], while other studies denied any kind such periodicity [16]. Our results prove the seasonal occurrence of the childhood lymphoid leukaemia in Hungary. Due to the controversial nature of the available international data, further studies should be carried out.

5. References

[1]   Box GER, Jenkins GM. *Time Series Analysis, Forecasting and Control.* San Francisco: Holden-Day, 1976.

[2]   Jenkins DM, Watts DG. *Spectral Analysis and its Applications.* San Francisco: Holden-Day, 1968.

[3]   Allard R. Use of time series analysis in infectious disease surveillance. *Bull World Health Organ* 1998: 76 pp: 327-333.

[4]   Helfenstein U. Detecting hidden relationships between time series of mortality rates. *Methods Inf Med* 1990: 29 pp: 57-60.

[5]   Helfenstein U, Ackermann-Liebrich U, Braun-Fahrlander C, Uhrs Wanner H. The environmental accident at 'Schweizerhalle' and respiratory diseases in children: A time series analysis. *Statistics in Medicine* 1991: 10 pp: 1481-1492.

[6]   Rios M, Garcia JM, Cubedo M, Perez D. Time series in the epidemiology of typhoid fever in Spain. *Med Clin* 1996: 18 pp: 686-9.

[7]   Fleming DM, Cross KW, Sunderland R, Ross AM. Comparison of the seasonal pattern of asthma identified in general practitioner episodes, hospital admissions and deaths. *Thorax* 2000: 8 pp: 662-5.

[8]   Saynajakangas P, Keistinen T, Tuuponen T. Seasonal fluctuations in hospitalisation for pneumonia in Finland. *Int J Circumpolar Health* 2001: 60 pp: 34-40.

[9]   Lani L, Rios M, Sanchez J. Meningococcal disease in Spain: Seasonal nature and resent changers. *Gac Sanit* 2001: 15 pp: 336-340.

[10] Cohen P. The influence on survival of onset of childhood acute leukaemia (ALL). *Chronobiol Int* 1987: 4 pp: 291-7.

[11] Harris RE, Harrel FE, Patil KD, Al-Rashid R. The seasonal risk of paediatric/childhood acute lymphocyte leukaemia in the United States. *J Chronic Dis* 1987: 40 pp: 915-23.

[12] Csaki P. ARMA processes. In: Tusnady G. and Ziermann M, eds. *Time Series Analysis.* Budapest: Technical Publishing House, 1986; pp. 49-84.

[13] Arato M, Benczur A. Exact distribution of the maximum likelihood estimation for Gaussian-Markovian processes. In: Tusnady G and Ziermann M, eds. *Time Series Analysis.* Budapest: Technical Publishing House, 1986; pp. 85-117.

[14] Arato M. *Linear Stochastic Systems with Constant Coefficients: A Statistical Approach.* Berlin: Springer, 1982.

[15] Vienna NJ, Polan AK. Childhood lymphatic leukaemia prenatal seasonality and possible association with congenital varicella. *Am J Epidemiol* 1976: 103 pp: 321-32.

[16] Sorenson HT, Pedersen L, Olse JH, et al. Seasonal variation in month of birth and diagnosis of early childhood acute lymphoblastic leukaemia. *J A M A.* 285 pp: 168-9.

6. Address for correspondence

Maria Kis
Böszörményi út 138, Debrecen, H-4032 Hungary
Department of Economic- and Agroinformatics, University of Debrecen
e-mail: kiss@thor.agr.unideb.hu

Connecting Medical Informatics and Bio-Informatics
R. Engelbrecht et al. (Eds.)
IOS Press, 2005

Bio-Health Information: a Preliminary Review of On-line Cystic Fibrosis Resources

Xia Jing, Stephen Kay, Nicholas R. Hardiker

Salford Health Informatics Research Environment (SHIRE), University of Salford,
Greater Manchester M6 6PU, UK

Abstract

The aims of this study are to determine, and to better understand, elements that are common across a range of bio-health information resources; and to characterize those resources in terms of search and display functionality. Our ultimate goal is to better define the role of bio-health information in clinical practice and in biological research. This paper reports our first step, which is to compare different web-based resources that describe cystic fibrosis. The resources came from PubMed, Nucleotide, EMBL-EBI, DDBJ, OMIM, MeSH, ICD-10, and the Cystic Fibrosis Mutation Database. We found obvious differences in terms of scope and purpose. However, while there were obvious similarities between related resources in terms of content, we also found differences among these resources in terms of display form, specificity of qualifiers, file format and the potential for computer processing. While our work is in its early stages, this study has clarified the nature of bio-health information resources and has allowed us to begin to characterize these resources in terms of their suitability in clinical practice and in biological research.

Keywords:
Medical informatics; Cystic fibrosis; Databases

1. Introduction

In the past decade there has been a rapid and large growth of biological information (bio-information), especially with respect to gene sequences. Certain bio-information is critical for describing the essence of disease. However, despite the increased pace of identification, many gene sequences remain poorly understood.

Cystic fibrosis (CF) has been studied for several decades and the body of knowledge is relatively mature. We seek to increase our understanding of bio-health information sources by investigating CF. We hope to do so by trawling and characterizing a number of web resources for CF. Anselmo [1] has reviewed CF-related web sites and assessed them systematically for adherence to the published AMA (American Medical Association) guidelines. Tebbutt [2] conducted similar research. Ours differs from these previous studies as it focuses on resources for clinical professionals.

CF is an autosomal recessive genetic disorder. The disease affects multiple systems: lung, pancreas, biliary system and sweat glands [3]. A defective gene causes the body to produce thick and sticky mucus that clogs the lungs and leads to severe lung infections. These thick secretions also clog the pancreas, preventing digestive enzymes from reaching the intestines to help break down and absorb food [4]. Symptoms can include weight loss, troublesome coughs, repeated chest infections, salty sweat and abnormal stools [5].CF is the most common life-shortening genetic disease in white populations. In the USA it occurs in around 1/3,300 white births, 1/15,300 black births, and 1/32,000 Asian-American births. CF is carried by approximately 3% of the white population [6].

2. Materials and Methods

We clarify the concepts of "tool" and "resource" in this paper. When we mention tool, we refer to the service and the database; when we mention resource, we refer to the content.
  In our study we consider different types of information about CF: scientific publications, gene sequence data, genetic information and concept descriptions. This is a preliminary study that will guide further research and we have been pragmatic in our choice of tools. Our inclusion criteria of tools were: (1) Domain coverage; (2) Free access; (3) Maintained by a recognised organization; (4) Evidence of updates [7, 8, 9].The exclusion criteria were: (1) protein data resources; (2) genome resources; (3) resources without qualifier for effective retrieval; (4) resources that can be processed further only by natural language processing; (5) resources for patients only; (6) commercial web sites.
  The tools selected include PubMed, Nucleotide, EMBL-EBI, DDBJ, OMIM, MeSH, ICD-10, and Cystic Fibrosis Mutation Database. PubMed, Nucleotide, OMIM and MeSH are all services provided by NCBI (National Centre for Biotechnology Information) in US; although they have a similar interface, the main content and focus are different. There was overlap between databases, for example between EMBL, Nucleotide and DDBJ.

2.1 Tools: an introduction

PubMed [10] is the most widely-used bio-health literature database; it is provided free by the US National Library of Medicine (NLM). The articles included in PubMed date back to the 1950's. There are many different formats and file types for entries selected by PubMed. Due to their strict inclusion criteria and restricted sources, literature selected by PubMed represents the most important outputs from the bio-health field.
  The **Entrez Nucleotides** database [11] is a collection of nucleotide and protein sequences from several sources, including GenBank, RefSeq, and PDB. The number of bases within the Entrez Nucleotides Database is growing at an exponential rate [11]. In April 2004, there were over 38,989,342,565 bases [12].
  EMBL-EBI [13], EMBL Nucleotide Sequence database is Europe's primary nucleotide sequence data resource. It is maintained by EBI (European Bioinformatics Institute) [14].
  DDBJ (DNA Data Bank of Japan)[15] began DNA data bank activities in earnest in 1986 at the National Institute of Genetics (NIG) in Japan[16].
  The Entrez Nucleotides database, EMBL-EBI and DDBJ are components of International Nucleotide Sequence Database Collaboration [8]. They represent the three main nucleotide sequence databases across the world.
  OMIM (Online Mendelian Inheritance in Man) [17] is a service provided mainly by University of Johns Hopkins and integrated with PubMed by NCBI. It is a catalogue of

human genes and genetic disorders. It contains textual information, copious links, sequence records, and additional related resources at NCBI and elsewhere [18].

Mesh (Medical Subject Headings) [19] is NLM's controlled vocabulary for indexing articles within MEDLINE/PubMed. Characteristics of MeSH such as multiple classifications of concepts and multiple entry terms allow for flexible searching.

ICD-10 [20], one of the World Health Organization's (WHO) family of classifications, is used to code and classify mortality and morbidity data in a number of countries worldwide. In many respects, ICD-10 could be seen as an international standard diagnostic classification for general epidemiology and health administration.

Cystic Fibrosis Mutation Database (CFMD) [21] is a collection of mutations in the cystic fibrosis transmembrane conductance regulator (CFTR) gene. It is currently maintained by the international CF genetics research community.

3 Results

3.1 Resources from PubMed

PubMed is a reliable tool to get the most important academic publications about CF. There are different qualifiers to limit literature searches. These include: fields, publication types, languages, subsets, ages, humans and animals, gender and publication date. By defining 'Cystic Fibrosis' to be the major MeSH topic, and restricting the search to 2 years, English, review and humans, we obtained 184 entries. It is possible to refine the queries further by using more specific qualifiers. There are 37 display styles and links for PubMed search results, including XML and ASN.1 file formats. The results can be sorted by author, journal and publication date. The results also can be sent to text, file, clipboard, or email.

3.2 Resources from MeSH

'Cystic Fibrosis' has 4 different positions in the MeSH hierarchy. On the MeSH search results page, there is an introduction to CF, subheadings, reference categories, modification history and a number of entry terms, which are automatically mapped to CF as entered terms. MeSH provides a general idea about the relationship of CF with other concepts.

3.3 Resources from ICD-10

In ICD-10 'Cystic Fibrosis', code E84, belongs to Chapter 4 Endocrine, Nutritional and Metabolic Diseases (E00-E90), within the range of Metabolic Disorders (E70-E89). Conventions within ICD-10 guide the user with respect to inclusion/exclusion. For example: there is an inclusion note under E84 Cystic Fibrosis 'Includes: mucoviscidosis'.

3.4 Resources from Nucleotide

There are descriptive definition, gene mutation types and location, keywords, source organism and its biological hierarchical category, reference related information, chromosome location, map location, molecular types and origin gene sequence. The constraints in the search page of Nucleotide include fields, molecular types, gene location, segmented sequences, source databases, and modification date. Nucleotide returned 23 entries when we selected 'cystic fibrosis' as our keyword. The results display page is similar to that of PubMed (there are 38 result display styles and links).

3.5 Resources from EMBL and DDBJ

There are detailed qualifiers in the advanced search pages of EMBL and DDBJ. When we limited 'cystic fibrosis' as the key word in EMBL and DDBJ, EMBL returned 23 target entries while DDBJ 22. The entries in DDBJ, EMBL and Nucleotide are almost the same except for one missing entry in DDBJ (Accession number: X16416). The complete entries view form of DDBJ and the GenBank display form of Nucleotide are the same.

3.6 Resources from OMIM

Search fields, MIM number prefixes, chromosomes, record sources, and modification dates can be used to limit searches in OMIM. With 'Cystic Fibrosis' as the keyword in the search field, OMIM returned 6 entries. There are 22 display styles and links for OMIM results. There is an 'authoritative overview' of genes and genetic phenotypes for every entry in OMIM [18]. The gene map locus, contributors, edits history and creation date are all included in the entry. If the entry includes clinical synopsis, there is a clinical feature description on the different systems involved and inheritance form.

3.7 Resources from Cystic Fibrosis Mutation Database

There are 8 qualifiers that can be used to limit searches within CFMD. The search results can be displayed in tabular form or as plain text. There are more specific qualifiers that can be used to limit searches in the advanced search page, such as mutation name, intron, exon, mutation types, submission date, etc. There is also a function for searching graphically for mutation, which returns an enlarged view and detailed description about particular mutations. A relative complete view about CF mutation can be obtained by using CFMD.

4. Discussion

There was a high-level of consistency across all resources with respect to gene name and location. The contents of EMBL, Nucleotide and DDBJ are almost identical. However EMBL differs in how it presents search results. Search results in EMBL are classified under a number of different categories: General, Description, References, Additional, Cross-references, and Sequence. In our experience, these higher-level categories serve to clarify the display form, thus improving readability. In terms of searching, the qualifiers in EMBL and DDBJ are similar to each other and more specific and detailed than in Nucleotide. For example there are 22 items in molecular types in EMBL's "Extended Query Form", 19 in DDBJ's "Advanced Search Page" and only 3 in Nucleotide.

   In OMIM, the entry includes 'authoritative' [18] textual descriptions for disorders, gene function and genotype/phenotype correlations, and clinical features. Resources in OMIM are different from others in the level of detail for these descriptions. However, the unstructured style makes them less suitable for computer processing.

   'Cystic Fibrosis' is represented in both MeSH and ICD-10. However, MeSH and ICD-10 have different aims. The ultimate aim for MeSH applications is to facilitate users to find all and only relevant articles. To facilitate this process 'Cystic Fibrosis' is classified along four different axes. ICD-10 is a statistical classification; there is a desire to avoid double-counting. Thus 'Cystic Fibrosis' appears in only one position in the ICD-10 hierarchy. Explicit inclusion notes guide the user to this unique position.

   CFMD is a database that contains detailed information, provided by the CF research community, about mutation of the CFTR gene. Each entry within CFMD has an associated mutation position, mutation type and nucleotide change. These are unique to CFMD. Within OMIM the description and annotation of phenotype contain greater detail than in other resources. Moreover, OMIM (and Nucleotide) includes XML and ASN.1 file formats. These formats increase the potential for computer processing. Table 1 compares the display items in the different resources with respect to CF; excluding PubMed, ICD-10 and MeSH.

Table1-Comparison of display items in a range of resources relevant to cystic fibrosis

	Nucleotide	DDBJ	EMBL	OMIM	CFMD
Locus	√	√	√	Gene map locus	√
Definition	√	√	Description	Allelic variants	Nucleotide change
Accession	√	√	√	√	√
Version	√	√	√	Edit history	--
Key words	√	√	√	--	--
Source/Organism	√	√	√	--	--
Reference	√	√	√	√	Contributor
Molecular type	√	√	√	--	--
Clone	√	√	√	Cloning	--
Note	√	√	√	--	√
Sequence length	√	√	√	--	--
Base count	--	√	√	--	--
db_xref	√	√	√*	--	--

Note: √ indicates presence of an item; -- absence;* there is 'Database Cross-reference' also in EMBL.

There are more CF resources on web [22-25], but we focus on CF's bio-health information. Galperin's [8] paper is a more complete molecular biology resources collection.

5. Conclusion

We believe that clinicians can enrich their practice if they use bio-health information conveniently and effectively. However, it is not easy for clinicians to familiarise themselves with genetic information, nor to gain the sense of it quickly and use it in routine practice. Of the diverse range of resources available on the web, OMIM, Nucleotide and EMBL would appear to be useful candidate tools for clinical professionals. The 'authoritative' description of gene, disorder and genotype/phenotype relationship in OMIM is presented in natural language; EMBL and DDBJ have more detailed and specific search pages than Nucleotide; and the results display pages in EMBL are structured to improve readability. The biological researchers focused more on genotype with some general notions of disease. So both OMIM and domain-specific databases such as CFMD might prove helpful.

This review is a first step towards finding common ground. Our present research is moving us a step closer to our final goal, i.e., how this bio-health information can be used more efficiently in solving clinical problems and what kinds of problems can be solved.

6. Acknowledgement

The authors wish to thank IHSCR the travel support. Thanks for Su Ellis's help and Miao Sun's counsel.

7. References

[1]   Anselmo MA, Lash KM, Stieb ES, and Haver KE. Cystic fibrosis on the Internet: a survey of site adherence to AMA guidelines. *Pediatrics* 2004:114(1):100-103.

[2]   Tebbutt SJ. Cystic fibrosis resources on the World Wide Web. *Mol Med Today* 1996: 2(4):148-149.

[3]   Cystic fibrosis's MeSH description. http://www.ncbi.nlm.nih.gov/entrez/query.fcgi?cmd=Retrieve&db= mesh&list_uids=68003550&dopt=Full [Accessed on May 20, 2005].

[4]   Cystic fibrosis foundation. http://www.cff.org/about_cf/what_is_cf/ [Accessed May 20, 2005].

[5]   Cystic fibrosis trust. http://www.cftrust.org.uk/scope/page/view.go?layout=cftrust&pageid=28 [Accessed May 20,2005]

[6]   The Merck Manual of Diagnosis and Therapy, section 19, chapter 267, cystic fibrosis. http://www.merck.com/mrkshared/mmanual/section19/chapter267/267a.jsp [Accessed   May 20,2005]

[7]   Criteria for assessing the quality of health information on the Internet. http:// hitiweb.mitretek.org/docs/criteria.pdf   [Accessed May 20,2005]

[8]   Galperin MY. The Molecular Biology Database Collection: 2005 update. *Nucleic Acids Res* 2005: 33: D5-D24.

[9]   Walton G, Booth A (eds). *Exploiting knowledge in health services*. London: Facet Publishing, 2004; 169.

[10] NLM. PubMed.   http://www.ncbi.nlm.nih.gov/entrez/query.fcgi?db=PubMed [Accessed May 20,2005]

[11] NLM. Nucleotide. http://www.ncbi.nlm.nih.gov/entrez/query.fcgi?db=Nucleotide [Accessed May 20,2005]

[12] Benson DA, Karsch-Mizrachi I, Lipman DJ, et al. GenBank. *Nucleic Acids Res* 2005:33: D34-D38.

[13] The EMBL Nucleotide Sequence Database. http://www.ebi.ac.uk/embl/ [Accessed May 20, 2005]

[14] Kanz C, Aldebert P, Althorpe N, Baker W, Baldwin A, Bates K, Browne P, van den Broek A, Castro M, Cochrane G, Duggan K, Eberhardt R, Faruque N, Gamble J, Diez FG, Harte N, Kulikova T, Lin Q, Lombard V, Lopez R, Mancuso R, McHale M, Nardone F, Silventoinen V, Sobhany S, Stoehr P, Tuli MA, Tzouvara K, Vaughan R, Wu D, Zhu W, and Apweiler R. The EMBL nucleotide sequence database. *Nucleic Acids Res* 2005:33: D29-D33.

[15] DDBJ. http://www.ddbj.nig.ac.jp/ [Accessed May 20, 2005]

[16] Tateno Y, Saitou N, Okubo K, Sugawara H, and Gojobori T. DDBJ in collaboration with mass-sequencing teams on annotation. *Nucleic Acids Res* 2005:33:D25-D28.

[17] NLM. OMIM. http://www.ncbi.nlm.nih.gov/entrez/query.fcgi?db=OMIM [Accessed May 20, 2005]

[18] Hamosh A, Scott AF, Amberger JS, Bocchini CA, and McKusick VA. Online Mendelian Inheritance in Man(OMIM), a knowledgebase of human genes and genetic disorders. *Nucleic Acids Res* 2005:33:D514-D517.

[19] NLM. MeSH. http://www.ncbi.nlm.nih.gov/entrez/query.fcgi?db=mesh [Accessed May 20, 2005]

[20] Cystic Fibrosis Mutation Database. http://www.genet.sickkids.on.ca/cftr/ [Accessed May 21, 2005]

[21] *International statistical classification of diseases and related health problems*. 10th edition. Geneva: WHO, 1992.

[22] CF foundation. http://www.cff.org/home/   [Accessed May 20, 2005]

[23] Cochrane Review. http://www.cochrane.org/cochrane/revabstr/CFAbstractIndex.htm [Accessed May 20, 2005]

[24] MedlinePlus.http://www.nlm.nih.gov/medlineplus/cysticfibrosis.html [Accessed May 20, 2005]

[25] Cystic Fibrosis Trust. http://www.cftrust.org.uk/index.jsp [Accessed May 20, 2005]

Address for correspondence

Xia Jing, SHIRE, Room PO30, Brian Blatchford Building, University of Salford, Greater Manchester M6 6PU, UK, Email, X.Jing@pgr.salford.ac.uk; URL: http://www. shire.salford.ac.uk/

Connecting Medical Informatics and Bio-Informatics
R. Engelbrecht et al. (Eds.)
IOS Press, 2005

27

Bioinformatics Meets Clinical Informatics

Jeremy Smith[a], Denis Protti[b]

[a]*Calgary Health Region, Alberta, Canada*
[b]*University of Victoria, British Columbia, Canada*

Abstract

The field of bioinformatics has exploded over the past decade. Hopes have run high for the impact on preventive, diagnostic, and therapeutic capabilities of genomics and proteomics. As time has progressed, so has our understanding of this field. Although the mapping of the human genome will certainly have an impact on health care, it is a complex web to unweave. Addressing simpler "Single Nucleotide Polymorphisms" (SNPs) is not new, however, the complexity and importance of polygenic disorders and the greater role of the far more complex field of proteomics has become more clear. Proteomics operates much closer to the actual cellular level of human structure and proteins are very sensitive markers of health. Because the proteome, however, is so much more complex than the genome, and changes with time and environmental factors, mapping it and using the data in direct care delivery is even harder than for the genome. For these reasons of complexity, the expected utopia of a single gene chip or protein chip capable of analyzing an individual's genetic make-up and producing a cornucopia of useful diagnostic information appears still a distant hope. When, and if, this happens, perhaps a genetic profile of each individual will be stored with their medical record; however, in the mean time, this type of information is unlikely to prove highly useful on a broad scale. To address the more complex "polygenic" diseases and those related to protein variations, other tools will be developed in the shorter term. "Top-down" analysis of populations and diseases is likely to produce earlier wins in this area. Detailed computer-generated models will map a wide array of human and environmental factors that indicate the presence of a disease or the relative impact of a particular treatment. These models may point to an underlying genomic or proteomic cause, for which genomic or proteomic testing or therapies could then be applied for confirmation and/or treatment. These types of diagnostic and therapeutic requirements are most likely to be introduced into clinical practice through traditional forms of clinical practice guidelines and clinical decision support tools. The opportunities created by bioinformatics are enormous, however, many challenges and a great deal of additional research lay ahead before this research bears fruit widely at the care delivery level.

Keywords:
Bioinformatics; Medical informatics; Clinical informatics; Genomics; Proteomics

1. Introduction

In their seminal paper, Maojo and Kulikowski compare and contrast medical informatics (MI) and bioinformatics (BI) and provide a viewpoint on their complementarities and potential for collaboration in various subfields [1]. They argue that the new field of biomedical informatics (BMI) holds great promise for developing informatics methods that will be crucial in the development of genomic medicine. In their view, the future of BMI will be influenced strongly by whether significant advances in clinical practice and biomedical research come about from separate efforts in MI and BI, or from emerging, hybrid informatics sub-disciplines at their interface.

What Maojo and Kulikowski fail to mention is that the field of bioinformatics has quickly become the focal point of the pharmaceutical industry. Where traditional biology and medical research has been practiced "in vivo" (in a living creature) or "in vitro" (in a glass container), increasingly research is being conducted "in silico" (in a computer) [2]. To accelerate drug development and create more effective treatments, pharmaceutical companies are finding it necessary to invest heavily in the computerization of their industry [3]. At the same time, the results of this research are helping to shift the approach to diagnosis and treatment from one of hypothesis and experimentation to one of direct analysis of underlying causes, prevention, optimal treatments, and analysis of both desired and undesired outcomes [4].

A great deal of work is already underway in the pharmaceutical and medical communities to bring together the clinical information of populations with the genetic profiles to enable scientists to conduct population-based research on the correlation between key genetic traits and the health status of the related individuals. Already, countries such as Iceland and Estonia are leading the way in merging electronic medical records for their population with their genetic profiles, and making this data available to researchers within tight codes of confidentiality and appropriate usage. With the advent of Canada Health Infoway and Genome Canada, both federally sponsored entities funded with a combined investment of roughly $1.5 billion, Canada could be poised to be on the forefront of this field in a few years' time [5]. The recent creation of a new Bioinformatics Centre at the University of British Columbia is one manifestation of this movement [6].

Yet another educationally oriented initiative occurred in 2002–2003, when the American College of Medical Informatics undertook a study of the future of informatics training [7]. The study members viewed biomedical informatics as an interdisciplinary field, combining basic informational and computational sciences with application domains, including health care, biological research, and education.

Finally, the use of clinical and genetic information for research is clearly receiving a great deal of focus and investment - and narrow, focused successes have at least partially proved its potential. What is less clear, however, is when, and how, the promise of genomics, proteomics, and their related fields will turn into useful clinical tools at the point of care on a widespread basis. This paper is intended to briefly address the state of this field of research, and identify areas of potential application to clinical informatics and the Electronic Health Record (EHR). In doing so controversial issues related to ethical, legal, and social concerns will be referenced but excluded from detailed analysis.

2. Background

To date, bioinformatics has had the greatest impact within the pharmaceutical industry. Drug companies are looking to bioinformatics to improve their speed to market, increase the efficacy of their products, and reduce complications related to those medications. Boston Consulting Group estimates that the average drug now costs $880m to develop and takes almost 15 years to reach the market [8]. Proponents believe that genomics and proteomics will have a tremendous and direct impact on direct care delivery. Others believe that the impact will be slower to materialize and will be less direct. Early evidence suggests that, regardless of when and how, bioinformatics will have a very positive impact on diagnostic practices, analysis of prognosis, prevention of disease, screening, and gene therapy.

Much focus to date has been on genomics, and the sequencing of the human genome.

Although this research shows promise, scientists are increasingly skeptical of the direct and widespread relevance to care delivery. The results of the human genome project have, however, highlighted the importance "single nucleotide polymorphisms" (SNP). SNPs are single-letter variations in DNA sequences that correlate to key differences between individuals – appearance, predisposition to disease, reactions to medications, etc. SNPs correlate to a set of conditions known as Mendelian diseases, or single gene disorders. Although these diseases are relatively easy to identify with genetic testing, they are, unfortunately very rare. The most common and expensive conditions, particularly chronic conditions, are far more complicated that Mendelian diseases – due to "polygenic" disorders - and therefore require far more complex analysis [9].

The weakness of genomics is that genes, although at the root of proteins and cells, do not generally have a one-to-one relationship with disease or human traits. They interact, and are affected by many biological and environmental factors. Proteins, on the other hand, have a much closer relationship with a person's health, as proteins themselves live within the cells of the body and regulate most of the functions of the human body. In fact, most drugs today act on proteins, not on genes, and proteins tend to show the first signs of ill-health, making them sensitive diagnostic tools.

To sequence the human proteome, however, is even harder than sequencing the human genome – if possible at all. Although the number of genes in the human genome is large (estimates vary between 35,000 and 150,000), the number of proteins expressed from those genes is far larger. A gene is made up of combinations of only four letters (AGCT). A protein, however, is made a string of 20 amino acids, making the permutations and combinations far more diverse. Furthermore, while only the linear sequence of the gene is relevant, proteins wrap themselves into 3 dimensional shapes which are just as relevant as the sequence of genes and amino acids within them. Most medications, for example, currently work by fitting into small gaps, grooves, or ridges in protein structures.

In addition, each type of cell has a different complement of proteins, and each of the 200 different types of cells in a human body has different protein patterns. For example, the proteins in the human brain are different from those of the pancreas. Furthermore, cells produce different protein structures over time, influenced by health, consumption of different foods, and other external factors.

The research does not, however, stop with genomics. Having succeeded in sequencing the human genome, researchers are turning to unraveling the multidimensional and dynamic collection of human proteins [10]. The goal of proteomics is to identify all the proteins, then understand their ranges of expression in different cell types, as well as characterize modifications, interactions, and structure. Though far from being fully mapped, the proteome is already yielding drug targets and information on disease states and drug response. Michael F. Moran, chief scientific officer of MDS Proteomics describes the proteomic challenge as "every state – plus or minus disease, plus or minus drug – is a different proteome [11].

The secret to unleashing both genomics and proteomics is high-throughput analytical devices. Gene chips contain thousands of probes, each of which fluoresces under different colors of laser light, showing which genes are present. The gene chips now have more than 500,000 interrogation points [12]. The biggest hurdle will be lowering the costs of these chips to a level that makes them viable for mass-market analysis. Due to the complexity and changing nature of proteins, the creation of "protein chips" is an even more challenging proposition. However a recent study revealed that a protein chip could be used to screen for a series of 16 prohibited drugs in urine samples [13].

3. Bringing Bioinformatics Research into Clinical Practice

There are two fundamental schools of thought regarding the translation of bioinformatics research into clinical practice. The proponents of genomics and proteomics believe that by combining large-scale databases of clinical data with the related individual genetic profiles, correlation analysis will permit the identification of key cause-and-effect relationships. This process is referred to as "bottom-up analysis" [14]. Others, however, believe that this approach will produce only minimal results due to the many interactions between genes and proteins, and the widely varying environmental factors. They, instead, believe that most significant findings will be identified by starting with known diseases and developing models which take into account the many related causal factors including genetics, environmental factors, etc. – known as "top-down analysis" [15].

In bottom-up analysis, pools of target genes are continuously evaluated against key diseases to establish relevance and test the ability to influence the disease with medications. This approach requires vast databases of medical records and genetic profiles, with the world's most powerful computer tools for correlation analysis [16]. In the diagram below, bottom-up analysis starts at the bottom row, with the genomic or proteomic sequences, and moves upward, trying to identify the impact of the particular gene or protein on the biology of the individual.

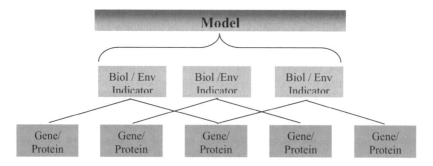

Top-down analysis uses the fact that a person with a particular condition will generally share a number of key traits with others who have the same condition, and develops models to describe the common patterns. In the diagram above, the process would start at the top, developing a model based on reliable biological and/or environmental indicators from the middle row. Genomic and proteomic profiles may, then be identified that are common to these individuals, and therefore become useful diagnostic tools [17].

According to a respected Canadian scientist:

> *"The main physiological pathways responsible for many diseases are probably identifiable with available data, top-down system analysis, and a tractable amount of experimentation (both virtually and clinically). The possible genes involved could be identified once the critical pathways are validated. However trying to do it from the bottom-up, starting at the genome level, without knowing which organ, which cell, and what time points, is like not even knowing which field and haystack to find a needle in. There will likely be relatively few diseases, and hence patients, that will be found to result from a single gene mutation/SNP. Most human diseases are likely to result from a combination of diet, multiple gene background, and their interaction" [15].*

Implications & Future Direction

Only recently, with studies on entire national populations such as those being carried out on the inhabitants of Iceland, are researchers beginning to overcome the problem of insufficient data [18]. Even in that case, however, the data is only applicable to the unique Icelandic population. Another project, in Estonia, is conducting similar research and since the Estonian population is far more heterogeneous, it should be easier to generalize the results [19].

The impact of genomics and proteomics on direct care delivery is starting to become clearer, however, the exact tools and information that will be required to support the individual care provider remain very unclear. If information about an individual's genomic or proteomic profile were known, clinical decision support tools could assist the physician with contraindications for prescriptions, however, these tools are likely to use "rules" that are not unlike those used in today's software [20]. Likewise, following the "top-down" approach, it is easily imaginable that the clinical practice guidelines used today will continue their role in brining clinical research to the hands of the front-line provider, but in the future they may be significantly more accurate, tailored to the individual, and/or include genetic or proteomic diagnostic tests and therapeutic substances. In the shorter term, more complex decision support tools may be used to avoid medication errors by mapping diagnostic, medication, and genomic/proteomic indicators that would point to efficacy or adverse reactions.

5. Acknowledgements

The authors would like to thank the following individuals for sharing their time, insights, and providing numerous sources for additional research: Dr. George Englebert, Chief Information Officer, MDS Diagnostics, Toronto, Ontario; Richard Ho, Director of Clinical Informatics, Johnson & Johnson Pharmaceuticals, San Diego, California; Roman Szumski, VP Science and Technology, MDS International, Toronto, Ontario; Dr. J. Hans van de Sande, Ph.D, University of Calgary Faculty of Medicine, Calgary, Alberta; and Dr. Janet Wood, Professor of Biochemistry, University of Guelph, Guelph, Ontario.

6. References

[1]   Maojo V and Kulikowski, CA. Bioinformatics and Medical Informatics: Collaborations on the Road to Genomic Medicine*? J Am Med Inform Assoc.* 2003;10:515-522

[2]   Ingenious medicine. *The Economist.* June 29, 2000.

[3]   Drugs ex machina. *The Economist.* September 20, 2001.

[4]   Ingenious medicine. *The Economist.* June 29, 2000.

[5]   Francis, Myrna. Personal Communication. August 14, 2002.

[6]   http://bioinformatics.ubc.ca/. Accessed December 30, 2004.

[7]   Friedman CP et al. Training the Next Generation of Informaticians: The Impact of "BISTI" and Bioinformatics-A Report from the American College of Medical Informatics. *J Am Med Inform Assoc.* 2004;11:167-172.

[8]   Ingenious medicine. The Economist. June 29, 2000.

[9]   Chakravarti A and Little P. Nature, nurture and human disease. *Nature.* 421, 412 – 414, 2003.

[10] Anonymous. Proteomics Emerges As The Next Frontier. *Chemical Engineering and News.* Volume 81, Number 49. December 8, 2003.

[11] Ezzell, C. Proteins rule. *Scientific American.* 286: 4, p 42-47, Apr 2002.

[12] The race to computerise biology. *The Economist.* December 12, 2002.

[13] Du H et al. Development of Miniaturized Competitive Immunoassays on a Protein Chip as a Screening Tool for Drugs. *Clinical Chemistry* 10.1373. Published online ahead of print November 24, 2004

[14] Szumski, R. MDS Diagnostics. Personal Communication. February 10, 2003.

[15] Ho R.. Johnson & Johnson Pharmaceuticals. Personal Communication. February 17, 2003.

[16] Koppal T. Genomic tools step up flow of drug pipeline. *Drug Discovery & Development. Highland Ranch*. December 2002.

[17] Stix G. Reverse-Engineering Clinical Biology. Scientific American. February 2002.
http://www.sciam.com/article.cfm?colID=6&articleID=000C4F01-FABE-1E19-8B3B809EC588EEDF

[18] Ingenious medicine. *The Economist*. June 29, 2000.

[19] eGreen Project. EGreen Summary.

Addresses for correspondence

Denis J. Protti
Professor, School of Health Information Science
Room A212, Human and Social Development Building
University of Victoria
Victoria, British Columbia, V8W 3P4 Canada
Tel: 250.721.8814, Fax: 250.472.4751, http://hinf.uvic.ca

Jeremy Smith
1436 Fairfield Road
Victoria, BC
V8S 1E5
Tel: 250-415-0516
jeremy@jeremysmith.ca

Connecting Medical Informatics and Bio-Informatics
R. Engelbrecht et al. (Eds.)
IOS Press, 2005

SITRANS: a Web Information System for Microarray Experiments

Frédérique Laforest[a], Anne Tchounikine[a], Tarak Chaari[a], Hubert Charles[b], Federica Calevro[b]

[a]UMR CNRS 5205 LIRIS Laboratoire d'Informatique en Images et Systèmes d'information
[b]UMR INRA 203 INSA de Lyon BF2I Biologie Fonctionnelle, Insectes et Interactions
INSA de Lyon, F-69621 Villeurbanne Cedex, FRANCE

Abstract

Microarray experiments aim at analyzing expression levels of genes using DNA probes. The amount of data managed for each experiment is very large. It is thus essential to provide electronic support for the capture and the management of information describing microarray experiments. We present here the SITRANS Web information system, the aim of which is to help research workers storing, browsing, sharing and publishing data.

Keywords
Information Systems, Microarray Analysis, World Wide Web

1 Introduction

Microarray analysis has become a widely used tool for the generation of gene expression data on a genomic scale. The amount of data managed for each experiment is very large. The steps used in a microarray experiment are numerous and various : optimization of probes positioning on the slide, preparation of slides surface, spotting, purification and labeling of messenger RNA, hybridization, washing, signal measurement, normalization and data analysis. The novelty of the technique makes that interesting data are also not well known nor normalized. The description of an experiment and moreover the comparison between experiments are thus difficult and often impossible. The reproduction of published experiments is also impracticable as many details are often not given or not precise enough. The MIAME model [1] has provided a big advance on the standardization for presenting and exchanging microarray data. But the fields it provides are not yet formatted (they are often textual descriptions) and the precision of information can thus differ from one MIAME description to the other.

The complexity of the process and the volume of data to be managed require the use of a computerized information system for the management of experiments, their publication and the exchange of results. In this context, the SITRANS project aims at answering three main objectives:

- Allow research workers to manage their experiments i.e. to have a history of each experiment step, from the microarray design to its analysis,
- Allow result publication in a standardized format (MAGE-ML [2]),

- Build a common database for all researchers of the platform in DTAMB (University Claude Bernard Lyon I) so that they can share both their know-how and their data.

To do so, we have developed and tested SITRANS, a Web information system that could be defined as a shared and electronic lab booklet. It does not include analysis tools, it is only dedicated to the storage and the retrieval of information about experiments. Data stored range from raw data on spotter configuration to scanned images, including results of normalization and analysis. It is based on a 4-tier architecture.

The next section presents the SITRANS information system. After a brief presentation of the technical architecture, we present the way we have defined the database schema and the functional view of the system. Section 3 then presents the navigation tool we have written, based on the topic maps theory.

2 The SITRANS information system

The SITRANS information system aims at capturing, storing, retrieving and publishing data on microarray experiments. The first and non trivial work has been to design the database schema. The second step has concerned the functional view of the application. We have collaborated al lot with end-users for these two first steps, and worked with simulations and demonstrators. We thus have designed the overall application architecture and developed it. The first subsection shows rapidly the technical environment we have chosen. The following subsections detail each step.

2.1 Technical environment

The SITRANS information system is a Web application. It is based on a multi-tier architecture. The database management system is PostgresQL. It interacts with EJBs on a jboss server. EJBs are divided into two layers: entity EJBs represent the database objects, while session EJBs represent the application functionalities. The user interface uses JSP pages that work in collaboration with session entities, using Data Transfer Objects (DTOs) [3]. As a matter of fact, as data exchanged between JSPs an EJBs are numerous, we have chosen to build DTOs that minimize the number of transfers (even if each transfer is heavier). JSP pages are managed by a tomcat server, coupled with an apache HTTP server that serves HTML pages to the end-user. HTML pages include some javascript code for captures validation before transfer to JSP pages.

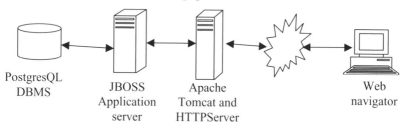

Postgresql DBMS   JBOSS Application server   Apache Tomcat and HTTPServer   Web navigator

Figure 1: Technical architecture of SITRANS

2.2 Database schema

The design of the database schema was initially developed in 2002 and has been made on two bases:

- first on the previous work made by Pr. Barbry Team in Nice, France (CNRS UMR 6097). His team gave us the database schema they built for their microarray experiments, called MedLab [4]. Their database relies on PCR microarrays.
- second on experiments done on the DTAMB platform located in Lyon. It has been designed in the objective to rapidly be accessible to the public research staff.

We thus have modified the Medlab database schema. The database we have built contains data on the experiment environment : it provides the list of scanners, spotters, analysis tools, experimental protocols and so on... that can be used on the DTAMB platform; it also manages the localization of new and used slides, allowing for a basic stock management. We have also modified the Medlab Schema so that it can manage both oligonucleotide-based and PCR-based experiments.

We have also defined the concept of project: a project concerns one or more experiments on the same slide model. A slide model defines the slide spots and their contents. Most projects use duplicated or quite similar slides that follow the same model, for validation purpose.

In this article, we cannot provide the database schema, as it contains 44 tables. It is available at the following address: http://liris.cnrs.fr/~sitrans/sitrans_v2.3_create.sql.The resulting schema conforms to the MIAME standard, and extractions to the MAGE-ML format will be automatized soon.

2.3 Functional view of the application

The functional view of the application has been built in close collaboration with end-users. We have proposed many different versions and discussed the overall functionning as well as details. Meetings made conclusions on the different pages to be shown, as well as their content, positioning of elements, navigation between pages and so on. We have concluded with a user interface organized as follows :

- The data capture menu follows exactly the steps of a typical project: project description, array design (slides, biochip/slide model and probes), target preparation (samples, extracted products, amplified products, labeled products), hybridization, and biochip analysis (raw images, raw data, and normalized data). We have thus designed a page for each step. Figure 2 shows on the left the list of available pages, and on the right a page being edited. A popup page allows for getting more details.
- Precedence rules have been defined for some steps, others may be filled in any desired order. The practice proved that the "logical" precedence of steps in a typical experiment are quite always followed. As soon as the data recording step is performed, a researcher has the possibility to "freeze" it, i.e. nobody can modify the project data anymore. A researcher may also "publish" project data, i.e. make them available to other end-users of the system.
- Each time it is possible, the hand-based capture is minimized. We have implemented it in two ways: first the integration and interpretation of robots description files (e.g. spotting map) with use of mediators, and second the choice of values in lists of available tools (protocols, machines and so on coming from the database itself).
- Lists of available tools are managed by the platform administrator, who can update them in function of the platform evolution. We have called them platform data, in

opposition to experiments data, that are created and managed by research workers themselves.

- We have defined 3 types of end-users: the platform administrator manages platform data ; the research worker creates and works on microarray projects, the visitor can explore published data.

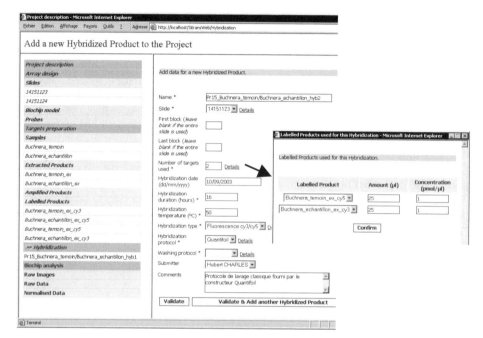

Figure 2: Capture page of an hybridized product

- The data consultation can be made in two ways. First a standard way allows for routing among capture pages of the different steps of the project. Pages are exactly the same ones as for capture: the only difference is that no data may be modified nor deleted. Second we have defined a navigation way, using a map of data. This is explained in more details in the following sub-section. No classical SQL-based querying has been implemented at the moment. As a matter of fact, end-users were first not able to define query forms embedding fixed SQL queries. Second, they are not enough familiar with the SQL language for writing themselves queries on the database

3 Data visualization using topic maps

Data visualization using capture forms is not flexible. That's why we have chosen to provide another visualization paradigm. It is based on navigation in a data map and has been developed as an applet. The data map is based on the topic maps theory [5]. In the navigation tab (see figure 3), we present topics to the end-user. In this first version, topics correspond to tables in the database schema, but logic predicates can be used to define topics as selections on the database [6]. Each topic is assorted with the number of corresponding occurrences in the database. The selected topic is also linked to other related topics. The values associated to the related topics provide the number of occurrences corresponding to the selected topics occurrences. Changing the selected topic is easy: a click on the desired topic centers it in the middle of the tab and provides its neighbor topics.

Changing to the "selection" tab, the end-user can make a selection of occurrences in the selected topic. The selection can be made on the list of occurrences or with constraints on columns values. The navigation tab then updates its occurrences counts in consequence.

A third tab ("history") provides the history of navigation. Buttons "precedent" (back) and "suivant" (next) allow for moving in the navigation history.

The data visualization is thus based on both navigation in topics and selection of instances.

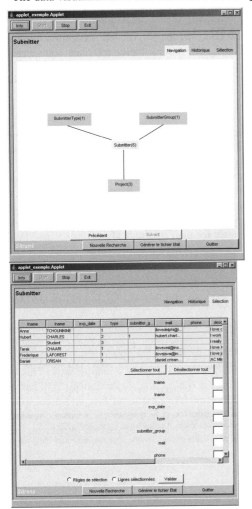

Figure 3: Applet for navigation in the data map

4 Conclusion

The SITRANS information system intends to help research workers, for them to organize, store and retrieve easily data on their microarray experiments. We have followed an agile development process [7] (including the client very frequently and at all steps) to ensure the appropriateness of the resulting work. This information system is operational since May 2004 on the intranet of the Lyon I University campus. Since then, tests with large real experiments have been conducted by research workers and the tool is thus validated. At the moment, SITRANS is on the private network of the university campus and cannot be accessed by external users. We intend to provide access soon on the Internet, on http://sitrans.insa-lyon.fr (name under creation).

For a larger use on a more efficient computer, we intend to provide it on the PRABI web site soon [8]. But before, we have to finalize the navigational consultation user interface, whose first beta version is under testing procedures at the moment. It is intended to be provided to local end-users for usability tests before end of February 2005.

Another point we have to rapidly implement concerns the MAGE-ML extraction of data. We intend to couple this extraction with the navigational consultation interface, so that end-users can select data to be extracted during a navigation process.

5 Acknowledgments

This work has been supported by the french Ministry of Research by the ACI IMPBio program of September 2003. Thanks to the support of INRIA to the Rhône-Alpes microarray platform, a computer science engineer (Daniel Crisan) has also worked on the project during one year from may 2003 to April 2004 for the design and the implementation of the information system. Students from the BioInformatics Department of INSA Lyon and from the Telecommunications Department of INSA Lyon also participated in prototyping and developments. We also want to thank the biologists and technicians working on the Rhône-Alpes microarray platform for their help and advice.

6 References

[1]   Bramsa et al. Minimum information about a microarray experiment (MIAME)-toward standards for microarray data, *Nature. Genetics*, 29(4), pp365-371, 2001

[2]   Paul T Spellman et al. Design and implementation of microarray gene expression markup language (MAGE-ML) *Genome Biology*, 3(9), pp. research0046.1-0046.9, 2002

[3]   Martin Fowler *Patterns of Enterprise Application Architecture*, Addison Wesley, 2002

[4]   Plate-forme microarrays/transcriptome de Nice/Sophia-Antipolis http://medlab.ipmc.cnrs.fr/. Last visited jan 11, 2005

[5]   ISO/IEC 13250:2000 Topic Maps: Information Technology -- Document Description and Markup Languages, Michel Biezunski, Martin Bryan, Steven R. Newcomb, ed., 3 Dec 1999

[6]   OUZIRI, Mourad. Utilisation des Topic Maps pour l'interrogation et la génération de documents virtuels : Application au domaine médical. Thèse : Institut National des Sciences Appliquées de Lyon, 2003, 220 p.

[7]   Scott W. Ambler, Ron Jeffries *Agile Modeling: Effective Practices for Extreme Programming and the Unified Process*, John Wiley & sons, 2002

[8]   Prabi web site http://www.prabi.fr/

7 Address for correspondence

Frederique Laforest
LIRIS, Bat Blaise Pascal
INSA de Lyon
F-69621 Villeurbanne Cedex
France
frederique.laforest@insa-lyon.fr

Connecting Medical Informatics and Bio-Informatics
R. Engelbrecht et al. (Eds.)
IOS Press, 2005

39

Practical Approaches to the Development of Biomedical Informatics: the INFOBIOMED Network of Excellence

Hans-Peter Eich[a]**, Guillermo de la Calle**[b]**, Carlos Diaz**[c]**, Scott Boyer**[d]**, A. S. Peña**[e]**,**

Bruno G. Loos[e]**, Peter Ghazal**[f]**, Inge Bernstein**[g] **and the INFOBIOMED Network**

[a]*Coordination Centre for Clinical Trials, Heinrich-Heine-University, Düsseldorf, Germany*
[b]*Artificial Intelligence Lab./Facultad de Informática, Universidad Politécnica de Madrid, Madrid, Spain*
[c]Biomedical Informatics Research Group, Municipal Institute of Medical Research - IMIM, *Barcelona, Spain*
[d]*AstraZeneca R&D Mölndal, Mölndal, Sweden*
[e]*Academic Center for Dentistry Amsterdam (ACTA), Universiteit van Amsterdam, Vrije Universiteit and VUmc Amsterdam, Amsterdam, The Netherlands*
[f]*Scottish Centre for Genomic Technology & Informatics,University of Edinburgh Medical School, Edinburgh, United Kingdom*
[g]*The Danish HNPCC-register, Surgical Department, Hvidovre Hospital, Hvidovre, Denmark*

Abstract

Biomedical Informatics (BMI) is the emerging discipline that aims to facilitate integration of Bioinformatics and Medical Informatics for the purpose of accelerating discovery and the generation of novel diagnostic and therapeutic modalities. Building on the success of the European Commission-funded BIOINFOMED Study, an INFOBIOMED Network of Excellence has been constituted with the main objective of setting a structure for a collaborative approach at a European level. Initially formed by fifteen European organizations, the main objective of the INFOBIOMED network is therefore to enable the reinforcement of European BMI at the forefront of these emergent interdisciplinary fields. The paper describes the structure of the network, the integration approaches regarding databases and four pilot applications.

Keywords:
Bioinformatics; Medical Informatics; Biomedical Informatics; Genomic Medicine; Research Networks; Data Integration; Ontologies

1. Background

Since the 1960s Medical Informatics (MI) has been established as an independent discipline, and some universities have consolidated specific departments and training programs. It was clear at the time that a new discipline was emerging, with professionals trained in fields outside classical medicine, e.g. computer science, decision analysis, engineering, or economics [1]. Computer scientists, mathematicians, and engineers joined MI to begin a professional career in this field. Such professionals, medical informaticians, began to merge models and techniques from computer science fields, like artificial intelligence, with knowledge about patient care. Later, the development of applications such as electronic health records, expert systems, hospital information systems, multimedia programs and many others have contributed to establish MI as a scientific discipline.

In the biological area, the consolidation of genetics as a scientific discipline, based on principles such as Mendel's Laws and the discovery of the physical structure of DNA led to an increasing amount of data and information that needed to be stored and analyzed. In the 1960s, this growth of data and the availability of computers led to the beginning of the discipline of computational biology [2]. A convergence appeared later, gathering topics from biology, biochemistry, engineering, and computer science, leading to Bioinformatics (BI). Some pioneers began to apply informatics methods and computer tools to molecular biology problems, even a decade before DNA sequencing was feasible. It was also shown that computers could dramatically speed up sequencing and determination of protein structures. Rapidly, BI began to develop. For instance, GENBANK, a DNA sequence database, was created in 1980 and SwissProt, for proteins, a few years later [3]. These and other computer systems led to the acceptance of BI as an independent discipline.

MI and BI have had problems in obtaining scientific recognition. Computer scientists considered that applied informatics is just a branch of computer science, and some biomedical professionals viewed informaticians as mere developers of computer programs without a real scientific merit. In this sense, advances in genomics might dramatically change this traditional perception. The techniques needed to advance genomic medicine might come from the intersection of these four areas: MI, BI, medicine and biology. That is the reason why a new area, Biomedical Informatics (BMI), is being brought at the intersection of both MI and BI to create a synergy between them. Only combined studies of gene interactions in humans and large epidemiological studies from many different populations can discover the complex pathways of genetic diseases. In such a postgenomic era, it is presumed that it will be easier to determine the risks of some specific populations in relation with certain diseases. Thus, personalized prevention and therapeutics could be established, with patient-customized pharmaceuticals or diet [4]. Therefore, a close collaboration between researchers in MI and BI can contribute to new insights in genomic medicine and towards the more efficient and effective use of genomic data to advance clinical care [5]. The need for integrated BMI efforts has been realized by different institutions. In this regard, the European Commission (EC) organized in 2001, in Brussels, a workshop to analyze the synergies between MI, BI and neuroinformatics. Later, efforts carried out at the EC and US institutions have led to various achievements. In Europe, the BIOINFOMED [6] study led to the publication of a White Paper about the challenges in BMI regarding genomic medicine. This study has led to launch the INFOBIOMED Network of Excellence (NoE) funded by the EC (6th Framework Programme) [7].

2. Research approaches in the network

In its initial phase, the NoE has carried out a comprehensive analysis of the state of the art in the areas of data models and ontologies, database integration, security, data mining and knowledge discovery, image analysis and processing, and decision support. These state of the art studies aim to provide basis for identifying the existing gaps and finding the best solutions that can be applied horizontally to the pilot applications. Although details cannot be fully reported in this paper, two areas - ontologies and data integration - have been considered as being crucial for the development of BMI solutions for common problems.

Ontologies were defined by Gruber as "explicit specifications of conceptualizations". They are much more than controlled taxonomies. They are conceived to represent the underlying meaning of a scientific domain or field. The OWL (Web Ontology Language), a proposed standard for developing and representing ontologies, linked to the concept of the

"Semantic Web", can be fundamental to link knowledge from many different and heterogeneous sources, including databases and documents accessible over the Web. The huge amount of data that biomedical genomic researchers must analyze generates important challenges that biomedical informaticians should address.

Bridges to overcome syntax and semantics gaps across different data sources are required for database integration. For instance, when the same concept is labeled with different names in different databases, it might be needed to map these names to the same concept within a specific ontology. In recent research approaches, specialized ontologies such as GeneOntology are used to create shared vocabularies, whose terms can be used to map terms from different database fields. For instance, the INFOGENMED project [8], funded by the EC, aimed to integrate public and private genomic and health databases to assist biomedical researchers in locating and accessing information over the Web.

Within the NoE, the use of ontologies in various areas related to database integration, data mining and information retrieval, is planned.

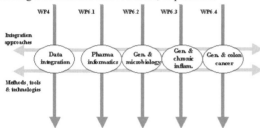

Figure 1-A diagram showing the horizontal and vertical integration approaches regarding database integration (WP 4), integration of tools, methods and technologies and the four pilot applications, WP 6.1 to 6.4

With respect to data integration, two different methods for heterogeneous database integration have been identified: data translation and query translation. In data translation approaches, data from heterogeneous databases at different sites are collected and placed in a local repository. In query translation approaches, queries are translated instead of data. Most recent approaches to database integration are based on a query translation approach.

Most approaches based on query translation can be classified into four categories: a) Pure mediation, using "mediators" and "wrappers". These are brokers between users and data resources; b) Single virtual conceptual schemas, using a unique semantic model to integrate the information available at the data sources. A broker module is responsible for retrieving, adapting, gathering and presenting the final results; c) Multiple virtual conceptual schemas, where each linked database is described with a different virtual schema; and d) Hybrid approaches, where a single schema is used to describe each data source. This schema is created using a shared vocabulary or ontology.

3. Pilot applications

The goal of the NoE is to be able to reuse BMI methods and tools within four pilot applications, showing the ability to carry out integrated ideas in different research domains.

Pharmainformatics, aimed at investigating the impact of BMI on the different stages of the drug discovery process, from target identification to clinical trials. The intensive use of new information technologies has been postulated as a way to accelerate and optimize the drug discovery process. To a large extent, information drives the development of new drugs, and the power of computers can be harnessed to sieve vast numbers of molecules with potential medicinal value. Computational procedures include the "in silico" creation, characterization and filtering of molecular libraries. Computer-based "virtual screening" experiments can automatically assess the fulfillment of drug-likeness criteria or pharmacophoric patterns, as well as perform the simulated docking of large series of compounds to 3D models of their potential targets. A recent extension of the virtual screening strategy is the chemogenomics approach, which aims to link both chemical and biological spaces by a joint analysis of libraries of selected ligands and related targets. Early virtual screening of ADMET properties is an computational task that is becoming crucial for optimizing the flow along the drug discovery pipeline. The aim of this pilot is therefore to extend the use of existing bioinformatic /chemogenomic approaches and to link them to clinical data relating either to a specific disease or adverse event. The activities in this pilot focus on carrying out two specific research examples of how software, database / format and work processes available within the NoE relate and contribute to the drug discovery process. The two examples are: Complex Regional Pain Syndrome (CRPS) and Nuclear Hormone Receptors (NHRs).

They will illustrate the information continuum from pathology to pathway to target to ligand/approved drug, but they will be approached from different directions. In the case of CRPS, a top-down approach will be used. The starting point will be the pathology, i.e. CRPS, and the end point will be possible ligands/approved drugs. In the case of NHRs, the starting point will be the ligands/approved drugs and the end point is pathology/adverse events. In both cases, the goal of this pilot application is to identify gaps in technologies and information that can be focus of further research to improve the drug discovery process. **Genomics and infectious disease**, focused on the study of host and pathogen genetic polymorphisms, protein interactions and transcriptional/translational control and how these impact on pathogen virulence and host immune responses to infection. To date in excess of 2000 viral and microbial genomes have been sequenced and genetic variation at the single nucleotide level of our genome is fast approaching eight figures. Comparative and functional genomic approaches combined with proteomic strategies are further helping to describe gene/protein interaction pathways. These recent advances are dependent on the use and development of novel BI tools. In medicine, the quantitative modeling of viral dynamics in patients treated with multi-drug regimes are gaining increasing effectiveness in treatment management. The determination of viral sequence variation for assessing escape mutants from therapeutic agents in individuals is fast becoming standard practice, e.g. in HIV infected patients. These advances require tools and new algorithm development in MI. Fundamental to the biology and virulence of an infection is a clear understanding of the host-pathogen interactions at the systemic and cellular levels and which opens new challenges and opportunities for advancing anti-infective therapies. These challenges and opportunities will require BMI approaches.

The general activities in this pilot are aimed at using pathway biology (of the interferon system) as a central hub for integrating BI and MI. Two distinct clinical relevant pathogens, HIV and Cytomegalovirus, will be used as exemplars in the pilot. Here, it will be necessary to further characterize a) the viral genome, load and dynamics at a given stage of disease and b) assess the host's genotype, e.g. polymorphisms in key genes defining the hosts innate resistance to viral infection and proliferation and those determining the efficacy of therapeutic drugs (and their combinations) in clinical use. Taking in account the higher complexity of the human genome, in this application the NoE concentrates on the interferon pathway, combining host and virus genotype data with clinical data in order to find new markers of host immunity and viral therapy resistance.

Genomics and chronic inflammation, aimed at investigating the complex susceptibility to adult periodontitis. About 10% of the adult population will develop severe forms of destructive, chronic periodontal disease (chronic periodontitis). This complex inflammatory disease is precipitated in susceptible subjects by infection of the periodontium (tooth supporting tissue) by Gram-negative, anaerobic, mostly commensal oral microorganisms. Moreover, the environmental factor smoking contributes importantly to disease severity. Modifying disease genes determine the susceptibility of periodontitis. However, still very little is known about the interplay and relative importance of genetic factors, bacterial pathogens and environmental determinants, like smoking and stress. There is a great need to gain more insight in the complexity of periodontitis, to design new treatment strategies and devise preventive measures. Periodontitis is an excellent model to study complex chronic inflammatory diseases because of its multifactorial etiology (genetics, bacteria, and environment), relative high prevalence and broad and easy access to diseased patients' and normal tissues, genomic DNA, and access to the history of infections and other relevant data through patient records. The aim of this pilot is to build a periodontitis data warehouse based on patient information coming from different sources: genetics, infection, environment, intermediate phenotype and disease phenotype. This data warehouse will be explored by data analysis and data mining tools from the various partners.

Genomics and colon cancer targets at accumulating knowledge useful for the planning and organization of screening in families with a high-risk of developing colon cancer and supporting research on the subject. HNPCC (Hereditary Non Polypose Colon Cancer) is a dominantly inherited colorectal cancer syndrome, with a lifetime risk up to 90% of developing colorectal cancer for carriers of the genes. Furthermore there is an increased risk of developing endometrial cancer or cancers in the urinary tract. The aim of this pilot is to build-up a general IT-infrastructure based on open XML standards for communication, to link different kinds of medical departments working together in an HNPCC register. These standards should meet HNPCC needs (e.g. transmission of pedigrees including geno-phenotype), the needs of related fields (e.g. other onco-genetic diseases) and should be usable in different countries. Existing international standards will build a basis (e.g. HL7) for this purpose. In a proof of concept, the IT-infrastructure of the Danish HNPCC register will be transformed from mainly isolated databases with paper-based communication amongst them to linked and interoperable databases with XML communication.

4. Network structure

This program of activities requires the participation of organizations with distinct profiles. The INFOBIOMED NoE gathers European research groups with a strong background and experience. Also technological groups that will ensure the application of state-of-the-art information tools and technologies (ontologies, web services, etc.) and their interoperability are included. Finally, biomedical research labs will offer real data and validate the network tools and methods in a number of biomedical research areas, as described above.

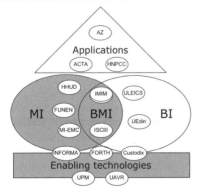

Figure 2-Profiles of the groups included in the network

The core of the INFOBIOMED NoE, formed by 15 renowned institutions that currently develop critical research in MI, BI and related fields, has been designed to offer the necessary critical mass to create a chain effect in the field at the European level that can foster the pursued integrative and structuring effort (figure 2): AstraZeneca R&D Mölndal (AZ), Academisch Centrum Tandheelkunde Amsterdam (ACTA), Danish HNPCC-Register (HNPCC), Heinrich-Heine University of Düsseldorf (HHUD), Municipal Institute of Medical Research (IMIM), University of Leicester (ULEICS), Danish Center for Health Telematics (FUNEN), University of Edinburgh (UEdin), Erasmus University Medical Center (MI-EMC), Institute of Health "Carlos III" (ISCIII), Informa S.r.l. (INFORMA), Foundation for Research and Technology – Hellas (FORTH), Custodix nv (CUSTODIX), Polytechnical University of Madrid (UPM) and the University of Aveiro (UAVR)

5. Conclusion

Following an initiative of the EC, INFOBIOMED offers an innovative networking approach that intends to exploit the potential synergies of already established scientific disciplines for the empowerment of an emerging one. This structuring effort seeks to deploy the promised benefits of the genomic revolution to society by combining the expertise and experience acquired through the, up to now, independent development of both BI and MI. Past and present integration initiatives in that respect suffer from an excessive isolation or only address the problem partially; INFOBIOMED represents the kind of global, integrative vision and joint effort required to overcome the obstacles that are delaying the development of true genomic medicine.

6. Acknowledgments

The present work has been funded by the European Commission (FP6, IST thematic area) through the INFOBIOMED NoE (IST-2002-507585).

7. References

[1]   Schwartz, WB. 1970. Medicine and the Computer: The Promise and Problems of Change. *New England Journal of Medicine*, 283:1257-1264.
[2]   Levitt M. 2001. The Birth of Computational Structural Biology. *Nat. Structural Biology*, vol 8, 5: 392-393.
[3]   Bairoch A. 2000. Serendipity in Bioinformatics, the Tribulations of a Swiss Bioinformatician through Exciting Times. *Bioinformatics* 16: 48-64.
[4]   Housman D. 1998. Why pharmacogenomics? Why now? *Nat Biotechnology* 16:492.
[5]   Knaup P., Ammenwerth E., Brander R., Brigl B., Fischer G., Garde S., Lang E., Pilgram R., Ruderich F., Singer R., Wolff A.C., Haux R., Kulikowski C. Towards Clinical Bioinformatics: Advancing Genomic Medicine with Informatics Methods and Tools. *Methods Inf Med*: 2004 43: 302-307.
[6]   Martin-Sanchez F., Iakovidis I., Norager S., Maojo V., de Groen P., Van der Lei J., Jones T., Abraham-Fuchs K., Apweiler R., Babic A., Baud R., Breton V., Cinquin P., Doupi P., Dugas M., Eils R., Engelbrecht R., Ghazal P., Jehenson P., Kulikowski C., Lampe K., De Moor G., Orphanoudakis S., Rossing N., Sarachan B., Sousa A., Spekowius G., Thireos G., Zahlmann G., Zvarova J., Hermosilla I., Vicente F.J. Synergy between Medical Informatics and Bioinformatics: Facilitating Genomic Medicine for Future Health Care. *J Biomed Inform*: Feb 2004 37(1): 30-42.
[7]   www.infobiomed.org / www.infobiomed.net
[8]   Babic A, Maojo V, Martin-Sanchez F, Santos M, and Sousa A. Ercim News. *Special Biomedical Informatics*. Jan 2005. n° 60. (www.ercim.org/publication/Ercim_News/enw60/)

Address for correspondence

Hans-Peter Eich, Coordination Centre for Clinical Trials, Heinrich-Heine-University Düsseldorf, Moorenstr. 5, 40225 Düsseldorf, Germany, Email: eich@uni-duesseldorf.de

Section 2

Computerized Patient Record

Connecting Medical Informatics and Bio-Informatics
R. Engelbrecht et al. (Eds.)
IOS Press, 2005

Quality Labelling and Certification of Electronic Health Record Systems

Morten Bruun-Rasmussen[a], Knut Bernstein[a], Søren Vingtoft[a], Christian Nøhr[b], Stig Kjær Andersen[b]

[a]MEDIQ – Medical Informatics and Quality Development, Copenhagen, Denmark
[b]Aalborg University, Denmark

Abstract:

The Danish Health IT strategy 2003-2007 demands implementation of Electronic Health Records (EHR) in all Hospitals based on common standards. The aim is to achieve integration and semantic interoperability between different EHR systems in order to support a better communication and coherence between the health care parties. The National Board of Health has developed a common model, which is a prerequisite for the development and implementation of interoperable EHR systems. The adoption of the common EHR model has been promoted and validated through a number of pilot projects in different Hospitals. The Danish EHR Observatory, which has been monitoring the development of EHR in Denmark since 1998, have developed a methodology for Quality labelling and certification of EHR systems. The methodology for certification of EHR systems has been used to validate EHR systems from different vendors to document to which extent the systems are based on the national requirements for EHR.

Keywords:
Electronic Health Record; Standards; Assessment; Quality labelling; Certification; Methodology; Interoperability.

1. Introduction

The Danish Electronic Health Record Observatory was launched in 1998 by the Danish Ministry of Health. The purpose of the EHR Observatory is to support the realisation of the National Health IT strategy by monitoring and assessing the dissemination and implementation of EHR applications in the Hospitals. The EHR Observatory is disseminating national and international experience and best practice to the EHR actors. The Danish EHR Observatory is funded by the Ministry of Interior and Health, the Association of Danish Regions and the Copenhagen Hospital Corporation.

The Danish Health Care system can in brief be characterised by:

- The National Health Service covers all 5.3 million citizens
- 3.500 GPs have 90% of all patient contacts
- More than 90% of GPs use EHR for clinical documentation
- GPs are largely publicly funded
- 65 hospitals are owned by 14 counties and the Copenhagen Hospital Corporation
- 4.6 million outpatient visits per year
- 22.000 hospital beds of which less than 100 are in private hospitals

- 1.3 million annual discharges
- 22 % of hospital beds are served by EHR (by mid-2004)

In 2003 the Ministry of Interior and Health approved a new national IT strategy for the Danish Health Care Service [1] for the period 2003 to 2007. The purpose of the National IT Strategy for the Danish Health Care Service is to establish a common framework for the full digitization of the health care service during the period 2003–2007. The fiscal agreement for 2003 between the government and the counties (i.e. the hospital owners) states as a common goal that electronic health records based on shared standards is to be implemented in all Danish hospitals by the end of 2005.

The aim of the shared standards and common concepts for health records and IT systems is that data can be shared and that they can efficiently support interdisciplinary high quality care. The purpose is also to enable communication of data between EHRs and other IT systems without forcing the involved parties in the health care service to utilize systems from the same vendor. In this way standards will support a free market as well as the desired degree of specialised applications

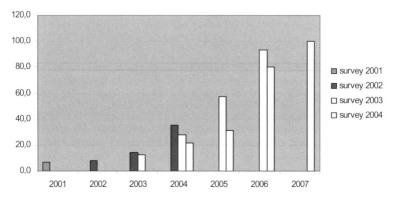

Figure 1 – EHR coverage 2001-2004

The ambitious goal that all hospitals must have EHR by the end of 2005 is a driving force for the EHR implementation in Denmark; however this rigorous schedule is now being eased. The dissemination of EHR is monitored and surveyed by the EHR Observatory using the number of beds covered by EHR as an indicator for the national coverage. In June 2004 the national average coverage was 22% [5][8], varying from 0% to 70% among the regions. The coverage in the previous years and the estimates for the next years are shown on figure 1.

A particularly important initiative of standardization is the national project "Basic Structure for Electronic Health Records" (BEHR)[2]. Based on standards elaborated by the National Board of Health, this project creates the foundation for a coordinated formation of concepts in EHRs in the hospital sector.

The "Basic Structure for Electronic Health Records" is a generic information model for clinical information systems published by the National Board of Health. This model sets the national standard for EHRs. It is characterized by using the clinical problem solving process as the structural backbone for all clinical information and it is designed to directly support continuity of multiprofessional health care across all environments of the entire health care service.

The Clinical Process is a specialization of the general method for problem solving and in the health care domain the BEHR model includes at a generic level: 'Diagnostic Consideration' leading to a set of 'Diagnosis', 'Planning' leading to a set of 'Interventions',

'Execution' of 'Interventions' leading to 'Outcome' and 'Evaluation' of 'Outcome' validated by 'Goal'.

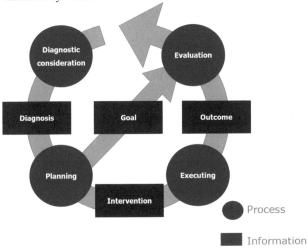

Figure 2 - Basic Structure for Electronic Health Records

1. Diagnostic Consideration

Diagnostic Consideration is a process of collecting and analysing facts in order to understand the patient condition and determine the problems faced. This process implies that the health professionals, describes the problems that are in focus. The documentation of the problems is expressed primarily as structured diagnoses by all kind of health professionals (doctors, nurses, physiotherapists). 'Diagnosis' is a clinical judgment where an actual or potential patient condition is in focus. Within the context of the conceptual model this professional judgment is defined in a much broader sense than a solely medical view.

2. Planning

Planning is a process during which interventions to be performed are outlined according to expected or desired outcomes. This process implies that health professionals add a number of concrete interventions for diagnostics, treatment, prevention, care, rehabilitation etc. The BEHR model requires that one or more diagnosis should be indicated for each intervention.

3. Execution

The interventions are executed and the outcome is documented. In this context, outcome is seen broadly as information about the patient's condition, i.e. results of examinations as well as different kinds of treatments and preventive actions e.g. medication, nursing, surgery, rehabilitation programmes etc.

4. Goal and evaluation

A goal in BEHR has to be operational and is the documentation of what is expected or desired outcome of intervention. If the expected outcome does not meet the expected goal, the health care professionals have to continue a new cycle in the BEHR model.

2. Materials and methods

An important aspect of the EHR implementation is that the EHR vendors use the common concept model in their solutions and that they participate in testing and the further development of BEHR. One of the tools to ensure a high degree of coherence when implementing BEHR has been addressed in the IT strategy by a specific action. The Danish National Board of Health launched in June 2003 a National BEHR project [6][7], with the objective to establish a number of reference implementation of the BEHR model in the Danish Hospitals. An important outcome of the project was to assess the actual use of BEHR and the clinical impact of using the BEHR model. The Danish EHR Observatory [3] has assessed the project within 3 areas:

- Certification: validate to what extend the EHR prototypes are based on the national BEHR model
- Exchange of information between EHR systems
- Assessment of the clinical impact by using BEHR.

The validation (certification) of to what extend the EHR prototypes was based on the BEHR model, was an important milestone in the project, to ensure that that the EHR system was compliant with the BEHR model when assessing the clinical impact of the systems.

This paper is only reporting the certification, where the prerequisite for the EHR prototypes in the project was:

- The EHR system has implemented the BEHR model, including the central use cases, the Reference Information Model (RIM) and the business rules.
- The EHR system is designed as a multi user system.
- The EHR system is user friendly and has an acceptable performance
- The EHR system is stable and includes all aspects of security

The BEHR model is specified in a number of documents and includes use-cases, business rules, RIM model, data descriptions and XML-schemas. The specifications include also a data set and data scenarios to validate if an EHR system is compliant with BEHR specifications. The data for validation is extensive and includes approximately 500 individual tests.

The EHR Observatory developed a methodology [4] to be used to validate to what extend an EHR system is compliant with the specifications as shown on Figure 3.

The test of an EHR system is done in two phases. In the first phase the test is done by the vendor of the system (self assessment). When the vendor finds, that the system is mature to pass the test, a new test is performed together with individuals from the EHR Observatory.

The purpose of the self-assessment phase is to allow the vendor to try out the methodology and ensure that the expected result of the assessment can be fulfilled. When the start for the self-evaluation is agreed with the EHR Observatory, the vendor has maximum 2 weeks to perform the self-assessment. During the self-assessment, the vendor documents the result of each individual test in a test protocol and a test log. In case the test protocol documents a result above an agreed threshold, the vendor requests the EHR Observatory to perform the final assessment.

The purpose of the assessment phase is to examine to what extent the EHR system is compliant with the BEHR specifications. The assessment process is fully documented and allows that parts of the test, which fails can be re-assessed later. The time for the assessment is scheduled to maximum 2 days and the EHR Observatory records the results of the individual tests in a test protocol. By the end of the assessment a report, which concludes the overall result of the test is prepared. The report is concluding whether the EHR system passed the assessment (Yes or No). If the EHR system did not pass the test it can be conditional approved which means that the vendor has to correct some minor errors. In case the result reveals considerable deviation from the BEHR specifications or that important elements are not implemented accurately, a new assessment is required. The assessment phase is finalised by the EHR Observatory and the vendor is signing the report.

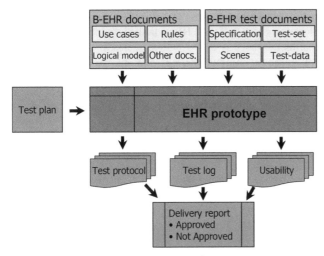

Figure 3 – Methodology for EHR certification

A prerequisite for running the assessment phase is that the vendor documents that the EHR installation and execution environment correspond to a real operational environment. This implies that the installation includes all necessary components and resources to avoid that the tests is not influenced by irrelevant causes.

Before the assessment phases are started, a set of criteria for passing the test has to be agreed upon. The criteria for the National BEHR project were stipulated by the National Board of Health:

- Minimum 90% of the test set can be demonstrated without any errors
- All use cases in the BEHR specifications can be demonstrated by the EHR system
- The 10% errors, which can be accepted, may not occur by excluding one or more use cases.

3. Results

In the National BEHR project the model was implemented in two main pilot projects, in Amager Hospital and in Aarhus County.

The first assessment took place in Amager Hospital the 24 and 25. February 2005. Before the assessment, the vendor had performed a self-evaluation, which documented that they had not performed all the required tests. By the EHR Observatory assessment, 50% of the 500 individual tests were tested and out of these, 50% was accepted. The result of the assessment was summarised in a report, which concluded that a new assessment should take place.

The 23. and 24. March 2004 a new assessment was performed. The starting point was to test the areas, which failed at the first assessment and continue with the individual tests which were not performed.

By the two assessments 90% of all tests were done and out of these test 55% was accepted.

Due to lack of resources in the pilot project the vendor had decided not to implement use cases for the tasks: "Manage relatives", "Monitor documentation" and "Error handling". If the test of these three use cases was excluded from the test protocol, the final result increased to 80%.

An analysis of the tests which was accepted showed that the EHR prototype had all the core parts of the BEHR model implemented and the EHR prototype was therefore approved as a basis for the clinical evaluation.

The second assessment took place in Aarhus the 12. and 13. April 2004. Before assessment the vendor had performed a self-evaluation, but the documentation was not forwarded to the EHR Observatory. At the EHR Observatory assessment, 100% of the 500 individual tests were performed and out of these 65% was accepted. In this pilot project the vendor had decided not to implement use cases for "Manage relatives", "Monitor documentation" and "Error handling". If the test of these 3 use cases was excluded from the test protocol the final result was increased to 85%. An analysis of the accepted tests showed that the EHR prototype had all the core parts of the BEHR model implemented and the EHR prototype was therefore approved as a basis for the clinical evaluation.

4. Discussion and conclusion

The assessment of the two EHR prototypes (Amager Hospital and Aarhus County) was performed in test environments, which, due to security reasons, was disconnected from the real operational environment. A prerequisite for the assessment was that the EHR installation and execution environment correspond to a real operational environment and that the installation had all necessary components and resources..

By the assessment of the two EHR prototypes a sufficient environment was established and the effort was concentrated on the task to assess to what extend the EHR prototypes had implemented the BEHR model.

As the assessment found a lot of errors in the EHR systems, which was not identified during self-assessment, the external assessment methodology can be used by the vendor to improve the quality of the system.

The same methodology can be used by the end-user as a part of the acceptance test when buying a new system.

Based on the result of the assessment, it can be concluded that the used methodology together with the BEHR specification is a systematic way to test to what extent an EHR system have implemented the BEHR model.

5. References

[1] Ministry of Interior and Health. National IT strategy 2003-2007 for the Danish Health Care Service. May 2003.
[2] Basic Structure for Electronic Health Records (BEHR). The National Board of Health, Denmark. Copenhagen.   URL: http://www.sst.dk/Informatik_og_sundhedsdata/Elektronisk_patientjournal/GEPJ.aspx - (Publication only available in Danish: GEPJ - Grundstruktur for Elektronisk Patientjournal).
[3] The Danish EHR Observatory. URL: http://www.epj-observatoriet.dk
[4] Assessment of EHR prototypes. The Danish EHR Observatory, M. Bruun-Rasmussen, K. Bernstein, S. Vingtoft, August 2004.
[5] Danish EHR Observatory - annual report 2004. C. Nøhr, S. K. Andersen, S. Vingtoft, M. Bruun-Rasmussen, K. Bernstein, October 2004.
[6] BEHR prototyping and clinical assessment (GEPKA), National Board of Health, 7. January 2003.
[7] The Danish National Health Informatics Strategy. S Lippert, A.Kverneland, *Stud Health Technol Inform*. 2003; 95:845-50
[8] Danish EHR Observatory - annual report 2003. M. Bruun-Rasmussen, K. Bernstein, S. Vingtoft, S. K. Andersen ,C. Nøhr, October 2003.

Address for correspondence

Morten Bruun-Rasmussen, mbr@mediq.dk, MEDIQ – Medical Informatics and Quality Development Østerled 8, 2100 Copenhagen O, Denmark,www.mediq.dk

Connecting Medical Informatics and Bio-Informatics
R. Engelbrecht et al. (Eds.)
IOS Press, 2005

Computerized Case History - an Effective Tool for Management of Patients and Clinical Trials

Nikita Shklovsky-Kordi[*1], Boris Zingerman[1], Nikolay Rivkind[2], Saveli Goldberg[3], Scott Davis[4], Lyuba Varticovski[5], Marina Krol[6], A M Kremenetzkaia[1], Andrei Vorobiev[1,] Ilia Serebriyskiy

[1]National Center for Hematology, Moscow, RF,
[2]Diagnostic Center N1, Bryansk, RF,
[3]MGH, Boston, MA, USA
[4]Fred Hutchinson Cancer Center, Seattle, WA, USA
[5]Tufts University, NEMC, Boston, MA,USA.
[6]Mount Sinai Hospital, New York, NY, USA.

Abstract

Monitoring diagnostic procedures, treatment protocols and clinical outcome are key issues in maintaining quality medical care and in evaluating clinical trials. For these purposes, a user-friendly computerized method for monitoring all available information about a patient is needed.
Objective: To develop a real-time computerized data collection system for verification, analysis and storage of clinical information on an individual patient.
Methods: Data was integrated on a single time axis with normalized graphics. Laboratory data was set according to standard protocols selected by the user and diagnostic images were integrated as needed. The system automatically detects variables that fall outside established limits and violations of protocols, and generates alarm signals.
Results. The system provided an effective tool for detection of medical errors, identification of discrepancies between therapeutic and diagnostic procedures, and protocol requirements.
Conclusions: The computerized case history system allows collection of medical information from multiple sources and builds an integrated presentation of clinical data for analysis of clinical trials and for patient follow-up.

Keywords:
Diagnosis; Clinical trials; Computerized case history; Standard protocols; Prevention of medical errors; Telemedicine

Introduction

Analysis of disease progression and treatment outcome in Hematology require primary data with reference to their temporary occurrence and causal connections. Therefore, there is a need for readily accessible unified instrument for management of clinical data with simultaneous access to clinical records and diagnostic material without compromising patient's privacy and safety. This instrument should be useful for real-time evaluation of clinical data based on primary evidence. Use of such an instrument will prevent bias in data interpretation and provide immediate access to new information on an individual patient as well as record storage in a database.

Advances in modern computer technology were helpful in design of various types of electronic patient records. Several studies suggest cost-effectiveness of electronic patient records [1, 2]. These computerized systems for storage of patient data were developed for such diverse fields as pediatric [3], drug rehabilitation [4], surgery [5, 6] diabetes treatment [7], radiology [8], nursing case [9] and others. Most existing systems are designed on a hierarchical basis or similar structured formats [10. 11], utilizing object-oriented (GEHR, Synapses, HL7 RIM) or other document-oriented methodologies (HL7 PRA)[12]. Although many systems are Internet-based, some use hospital-wide computer networks which may incorporate desktop systems [13, 14].

In our effort to create a computerized case history, we implemented the following principles:

- The system should be patient-focused. This led us to a common time-axis design rather than hierarchical structure for data analysis.

- The system should permit easy communications between health providers of different specialties. Thus, it has to accommodate different documents, such as text files, pictures, laboratory results, and others.

Materials and Methods.

We have taken advantage of an existing system used for logical structuring of data known as "temperature sheets" where leading parameters and therapeutic assignments on one sheet of observation have a common time axis. This approach is common in Hematology/Oncology units and, in our hospital, it has helped to develop clinical parameters for treatment of acute radiation (biological dosimetry, in particular), as well as to improve protocols for treatment of hematological malignancies [15, 16]. We used the following steps to generate this instrument:

1. Integration of data stored in different formats (text, tables, roentgenograms, microphotographs, videos etc.);
2. Compression of clinical data by highlighting important and urgent information;
3. Display of information in an integrated fashion on the same screen;
4. Automatic matching of entered data with stored timetables derived from established protocols for diagnostic procedures and treatment.
5. Generation of warning signs ("flags") wherever the data indicate divergence from specified protocols. Exit from the assigned limits of selected parameters is similarly controlled.

The data was plotted manually on the basis of standard case history (wherein the physician acquires medical or diagnostic information and enters it manually on a Page of Dynamic Observation (PDO)), or based on a computerized case history designed for TOMICH program (which provides a template of diagnostic criteria, current protocols and clinical management).

Manual method of entering data on PDO does not require additional devices or software besides a regular PC computer with Microsoft Office and a PDO template in an Excel format. PDO data entry form is an Excel spreadsheet, in which certain rows are reserved for specific type of information (i.e. clinical data, laboratory results, medications, etc.), and the far left column A contains row headings. The software contains a set of templates for widely used clinical protocols and a system for automatic detection of protocol violations.

PDO discription

Therapy: The appropriate medication is selected from a list. Drugs on each line can be selected by cursor for each day followed by pressing a button "therapy" which enters the dose for each specific medication.

Events: Significant events and diagnostic procedures are recorded by selection from a common list or by entering a descriptive term. The user marks the significance of each event by color coding and enters information on the given event. Files representing morphological images, roentgenogram, text documents, etc. can be attached to a specific time period by the indicating of the file's address. After filling the "event form", a cursor tags the event to a "window" for a brief description (i.e. CT scan description on Fig. 1). A double click opens a map of all pictures and text files linked to the event. All "windows" can be augmented or reduced for proper viewing.

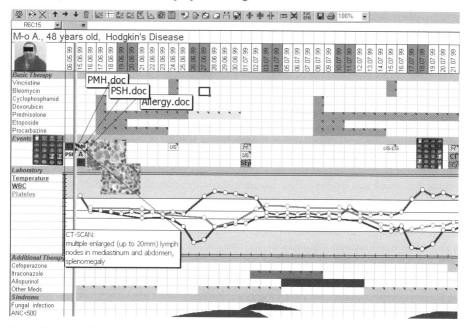

Fig.1. Example of the Page of Dynamic Observation of a patient with Hodgkin's Disease (HD) who underwent treatment with BEACOPP chemotherapy regimen. Some information presented as marks only, some as small windows. The dynamics of chosen parameters (Temperature, WBC and Platelet counts) are normalized and color-coded as described in Methods.

Laboratory data. All test results for a particular patient for each specific time are entered in this appropriate PDO field.

Normalization. All numeric clinical data is broken into normal, sub-normal and pathological range with values stored in PDO. This provides normalization of all parameters and presentation by using common axes. Division of the measured value by the accepted average value accomplishes the normalization. The calculation is executed separately for normal, sub-normal and pathological values. To define the range of sub-normal values, a team of experts empirically established the scope of "acceptable" (for the given diagnosis and selected method of therapy and, in some cases, for an individual patient) parameters. If a parameter stays within the defined sub-normal or normal range, no special action is required. The pathological range covers all the zone of possible values beyond the sub-normal values. In case of manual input, under the date of the analysis, the measured value should be entered. The cell on PDO is automatically converted to the color conforming its position on a scale of normal or pathologic range. If the specific value is out of the acceptance limits, the program generates an automatic alarm signal.

Transfusion: Transfusion data is entered into the PDO cell on a relevant line which includes patient's transfusion information, blood component and dosage for a particular date.

Complications: Complications are recorded on a specific line in PDO and serves to visualize the dynamics of patient's symptoms. After a symptom/syndrome is selected from a list, a window appears on the screen with a definition and criteria to assist in the diagnosis and management. Additional functions are available for further user assistance.

Presentation. The information on PDO presented in the spreadsheet can be automatically transformed in to a graph with the screen broken down into the three shaded zones: norm (white background), sub-norm (yellow) and pathological range (red). To the left of the graphics there is a list of parameters. The color of a title corresponds to color of a curve on the graphics. In each case, when the curves hinder perception of an important parameter, some data may be removed manually (Fig. 1).

Results and Discussion

TOMICH has a standard format for presenting key components of patient's medical record (the constant form of a positional relationship of the main (basic) semantic units of a case history), but also has the flexibility for adding new templates, as necessary for a specific diagnosis. These templates accumulate pre-defined lists of medications, required lab tests and syndromes, and define sub-normal and pathological range of values, as well as color palette for drugs and graphs. Also, the template may refer to the standard protocols for specific diseases or clinical trials stored in the database.

Using the steps outlined above, we developed a system of TOMICH the centerpiece of which is PDO. All information on PDO is structured and stored in sections briefly or graphically identified and interrelated in a time sequence. In addition, for every event, the user has an easy access to additional related information. All information on PDO is structured and stored in sections briefly or graphically identified and interrelated in a time sequence.

The beforehand constructed template permits standard recognized images for diagnosis and helps to discriminate general characteristics and specific features for an individual patient. For example, there are accepted criteria for decrease in platelets, leukocyte and hemoglobin in response to chemotherapeutic treatment. We found that these values express similar stability with a dose-dependent drop in leukocyte count after acute total body irradiation in doses between 50 and 600 cGr. Slower drop suggests a decreased dose; slower recovery indicates a poor bone marrow reserve, severe infection or other complications. We found that comparison of shapes of drug-dependent changes in blood counts is a valuable estimation of outcome.

In a real-time mode, TOMICH automatically performed data validation and notified a user when selected parameters were beyond acceptable ranges or when the timetable set by the protocol was not followed. These software features permit health care personnel to monitor and correct, when needed, individual actions taken by medical personnel. TOMICH links the actions of medical staff with requirements set by the protocols. Attention of physicians and staff is prompted by a color indicator and alarm signals and letter to the e-mail address of the individual in charge of the protocol management. Thus, the error is detected in real-

time and the system facilitates collective decisions for corrective action to avoid possible damage.
TOMICH has been successfully used for several years in the National Center for Hematology (NCH) in Moscow, Russia [17]. More recently, the system has been implemented in the Bryansk Diagnostic Center, Russia. The local users electronically transmit TOMICH files to NCH, where experts consult with Bryansk professionals by the means of telemedicine [18].

Conclusions

TOMICH is a convenient and easily automated method for entering all available information about a patient. It may be classified as a decision-support and expert – oriented system, which allows a physician to select a pre-entered template and to modify it for creating the most appropriate template for a particular patient. It provides easy access to primary data and allows generation of a common time-line axis format for multimedia presentation of a patient's record. The system links different medical images (pathology slides, EKG, x-rays, photos of patients, etc.) as well as text files (reports, notes, etc.) forming a recognizable image. This presentation allows real-time evaluation of disease and response to established protocols. Use of TOMICH facilitates the analysis of clinical course and compliance and reduces the probability of medical errors.

TOMICH was developed using a platform of Microsoft Windows with a standard interface and does not require re-training of users familiar with Microsoft Office. Modifications of Microsoft products, such as Word and Excel, will be instrumental for the further modifications of this program.

Acknowledgments:

This work was supported, in part, by a Grant 99-07-90314 of RFBR, Russia, Grant IBA812 of Institute for Open Society, Grant 0074821 from the NSF and by the Grant No 650 of the International Consortium for Research on the Health Effects of Radiation.

Bibliography

[1]   Thomas SM, Overhage JM, Overhage JM, McDonald CJ. A comparison of a printed patient summary document with its electonic equivalent: early results. Proc AMIA Symp. 2001;:701-5

[2]   Schmitt KF, Wofford DA. Financial analysis projects clear returns from electronic medical records. Healthc Financ Manage. 2002 Jan;56(1):52-7.

[3]   Gioia PC. Quality improvement in pediatric well care with an electronic record.   Proc AMIA Symp. 2001;:209-13

4]   Della Valle RM, Baldoni A, De Rossi M, Ferri F. SeCD electronic folder: CADMIO's application for the medical folder of a service for the care of drug addicts. Medinfo. 1998;9 Pt 1:237-41

[5]   Oyama L, Tannas HS, Moulton S. Desktop and mobile software development for surgical practice. J Pediatr Surg. 2002 Mar;37(3):477-81

[6]   Eggli S, Holm J. Implementation of a new electronic patient record in surgery Chirurg. 2001 Dec;72(12):1492-500

[7]   Hunt DL, Haynes RB, Morgan D. Using Old Technology to Implement Modern Computer-aided Decision Support For Primary Diabetes Care

[8]   Overhage JM, Aisen A, Barnes M, Tucker M, McDonald CJ. Integration of radiographic images with an electronic medical record. Proc AMIA Symp. 2001;:513-7.

[9]   Helleso R, Ruland CM. Developing a module for nursing documentation integrated in the electronic patient record. J Clin Nurs. 2001 Nov;10(6):799-805.

[10] Webster C, Copenhaver J. Structured data entry in a workflow-enabled electronic patient record. J Med Pract Manage 2001 Nov-Dec;17(3):157-61

[11] Bayegan E, Nytro O, Grimsmo A. Ranking of information in the computerized problem-oriented patient record. Medinfo. 2001;10(Pt 1):594-8

[12] Takeda H, Matsumura Y, Kuwata S, Nakano H, Sakamoto N, Yamamoto R.   Architecture for networked electronic patient record systems. Int J Med Inf. 2000 Nov;60(2):161-7

[13] Mangiameli R, Boseman J. Information technology: passport to the future. AOHN J. 2000 May;48(5):221-8.

[14] Chambliss ML, Rasco T, Clark RD, Gardner JP. The mini electronic medical record: a low-cost, low-risk partial solution. J Fam Pract. 2001 Dec;50(12):1063-5

[15] Vorobiev AI, Brilliant MD. WBC and Platelets dynamic during acute irradiation syndrome as biological dosimeter. (Russ.) Proc Conf. Institute of Biophysics, 1970, Moscow.

[16] Vorobiev AI, Brilliant MD. Experience of ambulance treatment of hemablastose patients. (Russ.) Arh.Sov.Med., 1977, 49(8):3-9.

[17] Shklovskiy-Kordi N., Goldberg S., Zingerman B. Time-oriented multi-image presentation of dynamic case history. Proc AMIA Symp. 1998:107.

[18] Shklovskiy-Kordi N., Freidin J., Goldberg S., et al."Standardization for Telemedical Consultation on a Basis of Multimedia Case History", Proc. 14th IEEE Symposium on Computer-Based Medical Systems 2001: pp. 535-540.

Address for correspondence

Nikita Shklovsky-Kordi, 1National Center for Hematology, Novozikovski Pr. No 4, Moscow, RF, 125167
Nikita@blood.ru

Connecting Medical Informatics and Bio-Informatics
R. Engelbrecht et al. (Eds.)
IOS Press, 2005

59

Information on Medication History - Basis for Improved Prescribing

Martina Zorko, Marjan Sušelj

Health Insurance Institute of Slovenia, Ljubljana, Slovenia

Abstract

The spectrum of applied pharmaceuticals, often interactive, persistently expands. In modern therapeutics, patients receive more and more drugs, cases of simultaneous administering of more than 10 different drugs are not seldom. The majority of drugs are prescribed by personal physicians, the rest by the secondary level service specialists, doctors on duty, doctors at the release from the hospital etc. Furthermore, patients keep in stock drugs prescribed in the past. In the Slovene practice of medication prescribing, a major setback is poor information linking between the doctor and the pharmacist, as well as between doctors at different levels of service. Thus, doctors have often raised the issue of timely and accurate informing on the administered drug. This issue became even more pressing upon the implementation of the scheme of substitutable drugs in 2003, allowing the pharmacist to substitute the prescribed drug for an equivalent less expensive one.

The paper outlines a project headed by the Health Insurance Institute of Slovenia (Institute) to facilitate the recording of issued drugs on the card. The information on drugs received by a patient in the past will in this way become readily accessible to the prescribing doctor as well as to the administering pharmacist. This objective requires a range of tasks to be completed: business/operational design of the system, introduction of a uniform drug information scheme at the national level, adjusting the functions of the health insurance card system, upgrading the software environment at the health care service providers, training doctors and pharmacists in applying the new information, and ensuring data security in conformity with regulations.

Keywords:
Medication; e-prescription; Health insurance card

1. Background

The health insurance card (HIC) system, introduced by the Institute in 2000, furnished the Slovenian health care system with an electronic insured person's document and established data interconnections between all insurance providers and health care service providers. The HIC system, which effectively combines the smart card technology and network services, consists of: insured person's cards, health professional cards, health care service providers' data processing environment, and an on-line network of self-service terminals.

As the owner and manager of the HIC system, the Institute has continually since the system's introduction in 2000 made efforts to enhance the functionality in order to extend the benefits and options for the card holders. Major such enhancements include:

- ordering of convention insurance certificates through self-service terminals, in 2001;

- recording of issued medical-technical aids on the card, in 2003;
- integration of a new voluntary insurance provider into the HIC system, in 2003;
- recording the commitment to posthumously donate organs and tissues for transplants, pilot implementation in one region in 2004, national scale implementation this year.

The infrastructure in place and experiences provide infrastructure for the extension of information technology to encompass professional medical work, which is the target of the next development steps.

2. Support to the Medication Management – Record of Drug History

The first step in medication IT management concerns the recording of issued drugs and providing this history to relevant processes. This enhancement is addressed by a project, managed and implemented by the Institute. In view of its national scope, the project is steered by the project board, which seats the representatives of the Ministry of Health and of competent institutions. The project also collaborates with a "counselling group", consisting of representatives of the professional chambers, the Office for Drugs and the Public Health Institute. With such a setup, the project aims at reaching the consensus in all competent bodies and in the medical and pharmacist profession. The project was launched in January 2004. According to the current time schedule, its pilot introduction will start in June 2005, and the national scale introduction early in 2006 [1].

In international perspective, a number of research studies have been undertaken and a host of data gathered concerning un-safe application of drugs, such as:

- Slovenia faces a safety and cost problem of stocks of left-over drugs at home, for it has been established (by a survey in March and April 2004) that of all the elementary drug packages, the users never use as much as 17.7%. [2]
- Experts estimate that, in the developed countries, the problems associated with dispensary prescribed drugs (un-safe or improper use - incorrect selection, administering not in compliance with instructions, incorrect metering, side effects, untreated indications, redundant treatment etc.) are the cause of 7.1 % of all hospital admissions, of which 4.3 % could be avoided. [3]
- It is estimated for the USA that ADR is the fourth most frequent cause of death, immediately following CVD, cancer and CVA. [4]

The objective of the project of recording issued drugs on the card is to set up professional, organisational and technological bases for the extension of the card dataset to include the record of issued drugs. The project aims to advance the level of safe use of drugs, to provide additional information to the prescribing doctors and to the issuing pharmacists, and to improve the information links between the different levels of the health care and between the doctors and the pharmacists (an even more important factor now, under the regime of substitutable drugs). The Institute further envisages the prescribing to be more rational and in this way to contribute to the containment of expenditure on medication, which is a rising trend in Slovenia, similar to other countries. In Slovenia, the expenditure on prescribed drugs from the compulsory health insurance funds is estimated to 61 billion Slovene tolars in 2004, which presents a rise of 1.8% in real terms compared to 2003.

The project ultimate goal is to provide integral support to the process of medication - embracing the prescribing, issuing and accounting of drugs; the recording of drugs on the card is the first step in this direction. In the second step, the HIC system will be enhanced with the e-prescription functionality and with an expert system to assist doctors in prescribing.

To summarise, the benefits for the different user groups include:

Insured persons:

- safer supply of medication (timely detection of potential incompatibilities with medication already administered).

Doctors, pharmacists:

- improved information links within the health care system;
- introduction of uniform drug information;
- first step towards information supported drug prescribing and issuing;
- in the regime of substitutable drugs, feedback information to the doctor on which drug has actually been issued in the pharmacy.

Insurance providers:

- rationalisation of medication expenditure at the national level;
- first step in the direction of e-prescription.

Since this is a pioneer work in the field of medication, the following risks and dilemmas need to be addressed and resolved in the scope of the project: the professional public is voicing a request to include the "opting-out" solution, to empower a patient to prohibit the inspection of drug record on the card to pharmacists and/or doctors. Here, consensus and support from the overall medical profession is required. Another challenge is to coordinate the project with similar projects unfolding at the Institute in relation to the drugs, i.e. the recording of allergies and hypersensitivity reactions to drugs on the HIC. Namely, the information on hypersensitivity reactions to drugs is essential for safe and quality prescription of medication, to avoid adverse reactions in the stage of prescription. The record of this information on the card will provide a systemic, user friendly and integral arrangement of this aspect. According to the draft concept, the card record of each established hypersensitivity reaction is to contain the data on the types of drugs involved, type of reaction, probability, and the indication of the author and the date of recording. Since the information on medication and allergies is sensitive medical information, the project shall observe high standards of the personal data protection regulations.

1.1   Design Solutions

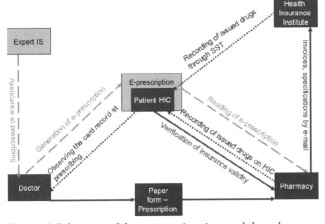

Figure 1-Schematic of the present situation, and the enhancements by steps

In the current arrangement, the doctor prescribes a drug on a paper prescription form, which then serves as a basis for the issuing of the drug in the pharmacy, after checking the HIC record of health insurance validity. The pharmacy reports the issued drug data to the Institute by email. (Fig. 1: solid arrow.)

The first step of enhancement, i.e. the recording of issued drugs on the card, will amend the procedures in the following ways (Fig. 1: dotted arrows):

- In the pharmacy, the issued drugs will be recorded in the card.
- The doctor will observe the record of issued drugs on the card at the time of prescribing new drugs.
- The data will be transmitted to the card (if data on issued drugs was not recorded on the HIC in the pharmacy – due to technical problems or if the patient did not have his/her HIC present) at the time of updating the card through the self-service terminal. Patients update their HIC themselves.

In the second step, i.e. e-prescription step, the system will be further enhanced with an expert system to assist the doctor at prescribing. Instead of the paper form, the doctor will apply electronic recording of the prescription on the HIC and will apply digital signature. In the pharmacy, the e-prescription record will be read from the HIC applying the public key infrastructure. (Fig. 1: dashed arrow.)

1.1.1   Which Data will be recorded on the Card?

For each issued drug, the following data are to be recorded on the card:
- drug operation code;
- issued quantity of the drug;
- date of issue;
- code of the prescribing doctor;
- code of the issuing pharmacy.

The card space allocated to the drug recording is 757b. With the above defined data set, this will allow the recording of 46 drugs. Upon filling up the file, a special algorithm will erase the old records and replace them with the new ones.

1.1.2   Uniform Drug Information - Prerequisite for the Drug Recording on the Card

At present, health care service providers and the pharmacies apply a variety of drug data collections. Accordingly, a prerequisite for the recording and reading of data to/from the card is the implementation of a uniform drug information. To this end, the Institute, in collaboration with the Public Health Institute, is setting up a modern technology based drug data collection with continuous updating from existing data sources, to be distributed to the users by the Institute.

1.1.3   Data Security

Information on received drugs is sensitive personal information, requiring the highest level of security. Card data security is ensured through the scheme of controlled access to different data segments by types of health professional card holders. In this scheme, access to the card drug record is granted to:
- doctors (read-only access); and
- pharmacists (read/write access).

1.1.4   Implementation in the User Environment

The implementation of the project will require upgrading of software in all the card system components and in all the environments of card application.

All the health insurance cards in circulation (close to two million cards) are already provided with the file structure to accommodate drug recording. The size of this file is to remain as original, while the internal file structure has been determined in the course of the project.

To allow the application of the new card file, upgrading of software libraries for all card reader types (desktop, keyboard integrated, portable) is required, as well as upgrading of all the card reader application platforms (DOS, Win 16, Win 32, Clipper, etc.). New library versions will be distributed by the Institute to all the users – 6000 work posts.

To support the recording of drugs through the self-service terminals, terminal software upgrading is required, including their card reader software libraries, for all the 296 terminals in the network.

The communication channel for the reporting and accounting data transfer between the pharmacies and the Institute is also in the process of reconstruction. The reconstruction will involve technology and the contents of communication (extended data set). The accounting reports from the pharmacies are the basis for the maintenance of the issued drug database at the Institute.

To allow reading of data at the doctors' offices and their writing in the pharmacies, software upgrades will be required in these environments, to integrate new software libraries, to allow the processing of issued drug card records and to allow the working with the drug data collection. Another important aspect is the training of doctors, medical nurses and pharmacists in the operation of the upgraded software. Since this is, in many cases, a premiere application involving the doctor's hands-on work with the computer, the training and informing will have to be extensive, carefully planned and professionally executed. A similarly important activity targets the acceptance among the users.

3.   Support to the Medication Management – e-Prescription

This is a second major step, based on and continuing the drug recording step. The e-prescription is an electronic document containing all the data of the present paper prescription form (or several such forms) stored on the patient's health insurance card. Alternative technical variant considered is to record the e-prescription on a server, with the patient card and the doctor's and pharmacist's health professional card serving as keys to access the e-prescription. The difference is only in the location of the storage of data, while for the user, the alternatives are virtually equivalent. The final decision will be made in the course of the project, according to the established conditions in the field as regards the technology and equipment.

The implementation of the e-prescription application depends on the introduction of the public key infrastructure. The introduction of the public key infrastructure is a vital upgrading need for the HIC system, to allow the recording of data requiring specific digital signature protection, among which the e-prescription is one example. In 2005, the Institute continues the preparatory activities, setting up of organisation and technology for phased introduction of the public key infrastructure in the HIC system. This will require the substitution of current health professional cards.

Along with the PKI activities, the project is to address different other aspects as well:
- further standardisation of the drug database;

- synthesis of all data (card, local database at the health care service provider, drug database) and expert SW tools into an integral expert system;
- development of universal interfaces for the integration in the local IT environments at the pharmacies and doctors' offices;
- informing and training of health care workers;
- upgrading IT equipment at the health care service providers - computers on the doctors' desks!

The e-prescription phase is a major step, introducing new technologies and functions into all the aspects of the national health care and health insurance system. We estimate it can be completed in 2 -4 years.

4. Conclusion

The recording of issued drugs on the card and the introduction of a uniform national drug database are to set information foundations for further development in the broad health care environment. Up-to-date and modern technology supported drug data will allow the development of tools to assist doctors in their decisions in the drug prescribing process. Positive effects, though, depend on the continual updating of professional guidelines for treatment and drug prescription, and on information support for these processes, which requires joint efforts by all the competent institutions at the national level. The new functionality will indirectly also promote equipping the health care environment with computer hardware and, in turn, propagation of other modern professional tools in the doctor's office.

The second step will extend the functionality in the direction of prescribing, including the application of the digital signature function. The digital signature functionality will open the way to a variety of other applications in the Slovene health care, dealing with sensitive health related data and subject to the provisions of the electronic commerce regulations in force.

5. References

[1] Health Insurance Institute of Slovenia: "Recording of Issued Drugs on the Health Insurance Card - Z-KZZ" project document file.

[2] Research study: evaluation of the home stocks of drugs in the safety and cost perspective; Faculty of Pharmacy, University of Ljubljana, September 2004

[3] AG, et al.: Preventable Drug-Related Hospital Admissions; The Annals of Pharmacotherapy, July-August 2002, No. 36: 1238-48

[4] Peter J. Zed: Drug-Related Hospital Visits. How Big is the Problem?, CSHP PPC, Feb 1, 2004

6. Address for correspondence

Martina Zorko
Health Insurance Institute of Slovenia
Miklošičeva 24, SI-1507 Ljubljana, Slovenia
martina.zorko@zzzs.si, www.zzzs.si

Connecting Medical Informatics and Bio-Informatics
R. Engelbrecht et al. (Eds.)
IOS Press, 2005

Users' Needs and Expectations of Electronic Medical Record Systems in Family Medicine Residence Settings

George Demiris [a], Karen L. Courtney [a], Steven E. Waldren[b]

[a] *University of Missouri-Columbia, Missouri, USA*
[b] *Center for Health Information Technology, American Academy of Family Physicians, USA*

Abstract

While physician informational needs have been examined in the literature, rarely do the findings have the specificity required to drive development of Electronic Medical Records (EMRs) features. Using Delphi methodology, a comprehensive list of desirable, ranked EMR features was developed for physician residency practices. The identified EMR features and implications for system development are explored in this paper.

Keywords:
Medical Record Systems; Computerized; Internship and Residency; Delphi Technique; Medical Informatics

1. Introduction

Informational needs of physicians have been studied in the scientific literature [1,2]. Many of these studies present needs at a more abstract or high conceptual level. What is lacking in the literature is an understanding of these needs at an *"implementable" level*. An implementable level is defined as the granularity or degree of detail sufficient for the developer of an Electronic Medical Record (EMR) system to devise a specification to meet that need. For example, stating that a user's need is to communicate with other users does not provide information at an implementable level. The developer must still decide whether this communication should take place in real-time or in an asynchronous matter and whether it may be text or voice based. In contrast, the need for secure messaging would be a possible implementable need; as the developer can infer that the communication will be text-based and asynchronous.

Partly responsible for this lack of design directives at this level, is the difficulty of defining and assessing users' needs and change over time. As individual physicians practice, their informational needs change, and medicine itself is constantly changing by introduction of new information. Another confounding factor is the heterogeneity of physicians. The needs of a primary care physician are not the same as those of a specialist. In addition, the practice setting can affect need, such as urban vs. rural or private practice vs. residency practice. The varied system requirements in different medical environments have been identified as a major barrier to adoption of Electronic Medical Record (EMR) systems [3], yet little is known about the unique system requirement of specific medical settings.

An EMR system can meet physicians' informational needs better than paper-based records[2]. In spite of the perceived benefits of an EMR and the recommendations of the Institute of Medicine[4], the use of EMR systems continues to be low. In a residency setting, where technology innovation is expected and physicians are trained for clinical practice [5], EMR usage was less than 20% in 1998 and was expected to be still less than 50% in 2000 [6]. Lenhart et al. also found non-EMR users viewed the capabilities of EMR systems significantly more optimistically than users[6], indicating many EMR systems fail to address users' expectations.

There is limited knowledge of physicians' needs and expectations of an EMR from the corpus of physicians at the level specified above. Less is known about the subgroup of physicians in a residency setting. Musham et al. studied the perceptions of family practice educators regarding EMRs [5]. They discovered that at a high level the users' needs were greater efficiency in delivering care, lowering costs, and improving quality of care. Their findings were not at an implementable level, which could empower user-driven EMR design for residency programs.

A residency practice has added dynamics that must be addressed on top of the issues of private practice. Residency practice encompasses almost all of the aspects of other practice settings, but it has different priorities. For example, research is of greater importance in a residency practice; also, the business model is different. Residencies are usually affiliated with a university and/or a large hospital and are frequently non-profit. This is in contrast to private practice where many are not affiliated with a university or hospital and if so, are profit-driven. On top of these aspects, other issues such as a more complex patient-provider model (e.g. a billing physician, a supervising physician, and a resident physician for a single patient visit) and resident education have an impact on informational needs. Once we have an understanding of physicians' informational needs at an implementable level, we can facilitate a user-driven EMR system design process.

The purpose of this study is to provide the framework for user-driven design of EMR systems for family practice residency programs that will bridge the gap between high-level informational needs and implementable features.

2. Methods

In order to determine family practitioners' needs and expectations of an EMR system, we conducted an extensive content analysis of published literature and a Delphi study with directors of family practice residencies.

Content Analysis

A literature review was performed to identify those articles that addressed EMR features or feature lists. The search strategy was a search of Medline from 1996 to March 2003 (week 1). We combined the MESH term "Medical Records Systems, Computerized" with the key words, "choosing", "feature", "attribute", and "resident." The articles were reviewed by title and abstract, if available, and those pertaining to EMR features were used. This resulted in ten articles[8-17]. The authors reviewed the articles and extracted features for an independently developed EMR feature list. These lists were then merged to form a new master feature list. Inter-reviewer reliability was not a concern since a comprehensive list was desired. This list was then used as the "designed questionnaire" for the Delphi method.

Delphi Method

A Delphi method "may be characterized as a method for structuring a group communication process so that the process is effective in allowing a group of individuals, as a whole, to deal with a complex problem." [7] Delphi methods can be separated into "blank questionnaire" or "designed questionnaire" approaches. The "blank questionnaire" approach presents the participants of the method with only the problem being addressed, in this case "what are the features of an EMR that satisfy your needs and expectations of an EMR." The "designed questionnaire" gives participants starting data about the problem, in this case a list of features from the literature. The main advantage of the latter approach is a lower level of effort on the part of participants. In our case, the participants did not have to originate a de novo list of features. The disadvantage of this approach may be a possible bias of respondents. In our case, the scientific approach of a content analysis for the "designed questionnaire" would limit this bias.

Directors of American Family Medicine residencies, who belonged to the Association of Family Practice Residency Directors' listserv, were asked to participate if they had an interest in EMR systems, products and/or design. The list contains approximately 330 unique email addresses. The number of unique directors or programs in the list is unknown. This listserv has been in existence for several years and has an active membership. The mode of communication with the individuals included email messages in addition to an initial face-to-face meeting with a subset of individuals [8]. This meeting was by convenience due to a previously scheduled directors' meeting by the American Academy of Family Physicians. The model consisted of three iterations. The first iteration started with a list of EMR features developed from the content analysis. Each individual was asked to add relevant features to the list and to remove irrelevant features. In order to increase face validity of the instrument, we asked several experts in health informatics, electronic medical records and questionnaire development to review the list. Content validity was addressed as the instrument was designed based on the content analysis of published literature. The questionnaire had a Flesch Reading Ease of 68% and a Flesch Kincaid Grade Level of 9.

After respondents provided us with suggestions to add new features and/or remove existing ones that they rated as irrelevant or of less priority, a new list of features was developed from these modified lists. For the second iteration, the new list was sent to each individual to rank each feature on the list on a scale of 0-5 (Table 1). To address unranked features, the average of all rankings for that feature was used for the missing rank score in order to correct the cumulative score. Features with a cumulative importance score being one standard deviation above or below the mean were extracted. In the third iteration, each individual was asked to comment on these features in order to confirm agreement with the classification of features with the highest and lowest importance.

Table 1 - Importance Scale

0	Would have a negative impact on the practice of medicine in a residency
1	Would have no impact on the practice of medicine in a residency
2	Would have little positive impact on the practice of medicine in a residency
3	Would have a big positive impact on the practice of medicine in a residency
4	Would be critical to practice medicine in a residency
5	Would be mandatory to practice medicine in a residency

3. Results

A total of 30 directors participated in the study. The types of residencies represented included: (1) community based, unaffiliated with a university, (2) community based, university affiliated, (3) community based, university administered, and (4) university based. The participating directors represented residency programs located throughout the United States.

The first iteration received a 37% (11 respondents) response rate; 5 of these 11 individuals proposed a modification of the list. Eight additional features included: (1) assignment of an attending and a resident as primary physician, (2) variable billing physician, (3) ability to generate consult letter from note, (4) digital signatures, (5) ability to import data into note, (6) resident reports, (7) ability to link information directly into the chart but not be part of the legal chart, and (8) document delinquency tracking. The feature removed was resemblance to a paper chart. This resulted in a new list of 74 features.

The second iteration received a 57% (17 respondents) response rate. The average importance score for all features was 3.57 (0.15 95% CI). The cumulative average score for all features was 60.44 with a standard deviation of 8.06. Eleven features were above one standard deviation of the mean and ten features were below (Table 2).

Table 2-Ranked Features

FEATURE	AVG	95%CI
Highest Importance Features		
Access for multiple, simultaneous users	4.88	0.17
System Reliability	4.82	0.20
Meets Regulatory Requirements	4.65	0.23
Rapid access to patient data	4.35	0.23
User-friendly (Intuitive user interface esp. for rotating residents and students)	4.35	0.29
Secure Remote access (Portability)	4.35	0.38
Decreased clinical errors	4.24	0.27
Digital Signatures (esp. to sign off resident notes)	4.18	0.35
Increased legibility	4.12	0.33
Compatible with existing computer systems	4.06	0.28
Integrated clinical reminders	4.06	0.31
Lowest Importance Features		
Allows add-on products	3.06	0.54
Open Source	2.94	0.48
Decreased doctor time per encounter	2.94	0.54
Import pictures and drawing capabilities	2.88	0.40
Support for develop of vocabulary	2.88	0.40
Available for multiple Operating systems	2.65	0.34
Voice recognition	2.65	0.39
Integrated consumer databases	2.59	0.50
Contract management	2.53	0.50
Available as Application Service Provider (ASP)	2.44	0.53

In the third iteration there was agreement on the features in the highest and lowest importance category (15 respondents). The two most common comments were (1) the need to define the features and (2) although features were in the low importance group, they have a place in the respondents' practice.

Individual features can be clustered into four logical groups: fast and easy access; research; EMR system properties; and low cost. The fast and easy access grouping is a cluster of features such as: access for multiple simultaneous users; secure remote access; PDA access; web-enabled access; rapid access; and user-friendly access. The access cluster has an average score of 3.39. The feature cluster labeled as Research with an average score of 3.53 is a composite of features such as data mining; data warehousing; support for clinical trials and increased opportunity for research. The feature relating to vendor or EMR system properties, which encompasses high vendor creditability, meets regulatory requirements, online support, high level of support, and system reliability, has an average score of 4.04. Low cost, which includes low implementation cost, increased staff efficiency, increased cost savings and profits, low hardware requirements, and low maintenance costs, has an average score of 3.55.

4. Discussion

The response rate was typical of Delphi methods except for the increase in the second iteration. This could be due to the relative lower effort needed of participants for the second iteration than the first. If so, this validates our choice of the "designed questionnaire" approach to increase response rates. The high average importance score implies participants believe all listed features are important.

The majority of highly ranked features can be categorized as core functionality of an EMR system. This implies that EMR design efforts should focus on improving core functionality instead of developing more "Bells and Whistles."

Musham et al. found high cost as a major concern for residencies [5], but those features which correspond to lowering cost (i.e. low implementation cost, increased staff efficiency, increased cost savings and profits, and low maintenance costs) were in the middle to lower half of the ranked list. The reason for this is uncertain. It could be the view of cost as a barrier and not a feature, or the fact that regardless of cost, an EMR system is perceived as not worth implementing if it does not possess important features.

Looking at the 95% confidence intervals for those features in the highest versus lowest categories, there is greater internal reliability with the highest importance features; however internal reliability of the lowest rated features was acceptable. Also the lowest importance features tended to be more technical in nature. We believe one reason for this could be a lack of knowledge about these technical aspects across all participants. As users' experience and knowledge of an EMR increases their needs and expectations will change.

5. Conclusion

These implementable features represent the needs and expectations of family practice residency users. These needs must be met for EMR systems to be adopted and utilized by users.

A major limitation in identifying important EMR features is the lack of a common terminology or ontology. Formal definitions, and in many cases one working definition, do not exist. This makes it difficult for individuals to discuss features and be confident that the other individual is thinking of the same functionality. There is a great need to develop such a terminology and ontology. [18]

Our data provides the ability for user-driven design of EMR systems for family practice residency programs. These data suggest that core functionality is of greatest importance for residency program users. Special attention to the underlying needs of the target user population is paramount. In the case of a family practice residency program, a complex patient-provider model and resident education tracking appear to be decision-driving factors. A Delphi method can be useful in delineating the feature list and underlying decision-making model for different target populations.

6. Acknowledgements

This work was supported in part by the National Library of Medicine Biomedical and Health Informatics Research Training Grant T15-LM07089-12.

7. References

[1] Strasberg HR, Tudiver F, Holbrook AM, Geiger G, Keshavjee KK, Troyan S. Moving towards an electronic patient record: a survey to assess the needs of community family physicians. *Proc AMIA Symp* 1998;230-234.

[2] Dumont R, van der LR, van Merode F, Tange H. User needs and demands of a computer-based patient record. *Medinfo* 1998; 9 Pt 1:64-69.

[3] Schoenbaum SC, Barnett GO. Automated ambulatory medical records systems. An orphan technology. *Int J Technol Assess Health Care* 1992; 8(4):598-609.

[4] Institute of Medicine Committee on Quality of Health Care in America. Crossing the Quality Chasm: A New Health System for the 21st Century. Hardcover ed. National Academy Press, 2001.

[5] Musham C, Ornstein SM, Jenkins RG. Family practice educators' perceptions of computer-based patient records. *Fam Med* 1995; 27(9):571-575.

[6] Lenhart JG, Honess K, Covington D, Johnson KE. An analysis of trends, perceptions, and use patterns of electronic medical records among US family practice residency programs. *Fam Med* 2000; 32(2):109-114.

[7] Linstone H, Turoff M. The Delphi Method: Techniques and Applications. *Addison-Wesley Publication Company*, 1975.

[8] Welch JJ. CPR systems: which one is right for your organization? *J AHIMA* 1999; 70(8):24-26.

[9] Ury A. Choosing the right electronic medical records system. *Cost Qual Q J* 1998; 4(1):4-6.

[10] Aaronson JW, Murphy-Cullen CL, Chop WM, Frey RD. Electronic medical records: the family practice resident perspective. *Fam Med* 2001; 33(2):128-132.

[11] Silver D. Doing away with paper. Part 2--Starting up your new system. *Aust Fam Physician* 2002; 31(6):527-531.

[12] DeBry PW. Considerations for choosing an electronic medical record for an ophthalmology practice. *Arch Ophthalmol* 2001; 119(4):590-596.

[13] Silver D. Doing away with paper. Part 1--Advice for setting up fully computerised medical records. *Aust Fam Physician* 2002; 31(6):521-526.

[14] Holbrook A, Keshavjee K, Langton K, Troyan S, Millar S, Olantunji S et al. A critical pathway for electronic medical record selection. *Proc AMIA Symp* 2001;264-268.

[15] Smith WR, Zastrow R. User requirements for the computerized patient record: physician opinions. *Proc Annu Symp Comput Appl Med Care* 1994;994.

[16] Shortliffe EH. The evolution of electronic medical records. *Acad Med* 1999; 74(4):414-419.

[17] Matthews P, Newell LM. Clinical information systems: paving the way for clinical information management. *J Healthc Inf Manag* 1999; 13(3):97-111.

[18] EHR Collaborative. Public Response to HL7 Ballot 1 Electronic Health Records. http://www.ehrcollaborative.org/EHR_Collaborative_Final_Report_082903.pdf . 2003. 9-24-2003.

Address for correspondence

George Demiris, PhD, University of Missouri – Columbia, 324 Clark Hall
Columbia, MO 65211   USA, demirisg@missouri.edu

Connecting Medical Informatics and Bio-Informatics
R. Engelbrecht et al. (Eds.)
IOS Press, 2005

Tracking Referents in Electronic Health Records

Werner Ceusters [a], **Barry Smith** [b]

[a] *European Centre for Ontological Research, Saarbrücken, Germany*
[b] *Institute for Formal Ontology and Medical Information Science, Saarbrücken, Germany and Department of Philosophy, University at Buffalo, NY, USA*

Abstract

Electronic Health Records (EHRs) are organized around two kinds of statements: those reporting observations made, and those reporting acts performed. In neither case does the record involve any direct reference to what such statements are actually about. They record not: what is happening on the side of the patient, but rather: what is said about what is happening. While the need for a unique patient identifier is generally recognized, we argue that we should now move to an EHR regime in which all clinically salient particulars – from the concrete disorder on the side of the patient and the body parts in which it occurs to the concrete treatments given – should be uniquely identified. This will allow us to achieve interoperability among different systems of records at the level where it really matters: in regard to what is happening in the real world. It will also allow us to keep track of particular disorders and of the effects of particular treatments in a precise and unambiguous way.

Keywords
Realist ontology; Unique identifier; Electronic health record; Universals and particulars

1. Introduction

Rector *et al.* have claimed that the information in the medical record consists of a collection of statements "*not about what was true of the patient but [about] what was observed and believed by clinicians*" [1]. They distinguish statements about direct observations concerning the patient (i.e. of what was heard, seen, thought, and done), and statements concerning the decision-making process and the clinical dialogue. In this way the authors seek to define the requirements to be satisfied by the EHR in order that it satisfies the criterion of "*faithfulness to the clinical history and care of the patient*". The requirements they list, however, refer exclusively to facilities for managing the statements inside EHR systems. Thus for instance they require that: "*the record should be capable of representing multiple instances of count nouns*". Count nouns are for example "fracture", "tumor", "leg" – nouns that can be pluralized (as contrasted with mass nouns like "urine"). The requirement is, therefore, as put forward by Rector *et al.*, that the record should be capable of multiple representations not of fractures, tumors, legs themselves, but of the corresponding *nouns*, or rather (though we are not sure what meaning to assign to this phrase) of *instances* of such nouns. Indeed the insistence by Rector *et al.* that the record be a record of what was *said* rather than of what actually happened, positively rules out that it should contain representations of fractures, tumors or legs – or more generally of all those disorders, activities, symptoms, etc. which, as we believe, are of primary relevance to the health record. But this very fact, we believe, deprives the other requirements listed by Rector *et al.* – such as the requirement that the record *allow conflicting statements* – of the possibility of coherent application to real cases, since there is no way in which the entities about which there is supposed to be a disagreement could be explicitly referred to.

Slightly more acceptable, in this respect, is the account proposed by Huff *et al.* [2], who take *"the real world to consist of objects (or entities)"*. They continue by asserting: *"Objects interact with other objects and can be associated with other objects by relationships … When two or more objects interact in the real world, an 'event' is said to have occurred."* They then, encouragingly, base their account upon the events themselves, rather than upon statements about events. Each event receives an explicit identifier, called an *event instance ID*, which is used to link it to other events (reflecting the goal of supporting temporal reasoning with patient data). This ID serves as an anchor for describing the event via a frame-representation, where the slots in the frame are name-value tuples such as *event-ID* = "#223", *event-family* = "diagnostic procedures", *procedure-type* = "chest X-ray", etc. The framework of [2] incorporates also explicit reference via other unique IDs to the patient, the physician and even to the radiographic film used in an X-ray image analysis event. Unfortunately, they fail to see the importance of explicitly referring also to *what was observed*. This is in spite of the fact that the very X-ray report that they analyse begins with the sentences: *"PA view is compared to the previous examination dated 10-22-91. Surgical clips are again seen along the right mediastinum and right hilar region."* Because they have no means to refer directly to those clips, they must resort to a complex representation with nested and linked event frames in order to simulate such reference. Even then, however, they are not able to disambiguate as between an interpretation in which (i) the surgical clips seen in the mediastinum are different from those seen in the hilar region and (ii) there is only one set of clips that extends from the mediastinum into the hilar region. The limitations of the event-based representation force them also to create a different event-frame for each location of the clips (though neither clips nor locations are themselves events). That this approach is questionable is seen in the fact that, while it is certainly possible, when looking at a chest X-ray, to see first a clip in the mediastinum (first event), and then by looking again (in a second event) to see a second clip, it is equally possible that just one glance suffices for the observer to apprehend all the clips at the same time, i.e. in one event. (To rule out this possibility would be tantamount to claiming that complex perceptions, e.g. of a tree, must involve the subject participating simultaneously in several thousands of distinct events of observation.)

Finally, we can mention Weed's *Problem Oriented Medical Record*, the central idea of which is to organize all medical data around a problem list, thereby assigning each indivi-dual problem a unique ID [3]. Unfortunately Weed proposes to uniquely identify only problems, and not the various particulars that cause the problems, are symptomatic for them, or are involved in their diagnosis or therapy. This is exemplified in Barrows and Johnson's model that suffers also from the ambiguity whether the unique IDs refer to the problems themselves or rather to statements about the problems [4].

2. Some ontological and epistemological aspects of introducing unique identifiers for particular entities in health records

We argue that the EHR should contain explicit reference, via unique identifiers, to the individual real world entities which are of relevance in such records – called "particulars" in what follows. These should be similar not only to the unique identifiers we already use to distinguish individual patients, individual physicians, individual healthcare organizations, individual invoices and credit card transactions, and even individual drug packages [5]. When I enter a hospital with a fracture of my left first metatarsal base, then I would like this particular fracture, which prevents me from dancing and causes me a lot of pain, and of which the clinician examining me can see an image on an X-ray, to receive a unique ID for further reference. Only in this way can this fracture be distinguished not just from a second fracture in the same metatarsal, but also from the fracture in the very same place from which I suffered two years earlier. The bunion, in contrast, which the clinician observes when examining my foot, and of which there is also an image on the X-ray, should not receive at that time its own unique ID. Reference to it should be effected, rather, by means of the ID it received already two years ago, when it was diagnosed at the same time as the first fracture. True, the bunion is now much bigger; but it is still the same entity as it was when first observed.

There are good reasons for the above. Coding systems such as ICD have labels such as "multiple fracture occurring in the same limb", "multiple fracture occurring in different limbs", and so forth. Statistics concerning the incidence of disorders would be erroneous if, because of unconstrained use of such labels, multiple observations of the same entity came to be counted as separate incidences of disorder. Few patients will care about such statistics, but they will care if having two fractures would make them eligible for cost reimbursement because of the different ways each fracture occurred. We would even like to go further: it is not just the particular fracture which should get an explicit ID, but also the particular bone in which it occurred. For it might happen that this bone is later transplanted into another patient, and becomes the cause of a malignancy in the recipient because tumor material in the bone was transplanted together with it [6].

What does it mean to assign identifiers to particulars in an EHR? First, we note that ontologies and terminologies have focused hitherto on what is general in reality, allowing particularization to occur almost exclusively where there is explicit reference to the *human beings* who are the bearers of named general attributes or to the *times* at which observations occurred or statements were made. The realm of particulars relevant to the health record is however vastly broader than this. Indeed, there are both particulars (tokens, instances), such as *this bone* of *that person*, and universals (types, classes), such as *bone* and *person*, throughout the entire domain of medical science. Thus there are the two particular fractures: the one from which I am now suffering, and one which occurred two years ago. But there is also the universal *basal fracture of left first metatarsal*, which is of course just as real as the particulars in which it inheres. There is the particular pain in my foot that I had two years ago, pain that was caused by that first fracture. And there is the pain from which I am suffering now, in the very same place. The pains may feel the same, but they are distinct entities nonetheless, though both are instances of the same universal. Universals and particulars exist in reality independently of our use of language. As such, they are distinguished from the *concepts* which are said to provide meanings for terms.

Second, assigning a unique identifier tells us that the particular exists (or has existed in the past), and that nothing else is that particular. The particular does not come into existence because we assign an identifier to it: it must have existed before it became possible for such an assignment to be made. The assignment itself is then an act comparable to the act of naming a fetus or newborn child (or ship or artwork).

Third, we would find in such an advanced EHR also statements about these assignment acts (and – to avoid the confusions one finds in the HL7 RIM [7] – these statements would be clearly distinguished from the acts they are intended to describe). We could then assign truth values to such statements, and we note that for such a statement to be true the particular referred to must exist (or have existed) and have no ID already assigned.

Fourth, the *use* of an ID in a statement does not entail that an assignment has already been made. If an X-ray is ordered, then the X-ray event does not exist, and so it cannot be *assigned* an ID. But it is perfectly possible to *reserve* such an ID in advance. This difference opens up interesting perspectives in the medico-legal context. If the X-ray that was ordered is carried out, and the images reveal a pathology, then the physician who issued the order can use this fact as a justification of the claim that his initial judgment about the case had been accurate. The mere fact of his having issued the order may protect him from a lawsuit, even when the X-ray is not carried out. Of course, the information relevant to such analyses can be extracted also from conventional records. The point here is that the framework here advanced would allow for the automatic analysis of such cases, and possibly even for the automatic prevention of associated medical mistakes or hazards.

Fifth, the mere fact of assigning an identifier to a particular does not imply that any statement is made about what *kind* of particular is involved. Such a statement is made only when one has grasped the relevant particular as an instance of some universal (such as "bone" or "fracture" or "pain"), and this often occurs only after the assignment or reservation of an ID. Statements of the given sort are then true only if the particular exists *and* is an instance of the claimed universal.

3. Towards and implementation of referent tracking

Let us go back to the emergency room of that modern hospital that I choose to be treated in because it has installed one of the new fancy EHR systems (EHRS) that allows careful and explicit reference to all my various problems and to the different kinds of entities associated therewith. Because of my story about what happened to my foot, and because of the pain the two attending physicians were able to induce by palpating my forefoot, both agreed that there was something wrong. That "something wrong" was given the ID #234, a meaningless consecutive number assigned automatically by the EHRS (and guaranteed to be unique according to some algorithm). The system at the same time also generated two statements, recording the assignment of #234 to that particular by each of the two physicians. These statements enjoy a high degree of positive evidence, since the referent-tracking database allows automatic checking to verify the absence of prior existing disorders of which my current problem might have been a continuation. It did find referent #15 for the left first metatarsal base fracture that I suffered from two years ago, but this – as witnessed by the X-ray image #98 taken half a year after the initial diagnosis – had since ceased to exist. The physicians also had good evidence that the referent-tracking database was complete in all relevant respects, since they knew that I never sought treatment elsewhere. The physicians' statements concerning the assignment were each time-stamped both for occasion of utterance and for point of appearance in the EHRS. Note that these time-stamps do not necessarily imply assertions about when #234 itself began to exist. Also, at this stage, no statement has been made about which universal disorder #234 is an instance of.

The physicians ordered and received three X-ray photographs taken of my foot from different angles. They both looked at the first (identified by the EHRS as #235 and stated to be an instance of the universal referred to by SNOMED-CT as "257444003: photograph"), but they saw nothing abnormal. Of course, they saw an image of my left first metatarsal bone, this image being identified as #286 (they did not bother to look for a SNOMED-CT code for such an image, knowing by experience that they would find nothing that comes close). They were at the same time aware that entity #286 is clearly different from entity #221, which is my left first metatarsal bone itself, and which they declared to be (i) an instance of the universal referred to by the SNOMED-CT concept "182121005: entire first metatarsal", further annotated with the side-modifier "left", and (ii) a part of #2 (me). On the second photograph (#236), both saw a thin hypodense line appearing towards the top of my left first metatarsal bone. They assigned that line in the image the label #287, and both stated it to be the image of some corresponding particular #288, thereby agreeing on the existence of #288 but disagreeing as to what universal it was an instance of – the one seeing it as a fracture line, the other as just a normal part of the bone somewhat less dense than the surrounding bony material. They agreed, however, that #287 was not an artefact, i.e. that it did indeed correspond to something in my body. On the third photograph (#237), both saw a clear fracture line, indisputably an image of a real fracture and identical with particular #288. They thereupon asserted that #234, i.e. the "something wrong" previously identified, was in fact an instance of the universal: *left first metatarsal base fracture*.

4. EHR architecture standards and health particulars

No current EHR architecture standards are to our knowledge able to deal with the tracking of all those types of referents that are required to support an implementation such as the one described above. The record architecture described in CEN prEN 13606-1:2004 draft [8] allows only a limited number of particulars to be referred to explicitly – i.e. without resorting to any external terminology – and as shown in Table 1 many of them (as we should expect, given what we observed in **1** above) are at the meta-level rather than at the level of direct care. Indirectly, it would be possible to use the "data item" construct as it is defined in CEN prEN 13606-1:2004 to refer to particulars – something that we strongly encourage, even though it would require an additional round of standardization.

Table 1-The different sorts of particulars that can be identified in CEN prEN 13606-1:2004

Direct care particulars	Meta-level particulars
1) the <u>subject of care</u> from whose EHR an extract is taken. This does not need to be the patient since an extract might contain data about an unborn child	4) the <u>EHR provider system</u> from which a record extract is being taken
	5) the <u>EHR</u> from which the extract is taken
	6) the different sorts of <u>components</u> involved in a record extract
2) the <u>healthcare agent</u> which participates in some interaction with the subject of care	7) <u>International Coding Scheme Identifier</u> (ICSI)
	8) <u>External Procedure Reference</u>: rather than referring to a real procedure that is carried out, this refers to a specific document in which a procedure is generically described
3) a <u>geographical location</u> for any person (i.e. subject of care or human healthcare agent) or organization referred to	9) The <u>software</u> used in the EHR extract transmission process

The HL7-RIM [9] is much worse in this respect. Particulars that are listed as "entities" can, it is true, be referred to by using the "Entity.Id" attribute: living subjects (either human or non-human), geographical places, organizations, and manufactured materials including devices and containers. Great care needs to be taken, however, since these labels are notoriously prone to inaccurate use. As an example, the class Person can be used to refer either to individuals or to groups, depending on how the attribute "Entity.Quantity" is set. As an example, a group with 60% females is to be represented as "*Person(quantity = 100) has-part Person(quantity = 60; sex = female)*". And similarly with HL7-RIM's notoriously problematic Act class. Perhaps (we do not know) the "Act.Id" attribute can be used to refer to concrete events. But then the Act class allows for "mood" (possible, planned, ordered, etc.) and "negation" attributes, so that a reference ID would sometimes need to be understood (in our terminology) as a *reservation* and sometimes as an *assignment*, though even this simple distinction is masked by layers of confusion. And in HL7-RIM, too, there is no room to refer to instances of body parts, of disorders, and so forth. The world of HL7, after all, is a world of Acts (Acts themselves being artefacts of the HL7 regime, rather than entities we could encounter in our everyday reality). Only a thorough reworking of the HL7-RIM, taking into account all aspects of reality, might solve these problems.

5. Conclusion

Nowadays, the medical informatics community prefers to restrict the use of ontology to the development of more or less well-structured vocabularies of general terms. Hardly at all does it care about the correct representation of particulars in reality – without which, of course, such vocabularies would be entirely superfluous. This is strange in an era in which the clinical community, i.e. the community that should be served by medical informatics, is focused so emphatically on Evidence Based Medicine. For on what should evidence be based, if not on real cases? The focus on what is general was perhaps defensible in an era of limited computer resources. Now, however, we argue that only benefits would accrue from inaugurating EHR systems which are able to refer directly and systematically to concrete instances along the lines proposed in the above. If a hospital database is able to store all the SNOMED-CT codes that apply to a particular patient, then adding an additional reference ID to the particulars that are the relevant instances of the SNOMED classes will hardly create massive storage problems. CEN prEN 13606-1:2004, too can be adjusted quite easily along these lines, though of course adapting actual EHR systems in an appropriate way would involve a more substantial effort. Considerable organizational issues would above all still need to be resolved – as witnessed by the problems encountered in establishing a Unique Patient Identifier in a safe and secure manner [10]. But the benefits, in terms of better patient management, supporting advances in biomedical science, health cost containment and more reliable epidemiological data, can be expected to be enormous. And just as pseudonymisation is an effective approach to the collection of data about the same patient without disclosing his or her identity, so also the mechanism of ID assignment to disorders, body parts, etc. would provide additional avenues for supporting anonymity and thus promoting more and better HIPAA compliant research.

6. Acknowledgments

The present paper was written under the auspices of the Wolfgang Paul Program of the Alexander von Humboldt Foundation, and the Network of Excellence in Semantic Interoperability and Data Mining in Biomedicine of the European Union.

7. References

[1]   Rector AL, Nolan WA, and Kay S. Foundations for an Electronic Medical Record. *Methods of Information in Medicine* 30: 179-86, 1991.
[2]   Huff SM, Rocha RA, Bray BE, Warner HR, and Haug PJ. An Event Model of Medical Information Representation. *J Am Med Informatics Assoc.* 1995;2:116-134.
[3]   Weed L. Medical Records That Guide And Teach. *N Engl J Med* 1968: 278: 593-600.
[4] Barrows RC, Johnson SB. A data model that captures clinical reasoning about patient problems. In: Gardner RM (editor). Proceedings of the 19th Annual Symposium on Computer Applications in Medical Care; New Orleans, LA; October 28 - November 1, 1995: pp 402-505.
[5]   Bell J. Drug firms see future in RFID technology. In: *Cincinnati Business Courier*, December 27, 2004.
[6]   Collignon FP, Holland EC, Feng S. Organ Donors with Malignant Gliomas: An Update. *Am J Transplant.* 2004 Jan;4(1):15-21.
[7]   Vizenor L. Actions in health care organizations: an ontological analysis. *Medinfo.* 2004;2004:1403-10.
[8]   CEN. Health informatics - Electronic healthcare record communication - Part 1: Extended architecture
[9]   Case J, McKenzie L, Schadow G. (eds.) HL7 Reference Information Model.
       (http://www.hl7.org/Library/data-model/RIM/C30202/rim.htm)
[10] http://www.hipaanet.com/upin1.htm.

Address for correspondence

Dr. W. Ceusters, European Centre for Ontological Research, Universität des Saarlandes, Postfach 151150, D-66041 Saarbrücken , Germany. www.ecor.uni-saarland.de.

Connecting Medical Informatics and Bio-Informatics
R. Engelbrecht et al. (Eds.)
IOS Press, 2005

The French Organ Transplant Data System

William Nigel Strang, Philippe Tuppin, Alain Atinault, Christian Jacquelinet

Agence de la biomédecine 1 avenue Stade de France 93212 SAINT DENIS LA PLAINE CEDEX France

Abstract

The Agence de la Biomédecine is a state agency dealing with Public Health issues related, among others, to organ, tissue and cell transplantation in France. The Agence maintains a national information system used to coordinate and administer organ procurement and transplant activities and to perform the evaluation of organ transplantation activities. This paper describes the core uses and functional requirements of Cristal, the donor, recipient and allocation software of the information system and its evolution in the new system.

Keywords:
Organ transplantation, Organ allocation, Decisional Information System, Health Planning, Government Agencies, Computer Communication Networks, Software

1. Introduction

Computer systems have been intimately associated with organ transplantation since its entry into mainstream medical practice in the 60's[1] evolving from recipient follow up through to the essential functions of waiting list administration, the coordination of procurement and the allocation of organs to patients on the waiting list. These activities create favourable conditions for the pre and post transplant follow up of patients since the mandatory identification of all transplant patients generates a cohort that includes the complete treated population[2] [3] .

The Agence de la Biomédecine is the state agency in charge of public health issues related to organ, tissue and cell transplantation and medically assisted procreation, embryology and human genetics in France. It is responsible for the registration of patients on and the management of the national organ transplant waiting list, the allocation of all organs retrieved in France or abroad the evaluation of these activities [4].

The Agence de la Biomédecine develops and maintains Cristal to record information concerning patients at registration, transplantation and pre and post transplantation follow-up as well as information concerning the coordination of donor procurement and organ allocation. This primary role, supporting the allocation of a scarce resource to patients, directly contributes to health care. Cristal is also the primary source of the accurate and controlled data used for the evaluation of organ retrieval and transplant activities that are published both in the annual report of the Agence de la Biomédecine and in the context of specific studies.

2. The transplantation process

Coordination of transplant and procurement activities in France is organised into six areas known as inter-regions. Decentralised departments of the Agence de la Biomédecine, the "Services de regulation et d'Appui"* (SRAs) are responsible for the control and coordination of organ procurement and allocation activities within each inter-region. [5] [6]

Hospital procurement coordinators, or other sources, inform the SRAs of potential brain dead donors. As the pre-procurement clinical, administrative and ethical procedures progress the available information can be† recorded in the potential donor's dossier within Cristal.

The SRA proposes the potentially available organs to transplant teams according to procedures defined in French legislation and following a hierarchy of local (the same hospital or network), inter-regional, national and international levels. Flows between the inter-regions are coordinated by the "Regulation Nationale" based near Paris as are exchanges with non-French organisations

Organs must first be proposed to recipients who benefit from a priority. In the absence of or after national or regional priorities, the order of the propositions (for organs other than the kidney) is based on a rota that permits local variation and practises. The propositions and the replies of the teams are recorded within Cristal. As soon as the organ of a donor is proposed to a team, the donor's dossier becomes available for consultation by the team via Cristal. Kidneys are currently proposed according to two procedures: a points score system similar to that proposed by Starzl [7] , or according to the number of mismatches, the waiting time and the degree of immunisation.

After the procurement and transplantation of the donor's organs the link between the donors' organs and the recipients is recorded in Cristal.

Donor records and data entry

The donor record is created early on the process by the SRA after initial contact with the hospital procurement coordinator. Hospital procurement coordinators gather the medical records of the donor and complete a standardised nationwide donor dossier. This document, preceded by essential documents (blood group, serologies) is faxed to the SRA who enters the data in Cristal.

Waiting list registration and the pre-transplant period.

130 organ transplant teams are active within the 30 teaching hospitals throughout France.

To benefit an organ transplant in France patients must be registered on the national waiting list by identified members of transplant teams, or their proxies.

Pre-transplant visit reports should be entered into Cristal every year for the kidney and every six months for the other organs.

Pre-transplant events should recorded in Cristal

- The patient may die. The patient may decide to leave the waiting list. The improvement or degradation of the patients state may render transplantation inappropriate. The transplant team may declare a temporary contra-indication. The patient may be accorded a priority.

---

* Literally the support and dispatch agencies
† If the information is not entered directly it is not available for consultation by the transplant teams, however, for operational reasons the system tolerates a deferred recording of the details of the donor dossier.

Transplantation

When a donor becomes available Cristal helps select the most eligible transplant patients via the implementation of the legal criteria in a series of programs that also take into account the ongoing regional and national priorities.

After transplantation the information that the patient has been transplanted with a specific organ of a specific donor is recorded in Cristal. A detailed report of concerning the peri-operative and 1 month post operative period should be recorded in Cristal.

The post transplant period

There are currently about 6500 patients on the waiting list in Cristal. The number of post transplant patients in Cristal is about 50 000. Post transplant follow up information should be entered into Cristal annually. The data entry confirms that the patient is living and indicates the occurrence of important episodes over the past year (complications, treatment changes).

3. Cristal: A centralised and integrated communications system

Cristal is a centralised system. A single copy of the software runs on a powerful, secure, computer based near Paris. For the time being users run a terminal emulation session on their computer and communicate over a modem-to-modem direct dial link with the central computer.

Cristal is integrated, that is to say Cristal is used to administer the national transplant waiting list, records patient details and pre and post transplantation follow up and is also used to record donor information, provides guidance concerning patient priority and emergency situations and records the proposition of organs to transplant teams (with their responses) as well as the final allocation of the organ.

Cristal can be appropriately viewed as a communication support infrastructure between the transplant teams and the organ allocation teams in the SRAs[8] .

Cristal Data Structures

Figure 1 illustrates a simplified vision of the data structures of Cristal. Each patient is identified in the table Patients and has one or more transplant dossiers containing pre and post-transplant information and a series of visit reports. At transplantation the donors' organs are linked to the various recipients in a transplants and organs table. The donor is recorded in the donor table and the donor's dossier is recorded as a set of data in an associated table.

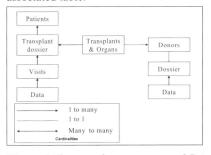

Figure 1 The core data structures of Cristal

Matching donors to recipients

Cristal helps match recipients to donors' characteristics according to the applicable legal dispositions. Given the age and blood group of the donor (and the HLA for kidney recipients) the donor matching program produces ordered lists of recipients and transplant centres that the regulators in the SRAs use to pilot the organisation of the procurement process.

4. Discussion and perspectives

Throughout the paper the conditional tense has been used whenever the data entry activities of transplant teams, beyond those that are obligatory for organ allocation have been described. As early as 1967 Murray and Barnes[2] identified that information gathering for transplant patient follow up and the completion of questionnaires for the then 'Human Kidney Transplant Register' was burdensome for the clinical staff, considered to be largely redundant and was carried out with variable assiduity. This state of affairs has worsened considerably over the last 40 years. Many reasons underlie this major obstacle to fully exploiting the potential of an exhaustive data set and we are addressing those that we can in the migration of Cristal.

Meeting the challenges

Functional migration

The Agence is also in charge of the Renal Epidemiology and Information Network (REIN) used for the follow-up of all patients treated by dialysis in France, linking the cohorts of dialysed and transplanted patients to offer a complete evaluation of end-stage renal disease treatment. The information system of the Agence is becoming a decisional information system supporting evaluation studies and decision making for public health policies in the field of organ failure, replacement therapies and transplantation. Due to individual and societal concerns, its use for organ allocation also requires an accurate evaluation process. To make relevant public health decisions, it is important to correlate temporal and geographical data related to health needs and their determinants (patients' data), to temporal and geographical data related to health supplies and their determinants (health care offer, organ retrieval). Providing statistics for deciders requires the integration of data coming from consolidated sources with Data-warehousing techniques.

This extension of Cristal to support the national dialysis information system (Diadem) will complete the description of the treatment of end-stage renal failure in France.

Attaining this objective leads to two key requirements:
- A reliable patient identification process
- Facilitating a complete and coherent patient follow up.

Software migration

Cristal is archaic – it used obsolete technology at its launch in 1996 (Oracle® Forms 3). Since 2001 the computer department has been modernising its technology and methods. In 2002 we installed secure internet platforms on which a series of applications related to Cristal were deployed in 2003 including a geographical referential and a meta-thesaurus 9,10,11. 2004 saw the first modules of Cristal for internet deployed – namely the Cristal Quality tools, used for the traceable correction by the quality monitors and a simple interface onto the transplant team directory. In 2005 the first medical module, Cristal

Immunology, was deployed for the HLA laboratories. Cristal version 2 uses a service based architecture (Figure 2)

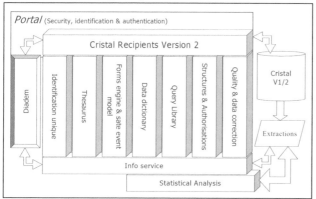

Figure 2 The services that are used to construct Cristal Version 2

Improving patient identification

Currently during patient identification Cristal checks for birth names and given names that are the same as, or that start with the entered name. This is insufficient and needs to be completed by phonetic searching, normalised string searching and other algorithms. These functions will be shared between Cristal and the software being developed for the end stage renal disease data system (Diadem).

Improving patient follow up

Five steps are being undertaken to improve patient follow up

- Human resources and financing

  Staff dedicated to gathering and entering the data are now associated with most transplant teams. The posts are directly financed by the administration and the financing mode has recently changed supporting and perpetuating these posts. The posts are directly attached to the regional health authority, but the national coordination centre of the Agence de la Biomédecine coordinates the work.

- Item review and the forms engine

  The items gathered in Cristal are under constant review whilst respecting the need for stability in the data analysed. The application used to the end stage renal disease data system includes a form engine that permits documented evolutions of the items gathered. This forms engine is destined for use by Cristal.

- Clinician appropriation and the forms engine

  Many transplants centres and groups of transplant centres set up their own data systems to observe their own cohorts of patients. Until the clinicians in the transplant centres perceive the national administrative system as a tool that they can use to meet their own then the data gathering for Cristal will continue to be a secondary activity. The forms engine aims to promote this appropriation of the system. It produces data collection forms using declarative descriptions of the data to be collected. The items, grouped in sections may be simple or complex. Items can be conditional on the basis of previous replies and may be repeatable. The values entered are verified by unitary controls and by more complex logic bringing implying multiple items and other data. It is also provides the possibility to gather information at the local, network centres, regional and national levels. as well as ad hoc questionnaires for logic driven transversal studies or longitudinal studies.

- Data integration

Much of the data typed into Cristal is already present in other computer systems, be they medical records, lab results, administrative information, clinical trial systems or other transplant recipient follow up systems. The long term intention of the Agence de la Biomédecine is to be able to integrate information from such disparate sources directly into Cristal.

- Towards a French consolidated end stage renal disease data system

The most powerful incentive towards the use of Cristal comes from its integration with the National Dialysis data system based on the work of Landais et al12,13. The ability to apprehend the complete illness and treatment history will hopefully bring considerable added interest to the participating clinicians.

5. Conclusion

The solution being developed for Cristal and Diadem is a specific instance of software of a generic type (patient identification linked to configurable follow up). The architecture retained during the migration of Cristal and its integration with Diadem, if proven to work by experience, provides a generic model and basis which could be used and extended to the patient registers in certain of the Agency's other domains of activity.

6. References

[1] Murray JE, Barnes BA. Introductory remarks on kidney transplantation with observations on kidney transplant registry. Transplantation. 1967 Jul;5(4):Suppl:824-30.
[2] US Renal Data System: Excerpts from the USRDS 2004 Annual Data Report. Am J Kidney Dis 45:S1–S280 (suppl 1)
[3] Cecka JM. The OPTN/UNOS Renal Transplant Registry 2003. Clin Transpl. 2003;:1-12
[4] Atinault A. Règles et organisation de la transplantation rénale du prélèvement. Encycl Méd Chir, Néphro-uro, 18-065-a-10,2001, 12p
[5] Desvaux C, Claquin J. Prélèvement d'organes et de tissus en France : modalités réglementaires. Objectifs soins, Avril 2003, n°115, pp 10-13
[6] Desvaux C, Atinault A, Claquin J. Législation des prélèvements et greffes d'organes. Objectif Soins Numéro 79, octobre 1999, pp 16-18 (1ère partie)
[7] Starzl A multifactorial system for equitable selection of cadaver kidney recipients. JAMA. 1987 Jun 12;257(22):3073-5.
[8] Smith T. Computerized kidney registry links transplant centers.Forum (Wash). 1977 Nov-Dec;1(2):36-7.
[9] Jacquelinet C, Burgun A, Strang N, Denis D, Boutin B, Le Beux P. Design considerations for an ontology in the domain of organ failure and transplantation. Stud Health Technol Inform. 2002;90:611-5.
[10] Jacquelinet C, Burgun A, Delamarre D, Strang N, Djabbour S, Boutin B, Le Beux P. Developing the ontological foundations of a terminological system for end-stage diseases, organ failure, dialysis and transplantation. Int J Med Inform. 2003 Jul;70(2-3):317-28.
[11] Jacquelinet C, Burgun A, Djabbour S, Delamarre D, Clerc P, Boutin B, Le Beux P. A contextual coding system for transplantation and end stage diseases.Stud Health Technol Inform. 2003;95:457-62.
[12] Landais P, Simonet A, Guillon D, Jacquelinet C, Ben Said M, Mugnier C, Simonet M.SIMS REIN: a multi-source information system for end-stage renal disease C R Biol. 2002 Apr;325(4):515-28.
[13] Ben Said M, Simonet A, Guillon D, Jacquelinet C, Gaspoz F, Dufour E, Mugnier C, Jais JP, Simonet M, Landais P. A dynamic Web application within an n-tier architecture: a Multi-Source Information System for end-stage renal disease. Stud Health Technol Inform. 2003;95:95-100

Address for correspondence

Nigel Strang, Direction des systèmes d'information, Agence de la biomédecine 1 avenue Stade de France 93212 SAINT DENIS LA PLAINE CEDEX France, Nigel.Strang@biomedecine.fr

Connecting Medical Informatics and Bio-Informatics
R. Engelbrecht et al. (Eds.)
IOS Press, 2005

Avoiding Doubles in Distributed Nominative Medical Databases: Optimization of the Needleman and Wunsch Algorithm

Loïc Le Mignot, Claude Mugnier, Mohamed Ben Saïd, Jean-Philippe Jais, Jean-Baptiste Richard, Christine Le Bihan-Benjamin, Pierre Taupin, Paul Landais

Université Paris-Descartes, Faculté de Médecine; Assistance Publique-Hôpitaux de Paris; Hôpital Necker, EA222, Service de Biostatistique et d'Informatique Médicale, Hôpital Necker, 149 rue de Sèvres, Paris, France.

Abstract

Difficulties in reconstituting patients' trajectory in the public health information systems are raised by errors in patients' identification processes. A crucial issue to achieve is avoiding doubles in distributed web databases. We explored Needleman and Wunsch (N&W) algorithm in order to optimize the properties of string matching. Five variants of the N&W algorithm were developed. The algorithms were implemented for a web Multi-Source Information System. This system was dedicated to tracking patients with End-Stage Renal Disease at both regional and national level. A simulated study database of 73,210 records was created. An insertion or suppression of each character of the original string was simulated. The rate of double entries was 2% given an acceptable distance set to 5 modifications. The search was sensitive and specific with an acceptable detection time. It detected up to 10% of modifications that is above the estimated error rate. A variant of the N&W algorithm designed as "cut-off heuristic", proved to be efficient for the search of double entries occurring in nominative distributed databases.

Keywords
Dynamic algorithm; Alignment; Edit distance; Pattern matching; End- Stage Renal Disease

1. Introduction

This work focused on character strings comparison between the user entry information and the stored information in a simulated national patient database. Our method is derived from the Needleman and Wunsch (N&W) algorithm developed in bio-computing [1] searching for similarities in amino acid sequences of two proteins and for the sequence of maximum match between two strings. An important implication of the N&W algorithm is the "distance" between two strings. The goal is to make the distance the smallest possible when one of the strings is likely to be an erroneous variant of the other under the error model in use. One error model is the edit distance, which allows deleting, inserting or substituting simple characters [2]. We considered that all operations have the same cost and we focused on finding the minimum number of insertions, deletions and substitutions to make both strings equals. A value of an "acceptable distance" between two strings is assigned while testing the N&W algorithm. If the minimal computed distance is equal or lower than acceptable distance, the information entered is considered as having a match in the system.

The objective of our work, based on the N&W algorithm, was to optimize a method that allows deciding whether, given two strings, one is produced from the other by a limited series of modifications. The experimental design was applied to a Multi-Source Information System including a dynamic web server for identifying doubles in a nominative national database of End-Stage Renal Disease (ESRD) patients

2. Material and Methods

Patients and organizational support

A Multi-Source Information System (MSIS-REIN) was dedicated to collect continuous and exhaustive records of all ESRD cases and their clinical follow-up in France [3]. It collates in a standardized representation a condensed patient record elaborated by health professionals. MSIS-REIN aimed to fulfil the following requirements: scalability, portability, reliability, accessibility, and cost effectiveness oriented toward open source software. The use of standard references, the respect of privacy, confidentiality and security of patient information were required as well.

The architecture of MSIS-REIN has been described elsewhere [4]. Briefly, it is based on an n-tier architecture. Via a web browser the client tier connects to a middle tier that is in relation with several databases: the identification database, the production database and the data warehouse. The middle tier supports client services through Web containers and business logic services through component containers. Business logic components in the middleware support transactions toward the databases. A Web server application interacts with the production database system, consisting of a collection of Web components: Java Server Pages™ (JSP), Servlets and other resources (graphics, scripting programs or plug-ins) organized in a directory structure. Web components interact within a Web container, Tomcat, which corresponds to a runtime environment providing a context and a life cycle management. MSIS REIN was authorized by the Commission Informatique et Libertés.

Description of the algorithms

Both strings are arranged in a two-dimensional matrix and paired for comparison with the same value for the concordance score as well as for the penalty of modifying inserting/deleting one character. Five variants of the N&W algorithm were implemented and tested, with different optimization attempts. These algorithms were all functionally equivalent. A cell $S(i,j)$, within the similarity matrix defined above, can be viewed as a distance between the two substrings , using the relation:

Distance (i, j) = maximum (i, j) – similarity (i, j)
The corresponding matrix of distances is defined by:

$$S(i, j) = \min \begin{cases} S(i-1, j-1) + dist(i, j) \\ S(i-1, j) + P \\ S(i, j-1) + P \end{cases}$$

Where: dist(i,j) = 0 if characters are equal,
dist(i,j) = 1 if characters are different,
P = 1: penalty score of inserting or deleting a character.
- Alg #1: Direct implementation of Needleman-Wunsch algorithm as described above. The full matrix is computed for each record.

- Alg #2, #3, #4: variations on the use of the acceptable distance as a loop breaker, exploiting the properties of the distances matrix ("cut-off" heuristic).
- Alg #5: Use of common prefixes in records to avoid redundant computations. With the growing of the patient table, more and more concatenated strings will be found to have common prefixes. With a sorted list, time can be spared by re-using part of the precedent matrix.

Implementation of the algorithm

Eliminating non ASCII character errors:

Non-alphanumeric characters (space, hyphen, apostrophe, etc) are eliminated and non-ASCII characters (é,è,ç,ô etc) are transformed into capital ASCII character sets, example: Jean-françois La Pérouse, male, born on December 1st, 1954 becomes:
"JEANFRANCOISLAPEROUSE1120154"

Eliminating mistyping, orthographic errors:

The score in case of deletion or substitution is represented on Figures 1.

The experiment was tested using a usual PC Intel-Pentium-III™ computer with 396 megabytes of random access memory. The software development refers to the same approach and environment as used for MSIS-REIN: a dynamic web application based on JSP/ Java™ servlets, a web container, Tomcat/Apache Jakarta open source projects and MySQL open source database system is used. A simulated study database of 73,210 records was created. The characteristics of the concatenated data set are presented on table 1.

```
      M U  G  N  I  E  R              M  U  G  N  I  E  R
M     0 1  2  3  4  5  6       M      0  1  2  3  4  5  6
U     1 0  1  2  3  4  5       A      1  1  2  3  4  5  6
N     2 1  1  1  2  3  4       G      2  2  1  2  3  4  5
I     3 2  2  2  1  2  3       N      3  3  2  1  2  3  4
E     4 3  3  3  2  1  2       I      4  4  3  2  1  2  3
R     5 4  4  4  3  2  1       E      5  5  4  3  2  1  2
                              R      6  6  5  4  3  2  1
```

Figure 1 – Deletion penalty (deletion of one character) on the left and substitution penalty (mismatch one character) on the right (distance = 1)

Table 1 – Characteristics of the tested data set.

Rows	Min length	Max length	Range	Average
73210	9	35	27	20.17

When a new patient name is entered, a Java™ program searches for an existing patient record in the database. It comprised two parts: a function, which directly searches for exact match between the concatenated stored data, and a calculated string derived from the entered information. In case of a match, a dynamic web page is generated. The user is asked for confirmation to create the patient record. If no match is found, a second program function implementing the dynamic programming algorithm of N&W is run and searches the concatenated data for a patient record with a spelling close to the user-entered information. The program selects potential matches depending on their maximum match score relevance in conformity with the implemented algorithm. In case of potential matches, a dynamic web page informs the user. They are displayed according to the user's profile and authorizations to access nominative data of patients he is in charge of, or not.

3. Results

Accuracy

A modification was simulated by the addition of a probability of change, insertion and suppression for each character of the initial string. Given an "acceptable distance" set to 5, the false positive rate, i.e. new names detected as double entries, was 2 % (figure 3). Since the matching probability depends on the acceptable distance, a sizeable distance will cause the algorithm to become incapable to differentiate new entries from doubles. Moreover, the greater a data set, the higher the probability that it contains a "close enough" record. The false positive rate is thus expected to increase with the number of records.

Specificity

We checked whether double entries were properly detected. Given the so-called "acceptable distance" set to 5, the detection rate of doubles is presented on figure 4 according to the probability of simulated errors at data entry.

Time consumption

Direct access to last record in the database was 472 milliseconds in case of perfect matching. Search for a record within the "acceptable" distance appears below:

Algorithm version	Answering time (seconds)
#1	2.684
#2	1.758
#3	1.454
#4	1.432
#5	1.472

Quality of the chosen method

The comparison of a sufficient number of different strings provides the general distribution of the matching scores, which constitutes our "research space". Then, by comparing a string with its twisted version (simulation of double entry) we get the average score of a "positive case". The quality of the method (in term of discriminative power) is given by the quantity Q estimated by the following ratio: $Q = |Sg - Sp|/Dg$, which compares the difference between "matching" and "no-matching" score to the standard deviation of the general score where: Sg is the average score for the overall distribution, Sp the average score for positive cases, Dg the standard deviation of the overall distribution.

We checked whether the method, originally conceived for random sequences, is still relevant for matching our concatenated strings (any two "real" strings being closer than any two random strings). As expected, the results presented on figure 5 show that a better quality of match is observed with randomly generated strings rather than with real names. In effect, the discriminative power appeared better when the similarity between 2 strings is low. It confirmed however that the power of the approach remained satisfactory for real strings in the region of interest.

Algorithm #3 designed as "cut-off heuristic", appeared well discriminative since it detected up to 10 % of modifications that is above the estimated error rates of generating doubles at data entry. As the database will grow, the method version #5 represents a potential interest.

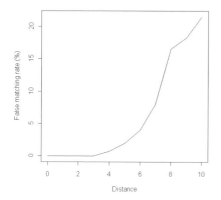

Figure 3-Rate of false positive (2%) as a function of the threshold of "acceptable" distance (distance = 5).

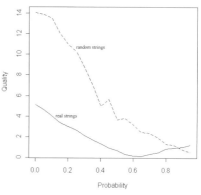

Figure 5-Quality of the method according to the probability of error (threshold set to 5) for strings based on random characters and for real strings (corresponding to names).

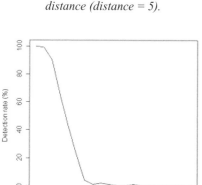

Figure 4-Detection rate of doubles (~100%) given the probability of error at data entry (10% of errors in a correct string).

A study is currently in progress to explore whether the same method can be used for patient linkage through year-by-year hospitalization database for 2002 and 2003 in Necker Hospital.

Preliminary results showed a correct linkage for 20,962 of 21,044 patients (99.6%), and caught attention on 0.68% of patients suspected to be double entries.

4. Discussion

We propose an updated implementation of the N&W algorithm adapted to the search of doubles in a web database. The original N&W algorithm was developed for computational biology. Other applications were also developed in the fields of signal processing or of text retrieval. Algorithms developed to approximate string matching were recently reviewed [3].

Identification of errors on names is crucial for medical databases. We adapted the N&W algorithm for a web database developed for End-Stage Renal Disease patients. We did not retain the Soundex algorithm despite its appreciable sensitivity [5]. However, its specificity

[6] is low and not adapted to nominative data for medical applications. It mainly consists in removing the vowels (plus H and W), merging the 18 consonants into 6 different numeric codes depending on their phonetic value, and then keeping 3 of the resulting digits added to the first letter of the word. By this way, the same code is used for many different words. For example, in a set of 30,000 names (distinct one from the others) a code is found to appear about 12 times on average. That is, for almost every new name entered, the algorithm would identify it as a double entry. It is therefore irrelevant in the case of our problem, unless another phonetic coding is defined.

The algorithm we used belongs to a family of algorithms derived from Levenshtein distance [7] such as Jaro-Winkler [8][9] or Smith-Waterman [10] algorithms. Smith-Waterman algorithm is dedicated to local subsequences matching: applied to characters strings, it may therefore be more relevant for search queries than for identity recognition where the whole signature string has to be matched. A recent work [11] presents an approach based on Porter-Jaro-Winkler algorithm, using weighting on identity items, and using similar items and string normalization. This work is focused on extracting identity aggregates in existing database, which is a different approach from our main objective.

The method we described proved to fulfil our goals. It provides a satisfactory answering time and specifity, in order to be easily accepted by the users. Moreover its high sensitivity avoids double entries in our database in accordance with our goal of detecting upstream a single new entry, quickly enough for the process to remain transparent to the end user.

6. References

[1]   Needleman S, Wunsch C. A general Method Applicable to the Search for Similarities in the Amino Acid Sequences of Proteins. J. Mol. Biol. 1970:48, 443-453.

[2]   Navarro G. A Guided Tour to Approximate String Matching. ACM Computing Surveys 2001: 33, 31–88.

[3]   Landais P, Simonet A, Guillon D, Jacquelinet C, Ben Said M, Mugnier C, Simonet M. SIMS REIN: a multi-source information system for end-stage renal disease. C R Biol. 2002 Apr;325(4):515-28

[4]   Ben Saïd M, Simonet A, Guillon D, Jacquelinet C, Gaspoz F, Dufour E, Mugnier C, Jais JP, Simonet M, Landais P. A Dynamic Web Application Within N-Tier Architecture : a Multi-Source Information System for End-Stage Renal Disease. In : Baud R, Fieschi M, Le Beux P, Ruch P, eds. Proceedings of MIE2003, Saint Malo:IOS Press, 2003;pp. 95-100.

[5]   The Soundex algorithm. D. Knuth. The Art of Computer Programming, vol 3. Sorting and searching. Addison-Wesley Pubs. Second printing 1975 pp 725.

[6]   Sideli RV, Friedman C. Validating Patient Names in an Integrated Clinical Information System. In: Clayton P, ed. Proceedings of the Fifteenth Annual Symposium on Computer Applications in Medical Care, Washington D.C.: McGrawHill, 1991; pp. 588-592.

[7]   Levenshtein V I. Binary codes capable of correcting deletions, insertions and reversals. Sov. Phys. Dokl. 1966;6:707-710.

[8]   Porter EH, Winkler WE. Approximate String Comparison and its Effect on an Advanced Record Linkage System. U.S. Bureau of Census. Research Reports Statistics #1997-02 (http://www.census.gov/srd/www/byyear.html)

[9]   Winkler WE, Approximate String Comparator Search Strategies for Very Large Administrative Lists. U.S. Bureau of Census. Research Reports Series Statistics #2005-02 (http://www.census.gov/srd/www/byyear.html)

[10] Smith TF, Waterman M.S, J Mol Biol (1981) 147:195-197.

[11] Paumier JP, Sauleau EA, Buemi A. Journées francophones d'informatique médicale, Lille mai 2005. (http://www.univ-lille2.fr/jfim2005/papiers/05-paumier-jfim2005.pdf)

Address for correspondence

Pr Paul Landais
Service de Biostatistique et d'Informatique Médicale, Hôpital Necker-Enfants Malades, 149, rue de Sèvres 75743 Paris cedex 15, e-mail : landais@necker.fr

Connecting Medical Informatics and Bio-Informatics
R. Engelbrecht et al. (Eds.)
IOS Press, 2005

Participatory Work Flow Analysis prior to Implementation of EPR: A Method to Discover Needs for Change

Pernille Bertelsen[a], Inge Madsen[b], Per Hostrup[c]

[a] *Department of Development and Planning, Aalborg University, Aalborg, Denmark*
[b] *Department of EPR Implementation, Aarhus University Hospital, Skejby Sygehus Aarhus, Denmark*
[c] *Department of Cardiothoracic Surgery, Aarhus University Hospital, Skejby Sygehus, Aarhus, Denmark*

Abstract

We need to know how clinicians' use their paper based medical records to secure a local participation in the implementation process of Electronic Patient Record (EPR). In what way their use of paper based medical records is related to, or dependent on, other people and artifacts. The research presented in this paper was done as part of a work flow analysis of the particular sequence of doing rounds at two distinct hospital departments, a thoracic surgical and a cardiology department. It was designed to develop a method that would let the hospital clinicians obtain knowledge on the daily use of the paper based medical records during rounds and thus make use of their local knowledge to start a discussion on changes in organization and knowledge before EPR can be successfully implemented.[1] The aim was to investigate how paper based medical records are currently used at two wards.

Keywords:
Electronic Patient Record; Implementation; Action research, Organizational change; Work flow analysis

1. Introduction

As the implementation of EPR systems penetrates the outlook of politicians, hospital management and system consultants, it becomes evident that implementation of EPR in Scandinavia offers tremendous opportunities for organizational change in the public hospitals covering more than 99% of the health services.

Among health informatics system developers in Denmark there seems to be consensus on the notion that EPR at Danish hospitals have to be more than "paper based medical records added IT-power". Full integration between data from different feeding pipes, and later on also from primary and secondary sectors, seamless care etc. are the new goals.

However, currently, the discussions at ward and department levels in hospitals are concerned with how implementation of EPR – or parts of EPR, changes the socio-technical use of medical records how it affects the quality of the work and further how to avoid negative effects for the patients.

---

[1] We are grateful to the following clinicians, Cathrine H. Foss, MD. Pauline Schrødder, MD. Morten Smerup MD and Niels Henrik Stålsen, MD and the medical director Børge H. Jensen, MD, Skejby Sygehus, Aarhus University Hospital for sharing their knowledge with us.

To support these discussions, we have chosen to investigate the work sequence when clinicians do rounds at ward level. Clinicians are known to have difficulties in giving up old habits and changing their routines. When it comes to documentation in medical records, which has not changed in Denmark during the last 25 years, we are up against a solid change of fundamental clinical documentation practice. We observe a need to raise awareness and discussion on how to make this staff category participate actively and benefit from the ICT changes that will take place in the hospital over the next few years [2]. The target group is staff involved in the implementation processes.

- How do we make sure that local EPR implementers pay attention to all the undocumented and non-verbal routines among clinicians and other clinicians categories?
- How do we make clinicians aware of the potential of EPR and their challenge for the traditional organizational context?

1.1 Research objective

The research objective was to be able to:

a) point out areas of practice where EPR will not be able to support current practice at the involved wards
b) point at possible difference between Medical and Surgical wards in their use of paper based medical records in clinicians' rounds
c) Develop a method that can be implemented at other wards.
d) Document how the paper records are being used and thereby make it possible to revisit the wards after the EPR have been implemented in order to see whether any change of practice can be observed.
e) Start a debate at the wards on how EPR challenge and change current practice.

2. Methods

The research project has developed an exploratory method that EPR implementers and super users can use to investigate what technical and organizational changes of routines that take place when a particular hospital ward changes from paper based medical records to EPR.

Our notion of the importance of developing a method to identify formal and informal work routines centered around the use of the paper based medical records is in line with the principles in Soft System Methodology and a ".... fundamental proposition that in order to conceptualize, and so create, a system which serves, it is first necessary to conceptualize that which is served, since the way the latter is thought of will dictate what would be necessary to serve or support it. "(Checkland and Holwell, 1998, p.10)

The method has been tested at a cardiology ward and a thoracic surgical ward at a University hospital. We have asked a number of clinicians – before the EPR system is being implemented at their hospital, - but after the decision to implement it has been made - to participate in an analysis of the objective and content of doing ward rounds and in particular to analyze the role of the paper based medical records in that particular classical work task. We focus on how the paper based medical records are being used during the ward rounds in order to be able to: Compare the different style of the individual clinician's use of the paper based medical records as well as b) Comparing two wards, each with a clinical specialty of its own.

2.1 Study design

The present research places itself in the Action Research tradition, in which research questions are made as collaboration between the researcher and the EPR implementation unit at the hospital. Action Research methods are highly clinical in nature and place the researcher in a helping role within the (hospital) organization that is being studied [3]. Action research merges research with practice and by doing so produces very relevant research findings. The social and organizational realities in a hospital and other health care organizations is a reality that is continuously being constructed and re-constructed in dialogue among the clinicians and in action which they take[4].

The actual study design chosen is inductive and interpretive. It does not considering the researcher as someone who is neutral, but influencing the result. We perceive the organization of work in a hospital as a social construction by human actors. Each ward or department has its own reality that we want to explore, not deduct. An explorative method is thus valuable when the objective is to break new ground and yield insights into a new topic [5]. Our study target was the individual clinicians and how they use the paper based medical records when they do rounds at the ward. The sample was selected by using what may be called a convenience or haphazard sampling method [6]. The informants were few, 2 clinicians in each ward, a medical and a surgery ward. We asked the administrative leaders to identify clinicians who did rounds on a regular basis. In order to test the method a pilot study with one clinician was done before start.

2.2 Participatory technology analysis

Each clinician was interviewed by the use of a semi-structured interview guide. An interview method which, in a participatory way, makes the informant explain and, in doing so, make an analysis of the technology in use exemplified as the sequence of doing rounds and the use of the paper based medical record.

We see the current change from paper based medical record to EPR as a change from the use of one technological system to another. The introduction of electronic devises is only a new technique which would never be successful without a simultaneous adjustment in two of the other three elements of the technology, namely in the organization, the knowledge. Changes in these three elements will finally affect the end result – the product, which in the case of paper based medical records, we defined as; timely, documented and accessible data ready for use by the health clinicians.

Our definition of technology influenced on the selection of subjects for the interview guide. We were interested in sociotechnical issues having to do with the organizational context among others: Focus area was when the clinicians do rounds; the objective of doing rounds, how rounds are organized at the particular ward, what inputs they use (artifacts and information), and what type of rounds the individual clinician does, the planning, the start and the end. We were also concerned with the following: who uses the paper based medical records, what they use them for, who have the legal responsibility, the informal responsibility, the content of the records and how the records at this hospital differ from records at other hospitals. At a later stage the participant observation method was used. We followed each informant on a workday when he/she did rounds, in order to observe and note how he/she used the paper based medical records. The informant was observed from when they met in the morning to they had finished doing their rounds. Notes were made of all their work tasks and how the records were used.

3. Result

The interviews revealed a distinct difference in the role the paper based medical records played at the surgery ward and at the medical ward. At the surgery ward the records were used to check up on special well-known standard events whereas at the medical ward the paper based medical records were the tool used to identify and monitor the diagnosis and plan for the cure of the patient. At both wards it was mainly the junior clinicians who did the rounds

In combination with the information obtained from the paper based medical records the clinicians' use a number of other artifacts and sources of information when they do their rounds:

- Department Conference
- Ward conference: briefing from the clinician on call
- x-ray conference
- The big whiteboard in the duty room (coordination room) outlining the placement of the patients etc.
- Information from nurses (based on their nurses record)
- light box at the ward
- The nurse
- Pharmacopeial
- private note book with important information relevant for this specific ward
- Small paper notes with things to remember
- Observation forms from nurses (pulse, blood pressure, temperature.)
- Internal telephone book
- Stethoscope
- Percussion hammer
- Pupil lamp
- Pens
- DICOM (Dictaphone)
- ECG
- printout of telemetry
- different order forms
- prescription pad
- medicine record
- Telephone

There were individual difference in whether the clinician prepares him/herself for all patients of the day together with the nurse or one patient at the time before visiting the patient. At the medical ward one of the clinicians always brought the paper record with her to the patient, whereas another clinician never brought the record with her to the patient. The nurses distribute the patients to the clinicians (3-5 to each) but the clinicians are of the opinion that it is their responsibility if they want to change the plan.

- At both wards they start at 9:00 after the morning and x-ray conferences.
- At the medical ward the work of doing rounds during the daytime finishes between 12:30 and 14:00. At the medical ward they finish between 10:00 and 12:00.
- All Clinicians only read the paper records in the ward never in their office.
- The paper based medical records are used by clinicians and nurses. Only one clinician also mentioned the physiotherapist. None of them mentioned the secretary.

The clinicians are responsible for what is written in the records. The secretaries are responsible for writing it as well as bringing it to and from the archives.

3.1 From the observation study

The nurse spends from 30 minutes to an hour during the preparation filling in the clinician with information on the patient from what she has in her written records.

Small "postIT notes", results from tests and other aspects the nurses or secretaries want the clinician to pay attention to are placed on the cover of the records with paper clips.

Clinicians waiting for an available phone line, seem to be a bottleneck.

Individual style with regard to whether the paper based medical records was taken into the patient or not, whether notes were made on paper or not during report from clinician on call.

The X-ray conference had participation of a large group of clinicians of whom only a few would do the rounds.

Medical wards more dependent on written documentation, different test results than surgery wards.

It became clear that the paper based journal was not used at the different conferences at all.

Structured information as well as non-structured information such as Pharmacopeial, private notebook and telephone book is not connected with the paper based journal.

4. Discussion

What do we do with the artefacts and sources of information – of which many cannot be replaced by the EPR? How do we create new routines known to all? Who has the formal and informal responsibility for domesticating the new routines? More studies on this subject are needed with involvement of local clinicians.

How do the clinicians change work routines that have been part of their work for many years. An example from the study could be the X-ray conference. Between 13 and 23 clinicians (different observations) participated in the conference. However, only a few of them needed the information for doing the rounds at the ward. Disregarding that the x-ray has been digitalized some years ago, and, therefore, the pictures are available electronically on monitors at all wards, the organisation of the conference was done in the same way as when the photos were developed into pictures only. From the interview we learned that the x-ray conference also served a social purpose. It was the only time of the day that the clinicians could talk informally to each other – on the way from the ward to the X- ray conference room. Therefore, though it seems apparent that organizational changes of old work routines could be needed; there may be unrecognised reasons as to why they are maintained. The above observation serves as an argument as to why interview and observation supplement each other.

How is non verbal communication going to be communicated and accommodated within use of EPR? There is at risk that we will lose important information. Today the nurses spend a lot of time filling in the clinicians with patient relevant information as preparation to the rounds. An interdisciplinary EPR system will change that work routine because the clinicians will be able to read the information on the screen themselves.

Not surprisingly the study revealed a difference in the role the records played for the treatment of the patients in the two wards. For this reason, the fear of not being able to carry out the work satisfactorily after implementation of the EPR was higher at the medical ward than at the surgery ward This difference will also appear at other wards, and it makes the local domestication of EPR to all departments and wards a job which can only succeed if the local clinicians and the knowledge they have are actively involved in the implementation process. In the two wards of the study have been studied it was mainly the young clinicians who did the rounds. This observation indicates that the group of senior clinicians may need extra attention in order to become accustomed to the EPR.

Will the EPR allow the same room for individual style in organisation of how the rounds are done? The hardware will determine whether the records can be brought to the patients or not. But whether the records are updated after each or all patients, and with or without participation of the nurse, are also at present a matter of individual style. The interesting issue is here to recognise that the individual style exists in a ward and to discuss whether or not that will have to change with EPR. However, EPR will also open up for new work routines like e.g. being able to read the paper based medical records in the office or elsewhere in the hospital. None of the clinicians did so today.

5. Conclusion

From our results we have developed a method to be used by healthcare informatics implementers and IT consultants in their daily practice. The model is designed to question daily routines as well as the local knowledge [8] and habits developed over time in a ward. It is meant to assist in creating ownership in a non normative way.

It is of great importance that clinical clinicians and the leadership are involved throughout the analysis, both to create possible solutions and to create ownership to the solutions.

Due to the fact that the methods do not focus on dataflow and redundant data, a work flow analysis is necessary.

It is also necessary to develop usable replacements for the artefacts that are not cared for in the design and use of the EPR otherwise important patient information will be lost.

8. References

[1] Andersen S.K, Nøhr C, Vingtoft S, Bernstein K, Bruun-Rasmussen M. (2002): The EPR Observatory Annual Report 2002and 2003, Aalborg, Virtual Centre for Health Informatics, 2002. Denmark

[2] Engsig-Karup M. & Rasmussen, JP. TEHRE conference, London 2002. Ugesk. laeger, 2003,September 9th vol. 36, Denmark (weekly magazine for Clinicians)

[3] Baskerville,R. and Wood-Harper, A.T. "Diversity in Information Systems (7:2) 1998, pp 90-107

[4] Checkland, P. and Holwell, S. (1998): Information, Systems and Information Systems. Making sense of the field. John Wiley & Sons Ltd. England. 1998.

[5] Babbie, E, (1998): The practice of social research. Eight edition. Chapman Univeristy. Wadsworth Publishing company.

[6] Bernard, H. R. (2002): Research methods in anthropology: qualitative and quantitative approaches 3rd edition, ALTAMIRA Press.

[7] Müller, J. (2003): in Kuada, John ed. Culture and Technological Transformation in the South pp. 27-41, Samfundslitteraturen, Denmark.

[8] Bertelsen, P. (2001) : Indigenous knowledge and IT Developments in Health Care. Rechnical Report No. 01-2. V.CHI – Virtuelt Center for Sundhendsinformatik, Denmark.

Connecting Medical Informatics and Bio-Informatics
R. Engelbrecht et al. (Eds.)
IOS Press, 2005

Use of Computer and Respiratory Inductance Plethysmography for the Automated Detection of Swallowing in the Elderly

Alexandre Moreau-Gaudry[a], **Abdelkebir Sabil**[b], **Pierre Baconnier**[b], **Gila Benchetrit**[b],

Alain Franco[a]

[a]*Department of Geriatric and Community medicine, University Hospital, Grenoble, France*
[b]*PRETA-TIMC-IMAG-CNRS Laboratory, Grenoble, France*

Abstract

Deglutition disorders can occur at any age but are especially prevalent in the elderly. The resulting morbidity and mortality are being recognized as major geriatric health issues. Because of difficulties in studying swallowing in the frail elderly, a new, non-invasive, user-friendly, bedside technique has been developed. Ideally suited to such patients, this tool, an intermediary between purely instrumental and clinical methods, combines respiratory inductance plethysmography (RIP) and the computer to detect swallowing automatically. Based on an automated analysis of the airflow estimated by the RIP-derived signal, this new tool was evaluated according to its capacity to detect clinical swallowing from among the 1643 automatically detected respiratory events. This evaluation used contingency tables and Receiver Operator Characteristic (ROC) curves. Results were all significant ($\chi2(1,n=1643)>100$, $p<0.01$). Considering its high accuracy in detecting swallowing (area under the ROC curve greater than 0.9), this system would be proposed to study deglutition and then deglutition disorders in the frail elderly, to set up medical supervision and to evaluate the efficiency of a swallowing disorder remedial therapeutic.

Keywords:
Frail elderly; Respiratory inductance; Plethysmography; Deglutition; Automatic data processing; Deglutition disorders.

1. Introduction

Swallowing disorders can occur at any age but are especially prevalent in the elderly [1]. They can have serious consequences [2,3]. The resulting morbidity and mortality are being recognized as major geriatric health issues. Ongoing research into swallowing disorders has highlighted inconsistencies in clinical evaluation and in instrumental decision making [4]. New tests were elaborated and evaluated for their effectiveness in predicting aspiration [5]. The relationship between breathing and swallowing has already been studied in healthy subjects and elderly adults using various instrumental methods [6].

Furthermore, instrumental evaluations are often not feasible in a frail population. In order to overcome these difficulties, a new system was developed. It combines the respiratory inductance plethysmography (RIP), a user-friendly, non-invasive bedside tool, and the computer, an objective tool, in order to detect swallowing by using an automated processing of the airflow signals obtained through RIP. If such is the case, this system affords a user-friendly objective bedside clinical tool for the detection and then the analysis of swallowing in the elderly. Its objective nature derives from the use of automated analysis elaborated specifically in this study.

2. Materials and methods

Materials

The RIP system used was the computer assisted Visuresp®. The sensor consisted of an elasticized jacket that could easily be worn by the patients over their usual clothing. The abdomen and rib cage signals obtained through RIP were combined to provide a volume signal. This latter was smoothed by low-pass filter and then differentiated to provide a valid estimation of the airflow signal [7]. A software was developed in order to analyze the airflow signal and detect swallowing automatically. This software, written in R (a language and environment for statistical computing and graphics) and in TCL/TK, consisted of two parts: the first part enabled the respiratory cycles to be delimited in an automatic way. In the second part, a test was elaborated to detect swallowing automatically. This test was based on the identification of a zero on the airflow signal (AS) as, during swallowing, the airflow is interrupted by a brief closure of the larynx, to protect the airway from the aspiration of ingested matter. In order to obtain this zero identification, a confidence interval of zero airflow was defined and totally determined by a cutoff value p. This confidence interval represented p percent ($0 \leq p \leq 100$) of the distribution of values of the airflow signal around zero airflow.

Clinical protocol

Swallowing was studied with this combined system in 14 patients aged 75-100 in a geriatric ward after obtaining informed written consent from each subject or their legal representative. Each patient, in a standardized but natural mealtime setting, wore the jacket in order for his or her breathing to be recorded continuously, and performed four swallowing: two swallowing of water, the first in a static mode (a 20 ml glass of water being given to the subject by the nurse), the second, in a dynamic way (the patient raised the 20 ml glass of water to his mouth to drink); two other swallowing of gelatinous water, with a little spoon, according to the same protocol. This clinical protocol was chosen in order to ascertain whether movement or the nature of the food would perturb the RIP signal. Each swallowing was carried out at our request after a regular respiratory rhythm had been observed. For each swallowing, the initial instant (when water or gelatinous water were placed in the mouth) and the final instant (the observed ceasing of larynx movement) were noted.

Test evaluation

The test was evaluated according to its capacity to detect the clinical Time-Marked Swallowing (TMS) from among the automatically detected respiratory cycles. Contingency tables were used. The test was performed for the two sets of respiratory cycles P1 and P2. The first, P1, was made up of elementary events. Each of these was in turn the set of respiratory cycles occurring during one TMS. The second, P2, was the set of respiratory cycles during which there was no TMS. Sensitivity, specificity, positive predictive value, negative predictive value, concordance rate and chi-square were computed for the test described above. Its accuracy was calculated by the area under the Receiver Operating Characteristic

(ROC) curve. The best zero AS confidence interval was determined from the best balance between sensitivity and specificity obtained from the ROC curve.

3. Results

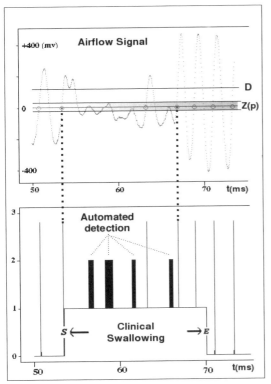

*Figure 1 - An example of the automated detection of a gelatinous water swallowing. **On the upper part**, the dotted curve represents the recording of the airflow signal during a swallowing of gelatinous water. The straight line D corresponds to the threshold used for the automated detection of respiratory cycles. Z(p) is the confidence interval of the zero airflow (p=10). **On the lower part**, S and E are the beginning and the end of the clinical swallowing of gelatinous water. The thin vertical lines represent the start points of each inspiration. A clinical swallowing is detected if and only if the parts of the airflow signal which lie in Z(p) are not monotonous (thick lines).*

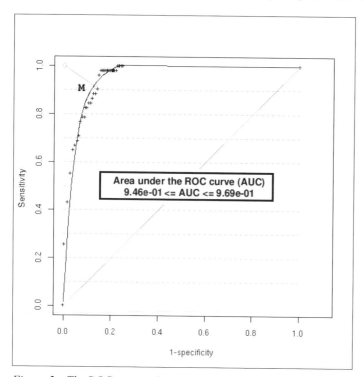

Figure 2 – The ROC curve is built from computed sensitivity and 1-specificity (cross-points). The area under the ROC curve (AUC) is greater than 0.9. The best balance between sensitivity and specificity is obtained for the M Point, where the optimal computed p-cutoff value is 18.05 with a sensitivity and a specificity at 91.37 and 87.20 percent respectively.

Among 56 swallowing, only 51 were correctly located in time. The recorded breathing period was 351.3 ± 93.7 seconds ranging from 189 to 583 seconds. 1592 respiratory cycles were automatically identified (see figure 1). Results for contingency tables computed for different values of the p-cutoff were all significant ($\chi^2(1,n=1643)>100$, p-value<0.01). The receiver operating characteristic (ROC) curve once computed (see figure 2), the accuracy of the elaborated test was calculated being the area under the curve (AUC): AUC > 0.9, which established its high accuracy [8]. At the best balance between sensitivity and specificity, the computed optimal p-cutoff was 18.05 with a sensitivity and a specificity at 91.37 and 87.20 percent respectively.

4. Discussion

There have been very few studies comparing airflow and RIP-derived signal under physiological conditions. The RIP-derived signal has been validated as providing an estimation of airflow acquired by pneumotachogram under physiological conditions and with varying postures [7].

We modified the water TMS from the water swallowing test [5] which serves as a method of evaluating the swallowing ability of patients. We also varied the type of swallowed food, as swallowing disorders may vary according to the ingested food texture. Indeed, the combination of water and food swallowing tests provided an enhancement in sensitivity for detecting swallowing dysfunctions.

We compared static and dynamic (movement of the arm) food intake, to ascertain if movement would perturb the RIP signal. We observed that the automated detection of swallowing was not impaired by change of food texture or movements of arms.

The present study was performed on only 14 patients. In order to obtain reliable data, the active participation of the patient is required. In addition, the patient should be capable of performing simple tasks. Although the AS analysis was possible with arm movements, it is difficult to carry out the protocol on restless patients.

Being solicited to take water or food could possibly induce stress in the patient, which might then affect respiratory events preceding swallowing, but not larynx closure during the swallowing. It was for this reason that zero airflow detection was used. This protocol differs from one where random swallowing is provocated [9].

The interplay of swallowing and breathing has been studied using other - and for these frailer patients - often unpleasant – methods (an electrode attached to the cheek, a throat microphone, a soft polythene tube inserted into a nostril, sub mental electromyography or a mouthpiece [9,10]). On the other hand the recording procedure used in this study was well accepted by the elderly, since the device consisted of a jacket worn over their usual clothing and the recordings were performed in their usual mealtime environment. Furthermore, the user-friendly nature of this equipment makes this method an appropriate bedside clinical tool. We have no knowledge of the existence of any study of a similar nature.

The detection of swallowing by means of automated recordings and analysis thanks to the computer was an essential prerequisite of an objective analysis. The use of the AS, time-derivative of the volume signal, providing zero airflow detection, made this automation possible.

Although the reliability of the automated detection appears to be sufficiently high in this study, as evidenced by the high sensitivity and specificity at the optimal p-cutoff computed, automated AS analysis may be refined by a more precise characterization of the events to be detected.

Because apnoeas are not specific to swallowing, the specificity of the detection will be reduced in a different experimental clinical context. Nevertheless, we prefer to attach greater importance to the sensitivity of the automated detection because of the serious, even fatal, consequences of dysphagia in the elderly.

We would tend to think that measurement of airflow could provide a valid method of detecting dysphagia. We suspect that when aspiration occurs, the recorded airflow will differ from that during a normal respiratory cycle, through being disrupted by the ingested material in the airway. Furthermore, we also suspect that the post-aspiration airflow will differ in a characteristic way (for example, post swallowing coughing) and that it will be possible, thanks to an automated signal analysis by the computer, to detect this difference among other physiological respiratory cycles.

However, as swallowing is only inferred from the respiratory recordings and not directly observed, it is essential for any detected dysphagia to be confirmed by means of a gold standard such as videofluorography.

We also intend to establish one-to-one relationships between the clinical events and the patterns of these events depicted on the AS. This opens up the possibility of monitoring swallowing by recording the airflow with the RIP and, using the recordings, to reveal certain swallowing disorders, as, for example, by identifying coughing during a meal. Such a tool would be very useful in enabling medical supervision [11] of swallowing to be put in place for acutely affected patients (e.g. recent cerebral stroke patients) or those with chronic diseases (e.g. Parkinson's disease) and also for monitoring the effectiveness of swallowing disorders therapy.

5. Conclusion

This study shows that the combined system developed enables swallowing to be detected in a non-invasive, convenient, bedside, automatic and objective way with high accuracy. To our knowledge, no other protocol exists offering such an approach to the detection. According to these results, this combined system will enable to study and monitor swallowing in order to detect certain swallowing disorders and so to prevent the frail elderly from their deleterious effects.

6. References

[1]   Domenech E, Kelly J. Swallowing Disorders. *Medical Clinics of North America* 1999;83(1):97-113

[2]   Feinberg MJ, Knebl J, Tully J. Prandial aspiration and pneumonia in an elderly population followed over 3 years. *Dysphagia* 1996;11:104-109

[3]   Siebens H, Trupe H, Siebens A, Cook F, Anshen S, Hanauer R, Oster G. Correlates and consequences of eating dependency in institutionalized elderly. *J Am Geriatr Soc* 1986;34:192-198

[4]   Mathers-Schmidt BA, Kurlinski M. Dysphagia Evaluation Practices: Inconsistencies in Clinical Assessment and Instrumental Examination Decision-Making. *Dysphagia* 2003:18;114-125

[5]   Tohara H, Saitoh E, Mays KA, Kuhlemeier K, Palmer JB. Three tests for Predicting Aspiration without Videofluorography. *Dysphagia* 2003;18:126-134

[6]   Smith J, Wolkove N, Colacone A, Kreisman H. Coordination of eating, drinking, and breathing in adults. *Chest* 1989;96:578-582

[7]   Eberhard A, Calabrese P, Baconnier P, Benchetrit G. Comparison between the respiratory inductance plethysmography signal derivative and the airflow signal. *Adv Exp Med Biol*. 2001;499:489-94.

[8]   Metz CE. Basic principles of ROC analysis. *Sem Nuc Med*. 1978;8:283-298

[9]   Nishino T, Yonezawa T, Honda Y. Effects of Swallowing on the Pattern of Continuous Respiration in Human Adults. *Am Rev Respir Dis* 1985 Dec;132(6):1219-1222.

[10] Selley WG, Flack FC, Ellis RE, Brooks WA. Respiratory patterns associated with swallowing : part 1. The normal adult pattern and changes with age. *Age Ageing 1989;* 18:168-172.

[11] Demongeot J, Virone G, Duchene F, Benchetrit G, Herve T, Noury N, Rialle V. Multi-sensors acquisition, data fusion, knowledge mining and alarm triggering in health smart homes for elderly people. *C R Biol*. 2002 Jun;325(6):673-82.

Address for correspondence

Alexandre Moreau-Gaudry, TIMC-IMAG-CNRS Laboratory, 38706 La Tronche, France.
Fax: +33 (0)4 56 52 00 55. Email: Alexandre.Moreau-Gaudry@imag.fr

Connecting Medical Informatics and Bio-Informatics
R. Engelbrecht et al. (Eds.)
IOS Press, 2005

Representing the Patient's Therapeutic History in Medical Records and in Guideline Recommendations for Chronic Diseases Using a Unique Model

Vahid Ebrahiminia[a], Catherine Duclos[a], Massoud E Toussi[a], Christine Riou[b], Regis Cohen[c], Alain Venot[a]

[a] *Laboratoire d'Informatique Médicale et Bioinformatique (LIM&BIO), UFR SMBH, University of Paris 13*
[b] *Laboratory of Medical Informatics, University of Rennes 1, France*
[c] *Department of Endocrinology, Avicenne Hospital, Bobigny, France*

Abstract

Computer-interpretable guidelines (CIGs) are more likely to affect the clinician's behavior when they deliver patient-specific and just-in-time clinical advice. CIGs must take into account the data stored in the patient's electronic medical records (EMR). For chronic diseases, the outcome of past and ongoing treatments (therapeutic history) is used in the clinical guidelines. We propose a model for the conceptualization of therapeutic history, facilitating data sharing between EMRs and CIGs and the representation of therapeutic history and recommended treatments in clinical guidelines.

Based on medical literature review and an existing treatment model, a core structure is first defined taking into account drug and non-drug treatment components and treatment type (e.g. bitherapy). These elements together with additional concepts obtained by analyzing a sample guideline relating to diabetes, are then organized into an object-oriented model, using UML formalism.

We show how this model can be used to store the patient's therapeutic history in the EMR, together with other attributes such as treatment efficacy and tolerance. We also explain how this model can efficiently code guidelines therapeutic rules.

We evaluated this model, using additional guidelines for hypertension, hypercholesterolemia and asthma. We found it capable for representing guideline recommendations in several domains of chronic diseases.

Keywords:
Computerized Medical Records; Computer Interpretable Guidelines; Decision Support Systems; Treatments; Models; Chronic Diseases

1. Introduction

Evidence-based clinical guidelines are developed to improve the quality of medical care but their impact depends on their optimal implementation in real practice. Studies have shown that computer interpretable guidelines are most likely to affect the behavior of a clinician if they deliver patient-specific and just-in-time clinical advice [1, 2]. Efforts have therefore been made to develop methods linking computerized guidelines to data concerning the patient stored in electronic medical records (EMR) [3]. However, few published studies have dealt with the automation of EMR-integrated guidelines for the management of chronic diseases [4-6]

Treatment decisions for chronic diseases depend on previous decisions and actions and the outcome of those actions [7]. Thus, automatic systems must be able to use the EMR to reconstitute previous treatments and their outcome, to trigger the new strategy recommended by a guideline. Therapeutic recommendations in the guidelines can be considered as rules composed of *conditions* and *actions* [8]. For chronic diseases, *conditions* are usually expressed as combinations of *clinical* and *therapeutic criteria* [9]. Two major aspects of patient's past or ongoing treatments (referred to hereafter as therapeutic history) are considered in *therapeutic criteria*: what has already been prescribed and the outcome of this treatment in terms of efficacy and tolerance. *Actions* in this context are sets of therapeutic options, generally expressed in terms of therapeutic classes, but sometimes expressed in other ways, as a particular type or group of therapeutic agents, for instance. An example of a therapeutic rule for type 2 diabetes management is, *"If oral monotherapy with maximal doses of sulfamide or metformin associated with lifestyle changes is not effective, then the monotherapy should be replaced by oral bitherapy."*

The automatic use of these kinds of rules in guideline-based reminders requires the correct and structured storage of outcome of the patient's treatments in the EMR. Drug prescriptions are often stored in the EMR as independent prescription lines without structured information concerning efficacy and tolerance. They do not help distinguish different treatments in a prescription (e.g. biotherapy for hypertension). Moreover, as seen in the example, specifying information concerning treatments in both *condition* and *action* parts of the guideline rules requires the use of terms or concepts in various levels of abstraction. The main challenge for reminder systems is therefore the integration, at the appropriate level of abstraction, of data from past prescriptions into the decision flow. If these systems are to produce reminders with the minimum human interaction, they should also compare, at an appropriate level of abstraction, the recommended action to the physician's prescription.

Several models and methods [8, 10] have been developed for the representation of medical knowledge, but they do not provide specific structures for representing and sharing treatment details in ways convenient for both EMRs and therapeutic rules.

During the two first phases of the ASTI project [11] , dealing with the implementation of guidelines for hypertension and diabetes, we looked for a generic representation of therapeutic history applicable to various therapeutic domains. We present here the main results of this research, in terms of the building and evaluation of an object-oriented model.

2. Materials and Methods

Building the conceptual model

Based on a preliminary review of several clinical guidelines [12] and using some concepts of the prescription model of Sene et al. [13] , we first defined the essential components of treatments and the major concepts required to describe information about those components. We then analyzed the recommendations of a sample guideline [14] and turned them into rules comprising *conditions* and *actions*. We identified the words or expressions describing therapeutic criteria as the rule *conditions* or proposing treatment in the *actions*. Based on methods used for the modeling of pharmacokinetics concepts [15], we grouped the terms on the basis of semantic similarity and linked them to general concepts. We then added labels characterizing their semantic content. This resulted in the formation of additional required concepts, elements or attributes, which were then reviewed and arranged into classes and objects. Relationships between the concepts and possible values of elements or attributes were then determined.

The obtained concepts and elements were finally organized according to classes, attributes, generalization, composition or association relationship, into an object-oriented model representation based on Unified Modeling Language (UML) formalism.

Preliminary evaluation of the model

We selected three guidelines covering various aspects of chronic diseases (hypertension, hypercholesterolemia and asthma) [16-18]. All guideline rules including conditions related to data about treatments or proposing therapeutic actions were extracted. The words or expressions delineating therapeutic criteria or treatment strategies were identified. Two physicians were then asked to determine whether they could be represented using the model.

We checked that all concepts from the guidelines could be structured into the model, ensuring that no concept was missed. The proportion of concepts included provided an assessment of the completeness of the model for representing guideline knowledge about treatments.

We then assessed the model comprehensibility by checking that all users converted the text into the model in the same way. We then calculated the ratio of the number of concepts identically modeled to the total number of concepts.

3. Results

We will first describe the core of the model representing information about treatment and will then show how the model can be used to store treatments and their outcomes in the EMRs or be used to represent guideline therapeutic recommendations.

The core of the model

As the model applies to management of chronic diseases, in which non-drug treatments such as diet and physical exercise are important therapeutic components, the treatment model must represent information relating to not only drugs, but also non-drug components (Figure 1).

The overall combination of drug and non-drug elements results in a treatment with a particular attribute *Treatment Type*, e.g bitherapy. Most guidelines predefine treatments in terms of several treatment types. Recommendations such as "prescribe bitherapy" can therefore be represented in the model, using this *Treatment Type* attribute. However, recommended treatments are sometimes addressed indirectly by specifying a strategy such as "replace monotherapy". We therefore introduced the attribute *Intended Strategy* into the treatment, enabling the direct transfer of the concept to the end user or to a calculating algorithm.

We also introduced, as *Treatment Objective*, attributes representing the *Reason* for treatment (e.g. hypertension), the goal to achieve (e.g. blood pressure under 14/9) and the estimated time to achieve the goal (e.g. 3 months).

The drug components of the treatment can be specified based on pharmacological group, therapeutic class, non-proprietary name or trade name. Dosage may be represented quantitatively (e.g. 1 g per day) or qualitatively (low, intermediate or high dose). The non-drug component, including any therapeutic lifestyle change that the patient is advised to make in addition to taking the prescribed drugs, has a denomination and an intensity (e.g. for representing moderate or intense physical exercise).

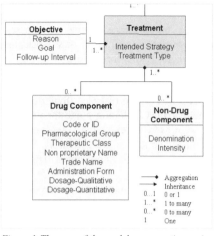

Figure 1-The core of the model, representing major concepts concerning a treatment

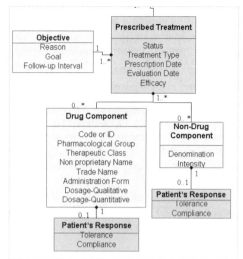

Figure 2 Model for storing prescribed treatments and their outcome in EMR

Using the model in EMRs

This core structure of the model can be used to store the therapeutic history of the patient in EMR (Figure 2). The distinction of treatments in a prescription according to therapeutic indication of each prescription line, makes it possible to attribute the outcome of the evaluation to the appropriate elements at every visit. As seen in figure 2, it is to the *Treatment* (i.e. the combination of related components) that *Efficacy* is attributed while *Tolerance* and *Compliance* are associated to each separate component.

We also added an attribute *Status*, with two values "past" and "ongoing" to make it possible to distinguish representations of treatments currently in use from those previously used.

Using the model to represent guideline recommendations

We can also use the same model to represent condition and action parts of guideline rules (figure 3). Based on the data from *Efficacy* and *Tolerance* of the ongoing treatment, characterized by *Therapeutic Criteria* in the condition part, new treatments are proposed in the action part. Treatment is usually specified in terms of the *Therapeutic Class* and/or international non-proprietary name (*INN*) of each component, but may also be expressed using high-level concepts such as *Treatment Type,* or *Intended Strategy.*

The action part of a recommendation may be the prescription or prohibition of a treatment. We therefore added the attribute *Proposition Type*, which may take the values "Prescribe" or "Do not prescribe".

Evaluation of the model for representing guideline rules

The model was found to represent therapeutic recommendations accurately in 99% of cases. For the very few terms that could not be entered directly into the model, a simple interpretation of the rule made representation entirely possible.

The ratio used to evaluate concordance between modeling results was found to have a value of 90 %. The main difficulty encountered was ambiguity in the text of the guidelines.

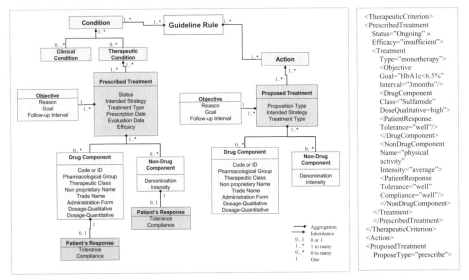

Figure 3 : Representing therapeutic history and proposed treatments in guideline rules
accompanied by an implementation example in XML

4. Discussions and Conclusion

We used an approach based on medical literature review and analysis of a guideline for diabetes, in which we thought that therapeutic history was likely to be extensively used and a variety of modifications were seen on the type, group, class or dose of the drugs as new treatment propositions. The demonstrated applicability of this model to other domains shows that this model has the potential to represent treatment concepts in medical knowledge in a generic manner.

Some of the concepts used in our model may already have been included in existing guideline models, but this model seems to facilitate the sharing and representation of data concerning treatment outcome and other details. It also facilitates switching between abstraction levels, making it possible to compare data at the appropriate level in automatic systems.

This model is based on the usual working practices of physicians, who tend to combine drug and non-drug components to obtain an efficient treatment. The physician then assesses at the next visit, the overall efficacy and evaluates the tolerance to each independent component of treatment. This representation corresponds to the most frequent cases, but it should be possible to find specific cases in which each drug component of a treatment is well tolerated by the patient when taken alone, but the combination of drug components is poorly tolerated. However, such situations do not appear to be frequent.

Dose description has been simplified by using qualitative rather than quantitative dose information, as they are generally specified in guidelines. This matter is also reported in other models [13].

A first-step translation of narrative guidelines by the model generates information in a format that can be processed by the computer. However, it can do little to resolve the ambiguity of paper-based guidelines, for which the resolution is left to the user.

Further evaluation of this model is required to confirm its generic nature. Chronic disease or other domains in which there are many different modes of treatment could be used for these subsequent evaluations.

5. Acknowledgements

ASTI project is partly supported by a grant from national fund of health assurance, the scientific council, in France, (CNAMTS, Conseil scientifique).

6. References

[1]   Shiffman RN, Liaw Y, Brandt CA, and Corb GJ. Computer-based guideline implementation systems: a systematic review of functionality and effectiveness. J Am Med Inform Assoc 1999; 6(2): 104-14.

[2]   Grimshaw JM, and Russell IT. Effect of clinical guidelines on medical practice: a systematic review of rigorous evaluations. Lancet 1993; 342: 1317-22.

[3]   Elkin PL, Peleg M, Lacson R, Bernstam E, Tu S, Boxwala A, Greenes R, and Shortliffe EH. Toward Standardization of Electronic Guideline Representation. MD Computing 2000; 17(6): 39-44.

[4]   Maviglia SM, Zielstorff RD, Paterno M, Teich JM, Bates DW, and Kuperman GJ. Automating Complex Guidelines for Chronic Disease: Lessons Learned. J Am Med Inform Assoc 2003; 10(2): 154–165.

[5]   Persson M, Bohlin J, and Eklund P. Development and maintenance of guideline-based decision support for pharmacological treatment of hypertension. Comput Methods Programs Biomed 2000; 61: 209-219.

[6]   Goldstein MK, Hoffman BB, Coleman RW, Musen MA, Tu SW, Advani A, Shankar R, and O'Connor M. Implementing clinical practice guidelines while taking account of changing evidence: ATHENA DSS, an easily modifiable decision-support system for managing hypertension in primary care. Proc AMIA Symp 2000: 300-4.

[7]   Johnson PD, Tu S, Booth N, Sugden B, and Purves IN. Using scenarios in chronic disease management guidelines for primary care. Proc AMIA Symp 2000: 389-93.

[8]   Peleg M, Tu S, Bury J, Ciccarese P, Fox J, Greenes RA, Hall R, Johnson PD, Jones N, Kumar A, Miksch S, Quaglini S, Seyfang A, Shortliffe EH, and Stefanelli M. Comparing computer-interpretable guideline models: a case-study approach. J Am Med Inform Assoc 2003; 10(1): 52-68.

[9]   Seroussi B, Bouaud J, Chatellier G, and Venot A. Development of computerized guidelines for management of chronic diseases allowing to position any patient within recommended therapeutic strategies. Medinfo 2004: 154-8.

[10] Shiffman RN, Karras B, Agrawal A, Chen R, Marenco L, and Nath S. GEM: a proposal for a more comprehensive guideline document model using XML. J Am Med Inform Assoc 2000; 7(5): 488-98.

[11] Seroussi B, Bouaud J, Dreau H, Falcoff H, Riou C, Joubert M, Simon C, Simon G, and Venot A. ASTI, a guideline-based drug-ordering system for primary care. In: Patel VL, Rogers R, Haux R, eds, Medinfo 2001: 528-32.

[12] Riou C, Dreau H, Seroussi B, Bouaud J, and Venot A. Recommandations de rédaction des guides de bonnes pratiques en vue de leur implémentation dans un système d'aide à la décision. In: Harmel A, Hajromdhane R, Fieschi M, eds. Informatique et Santé . Vol 16 France: Springer - Verlag 2004 .

[13] Sene B, Venot A, de Zegher I, Milstein C, Errore S, de Rosis F, and Strauch G. A general model of drug prescription. Methods Inf Med 1995; 34(4): 310-7.

[14] Stratégie de prise en charge du patient diabétique de type 2 à l'exclusion de la prise en charge des complications. ANAES, Mars 2000, available at: http://www.anaes.fr (Accessed Nov 2004)

[15] Duclos-Cartolano C, and Venot A. Building and evaluation of a structured representation of pharmacokinetics information presented in SPCs: from existing conceptual views of pharmacokinetics associated with natural language processing to object-oriented design. J Am Med Inform Assoc 2003; 10(3): 271-80.

[16] The Seventh Report of the Joint National Committee on prevention, detection, evaluation and treatment of high blood pressure (JNC 7). NHLBI, 2004., http://www.nhlbi.nih.gov/guidelines/hypertension (Accessed Nov 2004)

[17] Detection, evaluation and treatment of high blood cholesterol in adults. NHLBI, May 2001. available at: http://www.nhlbi.nih.gov/guidelines/cholesterol/atp3_rpt.htm (Accessed Nov 2004)

[18] Medical follow-up of patients with asthma - adults and adolescents. ANAES, Sept 2004. available at: http://www.anaes.fr (Accessed Nov 2004).

Address for correspondence

Vahid Ebrahiminia MD, Laboratoire d'Informatique Médicale et de Bioinformatique (LIM&BIO), UFR Santé, Médecine, Biologie Humaine, Léonard de Vinci, 74 rue Marcel Cachin 93017 Bobigny cedex, France. Email: vahid.nia@avc.ap-hop-paris.fr

Connecting Medical Informatics and Bio-Informatics
R. Engelbrecht et al. (Eds.)
IOS Press, 2005

mGen - An Open Source Framework for Generating Clinical Documents

Fredrik Lindahl, Olof Torgersson

Department of Computer Science and Engineering, Chalmers University of Technology, Sweden

Abstract

> As formalised electronic storage of medical data becomes more and more wide spread the possibility and need for creating human readable presentations for various purposes increases. This paper presents the mGen framework - a general framework for text generation, written in Java and in the process of being open-sourced, that has been developed within the MedView project[1]. The framework has been used for several years to generate literally thousands of clinical documents at an oral medicine clinic in Sweden.

Keywords
Computerized Medical Record Systems, Computerized Patient Records, Medical Records, Medical Informatics, Medical Informatics Computing, Natural Language Generation, Natural Language Processing, Clinical Documents, Dental Informatics, Dental Records, Oral Medicine

1. Introduction

As formalised electronic storage of medical data becomes more and more wide spread the possibility and need for creating human readable presentations for various purposes will increase as well [3]. In the medical field textual presentations, i.e., records, referral letters and patient information are ubiquitous. Thus, enabling simple and useful ways of generating text from medical data becomes very important.

Natural Language Generation (NLG) is the activity of generating text from some kind of sources. NLG has been applied within several projects in the medical domain. Overviews of results and problems can be found in [1][4].

Within the MedView project [5] text generation has been used for a number of years to generate literally thousands of medical documents, mostly patient records and referral letters, but also documents aimed at patient information and education [2]. Although rather simple from an NLG perspective, the generation system has been proved to be useful and stable enough for real-world everyday use.

Recently, Open Source software has started to attract the Medical Informatics community [6]. In the Open Source software distribution model users are typically allowed to use applications and libraries for free, without paying any license fee. Furthermore, they are given access to the source code and accordingly have the opportunity to examine, modify and incorporate it into their own system. Following these principles we have decided to make the document generation part of the MedView system, called *mGen*, available as an Open Source

---

[1] The work presented in this paper was supported by the Swedish Agency for Innovation Systems (VINNOVA)

project. Our motivation for this is 1) to provide others with a ready-to-use system for generating clinical documents, and 2) to attract interest for further development.

The aim of the present paper is to introduce the mGen framework and show how it can be used. For information on where and how to obtain the framework source code, please see our project webpage *www.cs.chalmers.se/proj/medview/website/medview/*.

2. The mGen Framework

The mGen framework, written in Java, provides developers with a complete ready-to-use system for text generation. In order to describe how the system can be used, we will present how it is used to generate a clinical document summarizing a small part of a fictive medical examination.

2.1 Case Study – The Examination Data

When a patient is examined at the clinic, various data describing the examination are gathered. Our framework works with *value-containers*, containing assignment of *values* to various medical concepts (which we call *terms*). An examination is thus represented by a value-container, containing the examination data in a concise and formal form. The framework does not provide any components for entry of examination data.

```
Patient_Identifier = FXX0006039771
Examination_Date = 2004-11-21
Patient_First_Name = Fredrik
Patient_Last_Name = Lindahl
Reason_Referral = pain in tooth
Care_Provider = Mats Jontell
Diagnosis = infection
Treatment_Action = extraction
Treatment_Date = 2005-01-12
```

Figure 1 – The examination value-container used in the case study

We now want to transform the concise, formal description of the data in the value-container to an informal one using our text generation system. First, we need a *template model*.

2.2 Case Study – The Template Model

A template model is comprised of *section models*, where each section model contains *term models*. Figure 2 shows this general hierarchical structure.

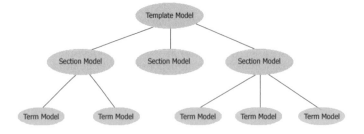

Figure 2 – Template model structure

The template model contains a document containing styled text. The section models and the term models are simply pointers to sections of this text, superimposing a logical structure upon the template text. Term models correspond to 'slots' in the template text where the values from a value container (after certain processing – see below) are inserted at generation time. The template model used in the case study is rather simple, an actual template model typically consists of several section models containing hundreds of term models. At generation time, you can choose which sections to include.

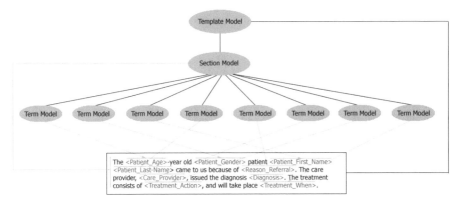

Figure 3 – An example of a template model structure along with text

An editor component used for working with template models is provided by the framework, providing the user with graphical highlighting of the concepts mentioned above. The editor stores and retrieves template models in XML. Figure 4 shows the component in use when editing the small template used in our example:

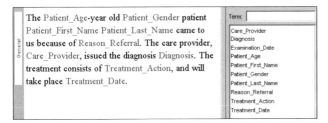

Figure 4 –Template editor component editing the template used in the case study

Now that we have the template model and the value-container containing the examination data, we need only one more component before the system is ready to convert the mappings to natural text. The last component is the translator model, responsible for translating the examination values to values fitting the template context.

2.3 Case Study – The Translator Model

As with the template model, an editor component is provided for creating and editing translator models. Just as the template model editor component, the translator editor component supports storage and retrieval of translator models in XML. A translator model contains translations for each value a term can obtain.

Diagnosis
Infection = infection of the oral mucosa
Plauque = $?$
Lichen planus = $?$
Nothing wrong = $NOLINE$
Patient_Gender
Male = $?$
Female = $?$
Reason_Referral
Pain in tooth = sensation of pain in a tooth
Sore tongue = a sore tongue
Pain in mouth = $?$
Treatment_Action
Extraction = extraction of tooth

Figure 5 – The translator model used in the case study

As can be seen in the figure, translations can consist of plain text or macros. The default macros provided by the framework are the $?$ and $NOLINE$ macros, where the $?$ macro is a placeholder for the actual value and the $NOLINE$ macro indicates that the line containing the slot with this value should be removed.

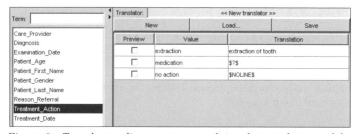

Figure 6 – Translator editor component editing the translator model used in our case study

Some terms found in the template are not included in the translator, these are terms that for some reason need not be translated. Also included in the framework is support for *derived* terms, i.e. terms whose values depend on the value of another term. In our example, the Patient_Age term is a derived term, whose value depends on the value of the Patient_Identifier term. For a Patient_Identifier value of FXX0006039771, it can be deduced (due to the format of the identifier – UUUNNNNNNNCYYG where G is gender (0 – female, 1 – male), YY is year of birth, and C is century of birth (9 – 1900, 0 – 2000)) that the age of the patient is 27 years and the gender is male. Additional derived terms and their handling can be added by extending appropriate handlers in the framework.

2.4 Case Study – The Result

Now that we have all components necessary for generation, we pass them to the *generator engine*. A default implementation of a generator engine is provided in the framework, and using it together with our components generates the text shown in Figure 7.

The 29-year old male patient Fredrik Lindahl came to us because of sensation of pain in a tooth. The care provider, Mats Jontell, issued the diagnosis 'infection of the oral mucosa'. The treatment consists of extraction of tooth, and will take place 2005-01-12.

Figure 7 – The resulting generated text

To summarize, a generator engine takes as input a template model, a translator model, and a value-container. As output, it generates a javax.swing.text.StyledDocument - Java's standard model for representing a styled text document which can be visualised using standard Java GUI components. The framework contains all necessary model components, a default generator engine implementation, and GUI components for creating / editing the models.

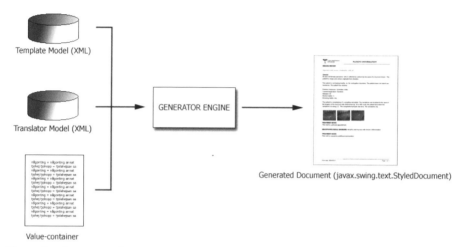

Figure 8 – Overview of generation process

3. Results

The text generation system, as described, has been in daily use at the clinic for several years now, and has been used to generate thousands of clinical documents. The generated documents are printed and primarily used as patient medical journals. The quality of the generated text is deemed sufficient and is, as previously stated, in actual use for the daily work at the clinic. This said, there have been occasions where clinicians have wished for higher quality of the generated text. Thus, even though we provide a fully functional generation system as-is, it is built as a general, extensible, framework, thus allowing for more refined text generation solutions to replace / extend the system.

4. Discussion

In the context of NLG systems, the text generation system can be described as a combination of of the SDE (structured data entry), canned text, and slot-and-filler approaches [2]. The translated values can be seen as canned text segments, though they are not intended to be self-contained, i.e. they are intended to be placed in the context of a template. The system decouples user-entered instance data (creation of value-containers) from output (the generated text), and provides clinicians with the ability to create their own templates and translators, and thus to have full control over the appearance of the generated document.

Lack of support for certain linguistic phenomena such as aggregation, anaphora, rhetorical relations and referential expressions, along with a very basic implementation of ellipsis and enumerative phrases, leaves some to be desired in the quality and fluency of the generated text. The open-sourcing of the text generation framework provides interested NLG researchers with the opportunity to study and improve on text generation in a framework which has been in practical use for several years.

5. Conclusion

The text generation system described here is deemed sufficient for daily use, though there is ample room for improvement in the quality of the generated text. It is our hope that the open-source initiative will attract researchers and projects within the NLG domain, and that our system provides an interesting platform on which to build more advanced text generation solutions.

6. References

[1]   D. Kraus. Text generation in clinical medicine - a review. Methods Inf. Med. 2003;42.

[2]   O. Torgersson and G. Falkman. Using text generation to access clinical data in a variety of contexts. Surjan, G., Engelbrecht, R. & McNair, P. (eds.): Health Data in the Information Society, vol 90 of Studies in Health Technology and Informatics, IOS Press, pages 460-465, 2002.

[3]   A. Belz, R. Evans and P. Piwek . INLG04 Posters: Extended abstracts of posters presented at the Third International Conference on Natural Language Generation, pp 22-27, 2004.

[4]   A. Cawsey. B. Webber and R. Jones. Natural Language Generation in Health Care, *Journal of the Medical Informatics Society*, 4, 1997.

[5]   Jontell M, Mattsson U, and Torgersson O. MedView: An instrument for clinical research and education in oral medicine. *Oral Surg. Oral Med. Oral Pathol. Oral Radiol. Endod.* 2005: 99, 55–63.

[6]   C J. McDonald, Gunther Schadow, Michael Barnes, Paul Dexter, J. Marc Overhage, Burke Mamlin and J. Michael McCoy, Open Source software in medical informatics--why, how and what, International Journal of Medical Informatics, Volume 69, Issues 2-3, March 2003, Pages 175-184.

7 Address for correspondence

Fredrik Lindahl, Computing Science, Chalmers University of Technology
SE – 412 96, Gothenburg, Sweden. Email: lindahlf@cs.chalmers.se

Connecting Medical Informatics and Bio-Informatics
R. Engelbrecht et al. (Eds.)
IOS Press, 2005

Comparing Different Approaches to Two-Level Modelling of Electronic Health Records

Line Michelsen, Signe S. Pedersen, Helene B. Tilma, Stig K. Andersen

Department of Health Science and Technology
Aalborg University, Denmark

Abstract

Electronic Health Record (EHR) systems are being developed to improve the communication of patient data. The health care domain includes many different types of data and concepts, of which some are constantly changing, and some are more lasting. This makes the development of an EHR a complex task. In order to improve the handling of this complexity, a new two-level modelling approach in EHR system development has emerged, using a concept of archetypes as the pivot in the representation of the health care knowledge. The key issue in this approach involves dividing the problem field into two separate models: A generic information model and a domain knowledge model. By analysis of how this layering has been carried out in two different two-level EHR systems – the OpenEHR (formerly the Australian GEHR, Good Electronic Health Record) and the EHR project of Aarhus County, Denmark. We have identified critical meta model parameters influencing the ability of the modelling paradigm to meet the expectation for easy handling of the development process (flexibility) and the capability to manage changing models (dynamics). The OpenEHR has defined the division line in such a way that it makes the generic model small and the domain model large. The opposite is the case of the Aarhus EHR system, where the information model is large, and the knowledge model is small. A small information model and a large knowledge model make more of the system changeable, but it also makes it less flexible to develop. The opposite is the case for a large information model and a small knowledge model.

Keywords:
Electronic Health Record (EHR); Two-Level Modelling; Archetype; EDD (Event Description Definition); Information Model; Domain Model; Generic Model, Meta Model

1. Introduction

An essential motive for implementing Electronic Health Records (EHR) is the desire to utilize the opportunities of information technology to support the work and development taking place within the health care sector. The fundamental reason for implementing an EHR is to improve the possibilities of providing better, coordinated care, and to create better documentation of the events as well as the composition and the quality of health care contributions.

There are many things to be considered when developing an EHR system. First of all, the EHR system must be designed for several types of users and hospital departments. The EHR system must therefore be flexible to fulfil the demands of the different users and departments and to cover a wide range of clinical domains. Secondly, the clinical domain is constantly encompassing new knowledge and improved technology. The process of modifying an EHR system should be flexible and dynamic.

The classical single-level model approach to develop an information system is to model domain concepts directly in software and database models. It is difficult to fulfil the demands of a flexible and dynamic EHR system with this single-level approach, as it uses one comprehensive information model. The single-level approach system can be seen as a snapshot of knowledge existing at the time the EHR system was developed. [1, 2]

A new approach has emerged in EHR development where the idea is to divide the problem field into two separate models: An information model and a knowledge model [2]. This approach is often called two-level modelling. The information model depicts stabile and generic concepts, whereas the knowledge model expresses the variability and dynamics of the problem field.

Terms like archetypes [2], event description definitions (EDD) [3], clinical templates [4], and clinical document architectures (CDA) [5] are used to describe concepts representing self-contained parts of domain knowledge, acting as building blocks in the knowledge model.

The purpose of the two-level model approach is to make it possible to change or extend the knowledge model without changing the basic functions of the system, as they are to remain static within the information model. The generic information concepts are steady in time, while the domain knowledge specific concepts express variability [1, 2]. The implementation of the dynamic aspect of the modelling process has to be sufficiently flexible to make it attractive in practice.

In this paper we have chosen to analyze how the division between the model layers has been carried out, and what the consequences are in two different EHR systems using the two-level approach: the OpenEHR [2] and the EHR project in Aarhus County, Denmark [3]. In these two examples we have identified critical meta model parameters which affect the ability of the modelling paradigm to meet the expectations for (1) easy handling of the development process (flexibility) and (2) the capability to manage changing models (dynamics).

2. Methods

Information about theories and principles of two-level modelling and the two EHR approaches is obtained from literature and websites of OpenEHR and Aarhus County, Denmark, and through semi-structured qualitative interviews and questionnaires. The analysis is a comparative study of the two EHR approaches, concentrating on their ontology structure and the division between the model layers. Moreover focus is chosen to be on three specific aspects: Version control, legislative requirements, and domain knowledge acquisition. Other aspects as economic circumstances, data security, structured querying, patient interaction, and use of terminologies are not treated in this analysis.

3. Two-Level Modelling and Archetypes

In the OpenEHR approach the term archetype is used, while the corresponding concept in the Aarhus EHR approach uses the term EDD. In the following description of two-level modelling and archetypes, the term archetype is used as a general concept covering both the term archetype used in the OpenEHR approach and the term EDD used in the Aarhus EHR approach. The essential concept in two-level modelling encompasses the separation of information and knowledge, where all clinical information is created in the image of appropriate knowledge structures [6].

The information model includes software object models and database schemas, while the knowledge model contains the domain specific concepts, consisting of terminologies and ontologies. Archetypes are used to express self-contained domain knowledge chunks, which are expressed by the terms of a constrained information model. The advantage of separating knowledge from information is the possibility to make domain experts model the knowledge model using archetypes and make technical developers model the information model.

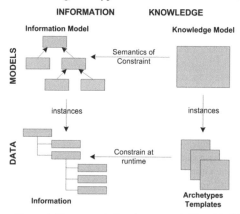

Figure 1-The concept of archetype modelling. Modified from [8, 9].

An archetype is a constraint model that defines interpretation restrictions for EHR information, for instance information about the composition of blood pressure measurement expressed in information model terms. The purpose of archetypes is to ensure that only data with a certain structure can be added to the EHR. As the archetype is developed from the underlying information model, the ability to add new archetypes over time is present without having to remodel the whole information model [7].

Archetypes are used to drive the runtime features of software in the information model, entailing that the data shown to the user is a combination of the data in the information model and the restrictions prescribed by the archetypes. This principle is illustrated in Figure 1. On the knowledge side to the right, the knowledge model is illustrated. This knowledge model constrains its underlying information model. Archetypes are instances of this model [8].

The actual information obtains its structure from the information model via the archetype. The knowledge model provides a sensible health domain information structure of the elements in the information model [2], shown on the left. The archetype assures that data acquisition is processed in accordance with the information model, so that data can be stored in databases.

4. Results

The OpenEHR and Aarhus EHR Approach

Ontology levels: In order to classify the clinical domain knowledge, the OpenEHR approach makes use of six different ontology levels to structure its information model. The ontology levels are used to find classes in the information model and to classify and compose archetypes. The six ontology levels are labelled: principles, descriptive, organizing, unit of work, historical, and communication [6]. Archetype is the crucial class in the information model from where the classes connected to the ontology levels inherit. This is illustrated in Figure 2.

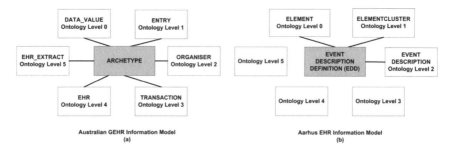

Figure 2 (a) The illustration shows the archetype class connected to all six ontology levels. (b) The illustration shows the EDD class connected to only three ontology levels.

To compare the two models we have arranged the model of the Aarhus EHR in accordance with the equivalent six ontology levels used in the OpenEHR. The result of the comparison is shown in Figure 2. The EDDs are not related to all six ontology levels, but only the first three levels of abstraction. In the Aarhus EHR information model, the fundamental class is the Event class [3] (not shown in Figure 2). Consequently, archetypes can represent a wider range of levels of abstractions than EDDs.

General structures: The OpenEHR approach is built completely as a two-level model, whereas the Aarhus EHR approach is built both as a two-level and a single-level model. The information model of the Aarhus EHR contains three main models: A process model, a logistic model, and a registration model [3]. The process model contains the classes shown in Figure 2 and is built according to the two-level modelling principles. The logistic and registration models are both single-level models. Figure 3 compares the general structure of the OpenEHR and the Aarhus EHR models.

Domain knowledge acquisition: In the Aarhus EHR and the OpenEHR, maintenance of the EHR systems is managed in different ways. The Aarhus EHR has a specific organization developing EDDs. This is a technical organization co-operating with the domain experts in creating the EDDs [10]. No EDD editor is available for the clinicians. In the OpenEHR an archetype editor is to be used by clinicians and developers [11]. The archetype editor is a modelling tool for creating and editing archetypes in accordance with the information model [12].

Legislative requirements: In the Aarhus EHR the development of EDDs is influenced by legislation about national reporting requirements and clinical databases. For this reason, to make the automatic reports, the structure of some EDDs must be stable and follow the requirements established by legislation [13].

The OpenEHR must follow the same legislation about national reports, but archetypes have not yet been modelled for report use. With regard to this, an advantage in the OpenEHR might be that archetypes can be made up of smaller archetypes and can be reused in one large archetype corresponding to a report [12].

Version control: The advantages of EDDs and archetypes are that they can be modified, which implies change management and version control. An EDD or an archetype may be changed due to omissions, legislation, technology, or traceability. The last point is due to the requirement that it must be possible to return to any previous version of the record [2, 6]. In the OpenEHR

each archetype has its own version with version control provided by the information model. In the Aarhus EHR the single EDD is not version controlled, but the whole collection of EDDs is version controlled. In both EHR projects there are more dimensions of version control than indicated above. The information models, the archetypes/EDDs, and the terminologies are all to be version controlled independently. What makes the task complex is that these three aspects depend on each other.

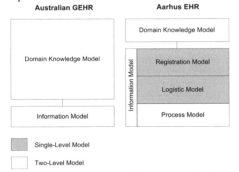

Figure 3-The OpenEHR model is built completely as a two-level model, while the Aarhus EHR model also contains single-level models.

5. Discussion and conclusion

The OpenEHR and the Aarhus EHR have defined the dividing line between the information model and the knowledge model differently. The dynamic part of the Aarhus EHR covers fewer modelling aspects than the OpenEHR approach, leaving fewer clinical concepts to be modifiable. Consequently the OpenEHR seems to be more future-proofed with regard to the amount of knowledge structure that can be changed, although it may be irrational to model persistent concepts such as professional groups, departments etc.

In the Aarhus EHR, EDDs are developed by one separate technical group in co-operation with clinicians. In the OpenEHR, the archetypes are to be developed by domain experts using an archetype editor. Archetypes may require a lot of insight into the information model in order to be able to model them. Modelling EDDs also requires domain knowledge and insight into the domain knowledge, and this might challenge the technical group of the Aarhus EHR.

Version control is performed on each archetype in the OpenEHR and on the complete knowledge model in the Aarhus EHR. It is therefore difficult to compare how archetypes and EDDs are version controlled. Version control is a non-trivial task in both cases. The essential problem in version control is granularity. Version control of archetypes might be more complex than version control of EDDs, due to the fact that archetypes have more structures. The Aarhus EHR is performing version control on the complete model. By using this solution the basic properties of the EDD, which are reducing redundancy, providing reusability, and being replaceable, are not obtained.

Due to external circumstances, the dynamics of the Aarhus EHR system is restricted. Conditions concerning legislation about national reporting mean that some EDDs have to be structured in a certain way to comply with the reporting rules. In the OpenEHR the same legislation exists, but there is no practical experience with archetypes and national reports.

Based on the analysis, our hypothesis is that the division between the model layers influences the flexibility and dynamics of the EHR systems. A small information model and a large knowledge model make more of the system changeable, but also make development less flexible. The opposite is the case for a large information model and a small knowledge model.

There are no fully implemented and evaluated EHR systems using the two-level approach. Therefore experiences regarding this hypothesis are sparse. The hypothesis can be utilized to analyze the flexibility and dynamics of other EHR projects using two-level modelling. HL7v3 and CEN ENV 13606 are both EHR projects using the two-level approach [4, 5]. In the CEN ENV 13606 pre-standard for EHR a generic model for the EHR architecture has been constructed, together with archetype-like templates. In HL7 a knowledge model has been developed with the purpose of representing semantics and relations between concepts for all data in a HL7-message.

6. Acknowledgements

We thank Mona Holm from the Virtual Hospital in Aarhus County, Trine Joergensen from Systematic Software Engineering A/S, and Inge Madsen from Skejby Hospital, Aarhus, for answering questions about the Aarhus EHR project. We also thank Thomas Beale and Sam Heard from Ocean Informatics for answering questions about the OpenEHR project.

7. References

[1]   Andersen SK, Nøhr C, Vingtoft S, Bernstein K, Bruun-Rasmussen M. *EPJ-Observatoriet : statusrapport 2002*. Aalborg Universitet; Center for Sundheds-telematik; MEDIQ. 2002.
[2]   Beale T. *Archetypes: Constraint-based Domain Models for Future-proof Information Systems*. Deep Thought Informatics. 2002. URL: www.deepthought.com.au/it/archetypes/archetypes_new.pdf, accessed December 2004.
[3]   The County of Aarhus. *Domaene Objektmodel*. 2000. URL: www.aaa.dk/aaa/dom_2.pdf, accessed December 2004.
[4]   *CEN/TC251 European Standardization of Health Informatics*. URL: www.centc251.org, accessed December 2004.
[5]   *Health Level Seven*. URL: www.hl7.org, accessed December 2004.
[6]   Beale T, Goodchild A, Heard S. *Design Principles for the EHR*. Rev. 2.4. The OpenEHR Foundation. 2004.
[7]   Bird L, Goodchild A, Tun Z. *Experiences with a Two-Level Modelling Approach to Electronic Health Records*. Journal of Research and Practice in Information Technology, 35(2), 121-138. 2003.
[8]   Beale T. *OpenEHR Modelling and Design Principles*. Rev. 0.3. The OpenEHR Foundation. 2003.
[9]   Beale T, Heard S. *Archetype definitions and principles*. Rev. 0.5. The OpenEHR Foundation. 2003.
[10]   Interview with M. Holm. September 2004.
[11]   DSTC Titanium. *Clinical Model Builder Software*. 2002. URL: titanium.dstc.edu.au/gehr/clinical-model-builder, accessed December 2004.
[12]   Mail Correspondence with T. Beale. December 2004.
[13]   Private Communication with T. Joergensen. November 2004.

Address for correspondence

Assoc. Prof. Stig Kjær Andersen, Ph.D., Virtuel Center for Health Informatics (V-CHI), Department for Health Science and Technology, Aalborg University, Fr Bajersvej 7 D, DK-9220 Aalborg, ska@hst.aau.dk

Connecting Medical Informatics and Bio-Informatics
R. Engelbrecht et al. (Eds.)
IOS Press, 2005

Introducing the Electronic Health Record in Austria

Wolfgang Dorda[a], Georg Duftschmid[a],
Lukas Gerhold[a], Walter Gall[a], Jürgen Gambal[b]

[a]*Core Unit for Medical Statistics and Informatics, Medical University of Vienna, Austria*

[b]*AustriaPro, The Austrian Federal Economic Chamber*

Abstract

The Austrian parliament has adopted legislation to introduce the electronic health record under the title ELGA. The present article first discusses several activities of other countries in this context. It then deals with the current situation of healthcare telematics in Austria and the next planned steps to introduce the life-long electronic health record.

Keywords:
Medical Records Systems, Computerized; Public Health Informatics; Computer Communication Networks; Standards

1. Introduction

Increasing specialization has given rise to substantial progress in modern medicine. At the same time, the requirements for multidisciplinary collaboration in patient care have become extensive. More and more data are collected for individual patients as novel measurement techniques are developed. These data have to be exchanged between the various physicians and facilities involved to allow efficient cooperation. Clinical information management has therefore become a key technology in modern healthcare.

The issue of consolidating all the information available on individual patients in a single electronic health record (EHR) has been extensively discussed within the medical informatics community over the past decade. Records of this type would enable physicians and nursing staff to access the complete medical history of a patient in a well-structured format. Introducing the EHR for all citizens of a country therefore has the potential of revolutionizing healthcare.

ELGA[1] is the name of an initiative that has recently been launched after legislation had been adopted by the Austrian parliament to reform the healthcare system in this country. The present article will first discuss several activities of other countries in the EHR domain. Subsequently it will outline the current situation of healthcare telematics in Austria and the next planned steps to introduce the EHR.

---

[1] German acronym meaning "life-long electronic health record"

2. National EHR initiatives

In 2004, the **European Commission** presented an *action plan for a European e-Health Area* [1]. It requires all member states to take measures to (a) support the interoperability of e-Health data records, e.g. by identifying an outlining EHR standards and through a common approach to patient identifiers until 2006; (b) offer EU citizens easier access to healthcare information and services, e.g. by supporting healthcare networks that provide services such as e-referral or e-prescription, or the use of electronic health insurance cards until 2008; (c) disseminate best practices, including the establishment of an e-Health monitoring institution that evaluates the progress made and develops recommendations for future e-Health measures until 2005.

In the **UK,** the NHS's *National Programme for IT* (NPfIT) [2] includes an initiative to implement the so-called *NHS Care Records Service* (NHS CRS), which shall provide a nation-wide EHR for all British citizens by 2010. A summary of each person's medical history, the *Spine*, will be held in a central database and build the basis of the EHR. The summary record will also contain links to more in-depth clinical information, which will be stored in local systems. EHR systems may only be acquired from a small number of selected providers, which have been particularly licensed for this purpose. Patients will have the possibility to access their own health records by means of a web-based service.

In **Denmark,** the *MedCom* initiative [3] was initiated in 1995 with the goal of setting up a message-based national healthcare data network. The implementation of MedCom is widely advanced today, which is underlined by the fact that, in April 2005 more than 60 % of healthcare communications in Denmark took place through the healthcare data network. A major issue addressed by MedCom since 2002 is the development of regional central EHR databases (the SUP project), which will be fed by standardized extracts from individual local EHR systems. The unified EHR extracts may then be accessed by means of a regular internet browser.

The **United States'** government has outlined a plan to provide most US citizens with EHRs until 2014 and created the *Office of the National Coordinator for Health Information Technology (ONCHIT)* [4] for this purpose. The ONCHIT has specified a "Strategic Framework", which describes a 12-step process for the implementation of this plan. Amongst others, it (a) demands certification of EHR systems' functionality; (b) plans to achieve nation-wide EHR interoperability by fostering "Regional Health Information Organizations" that enable local EHR data exchange and interconnecting them within a "National Health Information Network"; (c) plans to provide patients with access to their own EHRs. Approximately $4 billion will be spent for health information technology programs and initiatives in this context.

In **Canada,** an independent not-for-profit corporation was initiated (Canada Health Infoway Inc.) after the government had announced in September 2000 to accelerate the development and adoption of modern systems of information technology in healthcare. One of the immediate priorities of this corporation is to develop and implement effective interoperable EHR solutions [5]. It now has a total capital infusion of $1.2 billion (CDN) from the federal government. Infoway has embraced a seven-year plan to have interoperable EHRs in place across 50% of Canada's population by 2009.

In **Australia,** the government will provide $128 million over four years towards the implementation of the national health information network Health*Connect* [6]. The aim of this project is to collect, store and exchange EHRs via a secure network and within strict privacy safeguards. Currently, a trial is being conducted which seeks to evaluate whether the EHR architecture specified by the *open*EHR foundation [7] is suitable to meet the project's requirements.

3. Introducing the EHR in Austria (ELGA initiative)

3.1 Previous efforts related to healthcare telematics

In 1995, the Austrian Ministry of Health appointed the STRING[2] commission to advise the minister on all issues related to healthcare telematics.

The MAGDA-LENA framework: In 1998, the STRING commission developed MAGDA-LENA [8] as the governing framework for electronic exchange of patient-related data in Austria. MAGDA-LENA outlines the technical and organizational aspects governing the development of an Austrian healthcare information network that will allow EHR contents to be exchanged. A detailed description of MAGDA-LENA—including a comparison with the HIPAA regulations in the US [9]—was given in a previous communication [10].

A number of standardization projects have been conducted under the auspices of the STRING commission to facilitate implementation of the MAGDA-LENA framework by collecting experience in real-life environments, including a project on e-referral [11].

The key recommendations of MAGDA-LENA, relevant for introducing the EHR, are

(a) to promote the use of standardized message formats for exchange of healthcare data. MAGDA-LENA aims to achieve a high level of compatibility between healthcare messages by specifying a common methodology for the development of new message standards;

(b) to enable unique identification of patients, communicating parties and transmitted data via registered directories;

(c) to implement specific privacy and security measures for the communicating parties both within their own working environment and in their electronic communications with others.

The MAGDA-LENA framework has recently been incorporated into an Austrian law on healthcare telematics (see section 3.2).

Electronic index of Austrian healthcare providers: In 2001, the Austrian Medical Chamber established an electronic index of Austrian healthcare providers. This index is currently used to promote electronic exchange of clinical information by providing the necessary identification data for both automatized and individual queries.

Social-security chip card: In 1999, the Central Association of Austrian Social Insurance Authorities was commissioned by parliament to develop a social-security card system. The system consists of chip cards providing a non-forgeable key for patient identification and card-reading devices connected to computers. In early 2002, parliament expanded the functionality of this chip card to facilitate its use as a *citizen card*, including the option to store digital signatures and medical data on a voluntary basis. In December 2004, the first chip cards were distributed in a comprehensive field trial. The process of issuing these cards nationwide is to be completed by November 2005. Eight million Austrians are then expected to have the card, and around 12 000 physicians working for the Austrian social insurance authorities will have card-reading devices in their offices.

3.2 The ELGA initiative and legislation to promote healthcare telematics

In 2003, the STRING commission recommended that concrete plans be undertaken to introduce the EHR in Austria. This initiative was entitled ELGA.

ELGA was embraced by the ministry of health and incorporated into the measures aimed at reforming the Austrian healthcare system. The 2005 Healthcare Reform Act [12], adopted

---

[2] German acronym meaning "standards and guidelines for the use of informatics in healthcare"

by parliament in December 2004, therefore includes a regulation on healthcare telematics.

This law on healthcare telematics defines minimum standards to safeguard the confidentiality, reproducibility and non-manipulation of communication activities. Its provisions also include measures for healthcare information management and the establishment of an e-Health index to facilitate access to healthcare providers.

Furthermore, the Austrian parliament has made arrangements to introduce the EHR (ELGA initiative), has adopted general provisions to optimize the use of information and communication technologies in healthcare telematics, and has prepared the ground for e-prescription and e-reimbursement.

Based on these resolutions of the Austrian parliament, the STRING commission has specified the next work items in the implementation of ELGA:

- Contents and structure (which data should be contained in ELGA, to what extent should the structure be standardized, ...)
- Organisational measures (which processes will be supported, concept of privileges, ...)
- Legal basis (storage / access of patient data on voluntary or mandatory basis, ...)
- Technical standardization (central or federated local databases, communication standards, ...)
- Social and ethical issues (sensitive health data, technological impact assessment, ...)
- Economic aspects (cost / benefit, installation and maintenance of infrastructure, ...)
- etc.

A strategic framework to solve these open points will be developed by a professional consulting firm. The implementation will be coordinated on national and regional levels by a political steering board. The ministry of health has further started an e-Health initiative with the goal of integrating the industry.

To summarize, a number of legislative measures aimed at promoting healthcare telematics have been taken in Austria over the past few months, which notably include the introduction of the EHR.

4. Discussion and recommendations

In the authors' view, two issues related to the EHR need to be addressed as a matter of priority in Austria. These concern (i) the standardization and (ii) the confidentiality of EHR contents. A brief discussion follows.

4.1 Standardization of EHR contents

The objectives of the ELGA initiative are now being defined in greater detail and have been categorized in order to permit more accurate cost-benefit analysis. At the time of writing this paper, a final decision on how to prioritize the various objectives of the ELGA initiative has not been reached, and the roadmap for implementation has not been finalized. Definitive schedules for rapid implementation have, however, been defined for some projects such as e-prescription.

The next step will be to derive the concrete communication processes and data contents from the various objectives and user requirements involved and to standardize them. To avoid an isolated EHR solution in Austria, it will be necessary to rely heavily on international standards. With this consideration in mind, all relevant international efforts at EHR standardization (CEN, HL7, *open*EHR [13, 14, 7]) are closely monitored at the Core Unit for Medical Statistics and Informatics of the Medical University of Vienna. It is recommended and planned to incorporate the results of these efforts into the ELGA initiative wherever possible.

4.2 Confidentiality of EHR contents

The legal implications of data protection were a key concern of the STRING commission from the very outset. Therefore, a task force to address these issues was established immediately when the recommendation to launch the ELGA initiative was published in 2003.

Meanwhile, this task force has thoroughly analyzed the legal requirements for introducing the EHR. Special emphasis has been placed on the differences between voluntary and mandatory participation.

It concluded that a mandatory life-long EHR for all Austrians presumes the demonstration of a public benefit and an accurate definition of the data protection requirements involved so that the constitutional right to data privacy would not be violated.

5. Summary

From the authors' perspective, the situation of healthcare telematics in Austria and current activities for the introduction of the EHR can be summarized as follows:

Beginning in the mid-1990s, substantial efforts have been made to coordinate healthcare telematics. One result of these efforts has been the MAGDA-LENA framework for electronic data exchange. Furthermore, a number of standardization projects have been implemented.

Important steps have been made to promote the use of healthcare telematics as part of the ongoing healthcare reform. For example, parliament has adopted legislation

- on healthcare telematics
- to introduce the EHR (ELGA initiative)

This legislation has prepared the ground for extensive planning, which is currently under way to implement the concept of a life-long electronic health record in Austria.

6. References

[1]   e-Health - making healthcare better for European citizens: An action plan for a European e-Health Area, COM(2004) 356 final, http://europa.eu.int/eur-lex/en/com/cnc/2004/com2004_0356en01.pdf. 30.4.2004

[2]   NHS's National Programme for IT (NPfIT): www.connectingforhealth.nhs.uk/programmes/nhscrs/

[3]   MedCom initiative: www.medcom.dk

[4]   Office of the National Coordinator for Health Information Technology (ONCHIT): www.hhs.gov/healthit

[5]   Canada Health Infoway Inc.: http://www.infoway-inforoute.ca/home.php?lang=en

[6]   HealthConnect: A health information network for all Australians, http://www.health.gov.au/healthconnect

[7]   The openEHR foundation. http://www.openehr.org/

[8]   Burggasser H, Dorda W, Gambal J, Gell G, Ingruber H, Kotschy W, et al. Rahmenbedingungen für ein logisches österreichisches Gesundheitsdatennetz (MAGDA-LENA V2.0); 2000. http://www.akh-wien.ac.at/STRING/.

[9]   Health Insurance Portability and Accountability Act (HIPAA); 2004. http://www.hhs.gov/ocr/hipaa/.

[10] Duftschmid G, Wrba T, Gall W, Dorda, W. The strategic approach of managing healthcare data exchange in Austria. Methods Inf Med 2004; 43(2):124-132.

[11] Austrian Standards Institute, ÖNORM K2202. 1999. Medical informatics - Patient referral. http://www.on-norm.at/index_e.html.

[12] Gesundheitsreformgesetz : http://www.parlament.gv.at/portal/page?_pageid=908,731734&_dad=portal&_schema=PORTAL

[13] CEN/TC 251. Health informatics - Electronic healthcare record communication. European Prestandard: European Committee For Standardization; 2000. Report No.: ENV 13606. http://www.centc251.org/FinWork/greensheetpwd.htm.

[14] Beeler GW. HL7 version 3--an object-oriented methodology for collaborative standards development. Int J Med Inf 1998;48(1-3):151-161.

Correspondence to:

Wolfgang Dorda
Core Unit for Medical Statistics and Informatics, Medical University of Vienna
Section of Medical Information and Retrieval Systems
Spitalgasse 23
1090 Vienna, Austria
Phone: +43 1 40400 6699 (Phone); Fax: +43 1 40400 6697
e-mail: wolfgang.dorda@meduniwien.ac.at

Connecting Medical Informatics and Bio-Informatics
R. Engelbrecht et al. (Eds.)
IOS Press, 2005

125

Medical Record Linkage of Anonymous Registries without Validated Sample Linkage of the Dutch Perinatal Registries

Miranda Tromp, Nora Méray, Anita C. J. Ravelli, Johannes B. Reitsma,
Gouke J. Bonsel

Academic Medical Center, University of Amsterdam, Department of Clinical Informatics

Abstract

This paper describes the linkage of data from three Dutch Perinatal Registries: the Dutch National Midwife Registry, the Dutch National Obstetrics Registry and the Dutch National Pediatrics Registry, for the year of 2001. All these registries are anonymous and lack a common identifier. We used probabilistic and deterministic record linkage techniques to combine data from the mother, delivery and child involving to the same pregnancy. Records of singleton and twin pregnancies were linked separately. We have developed a probabilistic close method based on maximum likelihood methods to estimate the weights of individual linking variables and the threshold value for the overall weight. Probabilistic linkage identified 80% more links than a full deterministic linkage approach. External validation revealed an error rate of less than 1%. Our method is a flexible and powerful method to link anonymous registries in the absence of a gold standard.

Keywords:
Medical Record Linkage; Probabilistic linkage; Medical registries; Perinatal care; Perinatal

1. Introduction

In the Netherlands four different caregivers: midwifes, general practitioners, obstetricians and pediatricians are involved in perinatal care. All these four caregivers have their own anonymous registry: the registry of midwifes ("MR"), of general practitioners ("GR") of obstetricians ("OR") and of pediatricians ("PR"); given the Dutch two-tier system. As in 2001 no information from the general practitioners was collected, only the MR, OR and PR registries were available for our study. About 30 to 40% of the pregnant women are treated by both midwifes and obstetricians. 2% of the newborn children are admitted to the pediatrician. This means that information about the same mother/pregnancy/child often can be found in different perinatal registries. For studies focusing on outcomes of pregnancies (perinatal mortality and morbidity, etc.), it is essential that all information about mother, pregnancy, childbirth and child is available in one dataset. Linkage of the Dutch perinatal registries is therefore essential. Because of privacy laws in the Netherlands, no unique personal identifier exists that would enable linkage of records of different medical files.

 Medical record linkage is the most commonly used technique to link records of the same individual in different files without a common identifier. In full *deterministic MRL* the value of each linkage variables has to be identical in both records that are compared to be accepted as 'link' [1]. Deterministic linkage has a very high specificity, but low sensitivity. A refinement of deterministic linkage is the 'n-1 deterministic linkage', where one of the linkage variables is allowed to differ.

In *probabilistic linkage* a linkage weight is assigned to all independent linkage variables depending on the variable's discriminating power and reliability [1-3]. This linkage weight is positive (reward) if the variable agrees in two compared records and has a negative value (penalty) in case of disagreement. The more discriminating power the variable has, the higher the linkage weight is in case of agreement. If a variable contains fewer errors, disagreement is less likely to occur among two related records, hence a higher negative weight (higher penalty) For every record pair the weight of the individual linkage variables is summarized in a total weight. This total weight represents the ratio of the probability of finding a particular pattern of agreements and disgreements among two records belonging to the same person to the same probability among two unrelated records. A "threshold value", a total weight above which all records are accepted as links (and bellow which all pairs are considered as non links) has to be determined as well. The range around the threshold value is called 'uncertain region'. Probabilistic compared to deteministic linkage trades a, hopefully small loss in with a higher gain in sensitivity.

This paper describes how probablistic Medical Record Linkage (MRL) was applied to link the Dutch perinatal anonymous registries for the year of 2001. In absence of a golden standard we used additional information from original health care records to validate our approach.

2. Materials and Methods

Preparations prior to linkage procedure

Prior to linkage, the timeframe of the data files had to be defined. We chose for a birthday-based timeframe: all MR, OR and PR records where the child was (assumingly) born in 2001 were taken into account. In a second step the registries were cleaned from double entries by deterministic linkage. Prior to subsequent linkage procedures, the records of singletons and twins were separated in all three registries. Twins have the same mother and the same pregnancy information, often they are born on the same day and have the same gender, therefore linking records of twin pregnancies is complex. As a last step prior to linkage procedures, we reduced the number of pairs to compare by blocking either on birthday of the mother or on birthday of the child. This means that only pairs in which the two records agree on the blocking variable were compared. All records that were not linked with the first blocking variable were linked again with blocking on ZIP code of the mother to reduce the number of false negative links due to missing values and typing errors in the blocking variable.

Variable weights and the threshold value

In this study we further refined probabilistic linkage by allowing close values as well. This method is called the *probabilistic close linkage*. Close is where two records disagree on a variable but the difference is small and might be related to a typing error or a to a different way of measuring the same variable. In case of close agreement the linkage weight has still a positive value, but it's always lower than in case of full agreement. The range of values for close agreement was defined based on the data. Likelihood methods were used to estimate the weights associated with agreement and disagreement for each variable, and to obtain an optimal value for the threshold value (more details in [8]). First, we estimated the so called

m_i- and u_i-values which are the probability of agreement among matches (m_i) and among non-matches (u_i) for each linkage variable had to be calculated:

u_i = Pr(variable agrees | non matches)

m_i = Pr(variable agrees | matches)

where i = 1,2,...,k; k being the number of variables.

An estimate of the u_i- value was obtained by calculating the chance of agreement for the ith variable among all record pairs based on the marginal distribution of its values in the two files; a valid approach as long as the number of true matches is very small compared to the total number of pairs. Estimation of the m_i values is more difficult as it requires the true state of (a large sample) pairs to be known. In the absence of a validated sample, we estimated the m_i values by analyzing the observed patterns of agreements and disagreements among all pairs. If the outcomes of the comparisons are independent between variables, the total log likelihood can be written as:

$$\sum_p n(\gamma^p)\left\{\log\left(\pi\prod_{i=1}^{k} mf_i^{\gamma_i^p} mc_i^{\gamma_i^p}\left(1-mf_i-mc_i\right)^{1-\gamma_i^p} + \left(1-\pi\right)\prod_{i=1}^{k} uf_i^{\gamma_i^p} uc_i^{\gamma_i^p}\left(1-uf_i-uc_i\right)^{1-\gamma_i^p}\right)\right\} \quad (1)$$

Where mf_i is the probability of full agreement of the ith variable among matches, mc_i is the probability of close agreement among matches, uf_i is the probability of full agreement among non-matches, uc_i is the probability of close agreement among non matches, π is the proportion of true matches among all possible record combinations, $n(\gamma^p)$ the number of record pairs with pattern γ, γ_i^p is the outcome of the comparison of variable i in the pattern p, for i = 1,...,k and p = 1,...,2^k.

Using the m_i- and u_i-values that were estimated in equation 1, the variable weight of the "full agreement", "close agreement" and "disagreement" can be calculated as:

full agreement weight of the ith variable = $\log_2 \dfrac{mf_i}{uf_i}$,

close agreement weight of the ith variable = $\log_2 \dfrac{mc_i}{uc_i}$,

disagreement weight of the ith variable = $\log_2 \dfrac{1-mf_i-mc_i}{1-uf_i-uc_i}$.

If a variable was missing in one or both of the records, the linkage weight for this variable was arbitrary set to 0 for this record pair.

The linkage procedure

The actual linkage procedure takes up to 13 different steps. Table 1 gives an overview of the linkage procedures. All steps of the record linkage were done with SAS software using standard procedures and self-written algorithms.

External validation of MRL

Two types of errors arise from MRL: false negative links where two records belonging to the same person are not linked; false positive links where two records not belonging to the same person are linked together [1]. Because no golden standard was available, we used an external validation procedure to determine the specificity and sensitivity of our linkage method. A stratified sample of the linked and non-linked pairs was chosen. We sought additional information from caregivers for each pair to determine the true status using information from medical records, discharge letter, personal communication, etc.

Table 1-13 independent linkage procedures were necessary to link the three registries of 2001

		Type of linkage procedure	Aim of linkage procedure
data cleani	1	MR with MR, deterministic linkage	Finding administrative double entries
	2	OR with OR, deterministic linkage	
	3	PR with PR, deterministic linkage	
MR^OR^PR linkage	4	PR singletons with PR singletons, probabilistic linkage	Linkage of different hospital entries of the same child
	5	PR twins with PR twins, probabilistic linkage	
	6	MR singletons with OR singletons, probabilistic linkage	Linkage of midwife and obstetric records
	7	MR twins with OR twins, probabilistic linkage	
	8	MR non-link singletons with OR non-link twins, prob. link.	
	9	MR non-link twins with OR non-link singletons, prob. link.	
	10	(MR^OR linked) singletons with PR singletons, prob. link.	Linkage of the linked midwife and obstetric records with the neonatal care records
	11	(MR^OR linked) twins with PR twins, probabilistic linkage	
	12	(MR^OR linked) singletons with PR twins, prob. linkage	
	13	(MR^OR linked) twins with PR singletons, prob. linkage	

3. Results

Due to space limitation we only present the results of the MR^OR linkage involving singleton pregnancies. Other linkage procedures produce results similar in nature. Table 2 gives an overview about the linkage variable weights arising from the MR^OR linkage procedure.

Table 2-Full agreement, close agreement and disagreement weight of the matching variables for the MR^OR linkage

Matching variable	m_i-value	u_i-value	Linkage weight agree	disagree
Mother's date of birth	Blocking			
Mother's postcode	0.9608	0.000833	10.17	-4.67
Number of pregnancies	0.9474	0.3217	1.56	-3.69
Child's expected date of birth, fullmatch	0.8721	0.00267	8.35	-5.27
close (± 7 days)	0.1029	0.0345	1.58	-5.27
Child's date of birth, fullmatch	0.9719	0.00211	8.85	-5.26
close (± 1 day)	0.0175	0.00391	2.16	-5.26
Time schedule of birth	0.9736	0.0433	4.49	-5.18
Child's gender	0.9866	0.5003	0.98	-5.22
Child's birth weight, fullmatch	0.9308	0.00413	7.82	-4.48
close (± 10 gram)	0.0250	0.0103	1.28	-4.48

The total weight of a record pair: $W = \sum_i w_i$, where w_i is the (dis)agreement weight of the ith variable. The optimal threshold value for the MR^OR singleton linkage that minimised the overall error rate was estimated at 7.0. Therefore, every record pair with a total weight of more than 7 was classified as link.

Probabilistic close linkage of the MR and OR singleton records increased the number of links from 41,673 to 76,050 record pairs (Table 3).

Linkage procedure	Criterion	Number of Matches	
Full deterministic	All 8 linking variables must agree	41,673	**Table 3** Results of the MR^OR linkage with different linkage procedures
Deterministic (n-1)	At least 7 variables must agree	56,391	
Probabilistic	Only weight for agreement and disagreement	73,932	
Probabilistic close	**Also weights for close**	**76,050**	

To validate the results of our probabilistic close method, we obtained additional information from caregivers of a stratified sample of 524 record pairs. Because of lost As not all records could be found by the caregivers (we asked data from three years before), or because of non-response, finally 339 pairs could be analysed. 84 pairs were assumed 'certain links' (total weight above 12). 90 pairs were 'certain non-links' (total weight below 2). 165 pairs were from the uncertain region (total weight between 2 and 12), from which 69 pairs were right above the threshold value, 'just linked pairs', and 96 pairs were right below the threshold values, 'just non-linked pairs'. We have found 19 false negative and 2 false positive links in the uncertain region. There was 1 false negative link in the certain non-link region, which was caused by a combination of missing values and typing errors in the records. All record pairs from the certain links region proved to be correctly linked. Figure 1 shows the number of correct (non)links and false positive-, false negative links against the total linkage weight of the record pairs.

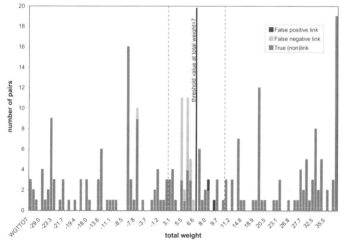

Figure - External validation of the linked MR^OR file of a stratified sample of links with a total weight > 12 (certain links) ; a total weight < 2 (certain non-link); a weight between 2 and 12 (grey zone)

Linkage of the MR and OR singleton records consists of comparison of more than 3 million record pairs, from which 3,080,264 pairs were found in the certain non-link region, 75,781 pairs in the certain links region (99.65 % of all linked pairs) and 1954 pairs in the uncertain region (1685 just non-links and 269 just links). Validation revealed 19+2=21 false links from the 165 validated pairs in the uncertain region, which means roughly (21/165) 13% false margin around the threshold value (about 254 pairs). Because only 0.35% of the linked pairs are in the uncertain region and only 0.055 % of the non-linked pairs, it means that our total linkage procedure has a less than 1 % margin of error.

4. Discussion

Linkage of the PR to find subsequent hospital entries of the same child and linkage of the PR registry with the linked MR^OR registry was based on the same method as described above. The main difficulty of these linkage processes was that while the pregnant woman is the determinator of the MR and OR registries, the PR registry has the child as determinator.

Data cleaning proved to be essential prior to all linkage procedures. Blocking was unavoidable in all cases, though we are aware that it always introduces false negative links. Linkage of twin records remains difficult because of the very limited number of discriminating variables of the brothers and sisters. Longitudinal linkage to link different pregnancies of the same mother is at this moment impossible because of the limited maternal identifying variables in the recent registries. For this type of linkage only the mother's birthday and her ZIP code could be used, but the later one often changes during the years due to moving.

5. Conclusion

We succeeded to link the anonymous Dutch perinatal registries in the absence of a golden standard. Probabilistic close linkage was the best linkage procedure. External validation proved more than 99% validity of the linked data. All information about pregnancy, child birh and postnatal period is now included in one record. The probabilistic method described here is useful tool for linking anonymous data from registries in the absence of a golden standard is present.

6. Acknowledgements

We gratefully acknowledge the support and funding of the SPRN (Foundation of the Dutch Perinatal Registry).

7. References

[1] Newcombe HB. Handbook of record linkage: methods for health and statistical studies, administration, and business. Oxford: Oxford University Press, 1988.

[2] Jaro MA. Probabilistic linkage of large public health data files. *Stat Med* 1995; 14: 112-121

[3] Fellegi IP, Sunter AB. A theory for record linkage. *J Am Stat Assoc* 1969; 64: 1183-1210

[4] Jaro MA. Advances in record-linkage methodology as applies to matching the 1985 census of Tampa, Florida.

[5] Winkler WE. Matching and record linkage. In: *Business survey methods.* New York: J Wiley, 1995: 355-384

[6] Belin TR, Rubin DB. A method for calibrating false-match rates in record linkage. *J Am Stat Assoc* 1995; 90: 694-707

[7] Grannis JS, Overhage JM, Hui S, McDonald CJ. Analysis of a Probabilistic Record Linkage Technique without Human. Review. *AMIA Symposium Proceedings* 2003; 259-263.

[8] Reitsma JB. Registers in Caridovascular Epidemiology. PhD thesis Academic Medical Center, University of Amsterdam, 1999. ISBN 90-9013206-6

8. Address for correspondence

Nora Méray & Anita Ravelli
Academic Medical Center, University of Amsterdam, Department of Medical Informatics, J1B-115-1
P.O. Box 22700, 1100 DE Amsterdam, The Netherlands
email: n.meray@amc.uva.nl & a.c.ravelli@amc.uva.nl

Connecting Medical Informatics and Bio-Informatics
R. Engelbrecht et al. (Eds.)
IOS Press, 2005

The Core Data Elements of Electronic Health Record in Finland

Kristiina Häyrinen, Kaija Saranto

University of Kuopio, Finland

Abstract

Delivery of good care, ability to communicate effectively about patient care and the decision-making during the care process depends on the quality of the information available to all professions and between sectors. The main purpose of an electronic health record is to support the multidisciplinary communication, cooperation and decision-making in the patient's care process. In addition, the data in electronic health records are used, e.g. in clinical research, health system management, the planning of health services and government reporting. A nationwide electronic health record will be introduced in Finland by the end 2007. Reaching this target has been a special part of the national health project. In a subproject of the introduction of a national electronic health record, core data elements of electronic health record have been defined through a consensus-based approach. The main elements are the patient identification information, the provider's identification information, care episode, risk factors, health patterns, vital signs, health problems and diagnosis, nursing minimum data set, surgical procedures, tests and examinations, information about medication, preventive measures, medical statements, functional status, technical aids, living will, tissue donor will, discharge summary, follow-up care plan and consent information. Furthermore, existing vocabularies, nomenclatures, classifications and codes were clarified. The HL7 Finland has defined the manner in which this information is expressed in the CDA R2 structure. The core information elements will be implemented in regional development projects which are partly funded by the Ministry of Social Affairs and Health. This paper presents the defining process of the national core data elements of electronic health record systems in Finland.

Keywords:
Medical Records Systems, Computerized; Standards; Medical Informatics; Nursing Informatics

1. Introduction

According to the Decision in Principle by the Council of State [1] on Securing the Future of Healthcare,"Nationwide electronic patient records will be introduced by the end of 2007". In this article, the term electronic health record is used according to the ISO (International Organization for Standardization) definition [2]. Implementation of a national electronic health record is one of the key issues in reforming the activities and the structures of health care. The Ministry of Social Affairs and Health coordinates the implementation of the National Electronic Health Record in Finland. The National Electronic Health Record Introduction project is a part of a national project to ensure the future of health care the aim of which is to evaluate the existing and threatening problems of the service system as well as to prepare a plan and action programme to eliminate the problems. The objective of the project is to ensure equal availability, quality and sufficiency of care in the different parts of the country.

The history of patient care documentation is long. The development of the documentation has changed from physician's notes to multi-disciplinary paper record. The need for collecting data from different professionals raise up when more people take part of patient's care. Therefore, the recommendations for a unified national manual patient record has been determined apart from specialized medical care [3] and primary health care [4] and used widely for more than 30 years. Electronic health records have been available for several years mostly in primary care [5]. The first electronic health record system, Finstar, was introduced in 1982. In primary care, 93.6 % of health centres and 82 % of private sector organisations used electronic health record in 2003. In addition 62 % of hospitals used electronic health record in some clinics. [6] However, there is a number of different computerized information systems and, also, the same software application can differ between organisations. Some of applications include, *e.g.* laboratory and radiology components but there are also separate departmental systems, *e.g.* laboratory, radiology reporting, intensive care, or maternity. Most of the present-day electronic health record applications are based on the idea of a paper-based record simply turned into an electronic form. Due to this, the possibilities of information and communication technology (ICT) are not fully utilized. These electronic health record systems are poorly structured, even if the core elements of the electronic health record have been determined [7]. They are also passive and inflexible and do not support the continuity of care, quality assessment, education, health care management or statistics automatically. Furthermore, the development of the electronic health record systems has taken place under the control of commercial software producers and has aimed only towards immediate practical solutions [5].

2. The National Project Organisation

The Ministry of Social Affairs and Health has set up a Working Group to guide the introduction of electronic health record documents. One task of the Working Group was to create a strategy [8] for promoting the introduction of interoperability into electronic health records within health care organisations. The aim of the strategy is to provide possibilities for required data exchange in interoperable electronic health records and to build infrastructure supporting the computerized information systems used within health care.

The vision of the national electronic health record introduction project (2003–2007) is that the minimum requirements for the electronic health records will be met in all electronic health record systems. The purpose is to give the health care organisations a means through which health care professionals, by using information systems, are able to deliver effective, safe, seamless and high-quality care and maintain the best quality of information. The data can be utilized among the organisations or used regionally which guarantees the continuity of care. Further, the electronic health record allows managers to plan better services with available high-quality data.

The national electronic health record introduction project includes many subprojects which address different issues, e.g. the core data elements, open interfaces, data security, document metadata, national code and terminology server, architecture and documentation of nursing care. The different subprojects are coordinated, and the results of subprojects are cross-utilized in other projects. The purpose of this paper is to report the first results of the core data elements subproject.

The national electronic health record introduction project has followed on-going international projects which aim to develop an infrastructure for national health care with an electronic health record at its core, for example, in Canada [9], Australia [10] and England [11] under way. Moreover, the work of standardization organisations ISO, CEN and HL7 has been followed. The common elements of these international projects are: 1) patients have access on their own health records and can control the use of information 2) need to define the core information 3) need to choose standards, nomenclatures, codes and vocabularies and their implementation 4) need to develop data security infrastructure and policies 5) aim to produce open, standard-based and interoperable solutions 6) need to divide the development work in subprojects. Further all these international projects focus on data exchange in interoperable electronic health records. However, the core information data varies between different countries.

3. The process of defining the core data elements of electronic health record

The aim of the project is to determine the core data elements and the structure of the electronic health record. The core data mean that the information required for data exchange between information systems uses a standardized form. The core data are defined as the data that can be standardized. The documentation of the core data requires the use of vocabularies, nomenclatures and classifications. Available terminologies have been defined if possible. The core information is the most significant information in the patient care process in the different health care sectors. It contains the health or disease information of patient. The core information is formed chronologically during the care of patient by different professionals. The aim of core information is to give a holistic view of the patient's health and disease history and the care and guidance given. [7] Further health information needs e.g. statistics, health policy and management should be take account. All these different purposes of data reuse should be considered in defining data elements.

As a basis, a list of items was formulated. The list of items was based on earlier broad definitions for the content of the whole electronic patient record [7] and on the Decree of the Ministry of Social Affairs and Health 99/2001 [12]. Delphi method was used to reach a national consensus of the data elements. The definitions of the core data elements and terminologies were founded on two consensus seminars and working group meetings. The definitions were also publicly available for comments through the Internet. The participants of the consensus seminars and working groups included health professionals, electronic health record vendors, representatives of health managers, and experts of hospital districts. The electronic health record vendors and the experts of hospital districts will be committed to implement definitions to electronic health record systems through the involvement in the definition process.

4. The core content of the electronic health record

The core data set of the electronic health record was determined in 2003 (Table 1). Furthermore, the existing terminologies and codes have been clarified for the use of the core data elements. The data can be exchanged between the health care organisations based on the consent of the patient during the caring process. The data can be used to generate reports for institutional, regional or national repositories. The referral and discharge letters can also be generated with the data in the electronic health record. The decision support systems can be connected, e.g. to support diagnosis making or choice of the treatment protocol.

Table 1 - Core data elements of the electronic health record in Finland

The core data element	Terminology/Code	Meaning and use of the core information
The patient identification data	ISO OID (Object Identifiers)	The data include, e.g. the patient's name, social security number, and address. The data are used to identify the patient and to contact the patient.
The provider's identification data	ISO OID	The data include, e.g. the name of the organisation and the health care professional. The data are used to identify the organisation and the health care professional
The episode of care	ISO OID	The data are used to identify the episode of care and link the data with certain episode of care.
Risk factors	ICD-10 (The International Statistical Classification of Diseases and Related Health Problems) ICPC (International Classification of Primary Care)	The data include, e.g. allergies and infectious diseases. The information is used to warn the health professionals about risks that require medical attention or that certain conditions must be met to allow a specific procedure during the current or future care process.
Health patterns	-	The information gives details relating to relevant lifestyle, e.g. smoking, and the use of alcohol. The information is needed during the current care.
Vital signs	LOINC (Logical Observation Identifiers Names and Codes)	The data include, e.g. height and blood pressure. The information is needed during current and future care. The numeric or graphic lists of vital signs could be drawn up by describing the variation of the sign. The vital signs could be connected to the guidelines.
Health problems and diagnosis	ICD-10 ICPC	Diagnosis lists and problem lists could be drawn up. The guidelines could be connected to the diagnosis.
The nursing minimum data set	Several national classifications, some of them based on international classifications, e.g. CCC (Clinical Care Classification)	The data include nursing diagnosis, interventions, outcomes, intensity and discharge summary. The data are gathered with a structured documentation during the nursing process. The information is used during future care.
Surgical procedures	National classification of surgical procedures	The information is used to assess the outcomes of procedures or complications. The information is needed for the health care professionals participating in current and future care. The information could be used to draw up procedure lists to complete the patient's medical history. The guidelines could be connected to the procedures or allocation of resources.
Tests and examinations	National nomenclature of laboratory tests and national nomenclature of radiological examinations and procedures	The information consists of the results of laboratory tests and imaging reports. The information is used to assess the given care. The information is needed for the health care professionals participating in current and future care. The guidelines could be connected to the test and examination results and, also, the information could be related to the allocation of resources.
Information of medication	ATC (Anatomic Therapeutic Chemical Code)	The information is used to assess the results of medication or complications. The information is needed for the health care professionals participating in current and future care. The information could be used to form medication lists to complete the patient's medical history. The guidelines could be connected to information concerning medication.
Prevention	ATC	The information describes the patient's methods of prevention, *e.g.* immunisation.

Medical Statement Medical Certificate	-	A medical statement is based on medical experts' assessment of the patient, *e.g.* for a court of law. A medical certificate is a structured written document on the patient's disease written by a physician, *e.g.* for the patient's employers.
Functional Status	ICF (International Classification of Functioning, Disability and Health)	The information describes the patient's present functionality. The information is needed for the health care professional and social workers participating in the patient's follow-up care.
Technical aids	SFS-EN ISO 9999 (International Classification of Technical Aids for Persons with Disabilities)	The information includes, *e.g.* the fact if the patient is using a wheelchair. The information is used in describing the technical aids the patient needs. The health care professionals participating in the patient's follow-up care and the health management personnel need this information.
Tissue donor will	-	The information is used to announce the patient's wish to donate his organs after death.
Living wills	-	A signed document in which the patient gives the health care professionals the permission to end the care when curing care is not available or the patient cannot express his will.
Discharge summary	-	A discharge summary is a description and an analysis of the events during the episode of care. The information is used by health care professionals in future care in the same organisation and in follow-up care in different organisations.
Plan for follow-up care	-	The information is needed for coordinating the follow-up care.
Consent information	-	The information is needed for announcing the consent of patient to give his documentation to another health care organisation.

5. Conclusion

This paper describes the development of the core data elements of the electronic health records in Finland. The information needs of different stakeholders are taken account. The definition of the core data elements is just beginning to be introduced into the nationwide electronic healthcare record by the year 2007. The core data elements will be implemented in the different electronic health record systems in the regional development projects. The terminologies (nomenclatures, vocabularies and classifications) and codes needed in the electronic health care record systems will be obtained from the national code server. The gaps in the related terminologies and codes are also identified. The need for further specifications of data elements for certain medical specialities has emerged, e.g. in occupational health care, psychiatry, and dental care. The implementation of the electronic health record has caused large behavioural and organisational changes. Thus, it is evident that educational activities must be included in the electronic health care introduction project.

There are many benefits which could be achieved after the core data elements have been implemented to the electronic health records. The structured and coded data elements of the electronic health records will facilitate the finding of the essential information when structured data work as a link to free text. The development of reminders and alerts in the electronic health record as well as links to medical knowledge is possible. The interoperability between different electronic health record systems is achieved, which guarantees the continuity of care. Structured data elements support the quality management, evaluation, benchmarking and statistics. And all of this benefits the patient.

6. Acknowledgements

The authors want to express their gratitude to the Cesar-group and all the actors who have been involved in work of defining the core data elements in the national electronic health record.

7. References

[1]   Ministry of Social Affairs and Health. Decision in Principle by the Council of State on securing the future of health care. *Brochures of the Ministry of Social Affairs and Health* 2002.

[2]   ISO/DTR 20514. Health Informatics- electronic health record- definition, scope, and context. 2004.

[3]   The Association of Hospitals. Health care record and patient record in special health care. 1974. Helsinki:Printel Oy. [In Finnish]

[4]   The Association of Finnish Local and Regional Authorities. Health care record: manual. 1982.[In Finnish]

[5]   Hartikainen K, Kuusisto-Niemi S, and Lehtonen E. Survey of Social and Health Care Information Systems 2001. Publications of the Network of Excellence Centers 1/2002. [In Finnish]

[6]   Kiviaho K, Winblad I, and Reponen J. The information systems which support health care processes in Finland. Survey and use analysis. 2004. *Publications of the Network of Excellence Centers* 8/2004. [In Finnish]

[7]   Hartikainen K, Kokkola A, and Larjomaa R. The Content Definitions for the Electronic Patient Record. 2000. *Publications of the Network of Excellence Centers* 4/2000. [In Finnish]

[8]   Ministry of Social Affairs and Health. National definition and implementation of the electronic patient record system. Working Group Memonrandum of the Ministry of Social affairs and Health. 2002. [In Finnish]

[9]   Canada Health Infoway. 2003. http://www.infoway-inforoute.ca/home.php?lang=en

[10]   HealthConnect.2004. http://www.healthconnect.gov.au

[11]   ERDIP 2002. http://www.nhsia.nhs.uk/erdip/pages/default.asp

[12]   Ministry of Social Affairs and Health. Decree of drawing up of patient documents and on keeping them and samples and models related care 99/2001. [In Finnish]

8. Address for correspondence

Kristiina Häyrinen
University of Kuopio, Department of Health Policy and Management
P.O.Box 1627
Fin-70211 Kuopio, Finland
kristiina.hayrinen@uku.fi

Connecting Medical Informatics and Bio-Informatics
R. Engelbrecht et al. (Eds.)
IOS Press, 2005

HealthInfoCDA: Case Composition Using Electronic Health Record Data Sources

Grace I. Paterson[a,b], Syed Sibte Raza Abidi[b], Steven D. Soroka[c]

[a]*Medical Informatics, Faculty of Medicine,*

[b]*Health Informatics Lab, Faculty of Computer Science,*

[c]*Department of Medicine (Nephrology), Faculty of Medicine,*
Dalhousie University, Halifax, NS Canada B3H 4H7

Abstract

HealthInfoCDA denotes a health informatics educational intervention for learning about the clinical process through use of the Clinical Document Architecture (CDA). We hypothesize those common standards for an electronic health record can provide content for a case base for learning how to make decisions. The medical record provides a shared context to coordinate delivery of healthcare and is a boundary object that satisfies the informational requirement of multiple communities of practice. This study transforms clinical narrative in three knowledge-rich modalities: case write-up, patient record and online desk reference to develop a case base of experiential clinical knowledge useful for medical and health informatics education. Our ultimate purpose is to aggregate concepts into knowledge elements for case-based teaching.

Keywords:
Medical Informatics Applications; Medical Records Systems, Computerized; Case Management; Nephrology; Artificial Intelligence; Boundary Object; Case-based Reasoning; Health Informatics Education; Medical Education; HL7 CDA

1. Introduction

The HealthInfoCDA project aims at providing an educational intervention to medical residents treating patients with kidney disease secondary to diabetes and hypertension. A key issue that is being investigated is achieving semantic interoperability among electronic health resources to not only support disease management but also for lifelong learning/education.

Medical schools are shifting from passive acquisition of knowledge to active learning in a clinical context. Problem Based Learning (PBL) is 'an educational method characterized by the use of patient problems as a context for students to learn problem-solving skills and acquire knowledge' [1]. PBL curricula endorse the use of Electronic Health Record (EHR) of actual patient problems as an educational resource depicting a clinical context for medical students to learn both clinical sciences and problem-solving skills. EHR can be regarded as the the glue for the clinical care, medical education and health informatics communities; each community enriches, interacts and leverages the EHR. Given the central nature of EHR in patient care—i.e. EHRs not only record operational patient data but also encompass the working behaviour and mental models of the practitioners generating it—they are a vital and rich source of medical/healthcare knowledge. We contend that episodic information contained in an EHR can function as 'learning objects' about action-related decisions for medical and health informatics education, in particular in a PBL paradigm [2]. PBL cases, derived from EHR, support experiential learning in clinical settings as follows: anchoring instruction in cases, actively involving learners, modelling professional thinking and action, providing direction and feedback and creating a collaborative learning environment [3]. Furthermore, there is a strong association between PBL and the computational reasoning paradigm of Case-Based Reasoning (CBR) [4] which is the motivation for this project.

The relevance of CBR-based knowledge representation with a PBL compliant teaching framework is grounded in the fact that CBR provide 'analogy-based' solutions to clinical problems by manipulating knowledge derived from similar previously experienced situations called *Cases*. According to the CBR methodology, a new problem is solved by finding similar past cases and reusing their problem-solving strategy to derive a solution to the new, yet similar, problem situation. Note that each case is described by a set of case-defining attributes and is associated with a solution (or decision) suggested by a medical practitioner [5]. For learning purposes we argue that for a medical student, learning to be a clinician is contingent on exposure to large repertoire of clinical experience. In this regard, CBR cases derived from actual patient information will provide an opportunity for learners to draw on prior knowledge and experience to learn about how to solve such problems in the clinical setting. Reasoning with CBR cases will also impress on the learner the dichotomy of theory and practice—i.e. clinical practice does not always follow theoretical norms. For a medical student, CBR cases will provide an opportunity to learn how experts conceptualize medical information in terms of constructs [6] and also to leverage on experiential knowledge accumulated in the EHR which is then translated into a CBR case.

In this project we aim to automatically generate PBL cases, in a CBR formalism, from narrative teaching cases and EHR. The intent is to anchor instruction in PBL cases that model professional thinking and action and to produce a case-based curriculum resource that is useful for medical and health informatics educators. In this paper we present a strategy to automatically (a) extract clinical concepts from narrative EHR using lexical analysis and natural language parsing techniques [7]; and (b) generate CBR-specific cases (akin to clinical documents) represented using the extended markup language (XML) for the Health Level 7 (HL7) Clinical Document Architecture (CDA) specification. HL7 Templates enable formal expressions of large portions of clinical documents without sacrificing semantic interoperability.

To achieve the above objectives, we present HealthInfoCDA that leverages health information standards, classification systems and templates as building blocks for a health infostructure in a PBL context. As stated earlier, a key issue is information exchange between these health information elements whilst ensuring semantic interoperability between the content and the information structures. Digital documents play a role as boundary objects for representing clinical activity across time and space and for achieving a shared understanding between caregivers [8]. Our approach is to regard these building blocks function as boundary objects, 'objects which are both plastic enough to adapt to local needs and the constraints of the several parties employing them, yet robust enough to maintain a common identity across sites' [9, p. 393]. They provide an opportunity for learning about the representation of clinical activity in computerized records and for building a shared understanding amongst the people who provide clinical care to patients, produce medical education resources and participate as health informaticians.

We use the CDA Release 2.0 to capture clinical activity associated with care [10]. CDA is a document specification standard produced by HL7—it defines a new target for clinical information exchange that is substantially easier to hit than one based on standards for discrete data. It delivers 80% of the value of the latter approach and, as such, hits the 80/20 sweet spot [11]. We argue that the encoding of medical information in a CDA document facilitates sharing and exchanging information between the EHR and CBR systems. More specifically, our focus is to capture and represent action-related decisions associated with renal care. We seek effective and efficient methods to represent the clinicians' experience with renal disease in a CDA form to improve health outcomes, disease management and lifelong learning/education.

2. Materials and Methods

The HealthInfoCDA project team developed an information flow model to document healthcare activities and patient care data collection. Storyboards, or use case paths, – the term preferred in the ISO 17113 Health Informatics standard [12]—are narratives that collect domain knowledge and describe processes pertaining to the interactions between people and the healthcare system. They help the reader understand the flow of information in the clinical environment.

For EHR creation, we started with a single clinical communication for the specific task of patient discharge. Our hypothesis is that we can improve the quality of discharge summaries for chronic kidney disease patients by using a template to prompt medical residents to enter relevant data. For our pilot test of the template, clinical educators produced CDA documents from a simulated chart. These were automatically scored against the gold standard CDA document produced by the investigators. The characteristics of the difference inform the case composition process. It may illustrate a record keeping gap that can be addressed in the case base for the CBR system [13].

For the longitudinal EHR, we used the chart of a patient with chronic renal failure secondary to hypertension and diabetes. This record spanned over 20 years and included clinical care communications originating from family physicians, specialists, surgeons, nurses, social workers, laboratory technicians, educators and pharmacists.

The EHR to HealthInfoCDA case transformation methodology is based on Abidi's case acquisition and transcription info-structure (CATI) methodology [5]. Phase I attempts to establish structural mapping and Phase II attempts to establish content mapping.

2.1 Phase I: Structural Mapping between CDA-based EHR and Case

The HL7 community of practice assigns unique identifiers to code sets and common templates available for reuse:

1. Metadata for case indexing using Object Identifiers (OID) for over 100 code sets
2. Templates for common concepts from the NHS Clinical Statement Model, including Allergy and Adverse Reaction, Blood Pressure, Height, Weight, Temperature, Smoking/Tobacco Consumption and Alcohol Intake [14]

The HL7 Reference Information Model (RIM) defines two classes specifically for CDA structured documents. The Class:Document is a specialization of the Act class and is used for attributes needed for document management. It has an attribute, Document:bibliographicDesignationText, defined as the 'citation for a cataloged document that permits its identification, location and/or retrieval from common collections' [15]. This attribute is useful for retrieval of a document from a specific electronic resource in the infostructure. CDA is used for clinical and reference documents in the HealthInfoCDA project.

The first step in identifying the situation-action content is the processing of a text corpus created from teaching cases, EHR instances and guidelines. The case entries and supporting tutor guides are from the Case-Oriented Problem-Stimulated (COPS) Undergraduate Medical Education curriculum, Dalhousie University. The goal for these cases is to enable the student to understand the manifestations, pathogenesis and management of common chronic metabolic disorders of diabetes mellitus and its associated complications which involve the renal system.

Our diabetic patient develops chronic kidney disease. He is followed for over 20 years. The patient's episode of care dictates the most appropriate site for care. The paper record includes care in multiple settings and exceeds 300 pages. We select a representative sample for use in this study (Table 1).

Table 1. Clinical Documents from Patient's Paper Chart

Form	Settings	Count	Dates
Discharge Summary	Community hospital	1	1982/05/28
	Acute care hospital	2	2002/11/12
			2003/06/14
Clinic Letter	Nephrology Clinic	4	2002/10/29
			2002/11/06
			2002/12/18
			2003/04/07
Protocols	Acute care-Erythropoietin	1	2003/04/01
Consultation	Community hospital	1	2003/07/29
Operative Report	Acute care hospital	1	2002/11/29
Diagnostic Imaging	Community hospital	1	2002/10/23

There are evidence-based marker therapies to prevent or retard kidney disease in patients with diabetes. Such knowledge about marker therapies is pivotal to the design of a health informatics educational intervention. We add electronic guidelines to our text corpus from two sources: 1) Diabetes: an Instant Reference, a web portal supported as a separate project in Dalhousie's Health Informatics Laboratory and updated in 2005 to reflect the changes in the most recent guidelines [16]; and 2) Therapeutic Choices [17] published by the Canadian Pharmacists Association on their e-therapeutics website.

To ensure inter-case matching accuracy, we define both a numerical and vocabulary domain for each HealthInfoCDA case attribute value, and standardize the EHR values with respect to the pre-defined case content. Phase 2 of our EHR to HealthInfoCDA transformation methodology deals with these tasks.

2.2 Phase 2: Content Equivalence

We utilize Unified Medical Language System (UMLS) MetaMap Transfer (MMTx) software to parse the narratives in the text corpus (EHR, teaching cases and therapeutic guidelines) and to map clinical concepts to unique UMLS concept identifiers. MMTx program takes an input sentence, separates it into phrases, identifies the medical concepts and assigns proper semantic categories to them according to the knowledge embedded in UMLS [18]. The MMTx program maps biomedical text in the clinical narrative to concepts in the UMLS Metathesaurus. We downloaded MMTx software from website, http://mmtx.nlm.nih.gov. We manually filter the output to select the best match for a clinical concept. The text corpus is also processed by SnoCode® from MedSight Informatique Inc. This natural language processing software encodes the clinical concepts in SNOMED International. SNOMED is the coding language of choice for the NHS clinical statement model. SNOMED has been added as a source vocabulary to the UMLS Metathesaurus in the 2005 version. The UMLS and SNOMED ontologies serve as semiotic vehicles for sharing medical knowledge and matching two concepts.

MMTx output consists of information on how the candidate concept matches up to words in the original phrase. There may be lexical variation in the matching. We use scoring criteria for coding accuracy ranging from 0 (no information found) to 4 (perfect matching) [19].

We use the XML-based HL7 standard, CDA, to standardize our case structure and link clinical documents to each other. Health care activity occurs within a context of who, whom, when, where, how and why. HL7 developed a service action model of healthcare processes which focused on context. The application of this model produced a simplification of the HL7 RIM [20]. When we transform the teaching cases and the actual patient record, the information should be readily represented as a set of actions in a longitudinal record. This identifies who did what and the target that the action influences. The information available about circumstances -- such as location, time, manner, reason and motive -- is entered into the CDA.

3. Results

We chose UMLS and SNOMED as the 'switching languages' between concepts in the case base and the knowledge resources. The mean accuracy score assigned to concept encoding in UMLS was 3.6. The text should be pre-processed to remove punctuation, such as hyphens, to improve the mapping.

The clinical documentation represented in CDA includes Laboratory Report, Physician Note, Referral Form Ambulatory Care, Consultation Letter, Clinic Letter, Operative Report and Discharge Summary. The relationships between the generic drug names in the teaching case and the brand names in the patient chart are made visible through online linkage to the Nova Scotia Formulary. For example, the patient is prescribed gemfibrozil, which is shown on the formulary with brand name Lopid®.

For EHR creation, the clinical educator uses a patient chart for the usual transcription and dictation process, and then uses the HL7 Template to try to express the same information. The HL7 Template provides a structure and concurrent coding to the data entry process. It supports pulling information from linked resources, such as the Nova Scotia Drug Formulary. The clinician enters the summary information as free text. Problems encountered in the pilot study are resolved with the clinical educators prior to recruiting medical residents to use the HL7 Template.

Health Informatics students access the case base through a web portal. It displays the EHR as a linked set of CDA documents with information presented in the same way as the hospital forms. Our added value is to integrate clinical concept definitions, links to reference resources, XML viewer and record linkage for longitudinal record for a patient. This makes visible the complexities of the clinical action-related decision process to the health informaticians.

The EHRs are real-life cases that depict both a clinical situation and an associated solution. They are a source of diagnostic-quality operable clinical cases. They contain knowledge about what clinical activities were done and in what context. SNOMED International and UMLS will be initially tested as the controlled vocabularies for querying the case base.

4. Discussion

A case base can serve to teach the clinical care process, healthcare delivery models, and the manifestations, pathogenesis and management of disease. A semantic analysis of the clinical discourse used for teaching, reference material and medical records can be used for thesauri discovery for a domain. Patient information is coded in EHRs. The ability to link from patient records to reference sources is affected by the choice of coding system. The digital case base can help bridge between the educational settings a student encounters. If a standardized terminology-architecture interface is achieved through an HL7 CDA specification, it will serve to support education as well as clinical care. Education cases that focus on chronic disease teach longitudinal record keeping. They are useful for teaching medical students the medical records management process and for illustrating to health informatics students the complexities of the clinical action-related decision process.

5. Acknowledgements:

We acknowledge content authors Sonia Salisbury, Meng Tan, Sarah Seaman, and Michael West; template designers Zhihong Wang and Ron Soper; funder of the server, HEALNet NCE; and scholarship funding from the Canadian Institutes of Health Research (CIHR) PhD/Postdoctoral Strategic Training Program in Health Informatics.

6. References

[1]   Albanese MA, Mitchell S. Problem-based learning: a review of literature on its outcomes and implementation issues. *Acad Med* 1993;68:52–81.

[2]   Patterson R, Harasym P. Educational instruction on a hospital information system for medical students during their surgical rotations. *J Am Med Inform Assoc* 2001:8(2):111-116.

[3]   Irby DM.Three exemplary models of case-based teaching. *Acad Med* 1994 Dec;69(12):947-53.

[4]   Eshach H, Bitterman H. From case-based reasoning to problem-based learning. *Acad Med* 1994 Dec;69(12):947-53.

[5]   Abidi SS, Manickam S. Leveraging XML-based electronic medical records to extract experiential clinical knowledge: an automated approach to generate cases for medical case-based reasoning systems. *Int J Med Inf.* 2002 Dec 18;68(1-3):187-203.

[6]   Patel VL, Arocha JF, Kaufman DR. A primer on aspects of cognition for medical informatics. *J Am Med Inform Assoc* 2001;8(2):324-343.

[7]   Evans DA, Ginther-Webster K, Hart M, Lefferts RG, Monarch IA. Automatic indexing using selective NLP and first-order thesauri. *RIAO'91,* April 2-5, 1991, Automoma University of Barcelona, Barcelona, Spain, 1991. pp. 624-644.

[8]   Shepherd M. Interoperability for digital libraries. *DRTC Workshop on Semantic Web.* 2003 December 8-10.

[9]   Star SL, Griesemer JR. Institutional ecology, translations and boundary objects: amateurs and professionals in Berkeley's Museum of Vertebrate Zoology 1907-39. *Soc Stud Sci* 1989:19:387-420.

[10]   Itälä T, Mikola T, Virtanen A, Asikainen P. Seamless service chains and information processes. *Proceedings of the 38th HICSS* 2005 January. Available at: http://csdl.computer.org/comp/proceedings/hicss/2005/2268/06/22680155b.pdf

[11]   Klein J. Bridging clinical document architecture across the chasm. In: *2nd International Conference on the CDA* 2004 October. Available at: http://www.hl7.de/iamcda2004/finalmat/day3/Moving%20Adoption%20of%20HL.pdf

[12]   Hammond WE. Method for the development of messages: a process for developing comprehensive, interoperable and certifiable data exchange among independent systems. *ISO Bulletin* 2002 August;16-19.

[13]   Cox JL, Zitner D, Courtney KD, MacDonald DL, Paterson G, Cochrane B, Flowerdew G, Johnstone DE. Undocumented patient information: an impediment to quality of care. *Am J Med.* 2003 Mar 15;114(3):211-6.

[14]   Bentley S. Representation of commonly used concepts within messaging P1R2 build 3. *NHS National Programme for Information Technology* 2005 January 7.

[15]   Beeler G, Case J, Curry J, Hueber A, Mckenzie L, Schadow G, Shakir A-M. *HL7 Reference Information Model.* Version: V 02-04. Available at: http://www.hl7.org/library/data-model/RIM/C30204/rim.htm

[16]   Canadian Diabetes Association Clinical Practice Guidelines Expert Committee. Canadian Diabetes Association 2003 Clinical Practice Guidelines for the Prevention and Management of Diabetes in Canada. *Can J Diabetes.* 2003;27(suppl 2). Available at: http://www.diabetes.ca/cpg2003/

[17]   Gray J.(Ed.) *Therapeutic Choices,* 4th Edition. Canadian Pharmacists Association, Ottawa, ON, 2004. Available at: http://www.e-therapeutics.ca

[18]   Aronson AR. Effective mapping of biomedical text to the UMLS Metathesaurus: The MetaMap Program. *Proc AMIA Symp.* 2001:17-21.

[19]   Strang N, Cucherat M, Boissel JP. Which coding system for therapeutic information in evidence-based medicine. *Comput Methods Programs Biomed.* 2002 Apr; 68(1):73-85.

[20]   Russler DC, Schadow G, Mead C, Snyder T, Quade L, McDonald CJ. Influences of the Unified Service Action Model on the HL7 Reference Information Model. *Proc AMIA Symp.* 1999:930-4.

7. Address for correspondence

Grace I. Paterson, Medical Informatics, Faculty of Medicine, Dalhousie University, 5849 University Avenue Halifax, NS Canada B3H 4H7, Email: grace.paterson@dal.ca,
URLs: http://informatics.medicine.dal.ca and http://healthinfo.med.dal.ca

Connecting Medical Informatics and Bio-Informatics
R. Engelbrecht et al. (Eds.)
IOS Press, 2005

143

Nursing Documentation in Occupational Health

Denise Tolfo Silveira [a] **, Heimar de Fátima Marin** [b]

[a] *Federal University of Rio Grande do Sul (UFRGS), Doctoral Candidate UNIFESP, Brazil*
[b] *Federal University of São Paulo (UNIFESP), Brazil*

Abstract

<u>Purpose</u>: *Traditionally, nursing documentation has been consistent with hospital standards and legal definitions of clinical nursing practice. Identify data and information nurses need to be recorded in order to maintain the continuity and quality of nursing care and the efficiency of nursing performance is a research question that is moving professionals around the world. This study objective is to describe the analysis of nursing documentation in the patient records.* <u>Methods</u>: *It is a retrospective study. The study was conducted in the ambulatory occupational health nursing; it was selected 111 patient records. Of these, in 106 we identified a total of 775 nursing records. The nursing records comprise the following dimension: identification, job history, health state, health and safety, psychological e socio-cultural, medical history, physical examination and nursing assessment.* <u>Results</u>: *In the data set elements found as documented in the subjective data and objective data, there was higher frequency of data elements related to the following nursing dimensions: health state, health and safety, physical examination and nursing assessment. The dimension of job history we found that 25% of the nursing records did not documented information about the current work status of the patient. In addition, the current job activity (20.77% of the records), working day (9.03% of the records), job process (8.13% of the records), worksite exposure (8.0% of the records), environmental works (6.19% of the records), occupation (5.81% of the records), job time (4.39% of the records), before job activity (4.13 % of the records), and work location (3.23% of the records) were not also documented.* <u>Conclusion</u>: *In conclusion, the present study was an attempt to highlight the importance of data to be documented and organized in the existing information systems in the specific area of occupational health care. The adequate data collected can provide the right information to improve nursing care in this care setting and enhance health population.*

Keywords:
Documentation; Nursing Records; Occupational Health Nursing; Nursing Informatics

1. Introduction

The American Nurses Association –ANA [1] defines nursing as the diagnosis and treatment of human responses to actual or potential health problems. To support nursing care practice in different countries and settings, the nursing process methodology have been used as a useful instrument of record to answer the retrieval of data improving individualized patient care, and patient needs for decision making. The ability of the nursing professional to make a difference in patient outcomes must be demonstrated in practice and reflected in the records in the documentation [2] [3] [4].

Traditionally, nursing documentation has been consistent with hospital standards and legal definitions of clinical nursing practice. The records and reports of nursing care are also considered a legal documentation in the patient records [4]. The clinical record is the vehicle of communication of patient information among the multi-professional direct care health team members. It is through this record that nurses, physicians and other professionals involved with care are able to guarantee the performance and continuity of proper treatment, enabling the adequate delivery of care and safeguarding ethical and legal aspects involved in it. [5] However, some studies demonstrate that manual nursing records of patient information is frequently inaccurate and incomplete.

It is also important to emphasize the adequacy by which the information is presented in those records; information must be objective, clear, complete, so that all members of the health team understand its context and meaning [5].

In Brazil, the nursing practice on outpatient unit is named as nursing consultation. It is the encounter between nurses and patient, the mean nurse uses to provide care to the patient in the ambulatory unit. It is regulated and legitimated by Decree n. 94.496, dated June 8, 1987 of the Law of Professional Practice n. 7.498, dated June 25, 1986 [6]. The nursing consultation is also based on the nursing process that is a systematized and scientific methodology to identify real or potential health needs of the patient in order to provide an effective care.

In occupational health, nursing consultation practice and record must include what is related to the workplace and its influence on the health-sickness process, aiming at measures of promotion, protection, and rehabilitation. With the establishment of systematic records, we can obtain essential information to generate individual or collective work-health-sickness process and to identify characteristics of the social groups where this process takes place, allowing for a better understanding of real or potential life and work conditions [7].

In nursing occupational health care, the protocol for nursing interview can comprises questions related to health history (survey on chronic-degenerative damages[1]) and occupational history (survey on occupational damages[2], occupational situation, work relations, work environment, ergonometric issues). Frequently, patient information is recorded based on: (a) **Subjective data** that comprises the data related to clients' complaints; (b) **Objective data** which refers to physical and clinical exams; (c) **Impression** that is the documentation of all considerations that nurses had about clients, problems, diagnosis and treatment), and (d) **Conduct** that refers to the actions and interventions of the nursing staff in the resolution of problems identified.

With the adequate information obtained and identified, nurses can implement interventions at the individual level as to:

- Nutritional reeducation;
- The adequate use of protection or spacing equipment, in cases of exposure to harmful factors;
- Orientation as to physical safety rules, that is, the importance of respecting the vertebral axis, maintaining balance, using the strength of legs, nearing to loads to be lifted, among others;
- Prevention and control of damages produced by mental and psychical loads of work; all of these should not be neglected in interventions.

---

[1] Chronic-degenerative damages are understood as: systemic arterial hypertension, diabetes mellitus, cardiopathy, obesity, dislipidemias, etc.
[2] Occupational damages are understood as: repeated effort lesions or osteomuscular diseases related to work, dermatoses, illnesses related to hearing, sight, the respiratory system, etc.

Considering *the increasing volume of information and the greater complexity of data,* the clinical records in its manual format, i.e., paper-based, *is an inefficient records* that can compromise the quality of nursing care [5]. Identify data and information nurses need to be recorded in order to maintain the continuity and quality of nursing care and the efficiency of nursing performance is a research question that is moving professionals around the world.

This study objective is to describe the analysis of nursing documentation in the patient records. The selected local is the nursing ambulatory of occupational health. It is our understanding that patient records are both a means of clinical documentation and a means of communication between providers involved in patients' care.

Background

The study was conducted in the teaching hospital of Federal University of Porto Alegre, Rio Grande do Sul, situated on the south region of Brazil. Since 1997, the hospital implemented a computer-based application system for management and clinical documentation, including admission, transferring and discharge, diagnosis and therapeutics' support service, surgery scheduling; drugs order, and patient management. In 2004, it was included the clinical documentation application. In such a system, nurses, physicians and professionals involved in the delivery of care, can record patient information. Nursing documentation is based on the nursing process. The institution staff designed the protocol for data collecting. The general format includes subjective data, objective data, impression and conduct.

2. Materials and methods

It is a retrospective study. The study was conducted in the ambulatory occupational health nursing of the teaching hospital of the Federal University of Porto Alegre, Brazil.

It was selected 111 patient records. Of these, in 106 we identified a total of 775 nursing records. The period of data collection was from August 1998 to August 2003.

The nursing records comprise the following dimension: identification, job history, health state, health and safety, psychological e socio-cultural, medical history, physical examination and nursing assessment. The data set elements selected are presented in the Table 1.

The analyses were done by SPSS (Statistical Package for the Social Sciences), according to the theoretical perspective of studies in nursing and informatics and its interrelations.

3. Results and discussion

Of the 111 patient records analyzed, 106 presented nursing information in occupational health. These records comprised several outpatient visits per patient in which we identified a total of 775 (N) nursing records.

The nursing record protocol is based on the phases of the nursing process that is recognized a method of obtaining patient information. It can combine data gathered from the history-talking interview, the physical examination, and data gathered from the results of laboratory/diagnostic studies.

In the data set elements found as documented in the subjective data and objective data, there was higher frequency of data elements related to the following nursing dimensions:

- Health state: food (93.03% of the records), hydration (89.42% of the records) and leisure activity (79.87% of the records);

- Health and safety: symptoms of disease/illness (86.45% of the records), current complaints (85.94% of the records), treatment (63.23% of the records) and medication (52.90% of the records);
- Physical examination: blood pressure (96.65% of the records), body weight (95.10% of the records) and behavioral (62,32 % of the records);
- Nursing assessment: adherence behavior nursing care (75.61% of the records).

Table 1 - Data set element of nursing records documentation

Dimension Identification	Dimension Job History	Dimension Physical Examination
Name	Job Activity (current)	Blood Pressure
Age	Job Activity (before)	Body Weight
Race	Job Process	Height
Sex	Job Time	Laboratory/diagnostic studies
Religion	Working Day	Pulse (palpation)
Hail from	Current Work Status	Glucometer
From	Worksite Exposure	Muscle Measures
Phone number	Work Location	Assessment Respiratory
Civil status	Environmental Works	Face
Occupation		Ears
	Dimension Health and Safety	Eyes
	Treatment	Neck
Dimension Health State	Health Medical History	Neuro/Muscular Assessment
Activity	Medical Diagnoses	Skin Integrity
Food	Medical Procedure and Surgical	Mucous
Hydration	Medication	Communication
Sleep/Rest	Familial Risk Factors	Behavioral
Leisure Activity	Symptom of Disease/Illness	Status Mental
Allergies	Current Complaint	Status General
Intestinal Elimination	Main Complaint	Emotional State
Urinary Elimination	Sexuality Revision	Body Balance
	Respiration Revision	Mobility
	Circulation Revision	
Dimension Nursing Assessment	Neurosensory Revision	
Difficulty managing therapy		
Need for information, knowledge health situation	**Dimension Psychological e Sociocultural**	
Adherence Behavior to Nursing Care	Alcohol/Drugs/Smoke	
	Relationship Familiar	
	Living With	
	Self Esteem	

The lower frequency of data elements related to physical examination was: height (29.94% of the records), laboratorial and other exams (28.77% of the records), emotional state (28.26% of the records), and neuro/muscular assessment (24.13% of the records).

The lack of data elements in the initial stage of the application of the nursing process in the records analyzed indicates an initial lack of information to support real and potential needs of patients. According to Marin, Rodrigues, Delaney, Nielsen and Yan [2] the subsequent stages of the process depend on the quality of the initial assessment and its respective documentation. In this study we verified that the initial stage of the process was not properly documented in the sample analyzed. For instance, related to the dimension of job history we found that 25%

of the nursing records did not documented information about the current work status of the patient. In addition, the current job activity (20.77% of the records), working day (9.03% of the records), job process (8.13% of the records), worksite exposure (8.0% of the records), environmental works (6.19% of the records), occupation (5.81% of the records), job time (4.39% of the records), before job activity (4.13 % of the records), and work location (3.23% of the records) were not also documented.

It can be said that a smaller frequency of data elements collection does not mean that it have not been collected, since this data is implicit in the nursing impression and conduct, where nurses record their diagnostic impression as well as actions and interventions they provided. Another interesting finding was that in around 6.0 % of all records analyzed, subjective and objective data, impression and conduct were not always interrelated, or were not even consistent when conduct and data collected in the anamnesis and physical examination were compared.

Florence Nightingale, in *Notes on nursing: what it is, and what it is not*, stated that the purpose of documentation such observations was to collect, store, and retrieve data so that patient care could be managed intelligently [8]. Moreover, the documentation is the evidence that nurse's legal and ethical responsibilities to the patient were met and that the patient received quality care [2] [8] [9].

Likewise, the documentation of phrases such as "there were no further alterations" (11.23% of the records), found in the subjective data, and "nothing further was observed" (21.42% of the records), found in objective data, are an ambiguous way of recording, for one cannot be sure whether elements were collected or not.

Marin states that *it is impossible to give continuity to quality care if documentation is inadequate, absent, unreliable, and incapable of supporting clinical decisions; (...) the health environment increases the demand for professional growth and for the development of efficient documentation systems to be used simultaneously by many health professionals.* [3]

4. Conclusion

Documented information is an essential element for the assessment of the quality of nursing care. Therefore, records must translate the application of the nursing process where action and delivery of care to the patients be assured and nursing ethical and legal aspects respected.

Developing a computer-based data collection to support nursing documentation is very important. Priority should be given to the design of interface and database. There is a real need of adequate methodological tools to provide not only the survey on health conditions and harmful occupational factors, but also the relation or association of elements that comprise the work-health-sickness process, taking into account both organizational and environmental aspects, as well as life conditions of workers.

Considering the scope of analyzed records, it is our understanding that:

a) Records must be kept in order to feed a database that guarantees the analysis of information to support and describe nursing practices in occupational health;
b) The terminology used must be adjusted in order to facilitate answers and avoid simple "yes" or "no" answers, making comprehension easier to achieve effective outcomes;
c) Question included on the patient interview protocols must be unambiguous in order to clarify its content in an accessible and pertinent way, facilitating the participation of providers.

In conclusion, the present study was an attempt to highlight the importance of data to be documented and organized in the existing information systems in the specific area of occupational health care. The adequate data collected can provide the right information to improve nursing care in this care setting and enhance health population.

5. References

[1] ANA (American Nurse Association). Standards of clinical nursing practice. 2nd ed. Washington, DC, 1998.

[2] Marin HF, Rodriguez RJ, Delaney C, Nielsen GH, Yan J, eds. *Building Standard-Based Nursing Information Systems*. Pan American Health Organization (PAHO), World Health Organization (WHO), Division of Health Systems and Services Development. Washington, DC: Pan American Health Organization, 2000.

[3] Marin HF. Os componentes de enfermagem do prontuário eletrônico do paciente. In: Massad E, Marin HF, Neto RSA, eds. *O prontuário eletrônico do paciente na assistência, informação e conhecimento médico*. São Paulo: H de F. Marin, 2003.

[4] McCargar P, Johnson JE, Billingsley M. Practice Applications. In: Saba VK and McCormick KA, eds. *Essentials of computers for nurses: informatics for the new millennium*.3rd ed. New York: McGraw-Hill, 2001. p. 233-247.

[5] Marin HF. Vocabulário: recurso para construção de base de dados em enfermagem. *Acta Paul Enf*, São Paulo, v.13, n.1, p.86-89, 2000.

[6] COFEN – Conselho Federal de Enfermagem. Código de ética dos profissionais de enfermagem. Rio de Janeiro, 1993.

[7] Silveira, DT. Consulta-ação: uma metodologia de ação em enfermagem na área da saúde do trabalhador. *Revista Gaúcha de Enfermagem*, Porto Alegre, v.22, n.1, p. 06-19, 2001.

[8] Saba VK. Historical perspectives of nursing and the computer. In: Saba VK and McCormick KA, eds. *Essentials of computers for nurses: informatics for the new millennium*.3rd ed. New York: McGraw-Hill, 2001. p. 09-45.

[9] Moen A. A nursing perspective to design and implementation of electronic patient record systems. *Journal of Biomedical Informatics*, 36 (2003) 375–378.

Address for correspondence

Denise Tolfo Silveira
Rua Guilherme Alves, 1130/419 – CEP 90680-000 Porto Alegre - RS / Brazil
F: 55 (51) 3339-6987 / 55 (51) 99642338
E-mail: dtolfo@denf.epm.br / dtsilveira@hotmail.com

Section 3

Decision Support and Clinical Guidelines

Connecting Medical Informatics and Bio-Informatics
R. Engelbrecht et al. (Eds.)
IOS Press, 2005
151

Structuring Clinical Guidelines through the Recognition of Deontic Operators

Gersende Georg, Isabelle Colombet, Marie-Christine Jaulent

Université Paris Descartes, Faculté de Médecine; INSERM, U729; SPIM, F-75006 Paris, France

Abstract

In this paper, we present a novel approach to structure Clinical Guidelines through the automatic recognition of syntactic expressions called deontic operators. We defined a grammar and a set of Finite-State Transition Networks (FSTN) to automatically recognize deontic operators in Clinical Guidelines. We then implemented a dedicated FSTN parser that identifies deontic operators and marks up their occurrences in the document, thus producing a structured version of the Guideline. We evaluated our approach on a corpus (not used to define the grammar) of 5 Clinical Guidelines. As a result, 95.5% of the occurrences of deontic expressions are correctly marked up. The automatic detection of deontic operators can be a useful step to support Clinical Guidelines encoding.

Keywords:
Clinical Guidelines; Deontic operators; Document processing; GEM.

1. Introduction

Clinical Guidelines are normalized documents which play an important role in the dissemination of standardized medical knowledge and Best Practice. In recent years, significant research has been dedicated to the computerization of Clinical Guidelines in order to facilitate their authoring or to promote their inclusion in Decision Support Systems [1]. An important aspect of that research has been the development of document processing tools that could support the encoding of textual guidelines. The most comprehensive approach is the Guideline Elements Model (GEM) [2], which is a model facilitating the translation of natural language guidelines into a standard, computer interpretable format based on XML markups. In this paper, we introduce a novel approach to the process of structuring textual guidelines, based on their actual linguistic content. Because guidelines are organized around recommendations, they tend to contain specific linguistic expressions which organize the medical knowledge they convey. Our initial hypothesis was that the automatic processing of such linguistic expressions could be used to automatically derive a document structure, while at the same time being tractable due to the limited number of these linguistic forms. This prototype is integrated into our G-DEE (Guideline Document Engineering Environment) environment, a document processing tool dedicated to the study of Clinical Guidelines. We conclude by presenting example results and analyzing system performance.

2. Material and Methods

Our source of inspiration was previous research in document processing, essentially for knowledge extraction from prescriptive texts, such as legal documents. These share many similarities with Clinical Guidelines at the linguistic level, both in terms of style and textual genre. Moulin and Rousseau [3] have described a method to automatically extract knowledge from legal texts based on the concept of *"deontic operators"*. They found that the contents of prescriptive statements are specified by "normative propositions", which in the French texts studied by Moulin and Rousseau manifest themselves through such verbs as *"pouvoir"* (to be allowed to or may), *"devoir"* (should or ought to), *"interdire"* (to forbid). Von Wright [4], who developed deontic logic, considered normative statements as "a statement to the effect that something ought to or may or must not be done. Deontic propositions have been found by Kalinowski [5] to be the most characteristic linguistic structures of normative texts. Moulin and Rousseau showed that knowledge extraction from legal texts based on deontic operators is a convenient way to resolve problems of knowledge acquisition from texts, without having to take into account the detailed meaning of recommendations, using them instead to structure the document.

The purpose of this research is to investigate the potential of automatic recognition of deontic operators to structure Clinical Guidelines. The automatic structuring of Clinical Guidelines can support their encoding through markup languages such as GEM, or the generation of IF-THEN rules from their contents [6].

Linguistic Analysis: Lexicometric Studies

To validate the above hypothesis on the role of deontic verbs in Clinical Guidelines we first carried a lexicometric analysis on a corpus of 20 Clinical Guidelines (in French) published by the ANAES[1], the French National Agency for Accreditation and Health Evaluation.

We first studied the frequency of deontic verbs for the set of 20 Clinical Guidelines collected. We used the statistical text analysis software *Tropes*[2] to analyze these documents, particularly words occurrences and lemmatized verbs. The corpus is composed of 280 pages containing 83 997 word occurrences. We counted 1137 occurrences of verbs indicating deontic modalities (for the verbs *"devoir"* (should or ought to), *"pouvoir"* (to be allowed to), *"recommander"* (to recommend) and *"convenir"* (to be appropriate)). We considered "to recommend" (*"recommander"*) as a deontic modality due to the fact that in medical texts it always expresses recommendations. These verbs account for 18 % of all occurrences of verbs in the corpus (7686 occurrences for the set of verbs), while deontic verbs only represent 3% of the verbs in the corpus vocabulary. We also noticed an important number of occurrences of verbs indicating deontic modalities, in individual texts (from 18 to 111 occurrences). Another property that needs to be investigated is the distribution of deontic operators throughout the text. Clinical Guidelines being a set of structured recommendations, one would expect deontic operators to be distributed in a way which is consistent with these documents' style. By analyzing the distribution of the principal verbs constitutive of deontic operators (i.e. in French *"recommander"* (to recommend)) in each guideline, we obtained several distribution patterns. All these patterns share two common features. The first one is the scope of distribution, which spans across the entire text. The second one is the recurrence of groupings of deontic verbs. The latter finding is an indicator of textual structure, namely the repetition of deontic operators within specific sections.

---

[1] http://www.anaes.fr
[2] http://www.acetic.fr/

Defining the Grammar of Deontic Operators

Our next step is to design a tool for the automatic recognition of deontic operators, which feature deontic verbs within specific syntactic structures. Those syntactic structures also relate the deontic operator to the remainder of the text, a property which will be used for automatic text structuring. To identify specific syntactic structures we have studied the occurrences of deontic verbs in context. In order to define a grammar for the recognition of deontic operators, we used a variant of our corpus, which comprises 17 documents, and also includes consensus conferences and medical teaching material (in the field of diabetes, hypertension, asthma, dyslipidemias, epilepsy, renal disease). This enables to collect examples of variability in the authoring of medical documents so as to improve coverage. We used the *"Simple Concordance Program (release 4.07)*[3]*"* to analyze these documents. This program provides scopes for each word in the corpus, as shown below deontic operators are: "is then recommended" (in French, *"est donc recommandée"*), "are not recommended" (*"ne sont pas recommandées"*), "should be proposed" (*"doit être proposé"*), "may then be advised" (*"peut être alors conseillé"*).

> *une insulinothérapie* ***est donc recommandée*** *lorsque l'HbA1C*
> *traitement oral* ***ne sont pas recommandées****, sauf en cas de*
> *traitant les addictions* ***doit être proposé*** *aux patients*
> *thérapeutique* ***peut être alors conseillée****. L'interrogatoire*

As previously described by Moulin and Rousseau, the first set of deontic operators is composed of *"pouvoir"* (to be allowed to or may) and *"devoir"* (should or ought to). By analyzing scopes of these deontic operators, we observed that these verbs are mainly followed by a verb in an infinitive form, which generally corresponds to a specification of the deontic operator. We also observed that deontic operators most often occur at the passive voice. In addition, we identified a set of deontic operators that appear to be specific to Clinical Guidelines. For example, in French *"recommander"* (to recommend), *"conseiller"* (to advise), or *"préférer"* (to prefer). By analyzing the scopes of these deontic operators, we observed that these verbs as well occur mostly in the passive voice (i.e. auxiliary followed by the past participle form of the verb). In order to define the coverage of a grammar recognizing these deontic operators from their surface form, we studied their expressions in our corpus, which led to the identification of 56 syntactic patterns for deontic operators corresponding to their various surface forms.

Automatic Recognition of Deontic Operators

The identification of deontic operators is based on a dedicated parser, which analyzes the whole document using our specialized grammar. We chose to use Finite-State Transition Networks (FSTN) [7] as a syntactic formalism. One reason was that they provide a convenient way to define specialized structures, including their morphological variants. Another rationale was their performance on certain Information Extraction (IE) tasks [8] (such as named entity recognition), which are similar to the recognition of deontic structures. Using results from our corpus analysis, we defined a complete set of FSTN to represent the surface forms of deontic operators. From the 56 syntactic patterns identified, we defined 546 FSTN to take into account morphological variants. An example of a FSTN is given in Figure 2 (deontic operators can contain negative statements as well, which means that the negation of a deontic operator does not have to be processed independently). Another aspect that needs to be represented is the relation between the operator and the surrounding text, in other words how the deontic operator actually structures the document. We defined, following Moulin and Rousseau [3], an operator's scope as that part of the

---

sentence to which the modal operator applies. A scope that precedes a modal operator is called *front-scope*, whereas the *back-scope* corresponds to a scope which follows the operator (see Figure 3). The actual parsing process identifies deontic operators in the guideline document and marks them up, together with the relevant text sections which constitute their *back-scope* and *front-scope* (Figure 1). It has been implemented as a two-stage process: the first stage is dedicated to the recognition and marking up of deontic operators in the textual document. The second stage uses the document marked up for deontic operators to specify their associated scopes.

Parsing Strategy

The FSTN grammar for deontic operators is contained in an external file which is loaded at the beginning of the automatic processing step (see Figure 1). Each sentence of the textual guideline is parsed in sequence by determining the relevant FSTN.

During parsing, FSTN are activated from the recognition of key vocabulary: once activated the corresponding text portion is parsed using generic parsing functions applied to the FSTN contents. Upon successful parsing the deontic operator is identified and marked up as such in the document (see Figure 4).

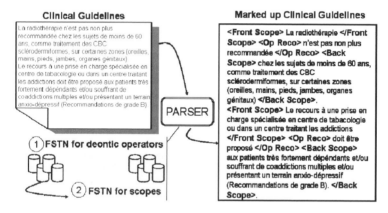

Figure 1 – Structuring of Clinical Guidelines through the recognition of deontic operators and their front- and back-scope.

A conflict resolution step determines the most relevant FSTN when several of them can be activated (for instance, due to shared patterns). By default, the most appropriate pattern is the pattern containing the largest number of concordances hence the more specific one. The application of a given FSTN recognizes a specific occurrence of a deontic operator in the text: it does not give raise to an instantiated representation but to the marking up of the textual occurrence of the specific operator recognized in the text.

Validation

We tested our FSTN parser on 5 randomly selected Clinical Guidelines among the 20 considered in our statistical analysis. None of these 5 texts has been used for the definition of our deontic operators' grammar. For this evaluation, we mainly focused on the correct identification of the following deontic verbs: *"recommander"* (to recommend), *"devoir"* *(should or ought to)*, *"pouvoir"* (to be allowed to or may) and *"convenir"* *(be appropriate)*. For each Clinical Guideline, we counted the number of correctly marked up occurrences of deontic verbs. As a preliminary result, 95.5% of documents in our test set (which contains

311 deontic operators) are correctly marked up (in terms of operator identification as well as *front-scope* and *back-scope* recognition). The 4.5% of errors identified arise from a few specific syntactic phenomena which had not previously been identified.

3. Example Results

We present two examples of marking up for the operator "*recommander*" (to recommend) and the operator "*devoir*" (should or ought to) (cf. Figure 4). The first occurrence of "*recommander*" (to recommend) illustrates the recognition of that operator expressed in the passive voice and in a negative form, using the FSTN of Figure 2. The second shows the direct recognition of the passive voice for "*devoir*" (should or ought to).

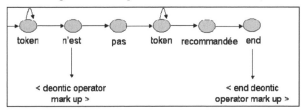

Figure 2 – FSTN for the recognition "is not recommended" deontic operator.

While the first step of document structuring marks up all occurrences of deontic operators, the second step identifies the operator's scopes. It does so by parsing the guideline previously marked up for deontic operators using another dedicated FSTN (Figure 3), which recognizes punctuation signs as well as markups inserted in the previous step.

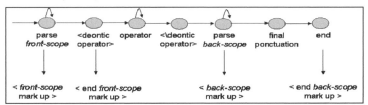

Figure 3 – FSTN for recognizing front- and back-scope for deontic operator previously recognized in Figure 2.

The final result is presented on Figure 4, which shows the kind of structuring produced on a portion of textual guidelines.

<Front Scope> La radiothérapie **</Front Scope>** **<Op Deont>** n'est pas non plus recommandée **</Op Deont>** **<Back Scope>** chez les sujets de moins de 60 ans, comme traitement des CBC sclérodermiformes, sur certaines zones (oreilles, mains, pieds, jambes, organes génitaux) **</Back Scope>**.[4]

<Front Scope> Le recours à une prise en charge spécialisée en centre de tabacologie ou dans un centre traitant les addictions **</Front Scope>** **<Op Deont>** doit être proposé **</Op Deont>** **<Back Scope>** aux patients très fortement dépendants et/ou souffrant de coaddictions multiples et/ou présentant un terrain anxio-dépressif (Recommandations de grade B) **</Back Scope>**.[5]

Figure 4 – Results of marking up deontic operators.

---

[4] **<Front Scope>** Radiotherapy **</Front Scope>** **<Op Deont>** is not recommended either **</Op Deont>** **<Back Scope>** for persons under 60 years of age, as treatment of sclerodermiforms CBC, or on certains body parts (ears, hands, feet, legs, genitals) **</Back Scope>**.

[5] **<Front Scope>** Referral to a specialized center treating addiction to tobacco **</Front Scope>** **<Op Deont>** should be proposed **</Op Deont>** **<Back Scope>** to the patients strongly dependants and/or suffering of multiple coaddictions and/or presenting an anxio-dependance context (Recommendations of grade B) **</Back Scope>**.

4. Conclusion

In this study, we discussed the role of deontic expressions in Clinical Guidelines and how these contribute to the textual structure of Clinical Guidelines. We showed that their automatic recognition using a dedicated FSTN parser supports the automatic structuring of the document. Our first prototype integrated into the G-DEE environment correctly marked up 95.5% of the occurrences of deontic expressions on a test set composed of Clinical Guidelines not used in the initial grammar definition. An analysis of recognition errors suggested that simple extensions of the recognition grammar could further improve the recognition score. The automatic detection of deontic operators can be a useful step to support Clinical Guidelines encoding in document-based approaches such as GEM. They can also serve as a pre-processing tool for knowledge acquisition from textual guidelines, where they would assist in the identification of expressions that could be converted into IF-THEN rules. A valuable extension of this approach would consist in the further processing of the textual contents of a deontic operator's *back-scope* and *front-scope*, which would identify relevant expressions, such as those denoting medical treatments. Such processing can be based on terminological recognition or information extraction methods such as named entity recognition.

References

[1]   Peleg M, Tu S, Bury J, Ciccarese P, Fox J, Greenes R, et al. Comparing Computer-Interpretable Guideline Models: A Case-Study Approach. *J Am Med Inf Assoc* 2003, 10(1):52-68.

[2]   Shiffman R, Karras B, Agrawal A, Chen R, Marenco L, Nath S. GEM: A Proposal for a More Comprehensive Guideline Document Model Using XML. *J Am Med Informatics Assoc* 2000, 7:488-498.

[3]   Moulin B and Rousseau D. Knowledge Acquisition from Prescriptive Texts. In: *ACM: 1990*; 1990: 1112-1121.

[4]   Von Wright G-H. "The Foundation of Norms and Normative Statements". *Philosophical Papers, Oxford, Blackwell* 1983:67-82.

[5]   Kalinowski G. La Logique Déductive. Presses Universitaires de France (in French); 1996.

[6]   Georg G, Séroussi B, Bouaud J. Does GEM-Encoding Clinical Practice Guidelines improve the Quality of Knowledge Bases? A Study with the Rule-Based Formalism. In: *Proceedings of the Amer Med Informatics Assoc: 2003; Washington, DC*; 2003: 254-258.

[7]   Roche E and Schabes Y. Finite-State Language Processing. MIT Press; 1997.

[8]   Pazienza M T. Information Extraction: A Multidisciplinary Approach to an Emerging Information Technology, vol. 1299: Springer-Verlag; 1997.

Address for correspondence

Gersende Georg
INSERM, U729; SPIM, 15 rue de l'Ecole de Médecine, F-75006 Paris, France.
Gersende.Georg@spim.jussieu.fr

Connecting Medical Informatics and Bio-Informatics
R. Engelbrecht et al. (Eds.)
IOS Press, 2005

Prototypical Cases and Adaptation Rules for Diagnosis of Dysmorphic Syndromes

Rainer Schmidt, Tina Waligora

Institut für Medizinische Informatik und Biometrie, University of Rostock
Rostock, Germany

Abstract

Since diagnosis of dysmorphic syndromes is a domain with incomplete knowledge and where even experts have seen only few syndromes themselves during their lifetime, documentation of cases and the use of case-oriented techniques are popular. In dysmorphic systems, diagnosis usually is performed as a classification task, where a prototypicality measure is applied to determine the most probable syndrome. These measures differ from the usual Case-Based Reasoning similarity measures, because here cases and syndromes are not represented as attribute value pairs but as long lists of symptoms, and because query cases are not compared with cases but with prototypes. In contrast to most dysmorphic systems our approach additionally applies adaptation rules. These rules do not only consider single symptoms but combinations of them, which indicate high or low probabilities of specific syndromes.

Keywords:
Dysmorphic Syndromes; Case-Based Reasonin;, Prototype;, Adaptation

1. Introduction

When a child is born with dysmorphic features or with multiple congenital malformations or if mental retardation is observed at a later stage, finding the correct diagnosis is extremely important. Knowledge of the nature and the etiology of the disease enables the paediatrician to predict the patient's future course. So, an initial goal for medical specialists is to diagnose a patient to a recognised syndrome. Genetic counselling and a course of treatments shall afterwards be established.

A dysmorphic syndrome describes a morphological disorder and it is characterised by a combination of various symptoms, which form a pattern of morphologic defects. An example is Down Syndrome which can be described in terms of characteristic clinical and radiographic manifestations such as mental retardation, sloping forehead, a flat nose, short broad hands and generally dwarfed physique [1].

The main problems of diagnosing dysmorphic syndromes are as follows [2]:

- more than 200 syndromes are known,
- many cases remain undiagnosed with respect to known syndromes,
- usually many symptoms are used to describe a case (between 40 and 130),
- every dysmorphic syndrome is characterised by nearly as many symptoms.

Furthermore, knowledge about dysmorphic disorders is continuously modified, new cases are observed that cannot be diagnosed (a special journal publishes nothing but reports of observed interesting cases [3]), and sometimes even new syndromes are discovered.

Usually, even experts of paediatric genetics only see a small count of dysmorphic syndromes during their lifetime.

So, we have developed a diagnostic system that uses a large case base. Starting point to build the case base was a large case collection of the paediatric genetics of the University of Munich, which consists of nearly 2.000 cases and 229 prototypes. A prototype (prototypical case) represents a dysmorphic syndrome by its typical symptoms. Most of the dysmorphic syndromes are already known and have been defined in literature. And nearly one third of our entire cases have been determined by semiautomatic knowledge acquisition, where an expert has selected cases that should belong to the same syndrome and subsequently a prototype has been generated, characterised by the most frequent symptoms of his cases. To this database we have added cases from "clinical dysmorphology" [3] and syndromes from the London dysmorphic database [4], which contains only rare dysmorphic syndromes.

1.1   Diagnostic systems for dysmorphic syndromes

The first systems to support diagnosis of dysmorphic syndromes have already been developed in the early 80ties. The simple ones perform just information retrieval for rare syndromes, namely the London dysmorphic database [3], where syndromes a described by symptoms, and the Australian POSSUM, where syndromes are visualised [5]. Diagnosis by classification is done in a system developed by Wiener and Anneren [6]. They use more than 200 syndromes as database and apply Bayesian probability to determine the most probable syndromes. Another diagnostic system, which uses data from the London dysmorphic database was developed by Evans [7]. Though he claims to apply Case-Based Reasoning, in fact it is again just a classification, this time performed by Tversky's measure of dissimilarity [8]. The most interesting aspect of his approach is the use of weights for the symptoms. That means the symptoms are categorised in three groups – independent of the specific syndromes, instead only according to their intensity of expressing retardation or malformation. However, Evans admits that even features, that are usually unimportant or occur in very many syndromes sometimes play a vital role for discrimination between specific syndromes.

In our system the user can chose between two measures of dissimilarity for concepts, namely one developed by Tversky [8] and the other one proposed by Rosch and Mervis [9]. However, the novelty of our approach is that we do not only perform classification but subsequently apply adaptation rules. These rules do not only consider single symptoms but specific combinations of them, which indicate high or low probabilities of specific syndromes.

1.2   Medical Case-Based Reasoning systems

Since the idea of Case-Based Reasoning (CBR) is to use former, already solved solutions (represented in form of cases) for current problems [10], CBR seems to be appropriate for diagnosis of dysmorphic syndromes. CBR consists of two main tasks [11], namely retrieval, that means searching for similar cases, and adaptation, that means adapting solutions of similar cases to a query case. For retrieval usually explicit similarity measures or, especially for large case bases, faster retrieval algorithms like Nearest Neighbour Matching [12] are applied. For adaptation only few general techniques exist [13], usually domain specific adaptation rules have to be acquired. In [14] we have presented an overview of medical CBR systems. For more recent developments see [15].

1.3   Prototypicality measures

In CBR usually cases are represented as attribute-value pairs. In medicine, especially in diagnostic applications, this is not always the case. Instead often a list of symptoms describes a patient's disease. Sometimes these lists can be very long, and often their lengths are not fixed but vary with the patient. For dysmorphic syndromes usually between 40 and 130 symptoms are used to characterise a patient.

Furthermore, for dysmorphic syndromes it is unreasonable to search for single similar patients (and of course none of the systems mentioned above does so) but for more general prototypes that contain the typical features of a syndrome. Prototypes are a generalisation from single cases. They fill the knowledge gap between the specificity of single cases and abstract knowledge in form of rules. Though the use of prototypes had been early introduced in the CBR community [16, 17], their use is still rather seldom. However, since doctors reason with typical cases anyway, in medical CBR systems prototypes are a rather common knowledge form (e.g. for antibiotics therapy advice in ICONS [18], for diabetes [19], and for eating disorders [20]).

So, to determine the most similar prototype for a given query patient instead of a similarity measure a prototypicality measure is required. One speciality is that for prototypes the lists of symptoms are usually much shorter than for single cases.

The results should not be just the one and only most similar prototype, but a list of them, sorted according to their similarity. So, the usual CBR methods like indexing or nearest neighbour search are inappropriate. Instead, rather old measures for dissimilarities between concepts [8, 9] are applied and explained in the next section.

2. Diagnosis of dysmorphic syndromes

Our system performs four steps. At first the user has to select the symptoms that characterise a new patient. This selection is a long and very time consuming process, because we consider more than 800 symptoms. However, diagnosis of dysmorphic syndromes is not a task where result are extremely urgent, but it usually requires thorough reasoning and afterwards a long-term therapy has to be started.

Since our system is still in the evaluation phase, secondly the user can select a prototypicality measure. In routine use, this step shall be dropped and the measure with best evaluation results shall be used automatically. At present there are three choices.

Since humans look upon cases as more typical for a query case as more features they have in common [9], distances between prototypes and cases usually consider the shared features.

The first, rather simple measure just counts the number of matching symptoms of a query patient (X) and a prototype (Y) and normalises the result by dividing it by the number of symptoms characterising the prototype. This normalisation is done, because the lengths of the lists of symptoms of the various prototypes vary very much. It is performed by the two other measures too. In the following formulae the function F is supposed to be the sum – exactly as we used it. However, in principle various weightings are possible.

$$D(X,Y) = \frac{f(X+Y)}{f(Y)}$$

The second measure was developed by Tversky [8]. It is a measure of dissimilarity for concepts. In contrast to the first measure, additionally two numbers are subtracted from the number of matching symptoms. Firstly, the number of symptoms that are observed for the query patient but are not used to characterise the prototype (X-Y), and secondly the number of symptoms used for the prototype but are not observed for the patient (Y-X) is subtracted.

$$D_{Tversky}(X,Y) = \frac{f(X+Y) - f(X-Y) - f(Y-X)}{f(Y)}$$

The third prototypicality measure was proposed by Rosch and Mervis [9]. It differs from Tversky's measure only in one point: the factor X-Y is not considered:

$$D_{Rosch,\,Mervis}(X,Y) = \frac{f(X+Y) - f(Y-X)}{f(Y)}$$

In the third step to diagnose dysmorphoic syndromes, the chosen measure is sequentially applied on all prototypes (syndromes). Since the syndrome with maximal similarity is not always the right one, the 20 syndromes with best similarities are listed in a menu (fig. 1).

Figure 1-Top part of the listed prototypes

Most similar prototypes:	
Names of the prototypes	Similarities
☐ SHPRINTZEN-SYNDROM	0.49
☐ LENZ-SYNDROM	0.36
☐ BOERJESON-FORSSMAN-LEHMANN-S.	0.34
☐ STURGE-WEBER-SYNDROM	0.32

2.1 Application of adaptation rules

In the fourth and final step, the user can optionally choose to apply adaptation rules on the syndromes. These rules state that specific combinations of symptoms favour or disfavour specific dysmorphic syndromes. Unfortunately, the acquisition of these adaptation rules is very difficult, because they cannot be found in textbooks but have to be defined by experts of paediatric genetics. So far, we have got only 10 of them and so far, it is not possible that a syndrome can be favoured by one adaptation rule and disfavoured by another one at the same time. When we, hopefully, acquire more rules such a situation should in principle be possible but would indicate some sort of inconsistency of the rule set.

How shall the adaptation rules alter the results? Our first idea was that adaptation rules should increase or decrease the similarity scores for favoured and disfavoured syndromes. But the question is how. Of course no medical expert can determine values to manipulate the similarities by adaptation rules and any general value for favoured or disfavoured syndromes would be arbitrary. So, instead the result after applying adaptation rules is a menu that contains up to three lists (fig. 2). On top the favoured syndromes are depicted, then those neither favoured nor disfavoured, and at the bottom the disfavoured ones. Additionally, the user can get information about the specific rules that have been applied on a particular syndrome.

In the example presented by the figures 1 and 2 the right diagnosis is Lenz-syndrome. The computation of the prototypicality measure of Rosch and Mervis Lenz-syndrome was the most similar but one syndrome. After application of adaptation rules, the ranking is not obvious. Two syndromes have been favoured, the more similar one is the right one. However, Dubowitz-syndrome is favoured too (by a completely different rule), because a specific combination of symptoms makes it probable, while other observed symptoms indicate a rather low similarity.

Names of the prototypes	Similarities	Applied rule
PROBABLE prototypes after application of the adaptation rules:		
☐ LENZ-SYNDROM	0.36	☐ REGEL-6
☐ DUBOWITZ-SYNDROM	0.24	☐ REGEL-9
Prototypes, no adaptation rules could be applied:		
☐ SHPRINTZEN-SYNDROM	0.49	
☐ BOERJESON-FORSSMAN-LEHMANN-S.	0.34	
☐ STURGE-WEBER-SYNDROM	0.32	
☐ LEOPARD-SYNDROM	0.31	

Figure 2. Top part of the listed prototypes after application of adaptation rules

3. Results

Cases are difficult to diagnose when patients suffer from a very rare dymorphic syndrome for which neither detailed information can be found in literature nor many cases are stored in our case base. This makes evaluation difficult. If test cases are randomly chosen, frequently observed cases resp. syndromes are frequently selected and the results will probably be fine, because these syndromes are well-known. However, the main idea of our system is to support diagnosis of rare syndromes. So, we have chosen our test cases randomly but under the condition that every syndrome can be chosen only once.

For 100 cases we have compared the results obtained by both prototypicality measures (table 1).

Table 1. Comparison of prototypicality measures

Right Syndrome	Rosch and Mervis	Tversky
on Top	29	40
among top 3	57	57
among top 10	76	69

Obviously, the measure of Tversky provides better results, especially when the right syndrome should be on top of the list of probable syndromes. When it should be only among the first three of this list, both measures provide equal results.

Since the acquisition of adaptation rules is very difficult and time consuming the number of acquired rules is rather limited, namely 10 rules. Furthermore, again holds: the better a syndrome is known, the easier adaptation rules can be generated. So, the improvement mainly depends on the question how many syndromes involved by adaptation rules are among the test set. In our experiment this was the case only for 5 syndromes. Since some syndromes had been already diagnose correctly without adaptation, there was just a small improvement (table 2).

Table 2. Results after the application of adaptation rules

Right Syndrome	Rosch and Mervis	Tversky
on Top	32	42
among top 3	59	59
among top 10	77	71

4. Summary

In this paper, we have presented our system to support diagnosis of dysmorphic syndromes. Our system, which is still under development, is not only based on single cases but mainly on meaningful prototypes. The diagnosis consists of two steps: first similar prototypes are calculated, and subsequently adaptation rules are applied.

For calculating similar prototypes, we have presented two sequential prototypicality measures. Our first test results do not show any significant difference between them.

For adaptation, our system still lacks of a sufficient number of adaptation rules. These rules are very difficult to acquire and it takes up a lot of our present work. The more a dysmorphic syndrome is studied, the easier it is for experts to express an adaptation rule. This is especially unfortunate, because the main idea of our diagnostic support program is to provide support for rare dysmorphic syndromes.

5. Acknowledgement

The project is funded by the German Research Society (DFG).

6. References

[1]   Taybi H and Lachman RS. Radiology of Syndromes, Metabolic Disorders, and Skeletal Dysplasia. Year Book Medical Publishers, Chicago, 1990

[2]   Gierl L and Stengel-Rutkowski S. Integrating Consultation and Semi-automatic Knowledge Acquisition in a Prototype-based Architecture: Experiences with Dysmorphic Syndromes. *Artif Intell Med* 1994: 6 pp. 29-49

[3]   Clinical Dysmorphology. www.clindysmorphol.com

[4]   Winter RM, Baraitser M and Douglas JM. A computerised data base for the diagnosis of rare dysmorphic syndromes. *Journal of medical genetics* 1984: 21 (2) pp.121-123

[5]   Stromme P. The diagnosis of syndromes by use of a dysmorphology database. *Acta Paeditr Scand* 1991: 80 (1) pp.106-109

[6]   Weiner F and Anneren G. PC-based system for classifying dysmorphic syndromes in children. *Computer Methods and Programs in Biomedicine* 1989: 28 pp. 111-117

[7]   Evans CD. A case-based assistant for diagnosis and analysis of dysmorphic syndromes. *Int J Med Inform* 1995: 20 pp. 121-131

[8]   Tversky A. Features of Similarity. *Psychological Review* 1977: 84 (4) pp. 327-352

[9]   Rosch E and Mervis CB. Family Resemblance: Studies in the Internal Structures of Categories. *Cognitive Psychology* 1975: 7 pp. 573-605

[10]   Kolodner J. Case-Based Reasoning. Morgan Kaufmann, San Mateo, 1993

[11]   Aamodt A and Plaza E. Case-Based Reasoning: Foundation issues, methodological variation, and system approaches. *AICOM* 1994: 7 pp. 39-59

[12]   Broder A. Strategies for efficient incremental nearest neighbor search. Pattern Recognition 1990: 23 pp. 171-178

[13]   Wilke W, Smyth B and Cunningham P. Using configuration techniques for adaptation. In: Lenz M et al., eds. Case-Based Reasoning technology, from foundations to applications. Springer, Berlin, 1998; pp. 139-168

[14]   Gierl L, Bull M and Schmidt R. CBR in medicine. In: Lenz M et al., eds. Case-Based Reasoning Technology, Springer, Berlin, 1998; pp. 273-297

[15]   Nilsson M, Sollenborn M: Advancements and trends in medical case-based Reasoning: An overview of systems and system developments. In: Proc of FLAIRS, AAAI Press, 2004; pp. 178-183

[16]   Schank RC. Dynamic Memory: a theory of learning in computer and people. Cambridge University Press, New York, 1982

[17]   Bareiss R. Exemplar-based knowledge acquisition. Academic Press, San Diego, 1989

[18]   Schmidt R and Gierl L. Case-based Reasoning for antibiotics therapy advice: an investigation of retrieval algorithms and prototypes. *Artif Intell Med* 2001: 23 pp. 171-186

[19]   Bellazzi R, Montani S, and Portinale L. Retrieval in a prototype-based case library: a case study in diabetes therapy revision. In: Smyth B and Cunningham P, eds. Proceedings of European Workshop on Case-Based Reasoning, Springer, Berlin, 1998; pp. 64-75

[20]   Bichindaritz I. From cases to classes: focusing on abstraction in case-based reasoning. In: Burkhard H-D and Lenz M, eds. Proceedings of German Workshop on Case-Based Reasoning, University Press, Berlin, 1996; pp. 62-69

Address for correspondence

Dr. Rainer Schmidt, Inst. für Medizinische Informatik und Biometrie, Universität Rostock, Rembrandtstr. 16/1, D-18055 Rostock,Tel.: +49.381.494.7307, rainer.schmidt@uni-rostock.de

Connecting Medical Informatics and Bio-Informatics
R. Engelbrecht et al. (Eds.)
IOS Press, 2005

Knowledge Discovery on Functional Disabilities: Clustering Based on Rules versus other Approaches

K Gibert[a], R Annicchiarico[b], U Cortés[c], C Caltagirone[b,d]

[a] Statistics and Operation Research Department. Universitat Politècnica de Catalunya.
[b] IRCCS Santa Lucia Foundation. Via Ardeatina 306. Roma, Italy
[c] Software Department. Universitat Politècnica de Catalunya
[d] Universit`a Tor Vergata, Roma, Italy

Abstract

In Europe senior citizens are a fast growing part of population, increasing proportion of disabled persons and that of persons with reduced quality of life. The concept of disability itself is not always precise and quantifiable. To improve agreement on it, the World Health Organization (WHO) developed the clinical test WHO Disability Assessment Schedule, (WHO-DASII) that includes physical, mental, and social well-being, as a generic measure of functioning. From the medical point of view, the purpose of this work is to extract knowledge about performance of the WHO-DASII using a sample of patients from an italian hospital.
This Knowledge Discovery problem has been faced by using clustering based on rules, an hybrid AI and Statistics technique introduced by Gibert (1994), which combines some Inductive Learning (from AI) with clustering (from Statistics) to extract knowledge from certain complex domains in form of tipical profiles. In this paper, the results of applying this technique to the WHO-DASII results is presented together with a comparison of other more classical analysis approaches.

Keywords:
Disability; Scale (clinical test); Assessment, Neurological Disease; Knowledge Discovery; Clustering based on Rules; Knowledge-based Applications in Medicine.

1. Introduction

The senior citizens represent a fast growing proportion of the population in Europe and other developed areas. Today [18], 629 million of persons aged 60 years or older is estimated to be around the world; it is expected to grow about 2 billion by 2050, when the population of older persons will be larger than that of children (0-14 years) for the first time in human history. The largest proportion (54%) of this people lives in Asia; Europe is the second (24%). This ageing population increases the proportion of individuals with physical and/or mental impairment that need any help for the daily tasks. According to Laselett [11], "*the human life span is now divided into four ages: the first is an age of dependency, childhood and education, the second is an age of indepen-dence, maturity, and responsibility, and although the third age is considered a period of fulfillment for physically and mentally fit people in retirement, the fourth age is associated with chronic diseases, disability and dependence*". A direct consequence is the increasing number of people affected by chronic diseases, such as heart disease, cancer and mental disorders, which are fast becoming the world's leading causes of death and disability. In fact, according to the *World Health Report 2001* [20], 59% of whole-world deaths relate to non-communicable diseases. In both developed and developing countries, chronic diseases are significant and costly causes of disability and reduced quality of life. Size and pattern of the fourth age is critical for the quality of life of elderly people but also for the use of health and social services [2]. Functional ability (FA), highly correlated with physical and mental health, is an important determinant of quality of life [17], and to measure it is increasingly important. Activities of Daily Living (*ADL*) rating scales are widely used for that [10]. However, disability scales typically including bathing, toileting, eating, dressing, and transferring from bed to a chair, like ADL, have been criticized. There is lack of consensus about measurement of FA [12]. The WHO, proposed a new reference classification (*ICF*) and an assessment instrument (*WHO-DASII*) [13] to complement the process (see bellow).

In this work, the functional disability degree of a neurological patients set is evaluated using *WHO-DASII*. First, extracting knowledge contained in the database to see how *WHO-DASII* provides information for identifying typical profiles of disabled patients. Afterwards relationships between *WHO-DASII* and other scales, like *SF36*, will be analyzed as well. Typical answers to *WHO-DASII* need first to be identified, together with the characteristics of the groups of patients providing each *type* of answers. This raises a clustering problem, but classical clustering cannot well recognize certain domain structures [7], producing some non-sense classes that cannot be interpreted by the experts. In fact, this happens with *ill-structured domains (ISD)* [4] [5], where numerical and qualitative information coexists, and there is relevant semantic additional (but partial) knowledge to be regarded.

Clustering based on rules (ClBR) [4] is especially introduced by Gibert to improve clustering results on *ISD*. It guarantees the semantic meaning of the resulting classes. Since an *ISD* is faced here, this work will show the advantages of *ClBR* vs other approaches.

Contents of the paper is: Introduction to the *WHO-DASII* scale, description of the target sample and the characteristics of the study, description of the analysis methodology, details on *ClBR*, results of applying *CLBR* to the sample and comparison with other approaches.

2. Methods

Scales and ontologies

The International Classification of Functioning

Regarding the controversy about disability, the *WHO* provided a common framework and language for the description of health and health-related domains. ICF (*International Classification of Functioning, Disability and Health*) defines components of functioning and disability, activities and participation [20]. It is a review of ICIDH-2 [19], moving from a classification of *consequences of disease* (1980 version) to a *components of health*; is the newest version of disability classification, systematically grouping different domains for persons in a given health condition (what a person with a disease or disorder can do or does). As f*unctioning* encompasses all body functions, participation and activities, *disability* encompasses impairments, activity limitations or participation restrictions. *ICF* lists environmental factors interacting with these constructs, allowing records of useful profiles of individuals' functioning, disability and health in various domains.

WHO-DAS II scale

WHO-DASII (*World Health Organization Disablement Assessment Schedule*) is a scale especially designed and proposed by the *WHO* [13], for assessing disability levels according to *ICIDH-2* (and with *ICF*). It includes mental health factors related to disability together with physical ones in the same set of instruments. It is a fully-structured interview measuring self-reported difficulty of functioning in six major domains considered important in most cultures: *Understanding & Communicating* (6 it), *Getting Around* (5 it), *Self Care* (4 it), *Getting Along with People* (5 it), *Life Activities* (8 it) and *Participation in Society* (8 it).

The *WHO-DASII* employs a 5 point rating scale for all items (1 is used for no difficulty and 5 for extreme difficulty or inability to perform the activity). Six *WHO-DASII* domain scores may be obtained by summing the answers in each domain, normalizing them on a 0 to 100 scale (expressing percentages) in such a way that higher values represent greater disability. Information related to the extent of disruption in life caused by these difficulties, extends of difficulties experienced in life and extends of dependence of assistive devices or other persons is considered as well. Items usually enquire about the last 30 days. Validation of *WHO-DASII* is in progress in international field trials (16 centers of 14 countries). Sample (1564) was drawn from population with physical, mental, drug, alcohol problems and general.

Experimental procedure

The target sample includes 96 neurological patients between 17 and 80 years, who were recovering at the *IRCCS Fondazione Santa Lucia di Roma* between October 1999 and February 2000. A control group of 20 healthy people, have also been enrolled.

Functional status and health-related quality of life of all patients was measured with *WHO-DASII* at admission. Patients were evaluated upon two other standardized clinical scales: Functional status was quantified using the *Functional Independence Measure (FIM)*. The *FIM* is a well-established measure for which reliability and validity have been proved. Patients' Quality of Life *(QOL)* was quantified using the *Short Form (SF-36)*, see [16].

Data analysis methodology

Here, a brief description of the whole proposed analysis methodology is presented: First, d*escriptive statistics of every variable* was done. Very simple statistical techniques [15] were used to describe data and to get preliminary information: histograms or bar charts to display variability, plots and multiple box-plots to observe the relationship between some pairs of variables, etc; classical summary statistics were also calculated. Next, *data cleaning*, including missing data treatment or outlier detection was performed. It is a very important phase, since the quality of final results directly depends on it. Decisions are taken on the basis of descriptive statistics and background knowledge of the experts.

Data was analyzed using three methods: *i)* Following the classical approach, the behavior of g*lobal WHO-DASII score* regarding the patient's pathology was studied. Since the global score is not normal, Kruskall-Wallis test was used to assess significant differences between groups. In case of rejecting null hypothesis, graphical representation is used for interpretation of differences. *ii)* Going into the multivariate approach, first a selection of *WHO-DASII* items was done, avoiding redundancies or inconsistencies. A hierarchical clustering was performed, using chained reciprocal neighbors method, with Ward criterion and the Gibert's *mixed metrics* [3], since both numerical and categorical variables were considered. *iii)* Finally, *clustering based on rules (ClBR)*, described bellow, was used on the same items selection. This paper does not go into mathematical details, just gives an intuitive idea of the method [5]. It was originally presented in [4]. It is a hybrid AI and Statistics technique combining inductive learning (AI) and clustering (Statistics) for KD in *ISD*. A *KB* is considered to properly bias clustering of the database. It is implemented in the software KLASS and it has been successfully used in several real applications. Our experience from previous applications [7] [8] [1] [14] is that using ClBR use to be better than using any statistical clustering method by itself, since an important property of the method is that semantic constraints implied by the *KB* are hold in final clusters; this guarantees interpretability of results, *meaningful* resulting classes. Also, it uses to be better than pure inductive learning methods, reducing the effects of missing some implicit knowledge in the *KB*. The general idea of *ClBR* is:

1. build a *Knowledge Base (KB)* with additional prior knowledge provided by the expert, which can even be a *partial* description of the domain
2. evaluate the *KB* on data for *inductive learning* of an initial partition on part of the data; put the data not included in this partition into the *residual class (RC)*.
3. perform one independent hierarchical clustering for every *rules-induced class (RIC)*.
4. generate prototypes of each *rules-induced class*.
5. build the *extended residual class* as the union of *RC* with the set of prototypes of *RIC*, conveniently weighted by the number of objects they represent.
6. use a hierarchical clustering for weighted clustering of the *extended residual class*.
7. in the resulting dendrogram, substitute every rules-induced prototype by its hierarchical structure, obtained in 3. This integrated all the objects in a single hierarchy.

For methods *ii)* and *iii),* clustering process can be graphically represented in a *dendrogram*. Final number of classes was determined on its best horizontal cut (where the largest gap exists). This identifies a partition of the data in a set of classes. *Interpretation of the classes* was based on conditional distributions of *WHO-DASII* items through the classes, displayed through multiple boxplots, and the corresponding significance tests to assess relevance of differences between classes (ANOVA, Kruskall-Wallis or χ^2 independence test, depending on the item). The aim is to extract qualitative information from the classes, to obtain a meaningful description for the user which indicates particularities of every class.

3. Results

In the sample, 58 patients were males (60.4%) and 38 females (39.6%). Average age was 56 years. Twenty patients had spinal cord injury (age 47.20, s= 17.6), 20 Parkinson (69.25, 6.53), 20 stroke (63.40,15.96), 16 depression (46.56,11.15) and 20 control (55.05,s=15.57)

i) Upon the classical approach, Kruskall-Wallis of *WHO-DASII* global score (GS) *versus* pathology showed signiffical difference ($p < 0.05$). Fig. 1 displays multiple boxplot of GS *vs* pathology: GS only allows distinction between non-disable and disable patients.

ii) With classical hierarchical clustering, 4 classes emerged. However, their interpretation was confusing and physicians could neither identify their *meaning* nor explain *why* depressed patients scattered along classes with other diseases fig.2.

iii) Using *ClBR*, 4 classes (and three outliers) of functional disabilities were found. Look-ing at different variables, a clearer conceptual interpretation of the classes is possible [9]:

Low (Cr93): no problems self-sufficient subjects, neither physical nor mental problems (includes all control patients and a few patients without apparent functional disability).

Intermediate-I (Cd52): moderate mental and/or cognitive disability and physical disability with a low to moderate degree of disability, physical and emotional, with perception of high disability but really showing lower level (e.g. on daily work or standing up to 30 minutes).

Intermediate-II (Cr89): moderate/severe disabilities with exclusive moderate physical disability related to autonomy (difficulties on toileting and dressing), non emotive problems.

High (Cd53): higher disability degree, physical and mental.

Relationship between discovered classes and global *WHO-DASII* score was studied and significant differences were found ($p < 0.05$). Fig. 3 shows increasing scores from group **Low** to **High**, according to the increasing degree of disability represented by the classes.

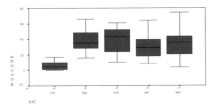

Figure 1 – Multiple boxplot of WHO-DASII Score vs pathology (i).

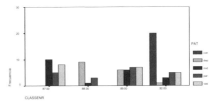

Figure 2 – Pathology versus classes with classical clustering (ii).

4. Discussion, Conclusions and Future Work

As said before, the study is mainly focused on identifying different kinds of responses to the *WHO-DASII* as well as to characterize the groups of respondents of any kind.

The (*i*) analysis only allows a trivial distinction between able and disable, missing the whole potential of *WHO-DASII*, which provides lot of information that, can sensibly enrich analysis. Facing a complex phenomenon as disability, concerned with a lack of consensus, requires a *multivariate approach* considering all the items of the test. Clustering techniques are suitable for detecting groups upon *WHO-DASII* responses. First, an standard clustering (*ii*) was used with Gibert's *mixed metrics*; results had confusing interpretation and the underlying clustering criteria was no clear. Although theoretical properties of solution could be clearly established, non-sense classes are useless in real applications. Patients with disabilities can be considered an *ISD*, as stated in [5] and clustering use to be unable to capture their complex structure by itself. *ClBR* is a more suitable approach (*iii*). Additional knowledge supplied by the experts for *ClBR* regards to emotional problems, since results of method (*ii*) show especially high confusion on this topic. Expressed by means of logical rules, it use to be a *partial* description of the domain (as usual for *ISD*, it is very difficult to make explicit a complete domain-*KB*, what is a great handicap for pure AI methods). Rules used for *ClBR* concern items of *WHO-DASII* regarding *emotive behavior*:

B4: *Rate your mental or emotional health in past 30 days?*
B9: *Worry or distress about your health in the past 30 days?*
S5: *Emotionally affected by your health condition?*
R2: *Have difficulties been caused by mental health or emotional problems?*

People providing values 4 or 5 to that questions should have any kind of emotive problem. So, the proposed *KB* for biasing cluster in method *iii*) is: **KB**={*r1:If B4 is in [4,5] then emotive-problems (EP), r2: If B9 is in [4,5] then EP, r3: If S5 is in [4,5] then EP, r4: If R2 is in [4, 5] then EP*}

ClBR was used with *KB* on the target sample. Rules divided the sample and clustering was done in the single *rules-induced part* (56 patients) as well as on the *extended residual class*, building a global hierarchy. None of the classical statistical methods support expert knowledge influencing the analysis. *ClBR* is a hybrid technique which sensibly improved results, regarding method *ii*) [9], by integrating clinical knowledge inside the analysis.

Finally, a set of 7 classes was recommended by the system. Three of them contain isolated patients that have outlier behavior; they were studied individually. Several tools were used to assist the interpretation of final classes. In case (*iii*), although rules proposed by experts represent partial knowledge on *FD*, the *KB* captured all the depressed patients (which are supposed to have emotive problems), but the clustering divided them into two main subgroups (Fig.3). This still follows understandable criteria: Cd53 has greater physical and mental problems (learning new computes, participating in community, concentrating, working) compared with Cd52; also Cd53 feel that difficulties (including toileting and dressing) affect much more to their life; on the contrary, Cd52 cannot stand up, while Cd53 can do; Cd52 can interact with other people and perform daily activities, while Cd53 cannot. Even with this subdivision, final classes fit on the semantic constraints expressed in *KB* (not to scatter patients with emotive problems along all the classes without criteria). *ClBR* identifies four disability profiles, representing a new taxonomy that contributes to improve the knowledge about Disability. Main group characteristics elicit that, from the medical point of view, groups indeed well correspond to 4 *different profiles* of *FD*, associated with increasing *WHO-DASII* global score; in consequence, they can be ordered according to increasing disability gravity, making even possible distinction between intermediate degrees, which are qualitatively different. The proposed profiles really face disabilities *from a functional point of view*. Furthermore, they are not directly associated with underlying pathology (fig.4), according to the geriatric approach, which regards functional improvement rather than medical aspect. There is no a group with high cognitive and no physical disability, probably owing to apraxia (impossibility of performing coordinate and finalized tasks) strongly related to severe degrees of cognitive impairment. Correlation between the gravity of the disability and the depression is being studied at present. Relationship with *FIM* and *SF-36* is also in progress.

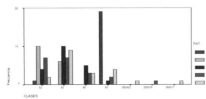 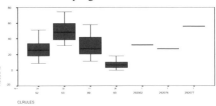

Figure 3 – Pathology vs classes with ClBR.   *Figure 4 – Multiple boxplot of GS vs classes of ClBR*

An appropriate analysis of assessment scales is critical to get good results; interpreted under a multivariate approach (considering the individual items of the scale) they are a rich source of information and produce a much more rich results than using the single global score. In this application *ClBR* produces meaningful classes and sensibly improves, from a semantics point of view, the results of classical clustering, according to our opinion that *hybrid* AI and Statistics techniques are more powerful for *KD* than pure ones, even in Disability.

5. Acknowledgements

To the EURO-MDSBL and WHO Assessment Classification and Epidemiology Group (WHO-DAS II designers).

6. References

[1] Comas J., *et al.* Knowledge Discovery by means of inductive methods in WWTP. *AICom* 01: 14(1): 45-62
[2] Fried, LP. *et al.* Disability in older adults: evidence regarding significance, ... *JAGS* 97: 45: 92-100
[3] Gibert, K., Cortés, U. Wheighing quantitative and qualitative variables in ... *Mathware* 97:4(7):251-266
[4] Gibert K.*et al.* Combining a KB system with a clustering method ... *LNCS* 1994:89:351-360.
[5] Gibert K. *et al.* ClBR and KD in ISD, *Computación y sistemas* 98: 1(4): 213-227.
[6] Gibert K. *et al.* Knowledge Discovery with Clustering Based on Rules. Interpreting *LNAI* 98: 510: 83-92.
[7] Gibert, K. and Z. Sonicki , Classification based on rules and medical ... *JASMDA*99: 15 (3): 319--324
[8] Gibert K. *et al.* Impact of Data encoding and Thyroids ... , *Technology and Informatics* 01:90: 494-503
[9] Gibert K. *et al.* Knowledge Discovery on functional disabilities using ClBR on WHO-DAS-III, *ITI* 2003
[10] Katz, S., *et al.* Studies of illness in the aged. The index of ADL: ... *JAMA* 1963: 185: 914-919.
[11] Laslett, P. A fresh map of life: the emergence of the third age. London: Macmillan Press, 1996.
[12] Ostir, G. V., *et al.* Summarizing amount of difficlulty in ADLs... *ACER* 2001:13:465-472.
[13] Rehm, J. *et al.* On the development and psychometric testing of the WHO... *IJMPR* 1990: 8(2): 110-122.
[14] Rodas J. *et al.* KDSM Methodology for KD from ISD presenting very short... *LNAI* 01:2504:228-238.
[15] Tukey, J.W Exploratory Data Analysis, Addison-Wesley, 1977
[16] Ware J.E., Sherbourne C.D. The MOS 36-item short-form health survey:.. *Medical Care* 92:30:473-481.
[17] Wilson, I. B. *et al.* Linking clinical variables with health-related quality of life...*JAMA*.1995.
[18] Second World Assembly on Ageing Madrid. 2002b. Building a Society for all Ages. Spain 8 -12 April.
[19] World Health Organization, ICIDH-2:International Classification of Functioning and Disability. 1999.
[20] WHO, The International Classification of Functioning, Disability and Health-ICF, Geneva

Address for correspondence

K. Gibert, Dep. Statistics and Operation Research, UPC. C5 CN. E-08028 Barcelona, karina.gibert@upc.edu.

Connecting Medical Informatics and Bio-Informatics
R. Engelbrecht et al. (Eds.)
IOS Press, 2005

Design of a Multi Dimensional Database for the Archimed DataWarehouse

Claudine Bréant, Gérald Thurler, François Borst, Antoine Geissbuhler

Service of Medical Informatics
University Hospital of Geneva, Geneva, Switzerland

Abstract

The Archimed data warehouse project started in 1993 at the Geneva University Hospital. It has progressively integrated seven data marts (or domains of activity) archiving medical data such as Admission/Discharge/Transfer (ADT) data, laboratory results, radiology exams, diagnoses, and procedure codes. The objective of the Archimed data warehouse is to facilitate the access to an integrated and coherent view of patient medical in order to support analytical activities such as medical statistics, clinical studies, retrieval of similar cases and data mining processes. This paper discusses three principal design aspects relative to the conception of the database of the data warehouse: 1) the granularity of the database, which refers to the level of detail or summarization of data, 2) the database model and architecture, describing how data will be presented to end users and how new data is integrated, 3) the life cycle of the database, in order to ensure long term scalability of the environment. Both, the organization of patient medical data using a standardized elementary fact representation and the use of the multi dimensional model have proved to be powerful design tools to integrate data coming from the multiple heterogeneous database systems part of the transactional Hospital Information System (HIS). Concurrently, the building of the data warehouse in an incremental way has helped to control the evolution of the data content. These three design aspects bring clarity and performance regarding data access. They also provide long term scalability to the system and resilience to further changes that may occur in source systems feeding the data warehouse.

Keywords:
Data warehouse; Medical Informatics; Database

1. Introduction

A data warehouse can be very simply defined as a copy of enterprise transaction data specifically structured, integrated, and organized for query, data analysis, and decision support applications [1,2]. In that regard, the architecture, the life cycle, and the end users of a data warehouse are profoundly different from those of transactional systems [1,2]. Data models and server technology that speeds up transactional processing may not be appropriate for query and reporting processing. It is therefore recommended to develop a data warehouse separately from the transactional environment. Its main requirement is to provide an intuitive, easy and performant access to enterprise wide data so that queries and reports can be quickly produced on a regular basis.

A hospital data warehouse organized around patient medical data involves integrating a wide variety of health data, including patient records, medical images, and genetic information, for the purpose of researching and improving the diagnosis and treatment of

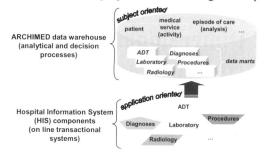

Figure 1 – The Hospital Information System components and the Archimed data warehouse

diseases. The objective is to use information technology to help achieve personalized health care by leveraging all the information and knowledge that exist about treated patients and, for instance, by studying how new patients compare with other patients with similar characteristics [3,4].

The development of the Archimed medical data warehouse started at the Geneva University Hospital in 1993. It has progressively integrated seven data marts (or *domains of activity*) archiving Admission/Discharge/Transfer (ADT) data, laboratory results, radiology exams, physiotherapy exams, clinical data relative to childbirth, diagnoses, and procedures codes. In the architecture of Archimed a data mart is simply a subset of the database for a specific domain of activity within the patient treatment workflow. As shown in figure 1, HIS operational systems are organized around applications managing for example ADT data or laboratory results. Archimed proposes a different organization of the data, which is dedicated to analytical activities such as medical statistics, clinical studies, retrieval of similar cases and data mining processes. As shown in figure 1, the Archimed data warehouse is organized around subject areas such as patient medical data, episodes of care, and medical specialties. End users can also access to the database through web-based applications [5].

This paper discusses three principal design aspects relative to the conception of the database of the Archimed data warehouse, towards the archiving and organization of patient medical data. The three following topics are described and discussed in the following sections:

1) the granularity of the database, which refers to the level of detail or summarization of data in the data warehouse,

2) the database model and architecture, describing how data will be presented to end users and how new data is integrated

3) the life cycle of the database, in order to ensure long term scalability of the environment.

The many other aspects of the Archimed system such as data source acquisition, end user applications, and meta data, can be found in [6,7].

2. The Archimed database records patient atomic data (or elementary facts)

The granularity of the data warehouse database refers to the level of detail or summarization of data in the data warehouse. The storage of atomic data (low level of granularity) versus storage of aggregated data (high level of granularity) is a major design issue since that it will affects the entire architecture of the data warehouse environment and more specifically the volume of the database and the type of query that can be answered. It is generally recognized that expressing the data at a low level of granularity will help to achieve a robust data warehouse, as it becomes resilient to changes and can easily accommodate new user needs. Moreover, when the fact tables are granular, they serve as the natural destination for operational data that may be extracted frequently from the operational systems.

The transactional hospital information system (HIS) creates and updates records describing most events occurring during patient in-patient or out-patient care. Events of interest for the Archimed data warehouse include encounters, observations, treatments, diagnosis and procedures. Relevant and validated facts such as encounter dates, laboratory results, radiology exams, diagnoses and procedure codes are transmitted to Archimed. The database has been designed to record patient medical data with that same level of detail under a format called *standardized elementary fact*. This offers many advantages over the storage of aggregated data. Indeed, whereas aggregated data already embeds the user queries, atomic data can be reshaped and presented in any format needed. Future unknown requirements or unusual queries can be accommodated, achieving flexibility of the system and reusability of the data.

Each *elementary fact* in the Archimed database is represented by its value (generally a numeric or a code), along with several additional properties describing the context of this value such as :

- patient/episode identification
  - patient identification number,
  - episode identification number,
- medical structures
  - service (medical responsibility),
  - medical unit (patient location),
- basic patient description to facilitate statistical queries
  - patient age,
  - patient sex,
- link to dictionaries and nomenclatures which are specific to each domain of activity
  - property name (laboratory result name, radiology exam, diagnosis or procedure description)

  Corresponding dictionaries are necessary for a correct interpretation of the fact at the time the value was produced. In that regard, historic versions of these dictionaries are managed if necessary.
- link to the time axis
  - date of the event that produced the value
  - date of archiving of the fact in the database.

Furthermore, elementary facts in Archimed are *standardized* the following way. Facts coming from different domains of activity are expressed using a common template, including a value and the set of corresponding properties. Basic properties are mandatory, additional ones are optional and their number may vary according to the domain of activity as shown in figure 2. The Archimed standardized elementary facts can therefore easily accommodate a new domain of activity.

The storage of aggregated data can be useful to speed up queries and optimize the database usage. They can be calculated from a group of selected facts from which can be applied aggregated functions (sum, average, count, etc.). The Archimed database doesn't currently store aggregated data; this area is however under consideration for future developments. Patient lengths of stay, indicators describing counts of diagnoses, or surgical procedures, and re admissions rates are some of the aggregates of interest.

The next section describes the database model used to structure these elementary facts.

Instanciated ADT fact		Instanciated Laboratory fact		Instanciated Procedure fact	
patient:	957688	*patient:*	345353	*patient:*	3345453
episode:	1000474	*episode:*	1000011	*episode:*	1190002
medService:	pediatric	*medService:*	INTERNAL MED	*medService:*	OBGYN
medUnit:	1-AL	*medUnit:*	7-AL	*medUnit:*	2-AL
patientAge:	7	*patientAge:*	46	*patientAge:*	34
patientSex:	M	*patientSex:*	F	*patientSex:*	F
property name:	out-patient	*property name:*	glucose	*property name:*	C-section
value:	regular entry	*value:*	6.8	*value:*	elected
dateOfFact:	2004-01-05	*dateOfFact:*	2004-02-23	*dateOfFact:*	2004-05-21
dateOfArchive:	2004-01-06	*dateOfArchive:*	2004-02-24	*dateOfArchive:*	2004-05-22
chief complaint:	accident	*unit:*	mml/L		additional
		material:	plasma		optional
		range:	4.2-6.0		properties

Figure 2 - Three instanciated Archimed facts according to the standardized elementary fact template

3. Patient medical data is organized using a multi dimensional approach

The Archimed database relies on a multi dimensional modeling approach. The dimensional model is a logical database design method particularly well suited to data warehouse databases [2]. In particular, it has the great advantage to allow data coming from various heterogeneous and independent sources, such as Archimed elementary patient facts, to be presented in an intuitive and standardized fashion. Contrary to the usual Entity/Relational data model used by transactional systems, it limits the number of tables to *fact* and *dimension* tables.

For instance, the multi dimensional model in Archimed for the Laboratory data mart includes:

- *one fact* table, recording the elementary facts produced by the operational system, namely the patient laboratory result values.
- a set of usually smaller dimension tables, each linked to the fact table through a primary key, and describing the context of interpretation of elementary facts. The dimension tables in the Laboratory data mart include tables describing patients, medical services, medical units, laboratory exams, laboratory ranges values, and units.

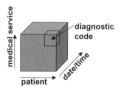

Figure 3 – Three dimensional data cube describing diagnostic codes
along three dimensions : patient, medical service, and time

Figure 4 shows the general *star schema* data model used for the representation of an Archimed data mart. The fact tables all contain zero or more facts that represent values (measurements) taken at each combination of the dimension key components. The fact table is also often represented by a data cube where each axis corresponds to one dimension, as shown in figure 3 [1,2].

As the Archimed data warehouse is composed of several data marts, the whole data model results in a set of inter connected *star schemas* including a collection of fact tables describing patient medical data (encounters, laboratory results, diagnoses and procedures,

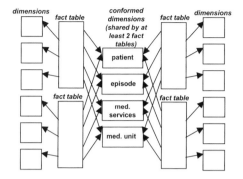

Figure 4 - Four Archimed data marts inter connected through conformed dimension tables

radiology exams and so on) and a set of dimension tables where some of them are shared by many facts tables. Indeed, the patient table or the medical services table record data meaning exactly the same thing in each data mart.

Dimension tables shared by several fact tables are called *conformed dimensions* [2]. Conformed dimensions constitute a very important and powerful aspect of the multi dimensional model. Indeed, the definition of conformed dimensions establishes the links between the data marts, providing an integrated view of the elementary facts. It builds the foundation for a simple and performant querying of the patient medical data as if it were initially part of the same database.

For example, the queries *'retrieve all medical data of patient of age 30-40 during its last hospitalization in the internal medicine department'* or *'retrieve all patients of the pediatric department having low hemoglobin and diagnosis of diabetes'* require many steps of laborious treatment when issued at the various hospital transactional database systems. It is however very simple to solve with the Archimed database model.

Establishing, enforcing, and maintaining, the dimension tables of the data warehouse Archimed are therefore important tasks respectively during the initial planning of the database architecture, during the integration process of a new data mart, and for the maintenance of the database overall coherence.

4. Implementation and life cycle of the Archimed database

The Archimed database was first developed using the Ingres database system before being recently migrated to the Oracle relational database system. In brief, the physical implementation of the database has required the definition of a physical data model, proper indexation of the tables, and definition of rules to consistently name tables and attributes.

Unlike classical transactional systems, a data warehouse is in perpetual evolution and cannot remain static. Indeed, its evolution must follow the changes occurring in the organization which it serves. User needs appear or change. New data sources become accessible and must be integrated in the warehouse.

The process of adding a new data mart to the architecture complies with the following steps. First, a detailed analysis of the source data provided by the transactional systems is carried out. Elementary facts are identified, setting the granularity of the fact table. Then, conformed dimensions are carefully highlighted; they define the links with the other data marts. Other dimensions are also identified which complement the definition of the elementary facts. A mapping between source data items and the data warehouse table attributes is established. Then, the physical table and index definitions can be derived and implemented.

The Archimed data warehouse has been built incrementally, in order to break the implementation task to manageable proportions. Each data mart has been successively implemented and connected to the overall architecture.

Moreover, the Archimed database was designed to anticipate changes and the evolution of existing data sources. As shown above, the data model accommodates the need for new descriptors and new dimensions without to have to change the database schema.

5. Conclusion

The planning, realization, maintenance and evolution of a large data warehouse database system can be overwhelming. Source data is complex, volumes are large, and portions of data will be dirty, erroneous, or hard to understand.

In the case of a data warehouse for medical data, we have discussed the three main design aspects of the Archimed database.

The organization of elementary facts (atomic) using the dimensional model has proved to be a powerful tool in order to integrate data coming from multiple heterogeneous database systems developed independently throughout the institution.   It brings clarity and performance regarding data access. It also provides scalability to the system and resilience to further changes that may occur in source systems feeding the data warehouse.

Moreover, the building of the data warehouse in an incremental way has helped to control the evolution of the data content

These design options constitute the main rules and act as a *road map* to follow when a new medical set of data (or data mart) is integrated to the system.   Sticking to these decisions has enabled to ensure the coherence of the integrated data, long term scalability, and to greatly simplify the access to data produced by tens of independent hospital wide operational databases.

These rules have been established progressively and result from more that 15 years of prior experience in providing information to hospital administrators and medical staff including departmental statistics, patient similar case retrievals, and clinical studies.

6. References

[1] Inmon WH, Building the Data Warehouse, Wiley; 3rd edition, 2002.

[2] Kimball R, Ross M. The Data Warehouse Lifecycle Toolkit, Wiley; 2nd edition, 2002.

[3] Kerkri R, Quantin C, Yetongnon K, Dusserre L.   Les entrepôts de données:application au suivi épidémiologique. Informatique et Santé, Springer-Verlag, France, Paris 1998(10):21-29.

[4] Ledbetter CS, Morgan MW, Toward best practice: leveraging the electronic patient record as a clinical data warehouse J Healthc Inf Manag. 2001 Summer;15(2):119-31.

[5] Lehner B, Thurler G, Bréant C, Tahintzi P, Borst F. Retrieval of Similar Cases using the ARCHIMED Navigator. *MIE*, 2003.

[6] Thurler G, Bréant C, Lehner B, Bunge M, Samii K, Hochstrasser D, Nendaz M, Gaspoz JM, Tahintzi P, Borst F. Toward a Systemic Approach to Disease. *Complexus*, 2003;1:117-122.

[7] Thurler G, Borst F, Bréant C, Campi J, Jenc j, Lehner B, Maricot P, and Scherrer JR. ARCHIMED: A network of Integrated Information Systems. Method Inform Med 2000; 39: 36-43.

Address for correspondence

Claudine Bréant HUG – Service d'Informatique Médicale   24, rue Micheli-du-Crêts   1211 Genève 14, Switzerland, claudine.breant@sim.hcuge.ch

Connecting Medical Informatics and Bio-Informatics
R. Engelbrecht et al. (Eds.)
IOS Press, 2005

Canonical Correlation Analysis for Data Reduction in Data Mining Applied to Predictive Models for Breast Cancer Recurrence

Amir Reza Razavi[a], **Hans Gill**[a], **Hans Åhlfeldt**[a], **Nosrat Shahsavar**[a,b]

[a] *Department of Biomedical Engineering, Division of Medical Informatics, Linköping University, Sweden*
[b] *Regional Oncology Centre, University Hospital, Linköping, Sweden*

Abstract

Data mining methods can be used for extracting specific medical knowledge such as important predictors for recurrence of breast cancer in pertinent data material. However, when there is a huge quantity of variables in the data material it is first necessary to identify and select important variables. In this study we present a pre-processing method for selecting important variables in a dataset prior to building a predictive model.

In the dataset, data from 5787 female patients were analysed. To cover more predictors and obtain a better assessment of the outcomes, data were retrieved from three different registers: the regional breast cancer, tumour markers, and cause of death registers. After retrieving information about selected predictors and outcomes from the different registers, the raw data were cleaned by running different logical rules. Thereafter, domain experts selected predictors assumed to be important regarding recurrence of breast cancer. After that, Canonical Correlation Analysis (CCA) was applied as a dimension reduction technique to preserve the character of the original data.

Artificial Neural Network (ANN) was applied to the resulting dataset for two different analyses with the same settings. Performance of the predictive models was confirmed by ten-fold cross validation. The results showed an increase in the accuracy of the prediction and reduction of the mean absolute error.

Keywords
Data Mining, Artificial Neural Network (ANN), Canonical Correlation Analysis (CCA), Dimension Reduction, Breast Cancer

1. Introduction

In recent years there has been an explosive increase in the amount of information stored in electronic documents. In medicine, information is saved in different forms such as registers. Large quantities of data are stored in registers for the purpose of monitoring and analysing health and social conditions in the population. Some registers in Sweden are nation-wide in scope and data have been collected for decades. These data are frequently utilised by a variety of users for research, evaluation, planning and other purposes [1]. Data mining methods can be applied to the data in order to find relationships between patients' states and their outcomes.

Artificial Neural Network (ANN) is a data mining method that has been used in the area of medicine for a long period of time. Before data are analysed by a data mining technique they should be pre-processed to remove or reduce noise and take care of missing values, relevance analysis should be performed to omit unnecessary and redundant data, and data should be transformed to higher-level concepts [2]. In order to produce a stable and accurate model of relationships, the sets of variables should be reduced to those that are relevant.

In this study, domain expert involvement and Canonical Correlation Analysis (CCA) were applied as pre-processing steps prior to ANN in order to reduce the number of variables to only those of importance.

Hotelling (1936) developed CCA as a method for evaluating linear correlation between sets of variables [3]. Our objective was to find a subset of variables with predictive performance comparable to the full set of variables [4].

After applying CCA and decreasing the number of predictors, the data were thus ready to be analysed more efficiently with Artificial Neural Network (ANN). In order to show the efficiency of CCA as a dimension reduction technique, ANN was also applied to the same database without pre-processing by CCA.

2. Materials and Methods

2.1. Dataset

In this study data from 5787 female patients, mean age 62.6 years, were analysed. The earliest patient was diagnosed in January 1986 and the last date of follow-up was June 2003. In order to cover more predictors and obtain a better assessment of the outcomes, data were retrieved from three different registers: the regional breast cancer register, the tumour markers register, and the cause of death register. After combining the information from these registers, the cases were anonymised for security reasons and to maintain patient confidentiality.

2.2. Predictors and Outcomes

There were more than 150 variables in the combined dataset. The first step in selecting appropriate variables was consultation with domain experts. In this step, sets of predictors and outcomes (Figure 1) were selected. Age of the patient and variables regarding tumour specifications based on pathology reports, physical examination and tumour markers were selected as predictors (Left side of Figure 1).

There were two variables in the outcome set, distant metastasis and loco-regional recurrence as observed at different time intervals after diagnosis, indicating early and late recurrence (Right side of Figure 1).

2.3. Data Cleaning

After retrieving information from different registers concerning selected predictors and outcomes, the raw data were cleaned and outliers and noises were removed by running scripts in SPSS. Cases that had missing values for any of the variables were omitted from the analysis.

2.4. Canonical Correlation Analysis

The fundamental principle behind CCA is the creation of a number of canonical solutions

[5], each consisting of a linear combination of one set of variables, which has the form:
$U_i = a_1 (predictor_1) + a_2 (predictor_2) + ... + a_m (predictor_m)$
and a linear combination of the other set of variables, which has the form:
$V_i = b_1 (outcome_1) + b_2 (outcome_2) + ... + b_n (outcome_n)$

The goal is to determine the coefficients (a's and b's) that maximize the correlation between canonical variates U_i and V_i. This creates a number of solutions equal to the number of variables in the smaller set. The first canonical correlation is the highest possible correlation between any linear combination of the variables in the predictor set and any linear combination of the variables in the outcome set.

The magnitudes of the structure coefficients (loadings) of the first solution are used to identify the most relevant variables. Using loadings as the criterion for finding the important variables has some advantages over weights [6]. As a rule of thumb for meaningful loadings, an absolute value equal to or greater than 0.3 is often used [7].

SPSS version 11 was used for transforming, handling missing values, and implementing CCA [8].

2.5. Artificial Neural Network

In this study, ANN was applied to two different sets of predictors and outcomes. First, ANN was applied to the reduced model resulting from CCA to achieve a predictive model for new cases. In the training phase of ANN, the resulting predictors in CCA with loadings ≥ 0.3 were used as input neurons. As the output neuron, two important outcomes with loadings ≥ 0.3 in CCA were combined into one dichotomous variable representing the recurrence of the cancer within a four-year period after detection of the disease.

Second, ANN was applied to the database without reducing the number of predictors, thus using all of the variables as input neurons, i.e. the same set of variables that was used as the predictor set for CCA (Left side of Figure 1).

In this analysis, any recurrence (either distant or loco-regional) at any time during the follow-up after diagnosis was used as output neuron.

ANN was carried out using WEKA, which is a collection of machine learning algorithms for data mining tasks [9].

2.6. Performance Validation

All cases were randomly re-ordered, and then the set of all cases was divided into ten mutually disjointed subsets of approximately equal size. The model then was trained and tested ten times. Each time it was trained on all but one subset and tested on the remaining single subset. The estimate of the overall accuracy was the average of the ten individual accuracy measures [10].

For comparing the performance of the two ANNs, i.e. with and without pre-processing with CCA , the accuracy, sensitivity and specificity were calculated [11].

In addition, the mean absolute error (MAE) was compared to see the average difference between actual and predicted values [12].

3. Results

CCA was applied to the dataset, and the loadings for each solution for predictor and outcome sets were calculated. The first solution with loadings (in parentheses) for variables is illustrated in Figure 1. In CCA, usually just the first solution is considered important. For this solution, the canonical correlation coefficient (rc) is 0.47 with a p value $\leq .001$. The important loadings for each variable are shown in bold type.

The reduced model after pre-processing by CCA is shown in Figure 2, where the important outcomes, i.e. DM and LRR for the first four years (Figure 1), are combined in a medically meaningful variable, i.e. Recurrence ≤ 4 years (Figure 2), which is used as a dichotomous outcome in ANN.

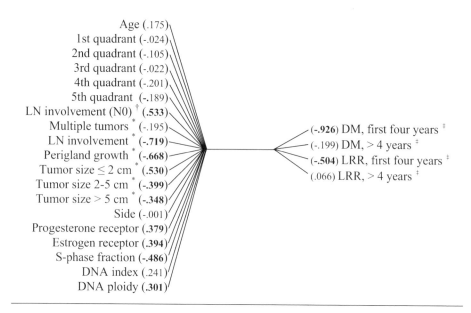

Figure 1- Canonical Structure Matrix for Predictor and Outcome Variates (LN: lymph node, DM: Distant Metastasis, LRR: Loco-regional Recurrence, †N0: Not palpable LN metastasis, * from pathology report, ‡ all periods are time after diagnosis).

The accuracy, sensitivity, specificity and mean absolute error for models with or without pre-processing by CCA are shown and compared in Table 1. It is seen that pre-processing by CCA improves accuracy, specificity and mean absolute error but the sensitivity is lower.

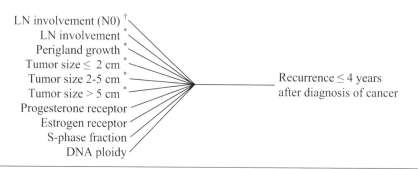

Figure 2- Extracted model from CCA in the pre-processing step (LN: lymph node ,†N0: Not palpable LN metastasis, * from pathology report).

4. Discussion

An important step in the data mining process is data preparation. This includes several steps, i.e. data cleaning, data integration, data transformation and data reduction, since most of the time real world data is incomplete and inconsistent [2]. Selection of relevant data is aimed at choosing a subset of features that is relevant to the target concept. Data reduction reduces the volume of the data, but it also produces a more stable model for a more efficient and faster data mining process. It is therefore essential to engage domain experts in the knowledge discovery and data mining process [13]. In registers with many variables, consultation with medical professionals in the area in question is needed to reduce the number of variables in the pre-processing step.

Artificial Neural Network (ANN) has many applications in medicine. It has been used in a wide range of applications such as predicting cancer occurrence and diagnosing tumours from X-rays [14, 15]. In some ANN applications, it is not clear what kinds of pre-processing techniques were used [16]. In most cases, the only pre-processing that was done was replacing missing values [17].

Table 1- Performance Validation Results.

ANN	Without pre-processing	With pre-processing
Accuracy	61%	71%
Sensitivity	75%	67%
Specificity	55%	72%
Mean Absolute Error	0.44	0.37

When applying ANN to registers with large numbers of variables, there is a repercussion that is called the curse of dimensionality [18]. This is the exponential growth of hyper-volume as a function of dimensionality, and it causes problems in ANN analysis.

In this study we used both domain experts and CCA for data reduction. Non-important variables were removed from the dataset by using CCA and considering loadings as criteria. Loadings are not affected by the presence of strong correlations among variables. In addition, CCA is useful in that it handles two sets of variables, while other data reduction techniques such as principal component analysis (PCA) treat just one variable set at a time. These are some of the advantages in using CCA [6].

After dimension reduction by CCA, the number of variables suggested by domain experts was reduced to 12 (10 + 2). These benefits are more apparent when the number of variables is much higher.

A comparison of the results of the two ANNs (Table 1) shows that the accuracy, specificity and MAE of the analysis with CCA prior to ANN are considerably better than the other ANN analysis, but the sensitivity has decreased. Reducing the number of variables results in models that are more accurate and stable, i.e. they are less sensitive to noise and outliers in the data and this reduces the risk for overfitting.

5. Conclusion

In this study, a new method for analysing the data for breast cancer patients is presented and examined using data from the registers in south-eastern Sweden. Applying CCA and consulting with domain experts are proposed for dimension reduction prior to ANN. CCA as an automatic method for dimension reduction prior to ANN results in better accuracy in predicting recurrence in breast cancer patients. ANN showed an increase in the accuracy of the prediction, reduced the MAE and decreased the processing time and resources needed for predicting the recurrence of breast cancer.

6. Acknowledgments

This study is supported by grant No. F2003-513 from FORSS (The Research Council of South-eastern Sweden). Special thanks to the South-East Swedish Breast Cancer Study Group for fruitful collaboration and support in this study.

7. References

[1]   Rosen M. National Health Data Registers: a Nordic heritage to public health. Scand J Public Health. 2002;30(2):81-5.

[2]   Han J, Kamber M. Data mining: Concepts and Techniques. San Francisco: Morgan Kaufmann Publishers, 2001.

[3]   Silva Cardoso E, Blalock K, Allen CA, Chan F, Rubin SE. Life skills and subjective well-being of people with disabilities: a canonical correlation analysis. Int J Rehabil Res. 2004 Dec;27(4):331-4.

[4]   Antoniadis A, Lambert-Lacroix S, Leblanc F. Effective dimension reduction methods for tumor classification using gene expression data. Bioinformatics. 2003 Mar 22;19(5):563-70.

[5]   Vogel RL, Ackermann RJ. Is primary care physician supply correlated with health outcomes? Int J Health Serv. 1998; 28(1): 183-96.

[6]   Dunlap WP, Landis RS. Interpretations of multiple regression borrowed from factor analysis and canonical correlation. J Gen Psychol. 1998, 125, 397-407.

[7]   Thompson, B. Canonical correlation analysis: Uses and interpretation. Thousand Oaks, CA: Sage publications, Quantitative Applications in the Social Sciences Series, No. 47; 1984.

[8]   SPSS for Windows, Rel. 11.0.1. 2001. Chicago: SPSS Inc.

[9]   Witten IH, Frank E. Data Mining: Practical machine learning tools with Java implementations. Morgan Kaufmann, San Francisco, 2000.

[10] Kohavi R. A study of cross-validation and bootstrap for accuracy estimation and model selection, in: International Joint Conference on Artificial Intelligence, San Mateo, CA, 1995, pp. 1137–1145.

[11] Delen D, Walker G, Kadam A. Predicting breast cancer survivability: a comparison of three data mining methods. Artif Intell Med. In press 2004.

[12] Sathe PM, Venitz J. Comparison of neural network and multiple linear regression as dissolution predictors. Drug Dev Ind Pharm. 2003 Mar;29(3):349-55.

[13] Babic A. Knowledge discovery for advanced clinical data management and analysis. Stud Health Technol Inform. 1999;68:409-13.

[14] Remzi M, Anagnostou T, Ravery V, Zlotta A, Stephan C, Marberger M, Djavan B. An artificial neural network to predict the outcome of repeat prostate biopsies. Urology. 2003 Sep;62(3):456-60.

[15] Joo S, Yang YS, Moon WK, Kim HC. Computer-aided diagnosis of solid breast nodules: use of an artificial neural network based on multiple sonographic features. IEEE Trans Med Imaging. 2004 Oct;23(10):1292-300.

[16] Samli MM, Dogan I. An artificial neural network for predicting the presence of spermatozoa in the testes of men with nonobstructive azoospermia. J Urol. 2004 Jun;171(6 Pt 1):2354-7.

[17] Ennett CM, Frize M, Walker CR. Influence of missing values on artificial neural network performance. Medinfo. 2001;10(Pt 1):449-53.

[18] Bellman RE. Adaptive Control Processes: A guided Tour. Princeton, NJ: Princeton Univerity Press, 1961.

Corresponding author:

Amir R Razavi, MD, Linköping University, Dept. of Biomedical Engineering, University Hospital, S-58185 Linköping, Sweden, Tel: +46-13-22 24 84, Fax: +46-13-10 19 02, E-mail address: amirreza.razavi@imt.liu.se

Connecting Medical Informatics and Bio-Informatics
R. Engelbrecht et al. (Eds.)
IOS Press, 2005

Tools for Statistical Analysis with Missing Data: Application to a Large Medical Database

Cristian Preda[a], **Alain Duhamel**[a], **Monique Picavet**[a], **Tahar Kechadi**[b]

[a]*Faculté de Médecine, France*
[b]*Department of Computer Science, University College of Dublin*

Abstract

Missing data is a common feature of large data sets in general and medical data sets in particular. Depending on the goal of statistical analysis, various techniques can be used to tackle this problem. Imputation methods consist in substituting the missing values with plausible or predicted values so that the completed data can then be analysed with any chosen data mining procedure. In this work, we study imputation in the context of multivariate data and we evaluate a number of methods which can be used by today's standard statistical software packages. Imputation using multivariate classification, multiple imputation and imputation by factorial analysis are compared using simulated data and a large medical database (from the diabetes field) with numerous missing values. Our main result is to provide a control chart for assessing data quality after the imputation process. To this end, we developed an algorithm for which the input is a set of parameters describing the underlying data (e.g., covariance matrix, distribution) and the output is a chart which plots the change in the prediction error with respect to the proportion of missing values. The chart is built by means of an iterative algorithm involving four steps: (1) a sample of simulated data is drawn by using the input parameters; (2) missing values are randomly generated; (3) an imputation method is used to fill in the missing data and (4) the prediction error is computed. Steps 1 to 4 are repeated in order to estimate the distribution of the prediction error. The control chart was established for the 3 imputation methods studied here, assuming a multivariate normal distribution of data. The use of this tool on a large medical database was then investigated. We show how the control chart can be used to assess the quality of the imputation process in the pre-processing step upstream of data mining procedures.

Keywords:
Statistical models; Databases; Data mining; Missing values; Imputation;

1. Introduction

Dealing with missing data is a major problem in Knowledge Discovery in Databases (KDD). This type of operation must be performed with caution in order to avoid deterioration in the performance of data mining procedures. The area has attracted much research interest over recent years and the mainstream statistical analysis software packages are starting to offer solutions (Celeux [1], Hox [2]). Dealing with missing data in the KDD process comprises three main strategies. The first consists in eliminating incomplete observations and has two major limitations. Firstly, the resulting information loss can be considerable if many of the variables have missing values for various individuals. Secondly, this method also runs the risk of introducing bias if the process behind the missing values is not completely random (Missing Completely At Random, MCAR [3]), i.e. if the subset analysed is not representative of the sample as a whole. The second strategy consists in using a method specifically adapted to the data mining algorithm employed (for example, CART [4]). These methods implicitly presuppose a MCAR mechanism and most have not been critically appraised. The third strategy is imputation: the missing data problem is tackled in the pre-processing step of the KDD process by replacing each missing value with a predicted value. This method is particularly well-suited to the KDD process, since the completed database can then be analysed with any chosen data mining procedure.

The goal of the present work is to compare different imputation methods according to their predictive power and as a function of the proportion of missing values in the database analysed. We consider here the case of quantitative variables and MAR-type missing data (Missing At Random [3]). One can say that the process is MAR if conditionally on observed data for certain variables X, the appearance of a missing value for Y is random. There are numerous imputation methods: single imputation using the mean, median or mode (Schafer [5]), regression-based methods (Horton [6]) and more complex methods such as those based on classification procedures (Benali [7]), the NIPALS algorithm (Tenenhaus [8]), multiple imputation (Rubin [9], [10], Allison [11], Donzé [12]) or association rules (Ragel [13]). Here, we studied three methods: multiple imputation, imputation via the NIPALS algorithm and imputation based on classification. These methods are suitable in cases where the missing values are present across several of the database's variables and can all be implemented easily with standard statistical software. Following a brief introduction to each method in section 2, section 3 introduces an indicator based on the mean square imputation error, which serves as a criterion for comparison. The methods are compared using simulated data and the large DiabCare medical database, generated under the auspices of the WHO for improving care provision to diabetic patients (section 4).

2. On multiple imputation, NIPALS and classification

2.1   Multiple imputation

One of the great disadvantages of single imputation (i.e. for a single value) is the fact that one is not aware of the uncertainty in predicting the unknown missing value. This can lead to significant bias - for example, systematic underestimation of the variance of the "imputed" variable. Multiple imputation enables this uncertainty to be taken into account when predicting the missing values. The basic idea, developed by Rubin [9], is as follows: (a) impute the missing values by using a suitable model which incorporates the random variation, (b) repeat this operation m times (3 to 5 times, in general) in order to obtain m complete data files. Statistical analyses are then carried out for each completed file and the results are combined in order to obtain the final model. In our simulation study (section 3), a missing value was predicted by the mean of the m predicted values generated in step (b). Different models can be used for imputation of the missing values, such as the MCMC model (Markov Chain Monte Carlo) and that based on the EM algorithm (Expectation–Maximization). Version 8.2 of SAS includes two new procedures which enable multiple imputations (MI and MIANALYZE procedures [14]). The MVA module (Missing Value Analysis) in SPSS only performs single imputation (m=1).

2.2   The NIPALS algorithm

The aim of the NIPALS (nonlinear iterative partial least squares) algorithm is to perform principal component analysis in the presence of missing data (Tenehaus [8]).

Given a rectangular data table of size $n \times p$, let us denote by $X = \{x_{ij}\}$, $1 \leq i \leq n$, $1 \leq j \leq p$, the matrix representing the observed values of the variables x_j for n statistical units. Next, if X is of rank a, then the decomposition formula for principal component analysis of X is

$$X = \sum_{h=1}^{a} t_h p_h', \text{ where } t_h = (t_{h1}, \dots, t_{hi}, \dots, t_{hn})' \text{ and } p_h = (p_{h1}, \dots, p_{hj}, \dots, p_{hp})'$$

are the principal factors and principal components, respectively. Therefore, the NIPALS algorithm estimates a missing value corresponding to the cell (i,j) as

$$\hat{x}_{ji} = \sum_{l=1}^{k} t_{li} p_{lj},$$

where k ($k \leq a$) is determined by cross-validation. Implementation of the NIPALS algorithm is very simple, since it is based only on simple linear regressions. The complexity of this algoritm is of order $O(a \times n \times p \times C)$, where C is the number of iterations required for convergence. The NIPALS algorithm is implemented in the SIMPCA-P software (release 10) but not yet in SAS. We programmed a C application which implements NIPALS and used it to compare the method with other approaches.

2.3   Imputation by classification

The principle is one of performing a classification of the data as a whole using a the k-means clustering method whilst taking into account the missing values in calculation of the distances via an appropriate metric (the FASTCLUS procedure in SAS). Each individual is assigned to a unique cluster and the missing value for the variable X is then replaced by the mean of X calculated from all the individuals in the cluster.

3. Comparison of imputation methods

Imputation quality depends on a range of different parameters, the most important of which are i) the number of missing data, ii) the distribution of the random vector which describes the data table and iii) the distribution of the missing values. Let us suppose the data are normally distributed with a zero-mean and covariance matrix S and that the missing values are uniformly distributed. In order to assess and compare the imputation methods as a function of the proportion of missing data, we suggest a method comprising the following steps:

Step 1. Using simulations, one generates a table T of n lines (individuals) and p columns (variables) representing n realizations of the random vector $X \sim N(0, S)$ (N designates a normal distribution). We chose n=100 so as to obtain a sufficiently large sample.

Step 2. One generates a fixed percentage p_m of missing values distributed uniformly within table T.

Step 3. The missing values are imputed by using the chosen technique (here, one of the three above-mentioned methods).

Step 4. In order to measure the precision of the imputation, one calculates the mean square error (MSE) defined by:

$$MSE = \frac{1}{n \times p \times p_m} \sum_{j=1}^{p} \left[\frac{\sum_{i=1}^{n} (x_{ij} - \hat{x}_{ij})^2}{\sum_{i=1}^{n} (x_{ij} - \bar{x}_j)^2} \right]$$

where n designates the number of individuals, p the number of variables and p_m the proportion of missing values. $\hat{x}_{ij}$ is the imputation of x_{ij} if x_{ij} is missing and $\hat{x}_{ij} = x_{ij}$ if not. $\bar{x}_j = \frac{1}{n}\sum_{i=1}^{n} x_{ij}$ is the mean of the variable X_j (prior to random selection of missing values).

In the MSE expression and for a given variable, the term between square brackets represents the ratio between the sum of squares of the imputation errors and the variable's variance (in order to take account of the measurement scale for each variable). We then calculate the mean square error by dividing by the number of missing data ($n \times p \times p_m$). In order to study the behaviour of the MSE as a function of the percentage of missing data, operations 1 to 4 are repeated K times for each percentage p_m from 1% to 15% in 1% steps. As with bootstrap methods, we set K to 1000. For each p_m, we thus obtain a series of 1000 MSE observations for which we calculate the quartiles and the mean.

Figure 1 presents the results obtained for imputation using the NIPALS algorithm (the two other methods gave similar results). The algorithm can be applied to any covariance matrix whatsoever. By way of an example, we chose the matrix S calculated from Fisher's Iris data [15]. This file (comprising 150 individuals and 4 numerical variables) is frequently used by statisticians to assess statistical methods. In order to assess the present method's robustness, we also applied the algorithm to Fisher's data: only step 1 is modified, and the corresponding table T thus refers to real data.

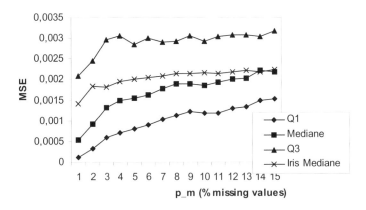

Figure 1: the NIPALS method. Change in MSE as a function of p_m (the proportion of missing values). Q1 and Q3 represent the first and third quartiles, respectively. The dotted curve represents the median MSE for the real data from the Iris file.

One can observe that as expected, the imputation error increases when the proportion of missing data increases. Even though the MSE is calculated with a hypothesis of multinormal distribution, the proximity of the two median curves (simulated data and Iris data) indicates a certain robustness for this indicator (the real Iris data do not follow a multinormal distribution). One can then use the MSE to predict the order of magnitude of the imputation error by simply using the covariance matrix for the observed data. Let us again take Fisher's Iris data as an example (150 subjects and 4 parameters = 600 data items and S, the covariance matrix). Let us then suppose that for each the 4 parameters, 12% of the data is missing: we must therefore impute 72 values. If we choose to impute with the NIPALS method, we use Figure 1, where the median MSE is 0.20%. If the variables were reduced (or if their variances were equal) the imputation would then introduce an error estimated at 0.20×72= 14.4% of the total variance. For each imputation method, steps 1 to 4 can be easily programmed so as to dynamically obtain a graph such as that shown in Figure

1. The algorithm's input parameters are the matrix S (that one can estimate from the available data) and the size n of the multinormally distributed sample to be generated.

4. Comparison of imputation methods using a large medical database

The imputation methods studied here were applied to the DiabCare database (40000 individuals, 250 variables) set up under the auspices of the WHO (the EuroDiabCare program) in order to assess quality care in diabetes. Our work follows one from the DATADIAB research program supported by the French Ministry of Research (ACI 2000) [16]. Here, we focussed on French type II diabetics (21419 individuals). The database suffers from missing values for numerous variables. Here, we present the results concerning 11 variables considered to be important for follow-up of diabetic patients. The variables and the corresponding proportions of missing values are as follows: age (1%), body mass index (5%), blood cholesterol level (9%), blood creatinine level (11%), time since diabetes onset (5%), glycated haemoglobin (7%), height (4%), blood triglyceride level (9%), weight (2%), diastolic blood pressure (5%) and systolic blood pressure (4%). In all, there are 13352 missing values, i.e. 5.7% of the data. The real values of the missing data are not available. We used the method described in section 3 for *a priori* estimation of the imputation error by supposing that the data follow a multinormal distribution. The table below gives the median MSEs. The covariance matrix S was estimated from the observed data.

Imputation method	NIPALS	Multiple	Classification
Median MSE (%)	0.00138	0.00146	0.00185
Estimated total error (% of the variance)	18.42	19.49	24.70

One can note that the NIPALS and multiple imputation methods give similar results, whereas imputation by classification seems less precise (results given by PCA on the imputation data: statistical units are the missing values, the variables being the imputation methods). We also compared the means, medians and variances calculated first for the available data (one just eliminates the variable's missing values) and then for the complete cases and finally after imputation by the 3 methods. The results obtained can be summarised in the following manner: for the mean, all the estimations are similar. In contrast, for the variance, calculations on complete cases led to systematic under-evaluation with respect to available cases, as expected. Imputation with the three methods produces variances close to those calculated using available cases, except for the creatinine variable. The latter included the highest proportion of missing data (11%) and the NIPALS method strongly overestimates the variance whereas classification underestimates it.

5. Discussion

We studied three imputation methods: multiple imputation (via the SAS procedure MI), imputation by classification (via the SAS procedure FASTCLUS) and imputation with the NIPALS algorithm. These methods have the advantage of being well-suited to MAR cases and of being practicable with mainstream software. Having compared the methods using both simulated and real data sets, none appeared to differ significantly from the others in terms of the quality of the results. One of the strong points of the MI procedure is that it is quick, easy to use and does not artificially decrease data variance. Imputation via the FASTCLUS procedure is based on a simple idea but one is obliged to choose a number of classes in order to optimize the estimations - and the cost in calculation time can be high for large databases. As for the NIPALS algorithm, it is easy to implement in standard programming languages (C, for example). Since this method is based on data reconstitution using PCA, NIPALS imputation takes into account the data's multivariate nature. It can be criticized for being poorly known to end users - except perhaps for fans of the PLS approach. Unsurprisingly, one observes a drop in performance for all methods when the proportion of missing values is high. We have thus developed a method which enables assessment of the imputation error as a function of the percentage of missing data. What we have, in fact, is a "control chart" for the *a priori* estimation of the quality of imputation of missing values for a given method and for a given covariance matrix table S. This "control chart" appears to us to be a highly valuable tool for use prior to statistical analysis of databases which may be completed with imprecise values.

We intend to continue this research by broadening the range of techniques used. An initial approach will consist in developing missing data processing techniques based on non linear tools such as the kernel methods widely used in statistical learning and neural networks. We have already developed a methodology based on a recurrent, multicontext neural network ([17]). This has been validated in different fields (notably for monitoring energy saving) and we believe that such an approach is very well-suited to missing data processing. Of course, imputation is only useful if analysis of the completed database with statistical methods or data mining procedures gives reliable results. This is why the methods' respective performances will be judged according to the results obtained with the completed database for the prediction of the macro- and microvascular complications of diabetes. We shall consider 2 types of validation criteria: mathematical criteria and the judgement of medical experts.

6. References

[1]   Celeux G, Le traitement des données manquantes dans le logiciel SICLA. Rapports Techniques n°102 1988, INRIA, France.

[2]   Hox J, A review of current software for handling missing data. Kwantitatieve Methoden 1999, 62: 123-138. http://www.fss.uu.nl/ms/jh/publist/misrevkm.pdf

[3]   Little RJA., Rubin DB, Statistical analysis with missing data, Wiley, New York 1987.

[4]   Breiman L, Friedman JH, Ohlsenn RA, Stone CJ, Classification and regression trees. Belmont, Wadsworth 1984.

[5]   Schafer JL, Imputation Procedures For Missing Data. USA Université de Pennsylvania 1999 : http://www.stat.psu.edu/~jls/session2.pdf

[6]   Horton NJ, Lipsitz SR, Multiple Imputation in Practice: Comparison of Software Packages for Regression Models With Missing Variables. Statistical Computing Software Reviews. The American Statistician 2001, 55(3). http://www.biostat.harvard.edu/~horton/tasimpute.pdf

[7]   Benali H, Escofier B, Nouvelle étape de traitement des données manquantes en analyse factorielle des correspondances multiples dans le système portable d'analyse de données. Rapports Techniques n°85 1987 ; INRIA, France.

[8]   Tenenhaus M, La régression PLS Théorie et pratique. Editions Technip 1998.

[9]   Rubin DB, Multiple imputation for nonresponse in surveys. New York: John Wiley 1987.

[10]   Rubin DB, Multiple imputation after 18+ years. Journal of American Statistical Association 1996; 91: 473-489.

[11]   Allison PD, Multiple Imputation for Missing Data : A Cautionary Tale. Sociological Methods and Research 2000, 28, 301-309, USA Université de Pennsylvania. http://www.ssc.upenn.edu/~allison/

[12]   Donzé L, Imputation multiple et modélisation : quelques expériences tirées de l'enquête 1999 KOF/ETHZ sur l'innovation. Ecole polytechnique fédérale de Zurich 2001. http://www.kof.ethz.ch/pdf/

[13]   Ragel A, MVC - A Preprocessing Method to deal with Missing Values, Knowledge Based System 1999;12: 285-291.

[14]   SAS institute INC., SAS Campus Drive Cary, NC 27513, USA

[15]   Fisher RA, The use of multiple measurements in taxonomic problems, Annals of Eugenics 1936, 7 : 179-188

[16]   Duhamel A, Nuttens MC, Devos P, Picavet M, Beuscart R, A preprocessing method for improving data mining techniques. Application to a large medical diabetes database, Studies in Health Technology and Informatics 2003 IOS press, 269-274

[17]   Huang BQ, Rashid T, Kechadi T, A new modified network based on the Elman network, Proceedings of IASTED International Conference on Artificial Intelligence and Application 2004, Innsbruck, Austria.

Address for correspondence

Cristian Preda, CERIM, Faculté de médecine, 1 Place de Verdun, F-59045 Lille cedex, France, cpreda@univ-lille2.fr

Connecting Medical Informatics and Bio-Informatics
R. Engelbrecht et al. (Eds.)
IOS Press, 2005
187

Diagnostic Support for Glaucoma Using Retinal Images: A Hybrid Image Analysis and Data Mining Approach

Jin Yu[a], **Syed Sibte Raza Abidi**[a], **Paul Artes**[b], **Andy McIntyre**[a], **Malcolm Heywood**[a]

[a]*Health Informatics Lab, Faculty of Computer Science, Dalhousie University, Halifax, Canada*
[b]*Department of Ophthalmology, Dalhousie University, Halifax, Canada*

Abstract

The availability of modern imaging techniques such as Confocal Scanning Laser Tomography (CSLT) for capturing high-quality optic nerve images offer the potential for developing automatic and objective methods for diagnosing glaucoma. We present a hybrid approach that features the analysis of CSLT images using moment methods to derive abstract image defining features. The features are then used to train classifers for automatically distinguishing CSLT images of normal and glaucoma patient. As a first, in this paper, we present investigations in feature subset selction methods for reducing the relatively large input space produced by the moment methods. We use neural networks and support vector machines to determine a sub-set of moments that offer high classification accuracy. We demonstratee the efficacy of our methods to discriminate between healthy and glaucomatous optic disks based on shape information automatically derived from optic disk topography and reflectance images.

Keywords:
Glaucoma, Confocal Scanning Laser Tomography, Moment Methods, Neural Networks, Support Vector Machines, Data Mining

1. Introduction

Glaucoma is an age-related disease that slowly and painlessly damages the optic nerve, causing loss of vision and potentially blindness. Glaucoma rarely causes symptoms until the later stages of the disease, and epidemiology surveys have shown that approximately 50% of cases are undetected. As yet there is no single diagnostic test that provides both high sensitivity and specificity, and epidemiological surveys in North America and Europe have shown that approximately half of all glaucoma cases remain undetected [1].

With modern imaging techniques such as Confocal Scanning Laser Tomography (CSLT), high-quality optic nerve images can now be speedily acquired for diagnostic purposes. The availability of CSLT image capture systems naturally provides the potential for the automated classification of optic nerve images into glaucoma and normal. Yet, to date, diagnostic analysis on optic disc profiles or contours requires human intervention—a trained professional defines the margins of the optic disc profile by manually outlining the optic disc of the patient (a process that is highly subjective in nature). Whilst CLST image analysis has tremendous potential to improve the detection of glaucoma, current methods for image analysis fail to detect optic nerve damage with sufficient accuracy to be reliable as diagnostic tools [2].

In this project, we aim to automate the interpretation of CSLT images by applying powerful image processing techniques to derive image data that can be applied to a suite of data mining algorithms to develop a *glaucoma diagnostic support system* as shown in Figure 1.

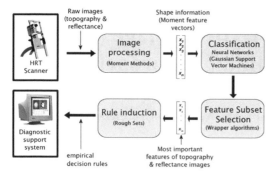

Figure 1: The functional diagram for a glaucoma diagnostic support system

In this paper we present research results concerning CSLT image analysis, feature subset selection leading to classification of the optic disk images. We present, the derivation of image-defining features from CSLT images using *Moment Methods* [3] and experiments involving neural networks and support vector machines to determine a sub-set of features that offer high classification accuracy. We demonstrate the efficacy of our methods to discriminate between healthy and glaucomatous optic disks based on shape information automatically derived from optic disk topography and reflectance images.

2. CSLT Image Analysis Methods

Segmentation of the CSLT image currently relies on the subjective definition of a contour line and is therefore subject to random and systematic error. Machine image analysis systems provide an objective mean to analyze CSLT images [4]. HRT devices capture the digital topographic optic disk image and pre-process it by compensation for shifts, tilt and rotation.

We use an image processing technique, referred to as Moment Methods, to extract features from CSLT images. The features are represented and analyzed in terms of orthogonal moments, in our case Zernike moments [5], which describe the image's properties by their order (n) and repetition (m) with respect to a digital image—the low order moments capture gross shape information and high order moments incrementally resolve high frequency information (representing detail) of the digital image. For a given order, n, there are a total of $(n / 2 + 1)(n + 1)$ Zernike moments, each of which is invariant to rotation in the digital image and which may be further normalized to effect invariance to image translation and scale.

An example of the reconstruction process for a CSLT topography images is illustrated in figure 2. In this example the upper left image is the original; the upper right is the result of an edge filter applied to extract the outline (or shape) of the original image; the lower left cell is the reconstructed image from Zernike moments (up to and including order 35 for figure 2); the lower right cell plots the original edge image overlaid on the reconstructed Zernike image for comparative purposes. Two attractive features of this analysis is that (a) moments can be made invariant to shifts, rotations and magnification changes; and (b) the optic disc is centered in the image, thus avoiding the requirement for an independent segmentation stage in which the object is explicitly identified.

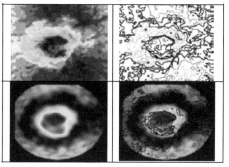

Figure 2: The transformation and reconstruction of a CLST image using moment methods

In our experiments, the moment order for the CSLT images ranges from 2 to 29. For each order n, the corresponding repetition m must meet the conditions (i) m <= n and (ii) m+n is always an even number. Finally, a total of 254 moment features are extracted for each image (shown in table 1). The combinations of different orders and repetitions are shown in table 2, where each moment is extracted from a unique order and repetition. For example, Moment1 is from order2 and repetition0; Moment254 is from order30 and repetition30. Out study is to select optimum moment feature subset to form an accurate classifier based on the data in table2.

Image #	Moment 1	Moment n	Moment 254	Order	Repition	Order	Repition
1	237417.84	...	30034.26	2	0, 2	3	1, 3
2	526288.12	...	38582.63	4	0, 2, 4	5	1, 3, 5
.....				...	...	...	...
N	233127.29	...	32372.43	29	1, 3, 5, 7, 9, 11, 13, 15,17,19, 21, 23, 25, 27, 29	30	0, 2, 4, 6, 8, 10, 12, 14, 16, 18, 20, 22, 24, 26, 28, 30

Table 1: A sample of moment values defining CSLT Images *Table 2: The order and repetition values for each CSLT image*

3. Feature Subset Selection from Moments

Given the set of 254 moments for each CSLT image, the next step is to determine a set of optimal moments that can provide a high value of classification accuracy. The rationale for feature subset selection is based on the observation that a large number of abstract moments tend to compromise the accuracy of supervised learning classifiers, the classification rules are difficult to understand and computational cost is high. To circumvent this problem, as a first step we attempt to determine N number of moments that can render a high classification accuracy.

Note that, low order moments capture gross shape information and high order moments represent finer details of the digital image [6]. For our experiments, high order moments can be regarded as noise because we are interested in the gross shape of the image which is essentially defined by lower order moments. So the feature selection problem is to determine the optimal value for N—i.e sufficent number of moments that can effectively determine the shape of the image. We use artificial neural network (ANN) and support vector machine (SVM) as the candidate classification methods used in tandem to determine the value of N.

3.1 Feature Selection Methodology

We list below the salient steps of our feature selection via classification methodology:

Dataset Selection: We had 1257 topography images spanning 136 subjects, of which 51 are healthy and 85 are glaucoma patients. Every subject has a series of images taken at different times. For our experiments, we considered the baseline image (i.e. the first image) for each patient. Hence, the dataset comprises 136 images reprsented as 254 moments each.

Dataset Partitioning and Normalization: For both ANN and SVM experiments, the dataset was randomly divided into 75% for training and 25% for testing data. The moment features were normalized in the range [-1, +1] using the following formula.

Moment Groups: Based on the moment extract algorithm, each image is represented as 254 moments that are subdivided into 29 groups based on their order (see table 2). For our experiments, we consider moments groups as opposed to individual moments.

Feature subset selection strategy: We employ a classifer based feature subset selection stragegy where the classifier is incrementally trained, where in each iteration the number of features is increased and the corresponding classification accuracy is determined. Given our understanding that high-order moments entail fine-grained image information, the assumption here is that when high-order moments are included in the training set the classification accuracy of the classifer will decrease and continue to decrease as additional high-order moments are subsequently included in the data-set. The point at which the classification accuracy starts to decrease can be deemed as the cut-off point for determining the optimal number of moments sufficent for representing the shape information of the CSLT image. For training the classifier, we start with the smallest group (i.e. moment order2), train and test the classifer. In the next step, the training data is supplemnetd with the next group of moments and the entire training cycle is repeated.

3.2 ANN Experimental Study

In our experiment, a three layer ANN employing the standard backpropagation algorithm is used [7]. The input layer corresponds to the number of moments in the training set and the output layer comprises one unit which represents the two classes—i.e. glaucoma (1) or healthy (-1). The backpropagation algorithm uses the tansigmoid function to adjust the weights.

Grp	Accur.	Grp	Accur.	Grp	Accur.
1	0.7197	11	**0.7393**	21	0.7390
2	0.7071	12	0.7224	22	0.7271
3	0.6868	13	0.7324	23	0.7179
4	0.7072	14	0.7294	24	0.7257
5	0.6769	15	0.7268	25	0.7176
6	0.6832	16	0.7241	26	0.7224
7	0.6762	17	0.7210	27	0.7257
8	**0.7400**	18	0.7359	28	0.7288
9	0.7297	19	0.7272	29	0.7144
10	0.7271	20	0.7235		

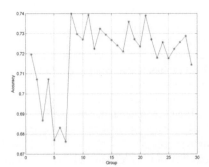

Table 3: Classification accuracy results for ANN   *Figure 3: Classification accuracy results for ANN*

As per our strategy, initially the input vector comprises group 1 moments (i.e. moment1 and moment 2). The classifer is trained 200 times, where each training instance represents a random initialization of the weights. The mean classification accuracy value is used as the final accuracy. The next training cycle includes the next group of moments and the training process is repeated. The classification accuracy results are shown in table 3 and the graph is shown in figure 3. It may be noted that high accuracies are achieved for momemts included between groups 8 and 11.

3.3 SVM Experiment Study

Feature subset selection is additionally pursued using a different learning method viz. SVM to get a comparable view of the classification accuracies with respect tomoment groups. We posit that a comparison of the experimental results for ANN and SVM will also us to determine the optimal number of moments for classiifcation purposes.

SVM is actually a linear machine and its goal is to find the particular hyperplane: $w^T x_i + b = 0$ for which the margin of separation is maximized. By using inner-product kernels to nonlinearly map an input vector into a high dimension space, SVM can find a linear separating hyperplane with maximal margin. In our experiment, RBF is chosen as the kernel function because of the following reasons:

1) RBF can handle cases when the relation between class labels and attributes is nonlinear. Linear perception and correlation analysis show our moments and class label are nonlinear.
2) Compared with polynomial kernel, it has less kernel parameter.
3) RBF has less numerical difficulties.

In order to use RBF, two hyper parameter C and γ need to be decided in advance. C is often one value among $2^{-5}, 2^{-3}, ..., 2^{15}$ and γ among $2^{-15}, 2^{-13}, ..., 2^3$. So a 5-fold cross validation is used to find a good pair of (C, γ) based on training data. We used the LIBSVM version 2.71 developed by National TaiWan University is used as our SVM experiment tool.

The training strategy for SVM is similar to that for ANN, where for each training cycle we increment the moments by the next group of moments and after training the classification accuracy is recorded. The experimental results are shown in table 4 and the graph is shown in figure 4.

Grp	Accu.	Grp	Accu.	Grp	Accu.
1	0.7618	11	**0.8696**	21	0.7985
2	0.7706	12	0.7676	22	0.7500
3	0.7529	13	0.7721	23	0.7912
4	0.7103	14	0.7941	24	0.7838
5	0.7250	15	0.7735	25	0.7662
6	0.7000	16	0.7662	26	0.7882
7	0.7147	17	0.8117	27	0.7941
8	0.7397	18	0.7853	28	0.7750
9	0.7162	19	0.7662	29	0.7941
10	0.7044	20	0.7750		

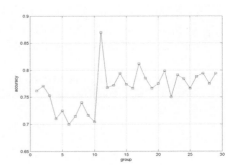

Table 4: Classification accuracy results for SVM

Figure 4: Classification accuracy results for SVM

4. Analysis and Conclusion

The classification accuracy, with increments of moment groups in the input vector, indicate a similar accuracy trends. When the feature subset comprises the first 11 groups of moments, both the SVM and ANN give a relatively high classification accuracy values of 86.96% and

73.93%, respectively. Also, it is noted that from group 12 and onwards the classification accuracy tends to decrease in both cases.

Based on this observation, we conclude that a feature subset comprising the first 11 moment groups represents the optimal number of features that are needed to produce high classification accuracy between normal and glaucoma patients. So moment group 11 is deemed as the cut-off point, such that moments 1 – 47 are used for training the classifiers. This is a significant reduction of the input space which originally comprised 254 moments.

We also note that the SVM based classifier typically produces comparatively higher accuracy values for similar moment groups than that produced by ANN on the same feature subset. We also note that SVM can produce more stable classification performance than ANN.

In conclusion, we have presented an alternate approach based on moment methods to analyze CSLT image for glaucoma detection. As a first step, we have demonstarted the application of machine learning algorithms on the rather unique data of moments to determine an optimal subset of moments using two methods, namely ANN and SVM. In the next step we plan to derive symbolic rules using a suite of rule induction algorithms to provide symbolic knowledge for diagnosing glaucoma which would be a step forward in the automation of decision support for glaucoma based on CSLT images.

5. References

[1] Nicolela MT, Drance SM, "Various Glaucomatous nerve appearances: Clinical Correlations," Ophthalmology. 103(4) pp 640-649, 1996.

[2] Teh CH, Chin RT, "On image analysis by the methods of moments," IEEE Trans. Pattern Anal. Machine Intell., 10(4), pp. 96-513, July 1998.

[3] Varma R., Steinmann W.C., Scott I.U., "Expert agreement in evaluating the optic disc for glaucoma," Ophthalmology. 99(2) pp 215-221, 1992.

[4] Castleman KR, "Digital Image Processing", Prentice Hall, Upper Saddle River, New Jersey 1996.

[5] Teague M, "Image analysis via the general theory of moments," J. Opt. Soc. Amer., 1980, Vol. 70(8), pp. 920-930.

[6] McIntyre A, Heywood MI, Artes PH, Abidi SSR, 'Toward Glaucoma Classification with Moment Methods," 1st Canadian Conference on Computer and Robot Vision (CRV'04), 2004.

[7] Khotanzad A, Her J, "Classification of invariant image representations using a neural network," IEEE Trans Acoustics, Speech, and Signal Processing, v. 38, pp. 1028-1038.

Connecting Medical Informatics and Bio-Informatics
R. Engelbrecht et al. (Eds.)
IOS Press, 2005

SVM Modeling via a Hybrid Genetic Strategy. A Health Care Application

Gilles Cohen[a], **Mélanie Hilario**[b], **Christian Pellegrini**[b], **Antoine Geissbuhler**[a]

[a] *Service of Medical Informatics, University Hospital of Geneva, 1211 Geneva, Switzerland*
[b] *Artificial Intelligence Laboratory, University of Geneva, 1211 Geneva, Switzerland*

Abstract

This paper addresses the model selection problem for Support Vector Machines. A hybrid genetic algorithm guided by Direct Simplex Search to evolves hyperparameter values using an empirical error estimate as a steering criterion. This approach is specificaly tailored and experimentally evaluated on a health care problem which involves discriminating 11 % nosocomially infected patients from 89 % non infected patients. The combination of Direct Search Simplex with GAs is shown to improve the performance of GAs in terms of solution quality and computational efficiency. Unlike most other hyperparameter tuning techniques, our hybrid approach does not require supplementary effort such as computation of derivatives, making them well suited for practical purposes. This method produces encouraging results: it exhibits high performance and good convergence properties.

Keywords
Machine Learning, Optimisation, Genetic Algorithm, Nosocomial Infection

1. Introduction

Support vector machines (SVM) are a powerful machine learning method for classification problems. However, to obtain good generalisation performance, a necessary condition is to choose an appropriate set of model hyperparameters (i.e. regularisation parameter (C) and kernel parameters) depending on the data. The choice of SVM model parameters can have a profound effect on the resulting model's generalisation performance. Most approaches use trial and error procedures to tune SVM hyperparameters while trying to minimise the training and test errors. Such an approach may not really obtain the best performance while consuming an enormous amount of time. Another common but more systematic and reliable approach is to decide on parameter ranges and then do an exhaustive grid search over the parameter space to find the best setting. Unfortunately, even moderately high resolution searches can result in a large number of evaluations and unacceptably long run times. Recently other approaches to parameter tuning have been proposed [1-3]. These methods use a gradient descent search to optimise a validation error, a leave-one-out (LOO) error or an upper bound on the generalisation error. However, gradient descent oriented methods may require restrictive assumptions regarding, e.g., continuity or differentiability. Typically the criterion, such as LOO error, is not differentiable, so approaches based on gradient descent are not generally applicable using cross-validation. Furthermore, they are likely to be trapped in a local minima. For such non differentiable criteria other approaches based on Evolutionary Algorithms have been investigated [4-6]. However, when applied to complex problems, such global approaches suffer from high computational cost due to their slow convergence. For Genetic Algorithms (GAs), a common method for dealing with this drawback is to combine GAs with a complementary local search technique [7, 8]. Such a hybrid approach combines the advantages of GAs with those of local search and explores a better trade-off between computational cost and the global optimality of the solution found.

To improve the convergence rate of a GA, we propose a hybrid approach that combines a GA with the Direct Simplex Search method of Nelder-Mead (DSS) and apply it to a medical problem. The main advantages of a hybrid GA (HGA) based strategy are (1) the increased probability of finding the global optimum within a reasonable convergence time, even where a large number of closely competing local optima may exist, and (2) the suitability for problems for which it is impossible or difficult to obtain information about the derivatives.

This paper is organised as follows. A brief introduction to GAs and DSS is followed by a short review on SVM and SVM model selection. We then describe our hybrid approach and the healthcare problem used as a testbed for assessing our method. Experimental results are presented to show the general applicability of the method. Finally, we close with a general conclusion and a preview of future work.

2. Materials and Methods

2.1   Genetic Algorithms

Genetic algorithms (GAs) are stochastic global search techniques and optimisation methods deeply rooted in the mechanism of evolution and natural genetics. GAs are attractive for their ability to avoid suboptimal solutions, freedom from derivatives and ease of parallelisation. By mimicking biological selection and reproduction, GAs can efficiently search through the solution space of complex problems. In GAs a population of possible solutions called chromosomes is maintained. Each chromosome, which is composed of genes, represents an encoding of a candidate solution of the problem and is associated with a fitness value, representing its ability to solve the optimisation problem and evaluated by a fitness function. The goal of GAs is to combine genes to obtain new chromosomes with better fitness, i.e., which are better solutions of the optimisation problem. Basically, a GA uses three operators, namely reproduction, crossover, and mutation. For a more thorough description of genetic algorithms the reader can refer to Goldberg (1989) [9].

2.2   Nelder-Mead Simplex Method

The Direct Search Simplex (DSS) of Nelder-Mead [10] is the most popular optimisation method that neither relies on derivatives nor requires the objective function to be smooth, it has been used to solve many problems, especially in chemistry, chemical engineering, and medicine. Although there are no theoretical results on the convergence of the algorithm, it works very well on a broad range of practical problems. The DSS method is based on successive transformations of a simplex, a geometric figure defined by $n+1$ vertices (real n-vectors). The method adapts itself to the local landscape, using four possible operations on the current simplex, each associated with a coefficient: reflection (ρ), expansion (ξ), contraction (γ), and shrinkage (σ), to locate the minimum. The simplex in n dimensions can be viewed as a creature with $n+1$ feet that tries to roll down into the global minimum. One foot is the starting estimate, and the others are generated randomly within the search space. The objective function is computed for each foot, and the creature decides to move its "worst foot" to a better position. The creature first attempts to reflect its worst foot through the centroid of the remaining feet (reflection). If the new position it lands on is better than the one it came from, it attempts to go further in that direction (expansion). If the position after reflection is worse, it attempts to place its foot in an intermediate position (contraction). If none of these moves gives a better solution than the worst leg, it attempts moving all its feet closer to the best one (shrinkage). The procedure is iterated until a stopping criterion is satisfied. Usually two stopping criteria are used: either the length of the edges of the current simplex becomes less than a prescribed positive number (the simplex becomes too small) or the function values at the vertices are too close. Figure (1) depicts the effect of the different operations.

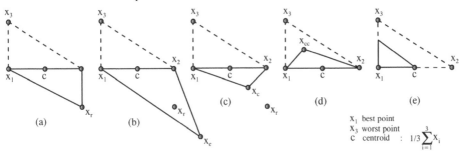

Figure 1 Nelder-Mead simplices after (a) reflection, (b) expansion, (c) outside contraction, (d) inside contraction and (e) shrinkage. The original simplex is drawn with a dashed line.

2.3   SVM Model Selection via Hybrid GA-DSS

2.3.1   Support Vector Machine

Support vector machines [11-12] (SVMs) are state of the art learning machines based on statistical learning theory. The basic idea is to map each data point of the training set onto a high dimensional space by some function ϕ and to seek for a separating hyperplane (w,b), with w the weight vector and b the bias, in this space which maximises the *margin* or distance between the hyperplane and the closest data points belonging to the different classes. When nonlinear decision boundaries are not needed ϕ is an identity function, otherwise ϕ is performed by a non linear function $k(.,.)$, also called a *kernel*, which defines a dot product in the feature space. We can then substitute the dot product $\langle\phi(x),\phi(x_i)\rangle$ in feature space with the kernel $k(x, x_i)$. Conditions for a function to be a kernel are expressed in a theorem by Mercer [13]. The optimal separating hyperplane can be represented based on a kernel function:

$$f(x) = sign\left(\sum_{i=1}^{n}\alpha_i k(x,x_i) + b\right) \qquad (1.1)$$

For a separable classification task, such an optimal hyperplane exists but very often, the data points will be almost linearly separable in the sense that only a few of the members of the data points cause it to be non linearly separable. Such data points can be accommodated into the theory with the introduction of slack variables that allow particular vectors to be misclassified. The hyperplane margin is then relaxed by penalising the training points misclassified by the system. Furthermore, to adapt to the case of unbalanced distributions the basic idea is to introduce different error weights C^+ and C^- for the positive and the negative class in order to penalise false positives and false negatives differently [4]. This induces a decision boundary which is more distant from the smaller class than from the other. Hence one variant of the algorithm consists of solving the following optimisation problem

$$\text{minimize} \quad \frac{1}{2}\|\mathbf{w}\|^2 + C^+ \sum_{i:y_i=+1} \xi_i + C^- \sum_{i:y_i=-1} \xi_i$$

$$\text{subject to} \quad y_i\left(\langle \mathbf{w}, \phi(\mathbf{x}_i)\rangle + b\right) \geq 1 - \xi_i, \xi_i \geq 0 \ \forall i : y_i = +1 \qquad (1.2)$$

$$y_i\left(\langle \mathbf{w}, \phi(\mathbf{x}_i)\rangle + b\right) \leq 1 - \xi_i, \xi_i \geq 0 \ \forall i : y_i = -1$$

where ξ_i is a positive slack variable that measures the degree of violation of the constraint. The penalties C^+ and C^- are regularisation parameters that control the trade-off between maximizing the margin and minimizing the training error.

2.3.2   Model Selection Criteria

To obtain good performance, some parameters in SVMs have to be selected carefully. These parameters include the regularisation parameters C and the parameters of the kernel function. These "higher level" parameters are usually referred to as hyperparameters. The model selection problem is to select the best model from a candidate set so that generalisation error is minimised over all possible examples drawn from an unknown distribution $P(x,y)$. As the data distributions P in real problems are not known in advance, generalisation error is not computable and one needs some reliable estimates of the generalisation performance. We estimate generalisation error via cross-validation using class weighted accuracy $CWA=w^*sensitivity+(1-w)^*specificity$, which assigns user-defined weights to sensitivity and specificity in order to compensate for class imbalance [14].

2.3.3   Hybrid Global-Local Search Method

Many studies have shown that GAs perform well for global searching because they are capable of quickly finding and exploiting promising regions of the search space, but they take a relatively long time to converge to a local optimum. Although best suited for hyperparameter tuning in which typical selection criteria exhibit multiple local optima [3], GAs are too expensive in terms of computational time [4] for this task. Hence, since GAs work well as a coarse global search technique we combine them with a local search method in order to increase the likelihood of reaching the global optima within an acceptable amount of time. In our proposed hybrid scheme the GA is used to find hills and DSS to climb them. In this way, the GA is used to optimise the search space and the hill climber is used to optimise the search locally in the discovered areas. This combination is done as follows: first GA is started, then DSS is turned on after a prescribed number of generations N_G. The connection between the GA and DSS is made by choosing the best solution of the optimised GA population. It is expected that DSS, starting from a pre-optimised solution could converge more quickly and more accurately.

2.4   Application to Nosocomial Infection Detection

We applied our hyperparameter optimisation method to a medical problem, the detection of nosomial infections. A nosocomial infection (from the Greek word *nosokomeion* for hospital) is an infection that develops during hospitalisation whereas it was not present or incubating at the time of the admission. Usually, a disease is considered a nosocomial infection if it develops 48 hours after admission. The University Hospital of Geneva (HUG) has been performing yearly prevalence studies to detect and monitor nosocomial infections since 1994 [15]. Their methodology is as follows: the investigators visit every ward of the HUG over a period of approximately three weeks. All patients hospitalised for

48 hours or more at the time of the study are included. Medical records, kardex, X-ray and microbiology reports are reviewed, and additional information is eventually obtained by interviewing nurses or physicians in charge. Collected variables include demographic characteristics, admission date, admission diagnosis, comorbidities, McCabe score, type of admission, provenance, hospitalisation ward, functional status, previous surgery, previous intensive care unit (ICU) stay, exposure to antibiotics, antacid and immunosuppressive drugs and invasive devices, laboratory values, temperature, date and site of infection, fulfilled criteria for infection.

After preliminary data cleaning with the help of hospital experts on nosocomial infections, the resulting dataset consisted of 683 cases and 49 variables. The major difficulty inherent in the data (as in many medical diagnostic applications) is the highly skewed class distribution. Out of 683 patients, only 75 (11%) were infected and 608 were not. This application was thus an excellent testbed for assessing the efficacy of the use of genetic algorithms to tune SVM hyperparameters in the presence of class imbalance.

3. Experimentation and Results

The experimental goal was to assess the hybrid GA for tuning SVM hyperparameters automatically and within a reasonable amount of time. We used 5-fold cross-validation to compare the quality of the HGA with pure GA in terms of performance and computational cost. To train our SVM classifiers we used a Gaussian kernel $k(x, x_i) = \exp(-\gamma|x-z|^2)$. Thus the hyperparameter set to tune was $\theta : (\gamma, C^+, C^-)$. Standard parameter settings from the GA and DSS literature were used: (a) for GAs, a constant population size of 20, a crossover of 0.6 and a mutation parameter of 0.001; (b) for DSS, the coefficient values $\rho=1$, $\xi=2$ and $\sigma=1/2$ were used for reflection, expansion and shrinkage respectively. Different values of N_G were tried. For CWA, a weight of 0.7 was assigned to sensitivity which is the priority goal in nosocomial infection surveillance. Table 1 shows the comparative results between our search method (HGA) and a simple GA for the nosocomial dataset. Final results were compared using McNemar's test which revealed no significant difference between the two approaches at the 95% confidence level. However, it is clear from the last column of the table that HGA incurred roughly half the number of function evaluations required by GA to find the best parameters (one function evaluation corresponds to building 5 SVM models).

Table 1 –Performance of SVMs using a Gaussian kernel with optimal parameter set (γ, C^+, C^-) found via GA and HGA. Computational load: number of function evaluations.

Methods	Performance							Computational load		
	C^+	C^-	γ	Acc.	Sens.	Spec.	CWA (w=0.7)	N_G	DSS (N. ev.)	N. fct eval.
Pure GA	14	0.1	10^{-3}	80	92	78.3	87.9	50	-	1000
HGA	30	0.15	26.10^{-3}	80.9	92.7	78.8	88.53	25	35	535

4. Conclusion and future work

We developed a hybrid algorithm in an attempt to blend the power of GA-based search with the speed of local search. The proposed hybridisation approach is fairly simple: a coarse-grained algorithm which first runs GAs to focus on a promising initial region, followed by DSS to quickly find the optimum in that region. This approach can reliably find very good hyperparameter settings for SVMs with Gaussian kernels in a fully automated way. Our experiments have shown that HGA outperforms pure GA in terms of computation time.

However, the performance value found is, at best, a small improvement over the ordinary GA; improvement of solution quality by means of HGA is not obvious and more extensive experiments on other problems must be done.

Another issue we would like to address is how to decide when the GA has reached the "right region". If the GA is terminated too late, it wastes potentially expensive function evaluations; if it is terminated prematurely the solution subsequently found by the local search algorithm finds will not be the global optimum. A potential solution could be to examine the current GA population at fixed intervals in order to determine useful characteristics concerning the topography of the area of the search space being explored. Based on this information, GA search is either pursued or terminated (and the local search algorithm is started). Finally, we plan to extend this work to other kernels with much more hyperparameters and to compare it with gradient-based hybridisation.

5. Acknowledgments

The authors are grateful for the dataset provided by the infection control team of the University of Geneva Hospitals.

6. Reference

[1]   Chapelle O., Vapnik V., Bousquet O., Mukherjee S. Choosing Multiple Parameters for Support Vector Machines. *Machine Learning* 2002;46:131-159.

[2]   Keerthi S.S. Efficient tuning of SVM hyperparameters using radius/margin bound and iterative algorithms. In: IEEE Transactions on Neural Networks; 2003; 2003. p. 1225-1229.

[3]   Chung K.M., Kao W.C, Sun C.L, Wang L.L, Lin C.J. Radius margin bounds for support vector machines with the RBF kernel. *Neural Comput.* 2003;15:2643--2681.

[4]   Cohen G., Hilario M., Geissbuhler A. Model Selection for Support Vector Classifiers via Genetic Algorithms. An Application to Medical Decision Support. In: Int Symp Biol Med Data Analysis; 2004.

[5]   Friedrichs F., Igel C. Evolutionary tuning of multiple SVM parameters. In: *12th European Symposium on Artificial Neural Networks (ESANN)*; 2004; 2004.

[6]   Runarsson T.P., Sigurdsson S. Asynchronous Parallel Evolutionary Model Selection for Support Vector Machines. *Neural Information Processing - Letters and Reviews* 2004;3:1065-1076.

[7]   Hart W.E. *Adaptive Global Optimization with Local Search.* San Diego: University of Calfornia; 1994.

[8]   Yen J., Liao J.C., Lee B., Randolph D. A hybrid approach to modeling metabolic systems using a genetic algorithm and simplex methods. *IEEE Trans. on Sys., Man, and Cybern.* 1998;28:173-191.

[9]   Goldberg DE. *Genetic Algorithms in Search, Optimization, and Machine Learning*: Addison; 1989.

[10] Nelder J.A., Mead R. A simplex method for function minimization. *Computer Journal* 1965;7:308-313.

[11] Cortes C., Vapnik V. Support Vector Networks. *Machine Learning* 1995;20:273-297.

[12] Vapnik V. *Statistical Learning Theory*: Wiley; 1998.

[13] Cristianini N., Taylor J.S. *An Introduction to Support Vector Machines*: Cambridge U. Press; 2000.

[14] Cohen G., Hilario M., Sax H., Hugonnet S. Data Imbalance in surveillance of nosocomial infections. In: *International Symposium on Medical Data Analysis*; 2003; Berlin; 2003.

[15] Harbarth S., Ruef C., Francioli P., Widmer A., Pittet D. Nosocomial infections in Swiss University Hospitals: a multicentre survey and review of the published experience. *Schweiz Med Wochenschr* 1999 (129):1521-28.

Address for correspondence

Gilles Cohen, University and Hospitals of Geneva, Service of Medical Informatics
24, rue Micheli-du-Crest, CH-1211 Geneva 14, Switzerland. gilles.cohen@sim.hcuge.ch

Connecting Medical Informatics and Bio-Informatics
R. Engelbrecht et al. (Eds.)
IOS Press, 2005

Improving Pathway Compliance and Clinician Performance by Using Information Technology

R Blaser[a], M Schnabel[b], O Heger[a], E Opitz[a], R Lenz[a], K A Kuhn[c]

[a]*Institute of Medical Informatics, Philipps-University Marburg, Germany*
[b]*Department of Trauma, Reconstructive and Hand Surgery, Philipps-University Marburg, Germany*
[c]*Institute of Medical Statistics and Epidemiology, Technical University Munich, Germany*

Abstract

To deliver patient-specific advice at the time and place of a consultation, to improve clinician performance and compliance by using computer-based decision support, and to integrate such IT solutions with the clinical workflow are important strategies for the implementation of clinical pathways. User acceptance plays a critical role: additional effort has to be balanced with enough benefit for the users. Experiences from routine use of an online surgical pathway at Marburg University Medical Center show that it is possible to successfully address this issue by seamlessly integrating patient-specific pathway recommendations with documentation tasks which have to be done anyway and by substantially reusing entered data to accelerate routine tasks (e.g. by automatically generating orders and reports).

Keywords:
Clinical Pathways; Clinical Decision Support Systems; Systems Integration; User Acceptance

1. Introduction

For more than a decade, studies on the incidence and nature of adverse events in medicine have shown that errors in medicine are not rare and may cause severe harm [1-3]. The nature and preventability of adverse events have been studied, and cognitive overload of physicians was found to be among the reasons. Evidence-based clinical guidelines or pathways can reduce variability in practice and improve patient care outcomes [4]. Implementation strategies for guidelines and pathways which deliver patient-specific advice at the time and place of a consultation are most likely to be effective [4, 5]. Computer-based decision support (e.g. reminder systems) can improve clinician performance and guideline compliance [6, 7]. Such a capability depends on the availability of the data to make the appropriate recommendations [8]. Suitable interaction mechanisms for data entry during consultation and for the representation of patient-specific recommendations and warnings are needed. These IT solutions should be integrated with the clinical workflow and give back to the user something of value in order to minimise and to offset the inconvenience of using the system [5, 8].

  In 2003 we analysed quality problems with discharge letters at the Department of Trauma, Reconstructive and Hand Surgery at University Medical Center, Marburg, Germany. Based on this analysis we systematically elaborated easy to implement IT solutions which have the potential to prevent treatment errors and to improve the documentation quality by using structured data entry and reminders [9]. We used these interaction mechanisms not only to increase the quality of our discharge letters by implementing a kind of a "mini-pathway" for the letter writing process, but also to support the online implementation of major parts of clinical pathways by integrating the routine documentation process with patient-specific advice in the context of the clinical pathway.

In this paper we describe our computer-based implementation of a surgical pathway at the Department of Trauma, Reconstructive and Hand Surgery at Marburg University Medical Center, and we report on first experiences from routine use.

2. Background

Setting

In 2001/2002 the care process for patients with proximal femoral fracture at the Department of Trauma, Reconstructive and Hand Surgery was analysed and weak points were identified (e.g. delays in timing the operation, clarification of osteoporosis) by a prospective study on 169 patients with a one year follow up (96.6% survivors). Based on the process analysis, a formal barrier analysis, and a literature and guideline research a target pathway was defined. The pathway was finalised through a multi-tiered consensus process and adopted by the board of directors. Figure 1 shows a simplified diagram of the pathway. For each step in the pathway there exists a detailed description with recommendations, e.g. for indicated X-ray examinations or appropriate medication.

In order to train the clinicians and to integrate the clinical pathway into daily routine, academic detailing and pathway controlling are used as implementation strategies. The integration of an online model of core parts of the pathway into the Marburg Health Information System was aimed at to get active decision support at the time and place of a consultation and to receive additional benefits for the clinicians from data reuse.

IT infrastructure

Marburg University Medical Center has established a responsive IT infrastructure and a holistic Health Information System (HIS) on the basis of a commercially available product, which is in widespread use in Germany, Austria, and Switzerland: the Orbis®/OpenMed-system. The Marburg HIS represents one of the most advanced installations of this system, and significant impulses for improving the system have resulted from the Marburg project [10, 11]. The system offers functionality for business/financial purposes and patient data management, as well as basic clinical functionality (e.g. ICD/ICPM and reports), and comprises an integrated CASE1 tool for rapid implementation of integrated clinical modules ("generator tool"). This generator tool is part of a vendor-specific application framework which allows to incrementally add new application modules or to adapt generic applications to specific requirements, and thereby provides the fundamentals for a responsive IT-infrastructure and demand driven software development. A detailed description of the implementation of the generator tool can be found in [11]. We have also developed an adapted software engineering process which is primarily intended to achieve an IT-alignment to healthcare process requirements [10, 12].

---

[1] CASE: Computer Aided Software Engineering

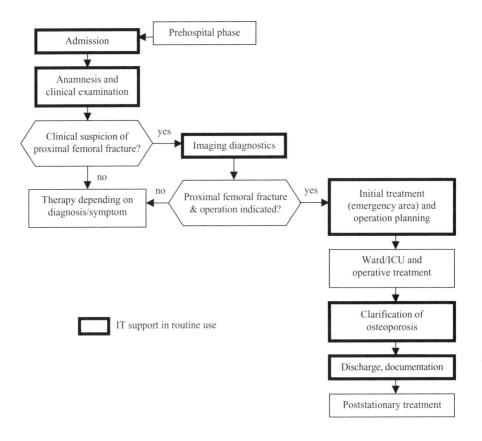

Figure 1: Clinical pathway for proximal femoral fracture (simplified

3. Materials and methods

Our intention was to utilise the potential of our responsive IT-infrastructure and our adapted software engineering process to develop an IT-supported pathway that is aligned to the clinical work process. Based on the results from pathway controlling, those core parts of the clinical pathway were identified for which computer-based decision support could be used effectively or necessary data should be entered. The clinical pathway model and other results from the pathway development process (e.g. quality affecting factors from the formal barrier analysis) as well as the experiences from pathway controlling and from our previous work described in [9] flowed into the specification of user-defined forms for structured data entry and of rules for recommendations and warnings.

According to our adapted software engineering process the users were intensively involved in the development of the application aligned to their requirements and integrated with the clinical workflow. The generator tool was used to rapidly develop and iteratively refine prototypes of the application directly based on the common database of the Marburg HIS. Feasibility and usability analyses were performed to test the interaction design and different mechanisms for the representation of rules.

After the application was intensively tested and approved by the key users, it was activated in the routine system at the end of August 2004. IT-support for further parts of the pathway (clarification of osteoporosis and generation of discharge letters) followed in April 2005. Feedback from the clinicians is used to continuously improve the application resulting in two minor updates since begin of routine use.

4. Results

Figure 1 shows the parts of the clinical pathway which are supported by IT. The application consists of 10 forms for structured data entry and decision support:

- Structured entry of data from *admission*, *anamnesis* and *clinical examination*;
- Selection of procedures for *imaging diagnostics* with rule-based recommendations derived from previously entered data; online orders of the selected procedures to the radiology department can be placed (previously entered patient data is reused);
- Documentation of the *principle diagnosis* and *other diagnoses* (ICD codes and additional medical description);
- Selection of procedures and medication for the *initial treatment* in the emergency area, and *operation planning* (e.g. selection of appropriate implant) with rule-based recommendations and warnings derived from previously entered data;
- Structured entry of *instructions for the ward*;
- Structured data entry for *clarification of osteoporosis*.

A *report* for further treatment on the ward can be generated from previously entered data, and these data also can be reused for other routine documentation (e.g. *discharge letters*).

As an example, figure 2 shows the form for initial treatment. Patient-specific pathway information is given by preselected medication and procedures. Those selections which correspond with an existing pathway recommendation are marked with a superscript "p". Deviation from the pathway is possible but needs to be documented (variance documentation). The user can navigate through the forms in the predefined order ("previous" or "next") or he can jump directly to the desired form.

So far, the application contains about 20 rules e.g. for medication, for X-ray recommendations based on the age of the patient and documented diagnoses, and for warnings, e.g. if a documented allergy contraindicates the use of the selected implant. These rules are represented by using catalogues (e.g. for diagnoses and for X-ray examinations) and correlations between the catalogue entries.

During eight months of routine use, the online pathway was successfully used for 84% of the patients with proximal femoral fracture (n = 123). User feedback was very positive and additional effort for data entry was accepted as enough benefit from data reuse was given back to the users (e.g. generation of online orders and reports).

5. Discussion and Conclusion

More detailed studies on user satisfaction by means of standardised questionnaires and on pathway compliance are about to follow, but user feedback already shows that this clinical module is acceptable and usable in the daily routine.

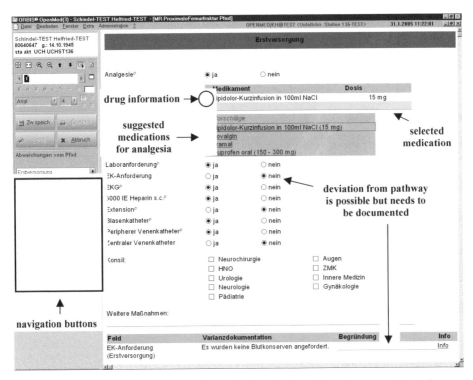

Figure 2: Form for initial treatment with preselected medication and procedures according to the recommendations in the clinical pathway as well as variance documentation.

To deliver patient-specific advice at the time and place of a consultation, to improve clinician performance and compliance by using computer-based decision support, and to integrate such IT solutions with the clinical workflow are important strategies for the implementation of guidelines and clinical pathways [5-8]. Our solution can reach this goal by seamlessly integrating patient-specific pathway information into the routine documentation. Data is made available through structured data entry during consultation, and rule-based recommendations are given to the users in an unobtrusive way by means of preselected medication or procedures. The integrated generator tool and our software engineering process [10-12] make it possible to integrate the IT solution with the clinical workflow and to rapidly adapt it to the users needs.

These approaches also can cause negative effects which have to be considered. Interaction mechanisms for recommendations have to be designed carefully to avoid biases or errors, and it is important to intensively involve the physicians [13]. User acceptance plays a critical role and is one of the major obstacles on the way to online guidelines and pathways [5,8]. Additional effort (e.g. from data entry) has to be balanced with enough benefit for the users. We address this issue by integrating parts of the online pathway with documentation tasks which have to be done anyway and by substantially reusing entered data to accelerate routine tasks (e.g. by automatically generating orders and reports). It is important to concentrate on core parts of the pathway and to keep the online implementation as simple as possible. So far, comparatively simple methods for the representation of rules and for workflow support sufficed for our implementation. In order to be able to implement more complex rules and workflows, if needed, we are testing the ARDEN engine and the workflow engine which are incorporated into the generator tool.

The effectiveness of our approach is continuously being evaluated and improved. Presently adaptations of the interaction mechanisms are being discussed to further increase user benefit and user acceptance.

6. References

[1] Leape LL, Brennan TA, Laird N, Lawthers AG, Localio AR, Barnes BA, Hebert L, Newhouse JP, Weiler PC, Hiatt H. The nature of adverse events in hospitalized patients. Results of the Harvard Medical Practice Study II. *N Engl J Med* 1991; 324(6):377-384.

[2] Thomas EJ, Studdert DM, Burstin HR, Orav EJ, Zeena T, Williams EJ, Howard KM, Weiler PC, Brennan TA. Incidence and types of adverse events and negligent care in Utah and Colorado. *Med Care* 2000; 38(3):261-271.

[3] Wilson RM, Runciman WB, Gibberd RW, Harrison BT, Newby L, Hamilton JD. The Quality in Australian Health Care Study. *Med J Aust* 1995; 163(9):458-471.

[4] Grimshaw JM, Russell IT. Effect of clinical guidelines on medical practice: a systematic review of rigorous evaluations. *Lancet* 1993;342:1317-22.

[5] Shiffman RN, Liaw Y, Brandt CA, Corb GJ. Computer-based guideline implementation systems: a systematic review of functionality and effectiveness. *J Am Med Inform Assoc* 1999; 6(2):104-114.

[6] Johnston ME, Langton KB, Haynes RB, Mathieu A. Effects of computer-based clinical decision support systems on clinician performance and patient outcome. A critical appraisal of research. *Ann Intern Med* 1994; 120(2):135-142.

[7] Elson RB, Connelly DP. Computerized decision support systems in primary care. *Prim Care* 1995; 22(2):365-384.

[8] Zielstorff RD. Online practice guidelines: issues, obstacles, and future prospects. *J Am Med Inform Assoc* 1998; 5(3):227-236.

[9] Blaser R, Schnabel M, Mann D, Jancke P, Kuhn KA, Lenz R. Potential Prevention of Medical Errors in Casualty Surgery by Using Information Technology. In: Haddad HM, Papadopoulos GA, Omicini A, Wainwright RL, Liebrock LM, Palakal MJ, Andreou A, Pattichis C, eds. *Proceedings of the 19th ACM Symposium on Applied Computing (SAC 2004)*. New York: ACM, 2004; pp. 285-290.

[10] Kuhn KA, Lenz R, Elstner T, Siegele H, Moll R. Experiences with a generator tool for building clinical application modules. *Methods Inf Med* 2003; 42(1):37-44.

[11] Lenz R, Elstner T, Siegele H, Kuhn KA. A practical approach to process support in health information systems. *J Am Med Inform Assoc* 2002; 9(6):571-585.

[12] Lenz R, Kuhn KA. Towards a Continuous Evolution and Adaptation of Information Systems in Healthcare. Int J Med Inf 2004; 73(1):75-89.

[13] Anderson JG. Clearing the way for physicians' use of clinical information systems. *Communications of the ACM* 1997; 40(8):83-90.

Address for Correspondence

Rainer Blaser
Institut für Medizinische Informatik
Klinikum der Philipps-Universität Marburg
D-35033 Marburg
GERMANY
e-mail: blaser@med.uni-marburg.de

Connecting Medical Informatics and Bio-Informatics
R. Engelbrecht et al. (Eds.)
IOS Press, 2005

Decision Support for Diagnosis of Lyme Disease

Ole K Hejlesen[a], Kristian G Olesen[a], Ram Dessau[b], Ivan Beltoft[a], Michael Trangeled[a]

[a]Aalborg University, Aalborg, Denmark, [b]Næstved Hospital, Næstved, Denmark

Abstract

This paper describes the development of a Bayesian model for diagnosis of patients suspected of Lyme disease, and the integration of such a model into a medical information system. A Bayesian network incorporating the clinical history and laboratory results has been constructed. Because many of the symptoms are not exclusive to Lyme disease and they develop over time, the clinical history is important for making the correct diagnosis. The model is based on time slices, where each time slice contains the observed pathological picture from one consultation with for example, the general practitioner. Since the time intervals between consultations typically are not equivalent, we have developed a novel method that can handle non-equivalent time intervals between the time slices in the network. The method is based on a description of the general development pattern of Lyme disease, which is implemented in a model that states the conditional probabilities of experiencing a certain pathological picture given time since infection. The model has been integrated into a web-based medical information system, called Borrelia Systems, which has enabled us to evaluate the model during a progressive diagnostic process. The integration has been accomplished through the development of a Bayesian Application Framework. This framework specifies a communication data structure in XML providing a graphical user interface and database components, which can be used when developing systems that are based on Bayesian networks. The framework generalizes the integration of Bayesian networks so that it is possible to switch network without manually having to update or change the system.

Keywords:
Lyme disease; Borrelia; Bayesian networks; Decision Support

1. Introduction

Lyme disease, or Lyme Borreliosis (LB), is the most commonly reported tick-borne infection in Europe and North America. The disease can affect many types of organs including the skin, nervous system, joints and in rare cases other organs. Lyme disease was named in 1977 when arthritis was observed in a cluster of children in and around Lyme, Connecticut, USA. Subsequent studies led to the isolation from the deer tick, Ixodes scapularis, of a gram-negative spirochaete, which was named Borrelia burgdorferi. These bacteria are transmitted to humans by the bite of infected ticks.

Lyme disease, or Lyme Borreliosis (LB), is divided into three stages, named early localized LB (stage 1, 2-30 days after initial infection), early disseminated LB (stage 2, few days - 3 months after initial infection) and late (chronic) LB (stage 3, from 3 months after initial infection). The stage of Lyme disease is decided from the symptoms that the patient is experiencing. In some cases the patient does not develop symptoms of a certain stage or the symptoms are not detected. Therefore, the patient does not always experience earlier stages of Lyme disease. The duration of the stages also varies substantially from case to case and it is therefore difficult to determine the stage of the disease, even though the time since the bite is known.

It is important to make the correct diagnosis of Lyme disease in an early stage, because the complications in the later stages can cause irreversible injuries, if not treated with antibiotics. If Lyme disease of an early stage is diagnosed and treated, almost all cases will recover completely.

The symptoms of Lyme disease are not exclusive for Lyme disease, and it is therefore important to include all parameters when the diagnosis is made. These are the clinical findings, the clinical history, the risk exposure history, and laboratory evidence [1, 2].

Clinical Findings

Erythema Migrans (EM) (stage 1) is the most frequent clinical manifestation of LB and is found in approximately 60% of the cases with LB. EM is characterized by a red rash spreading from the site of a tick bite, as illustrated in Figure 1. The lesion evolves in a circular shape from the centre of the tick bite and out, and can reach from a few centimetres up to 75 cm in diameter. The incubation time is between 2-30 days after the tick bite with a median of 10 days. EM occurs at any age and in both sexes.

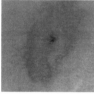

Figure 1 - Erythema Migrans (EM)

Borrelial Lymphocytoma (stage 2) presents as a bluish-red tumour skin infiltrate, up to a few centimetres in diameter, which may occur in some patients. The lesion may develop several weeks to months after a tick bite. The preferred sites are the ear lobe, ear helix, nipple or scrotum in children, and nipple in adults. The lesion may be preceded by EM or occur simultaneously with it. The lesion heals spontaneously but can persist and even grow for several months. Borrelial lymphocytoma is not found in North America.

Acrodermatitis Chronica Atrophicans (ACA) (stage 3) is a progressive skin condition that is most commonly found on the lower leg, but also the soles and palms, toes, fingers, and knees can be involved. The initial signs of ACA are a bluish discoloration and swelling of the skin. ACA does not heal spontaneously and if the patient does not seek medical attention, fibrous thickening may develop over, or close to joints, and after years of progression the skin lesion will gradually become thin shiny and papery.

Early neuroborreliosis (stage 2) is one of the clinical manifestations of Lyme disease that affects the nervous system and is also known as the Bannwarth syndrome. It affects all age groups with a median at the fifth decade. The incubation period of the Bannwarth syndrome is from few weeks to 2 months in adults, but shorter in children. The main manifestations are radicular pain, peripheral pareses and most often facial palsy. It begins with severe radicular pain that have been described as burning, tearing and migrating. The pain continues for approximately two weeks, but has been seen to last up to 25 weeks before complete recovery. Patients with radicular pain may experience depression, agitation, restlessness, sleeplessness, and anxiety. The majority of cases of early neuroborreliosis occur between July and November with the most cases observed in August.

Chronic Neuroborreliosis (stage 3) is very rare and should not be diagnosed without clear laboratory evidence of B. burgdorferi infection, because the symptoms could be caused by other non borrelia related manifestations as neurosyphilis, fungal meningoencephalitis and brain tumours. The major manifestations of chronic neuroborreliosis are encephalitis, radiculomyelitis, transverse myelitis, stroke-like disorders and cranial nerve deficits. It can result in the patient having memory loss, depression, and spastic paraparesis.

Lyme arthritis (stage 2 and 3) is the major clinical manifestation affecting the joints. The knees are most often affected, together with other major joints as ankle, wrist and elbow. 50% of the cases of LB in North America develop arthritis posterior to untreated EM. The problem is not as common in Europe, which is thought to be because of the variations in the distribution of the different species of the bacteria in different parts of the world. Lyme arthritis may occur within several months after an unrecognized primary infection and last for several years. It affects most age groups, but is most likely found in the fourth decade, and older children are more affected than younger.

Acute cardiac involvement (stage 2) is a rarely observed manifestation. The symptoms are conduction disturbances and rhythm disturbances.

Laboratory Evidence

With the exception of typical EM, diagnosis of Lyme disease should always be confirmed by laboratory evidence. In clinical practice indirect methods of detecting borrelial infection is widely used. The method consists of determination of *IgM and IgG antibodies* by e.g. an enzyme linked immunosorbent assay test (ELISA). One of the major advantages of the ELISA test is its ease of use in large scale testing and the avoidance of subjective interpretation. Determining antibodies should be done with caution, as the correlation of results from different laboratories may be poor. This means that clinicians should understand the sensitivity and specificity of ELISA, and be aware of the predictive values for certain clinical manifestations.

A large proportion of the EM patients may have no antibody response. For all other clinical manifestations of LB, laboratory evidence of infection is essential for the diagnosis.

IgM antibodies directed against Borrelia burgdorferi antigens usually appear within three weeks of infection, and peak between four and six weeks post-infection, when IgG antibodies are also likely to be present. The IgG test can show negative until 2-3 months after the infection. The IgG level normally peaks after 4-6 months. Although antibodies tend to wane, they may remain detectable for months or years, with or without treatment, and serology has no role in measuring the response to treatment. The progress of the antibody response is illustrated in Figure 2. Not all patients follow this typical pattern.

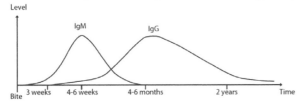

Figure 2 – Typical IgM and IgG development after infection

Epidemiology

LB affects all age groups, but the rate of disease incidences is bimodal with the highest rates found in children less than 15 years of age and in adults older than 35 years of age, and there are slightly more males than females reported with Lyme disease. Disease incidence rates are increased in certain occupational groups, e.g. forestry workers, in some recreational groups such as orienteers and in tourists to high-endemic areas. The majority of the reported cases of LB experience disease onset in June, July, or August, which account for about 70% of the total number of reported cases, and with neuroborreliosis peaking approximately one month later in August.

2. Materials and methods

As described, the disease, i.e. its history, clinical manifestation, time course, serology, and epidemiology, is very variable and has a high degree of uncertainty. Bayesian networks are specifically suited to handle such problems [3, 4] and have also been used in earlier versions of our Borrelia model [5], which were however, not able to handle a history with repetitive clinical examinations. The present version of our system explicitly models the clinical history with one or more consultations with the clinician, and based on this information, it *calculates the probability of Lyme disease*. It should be noted that he present model is tuned to match the European variant of Lyme disease.

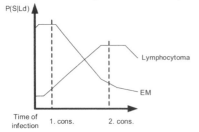

Figure 3 - The concept of modelling the clinical history by comparison with the general development pattern of Lyme disease over time

A normal procedure, when the diagnosis on Lyme disease is uncertain, is to ask the patient to return for a later examination in order to check if the disease develops as the typical pattern of Lyme disease. Thus, the clinical history is an important parameter when a diagnosis on Lyme disease is made and therefore, the Bayesian model also has to include the clinical history as one of its parameters.

The *concept of modelling* the clinical history is based on a description of the development pattern of Lyme disease over time. The development of Lyme disease begins at the time of the infection and then it progresses with the development of the different symptoms as time passes. The patient typically first discovers the infection some time after the bite incident and perhaps first when consulting the doctor. The concept of modelling the clinical history is to find out if the clinical findings at the time of the consultation match the general development pattern of Lyme disease. This concept is illustrated in Figure 3, where the horizontal axis represents the time, starting at the time of infection, and the vertical axis represents the probability of having a symptom (S) given that the patient suffers from Lyme disease, $P(S \mid Ld)$. The development of the stage 1 symptom Erythema migrans (EM) and the stage 2 symptom Lymphocytoma over time is shown: Typically, EM appears within a few days after

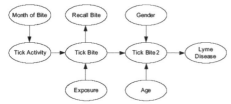

Figure 4 - The exposure risk history model

the infection and is likely to be found up to one month after. The highest probability of observing EM is therefore, found in this period. Typically, lymphocytoma appears in the period from two weeks to two months after the infection, and the probability therefore peaks within this period. The concept of the development pattern illustrated in the figure, describes the probability of experiencing a time dependant variable at different times after the infection.

First stage of the Bayesian model is the *exposure risk history* model, which can be seen in Figure 4. The arrows in a Bayesian model represent causal relations, and for example, the tick activity is dependant on the month of the year and the probability of a tick bite is

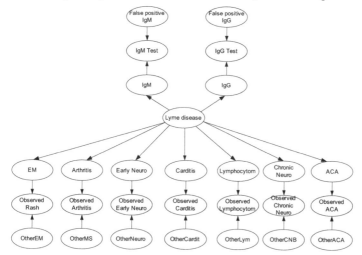

Figure 5 - The clinical findings and laboratory evidence model

dependant on the tick activity. Likewise, the patient's ability to recall a tick bite is dependent on the actual occurrence of a tick bite. The two separate tick bite variables, Tick Bite and Tick Bite 2, is just a result of a design trick ('divorcing parents') helping to avoid too many dimensions in the conditional probability tables in the model. The other variables represent other epidemiological aspects described previously.

The following stages of the model are blocks of the *clinical findings and laboratory evidence model*, which can be seen in Figure 5. For example, it can be seen how a positive result of an IgM test can be caused by both a rise in IgM caused by Lyme disease (i.e. a true positive) and by other reasons (i.e. a false positive). Likewise an observed rash can be caused either by Erythema migrans (EM), which again is caused by the Lyme disease, or by other reasons. The conditional probability tables for the variables directly dependant of the Lyme disease variable, e.g. IgM and EM, are calculated dynamically by the method illustrated in Figure 3. The model can handle any number of clinical consultations as illustrated by Figure 6, where the blocks are connected by causal relations between the Lyme disease variables; i.e. the probability of Lyme disease at a given consultation is dependent on the occurrence of the disease in the previous block.

The model has been integrated into a system by developing a Bayesian Application Framework. This framework specifies a communication data structure in XML providing a graphical user interface and database components, which can be used when developing systems that are based on Bayesian networks. The framework generalizes the integration of Bayesian networks making it possible to switch network without manually having to update or change the system.

Both the model and the total system have been tested along commonly accepted guidelines proposed by Jeremy Wyatt and David Spiegelhalter [6] and by Jacob Nielsen [7]. The results are summarised in the following section.

3. Results

Two expert microbiologists tested the model behaviour with a single consultation and with multiple consultations. The results show that the model with a single consultation, in general behaves as previous models. With multiple consultations it was concluded that the new time sliced model behaves as intended when the clinical history is incorporated. Also with an atypical course of the disease, the model in general behaves as expected.

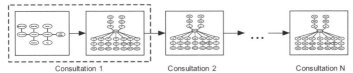

Consultation 1   Consultation 2   Consultation N

Figure 6 - The full model combining the risk history model with one or more clinical findings and laboratory evidence models

The *usability evaluation of the full system* was performed by five general practitioners (GPs) who answered the 3 questions: 'is it pleasant to use?', 'does it say sensible things?' and 'is it wanted?'. In general, the GPs found that the system is simple and has a good layout, and the layout was found to be logical and to have a good overview of the details. When entering different pathological pictures, the GPs in general found that the results were consistent with what could be expected, even though most of them found it difficult to evaluate an estimated probability of Lyme disease. In general, the GPs did not want a stand-alone system to handle Lyme disease, but suggested that the system, if it is to have any chance of success, has to be integrated into the general GP IT solution.

4. Discussion

From the analysis of Lyme disease it was evident that a decision support model for diagnosis of Lyme disease needs to incorporate the clinical history, which was not the case in previous models. Based on the evaluation of the present time sliced model it can be concluded that the method proposed for handling non-equivalent time intervals in order to incorporate the clinical history works as expected by expert microbiologists. Even though the general practitioners found that the system was pleasant to use, and was providing sensible information, they felt that the system in order to fit into daily routines, has to be integrated into their general IT systems. It is therefore concluded that in addition to more testing of the models performance on clinical cases, more work also has to go into improving the usability, i.e. the functionality in daily clinical practice.

5. Acknowledgments

The authors wish to thank Virtual Centre for Health Informatics, Denmark, for financial support.

6. References

[1] Gray JS, Kahl O, Lane RS, and Stanek G. *Lyme Borreliosis: Biology, Epidemiology and Control.* Cabi Publishing, 2002.
[2] Smith M, Gray J, Granström M, Revie C, and Gettinby G. *European Concerted Action on Lyme Borreliosis.* http://vie.dis.strath.ac.uk/vie/LymeEU, read 30-01-2005.
[3] Jensen FV. *Bayesian Networks and Decision Graphs.* Springer-Verlag, 2001.
[4] Hugin Expert. *Hugin.* http://www.hugin.com, read 30-01-2005.
[5] Dessau RB, Andersen M-BN, Hejlesen OK. Diagnosis of Lyme disease. Calculating the pre- and post-test probability with a probabilistic belief network. In: *Proceedings of MIE2003, St. Malo, France,* 2003, 5pp.
[6] Wyatt J, and Spiegelhalter D. Evaluating medical decision-aids: what to test, and how? *Medical Informatics* 1990: 15 piii: 205-217.
[7] Nielsen J. *Usability Inspection Methods.* John Wiley & Son, 1994.

Address for correspondence

Ole Hejlesen, Ph.D., Associate Prof. , Head of Med. Inf. Group, Dept. of Health Science & Technology, Aalborg Univ., Fredrik Bajersvej 7 D1, DK-9220 Aalborg, +4596358808/+4520459779, okh@hst.aau.dk.

Connecting Medical Informatics and Bio-Informatics
R. Engelbrecht et al. (Eds.)
IOS Press, 2005

211

Towards a Generic Connection of EHR and DSS

Helma van der Linden[a], Sjoerd Diepen[b], Gerrit Boers[a], Huibert Tange[a], Jan Talmon[a]

[a]*Dept. of Medical Informatics, University Maastricht, Maastricht, The Netherlands*
[b]*Dept. of Electrical Engineering, Eindhoven University of Technology, Eindhoven, The Netherlands*

Abstract

Decision Support Systems (DSS) are typically integrated in Electronic Health Record systems (EHR). By removing this integration full reuse of a DSS system is possible. The connection between the EHR and the DSS system should be standards-based and generic. We intend to demonstrate the viability of this setup by implementing it using PropeRWeb as EHR system, Gaston as DSS system, HL7v3 messages and the SOAP protocol.

Keywords:
Decision Support Systems, DSS, EHR, standards, HL7, distributed connection

1. Introduction

Decision support systems (DSS) are traditionally implemented either as a stand-alone system or as a component that is highly integrated in a specific Electronic Health Record (EHR) system[1, 2]. Since there is a trend to build information systems in general and health information systems in particualr from components there is a need for other approaches to link the EHRs with DSS. Till now combinations of EHR and DSS systems in an open environment hardly exist.

Our PropeR project studies the use of decision support combined with an EHR system and focuses on a generic connection in an open environment between these two components. We developed an extendable, generic EHR system, PropeRWeb [3, 4]. This system is currently in use by two groups of users for testing.

We are now working on extending the functionality of PropeRWeb by including a generic connection to an independent DSS system.

In this paper we will describe the requirements necessary to implement this connection.

2. Design considerations

The costs and effort of implementing guidelines in DSS systems are high [5]. Many projects have therefore focused on defining reusable DSS components and/or reusable guideline implementations.

Guidelines are typically defined for a specific medical specialism or disease. Some will be used as is, while others will be localized to incorporate the work process of the implementing institution. Reusable guidelines in local DSS systems (i.e. systems closely coupled to the EHR system that contains the data) have a drawback: the process of installing the guidelines have to be repeated in each institution that wants to use the guideline. The same holds for the management of updates. This is inevitable for the localized guidelines, but the former two categories would benefit from a centralized service where implementation and maintenance are combined.

A possible future configuration is shown in Figure 1 as an illustration. There may be a national authority which provides a DSS for drug interactions, while a national institute for cardiology provides a DSS with cardiology guidelines. General practitioners use a regional DSS which contains relevant guidelines, while the hospital also uses a dedicated DSS for guidelines modified to the local situation.

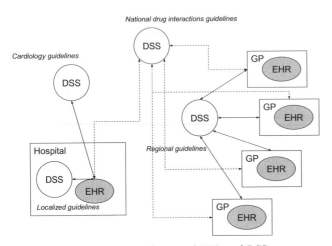

Figure 1: Distributed setup of EHR and DSS

For a generic connection between an EHR system and a DSS system, each system has to be regarded as a black box, communicating through standards-based messages.

When a set of messages is defined and widely adopted, it becomes possible to build a distributed support system that is maintained by various parties.

2.1. Guideline execution

Computer interpretable formats for guidelines such as GLIF [6], EON [7], and PROforma [8], basically have a similar structure.

A guideline is usually broken down in steps which include multiple decisions. To support a decision the DSS system needs information that can either be formalized, and therefore retrieved from the EHR data source (e.g. lab results), or it cannot be formalized and needs to be requested from the user (e.g. the current patient state). The result of a decision can lead to a message (reminder or alert) to the user1.

In current configurations (e.g. GLEE [9] and SAGE [10]) a DSS has direct access to both the EHR data and the user interface. In a distributed configuration however, there is no direct connection between the DSS and the EHR data or between the DSS and the user. All information has to be provided by the EHR system, since it is the only system with access

---

[1] For the sake of simplicity, we will use the term reminder in this article to refer to both reminders and alerts.

to the EHR data and also the only system to communicate with the user. This will lead to three types of messages:
    messages from the DSS to the EHR requesting data;
    messages from the DSS to the EHR requesting user information;
    messages from the DSS to the EHR to remind the user.
A generic connection should support this pattern.
Since the EHR system is the entry point of new patient data, it is also responsible for initiating the communication with the DSS.

3. Implementation design

3.1. Communication states and channels

The communication between an EHR and a DSS starts from the moment decision support is requested for a specific patient. This can either be actively initiated by the EHR user or automatically initiated by the EHR through configuration according to institutional regulations.

The communication is ended when the end of the guideline is reached. The latter can be because (1) the last step of the guideline is executed, (2) the user has indicated that no guideline support is necessary or (3) the user has deviated from the guideline and it is not possible to continue execution of the guideline. In all cases the DSS can signal the EHR that the communication is ended.

During the communication, multiple messages are exchanged between the EHR and the DSS.

A period of communication regarding one guideline for one patient is called a channel. The lifetime of a channel spans the execution of one guideline. The channel is a virtual concept to simplify the administration of the communication.There can be multiple channels open at one point in time.

There are two states for a channel: open and closed. The initial state is always closed. The state is changed to open after a request from the EHR to the DSS for guideline support. We call this the "establish channel request". While the guideline steps are executed one or more message pairs are exchanged (see below). When the DSS finishes processing the last step in the guideline, it notifies the EHR with a "shutdown call". This changes the state of the channel to "closed".

These state changing messages are responded to only by an acknowledgment.

3.2. Message types

Looking at the message types, two situations can be discerned. The DSS sends a request for data. If the data are available in the EHR, they will be retrieved; otherwise the request will be presented to the user for answering. The EHR will send the result as response to the DSS.

The DSS can also send a request for user interaction. This is typically a question with one or more predefined answers. A reminder can be modelled as a question with one answer. The EHR will present this question/answer pair to the user and return the selected answer to the DSS. In case of a reminder, either the EHR or the DSS can choose to ignore the answer based on configuration settings.

All DSS requests and the user responses are logged in the EHR.

3.3. Responsibilities

In a peer-to-peer connection between two independent systems, there should be a clear definition of the responsibilities of each system. In our approach, the overall responsibility for the communication lies with the EHR system. It is the only system with access to the clinical data and the applicable authorization rules. It also maintains the user interface.

  The EHR system should initiate the communication with the DSS, handle requests for data and user interaction, and log all activity pertaining to this communication (i.e. the requests from the DSS as well as the user responses).

4. Requirements

4.1. Message content

The communication messages must have a standard format and must use a terminology and domain model that is either the same for the EHR and the guideline or can be mapped to the terminologies used in either system. HL7v3 provides a format and a method to define these messages [11]. HL7v3 messages require definition of coding schemes and other terminological origins. This made us decide to move the terminology mapping to the EHR system, i.e. the EHR system is responsible for mapping the HL7v3 messages to the internal representations.

  Although there are currently no specific messages defined for this communication, HL7v3 specifies how to define such messages based on the domain model. This allows us to define our own messages with a reasonable guarantee that the implementation is future-proof, i.e. only the structure of the message itself will be subject to change, not the overall structure.

4.2. Requirements for the EHR

Following the design explained above, an EHR system capable of communication with a DSS needs to be able to:

- handle the communication, i.e. it needs a communication interface;
- map the message domain model to the internal domain model;
- map terminology to internal terminology;
- handle requests for user interaction;
- log the actions resulting from the communication;
- (in future) handle multiple requests from different DSS systems.

4.3. Requirements for the DSS

  The DSS system needs to be able to:
- handle the communication, i.e. it needs a communication interface;
- map the message domain model to the internal domain model;
- (in future) handle multiple requests from different EHR systems;

5. Current state

The approach outlined, is currently under development using the PropeRWeb EHR system and the Gaston guideline execution engine [12]. As guideline we use a treatment protocol for AML patients [13] as it is currently in use in the hematology department in the University Hospital Maastricht (azM).

The first version will be a simple setup of a direct connection between EHR and DSS system. To stay as much as possible with current common, standardized approaches, the connection between the EHR system and the DSS system will be implemented as a peer-to-peer connection of two web services using SOAP [14, 15] over TCP/IP with HL7v3 messages.

Subsequent versions will add complexity such as security, multiple protocols, multiple EHR systems and multiple DSS systems.

6. Discussion

The approach outlined has several drawbacks. First of all, there are more significant security issues when communication involves two independent systems compared to one system containing a specialized component. Separating knowledge into dedicated DSS systems and EHR systems will inevitably raise questions as to what goes where. Solving these issues (security and knowledge separation) will also result in a precise specification of either system and therefore enhance the quality of both systems.

Using technological standards that are currently under development (such as service oriented architecture (SOA) [16] and HL7v3 messages) will add a challenge to the implementation. This approach also differs from the current CORBA/archetype based approach we followed in the development of the PropeRWeb EHR system. We changed approach due to the fact that HL7v3 is the preferred standard of communication, which also specifies the use of SOAP and webservices as preferred standard.

Only after implementation, the specifications of standards show their strengths and weaknesses. This will give enough information to compare both approaches.

The content of the messages in this communication is strongly defined by the guideline domain. Yet, the request for data might show a significant overlap in domains (e.g. medication, lab results). This justifies the use of generic messages that are independent of the guideline. Implementing multiple guidelines from different domains should prove the correctness of this assumption.

A configuration where an EHR system and a DSS system are not intricately connected will severely influence the performance. However, the Internet has multiple examples of web servers handling high volume request rates with good performance. We anticipate no serious performance problems.

A complex setup with multiple EHR systems and multiple DSS systems, such as presented in figure 1, could benefit from a broker system where DSS and EHR systems register their services and support requests respectively. This broker system could also resolve timeout problems and provide message persistence and even interfaces to dedicated terminology servers.

7. Acknowledgments

The PropeR project is funded by a stimulation program for ICT in healthcare (ICZ) of the Netherlands Organisation of Scientific Research (NWO).

8. References

[1]   Kawamoto K, Houlihan CA, Balas EA, Lobach DF. Improving clinical practice using clinical decision support systems: a systematic review of trials to identify features critical to success. *Bmj* 2005;330(7494):765.

[2]   Shiffman RN, Liaw Y, Brandt CA, Corb GJ. Computer-based guideline implementation systems: a systematic review of functionality and effectiveness. *J Am Med Inform Assoc* 1999;6(2):104-14.

[3]   van der Linden H, Tange H, Talmon J, Hasman A. PropeR revisited. *Stud Health Technol Inform* 2003;95:346-51.

[4]   van der Linden H, Boers G, Tange H, Talmon J, Hasman A. PropeR: a multi disciplinary EPR system. *Int J Med Inform* 2003;70(2-3):149-60.

[5]   Johnson P, Tu S, Jones N. Achieving reuse of computable guideline systems. *Medinfo* 2001;10(Pt 1):99-103.

[6]   Peleg M, Boxwala AA, Ogunyemi O, Zeng Q, Tu S, Lacson R, Bernstam E, Ash N, Mork P, Ohno-Machado L, Shortliffe EH, Greenes RA. GLIF3: the evolution of a guideline representation format. *Proc AMIA Symp* 2000:645-9.

[7]   Musen MA, Tu SW, Das AK, Shahar Y. EON: a component-based approach to automation of protocol-directed therapy. *J Am Med Inform Assoc* 1996;3(6):367-88.

[8]   Fox J, Johns N, Rahmanzadeh A. Disseminating medical knowledge: the PROforma approach. *Artif Intell Med* 1998;14(1-2):157-81.

[9]   Wang D, Peleg M, Tu SW, Boxwala AA, Ogunyemi O, Zeng Q, Greenes RA, Patel VL, Shortliffe EH. Design and implementation of the GLIF3 guideline execution engine. *J Biomed Inform* 2004;37(5):305-18.

[10] Ram P, Berg D, Tu S, Mansfield G, Ye Q, Abarbanel R, Beard N. Executing Clinical Practice Guidelines Using the SAGE Execution Engine. *Medinfo* 2004;2004:251-5.

[11] anonymous, Health Level 7 Ballot 8 (only available to members), http://www.hl7.org, 2004, Last accessed: Jan 2005

[12] De Clercq PA, Blom JA, Hasman A, Korsten HH. GASTON: an architecture for the acquisition and execution of clinical guideline-application tasks. *Med Inform Internet Med* 2000;25(4):247-63.

[13] HOVON, HOVON 42 AML / SAKK, http://www.hovon.nl, 2001, Last accessed: Jan 2005

[14] anonymous, Web Services Activity site, http://www.w3.org/2002/ws/, Last accessed: Jan 2005

[15] Gudgin M, Hadley M, Mendelsohn N, Moreau J-J, Nielsen HFN, SOAP Version 1.2 Part 1: Messaging Framework, http://www.w3.org/TR/soap12-part1/, 2003, Last accessed: Jan 2005

[16] He H, What is Service-Oriented Architecture?, http://webservices.xml.com/pub/a/ws/2003/09/30/soa.html, 2003, Last accessed: Jan 2005

Address for correspondence

H. van der Linden
Dept. Medical Informatics,
University Maastricht
POBOX 616
6200 MD Maastricht
The Netherlands
h.vanderlinden@mi.unimaas.nl

Connecting Medical Informatics and Bio-Informatics
R. Engelbrecht et al. (Eds.)
IOS Press, 2005

217

Using Blood Glucose Data as an Indicator for Epidemic Disease Outbreaks

Eirik Årsand[a], Ole Anders Walseth[a], Niklas Andersson[a], Ruchith Fernando[b],
Ove Granberg[c], Johan G. Bellika[a], Gunnar Hartvigsen[ac]

[a]*Norwegian Centre for Telemedicine, University hospital of North Norway, Tromsø, Norway*
[b]*Computer Science and Engineering Department, University of Moratuwa, Sri Lanka*
[c]*Department of Computer Science, University of Tromsø, Tromsø, Norway*

Abstract

In the future, transfer of vital sensor data from patients to the public health care system is likely to become commonplace. Systems for automatic transfer of sensor data are now at the prototype stage. As electronic health record (EHR) systems adapt such functionality, widespread use may become an actuality in the foreseeable future.

To prevent spreading of diseases, an early detection of infection is important. At the time an outbreak is diagnosed, many people may already be infected due to the incubation period. This study suggests an approach for detecting an epidemic outbreak at an early stage by monitoring blood glucose data collected from people with diabetes. Continuous analysis of blood glucose data may have the potential to prevent large outbreaks of infectious diseases, such as different strains of Influenza, Cholera, Plague, Ebola, Anthrax and SARS.

When a person gets infected, the blood glucose value increases. If the blood glucose data from a large number of patients with diabetes are collected in a central database, it may be possible to detect an epidemic disease outbreak at an early stage. Advanced data analysis on the data may detect predominant numbers of incidences, indicating a possible outbreak. This gives the health authorities the possibilities to take actions to limit the outbreak and its consequences for all the inhabitants in an affected area.

At the Norwegian Centre for Telemedicine, a mobile system for automatic transfer of blood glucose values has been constructed. By using wireless communication standards such as Bluetooth and GSM, the system transfers blood glucose data to an electronic health record system. Combined with a system accessing and querying data from EHR systems for patient surveillance we are extending our work into an Epidemic Disease Detection using blood Glucose (EDDG) system.

Keywords:
Epidemical diseases, diabetes; Blood glucose data; medical informatics; Geographic Information Systems (GIS); Software agent technology; Fuzzy logic.

1. Introduction

The spreading of infectious diseases is generally difficult to predict, and it is of great importance to detect an outbreak as early as possible to reduce further spreading and simplify treatment of people infected. Examples of diseases involving infections are various strains of Influenza, Cholera, Plague, Ebola, Anthrax and SARS.

The International Diabetes Federation estimates that there are currently some 194 million people around the world with diabetes [1]. Monitoring and control of blood glucose levels is critical in the management of Type 1 and Type 2 diabetes. The patients measure their blood glucose levels up to several times a day to minimize long-term complications [2,3].

The basis for this proposed system is the fact that people with diabetes experience an increase in their blood glucose value when they get an infection [4]. If values from all diabetes patients in a region were instantly accessible, it would provide a foundation for extended data analysis. Extreme accumulations of high values in specific areas could be spotted, and the national health care service could monitor and act on such signals. In this way data from patients with diabetes could provide early warnings of an outbreak in the population. This would give the health care services possibilities to take action to limit the outbreak and its consequences for all the inhabitants in the affected area. Typical actions will be advice, vaccination and even isolation in serious cases.

The routines and strategies for storing and maintaining patient information such as blood glucose data vary between different diabetes teams and health services today. The information may be stored on paper-based health records, in electronic health record (EHR) systems or both. Most Norwegian general practitioners (GPs) and hospitals store information electronically in EHR systems, and the expansion of health networks enable communication and collaboration between hospital - hospital and hospital - GPs.

2. Materials and methods

The system described in this paper is based on the methodology and results of previous projects undertaken by the Norwegian Centre for Telemedicine (NST), especially the projects "Automatic transfer of blood glucose data" [5] and "Wireless Health and Care" [6]. One essential element from the former is a system that automatically transfers data from blood glucose sensors to a database. A wireless system that transfers blood glucose data to a relative's mobile phone as an SMS was developed and tested on a small-scale (n=15) intervention [5] from 2004. The transfer of the blood glucose data into the EHR system "DIPS" (from *DIPS ASA Norway*) was implemented as a prototype in the "Wireless Health and Care" project. The significance of this prototype for patients and health care personnel is described in proceedings [6] from 2004.

The system proposed in this paper involves immediate transfer of patient-initiated blood glucose samples into one or more national or international databases. Using geographic information systems, software agent technology and fuzzy logic, this will enable an analysis for detecting infectious disease outbreaks at an early stage.

One example of a "Real-time Outbreak and Disease Surveillance system" (RODS) is in use in Western Pennsylvania [7]. This system and others like it capture clinical data from health systems, not from the patient in her daily environment as we suggest.

3. Results

The main components of the Epidemic Disease Detection by blood Glucose (EDDG) system and how they in a future implementation will interact with each other are described below.

Data sampling

Our starting point is an application implemented using a programmable mobile phone, communicating wirelessly with a blood glucose meter using the short-range communication standard Bluetooth. The glucose meter is attached to a Bluetooth adapter through the serial port, and the mobile phone is equipped with a built-in Bluetooth chip. The mobile phone (Nokia 7650) is programmed to send the measurement result automatically, by means of an SMS to a distant mobile phone or a database server using GSM, see figure 1.

The process is seamless and invisible to the user, and the elements are being refined in concurrent projects at NST. Implementing the proposed system requires capturing of the user ID, blood glucose value and geographical location. Even though the blood sampling process is manual and invasive for persons with diabetes today, in future this process will become fully automatic using implantable and non-invasive sensors. The Institute of Nanotechnology in the UK characterises "Body friendly implants" and "Sensors (bio and chemical)" as areas where nanotechnology will have an impact in the short term [8].

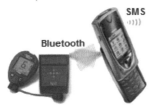

Figure 1 - Wireless blood glucose transfer system.

Data repository

After the data have been sampled and stamped with user ID, time and location, data is sent to a data repository. Depending on the size of the area in which the system is to be implemented, it must be considered whether data is to be transferred to one or more repositories. The system will potentially operate in both narrow and wide geographical areas. When the system covers a large area, software agents will be used for transferring and processing tasks across repositories.

Our research team has developed a prototype where blood glucose data is sent to the electronic health record system "DIPS". This process is automated to the extent that the blood glucose value, sample time and user ID are automatically sent and stored in the repository after the user has taken a blood sample. People with Type 1 diabetes take blood samples several times a day, while those with Type 2 often take daily or weekly samples.

Considering where the competences of specific local epidemic disease characteristics are located, it seems introductorily natural to store data at the nearest regional county hospital's EHR system.

Geographic location

There is a need both to record the geographic location of where each blood sample is taken, and to process the data with respect to its geographic location after the data acquisition. Using Geographic Positioning Systems (GPS) integrated into the sensor system is not an alternative due to factors such as battery consumption, reduced service inside buildings and costs. Since the proposed EDDG system is based on an implementation including a mobile phone as the data transport unit, we propose to use the information transmitted from GSM/3G network nodes for adequate positioning. For the purpose of discovering congestions of high blood glucose values in a town or village, this precision is assumed to be adequate, but needs further investigation and is not yet implemented.

Once all blood glucose sample data are stamped with their geographic position, a tool for analysing the trend in the spatial dispersion of the data is required. Geographical Information Systems (GIS) are one kind of tools which would support this task (traditionally cartographically tasks), and are also used for health and epidemiology issues in a growing number of cases. An example of this is the RODS in Western Pennsylvania mentioned earlier, which uses GIS as one of the tools in analysing the data for suspicious trends [7]. The role of GIS as an important component in epidemiology is documented in a review by Clarke, McLafferty and Tempalski [9].

Software agent technology

The role of software agents in an implemented system will be to collect both dynamical and static background data such as geographic information, climate, air pollution, human-related activities and infrastructures, and specific patient data, to be entered into the epidemic disease detection system. Depending on the size of the area, the EDDG system will benefit from offering two or more levels of analysis. Briefly, the analysis will be based on the blood glucose values and other relevant data, ending with a computation of geographic dispersion and a conclusion on whether there are indications of outbreak of infectious diseases or not. An increase in relevant data used in the computations can give a more holistic picture of the result from the detection system.

If the area object for an EDDG system is large, i.e. an international extension of the system, data may have to be processed at several sites and coordinated. It may therefore be expedient to divide inhomogeneous geographic areas into segments, depending on the characteristics of the access to health registers, population, climate and/or infrastructure, before performing the final analysis. Then, for this second-level analysis, multi-agent technology may be needed for coordinating data from all sites in the EDDG system into a central international risk analysis. Multi-agent technology is characterised by cooperation between individual agents for achieving a common goal [10], which may be necessary in epidemic disease detection for a large area.

The Epidemic Disease Detection using blood Glucose (EDDG) system

The EDDG system and its decision algorithms do need to handle a kind of fuzziness. Fuzzy logic handles the concept of partial truth – truth values between "completely true" and "completely false", e.g. Horstkotte [11]. Fuzzy logic has proved to be particularly useful in expert systems, systems having a collection of membership functions and rules [12], considering parameters such as those mentioned above. The proposed EDDG system will use the concept of fuzzy logic in its analysis process when considering the impact the background data, together with the main data source: blood glucose measurements from people with diabetes. The result of the analysis will end up as outputs that indicate whether there are any tendencies towards infectious diseases. This output only needs to be sent to health care surveillance authorities if the result needs to be investigated further.

The main elements of an implemented EDDG system will be the blood glucose sensor, sensor adapter for wireless communication of data, personal communication unit (e.g. smartphone), EHR import routines, geographic positioning solution, geographic information system element, software agent technology, fuzzy logic algorithms and routines for detecting and handling potential alerts. Half of the elements are implemented while the second half are part of ongoing projects and research thesis.

4. Discussion

An agent-based distributed information system called NZDIS in New Zealand [10] uses asthma incidence as the disease case. Software agents are used for processing the asthma incidence with geographic location and climatological information in queries. Our plan for the EDDG system is to provide indicators of infectious disease incidences (clusters of high values of blood glucose) in real time to intelligent agents. The agents must always be ready to consider new values that enter the system. This requires high demands for coordination, processing and stability in the elements that form such a system.

In Norway, the yearly influenza spreads the most in winter. Five to ten percent of the population are then infected, i.e. between 200,000 and 450,000 persons [13]. This highlights the fact that background data such as seasonal variations and average spreading numbers must form part of the detection system. This also implies a need for input from, and communication with, updated sources for the background information, something that implies coordination with health registers and other registers. Our work is now continued in a project where also use of "sensors" in the form of software systems distributed to places where patients show up, i.e. deploying the results and principles from Bellika et al.'s SNOW Agent system [14].

In Norway alone, the National Insurance Administration records that in the year 2003 reimbursement was given for 36 million blood glucose measurement strips, with a total value of EUR 36 million [15]. This large sum of money for a country as small as Norway with a population of 4.6 million, results today only in the patient's one-time use of the blood glucose measurements. No data is transferred to the health care services, even though there ought to be very good health- and economically reasons for this in the long-term. We are aware that we are proposing a futuristic use of the sensor data for an epidemic disease detection system, and our aim is to increase awareness of the possibilities: technically, health-related and economically.

5. Conclusion

Most of the prerequisite of the EDDG system are prepared and an implementation is started as a cooperative project between the Norwegian Centre for Telemedicine and the University of Tromsø, Norway. Through the work with the previous mentioned projects and studies, the system specifications are considered to be acceptable. In this paper, we have outlined the architecture of a system and indicated the effects of using blood glucose data for this epidemical disease detection purpose.

The work that has already been done on this approach, confirms that it is possible to achieve a fully automated system for the transfer of blood glucose data from the patient into an EHR system.

The remaining technical issues to solve are mainly at the receiving side of the system. This involves merging all elements together in a functioning system, which includes an analysis of the aggregated data, executed in decision support management modules to provide the national or international health care surveillance authorities with justified information related to epidemic disease outbreaks.

6. Acknowledgments

Diabetes has been the theme of several projects initiated by the Norwegian Centre for Telemedicine in the period 2001-2005. We wish to thank all our cooperating partners in these projects, including everyone in the internal "diabetes project team" at NST.

7. References

[1] International Diabetes Federation. (2003). Diabetes Prevalence, [Homepage of International Diabetes Federation], [Online]. Available: http://www.idf.org/home/index.cfm?node=264 [2005, January 13].

[2] Prospective Diabetes Study (UKPDS) Group. Intensive blood-glucose control with sulphonylureas or insulin compared with conventional treatment and risk of complications in patients with type 2 diabetes (UKPDS 33). Lancet North Am Ed. 1998;352 (9131):837-853.

[3] Prospective Diabetes Study (UKPDS) Group U. Effect of intensive blood-glucose control with metformin on complications in overweight patients with type 2 diabetes (UKPDS 34). Lancet North Am Ed. 1998;352(9131):854-865.

[4] Chase HP. Long-term Complications of Diabetes. Harris S. Understanding Diabetes. 10th edn. Denver, Colorado: MGM Consumer Products, 2002: Available at URL: http://www.uchsc.edu/misc/diabetes/udchap22.html. [2005, January 11].

[5] Norwegian Centre for Telemedicine. (2004). Automatic transfer of blood glucose data from children with type 1 diabetes. [Homepage of Norwegian Centre for Telemedicine], [Online]. Available: http://www.telemed.no/cparticle44523-4357b.html. [2005, January 10].

[6] Årsand E, Walseth OA, Skipenes E. Blood glucose data into Electronic Health Care Records for diabetes management. Øystein Nytrø. In Proceedings of the second HelsIT Conference at the Healthcare Informatics week in Trondheim, Norway, 21-22 September. Trondheim: Norwegian Centre for Electronic Patient Records; 2004;19-23.

[7] Gesteland PH, Wagner MM, Chapman WW, Espino JU, Tsui F-C, Gardner RM, Rolfs RT, Dato V, James BC, Colecchia TJ, and Haug PJ. Rapid Deployment of an Electronic Disease Surveillance System in the State of Utah for the 2002 Olympic Winter Games. In Proceedings of the 2002 American Medical Informatics Association (AMIA) Symposium, San Antonio, 9-13 November 2002. San Antonio: Conference Organising Committee, 2002;285-9.

[8] The Institute of Nanotechnology. Nanotechnology in the UK, Report from 2004. [Homepage of The Institute of Nanotechnology], [Online]. Available: www.nano.org.uk/Reports2004/UK_Sample.pdf [2005, January 7].

[9] Clarke KC, McLafferty SL, Tempalski BJ. On Epidemiology and Geographic Information Systems: A Review and Discussion of future Directions. Emerg Infect Dis. 1996; 2(2):85-92.

[10] Purvis M, Cranefield S, Bush G, Carter D, McKinlay B, Nowostawski M and Ward R. The NZDIS Project: an Agent-Based Distributed Information Systems Architecture. In Proceedings of the Hawai'i International Conference On System Sciences. Maui, Hawaii, 4-7 January 2000. Hawaii: IEEE Computer Society; 2000; 1-10.

[11] Horstkotte E. (2000). Fuzzy Logic Overview [Homepage of Austin City Links], [Online]. Available: http://www.austinlinks.com/Fuzzy/overview.html [2005, January 11].

[12] Horstkotte E. (2000). Fuzzy Logic Overview [Homepage of Austin City Links], [Online]. Available: http://www.austinlinks.com/Fuzzy/expert-systems.html [2005, January 11].

[13] Helsedepartementet/Ministry of Health and Care Services. (2004). Folkehelserapporten 2002 Vedlegg 1/ Health report 2002 Annex 1 [Homepage of Ministry of Health and Care Services], [Online]. Available: http://odin.dep.no/hod/norsk/dok/regpubl/stmeld/042001-040003/ved001-bn.html [2005, January 7].

[14] Bellika JG, Hartvigsen G. SNOW Agents: Simple Network Of Working Agents. Øystein Nytrø. In Proceedings of the second HelsIT Conference at the Healthcare Informatics week in Trondheim, Norway, 21-22 September. Trondheim: Norwegian Centre for Electronic Patient Records; 2004; 25-29.

[15] National Insurance Administration / Price negotiation office Norway. (2003) Statistikk diabetesutstyr for 2003 (eng.: Statistics regarding equipment within diabetes for 2003). [Report] Available as e-mail 2004, May.

8. Address for correspondence

Eirik Årsand
Norwegian Centre for Telemedicine
University hospital of North Norway
E-mail: eirik.arsand@telemed.no.
Phone +47 992 43 592.

Connecting Medical Informatics and Bio-Informatics
R. Engelbrecht et al. (Eds.)
IOS Press, 2005

Ontology Driven Construction of a Knowledgebase for Bayesian Decision Models Based on UMLS

Sarmad Sadeghi[a], Afsaneh Barzi [b], Jack W Smith [a]

[a] The University of Texas Health Science Center at Houston, Houston, TX, USA
[b] The University of Texas Medical Branch, Galveston, TX, USA

Abstract

All decision models use some form of language to describe domain elements and their interactions. The terminology is often specific and even unique to the algorithm and is a choice of designers. Nevertheless the domain elements and concepts of any decision problem are almost never unique and are used and reused in many other decision problems. The same is true about the information about those elements in the context of different decision problems. Put together, the information about any given element forms our knowledge about the element and if stored properly in a knowledgebase, can be used and reused as necessary without the need for duplication.

In this paper we discuss creation of an ontology using UMLS vocabulary and semantic network that provides an abstract understanding of elements (or objects) in the problem domain. Based on this ontology, a knowledgebase will be constructed that provides further information about the object in relation to another object or objects as described in the semantic links.

A knowledgebase structured as such will have the benefit of problem-independence. It can be expanded as needed to include other objects that are used in a different series of problems and therefore, will have a one to many mapping between knowledgebase and decision models. Updating the knowledgebase will update the decision models seamlessly and maintenance will be less of an issue across decision models and within the knowledgebase. We are using this approach in building Bayesian decision models using Bayesian networks; however, this approach is not limited to Bayesian networks and has been and can be used for other decision making purposes.

Keywords:
Ontology, Bayes' Theorem, Decision Making, Artificial Intelligence, UMLS

1. Introduction

Using ontology to describe the elements of a domain and their interaction inherently overlaps with decision modeling. In fact, whether formally referred to as ontology or not, every decision making model has within its design a naming convention and interaction definition that forms an ontology for the problem. These ontologies are usually context specific and cannot be reused in another decision model, even though the elements are the same. The knowledge stored in the decision model is also context specific and is usually not reusable for another decision model.

This representation problem has been dissected into creation of vocabulary sets, thesauri, and semantic networks (UMLS), design of ontology and knowledge management tools, Protégé[1-5] (including OWL plug-in which is our choice tool) and finally, guideline management tools (GLIF)[6-8]. Although these components are each described in detail, a clear path towards building decision models that use artificial intelligence is not described in as much detail.

It has been argued that creation of an ontology for a localized area of the medical subject matter would help with construction of one or several decision models that use the elements of the ontology and allow for modeling their interactions according to the ontology[5;9].

In this paper we propose using a well defined vocabulary and semantic network to create a finite, well defined, and abstract model of a problem domain in medicine. Then we use this ontology to create a Bayesian network based decision model. In doing so, we can use the model to identify what information is needed for the Bayesian network; in effect creating a knowledge acquisition tool. The information elicited in this manner will be stored in a knowledgebase model according to the ontology. This knowledgebase can be expanded to accommodate other problem domains and be reused. This approach allows for a separation of the ontology and decision modules[4], which will allow for reusable ontology elements and will reduce maintenance.

2. Methods

We use an iterative and incremental approach to building the knowledgebase. The initial objective is to create an ontology that encompasses one single decision domain and grows as more decision domains are added. The vocabulary used for naming objects in the ontology as well as the semantic types and relations are based on UMLS.

An ontology model specific to the problem domain at hand could be developed based on what is available in UMLS. For example, *"chest pain on exertion"* is of semantic type *"sign or symptom"* and can have a semantic relation *"associated_with"* to *"myocardial infarction"* which is in turn of semantic type *"disease or syndrome."* A domain expert could determine what other diseases he/she wishes to consider in his/her evaluation of a complaint of *"chest pain on exertion."* Then, the related evidence that needs to be weighed in the evaluation of the symptom is also included, all using the appropriate terms from UMLS. At this point we have created an ontology that describes the domain for the *"chest pain on exertion"* evaluation decision model. This ontology could be used to prepare a lay out of a Bayesian network, based on a single fault assumption. Finally, based on this layout it can be determined what information is needed to complete the conditional probability tables of the network, which in turn will be abstracted into the knowledgebase.

1. The above example, although simple, captures the essence of this approach:
2. Build the ontology
3. Implement the Bayesian network model
4. Acquire the knowledge
5. Build the knowledgebase.

As the problem domain is extended or new domains are needed, the ontology could be extended as well by adding objects as needed; however, objects that already exist need not be created again and will be reused. This allows for reusing the modeling that was previously done and will make the information in the knowledgebase available to the new or extended domain. Figure 1 depicts the process as detailed in the following paragraphs.

Building the ontology

The UMLS Knowledge Sources have already amassed a wealth of information on medical descriptions. The components of the UMLS that are of importance to this approach are the:
Metathesaurus
Semantic Network

As stated previously, we start our iterative and incremental approach by building the ontology that models a decision domain for the problem at hand. It is important to remember that we are not duplicating UMLS; in its current form (2004AC), UMLS does not include adequate information on relationships between sets of semantic types. For instance, the concept "*nausea*" with semantic type "*Sign or Symptom*" does not have semantic relations to any concept under "*Disease or Syndrome.*" Our ontology needs to include this information so that a meaningful description of the decision problem domain is assembled.

Although the relationships between many concepts are not part of UMLS, the semantics needed to define those relationships do exist in UMLS. For instance, "*clinically_associated_with*" and "*co_occurs_in*" adequately describe the observations as far as symptoms, signs, lab, and imaging findings in the context of a decision problem.

Implementation of the Bayesian network model

Various methods have been described for representing domain knowledge in the structure of a Bayesian network[10-12]. We propose to use the descriptive information captured in the ontology to construct a Bayesian network. Once the ontology is constructed as described above, it can be used to construct a decision model using Bayesian networks. Given the information in the ontology and the fact that ontology was specifically created to model a decision problem, with certain assumptions, a simple lay out for the structure of a Bayesian network could be generated. The most important assumption is that one hypothesis (or disease) could explain the states of evidence observed in the domain. This assumption allows all concepts that are of semantic type "*Disease or Syndrome*" that are not directly and independently observable to be grouped together in one node, optionally called hypotheses node here. It is important to note that there could be other concepts in the domain that are of semantic type "*Disease or Syndrome*" which function as risk factors in the decision being modeled. An example is diabetes mellitus, a disease that is also a risk factor in evaluation of chest pain. These concepts that are not among the hypotheses will be treated according to the function they have in the decision model.

Of course, it does not mean that more sophisticated and complex networks that are not constrained by these assumptions cannot be built. However, for most cases these assumptions do not interfere with decision making process and make automatic modeling of the Bayesian network layout possible.

Knowledge acquisition

Earlier we showed that once the hypotheses are selected, other evidence in the domain that will have an effect on the state of hypotheses can be identified by searching the ontology. A Bayesian model of hypotheses and relevant evidence can be constructed automatically and the layout for conditional probability tables can be set up. The next step is knowledge acquisition. At this stage user can be prompted to provide information that is not available in the knowledgebase. This process is referred to as probability elicitation and has been studied in the literature[13-16].

A Bayesian network processes probabilities using probability calculus; there is no estimation involved in this part. However, finding probability values that accurately reflect the domain characteristics and incorporating them into the networks involves estimations. There are few references in the literature on how these probabilities can be extracted from literature[12]. Customarily, the probability values required for the tables of a Bayesian network can come from the literature and/or domain experts. Using the concepts of Bayes' theorem it can be shown that probabilities could be found and estimated from these two sources even if they are not explicitly drawn from the statistical reports[17].

It has been argued that experts come up with numbers based on predictiveness rather than normative probability but fortunately that doesn't change the reliability of the numbers for the final decision[18]. Domain experts' knowledge can be used for estimating the probabilities and building the system[19]as well as testing the model against simulated cases, and discovering problems in the model and offering solutions.

Methodology for construction of a Bayesian network based on datasets from observations already has been described in the literature[20;21] and used in real designs[22]. If the structure of a network can be determined based on the ontology, then datasets from observations could be used to train the network and generate tables that are compatible with outcomes. This can complement the supervised network construction and probability elicitation methods.

More advanced design issues such as creation of intermediary nodes are not automated but it is conceivable that when a node has too many parents, the design could benefit from insertion of an intermediary node changing the child into node a "*grandchild*" node. An example would be the evidence set hypertension, hypercholesterolemia, family history of heart attack, and previous heart attack, which ordinarily should parent the hypothesis node for causes of chest pain. However, it would simplify the architecture and knowledge acquisition considerably, if we have those nodes parent an intermediary node "cardiovascular disease risk" which can in turn parent the hypotheses node.

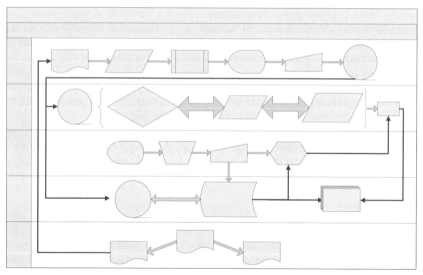

Figure 1

Once the structure is determined, the information acquired to fill the conditional probability tables as described above will be stored in the knowledgebase. The best way to do this will be to create abstract methods for capturing the essence of this information. For example, instead of storing the actual numbers for frequencies (or probabilities) it is best to store them in qualitative measures that could be used for translation back to quantitative measures. With such a classification, searching the ontology will be more intuitive, dealing with descriptive adjectives rather than absolute numbers. This will be a safe assertion as previous research has shown that Bayesian networks are forgiving when it comes to approximation on numerical values[19].

3. Discussion

As part of decision modeling, whether implicit or explicit, an ontology is also produced which describes the concepts of the domain and their interaction. As usually there is no further use for this ontology in sight, knowledge engineers and domain experts have grown used to arbitrary naming conventions and ad hoc classifications according to the specific needs of the task at hand. As new domains are introduced and concepts that are common between two or more domains are re-implemented in the newly built problem specific ontologies, maintaining consistency, updating the models, and portability from one ontology to another becomes an issue. It has been recognized that using a universal vocabulary and semantic model will help address some of these issues. Additionally, ontologies and the way concepts are defined and organized can become too context dependent. Keeping it concept oriented and not task oriented or objective oriented can make it more flexible.

Using UMLS is appropriate since it is regularly maintained an updated. It includes several instances of medical ontologies previously built, namely, Clinical Problem Statements[23], and SNOMED[24;25]. In its current form UMLS (2004AC) accumulates all and is perhaps the best choice for this purpose.

In our experience we have noticed that there are shortcomings in UMLS; we have addressed each instance by adding new terminology or semantic type or relationship. This is inevitable as there is no promise of comprehensiveness on the part of UMLS and there is always room for adding to the database. So far this has not caused us any problems, as we have maintained a singular instance of our ontology for a few decision models.

The preliminary Bayesian network structure built using this approach is usually close to the optimal representation. However, before the probability elicitation stage can begin, a knowledge engineer or domain expert must review the structure and modify it as needed.

We cannot comment on the escalation of this method to large Bayesian networks and complex problems. However, most of day to day practice and therefore decision support needs involve small and well defined problem domains. As a result, this methodology could be reliably used to construct small to medium size Bayesian networks.

We will further report on the success and modification of this methodology as the project advances.

4. References

[1]   Tu SW, Eriksson H, Gennari JH, Shahar Y, Musen MA. Ontology-based configuration of problem-solving methods and generation of knowledge-acquisition tools: application of PROTEGE-II to protocol-based decision support. Artif Intell Med 1995 Jun;7(3):257-89.

[2]   Tu SW, Musen MA. Modeling data and knowledge in the EON guideline architecture. Medinfo 2001;10(Pt 1):280-4.

[3]   Noy NF, Sintek M, Decker S, Crubezy M, Fergerson RW, Musen MA. Creating Semantic Web contents with Protege-2000. IEEE Intelligent Systems & Their Applications 2001 Mar;16(2):60-71.

[4]   Musen MA. Domain ontologies in software engineering: use of Protege with the EON architecture. Methods Inf Med 1998 Nov;37(4-5):540-50.

[5]   Biolchini J, Patel VL. From thesauri to ontology: knowledge acquisition and organization. Medinfo 2004;2004(CD):1525.

[6]   Boxwala AA, Peleg M, Tu S, Ogunyemi O, Zeng QT, Wang D, et al. GLIF3: a representation format for sharable computer-interpretable clinical practice guidelines. J Biomed Inform 2004 Jun;37(3):147-61.

[7]   de Clercq PA, Blom JA, Korsten HH, Hasman A. Approaches for creating computer-interpretable guidelines that facilitate decision support. Artif Intell Med 2004 May;31(1):1-27.

[8]   Mailhot M, Lenert L, Patrick K, Norman G. Use of GLIF to model a behavioral intervention. AMIA Annu Symp Proc 2003;924.

[9]   Hajdukiewicz JR, Vicente KJ, Doyle DJ, Milgram P, Burns CM. Modeling a medical environment: an ontology for integrated medical informatics design. Int J Med Inform 2001 Jun;62(1):79-99.

[10]   Jensen FV. An introduction to Bayesian networks. New York: Springer; 1996.

[11]   Pearl J. Probabilistic reasoning in intelligent systems networks of plausible inference. Rev. 2nd print ed. San Francisco, Calif: Morgan Kaufmann Publishers; 1988.

[12]   Taroni F, Biedermann A, Garbolino P, Aitken CG. A general approach to Bayesian networks for the interpretation of evidence. Forensic Sci Int 2004 Jan 6;139(1):5-16.

[13]   Achour SL, Dojat M, Rieux C, Bierling P, Lepage E. A UMLS-based knowledge acquisition tool for rule-based clinical decision support system development. J Am Med Inform Assoc 2001 Jul;8(4):351-60.

[14]   Achour SL, Dojat M, Rieux C, Bierling P, Lepage E. Knowledge acquisition environment for the design of a decision support system: application in blood transfusion. Proc AMIA Symp 1999;:187-91:187-91.

[15]   Druzdzel MJ, van der Gaag LC. Elicitation of Probabilities for Belief Networks: Combining Qualitative and Quantitative Information.: Morgan Kaufmann, San Francisco, CA.; 1995 p. 141-8.

[16]   Harmanec D, Leong TY, Sundaresh S, Poh KL, Yeo TT, Ng I, et al. Decision analytic approach to severe head injury management. Proc AMIA Symp 1999;:271-5:271-5.

[17]   Shortliffe EH, Perreault LE. Medical informatics computer applications in health care and biomedicine. 2nd ed ed. New York: Springer; 2001.

[18]   Lagnado DA, Shanks DR. Probability judgment in hierarchical learning: a conflict between predictiveness and coherence. Cognition 2002 Feb;83(1):81-112.

[19]   Zagoria RJ, Reggia JA. Transferability of medical decision support systems based on Bayesian classification. Med Decis Making 1983;3(4):501-9.

[20]   P.Spirtes, C.Glymour, R.Scheines. Causation, Prediction, and Search. 2nd edition ed. MIT Press; 2000.

[21]   Lauritzen SL. The Em Algorithm for Graphical Association Models with Missing Data. Computational Statistics & Data Analysis 1995 Feb;19(2):191-201.

[22]   Cao C, Leong TY, Leong AP, Seow FC. Dynamic decision analysis in medicine: a data-driven approach. Int J Med Inform 1998 Jul;51(1):13-28.

[23]   Brown SH, Miller RA, Camp HN, Guise DA, Walker HK. Empirical derivation of an electronic clinically useful problem statement system. Ann Intern Med 1999 Jul 20;131(2):117-26.

[24]   Rothwell DJ, Cote RA. Managing information with SNOMED: understanding the model. Proc AMIA Annu Fall Symp 1996;80-3.

[25]   Rothwell DJ. SNOMED-based knowledge representation. Methods Inf Med 1995 Mar;34(1-2):209-13.

Address for correspondence

Sarmad Sadeghi
7000 Fannin St. , Suite 600
Houston, TX 77030
Sarmad.Sadeghi@uth.tmc.edu

Connecting Medical Informatics and Bio-Informatics
R. Engelbrecht et al. (Eds.)
IOS Press, 2005

229

Estimation of Sex-Age Specific Clinical Reference Ranges by Nonlinear Optimization Method

Takeo Shibata[a], **Yoichi Ogushi**[a], **Teppei Ogawa**[b], **Takashi Kanno**[c]

[a]*Tokai University, Kanagawa, Japan*
[b]*Joto Hospital, Yamanashi, Japan*
[c]*Hamamatsu Medical Corporation, Shizuoka, Japan*

Abstract

Most reference ranges are not considered sex-age specific differences. We collected about 700,000 health examination data with 24 items to estimate sex-age specific clinical reference ranges. We proposed nonlinear optimization method as a new method compatible with NCCLS guideline. All items showed sex-age specific differences of reference ranges. Especially, hepatic functions in young aged men and all aged women, diabetic functions in young aged people, blood pressures in older people, and total cholesterol in all aged people might have serious problems. Some abnormal individuals might not be detected using established reference ranges, on the other hand, some normal individuals might be treated excessively.

Keywords:
Sex-age specific clinical reference ranges; Nonlinear optimization method; NCCLS guideline

1. Introduction

Recently, sex-age specific differences in medicine have been attracted attentions. But most reference ranges are not considered sex-age specific differences. Many guidelines defined reference ranges by the results based on patient's data [1,2]. To determine health examination values, the reference ranges should be defined based on pure normal individuals. So we collected about 700,000 health examination data to estimate sex-age specific reference ranges.

NCCLS (National Committee for Clinical Laboratory Standards) developed a guideline to define and determine reference ranges for clinical laboratory data in 2000 [3]. It would be a standard method to determine reference ranges, because the basis of the guideline is compliant with the committee of IFCC (International Federation of Clinical Chemistry) and ICSH (International Council for Standardization in Haematology). This guideline includes the methodological approaches and the procedure which is recommended to establish reference ranges.

But it is hard to apply NCCLS guideline for a determination of clinical reference ranges, because in-depth exclusion criteria and many partitioning factors are required, and selected individuals might be less than 5% of original individuals.

So we proposed a new method to establish sex-age specific clinical reference ranges which found a normal distribution mathematically. Our new method does not require any exclusion criteria and partitioning factors, and most individuals are used in a calculation of reference ranges. A confirmation of a compatibility with NCCLS method is require to verify a validity of our methods.

2. Materials

2.1. Data collection

Health examination data was collected between April 1 2002 and March 31 2003 with 45 institutions retrospectively in Japan. 45 institutions participated our study, and about 700,000 cases were collected. 24 items were collected for each institution (Table 1).

Table 1 - 24 items for estimation of sex-age specific reference ranges

BMI(upper & lower)	Systolic Blood Pressure	Diastolic Blood Pressure	
Total Protein	Albumin		
AST(GOT)	ALT(GPT)	G-GTP	Total Bilirubin
LDH	Alkaline Phosphatase		
TC(upper & lower)	Triglyceride	HDL cholesterol	LDL cholesterol
Fasting Blood Glucose	HbA1c		
Creatinine	Uric Acid		
Red Blood Cell	Hemoglobin	Hematocrit	
White Blood Cell	Platelet(upper & lower)		

Measuring methods had been standardized by JSCC (Japan Society of Clinical Chemistry), and all items could be categorized by one or two methods.

Cache' ver.5.0 was used to make database and to calculate reference ranges.

2.2. Data integration

The data were separated by measuring methods, sex and each 5 years old between 20 and 79 years old. At first, reference ranges were calculated for men aged between 50 and 54 by each institution to confirm if the measuring methods were right, because that age group had the biggest number of individuals.

To integrate all data, a random sampling technique was used to reduce the number and make no influence for a particular institution when the sample had more than 2,000 cases.

3. Methods

3.1. NCCLS method

NCCLS (National Committee of Clinical Laboratory Standard) provided a guideline to define and determine reference intervals in the clinical laboratory in June 2000. NCCLS guideline defines an exclusion criteria and partitioning factors to select reference individuals. To calculate reference ranges being compliant with NCCLS guideline, in-depth data with unified formats is required. It is hard to collect those exclusion criteria and partitioning factors.

3.2. Normal distribution test

Reference ranges are calculated as 95% confidence intervals of a normal distribution. If the distribution is not shown a normal distribution, the clinical laboratory test data is generally transformed as log, square, third power, square root, and third root. Chi-square test was used to test a normal distribution. At first, histograms were drown. Then the expected value as a normal distribution was calculated by each histogram. Chi-square test compared the number of individuals and the expected value. If a distribution of original data is not shown as a normal distribution, the data which has the smallest p value of chi-square test is selected.

If a distribution without any transformations shows a normal distribution, the original data is used to calculate the reference ranges. Then 2.5 percentile and 97.5 percentile are used as the reference interval.

3.3. Nonlinear optimization method [4]

In this study, NCCLS method was used to estimate the reference ranges first. But reasonable results were not estimated, because the data of exclusion criteria and partitioning factors were not enough to refine a pure normal group. So a nonlinear optimization method was used to estimate clinical reference ranges. The procedure of this method is as follows; (1) separate data by sex and each 5 years old in original data (without any transformations), (2) search linear areas on Q-Q plot, (3) make fitting a normal distribution to histogram between the linear areas data (4) calculate 95%CI of the fitted normal distribution.

To confirm the compatibility with NCCLS method, we used the data of Tokai University Health Checkup Center, because they contain detailed questionnaires. After separation of the data by sex and age, we selected the reference individuals by questionnaire data based on NCCLS method. Then we examined if the distribution shows a normal distribution. We compared histograms and 95%CIs between NCCLS method and those by our new method. Results of hepatic function tests were used to compare these two methods, because they had high abnormal rates.

On the other hand, we performed simulation of random walks with recovery force to confirm that a pure normal group shows a normal distribution. To examine the influence of abnormal rates, artificial data which had abnormal rates from 0 to 40 percentages were generated by a boot-strap method. Then the reference ranges calculated by the new method were compared.

3.3.1. Searching a linear area on Q-Q plot

Figure 1 shows a Q-Q (quantile-quantile) plot of HbA1c in the cases with men aged between 50 and 54. If a distribution is a normal distribution, Q-Q plot shows a linear line. A linear area including median on Q-Q plot means a pure normal area. So a linear area is searched on Q-Q plot.

The procedure to search a linear area as follows; (1) calculate and draw a regression line including the point of median, (2) take the higher intersection point, (3) narrow the targeted area to the intersection point and recalculate a regression line, (4) compare the intersection point and the previous one. Then if they are not corresponded, go back to (3), and if they are corresponded, (5) determine the higher edge of the linear area as the point which has no changes with the previous point, (6) go back to (1) and take lower intersection point on the procedure (2) to determine the lower edge (Figure 2).

3.3.2. Estimation reference ranges by nonlinear optimization method

The histograms ranged by the linear area are used to estimate reference ranges. A normal distribution curve is fit the histogram by nonlinear optimization method. Figure 1 shows an original histogram and a pure normal distribution curve. Reference ranges are calculated as 95% C.I. using the mean and the standard deviation of the pure normal distribution.

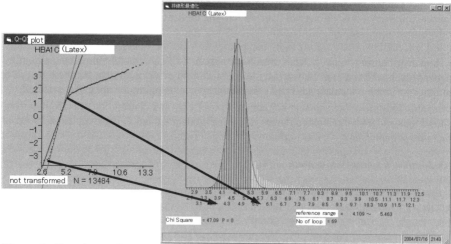

Figure 1 - Searching a linear area and nonlinear optimization method

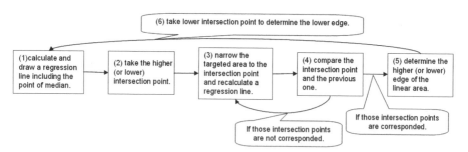

Figure 2 – Procedure of searching a linear area on Q-Q plot

4. Results

4.1. Compatibility with NCCLS method

The AST(GOT) data of 60s men who were selected as reference individuals showed a normal distribution. And the histogram and the 95%CI by our new method were coincident with NCCLS method. Our new method without any questionnaire data can estimate sex-age specific clinical reference ranges coincident with NCCLS method.

4.2. Simulation of a pure normal distribution

A random walk simulation proved that pure normal individuals show a normal distribution where they are affected with some noises and have recovery forces.

4.3. Estimatin of sex-age specific reference ranges

All items showed sex-age specific differences of reference ranges. The sex-age specific reference renges is shown on the following URL:
http://www.mi-tokai.com/defaulte.htm or http://mi.med.u-tokai.ac.jp/defaulte.htm

Though reference ranges have been separated by sex among some items, strong dependences with age are shown. Many reference ranges were similar with the ranges of middle aged men. A menopause had a potent influence on reference ranges in women.

Hepatic functions show potent influences by sex and age (Figure 3). Total cholesterol shows a crossover by sex and a potent influence by age and sex (Figure 4). Systolic blood pressure shows a linear upward influence by age (Figure 5). HbA1c shows a linear upward influence by age, and fasting glucose also shows a potent influence by sex. Albumin shows a linear downward influence by age and a clear menopausal effect in women (Figure 5). Alkaline Phosphatase and LDH show clear menopausal effects.

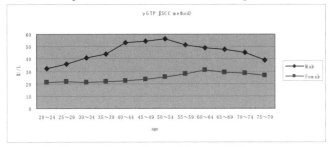

Figure 3 - Potent influence by sex (Gamma GTP)

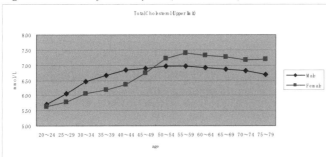

Figure 4 - Crossover by sex (Total Cholesterol)

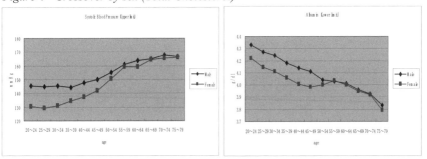

Figure 5 - Rise up by age (Systolic Blood Pressure) and down by age (Albumin)

4.4. Compliation of pure normal distributions and influence of abnormal rates

Though sex-age separated data selected as normal individuals showed a normal distribution, sex-age mixed data were not shown even if normal individuals were selected. The data with abnormal rate less than 40% had no problem to determine clinical reference ranges using our new method.

5. Conclusion

Nonlinear optimization method was able to estimate reference ranges without exclusion of abnormal individuals, and it has compatibility with NCCLS method. It also means that our new method is able to calculate reference ranges using many individuals. Some simulations reconfirmed the validity of our new method. So our new method is more useful than NCCLS method, because detailed exclusion criteria and partitioning factors are not necessary and more cases are effective for the calculation. It is the most important to separate by age (deservedly by sex), and many studies have been shown age specific diferences of clinical laboratory data [5,6]. NCCLS method also includes age and sex as partitioning factors.

Sex-age specific reference ranges by nonlinear optimization method shows interactions between sex and age in all items. Those reference ranges should be considered with the influence with sex and age. Especially, hepatic functions in young aged men and all aged women, diabetic functions in young aged people, blood pressures in older people, and total cholesterol in all aged people might have serious problems. Some abnormal individuals might not be detected using established reference ranges, on the other hand, some normal individuals might be treated excessively.

In this study, sex-age specific and "health associated" reference ranges were established. But some items might not be used for clinical decision making, because high risk people should be made decision by the ranges for high risk group.

6. References

[1] World Health Organization. 2003 World Health Organization (WHO) / International Society of Hypertension (ISH) statement on management of hypertension. *J Hypertension*, 2003; pp. 1983-1992.

[2] National Health Institute, National Heart, Lung, and Blood Institute. The Seventh Report of the Joint National Committee on Prevention, Detection, Evaluation, and Treatment of High Blood Pressure. NIH publication, 2003.

[3] Sasse EA, Doumas BD, Miller WG, et al.: How to Define and Determine Reference Intervals in the Clinical Laboratory; Approved Guideline – Second Edition. NCCLS, 2000.

[4] Kowalik J, Osborne MR. *Methods for unconstrained optimization problems.* Elsevier, 1968.

[5] Kannel WB, Castelli WP, Gordon T, et al.. Serum Cholesterol, Lipoproteins, and the Risk of Coronary Heart Disease. *Ann Int Med,* 1971; pp. 1-12.

[6] Morgan TO, Jacobsen ST, McCarthy WF, et al. Age-specific reference ranges for serum prostate-specific antigen in black men. *N Eng J Med,* 1996; pp. 304-10.

Address for correspondence

259-1193 Boseidai, Isehara, Kanagawa, Japan., Department of Medical Education and Informatics, School of Medicine, Tokai University, E-mail : tshibata@is.icc.u-tokai.ac.jp

Connecting Medical Informatics and Bio-Informatics
R. Engelbrecht et al. (Eds.)
IOS Press, 2005

Comparison Efficiency of the Artificial Intelligence Methods for the Diagnosis of Acid - Base and Anion Gap Disorders

Edward Kacki [a], Andrzej Małolepszy [b]

[a] *College of Computer Science in Lodz, Poland*
[b] *Institute of Computer Science, Technical University, Lodz, Poland*

Abstract

Diagnosis of the most complicated disorders in acid-base status and accompanying electrolyte balance creates a lot of troubles for practicing physicians. The purpose of our study was to create and compare: 1) an artificial neural network, 2) genetic program, 3) fuzzy-neural system that can diagnose acid-base disorders, based on a set of laboratory gasometric and electrolyte measurements. We took into account 7 single acid-base disorders, 11 double acid-base disorders and 6 triple complicated disorders with accompanying anion gap alterations. We prepared a set laboratory measurements consisting of 250 results for training and the same number of results for testing the program. Finally, the efficiency of presented artificial intelligence (AI) methods has been described and compared.

Keywords:
Artificial Intelligence; Medical Informatics; Diagnosis;

1. Introduction

Diagnosis of patient's acid-based disorders requires on appropriate interpretation of the relationship between electrolyte and arterial blood gas values.

In practice a consultant considers a diagnosis, rather than only a single diagnosis, the computer should then do likewise, especially since one of its strengths is its completeness, also taking into account all gasometric and electrolyte laboratory values. The human consultant also considers clinical observations about the patient, as well as any previous therapies that the patient may have received, such as medicaments or artificial respiration. The computer program must rapidly communicate about the diagnosis of the most complicated disorders in acid-base status and of the accompanying electrolyte balance, and must be helpful in most difficult parts of diagnosis which create problems for practicing physicians.

The purpose of our study was to compare the correctness of diagnosing made by:

- an artificial neural network described by the authors in [1],
- a computer program, obtained with use of genetic programming presented at the MIE2000 [2] and MIE2003 [3],
- the fuzzy-neural system which has not yet been presented.

2. Materials and Methods

In clinical practice, a physician can identify 24 acid-base disorders, basing on the values of serum pH, partial pressure of carbon dioxide (pCO_2), bicarbonate, base excess, sodium, potassium, chloride and anion gap as is shortly shown in Table 1.

Table 1 - Acid-Base disorders

1. Normal acid-base status
2. High anion gap metabolic acidosis
3. Normal anion gap metabolic acidosis
…
24.   Normal anion gap metabolic acidosis and metabolic alkalosis and respiratory alkalosis
25.   Normal anion gap metabolic acidosis and metabolic alkalosis and respiratory acidosis

Apart from normal acid-base status, we can identify 7 single acid-base disorders, 11 double acid-base disorders and 6 triple complicated acid-base disorders and accompanying anion gap alterations. We prepared a set of laboratory measurements, divided into 2 subsets of equal length. One subset consisted of 250 cases and was used in training of three different types of AI systems, and the second one also consisted of 250 results, used in testing of those AI systems.

Our sets of laboratory data consisted, apart from the gasometric values, used by Horn and coworkers [4], of the base excess (BE), calculated, using following equation:

$$BE = (1- 0.014 \, Hgb) \, (HCO_3 - 24) + 1.43 \, (Hgb + 7.7) \, (pH - 7.4)$$

Table 2 presents our example of four patients, suffering from normal anion gap metabolic acidosis, used to train the artificial neural network, to evaluate genetic programming and in fuzzy-neural system.

Table 2 - Normal anion gap metabolic acidosis

Patient's number	PH	pCO_2 mm Hg	HCO_3 act. mmol/l	BE mEq/l	Sodium mmol/l	Potassium Mmol/l	Chloride mmol/l	Anion gap mEq/l	Diagnosis' number
21	7,33	36	19	-5,5	131	4	100	16	3
22	7,31	36	18	-6,5	130	4	100	16	3
23	7,29	35	17	-7,0	120	5	97	12	3
24	7,25	36	16	-9,0	124	4	98	14	3

All the values of gasometric parameters are arterial values and, in case of venous blood, 0,03 should be added to receive arterial values of pH, according to Goldberg and coworkers [5].

3. Artificial neural network

The presented problem is that of the input pattern classification. During the training process different structures of a multilayer feedforward networks were examined. The network, examined first, had 5 inputs, and raw laboratory data (scaled to the range <-1, 1>), namely: pCO2 (mm Hg), HCO3 act.(mmol/l), Sodium (mmol/l), Potassium (mmol/l), Chloride (mmol/l) were used. The second network had three inputs more, to which three additional calculated values, i.e., pH, BE (mEq/l) and Anion gap (mEq/l). were presented to possibly improve the quality of classification. The hidden layer had a variable number of neurons, an output layer had 25 neurons. It is expected that, after the training process, only one output neuron should generate a high level signal as an answer to the input data. The quality of learning was estimated in two ways: first, with the MSE error during the learning process and then, with the use of a confusion matrix generated at the end of the process. The networks were taught, using the backpropagation method. Both the teaching set and the testing set contained 250 elements each, which means that 10 examples were associated with each disease unit. It turns out that the network with 5 inputs and 25 neurons in the hidden layer is the best of all the tested networks.

The confusion matrix is a very useful tool in classification problems. It is a square matrix 25x25 (in our case) built as follows. Each cell[i, j] (i – row number, j – column number) contains the number of diagnoses of the disorder number i, which the network identifies as disorder number j. The perfect confusion matrix is a diagonal matrix, each cell on diagonal contains the number 10, the other cells contain 0 and it means that the system made proper classification for all data from testing set. In our case, for the best neural network, we obtained the confusion matrix which is shown in Table 3.

Table 3 - Confusion matrix for neural network (testing set)

	1	2	3	4	5	6	7	8	9	10	11	12	13	14	15	16	17	18	19	20	21	22	23	24	25
1	10	0	0	0	0	0	0	0	0	0	0	0	0	1	0	0	0	1	0	0	0	0	0	0	0
2	0	10	0	0	0	0	0	0	0	0	0	0	0	0	0	0	0	0	0	0	0	0	0	0	0
3	0	0	10	0	0	0	0	0	0	0	0	0	0	0	0	0	0	0	0	0	0	0	0	0	0
4	0	0	0	8	0	0	0	0	0	0	0	0	0	0	0	0	2	0	0	0	0	0	0	0	0
5	0	0	0	0	10	0	0	0	0	0	0	0	0	0	0	0	0	0	0	0	0	0	0	0	0
6	0	0	0	0	0	8	0	0	3	0	0	0	0	0	0	0	0	0	0	0	0	0	0	0	0
7	0	0	0	0	0	0	10	0	0	0	1	0	0	0	0	0	0	0	0	0	0	0	0	0	0
8	0	0	0	0	0	0	0	5	0	2	0	0	0	0	0	0	0	0	0	0	0	0	0	0	0
9	0	0	0	0	0	0	0	0	9	0	0	0	0	0	0	0	0	0	0	0	0	0	0	0	0
10	0	0	0	0	0	0	0	4	0	3	0	0	0	0	0	0	0	0	0	0	0	0	0	0	0
11	0	0	0	0	0	0	0	0	0	0	10	0	0	0	0	0	0	0	0	0	3	0	0	0	0
12	0	0	0	0	0	0	0	0	0	0	0	10	0	0	0	0	0	0	0	0	0	0	0	0	0
13	0	0	0	0	0	0	0	0	0	0	0	0	10	0	0	0	0	0	0	0	0	0	0	0	0
14	0	0	0	0	0	0	0	0	0	0	2	0	0	4	0	0	0	0	0	5	0	0	0	0	0
15	0	0	0	0	0	0	0	0	0	0	0	0	0	0	9	0	0	0	0	0	0	0	0	0	0
16	0	0	0	0	0	0	0	0	0	0	0	0	0	2	0	6	0	0	0	0	0	0	0	0	0
17	0	0	0	1	0	0	0	0	0	0	0	0	0	0	0	0	9	0	0	0	0	0	0	0	0
18	0	0	0	0	0	0	0	0	0	0	0	0	0	0	0	0	0	10	0	0	0	0	0	0	0
19	0	0	0	0	0	0	0	0	0	0	0	0	0	0	0	0	0	0	8	0	1	0	0	0	0
20	0	0	0	0	0	0	0	0	0	0	1	0	0	1	0	0	0	0	0	7	0	0	0	0	0
21	0	0	0	0	0	0	0	0	0	0	0	0	0	0	0	0	0	0	0	0	10	0	0	0	0
22	0	0	0	0	0	0	0	0	0	0	0	1	0	0	0	0	0	0	0	0	0	10	0	0	0
23	0	0	0	0	0	0	0	0	0	0	0	0	0	0	0	0	0	0	0	0	0	0	10	0	0
24	0	0	0	0	0	0	0	0	0	0	0	0	0	0	0	0	0	0	0	0	0	0	0	10	0
25	0	0	0	0	0	0	0	0	0	0	0	0	0	0	0	0	2	0	0	0	0	0	0	0	8

The confusion matrix presented above shows, that our neural network has the serious problems with diagnosing of the disorder number 8, 10 and 14. We wanted to improve obtained results with help of the other method of AI described in the next paragraphs.

4. Genetic programming paradigm

The second attempt to solve the problem of diagnosis of acid-base and anion gap disorders was made with the use of methods of genetic, automatic programming. The goal of automatic programming is an automatic creation of a computer program that enables a computer to solve a problem. Genetic programming [6] is a domain-independent approach to automatic programming, in which computer programs are evolved to solve, or approximately solve, problems. In the genetic programming paradigm, populations of computer programs are genetically bred, using Darwinian principle of survival of the fittest and using the genetic crossover (recombination) operator, appropriate for genetically mating computer programs. Each individual computer program in the population is measured in terms of how well it performs in the particular problem environment.

The target classification system consists of twenty-five (25) independent genetic programs, from GP1 to GP25, automatically created. Each of these programs is responsible for diagnosing one disorder, so, finally, after presenting data into the input of the system, only one of these programs should generate high-level output, outputs of the other programs should be in low-level status.

This method is described in details in [3] so below we simply present in Table 4 the final result in form of the confusion matrix for testing data set. In this table are shown only the rows for which the number of the proper answers is less than 10.

Table 4 - Confusion matrix for GP (testing set)

	1	2	3	4	5	6	7	8	9	10	11	12	13	14	15	16	17	18	19	20	21	22	23	24	25
4	0	0	0	9	0	0	0	0	0	0	0	0	0	0	0	0	3	0	0	0	0	0	0	0	0
6	0	0	0	0	0	9	0	0	0	0	0	0	0	0	0	0	0	0	0	0	0	0	0	0	0
7	0	0	0	0	0	0	0	9	0	1	0	0	0	0	0	0	0	0	0	0	0	0	0	0	0
8	0	0	0	0	0	0	0	0	1	2	0	0	0	0	0	0	0	0	0	0	0	0	0	0	0
10	0	0	0	0	0	0	0	0	7	0	8	0	0	0	0	0	0	0	0	0	0	0	0	0	0
11	0	0	0	0	0	0	0	0	0	0	5	0	0	0	0	0	0	0	0	0	0	0	0	0	0
14	0	0	0	0	0	0	0	0	0	0	2	0	0	5	0	0	0	0	0	3	0	0	0	0	0
17	0	0	0	1	0	0	0	0	0	0	0	0	0	0	0	0	7	0	0	0	0	0	0	0	0
20	0	0	0	0	0	0	0	0	0	0	1	0	0	5	0	0	0	0	0	5	0	0	0	0	0

This GP solution has diagnosing problems with disorders number 8, 11, 14 and 20 so it is seemed to be worse to the neural network. The advantage of the presented GP method is possibilities obtaining solutions in form of the Boolean expressions, which may be theoretically analyzed by physicians.

5. Fuzzy-neural network

In spite of the satisfying results, obtained with artificial neural networks and genetic programming, we decided to try fuzzy sets and fuzzy logic to eventually further improve the accuracy of diagnosing disorders. In our attempts, we connected the possibilities of the fuzzy controllers and artificial neural networks. The fuzzy-neural controller is a fuzzy controller the shape of a multilayer, feedforward network, which is taught by the modified error-backpropagation method.

The typical fuzzy controller is presented in Figure 1. It consists of four main elements: rule base, fuzzification block, inference engine, defuzzification block.

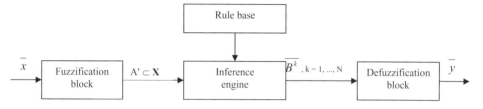

Figure 1 - Fuzzy controller

The conclusion system, which is based on the fuzzy controller and which uses neural network may be presented as a four-layer neural network [7]. The L1 layer performs fuzzification process, layer L2 is a conclusion block, layers L3 and L4 perform defuzzification of the output data.

A controller with the following parameters was chosen for our research:

- Five inputs: pCO2 , HCO3 act., Sodium, Potassium, Chloride,
- Fuzzification – singleton,
- Inference engine – Larsen rule,
- Defuzzification - center average (CA)
- The number of membership functions in fuzzification block – 15, the empirical value,
- 25 outputs.

Fuzzy-neural controllers usually have only one output. In the considered problem, we need a net with 25 outputs and, to obtain this kind of architecture, we joined 25 independent controllers into one net. The fuzzy-neural controllers have common inputs, but each of them may be taught individually.

As previously, after finishing the learning of the system, we constructed a confusion matrix for testing data set. This confusion matrix is presented in Table 5.

Table 5 - Confusion matrix for fuzzy-neural net (testing set)

	1	2	3	4	5	6	7	8	9	10	11	12	13	14	15	16	17	18	19	20	21	22	23	24	25
3	0	0	9	0	0	0	0	0	0	0	0	0	0	0	0	0	0	0	0	1	0	0	0	0	0
4	0	0	0	9	0	0	0	0	0	0	0	0	0	0	0	0	0	0	0	0	0	0	0	0	0
8	0	0	0	0	0	0	1	7	0	2	0	0	0	0	0	0	0	0	0	0	0	0	0	0	0
10	0	0	0	0	0	0	0	2	0	8	0	0	0	0	0	0	0	0	0	0	0	0	0	0	0
14	0	0	0	0	0	0	0	0	0	0	0	0	0	9	0	0	0	0	0	1	0	0	0	0	0
17	0	0	0	1	0	0	0	0	0	0	0	0	0	0	0	0	9	0	0	0	0	0	0	0	0
18	0	0	0	0	0	0	0	0	0	0	0	0	0	0	0	0	0	9	0	0	0	0	0	1	0
24	0	0	0	0	0	0	0	0	0	0	0	0	0	0	0	0	0	1	0	0	0	0	0	9	0
25	0	0	0	0	0	1	0	0	1	0	0	0	0	0	0	0	0	0	0	0	0	0	0	0	7

6. Conclusions

The aim of this paper is presentation and comparison of three different artificial intelligence methods for the diagnosis of acid - base and anion gap disorders. Table 6 below shows the number of proper diagnoses for: neural network, genetic programming and fuzzy-neural system.

Table 6 - Proper diagnosis for each kind of AI system

Diagnosis' number	1	2	3	4	5	6	7	8	9	10	11	12
Neural Network	10	10	10	8	10	8	10	5	9	3	10	10
Genetic Programming	10	10	10	9	10	9	9	1	10	8	5	10
Fuzzy-Neural Net	10	10	9	9	10	10	10	7	10	8	10	10

Diagnosis' number	13	14	15	16	17	18	19	20	21	22	23	24	25
Neural Network	10	4	9	6	9	10	8	7	10	10	10	10	8
Genetic Programming	10	5	10	10	7	10	10	5	10	10	10	10	10
Fuzzy-Neural Net	10	9	10	10	9	9	10	10	10	10	10	9	7

The presented AI methods have similar possibilities to aid physician in diagnosing this kind of disorders, but fuzzy systems seem to be closer to the real world. The genetic programming, in presented forms, allows obtaining Boolean expressions which describe disorders, and which may be helpful in physician research work but the system of diagnosis of the acid - base and anion gap disorders should employ fuzzy-neural controllers which proved to be the best in this type of diagnosing challenge. It should be pointed out that all methods are useful in diagnosing the triple complicated acid-base disorders and accompanying anion gap alterations (diagnosis number 20 ÷ 25), for which diagnosis is very difficult for physicians.

7. References

[1]   T. Bogdanik, E. Kacki, A. Malolepszy: Application of an Artificial Neural Network for the Differential Diagnosis of Acid-Base and Anion Gap Disorders, Proc. of the Fifth Conf "Computers in Medicine", Lodz, Poland, 1999, pp. 75-80

[2]   A. Małolepszy, E. Kącki, T. Bogdanik: Application of Genetic Programming for the Differential Diagnosis of Acid-Base and Anion Gap Disorders in Medical Infobahn for Europe, Proc. of MIE2000, IOS Press Ohmsha, Washington, USA, pp. 388-394

[3]   A. Małolepszy, E. Kącki: Genetic Programming In Medical Diagnosis, The New Navigators: from Professionals to Patients, Proc. of MIE2003, IOS Press Ohmsha, Washington, USA, 2003, pp. 44-49

[4]   D.L. Horn, J. Radhakrishnan, S. Saini, et al., Evaluation of a computer program for teaching laboratory diagnosis of acid-base disorders. Comp. Biomed. Research, 1992, vol. 25, pp. 562-568

[5]   M. Goldberg, S.B. Green, M.L.Moss., et al., Computer-based instruction of acid-base disorders. JAMA, 1973, vol. 223, pp. 269-275

[6]   J. R. Koza, The Genetic Programming Paradigm: Genetically Breeding Population of Computer Programs to Solve Problems in Dynamic, Genetic and Chaotic Programming, New York, John Wiley, 1992

[7]   D. Rutkowska, M. Piliński, L. Rutkowski, Neural Networks, Genetic Algorithms and Fuzzy Systems, in Polish, PWN, Warsaw, Poland, 1999

Address for correspondence

Piotrkowska St. No. 182 ap. 473, 90-368 Lodz, Poland, e-mail: e25kacki@cosmosnet.pl

Connecting Medical Informatics and Bio-Informatics
R. Engelbrecht et al. (Eds.)
IOS Press, 2005

Outcome Prediction after Moderate and Severe Head Injury Using an Artificial Neural Network

Min-Huei Hsu[a,b], Yu-Chuan Li[c], Wen-Ta Chiu[d], Ju-Chuan Yen[e]

[a]*Department of Neurosurgery,* [e]*Department of Ophthalmology, Taipei City Hospital, Zhongxiao Branch*
[b]*Graduate Institute of Medical Sciences,* [c]*Graduate Institute of Medical Informatics, Taipei Medical University*
[d]*Taipei Municipal Wanfang Hospital (Managed by Taipei Medical University)*

Abstract

Many studies have constructed predictive models for outcome after traumatic brain injury. Most of these attempts focused on dichotomous result, such as alive vs dead or good outcome vs poor outcome. If we want to predict more specific levels of outcome, we need more sophisticated models. We conducted this study to determine if artificial neural network modeling would predict outcome in five levels of Glasgow Outcome Scale (death, persistent vegetative state, severe disability, moderate disability, and good recovery) after moderate to severe head injury. The database was collected from a nation-wide epidemiological study of traumatic brain injury in Taiwan from July 1, 1995 to June 30, 1998. There were total 18583 records in this database and each record had thirty-two parameters. After pruning the records with minor cases (GCS 13) and missing data in the 132 variables, the number of cases decreased from 18583 to 4460. A step-wise logistic regression was applied to the remaining data set and 10 variables were selected as being statically significant in predicting outcome. These 10 variables were used as the input neurons for constructing neural network. Overall, 75.8% of predictions of this model were correct, 14.6% were pessimistic, and 9.6% optimistic. This neural network model demonstrated a significant difference of performance between different levels of Glasgow Outcome Scale. The prediction performance of dead or good recovery is best and the prediction of vegetative state is worst. An artificial neural network may provide a useful "second opinion" to assist neurosurgeon to predict outcome after traumatic brain injury.

Keywords:
Head injury; Artificial neural network; Outcome prediction

1. Introduction

Considerable effort has been devoted to improving our ability to predict outcome after traumatic brain injury (TBI). More reliable prediction of outcome would be helpful for clinicians as an important aid to decision making about management and for communication with relatives and other healthcare professionals.

Mathematical and statistical methods have been used to develop models for outcome prediction. The most commonly used methods include Bayes' theorem [1], logistic regression and neural networks. [2]

A artificial neural network is a computerized construct consisting of input neurons (which process input data) connected to hidden neurons (to mathematically manipulate values they receive from all the input neurons) connected to output neurons (to output a prediction). Artificial neural networks have been successfully used for pattern recognition and outcome prediction in several clinical settings. The advantage of a neural network is the ability of the model to capture nonlinearities and complex interactions between factors related to the outcome of interest. Neural networks differ from other decision support systems in that the learning occurs by example through training and not by programming or pre-defined rules.

We conducted this study to determine if artificial neural network modeling would predict outcome using five levels of Glasgow Outcome Scale [3] (death, persistent vegetative state, severe disability, moderate disability, and good recovery) after moderate and severe head injury (initial Glasgow Coma Scale-Score of 3-12)

2. Materials and methods

This study was conducted using data collected from a nation-wide epidemiological study of traumatic brain injury in Taiwan from July 1, 1995 to June 30, 1998. One hundred and sixteen large to medium-sized teaching hospitals with qualified neurosurgeon participated in this study. There were total 18583 records in this database. The causes of head trauma were traffic crashes (14354 cases, of whom more than 65% were motorcycle crash victims), falls (2534 cases), and others (1695 cases). The mean age of the victims was 36.5 +/- 15.3 (SD), range 1 to 85 years old. In 7.8% of the cases, the victims were older than 60. The male to female ratio was about 3:1.

One hundred and thirty-two parameters including age, gender, causes of head trauma, GCS scores at the emergency department, CT findings and craniotomy for intracranial hematoma were recorded for each patient. The outcome was estimated by the Glasgow Outcome Scale (GOS), and was assessed as longer as 12 months after injury if possible.

After pruning the records with mild cases (GCS 13) and missing data in the 132 variables , the number of cases decreased from 18583 to 4460. In the second step, a step-wise logistic regression was applied to the remaining data set and 10 variables (Table 1) were selected as being statically significant ($p < 0.05$) in predicting of the dependent variable (Glasgow Outcome Scale).

From the 4460 cases, 75% were randomly selected as the training group (n=3345) in the development of the neural network models. The validation group (n=1115) was used to test the performance of this model. Generalized regression neural network software was used (NeuralShell Classifier Version 2; Ward Systems Group; Frederick, MD).

The accuracy, sensitivity and specificity are used to describe the performance of the predictive model.

Table 1 Variables as input neurons in the ANN model

Age
Number of nonreactive pupils
Score of motor resonse
Score of verbal response
Score of eye opening
Use of helmet in motorcycle crash
Intracerebral hematoma on CT
Subdural hematoma on CT
Craniotomy for intracranial hematoma
Alcohol-related traffic accident

Table 2 Actual and predicted outcome for 1115 patients

	Actual "1"	Actual "2"	Actual "3"	Actual "4"	Actual "5"	Total
Predicted as "1"	134	10	17	12	23	196
Predicted as "2"	2	12	3	5	1	23
Predicted as "3"	0	0	66	7	9	82
Predicted as "4"	20	2	14	132	19	187
Predicted as "5"	18	1	3	31	574	627
Total	174	25	103	187	626	1115

1=death, 2=vegetative, 3= severe disability, 4= moderate disability, 5=good recovery

Table 3 The sensitivity and specificity of prediction

	1	2	3	4	5
Sensitivity	77.01%	48.00%	64.08%	70.59%	91.69%
Specificity	93.41%	98.99%	98.42%	94.07%	89.16%

1=death, 2=vegetative, 3= severe disability, 4= moderate disability, 5=good recovery

3. Results

The prediction results from the ANN are shown in Table 2. As can be seen from the diagonal cells in the contingency table, Overall, 75.8% of predictions were correct, 14.6% were pessimistic (outcome better than predicted), and 9.6% optimistic (outcome worse than predicted). For patients with good recovery, 91.6 % of predictions were correct. For patients with moderate disability, 70.5% of predictions were correct. For patients with severe disability, 64.0% of predictions were correct. For death, 77.0% of prediction were correct but for vegetative state only 48.0% of prediction were correct. The sensitivity and specificity for each level are shown in Table 3.

4. Discussion

Approaches to developing prognostic models vary from using traditional probabilistic techniques, originating from the field of statistics, to more qualitative and model-based techniques, originating from the field of artificial intelligence (AI).

Until recently, attempts to predict outcome have focused on dichotomous result, such as alive vs dead or good outcome vs poor function. [4,5] The use of single variables, such as GCS [6], image finding [7], intracranial pressure [8] or cerebral blood flow [9], has allowed for a reasonable degree of accuracy in predicting those outcomes. With increased interest in predicting more specific levels of function, however, more sophisticated models are required. Such models require inclusion of multiple variables and better algorithm.

The neural network model developed in this study provided acceptable performance of overall outcome prediction. However it demonstrated a significant difference of performance between different levels of prediction. The prediction performance of dead or good recovery is best and the prediction of vegetative state is worst. This may be due to the small case number of the vegetative group in this study.

In most outcome prediction studies of TBI patients, death and vegetative state are combined as a single level (poor outcome). However, these two states have significant difference for clinicians and patient's relatives. Some people even think survival in a persistent vegetative state is worse than death. Any model could predict persistent vegetative state in early stage would be very helpful for clinicians in assisting treatment limiting decisions. But the predictive power of our model is still not good enough for that purpose.

We excluded the mild cases in our study, because most these patients will have a good recovery. Including mild cases could let prediction models have better performance without clinical significance.

Many other authors have shown age [10,11], GCS score, pupillary responsiveness [12,13] and findings of computed tomography (CT) to be significant predictors of outcome after traumatic brain injury. In our study, use of helmet in motorcycle crash was a significant outcome predictor. Before implementation of the motorcycle helmet use law, motorcycle collisions accounted for 74% of the traffic accidents in Taiwan, and most of the motorcycle riders were not helmet users. The motorcycle-related deaths have reached 48 percent of all motor vehicle-related deaths. [14] After implementation the helmet law in Taiwan on June 1, 1997, the mortality and morbidity from motorcycle-related head injuries decreased effectively in Taiwan. [15]

Although the ANN is a valuable method for outcome prediction, some of its nature should be noted before it can be widely applied. One is the `black box' nature of the ANN, which means that the logical procedure of how networks determine a prediction cannot be observed. Hart and Wyatt

believe that this "black box" aspect is a major obstacle to the acceptance of neural nets as part of medical decision support systems. [16]

Accurate prediction of outcome in the individual patient remains difficult to achieve for both clinicians and computer program. Our research indicates that an artificial neural network may provide a useful "second opinion" to assist neurosurgeon to predict outcome after traumatic brain injury.

5. Reference

[1]   Barlow P, Teasdale GM, Jennett B, et al. Computer assisted prediction of outcome of severely head-injured patients. Journal of Microcomputer Applications 1984;7:271-7.

[2]   Lang EW. Pitts LH. Damron SL. Rutledge R. Outcome after severe head injury: an analysis of prediction based upon comparison of neural network versus logistic regression analysis. Neurological Research. 19(3):274-80, 1997 Jun.

[3]   Jennett B, Bond M: Assessment of outcome after severe brain damage. A practical scale. Lancet 1:480, 1975

[4]   Hsu MH, Li YC. Predicting cranial computed tomography results of head injury patients using an artificial neural network. AMIA Annu Symp Proc. 2003; 868.

[5]   Jennett B. Teasdale G. Braakman R. Minderhoud J. Knill-Jones R. Predicting outcome in individual patients after severe head injury. Lancet. 1(7968):1031-4, 1976 May 15

[6]   van Dongen KJ, Braakman R, Gelpke GJ: The prognostic value of computerized tomography in comatose head-injured patients. J Neurosurg 59:951, 1983

[7]   Benzer A, Mitterschiffthaler G, Marosi M, et al. Prediction of non-survival after trauma. Lancet 1991;338:977-8.

[8]   Czosnyka M. Guazzo E. Whitehouse M. Smielewski P. Czosnyka Z. Kirkpatrick P. Piechnik S. Pickard JD. Significance of intracranial pressure waveform analysis after head injury. Acta Neurochirurgica. 138(5):531-41, 1996.

[9]   Kelly DF. Martin NA. Kordestani R. Counelis G. Hovda DA. Bergsneider M. McBride DQ. Shalmon E. Herman D. Becker DP. Cerebral blood flow as a predictor of outcome following traumatic brain injury. Journal of Neurosurgery. 86(4):633-41, 1997 Apr.

[10] Luerssen TG, Klauber MR, Marshall LF: Age and outcome from head injury: A longitudinal prospective study of adult and pediatric head injury. J Neurosurg 68:409, 1988

[11] Vollmer DG, Torner JC, Jane JA, et al: Age and outcome following traumatic coma: Why do older patients fare worse? J Neurosurg 75:S37, 1991

[12] Price DJ, Knill-Jones R: The prediction of outcome of patients admitted following head injury in coma with bilateral fixed pupils. Acta Neurochir Suppl 28:179, 1979

[13] Jennett B, Teasdale G, Braakman R, et al: Predicting outcome in individual patients after severe head injury. Lancet 1:1031, 1976

[14] Chiu WT. The motorcycle helmet law in Taiwan. JAMA. 274(12):941-2, 1995 Sep 27.

[15] Chiu WT. Kuo CY. Hung CC. Chen M. The effect of the Taiwan motorcycle helmet use law on head injuries. American Journal of Public Health. 90(5):793-6, 2000 May.

[16] Hart A, Wyatt J. Evaluating black-boxes as medical decision aids: issues arising from a study of neural networks. Med Inform 1990; 15: 229-36.

Address for correspondence

Min-Huei Hsu, M.D.
Address: 3F, No9, Lane 176, Sec1, Ta-An Road, Taipei, Taiwan
E-mail address: 701056@tmu.edu.tw

Section 4

Educational Technologies and Methodologies

Connecting Medical Informatics and Bio-Informatics
R. Engelbrecht et al. (Eds.)
IOS Press, 2005

Computer-based Training in Medicine and Learning Theories

Martin Haag[a], Matthias Bauch[a], Sebastian Garde[b], Jörn Heid[a],
Thorsten Weires[a], Franz-Josef Leven[a]

[a]*University of Heidelberg, Germany*
[b]*Central Queensland University, Australia*

Abstract

Computer-based training (CBT) systems can efficiently support modern teaching and learning environments. In this paper, we demonstrate on the basis of the case-based CBT system CAMPUS that current learning theories and design principles (Bloom's Taxonomy and practice fields) are (i) relevant to CBT and (ii) are feasible to implement using computer-based training and adequate learning environments. Not all design principles can be fulfilled by the system alone, the integration of the system in adequate teaching and learning environments therefore is essential. Adequately integrated, CBT programs become valuable means to build or support practice fields for learners that build domain knowledge and problem-solving skills. Learning theories and their design principles can support in designing these systems as well as in assessing their value.

Keywords:
Computer-Assisted Instruction; Problem-Based Learning; Medical Informatics

1. Introduction

For students of medicine or nursing, learning means to become familiar with clinical cases and problems. The best way to do this is to directly involve the students in the delivery of health care. But "real" patients with a particular disease are not always available. Often an appropriate patient is missing or can not be demonstrated to all students because of practical or ethical problems. Computer-based training (CBT) programs, which are available at any time and place possibly offer a solution to these problems. Therefore, the University of Heidelberg, Germany, developed CAMPUS, a web-based learning shell system to provide flexible, simulative real medical multimedia cases for use by educators, students, and physicians at different levels. It consists mainly of a user friendly authoring system as the tool for case-data input and a player component as the learner's front-end (Figure 1). The CAMPUS system features different kinds of case presentations in accordance to the level of professionalism of the user and the scenario the program is used in. The main screen represents a situated learning environment with familiar medical images and elements that provide an easily understandable, realistic, user interface. While working through a

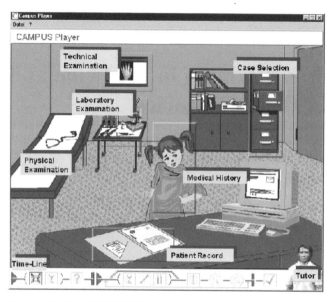

Figure 1 - The CAMPUS Player – main screen

case, the learner is able to consult the patient record for results. The tutor gives expert comments and asks questions. With the aid of this interface, the user tries to solve a medical case in a simulative manner, which means that he/she can do just about everything he/she wants to do (as in real life, e.g., anamnesis, physical and technical exams, lab tests). The learner can do a physical exam by choosing the kind of exam (e.g., auscultation) and pointing to a specific body region. To provide didactic elements, the case author can define expert comments and knowledge questions. At each feedback point the user gets feedback with respect to his/her decisions by presenting a comparison between his measures and the procedures which the author of the case considers to be right, distinguished by different colours. The feedback provided is neutral without messages like "very good" or "bad answer". CAMPUS avoids such messages because of the different possible ways of solving a case, that is, the teacher or system's role is not directive.

This paper outlines current learning theories, demonstrates their relevance to computer-supported learning and shows on the basis of CAMPUS that these theories can successfully be applied in computer-based training.

2. Materials and methods

Current theories of learning acknowledge that learning is a wilful, intentional, active, conscious, constructive activity that requires reciprocal intention-action-reflection cognition. The theories therefore emphasize the importance of learner-centred, active, authentic environments for meaningful knowledge construction (constructivism). The fundamental shift to constructivist-oriented learning theories asserts that learning is a process of meaning making, not of knowledge transmission, and that it is a social-dialogical process influenced by communities of practice. The movement to a constructivist-learning paradigm has influenced the design and development of open-ended learning environments like problem-based learning [1] and goal-based scenarios [2].

Computerized case-based learning systems can efficiently build or support practice fields for learners to build domain knowledge and problem-solving skills and to support contextualized transfer of knowledge and skills to professional practice [3]. Computer-based learning systems can facilitate this "constructivist" type of transfer by bringing real world problems into the learning space and by providing performance feedback and opportunities for meta-cognitive reflection tied to authentic problems [4].

2.1 Bloom's Taxonomy

Bloom developed a classification of levels of intellectual behaviour [5]. The classification features 6 levels of intellectual behaviour: Knowledge, Comprehension, Application, Analysis, Synthesis and Evaluation. It is important for learning to be challenged on all levels of intellectual behaviour. Although not developed in light of constructivism, Bloom's Taxonomy is still often used e.g. to assess difficulties in exams or assessments.

2.2 Practice Fields

In practice fields [6] students engage in the kinds of problems and practices that they will encounter outside of school. Preparing practice fields involves creating circumscribed realistic activities or experiences for the learner. These activities must be authentic; they must present most of the cognitive demands the learner would encounter in the real world to foster authentic problem solving and critical thinking in the domain. Problem-based learning is one example of practice fields. Problem-based learning during the professional preparation years is more than practicing future skills; it builds domain knowledge and problem-solving skills in realistic situations. To maximize the usefulness of practice fields, design principles have been introduced by [7]. These principles are summarized in Table 1.

Table 1: Design principles for practice fields as proposed by [7]

Principle 1: Doing domain-related practice	Learners must be actively doing domain-related practice, not listening to the experiences or findings of others.
Principle 2: Ownership of the inquiry	Learners must see the dilemma as worth investing their efforts. They must feel they are responsible for the solution.
Principle 3: Coaching and modeling of thinking skills	The instructor's job (a real instructor or the learning system) is to coach and model learning and problem solving by asking questions that learners should be asking themselves.
Principle 4: Opportunity for reflection	Reflection provides individuals with the opportunity to think about why they are doing what they are doing and even to gather evidence to evaluate the efficacy of their decisions. The reflective process is essential to the quality of learning.
Principle 5: Dilemmas are ill-structured	Dilemmas in which learners are engaged must be either ill-defined or loosely structured so that learners can impose their own problem frames.
Principle 6: Support the learner rather than simplify the dilemma	The dilemmas that learners encounter should reflect the complexity of the thinking and work that they are expected in the real world.
Principle 7: Work is collaborative and social	Meaning is a process of continual negotiation. The quality and depth of this negotiation and understanding can only be determined in a social environment where ideas are discussed.
Principle 8: The learning context is motivating	Learners must be introduced to the context of problems and their relevance, and this must be done in a way that challenges and engages the learner.

3. Results

CAMPUS offers learning on all levels of Bloom's taxonomy. The following enumeration gives some examples:

1. Knowledge: Answer knowledge questions added by the case author.
2. Comprehension: Interpret single lab test results (e.g. a value is extremely high)
3. Application: Conduct efficient medical history taking and efficient physical examination
4. Analysis: Analyse lab results and draw conclusions; analyse physical examination and draw conclusions
5. Synthesis: Analyse lab results *and* analyse physical examination and draw conclusions, e.g. diagnosis and prognosis
6. Evaluation: Evaluate your own behaviour when comparing it with the case expert's "solution"; assess value of external medical knowledge found.

Below we analyse how far CAMPUS as an example for CBT fulfils the design principles of practice fields. Table 2 summarizes the findings.

Table 2: Design principles of practice fields and how they are fulfilled in CAMPUS.

Principle 1: Doing domain-related practice	Because of the simulative and interactive nature of the system, the workout of a case is domain-related learning by doing, not listening to the experiences or findings of others. Further, certain technical examinations might not be available at a given point of time, so that the student has to improvise – just as in real life.
Principle 2: Ownership of the inquiry	A feeling of ownership is achieved by using real medical cases. Patient images and videos intensify this effect. Because of the simulative format and use of neutral feedback, students can develop their own solution.
Principle 3: Coaching and modeling of thinking skills	Coaching of thinking skills is dependent on the program's author. She/he can create expert comments that are shown on demand or guide by asking the right questions or displaying the right hints. It is the author's responsibility to use this capability in the right way to coach the learner.
Principle 4: Opportunity for reflection	CAMPUS supports reflection in several ways: • By ordering single examinations and getting specific results, the user has to think about the results and decide on the next step to proceed. • Users must reflect in the feedback components where a comparison between the author's solution and their own is given. • Knowledge questions and expert commentary and hints can be used to prompt the student to think about special parts of the case.
Principle 5: Dilemmas are ill-structured	CAMPUS supports ill-structured and complex dilemmas by offering the user maximum and case-independent possibilities of examinations, diagnoses, and therapies. Again, the neutral feedback is important in this context. Without neutrality, the user would wait for feedback after each action and individual problem-solving approaches would not develop.
Principle 6: Support the learner rather than simplify the dilemma	CAMPUS supports the learner in several ways. Apart from the aforementioned knowledge-on-demand expert comments, questions, and hints, CAMPUS also provides more systematic knowledge: easy accessible integrated digitized textbook knowledge and access to online libraries in a context-sensitive manner.

Principle 7: Work is collaborative and social	CAMPUS offers important views of others by providing a comparison between the author's and the learner's solution. Other collaborative and social tenets are mainly system-independent and learning-scenario-dependent. An example of an appropriate scenario is that of students working on several cases in groups of two to three persons per computer as recommended through different studies, e.g., [8], assisted by a tutor. After completion, all students discuss the case together with the tutor. CAMPUS also can be integrated into learning management systems (LMS) such as .LRN. Within the LMS, students can learn collaboratively by discussing the CAMPUS cases.
Principle 8: The learning context is motivating	Because the aim of CAMPUS is to integrate real cases into training, these problems engage the learner. The web-based approach and case repositories offer rich opportunities for using CAMPUS in communities of practice. In such communities, students as well as teachers can easily contribute interesting, community-concerned cases via CAMPUS' authoring system and discuss them.

While CAMPUS fulfils principle 1 and 5 independent from the teaching and learning environment to fulfil the other principles in addition a good teaching and learning environment is mandatory.

4. Discussion

Many of the current learning theories focus on authentic, student-centred learning environments. As Jonassen and Land stated [3], the past decade "has witnessed the most substantive and revolutionary changes in learning theory in history". In fact, newer theoretical learning foundations – such as socially shared cognition, situated learning, everyday cognition and reasoning, activity theory, ecological psychology, distributed cognition, and case-based reasoning – share many of the beliefs and assumptions of constructivism.

Good educational practice principles are independent of the domain (e.g. medicine) and the degree of technology supporting the learner or teacher. In this context, practice field principles and Bloom's Taxonomy are a valuable means to assess the teaching provided. As shown in this paper, all of the practice field principles are achievable with interactive CBT systems. Some of these principles, however, cannot be fully fulfilled by the application program alone but are partially dependent on how the teaching and learning environment is designed and on the quality and suitability of the cases designed by case authors.

Bloom's Taxonomy – defining levels of intellectual behaviour – helps in determining on which levels the student is intellectually challenged. As shown in this paper, properly designed CBT programs can challenge the student on all levels of Bloom's Taxonomy. In CAMPUS the challenges on the different levels are interwoven – this reflects the real world situation of health professionals who do not have the luxury of being able to obtain a comprehensive knowledge of medicine.

Two evaluation studies have shown that the CAMPUS concept is regarded as useful by medical students. Evaluation results are described elsewhere in detail [9], but in summary 80.7% (176 out of 218 students who participated in a pediatric internship at the Heidelberg Medical Centre) liked learning with CAMPUS; 72% (157) rated learning with CAMPUS as effective; 73.5% (160) said that learning with CAMPUS was motivating for further learning.

5. Conclusion

Constructivism and CBT programs are valuable means for modern teaching and learning environments. Learning theories and their design principles can support in designing these systems as well as in assessing their value. As shown in this paper these design principles can be fulfilled by integrated computer-based training teaching and learning environments.

6. References

[1]   Hmelo C (1998): Problem-based learning: Effects on the early acquisition of cognitive skill in medicine. *Journal of the Learning Sciences*, 7, 173-208.

[2]   Schank R, Fano A, Bett B, Jona M (1994): The design of goalbased scenarios. *Journal of the Learning Sciences*, 3, 305-345.

[3]   Jonassen D (2000): *Mindtools for schools: Engaging critical thinking with technology* (2nd ed). Columbus, OH: Merrill/Prentice-Hall.

[4]   National Research Council (2000): *How people learn: Brain, mind, experience, and school*. Washington, DC: National Academy Press.

[5]   Bloom BS, Ed. (1956): *Taxonomy of educational objectives: The classification of educational goals: Handbook I, cognitive domain*. New York ; Toronto: Longmans, Green.

[6]   Senge P (1994): *The fifth discipline fieldbook: Strategies and tools for building a learning organization*. New York: Doubleday.

[7]   Barab S, Duffy T (2000): *From practice fields to communities of practice. Theoretical foundations of learning environments*. Mahwah, NJ: Lawrence Erlbaum.

[8]   Johnson DW, Johnson RT (1992): *Positive interdependence: Key to effective cooperation. Interaction in cooperative groups: The theoretical anatomy of group learning*. New York: Cambridge University Press.

[9]   Riedel J, Fitzgerald G, Leven FJ, Tönshoff B (2003): The Design of Computerized Practice Fields for Problem Solving and Contextualized Transfer. *Journal of Educational Multimedia and Hypermedia*, 12, 377-398.

7. Address

Martin Haag
Laboratory Computer-Based Training in Medicine, University of Heidelberg
Im Neuenheimer Feld 324, 69120 Heidelberg, GERMANY
martin.haag@fh-heilbronn.de
http://www.medicase.de

Connecting Medical Informatics and Bio-Informatics
R. Engelbrecht et al. (Eds.)
IOS Press, 2005

Instructional Technology Adoption of Medical Faculty in Teaching

Neşe Zayim[a], Soner Yıldırım[b], Osman Saka[a]

[a]*Akdeniz University, Antalya, Turkey*
[b]*Middle East Technical University, Ankara, Turkey*

Abstract

Despite large investment by higher education institutions in technology for faculty and student use, instructional technology is not being integrated into instructions in the higher education institutions, including medical education institutions. While diffusion of instructional technologies has been reached a saturation point with early adopters of technology, it has remained limited among mainstream faculty. This study explored technology adoption patterns and perceptions of medical faculty about barriers and incentives to technology adoption in teaching.Complete data was obtained from 155 participants by using survey methodology and analyzed on the basis of theories of diffusion of innovation.
Findings provided evidence for limited adoption of relatively new tools associated with instruction into mainstream faculty. Inadequate hardware for students and faculty, lack of reward structure, insufficient traing oppurtunites were identified as major barriers to faculty technology adoption.

Keywords:
Medical Education, Instructional Technology, Diffusion of Innovations

1. Introduction

During the past two decades, a number of reports have called on medical schools to incorporate instructional technology into their educational program in order to meet challenges of medical education [1,2]. Even though the reports of such organizations encourage medical school decision makers to initiate instructional technology programs, medical schools had made limited progress in accomplishing the recommend educational technology goals [3,4].

There are many reasons both technical and societal, why innovative technologies have not been widely adopted, however, the major reason for this lack of utilization is that most university-level technology strategies ignore the central role that faculty play in the change process [5]. Much of the conversation about technology in education continues to focus on products: computers, software, networks and instructional resources [6]. Certainly, adequate technology infrastructure use is a necessary condition for IT integration but major problem is getting faculty to adopt these technologies once they are made available.

Research findings indicate that there are variety factors involved in faculty members' decision to adopt or reject instructional technology in teaching and learning. According to Green's Annual Campus Computing Survey, user support and instructional integration is the most important of all issues surrounding the adoption of instructional technology for teaching and learning [6]. The interview results with faculty at a mid-sized university in USA indicate that faculty members' attitude and perceived value of IT are the most important factors in faculty member's decision to use or not to use instructional technologies [7]. Results of the study conducted in a medical school also indicate that lack of knowledge, lack of resources, reward systems, faculty development oppurtunities, financial supupport are few of the the barriers that medical faculty face in IT adoption [3].

Diffusion research investigates the factors that influence the diffusion process. Studies of diffusion and adoption help to explain the what, where, and why of technology acceptance or rejection in education [8]. Therefore, Rogers' theory of the diffusion of innovations provides a theoretical framework for present investigation [9].

Diffusion of an Innovation

Rogers' defines an innovation as "an idea or practice or object that is percieved as new by the individual", and diffusion as "the process by which an innovation is communicated though certain channels over time among the members of a social system"[9, p.5].

According to Rogers, an individual's decision about an innovation is not an instantaneous act, rather "the process through which an individual (or other decision-making unit) passes from first knowledge of innovation, to forming an attitude toward the innovation, to a decision to adopt or reject, to implementation of the new idea, and to confirmation of this decision"[9, p.163]. Rogers' states that individuals in a social system do not   adopt an innovation at the same time, a certain percentage of individuals are relatively earlier or later in adopting a new idea. On the basis of innovativeness-the degree to which an individual is relatively earlier in adopting new ideas than other members of a social system, Rogers categorizes adopters into five groups: Innovators, Early Adopters, Early Majority, Late Majority and Laggards (Figure 1).

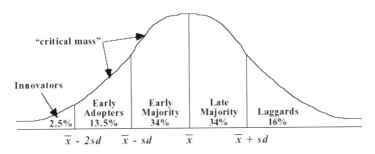

Figure 1. Adopter Categorization on the Basis of Innovativeness (Rogers, 1995)

2. Methodology

The present investigation surveyed medical school faculty members in a state university , who teach in the basic science and clinical science curriculum. Data was gathered about technology use patterns, computer experience, technologies used in teaching, percieved value of IT in medical education, barriers and   incentives to adoption, using a survey instrument. Survey items adopted or selected from previous investigations of faculty adoption patterns, teaching and learning with technology [10.11].

The survey was distributed to all faculty members(308) and 50,3 % (155) of the faculty members responded. Of the respondents, 112(72,7%) male and 42(27,3%) female, hold various academic raks (i.e. 32,7%(50) proffesor, 19,6%(30) Assoc. Proffesor, 22,1%(36) Asst.Proffesor and and 25,6%(39) others and had an avarage 10 years teaching experience. While 23,2%(36) of the respondents teaching in basic science curriculum, the largest group(76,8%(119)) teaching in clinical science. While the average age was 41 years, the largest group(≈55%(85) was in between 31-40 years range.

3. Results

Computer Ownership and Amount of Daily Computer Use

Faculty members were asked to indicate if they had a personal computer and internet access at home and at office, and how much time per day they used a computer. Althouh most of the participants (92,5%(135)) have computer at home and at office, only 21,5%(46) indicated that they spent more than 3 hours per day, 13,7%(20) spent less than one hour per day, and 54,8%(80) spent 1 to 3 hours per day.

Faculty Expertise in Technology Use

The faculty rated their level of expertise on eleven types of computer software and tools by using five-point likert-type scale (i.e., 1 for Extensive, 2 for Good, 3 for Fair, 4 for Novice, 5 for None). The majority of faculty (over %90) rated their skills at fair or higher at word proccecessing, presentation software, electronic mail, library and database searching, search engines and medline . Most faculties reported their skills at web page creation (76,1%) and statistics packages (54,2%) at novice or none. These findings indicate that faculty mostly use communication and research related tools. Relatively new tools associated with instruction (e.g.Web page creation) were not adopted by majority faculty.

Technologies Used in Teaching

Medical school faculty were asked to indicate which of the 12 instructional technologies they use in teaching-learning process. The mean number of technologies used in teaching is 4,56 with a standard deviation of 1,94. Based on Rogers' adopter categories, the descriptive results indicate that of the 12 instructional technologies, 9 have been used in teaching by more than 16% of the faculty, which means that these technologies have diffused into the Mainstream Faculty(MF). Of the 9 technologies that have been used by Mainstream Faculty(MF), 4 are used by more than 50% of the faculty(i.e. computer+projection 95%, slide projector 75%, overhead 71%, blackboard 66,5%) which indicate that these technologies have diffused into Late Majority(LM). The other 5 technologies have diffused into Early Majority(EM) which represents the segment between 16 and 50 percent of the Rogers' diffusion curve (i.e. Web resources 18,3% ,Video 20,9%, Special Laboratory 22,2%, word processors 33,3%, presentation software 32,7%)(Figure 2).

Percieved Value of IT

The participants used a five-point scale (i.e., 1 for Strongly Agree, 2 for Agree, 3 for Neutral, 4 for Disagree, 5 for Strongly Disagree) to rate their level of agreement on 9 statements about value of IT in medical education. A composite score for each individual faculty was calculated by summing the level of agreement indicated for each of the 9 statement about value of IT. The mean score for Perceived value of IT scale is 11,75 with a standard deviation of 3,4 which indicates that faculty have high level agreement on value of

IT use in medical education. The mean and standard deviation of each item in Perceived Value of IT Scale is presented in Table 1.

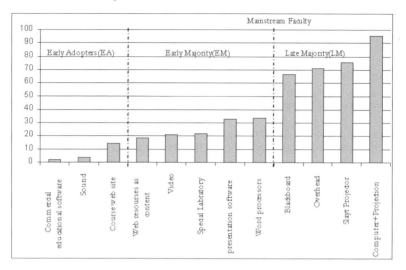

Figure 2. Technologies Used in Teaching

The mean score for Perceived value of IT scale is 11,75 with a standard deviation of 3,4 which indicates that faculty have high level agreement on value of IT use in medical education. The mean and standard deviation of each item in Perceived Value of IT Scale is presented in Table 1.

Percieved Value of IT

The participants used a five-point scale (i.e., 1 for Strongly Agree, 2 for Agree, 3 for Neutral, 4 for Disagree, 5 for Strongly Disagree) to rate their level of agreement on 9 statements about value of IT in medical education. A composite score for each individual faculty was calculated by summing the level of agreement indicated for each of the 9 statement about value of IT. The mean score for Perceived value of IT scale is 11,75 with a standard deviation of 3,4 which indicates that faculty have high level agreement on value of IT use in medical education. The mean and standard deviation of each item in Perceived Value of IT Scale is presented in Table 1.

Table 1. Means and Standard Deviations of Perceived Value of IT Subscale

Items	Mean	SD
Technology enables me to address different learning styles of students	1,57	0,61
ch as e-mail, enhance my contact with students	1,56	0,69
I think that technology enables learning more effective	1,40	0,58
Technology using increase motivation of students	1,59	0,71
Technology enables me update instructional materials easily	1,29	0,47
Using technology enables me to use my lecture time efficiently.	1,55	0,65
Using technology increase quality of my teaching	1,53	0,59
Using technology increase my productivity as an instructor	1,55	0,65
Technology enables me to reach instructional resources.	1,27	0,47

Perceived Barriers and Incentives to Adoption

In explaining faculty limited adoption of instructional technology, Jacobsen state that "explanation for limited adoption may be found in the many barrier that still constrain use by enthusiastic beginners" [12, p.2].

For the purpose of gathering data about perceived barriers to technology adoption, medical faculty were asked to rate their level of agreement on 20 statements about barriers to adoption. Six factors which were identified as a major barrier to adoption of instructional technology by over 50% of the faculty are 1) lack of computers for students , 2) lack of support service for students, 3) lack of reward structure, 4) lack of computers for faculty, 5) lack of peripherals for faculty and 6) lack of training opportunities (Table 2).

Table 2. Faculty Agreement on Items about Barriers to Adoption.

(SA=Strongly Agree, A=Agree, N=Neutral, D= Disagree, SD=Strongly Disagree)

Items	SA+A (%)	N (%)	SD+D (%)
There is too few computers for students.	68,0	22,0	10,0
There is not enough support for supervising student computer use.	68,5	22,8	8,8
There is no reward structure that recognizes faculty for using technology in teaching and learning.	67,1	19,5	13,4
There is lack of printers and/or other peripherals to effectively use computers for teaching and learning.	61,9	9,0	29,1
There are too few computers for individual faculty.	56,2	9,8	34,0
There are lack of / not enough training opportunities for faculty members to acquire new computer knowledge and skills.	50,6	18,2	31,2

Incentives to Adoption

According to Anderson, Varnhagen & Campbell, "Related to barriers are incentives that help faculty overcome barriers"[10]. In order to explore incentives that motivate faculty for technology use, faculty were asked to rate importance level of 5 statements about incentives for adoption.Items related to investment in infrastructure, training and support, policy and plans of university, and financial support for material development were rated important incentives by over 96% of the faculty. It is interesting to note that only 31,6% of the faculty agreed on that lack of time is a barrier, 71,6% of the faculty rated the item related to providing development time by reducing teaching load as an important incentive. As consistent with agreement on that reward structure is a barrier, 68,4 % of the faculty rated the reward structure recognizing the technology use as an important incentive.

4. Discussion

The findings of this study indicated that even though majority of the medical faculty percieved instuctional technology valuable for teaching and learning, adoption of instructional technology failed to cross mainsteam faculty. Findings provides evidence for widespread adoption of communication and research tools into late majority, and adoption of relatively new tools associated with instruction into early majority.

As stated by Surry, diffusion and adoption can not be base solely on the worth or quality of the innovation rather should be based on the culture, the needs and the demands of the faculty [13]. The medical school faculty in this investigation identified inadequate harware for students and faculty, lack of reward structure, insufficient traing oppurtunites as major barriers to their technology adoption. Related to the barriers, investment in infrastructure, training and support, policy and plans of university, financial support for material development, reward structure are identified as important factors for a motivating environment in their technology adoption.

5. Conclusions

Medical institutions today confronted with instructional technology innovation, which is transforming the way in which faculty and students interact and the roles they take. If the goal of a medical education institution is the integration of technology for a transformative change, then rather on technology itself, there must be a clear focus on the faculty who use technology. It is essential for administrators, policy makers and anyone interested in an effective teaching and learning in medical education to understand adoption patterns of faculty and how these patterns influence the adoption and diffusion of instructional technology in medical education institution.

6. References

[1]   ACME-TRI Report. Educating medical students:assessing change in medical eduction-the road to implementation .*Academic Medicine*.1993;68(6 Suppl.).
[2]   Association of American Medical Colleges. Report II: Medical school objectives project. Washington, DC, June 1998.
[3]   Lichty, M.. *The innovation-decision process and factors that influence computer implementation by medical school faculty*.[Dissertation]. Instructional Technology. Wayne State University; 2000.
[4]   Moberg TF, Whitcomb ME. Educational technology to facilitate medical students' learning: background paper 2 of the medical school objectives project. *Acad Medicine* 1999 Oct;74(10):1146-50.
[5]   Surry, D.W., Land, S. M. Strategies for motivating higher education faculty to use technology. *Innovations in Education and Training International* 2000; 37(2): 145-153.
[6]   Green, K. C.. The 1999 National Survey of Information Technology in Higher Education. c1998-1999 - [cited 2004 March 20]. Available from: http://www.campuscomputing.net/summaries/1999.
[7]   Spotts, T.H. Discriminating factors in faculy use of instructional technology in higher education. *EducationalTechnology and Society* 1999;2(4).
[8]   Holloway, R.E. Diffusion and Adoption of Educational Technology: A Crituque of Reseach Design. In David H. *Handbook of Reseach For Educational Communications and Technology*, New York: Simon& Schuster Macmillan;1996.
[9]   Rogers, E. M. *Diffusion of innovations* . (4th ed.). New York: Free Press;1995.
[10] Anderson, T., Varnhagen, S., Campbell, K.(1998). Faculty adoption of teaching and learning technologies:contrasting earlier adopters and mainstream faculty.*The Canadian Journal of Higher Education*. 1998; 28(2-3): 71-98.
[11] Jacobsen,D.M.. *Adoption patterns and characteristics of faculty who integrate computer technology for teaching and learning in higher education*.[Dissertation].Educational Psychology. University of Calgary;1998.
[12] Jacobsen, D. M. Examining technology adoption patterns by faculty in higher education. *Proceedings of ACEC2000: Learning Technologies, Teaching and the Future of Schools;* 2000 July 6 - 9, Melbourne, Australia.
[13] Surry, D.W. Diffusion theory and instructional technology. The *Annual Conference of the Association for educational Communications and Technology* (AECT); 1997 February 12-15; Albuquerque, New Mexico.

Contact Information

Dr.Neşe Zayim, Akdeniz Universitesi, Tıp Fakültesi, Biyoistatistik AD., Kampüs Antalya 07059 Turkey, E-mail: nzayim@akdeniz.edu.tr

Connecting Medical Informatics and Bio-Informatics
R. Engelbrecht et al. (Eds.)
IOS Press, 2005

Postgraduate Studies in Health Informatics in Greece

John Mantas

Laboratory of Health Informatics, Faculty of Nursing, University of Athens, Greece

Abstract

Health informatics is a well established and important multi-disciplinary and inter-disciplinary field that not only involves informatics but also medicine, nursing, engineering, biology and other-related subjects. A co-ordination of this field at a postgraduate level has become an important issue now in Europe where other European Community programs such as the Telematics for Health Care will require during the Fifth and Sixth Framework Programmes (2000-2006) adequate human resources of higher potential and knowledge. A European M.Sc. course met all the above objectives. The curriculum was developed according to previous experiences in similar programmes. Recently the course has been organised on the basis of an Inter-University nature with the participation of 5 Greek Universities. The paper aims at providing a current description of the academic programme and a brief evaluation of the implementation phase.

Keywords:
Health informatics; Inter-University academic Programmes, health telematics education

1. Aim and Objectives of the Course

The aim of the course is to give those working or intending to work in the health service and related activities, a broad advanced postgraduate education in health informatics [1] in order to develop the ability to understand and evaluate in detail the theoretical and practical requirements of informatics in medicine, nursing and health care and to solve information related problems arising from the dramatic advancement of technology as it is being applied in health care across the European Union member states.

The course [2] is relevant to those holding a degree in one of clinical sciences, life sciences or physical sciences like: medicine, nursing, dentistry, pharmacology, physiology, pathology, biochemistry, biology, biophysics, pharmacy, sociology of health, engineering, computer science, mathematics, microbiology, clinical chemistry and health economics, as long as they are all University graduates.

The graduate acquires:

- A good theoretical background in relevant aspects of basic scientific and health disciplines which interact with the application of information science and technology to the acquisition, processing, interpretation, storage and communication of health data, in both health education and research and in patient care.

- •A thorough training in the scientific method so that a problem may be assessed, experimental studies designed, available systems evaluated and a scientific or technical report prepared.
- An ability to understand the scientific basis of clinical and engineering problems encountered in medical, nursing and health care fields and a better understanding of the use of computers and knowledge-based computing methods.
- An ability to investigate advanced problems and to undertake research in health informatics.

2. Entry Requirements

Entrance to the course can be gained by those university graduates holding degrees in medicine, nursing and other health-care related professions, as well as in engineering and computer science who wish to work in the health service area. Graduates of any medical, nursing or health-related discipline, engineering, computer science or natural science may apply. Relevant experience in the health sciences will be taken into account for non-health related educational background. Applicants should demonstrate excellent command and knowledge both oral and written of the English language.

The following Greek Universities actively participate in the course by sending distinguished professors as well as enrolling students to the course: National and Kapodistrian University of Athens (Department, of Informatics, Department of Economics, Faculty of Nursing), Aristoteleion University of Thessaloniki (General Department of the Engineering School), University of Ioannina (Department of Medicine), Economics and Business University of Athens (Department of Informatics), University of Piraeus (Department of Production Technology, Department of Informatics). In addition, visiting scientists and visiting professors were invited to teach in the course. Until today professors came from the following institutions: University of Leuven, University of Madrid, University of Patras, National Technical University of Athens, King's College and London School of Economics of the University of London, City University, University of Manchester, University of Maastricht, and the University of Amsterdam.

3. Course Pattern

The course is available for full-time students and will subsequently lead to the award of the M.Sc. in health informatics. Full-time students will attend for one full calendar year. Lectures and laboratory exercises will be held from Mondays to Fridays at the School of Health Sciences Campus of the University of Athens as well as for certain modules in the cooperating Universities.

The course comprises a total of 370 formal contact hours (lectures and laboratory exercises). Lectures and laboratory exercises start on the first week of October and finish at end of May. The successful students need a further term (summer term) to complete the research project and submit the dissertation.

In case the student wishes to take the course in part-time he/she will need a two-year period. Appropriate management of the course programme will be required to select the modules need to be able to graduate in the two-years period.

4. Lecture Course

The academic programme is modular and comprises of 370 of formal lectures given by distinguished professors and lecturers of the participating universities [2], [3]. The course is organised in 10 compulsory modules and in 7 optional modules (from which 5 should be selected). The lecture material is distributed to all students before the start of each module. A total of 3000 pages of courseware and didactic material has been already prepared and is ready for distribution to the students. The students are encouraged to seek for bibliography and textbooks in the Universities Libraries. The content of the course is organised in such a way in order to give to the students, competence in making decisions in solving healthcare problems related to informatics. To fulfill this the students must acquire an amount of knowledge, skills and attitudes. Therefore, an important principle of the course is to develop the ability for life-long independent learning and understand the principles of health informatics as they are applied to the informatics field. Such competence means that the student shall be able to:

- Identify his/her learning needs.
- Evaluate critically different sources of information.
- Evaluate his/her learning in relation to the needs.

The educational methods used in the M.Sc. course have been chosen to train the students in the skills listed above. The learning is directed by objectives. The students have the main responsibility for reaching the competence set and have great freedom to choose between various learning resources offered in the laboratory of health informatics at the University of Athens as well as to the other laboratories of the participating Universities. Teaching staff will stimulate and guide such an active learning in various ways. The studies are problem-based to a large extent. Computer-based cases are used to focus on problems raised in the different modules. The structure of the modules is the following:

A. Obligatory modules:

- Introduction to health informatics.
- Introduction to health sciences.
- Health research methods.
- Hospital Information Systems.
- Management and Administration of Health care systems.
- Database Management Systems.
- Security of healthcare systems
- Methods in developing information systems
- Networks
- Electronic Patient Record Systems

B. Optional modules

- Knowledge-based systems
- Telemedicine.
- Language engineering in healthcare
- Object-oriented programming – Java
- Signal processing and medical imaging
- Managing health technology - Biomedical engineering.

- Electronic data interchange (EDI)
- Knowledge Management

5. Laboratory Exercises

Strong emphasis has been given to the provision of proper technological infrastructure in the students facilities and laboratories. The health informatics laboratory of the University of Athens comprises of 40 computer systems connected in a Local Area Network. All students can work under Windows and/or Unix environment. Related health informatics applications and computer-assisted learning software is available to the students. International computer networks (Internet) can be reached through the high-speed link to the main computer network of the University of Athens, which in turn is connected to the main highway of the Greek Universities Network (GUNET). The multimedia laboratory adjacent to the health informatics laboratory offers a CD-ROM based library access to rich resources of reference information and didactic material. The newest strategy used in the M.Sc. course includes the use of the local Intranet to support the student in his/her preparation of reports and essays. Most of the modules require the preparation of small projects/essays. The student is offered also with all Internet facilities (access to international sites, libraries, e-mail accounts, etc.). Printing facilities are also available through laser printers (both colour and monochrome). The laboratory facilities of the other departments and universities are also available to students when needed.

6. Research Project

All students will undertake a research project as part of the M.Sc. course. The aim of the project is to provide the student with an opportunity to undertake research work applying appropriate concepts, methods and techniques of health informatics to a particular problem. The research work can be carried out at each of the participating Universities. The process would be that the student selects a research topic from those available within the programme and under the supervision of one of the Professors works on the subject, prepares, finalises and submits the dissertation to the examinations committee.

7. Examinations

Each module is examined by a 2-hour examination paper. The examinations are held in February and June of each academic year. All examination papers are considered of equal importance. In case of failure the student can take a re-sit examination in September. If he/she fails in more than 4 examinations in the February and June examinations then the student is dropped from the course.

In the end the M.Sc. degree is awarded to students who meet the following requirements:

- Obtain a minimum of 50% in each of the examination papers.
- Obtain a minimum of 50% in the dissertation during the oral defence in from of a committee of three examiners.

8. Course Evaluation

During the 12 years of running the course under the previous structure [2], the number of enrolled students amounted to 200. Students came from different European countries, such as Greece, UK, the Netherlands, Spain, Belgium, Ireland, Finland, Sweden, even from Romania and Republic of China. The students showed an active interest in supporting the various learning experiences offered by the course and were actively involved in several social and cultural events in Greece provided by the co-ordinating University. Despite the usual problems, which arise in such courses (i.e. different educational backgrounds mixed in, different cultural behaviours and customs) a spirit of active cooperation, focused determination and groupware effort prevailed in the end.

During the recent year of running the course under the structure presented above the students enrolled were 20. Since the course is full-time few working students (4) found difficult to participate with full attendance, therefore, they had to leave the course. An additional problem encountered was the number of reports/essays given to the students as assignments increasing the burden to the students. However, even if the full academic year is not finished, it should be reported that the students were very much satisfied with the course and expressed their gratitude to the high level of teaching and facilities encountered in all participating universities they had to attend lectures.

Only for the academic years in which the course operates as an InterUniversity – Co-operational Postgraduate program, 80 students in total have been accepted, and 50 of them have been graduated. Most of the remaining 30 have not completed yet their lecture courses (have been accepted in the present academic year) or they are undertaking their project's dissertation (have been accepted in the previous academic year).

8.1 Evaluation by Students

The lecturers of each of the modules are encouraged to seek feedback from the students as an evaluation of the modules, both in terms of content and delivery. This has been achieved by a questionnaire and by direct feedback from the students to the members of staff. Student evaluation is taking place both during the course and after its completion per year. The evaluation was a major way of receiving feedback by the students, improving, thereafter, the course contents and delivery.

8.2. Evaluation by Staff

Members of staff provide course evaluation both by written comments and by discussion with members of the Steering Committee. The Steering Committee consists of one representative from each of the participating Universities. The Co-ordinating University of Athens is chairing the Steering Committee.

9. Conclusion

The M.Sc. course aiming to fulfill the above objectives will continue to operate in the following years. The course has been supported financially till recently with funds from the Greek Ministry of Education interlinked with the new EU initiatives of the structural funds and the SOCRATES/ERASMUS programmes. During the two recent academic years fees have been introduced to keep the momentum of the course as the initial financing by the ministry has ended. We have not observed any reduction of the number of applicants to the course due to the introduction of fees. Regarding the jobs that the graduates can find, we have noticed recently a large need in the medical software houses and in the hospital EDP centers. The numbers are now accumulated and results can be announced soon.

The course overall in the forthcoming years has to adapt to the changes introduced by technology advancement and globalisation [4]. The course organisers are willing to undertake this challenge.

10. References

[1] Hasman, A. (1997). State of the art report on Education and Telematics in the health care sector. In: J. Mantas (Ed.) Health Telematics Education (pp. 3-6). Amsterdam, IOS Press.

[2] Diomidus, M., Mantas, J. (1997). Erasmus master of science in health informatics. In: J. Mantas (Ed.), Health Telematics Education (pp. 33-37), Amsterdam, IOS Press.

[3] Mantas, J. (1998). NIGHTINGALE – A new perspective in nursing informatics education in Europe. In: J. Mantas (Ed.), Advances in Health Telematics Education – A NIGHTINGALE perspective (pp. 102-113). Amsterdam, IOS Press.

[4] Hovenga EJS and Mantas J. (Eds), Global Health Informatics Education, IOS Press, Amsterdam, 2004.

Address for correspondence

Laboratory of Health Informatics,
Faculty of Nursing,
University of Athens,
123 Papadiamantopoulou Street, Goudi,
GR-11527 Athens, Greece
Tel: +30 210 746 1460
E-mail: jmantas@cc.uoa.gr

Connecting Medical Informatics and Bio-Informatics
R. Engelbrecht et al. (Eds.)
IOS Press, 2005

267

Distance Learning at Biomedical Faculties in Bosnia & Herzegovina

Zlatan Masic[a], Ahmed Novo[a], Izet Masic[b], Mensura Kudumovic[b], Selim Toromanovic[c], Admir Rama[b], Almir Dzananovic[b], Ilda Bander[b], Mirza Basic[b], Emir Guso[b], Eldar Balta[b]

[a]*Technical University Vienna, Austria*
[b]*Cathedra for Medical Informatics, Medical Faculty, University of Sarajevo, Bosnia and Herzegovina*
[c]*Health centre Cazin, Bosnia and Herzegovina*

Abstract

Increase and development of distance learning technologies over the past decade has exposed the potential and the efficiency of new technologies. Benefit and use of contemporary information technologies is the area where medical informatics got the most on understanding and importance. Definition of distance learning as "use of technologies based on health care delivered on distance" covers areas such as electronic health, tele-health (e-health), telematics, telemedicine, tele-education, etc. For the need of e-health, telemedicine, tele-education and distance learning there are various technologies and communication systems from standard telephone lines to the system of transmission digitalized signals with modem, optical fiber, satellite links, wireless technologies, etc. Tele-education represents health education on distance, using Information Communication Technologies(ICT), as well as continuous education of a health system beneficiaries and use of electronic libraries, data bases or electronic data with data bases of knowledge. In this paper authors described activities on introduction of distance learning in teaching process at Medical faculty, University of Sarajevo, Bosnia and Herzegovina. Internet was not really meant to be a means of human communication at first; but the clearly the Net become a main piece of human communication.

Keywords:
Distance learning; Tele-education, Telemedicine, E-health,

1. Introduction

Distance learning is conventionally defined as: any educational or learning process or system in which the teacher and instructor are separated geographically or in time from his or her students; or in which students are separated from other students or educational resources (1,2,3). The most important factor which influences the changes occurring in education has been the installation and development of the Internet and electronic multimedia techniques. Contemporary tele-education or distance learning is affected through the implementation of computer and electronics technology to connect teacher and student in either real or delayed time or on an as-needed basis. Content delivery may be achieved through a variety of technologies, including satellites, computers, cable television, interactive video, electronic transmissions via telephone lines, and others. Distance learning does not preclude traditional learning processes; frequently it is used in conjunction with in-person classroom or professional training procedures and practices.

Distance learning is used for self-education, tests, services and for the examinations in medicine, i.e. in terms of self-education and individual examination services .the possibility to work in the exercise mode will image files and questions is an attractive way for self-education (4,5,6,7). The standard format of the notation files enables to elaborate the results by commercial statistic packets in order to estimate the scale of answers and to find correlation between the obtained results. The method of multi-criterion grading excludes unlimited mutual compensation of the criteria, differentiates the importance of particular courses and introduces the quality criteria. By using computers and teleconferencing technology and through partnerships with local communities, institutions and the private sector, an open, effective, virtual learning community is now in place. Sites are located in college and university campuses, hospitals, schools, libraries, community centers and private companies. Courses are also being delivered to private homes.

For the need of e-health, telemedicine, and tele-education there are various technologies and communication systems from standard telephone lines to the system of transmission digitalized signals with modem, optical fiber, satellite links, wireless technologies, etc. There is no doubt that Internet causes "revolution" in all above, and the latest its possibilities are distribution of virtual medical instruments and medical data in real time and possibility of use in primary health care, even for some diseases with bed prognosis. This revolution how information is stored, transmitted and accessed has extremely important implication for the health sector, especially now when embarking on a global effort to renew the tenets of Health for All based on primary health care and disease prevention, health promotion and costumer education, in the context of service delivery guided by the equity, quality, effectiveness and efficiency (7). According to Grimson at al in Dublin, "the need to participate in continuing professional development or continuing medical education is considered to be at the very least highly desirable and more likely mandatory. The use of Information Communication Technologies (ICT) is one way by which this can be facilitated in a timely and cost-effective manner" (8).

2. Distance Learning

2.1. Traditional way of learning and learning from the distance

The latest researches shows that the format of instructions itself has no important influence on the students' achievements if access and availability to information technologies is assured as well as usage of the adequate content of education. In the assessment of the authentic situation the following issues should be addressed:

- Results of different tests prepared by lectors has trend to show advantages in comparison with traditional learning methods and there is significant distinction in affirmative attitude to educational materials between distance and traditional learning
- Traditional methods demonstrate better organization and they are clearer in respect to distance learning
- Organization and needs for more efficient influence of distance learning very often improve traditional methods by teachers
- Future research should be focus on critical factors in determining student involvement in development of educational process.
- The variety of teaching and learning options provided by technology allows education to be provided in an appropriate manner to a broader student demographic then ever before.

2.2. e-Health

Although new technologies are widely used by European healthcare professionals and consumers, information about the value of distance learning and e-Health in improving quality of core is little. For some people, the term "e-Health" still conjures up a reference to the self medicine. But e-Health as a field is much broader and describes the application of information and communication technology across the whole range of functions that effect health. It is all about delivering healthcare tailored to the need of citizen. E-Health refuses to the use of modern information and communication technologies to meet needs of citizens, patients, healthcare professionals, healthcare providers, as well as policy makers (9).

2.3. Facts about distance learning and tele-education

Distance learning enables permanent learning (lifelong learning), students can improve themselves professionally and independently, at their own tempo, at place and time that they choose by themselves, they can choose great deal of subjects which offer different institutions, teachers-individuals; students go through materials for learning by speed of their own and as many times as they want. The place can be chosen – it depends on media which is used for learning material (they can learn at work or from home). Themes access which are not offered by studies in that field – students find and attend the programs which they are interested in, although they are not offered by educational or business institutions in place where they live in or work. Taking part in top-quality and most prestigious programs – student can "attend" at least some studies at the top-quality institutions or studies held by lecturers that are very famous experts without changing their place of living. Choosing this way of learning – active or passive learning, different kinds of interaction: "Classical" written material and writing down their own lecture notes, interactive simulations, discussion with other students (e-mail, tele-conferences).

Practical work with different technologies – they get not just information about that they learn, but additional knowledge and skills about using computer, CD players, video recorders. Independent learning – teachers learn too from students who independently ask for information source.

The meaning of education (learning) to distance can be expressed by the definition: That is a form of education which is in process permanently, or most of the time, all or most of the tasks of teaching and learning separately during the time and space between teacher and student.

Pedagogical and organizational improvements have fundamental importance. It is in use both interaction teacher – student and interaction student – student. Phases of synchronized and synchronized learning are combined. Individual and group works are also combined. If all these forms are involved in educational process, they mutually supplement each other, as a last resort. Traditional education as well as contemporary education is supported by informatics technologies in unique system of flexible education. In order to use advantages of flexible education, it is necessary to combine different forms of learning, during the preparation phase and development of every educational course in appropriate way.

Fundamental advantages of flexible education in terms of classical education are:

- More efficiency
- Increase capacities of educational institutions
- Education can be easily adopted to the needs of education on-the-job
- Costs of educational process are smaller

- It is possible to distribute the education uniformly, thus the new educational programmes are available for fields outside of educational and economic centers
- It enables the possibility of access to the foreign educational resources to the various institutions
- Superior quality of the knowledge gained.

Distance learning is not simply a set infrastructure, but rather a concept of learning that incorporates different technologies and learning media. Within the province, different video, audio and computer teleconferencing systems, along with Computer Based Training, Computer Managed Instructional systems and other media are being integrated technologically, instructionally and organizationally. The Tele-education concept crosses all jurisdictions among institutions both within and outside the province, public and private, at any level of education, to anywhere including institutions, workplaces and the home. Tele-education, Tele-teaching, Tele-training, Tele-mentoring, and Tele-accreditation have been clearly demonstrated and are now common practice.

2.4. Distance learning in medical curriculum and implementation of distance learning at Medical Faculty, University of Sarajevo, Bosnia and Herzegovina

The Internet is case of point. What in 1970s began as a small, restricted network, linking three Unites States universities growth into gigantic, worldwide "network of the networks". By late 1994, the Internet encompassed same 3.2 million computer nodes spread across more than 57,000 institutions in more then 80 countries, with an estimated 30 million users. By the end of the century the Internet linked more then 400 million persons.

The 2002 Eurobarometer survey showed that an average of 78% of EU medical GPs were online, with at the highest level – 98% in Sweden and 97% in United Kingdom. Number of "online patients" growing every day as well. The 2003 Eurobarometer survey on health information sources shows that 23% of Europeans use Internet for health information and that 41% of the European population considers that Internet is a good source of information on health (8).

In October 2003, University of Sarajevo began with Distance learning education, opening University Distance Learning Centre. Opening the University Distance Learning Centre, as coordination body and leader in all activities in connection to Distance learning, has provided opportunity for development and growth of this kind of lifelong education.

In correlation with above project conducted by the University Tele-information Centre (UTIC) and as continuation of two-year project Possibilities of introduction of Distance learning in Medical curriculum, the Cantonal Ministry approved and supported a new project; Introduction and implementation of Distance learning in medicine.

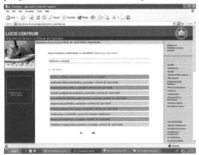

Figure 1-Uploaded materials for subject Medical Informatics

On UTIC web site, seven students enrolled from Medical faculty, for the subject Medical Informatics are able to learn from the distance location. So far, teaching staff uploaded eleven lectures at the web site: Hardware and software, Medical documentations, Medical informatics, Methods of data manipulation, Nomenclatures and classification systems, Data organization, Data, information and knowledge, Lectures 1, System and communication, Structure and data organization and Expert systems. Beside the materials it is possible to upload and download the following: Practical works, Seminar work, Information, Recommended links, Plan and programs, Quiz, Schedule, Recommended readings, Examination schedule and Examination results.

Basically software application has two interfaces: teacher and student interface. Access from any of these is very simple and fast.

3. Age of Information

The rise of IT as an artefact of everyday life in the modern world has brought with it the dawn of a new era, often dubbed the "Age of Information". These technologies are changing the way we perceive the world, how wee think and communicate with another. Established cultures are being transformed and new cultures are forming. New virtual environment affects the way we build our sense of who we are.

Some characteristics of the Internet:

- Large volume of users and potential users,
- Lack of physical boundaries which allows for the manipulation of time and space,
- Information can be accessed in a concurrent fashion using different media,
- Concept of redundancy.

In the virtual environment we are applying for information in a way that is expanding our senses and one must to take into account that experience is occurring in the context of the virtual environment. Information without a context has no meaning.

Expected outcomes of the project Introduction and Implementation of Distance learning in medicine are:

- Development and integration of informatics-computer technologies in medical education
- Creation of flexible infrastructure which will enable access to e-Learning by all students and teaching staff
- Improvement of digital literacy of academic population
- Ensure high educational standards to students and teaching staff and
- To help medical staff to develop "Lifelong learning way of life".

The health sector is one of the most evident potential beneficiaries of the Internet revolution and World Wide Web resource in the present and in the future, when the tools now available and the system's reliability and efficacy as a whole will be further incremented and improved.

Distance learning in medicine has impact on telemedicine and practicing medicine as well. Basic skills of the use of computers and networks must be a part of all future medical curricula. The impact of technical equipment between patient and the doctor must be understood, and the situation where the diagnosis based on live voice or picture is different from a normal doctor-patient contact (10). In some areas telemedicine requires unique techniques. Tele-robotical guaranties differ from what surgeons normally learn. Telemedicine, and distance learning as a prerequisite for it, is lest suited for doctor-to-doctor consultation, and the first contact to a doctor should always be a face-to-face consultation.

4. References

[1]   Engelbrecht R, Ingenerf J, Reiner J. Educational standards - terminologies used. *Stud Health Technol Inform.* 2004;109:95-113.

[2]   Masic I, Ramic-Catak A, Kudumovic M, Pasic E. Distance learning in the medical education in B&H: *E-Health & Education Proceedings*, Zagreb, 2002: 17

[3]   Masic I, Bilalovic N, Karcic S, Kudumovic M, Pasic E. Telemedicine and telemetric in B&H in the war and Post war Times. *European Journal of Medical Research*, 2002; 7(supl.1): 47.

[4]   Hovenga J. Bricknell L. Current and Future Trends in Teaching and Learning. *Stud Health Technol Inform.* 2004;109:131-142.

[5]   Mantas J. Future Trends in Health Informatics – Theoretical and practical. *Stud Health Technol Inform.* 2004;109:114-127.

[6]   Mantas J. Comparative educational systems. *Stud Health Technol Inform.* 2004;109:8-17.

[7]   Sosa-Iudicissa M, Oliveri N, Gamboa CA, Roberts J. Internet, Telematics and Health. IOS Press, 1997; 36: 1-530

[8]   Silber D. The case for eHealth. *E-Health,* IOS Press 2004; 3-27

[9]   Ministerial declaration. *eHealth 2003 conference*. Brussels, 22 May 2003.

[10] Aarimaa M. Telemedicine, *Contribution of ICT to Health*. IOS Press 2004, 111-6

Connecting Medical Informatics and Bio-Informatics
R. Engelbrecht et al. (Eds.)
IOS Press, 2005

Combining Advanced Networked Technology and Pedagogical Methods to Improve Collaborative Distance Learning

Pascal Staccini[a], **Jean-Charles Dufour**[b], **Hervé Raps**[a], **Marius Fieschi**[b]

[a]*Département STIC Santé, UFR Médecine, Université Nice-Sophia Antipolis, France*
[b]*LERTIM, UFR Médecine, Université de la Méditerrannée, France*

Abstract

Making educational material be available on a network cannot be reduced to merely implementing hypermedia and interactive resources on a server. A pedagogical schema has to be defined to guide students for learning and to provide teachers with guidelines to prepare valuable and upgradeable resources. Components of a learning environment, as well as interactions between students and other roles such as author, tutor and manager, can be deduced from cognitive foundations of learning, such as the constructivist approach. Scripting the way a student will to navigate among information nodes and interact with tools to build his/her own knowledge can be a good way of deducing the features of the graphic interface related to the management of the objects. We defined a typology of pedagogical resources, their data model and their logic of use. We implemented a generic and web-based authoring and publishing platform (called J@LON for Join And Learn On the Net) within an object-oriented and open-source programming environment (called Zope) embedding a content management system (called Plone). Workflow features have been used to mark the progress of students and to trace the life cycle of resources shared by the teaching staff. The platform integrated advanced on line authoring features to create interactive exercises and support live courses diffusion. The platform engine has been generalized to the whole curriculum of medical studies in our faculty; it also supports an international master of risk management in health care and will be extent to all other continuous training diploma.

Keywords:
Learning; Education, Distance; Models, Educational; Computer systems; Internet; Health Education

1. Introduction

Distance learning has become a topic of intense interest. Since 2000, the French Ministry of Higher Education and Research has issued numerous calls for projects in order to encourage universities and teachers to publish French academic resources on the web. Among the projects that have been granted, three categories can be identified [1]: production of high quality hypermedia resources, implementation of web services to distribute pedagogical resources, and distance learning applied research projects. The Information Technology Department of the School of Medicine of Nice submitted a project called "ESSQU@D" (Enseignement Santé, Sécurité et Qualité à Distance). It also joined the French Virtual Medical University team project (UMVF), in connection with the Medical Information Research Laboratory of the School of Medicine of Marseille. The purpose of "ESSQU@D" was to offer a master degree in the area of quality improvement and risk management in health care services. The aim of our involvement into the French virtual medical university was to develop a remote control prototype for live course acquisition and publishing through the Internet. In order to combine these objectives and integrate a web-based authoring tool to support the creation of pedagogical material, we concentrated on pedagogical methods, and problems that may occur, when using distance learning technologies [2,3,4]. Some issues were highlighted: How can one assist teachers to create modular and reusable training schemes? How can one motivate students to use on line resources to learn? How can one guarantee them the effectiveness of distance training as compared to the traditional teaching process, and what could be the importance of a collaborative approach to support web mediation? On the basis of this analysis, the project consisted of: 1) integrating constructivist principles and teaching engineering in order to provide users with efficient collaborative tools; 2) analysing and offering a tutoring model; 3) analysing and implementing techniques for the acquisition and publishing of course contents, while using open source standards. The aims of this paper are: 1) to detail and discuss the lesson data model we deduced from the study of educational methods and 2) to analyse the way we implemented this model in a web-based collaborative and object-oriented programming environment (platform J@LON : Join And Learn On the Net).

2. Materials and Methods

Building a course requires teachers to adapt to the specificities of a heterogeneous audience. Teachers ask questions, invite students to contribute, and provide them with handouts. They encourage students to work together, or have them perform self-assessment. It can be argued that any live lesson is based on a scenario that teacher adapts according to the audience. As regards student learning processes, teachers do not convey knowledge. Rather, they deliver, in a pedagogically relevant way, sets of information, through situations and activities with which students will build up their own knowledge according to their own mode of training [5]. Students organize their paths of learning according to their own mind-frame. The individual student is the centre of the learning process. The ways information is organized and the sample situations submitted to him/her are key elements. An effective training situation must be organized in the context of the target environments, namely, those in which student will later have problems to solve [6,7]. The design of a lesson must observe some key principles [8,9]: 1) the understanding of a concept requires the gathering and organization of information; 2) cognitive skills require the resolution of problem and critical appraisal; 3) psychomotor skills require real practice and experience; 4) changes of attitude require role games. Thus, the teaching scenario will endeavour to combine the trainings to be acquired with activities, at least those available on Internet [10]: 1) the reading of and active listening to multimedia documents, more or less enriched with hypertext links for explanatory matter or for further inquiry; 2) interactive analysis of iconographic items; 3) creative activities involving the writing of notes, solving exercises, answering a set of questions; 4) experimental trial and error activities; 5) simulation and, 6) self-evaluation or tutor-based evaluation. As regards the scenarisation of contents, the model must achieve a compromise between the use of the main teaching modes and functional screen ergonomics. We defined a minimum model to answer the main teaching modalities (deductive, inductive, procedural and meta-cognitive modes of learning). We analysed the part of collaborative features for each teaching modalities and defined the ways students and teachers could view their use of the platform and their progress.

3. Results

Based on the analysis of pedagogical requirements needed to provide students with a structured and consistent method to access digital resources, we defined the object model of the components the environment (figure 1) [11]. The main object class is a lesson offering a synthesis of six components: objective, sequence, download, "know more", a glossary and a quiz. A lesson forms part of a learning unit. A curriculum is hierarchically composed of specific lessons and learning units. The sequence component can display the content of a local stored file or the content of a remote resource (URL). Sequences can be arranged in order to guide the student's progression. The glossary and the quiz components comprise a set of terms or questions.

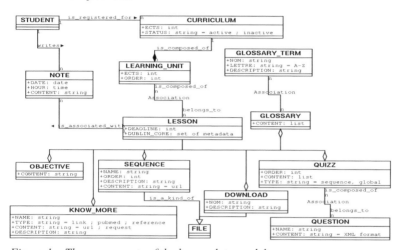

Figure 1 – The components of the lesson data model

We identified the roles and their associated work spaces (figure 2). A private directory is available for each user and sharable spaces can be browsed such as: news, diary, history of updates, glossary, and comments per lesson. Discussion tools have been designed to allow global or specific exchanges between users.

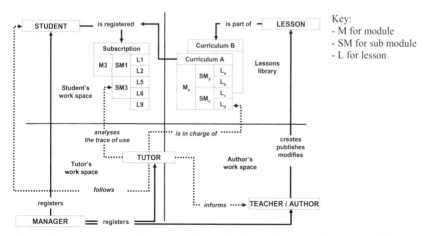

Figure 2 – Interrelations between roles and objects: the central position of the tutor

We wanted students to be guided to "read" lesson content, but they may choose other paths, for example, direct access to the global self-assessment part of the lesson. However, within a lesson, one node is systematically displayed before any action, the "home page" of a lesson with a reminder of the learning objectives defined by the teacher. This navigation logic is closely related to the level of granularity a teacher wants to give to a lesson. Each sequence follows a structure with a set of explanatory pages ending with a summary page and a short self-assessment quiz. Cases can also form part of a lesson and are considered as specific sequences. These are built in order to introduce the subject of the lesson to the student using a short practical example to illustrate to him/her why the subject has been selected.

The method of implementation of the platform consisted of three steps: 1) the programming of the lesson components and its workflow characteristics (published, retracted, read); 2) the programming of the databases to store the description and the composition of curricula, and the tracking students' data; 3) the customisation of the learning space according to the roles. An object-oriented Content Management System (CMS) has been chosen which combines the Zope platform [12] and a workflow generic product named Plone [13], full Dublin core compliant [14] and providing RSS feeds. The architecture of the system is composed of four parts: 1) a library of components (lessons, questions, cases, glossary terms) stored in the Zope object-oriented database; 2) relational tables to store the hierarchy of curricula and students' data (PostgreSQL database management system); 3) a user interface layer to access the data/objects management functions; 4) a portal customisation layer which is based on the Plone product. A specific tool has been included to allow the creation of interactive questions (simple/multiple choice questions, questions using clicking or 'drag and drop' areas); questions can also be imported into the platform using an XML grammar [11,15]. External libraries are available, for example, a video library containing movies of the original courses (Real format) and "rich media" courses (Smile standard).

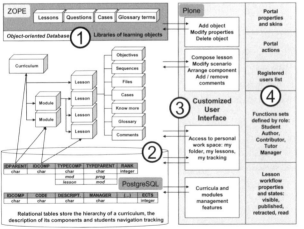

Figure 3 – Technical architecture of the platform

A specific workflow has been implemented to trace the different states of a lesson. A lesson is created by the author in his/her private space. When it is published, the lesson object is physically moved to a public space. When reading a lesson, students can add a short comment and indicate for themselves that they have completed it (workflow state attribute). This information is stored in the student's tracking table. Viewing features of this table have been implemented in order to provide students with individual feedback. When needed, an author can retract a lesson from the published lessons folder, modify it and publish it again.

For each lesson, the whole history of the publishing process can be read. Students access the lessons they are registered for by choosing one in a hierarchical list. Authors access the lessons they have created by choosing in a list that distinguishes between published lessons, "in process" lessons and co-authoring ones. Students and authors can read global and role-related news. Each author can complete and publish a "personal home page" that students can access when reading their lesson or browsing other libraries of pedagogical resources. Dialog between users is available by means of a forum and a private chat channel.

5. Discussion

While normative approaches and standards are emerging to structure pedagogical resources [15], we only used the Dublin Core metadata set [14]. We looked forward to complying with national principles edited by the referencing working group of the UMVF [16]. We focused the project on integrating a true pedagogical method to help teachers to build and organize materials. We wanted them first to think about the quality of the selection, the description and the arrangement of the resources. A specific training-course was organized to help them understand constructivist learning principles, to allow them to comply with the pedagogical working framework and to show them how to design a lesson bearing in mind that emphasis. This method also provides students with relevant, selected and classified learning materials, combining traditional text-based documents, annotated images, and appropriate keywords or links to find other resources available on Internet. The strength of this model and this collaborative approach lies in the fact that, whatever the teacher, whatever the content of a lesson, a same navigational pattern is offered to the students while bearing in mind pedagogical imperatives [17]. While the efficacy of such techniques of knowledge acquisition remains difficult to measure, we anticipate that this kind of pedagogical ergonomics will enable teachers to improve content quality and students to avoid wasting seeking unhelpful information [18]. Our project addresses the challenges of high-performance web-site development and maintenance. Among the current available content management products, Zope has been chosen. This development framework controls the construction of objects to enforce consistency across an entire site. Zope implements a comprehensive system of permissions and roles to ensure that projects develop in harmony. The Plone layer reinforces these basic features and brings additional ones such as object workflow, new data objects indexing and management functions, and members' work spaces. The content lesson product we implemented (in Python language) acquires basic properties from the Plone layer (Dublin Core metadata set) and encapsulates its own methods (such as add/modify/view methods, combine/remove sub-components and workflow states). The modular architecture allows direct access to objects in libraries and answers the problem of creating modular curricula. The design of this lesson object according to the data model is generic enough to allow the integration of new kinds of resources. In fact, a sequence is a link to a single local file (doc, xls, pdf, swf, ppt, etc.) or a link to a remote resource (especially streaming video resources). The way the user navigates through resources is partially traced but the system does not store the complete student's profile in order to provide him/her with adaptive learning features. From a pedagogical point of view, this tool can be considered to be the first step to preparing students and teachers to work, learn and teach within virtual, collaborative environments. This tool supports the entire program of medical curriculum in our faculty in order to prepare the national pre-residency exam. All teachers can access the platform to upload files or create quizzes and cases on line by their own. They are invited to describe the modifications they made before publishing a lesson. The whole glossary is available and teachers can read the definitions and their author. The same feature has been set up for questions and any teacher may use one or more in his own lessons. We intented to promote collaborative interactions between teachers in order to improve the quality of resources they provided to students. Two implementations of the J@LON platform can be reached at: http://www.essquad.org and http://www.internatice.org.

6. Acknowledgements

The ESSQU@D project and the J@LON collaborative tool have received a grant from the French Ministry of Higher Education and Research as a "Campus numérique 2000" project and are supported by the French Medical Virtual University project (RNTS 2002).

7. References

[1]   Educnet. Les campus numériques français. http://www.educnet.education.fr/superieur/campus.htm (last visited: 01/15/2005)

[2]   Burge Z. New Roles for Learners and Teachers in Online Higher Education. In: Graeme Hart, ed. *Readings and resources in Global Online Education*. Whirligig Press, Melbourne, 2000; 4.

[3]   Prendergast   GA.   Successful   introduction   of   computer   mediated   learning. http://www.globaled.com/articles/PrendergastGerard2000.pdf (last visited: 01/15/2005).

[4]   Zaina LAM, Bressan G, Silveira RM, Stiubiener I, Ruggiero WV. Analysis and comparison of distance education environments. International Conference on Engineering Education, Oslo, August 6-10,2001;7E8:19-24

[5]   Eskola EL. University students' information seeking behaviour in a changing learning environment. http://www.shef.ac.uk/~is/publications/infres/isic/eeskola.html (last visited: 01/16/2005).

[6]   Kolb DA. *Experiential learning*. Englewood Cliffs, New Jersey: Prentice-hall, 1984.

[7]   Lebow D. Constructivist Been worth for Instructional Systems Design: Five Principles Toward has New Mindset. *Educational Technology Research and Development* 1993; 41(3):4-16.

[8]   Florida GULF Coast University. Instructional design. http://www.fgcu.edu/onlinedesign/designDev.html (last visited: 01/15/2005)

[9]   King JW. Seven principles of good teaching practice. http://www.agron.iastate.edu/nciss/kingsat2.html (last visited: 01/15/2005)

[10] Bearman M, Kidd M, Cesnik B. Methodology for developing educational hypermedia systems. In: Cesnik B, McCray AT, Scherrer JR, eds. *Medinfo'98*. Amsterdam: IOS Press, 1998; pp. 720-6

[11] Staccini P, Dufour JC, Joubert M, Michiels JF, Fieschi M. A full XML-based approach to creating hypermedia learning modules in web-based environments: application to a pathology course. *AMIA Annu Symp Proc.* 2003;:619-23.

[12] Spiklemire S, Friedly K, Spiklemire J, et al. Zope: *Web Application Development and Content Management*. New Riders Publishing, 2001; 480p

[13] Plone. http://www.plone.org (last visited: 01/15/2005)

[14] Dublin Core qualifiers. http://dublincore.org/documents/2003/03/04/dcmi-terms/ (last visited: 01/15/2005)

[15] El Saddik A, Fischer S, Steinmetz R. Reusability and adaptability of interactive resources in Web-based educational systems. *ACM Newspaper of Educational Resources in Computing* 2001;1(1):1-19

[16] Darmoni SJ, Leroy JP, Baudic F, Douyere M, Piot J, Thirion B. CISMeF: a structured health resource guide. *Methods Inf Med.* 2000;39(1):30-5

[17] Honebein P. Seven goals for the design of constructivist learning environments. In: B Wilson, ed. *Constructivist learning environments: Put studies in instructional design*. New Jersey: Educational Technology Publications, 1996; 11-24.

[18] Mallinen S. Teaching effectiveness and online learning. In: John Stephenson, ed. *Teaching and Learning Online, pedagogies for New Technologies*. Kogan Page, London, 2001; 141.

8. Address for correspondence

Pascal Staccini
Département STIC-NTIC Santé – UFR Médecine – 28 av. de Valombrose – 06107 Nice cedex 2 – France
email: pascal.staccini@unice.fr
url: http://wwwmed.unice.fr – url: http://www.essquad.org – url: http://www.internatice.org

Connecting Medical Informatics and Bio-Informatics
R. Engelbrecht et al. (Eds.)
IOS Press, 2005

An Improved Publication Process for the UMVF

Jean-Marie Renard[a], Jean-Marc Brunetaud[a], Marc Cuggia[b],
Stephan Darmoni[c], Pierre Lebeux[b], Régis Beuscart[a]

[a] CERIM, faculté de médecine, Université Lille2
[b] LIM, Rennes
[c] Université de Rouen

Abstract

The "Université Médicale Virtuelle Francophone" (UMVF) is a federation of French medical schools. Its main goal is to share the production and use of pedagogic medical resources generated by academic medical teachers. We developed an Open-Source application based upon a workflow system which provides an improved publication process for the UMVF. For teachers, the tool permits easy and efficient upload of new educational resources. For web masters it provides a mechanism to easily locate and validate the resources. For both the teachers and the web masters, the utility provides the control and communication functions that define a workflow system.
For all users, students in particular, the application improves the value of the UMVF repository by providing an easy way to find a detailed description of a resource and to check any resource from the UMVF to ascertain its quality and integrity, even if the resource is an old deprecated version. The server tier of the application is used to implement the main workflow functionalities and is deployed on certified UMVF servers using the PHP language, an LDAP directory and an SQL database. The client tier of the application provides both the workflow and the search and check functionalities and is implemented using a Java applet through a W3C compliant web browser. A unique signature for each resource, was needed to provide security functionality and is implemented using the MD5 Digest algorithm. The testing performed by Rennes and Lille verified the functionality and conformity with our specifications.

Keywords:
Web publishing; Indexation; UMVF; Workflow management; Medical pedagogy; Resource searching, Cryptographic digest.

1. Introduction

The " Université Médicale Virtuelle Francophone " (UMVF) is a federation of French medical schools. Its main goal is to share the production and use of pedagogic medical resources generated by academic medical teachers. The resources provided by each school are located on the web sites of the individual medical schools. In order to help the students to find the specific resources they were seeking, the UMVF decided to use a search engine developed in Rouen, "DocCisMef" [1].

This search engine depends on manual indexation performed by librarians, rendering it very difficult for the Rouen team to keep up with the increasing flow of information coming from the individual schools. The solution to this problem was to associate with each new document a standardised description. This "UMVF-notice", SCORM compliant

[2], provides all the information needed for an automatic and immediate pre-indexation by the Rouen team, the full indexation remaining manual. The group in Rennes then developed a specific application to fill in this "UMVF-notice ". However, the questions remained: who would fill in this notice and who would verify its quality?

The documents referenced on the UMVF web site are widely circulated by a variety of means, such as downloading, and distribution on CDs and disks. The students experienced considerable difficulties determining the author, date of publication and origin of the information, its validity and its accuracy. Without this information, the students were unable to determine whether the document they had in hand was the most current version, nor were they are able to assess the quality of information therein.

For the instructors the problem was how best to submit to the central office the details of their resources. In the absence of a formal submission mechanism these details might be sent in a variety of ways with no standardization of mechanism of submission, details, version numbers, dates or authors. At the same time, in the absence of standardization, the personnel in Rouen had great difficulties posting the information in a timely fashion.

We thus sought to create an application which would ensure standardized data entry, assist the webmaster in validating the data, and render the entry of the data into the database more efficient and thus faster. With such an application, the work would be easier for the teachers, the webmasters and the personnel in charge of the final manual indexation.

2. Specifications

To build our application we defined specifications which provided the functionality necessary to solve the identified problems. Some of these were related to the solutions we chose, others were related to UMVF organizational constraints.

2.1- The publication process

For teachers: The tool had to permit easy and efficient upload of new educational resources; these were designated as "primary resources" in this process. It had to be usable from behind hospital network firewalls. The required base functionalities were the ability to add, modify or delete the file of pedagogic medical resources on the UMVF web sites. The tool also had to assist the teacher in filling out the UMVF-notice of the resource, by pre-filling fields such as file name, medical school, and date.

For webmasters: the tool had to provide a mechanism to easily locate new uploaded files, to associate them with their author and to validate them, if necessary after having modified their style settings.

These (possibly modified and validated) files were designated "secondary resources" in this process. The web master must add the URL for the resource to the UMVF-notice, (which was pre-filled by the software and completed by the original author). He must then validate the notice and send it to the indexation centers in Rouen and Rennes.

For both the teachers and the web masters, the utility had to provide the control and communication functions that define a workflow system [3]. Each user had to have a simple view of the status of the data, resources and associated UMVF-notices for which he was responsible. The teachers needed to be able to see if their data were in stand-by mode, rejected, validated or published; the webmasters had to be able to determine if the author had made any changes to their submissions or corrections to rejected data. And if more information were needed, the workflow system had to allow the webmaster to easily communicate by e-mail with the author, including references to the data with problems.

2.2- Security of resources

A very important functionality for students was the ability to verify the validity and integrity of the resources they had downloaded or received from friends. It was thus necessary to provide a simple means for students to search for the original UMVF-notice from a resource they had in hand. We needed a unique signature for each resource, easy to rebuild from the resource itself, and incorporated into the description. The student's tool should compute the signature of the resource in hand, and use it to search for the corresponding UMVF notice [4, 5]. Armed with this description the student would then be able to access the information collected by the indexation team such as key words, topics, versions authors, dates of revision, etc. If the student's copy of the resource was either corrupted or not a valid UMVF notice, the software should identify this fact.

2.3- UMVF organisational constraints

We inherited some constraints directly from the UMVF organisation [6]. One was related to the heterogeneity of UMVF users' computers (PC-Windows, PC-Linux, Mac-Macintosh); the application had to run on disparate architectures and operating systems. Another constraint stemmed from national Education Ministry specifications : we were required to use an external directory for authentication and access control, conformant with the university directory specification (SUPAN). A third constraint was a result of the nature of the information system, which is a distributed system in which the resources are distributed across multiple different medical school web sites. A further constraint was the use of the extant on-line description editor provided by the medical school of Rennes. This is the means by which a uniform description of the resources is obtained from each medical school. Changes made in these descriptions should affect the application only if the fields used specifically by the workflow application are changed. A final constraint was the need to send the description both to Rennes and Rouen where the two search engines of the UMVF are located.

3. Results

We developed two applications. The first is the workflow application and the second is the security application

3.1- The workflow application:

The language used was PHP and the development was done by our private partner, Archimed, Lille, France.

The authentication and the profiles are managed in an external LDAP directory which is SUPAN compliant.

We implemented the application on Microsoft-Windows and GNU-Linux servers with IIS or Apache web server running PHP v5 , OpenLDAP Directory and MySQL Database engine. In the validation sub-process, a signature is computed as an MD5 sum digest and is inserted into the resource description. Our application is conformant with Open-Source GNU licencing.

3.2-The security application

The application was built as a Java applet downloadable from the main UMVF web site (http://www.umvf.org/). The user selects the resource he wishes to check. The applet then computes the MD5 digest of the resource and submits it to the description search engine hosted by Rennes. If a description related to the resource is found, the content of the description is displayed, in particular the version of the resource. If no description corresponding to the digest is found, it indicates that the resource is either corrupted or is not referenced by the UMVF.

3.3- Tests

Testing was performed by Archimed on the Windows platform and by Lille and Rennes on GNU-Linux.

6. Discussion

This application improves the value of the UMVF repository by providing an easy way for all users, teachers and students to find a detailed description of a resource such as the dates of publication or revision, the authors, the content of the resource and the course to which it refers. Of more importance, it provides an easy way to check any resource from the UMVF to ascertain its quality and integrity, even if the resource is an old deprecated version. In such a case, the description provides a link to the accurate version. This functionality is very important because students use these resources in preparing for their exams and certifications. The wide distribution of the resources across multiple medical schools renders it very difficult for the students to be certain of the validity of the information [7]. The ability to verify the content distinguishes the UMVF search engine from the usual search engines such as Google, constituting a critical improvement in this context.

Our application depends on only a small specific subset of the fields from the UMVF notice. As long as these fields are not changed, no modifications to the record in our application are needed. Changes to those fields which are outside our application continue to be solely the responsibility of the teams in Rouen and Rennes, and are reflected in our application with no further intervention. By contrast, changes to any of the specific fields which are used directly by our application require specific modification in our application also.

- For the teachers, this application is of considerable help by providing management reports giving a quick and easy view of the status of all submissions they have made. They can readily distinguish the old from the new submissions, and the validated from the rejected ones.

- For the web master, the application provides a display of the status of all active files, permitting rapid and easy task management, as well as a search function for retrieving any resource according to its parameters, names, dates, or keywords.

- For both teachers and web masters, the application provides some communication facilities for informing the other of the status of the resources for which they are responsible. If more information must be sent between users, the application provides a link with a conventional e-mail system.

- For the indexation centres of Rouen and Rennes, this application is designed to help cope with the increasing flow of new resources created by all the medical school teachers of the French-speaking medical universities by providing validated base descriptions for their indexation work. At the same time, the application is designed to be as independent as possible from the description editor used for indexing. In general, changes and additions made to the UMVF notices by the indexers have no impact on our application; only if they involve the few specific fields used for reference between the two applications is it necessary to modify our application also.

With respect to security, a limitation to the use of the MD5 digest keys is the fact that they are not encrypted. Consequently, the digest search engine must be implemented only on a certified server. An improvement would be to encrypt the digest incorporated in the notice by certificate assigned to the web masters. Such an improvement would require the building of a public key infrastructure (PKI) for the UMVF [8].

7. Conclusion

The testing performed by Archimed, Rennes and Lille verified the functionality and conformity with our specifications. We now have to deploy the application to all the UMVF members.

12. Acknowledgments

We are very grateful to David Maxwell for his help with the English text.

13. References

[1] Darmoni SJ, Thirion B, Douyere M, Dahamna B, Weber J. A Quality-controlled Health Gateway to Disseminate French Pre-residency Examination Program Teaching Resources on the Internet. *Medinfo. 2004*; 2004(CD):1566.

[2] Mougin F, Cuggia M, Le Beux P., Development of an indexing search engine for the UMVF: proposal for an indexing method based on Dublin Core and XML. *Stud Health Technol Inform.* 2003;95:727-31.

[3] http://www.wfmc.org/ Workflow Managment Coalition *web site*, 2005.

[4] Menezes A. J., van Oorschot P. C., Vanstone S. A., Hash Functions and Data Integrity, in Handbook of Applied Cryptography, Chap 9, p321-383, CRC Press 2001.

[5] Menascé D. A., Security Performance, *IEEE INTERNET COMPUTING* Vol. 7 No. 3; MAY/JUNE 2003, pp. 84-87.

[6] Beux P, Duff F, Fresnel A, Berland Y, Beuscart R, Burgun A, Brunetaud JM, Chatellier G, Darmoni S, Duvauferrier R, Fieschi M, Gillois P, Guille F, Kohler F, Pagonis D, Pouliquen B, Soula G, Weber J. The French Virtual Medical University., *Stud Health Technol Inform.* 2000;77:554-62.

[7] Darmoni SJ, Dahamna B, Roth-Berghofer TR. Related Articles, Seal of transparency heritage in the CISMeF quality-controlled health gateway.BMC Med Inform Decis Mak. 2004 Sep 14;4(1):15.

[8] Thompson M. R., Essiari A., Mudumbai S., Certificate-based authorization policy in a PKI environment, *ACM Transactions on Information and System Security (TISSEC)* Volume 6 , Issue 4 (November 2003) Pages: 566 – 588.

Address for correspondence

Dr Jean-Marie RENARD
CERIM, 1 place de Verdun
59045 Lille CEDEX
FRANCE – EUROPA
e-mail: jm.renard@univ-lille2.fr

Connecting Medical Informatics and Bio-Informatics
R. Engelbrecht et al. (Eds.)
IOS Press, 2005

A Multimedia Educational System to Teach Epidemiology

Marianna Diomidous

Department of Public Health, Faculty of Nursing, University of Athens, Greece

Abstract

An educational system has been developed which consists of a module to help both teachers to design courses with different levels of knowledge regarding epidemiology and students to get acquainted with the field of epidemiology.

The software development product Director was used to develop the software application. The capacity required to install the software is 130MB although each individual component is not greater than 1.2 megabytes in order to facility its handling. The user interface of the system employs colour, text, complementary voices and animation. Moreover, exercises have been designed to facilitate the learning process and to allow students and teachers to interchange information with it.

The system has been evaluated by a number of 65 students both graduate and undergraduate. Half of them were attending the undergraduate course in Nursing. The rest were graduate students attending a Master's Course in Health Informatics and Health Management. The first group of students had some prior knowledge of Epidemiology. The latter group had different levels of knowledge (none, little prior knowledge or an intermediate level of knowledge), of Epidemiology. The scope of this research is to prove the efficiency of Multimedia in teaching the rather difficult subject of Epidemiology.

Keywords:
Epidemiology, Education, Multimedia

1. Introduction

The description of multimedia by Professor Stephen Heppeli is note worthing for its attention on the potential for choice "Multimedia is a single word invented comparatively recently to describe the possibility that a computer might finally deliver all the elements that we take for granted during our everyday lives such as speech, text, graph, video, music, sounds, and data" [1]..

The term "multimedia" describes the opportunity to use a choice of media delivered via a range of information and communication technologies including electronic networks, touch screen, CD-ROM's, cable and satellite [2],[3].

Educational multimedia is not a new concept. However, it has only become a realistic means of delivering educational materials over the last few years. Technology is now sufficiently powerful and appropriately priced to deliver multimedia to desktop and portable computers.

Multimedia presents great opportunities for education and holds much more potential than merely providing access to large quantities of information. It can be used to support the "process" of learning by engaged learners in two-way communication with the computer that is driven by personal learning needs.

Multimedia can also help visualize and relate information in new ways to increase depth of understanding and the communication of ideas and concepts. At best, interactive multimedia offers an individual not threatening environment in which learners can question, offer solutions and test and develop ideas. This type of multimedia and be used for formal and informal education for both children and adults of all ages.

Therefore, educational multimedia can provide to learners, access to a wide range of learning resources through the internet and CD-ROM. Thus learners can use multimedia programs to:

- Monitor personal preferences and progress
- Learn new material
- Brainstorm ideas and real-life clinical scenarios
- Take self-assessment tests
- Develop learning agendas related to personal strengths and weaknesses
- Communicate with other students/tutors from around the world
- Graphically map learning needs and plans (i.e. using initial maps)
- Manage organize and plan learning

Based on the above mentioned assumptions and the importance of informing health professional of current practice future opportunities, a multimedia educational system has been developed in the Laboratory of Health Informatics at the Faculty of Nursing of the University of Athens. The main scope of the system developed consists of an effort to prove that education with the use of multimedia voices and animation is more efficient than the traditional way of teaching with a single tutor. The educational software developed, has been designed to provide and intermediate level of knowledge in epidemiology both to undergraduate and to graduate students in the field of Health Care Sciences and to help teachers to design courses with different levels of knowledge regarding Epidemiology.

With the developments of this system the following objectives can be achieved:

- To describe the structure and the characteristic of a population and its relationships with a health problem.
- To compute simple analysis of morbidity and mortality according to gender, race, place and time.
- To compute different types of ratios by age and gender.
- To investigate different types of hypotheses, different aspects of causality and a variety of diagnostic processes.
- To study the different types of epidemiological designs and results of epidemiological research
- To read epidemiological and medical/nursing publications in order to identify possible bases with methodology and data analysis.

2. Characteristics of the System

Director was used to develop the application software. The capacity required to install the system is 130 MB although each individual component is not greater that 1.2 Megabytes in order to facilitate it's handling. The system has more than two hundred screens voices and animations. The screens have different kinds of fonts and styles of letters in order to distinguish different aspects. As a matter of fact, bold letters were used to emphasize same concepts, grey characters to indicate a voice animation or additional information in other chapters etc. The fonts used have been brush script to display concepts and Helvetica narrow to display examples. The advantages of the system are to facilitate the learning process through text, colours, complementary voices animation. Moreover, exercises have been designed to allow students to interchange information with it. (1).

Future plans include the following:

a. design a www version to allow students to manage this system through internet.

b. design a virtual reality classroom to allow people to follow a regular course from the workplace or from home. The virtual classroom teaching can be completed with a discussion by using a list of different subjects and with an interchange of information and ideas with professionals and other specialists in the field of Epidemiology and Public Health.

3. Interface of the system: the multi-windows environment

This interface is justified for:

a. providing a powerful interface to let users to handle easily and quickly the system

b. separating different tools of the system since all components are not necessarily presented simultaneously

c. making use of the size of monitors since it is possible to display some windows thus increasing visualization surface

4. The Electronic Book

The electronic book has three components:

- Index
- Chapters
- Glossary

Index I

Chapters of the Electronic Book of Epidemiology:

1) The definition of Epidemiology
2) Causation in Epidemiology
3) Prevention in Epidemiology
4) Statistics in Epidemiology
5) Indices in Epidemiology (Measuring Health and Disease)
6) Design of Epidemiological Research
7) Data Collection
8) Data Analysis
9) Biostatistical methods for comparing the results of different epidemiological studies
10) Possible errors in the results and methods to avoid them
11) Validity, generalization and confidentiality
12) Clinical Epidemiology

In each chapter, there are sub-chapters and sub-topics. For example in chapter 5 indices in Epidemiology five sub-topics and five windows with suitable animations are presented. These include the following:

a. Definitions of Health and Disease
b. Measures of disease frequency
c. Use of available information
d. Comparing disease occurrence
e. Study questions

5. Glossary

The Glossary has three areas sensible to mouse. The big one is a scrolling field where a list of terms is displayed. When one of them is selected, section numeric i.d. it appears at the "items" column then section title at the bottom line, and with a double click is possible to go to the selected section.

6. Bibliography module

This module is compounded of two databases. These are the following:
a. Description of a main book and journals of Epidemiology and Public Health
b. References used to develop each chapter of the electronic book.

7. Additional Modules

The system has two additional modules: one with exercises that help the students to understand the theoretical part and acquire hands on experience, and the other is a help module.

1. There have been designed numerous exercises and different methods have been used to explain the concepts presented in each chapter. In some of them students were able to use their own data.

2. A help module to explain the different aspects of the system: types of characters, text-styles, buttons, etc, has also been developed.

The contents of window 5.2, for example, include the following:

5.2.1 Population at risk	5.2.10. Life expectancy
5.2.2. Prevalence and incidence	5.2.11. Standardized rates
5.2.3. Prevalence rate	5.2.12. Morbidity
5.2.4. Incidence rate	5.2.13. Disability
5.2.5. Cumulative incidence rate	5.2.14. Comparing disease occurrence
5.2.6. Case fatality	5.2.15. Risk difference
5.2.7. Interrelationships of the different measures	5.2.16. Attributable fraction
	5.2.17. Population attributable risk
5.2.8. Mortality	5.2.18. Relative comparison
5.2.9. Mortality before and just after birth	

In each step users are able to join any part of the chapters with a "double click".

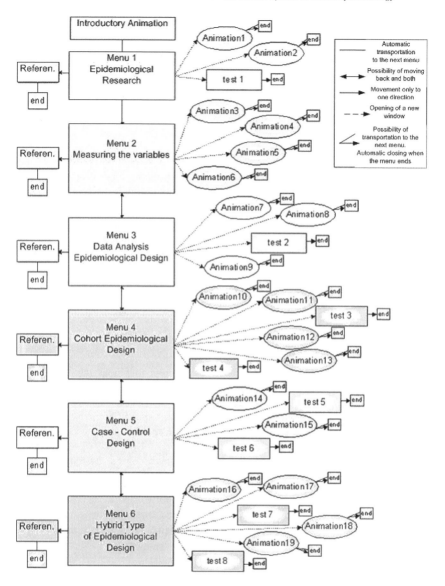

Figure i : Educational Software in Epidemiology

8. Evaluation

The system developed has been evaluated in the use of a questionnaire with 43 questions by 65 undergraduate and graduate students. The first section of the questionnaire was comprised of 23 questions and was focused on the evaluation of the level of knowledge and the general understanding of the concepts and principles of the subject of Epidemiology. The rest of the questions had their main focus on the friendliness and the general usability of the educational system developed. Chi-square, F-test and analysis of variance were used to statistically analyse the results of the data collected.

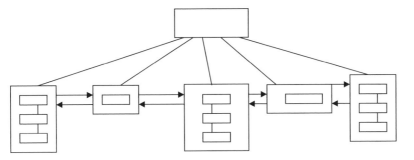

Figure 2 - Global structure of a chapter

From the analysis of the data the following results were recognized:

a. The use of computers and especially the use of multimedia in the teaching process may enable a great deal the understanding of the concepts and principles of the difficult subject of Epidemiology.

b. The existence of prior knowledge of the above mentioned subject was a major plus for the conceptualization of the basic ideas and principles of Epidemiology.

c. There was little or no difference between the undergraduate and the graduate students in terms of understanding the basic concepts of Epidemiology.

d. The existence of prior knowledge of the use of computers was helpful but not determinant factor.

e. Correspondingly there was little or no difference between the two categories of students in terms of being able to use efficiently the system.

f. The software used for the development of the educational system was proved to be user friendly and interesting to work with.

g. Finally, the majority of the students (85%) expressed the opinion that the educational system developed helped them a great deal to understand the subject presented even without the presence of a tutor in the classroom.

9. Conclusions

A multimedia system teaching epidemiology has been developed and evaluated by a number of students with positive results concerning the usability of the software package. Further study is under development to evaluate the usefulness of the application for teachers.

10. References

[1] Carlos de Castro, J.A Ramos, Dormido S," Open Hypermedia System for Automatic Control Teaching', ELDEN, 94

[2] Mean M., Roger M., Dannenberg B,, Multimedia Interface Design", ACM. Press Frontier Series

[3] Schank R.C.Active Learning through Multimedia", Multimedia , Spring 1994, 60-78

11. Address for correspondence

Department of Public Health, Faculty of Nursing, University of Athens, 123, Papadiamantopoulou Street, Goudi, GR-11527 Athens, Greece, Tel: +30 210 746 1448

290

Connecting Medical Informatics and Bio-Informatics
R. Engelbrecht et al. (Eds.)
IOS Press, 2005

Trends in free WWW-based E-learning Modules seen from the Learning Resource Server Medicine (LRSMed)

Jürgen Stausberg[a], Martin Geueke[b], Kevin Bludßat[a]

[a]*Institute for Medical Informatics, Biometry and Epidemiology, Medical Faculty,*
University of Duisburg-Essen, Germany
[b]*ClinResearch GmbH, Cologne, Germany*

Abstract

Despite the lost enthusiasm concerning E-learning a lot of material is available on the World Wide Web (WWW) free of charge. This material is collected and systematically described by services like the Learning Resource Server Medicine (LRSMed) at http://mmedia.medizin.uni-essen.de/portal/. With the LRSMed E-learning modules are made available for medical students by means of a metadata description that can be used for a catalogue search. The number of resources included has risen enormously from 100 in 1999 up to 805 today. Especially in 2004 there was an exponential increase in the LRSMed's content. Anatomy is still the field with the highest amount of available material, but general medicine has improved its position over the years and is now the second one. Technically and didactically simple material as scripts, textbooks, and link lists (called info services) is still dominating. Similar to 1999, there is not one module which could be truly referred to as tutorial dialogue. Simple material can not replace face-to-face-teaching. But it could be combined with conventional courses to establish some kind of blending learning. The scene of free E-learning modules on the WWW is ready to meet current challenges for efficient training of students and continuing education in medicine.

Keywords:
Computer assisted instruction; E-learning; Learning; World Wide Web

1. Introduction

E-learning has disappeared from the political agenda of strategically important topics [1]. This is due to the fact that expectations and promises have failed; unrealistic enthusiasm is followed by deep frustration. According to Jennett [2] E-learning stands in a critical phase of new technologies' life cycle. Promising reports had been followed by professional adoption and public acceptance. Now we can notice a phase of professional denunciation and it is not clear, whether E-learning will reach the status of a standard procedure in medical studies and continuing medical education.

In Germany, current regulations for medical education offer new chances for a revival of E-learning. On the one hand, conditions for education of medical students have been revised [3]. Education at medical faculties should be more oriented to health practice and health care system requirements. Ex-cathedra teaching becomes less important, the role of seminars and teaching small groups of one to three students has grown. As consequence lecturers are confronted with a dramatically increase in hours needed for education, which have been gained from time used for research and patient treatment. On the other hand continuing medical education becomes mandatory for physicians in outpatient care [4]. Within 5 years practitioners have to collect 250 points in certified courses to keep their licence and to avoid financial restrictions.

Both requirements, new regulations for medical education and mandatory continuing medical education, create new hopes and options for E-learning. Especially material offered on the World Wide Web (WWW) support the required efficiency in education and training through following advantages [5].

- Independence from local connections because the Internet allows access from all over the world with a low cost technical infrastructure.

- Independence from time restrictions because the material is available 24 hours 7 days a week without any technical necessity for downtime.

- Independence from the availability of teachers at the time of learning because their knowledge is integrated in learning modules.

- Easy and fast updating because all content is localized on the WWW-server.

A lot of useful material for WWW-based E-learning had been developed world-wide during the last 5 to 10 years of professional adoption. Especially material that is offered free of charge via a WWW-Browser is made accessible on demand by special catalogues in medicine. Well known academic services include:

- Computer aid learning reviews (CAL reviews) - http://axis.cbcu.cam.ac.uk/calreviews, a project of the Clinical & Biomedical Computing Unit at the University of Cambridge, UK, started September 1997.

- Commented database for E-Learning: Medicine (in German: Kommentierte E-Learning Datenbank: Medizin, KELDAmed) - http://www.ma.uni-heidelberg.de/bibl/KELDAmed/, offered by the University Hospital of Mannheim and the Heidelberg University, Germany.

- Learning Resource Server Medicine (LRSMed) - http://mmedia.medizin.uni-essen.de/portal/, developed and maintained by the Institute for Medical Informatics, Biometry and Epidemiology of the University Duisburg-Essen, Germany, started in 1997.

Being responsible for the LRSMed we are able to analyze the trend of free WWW-based E-learning modules over the last decade. In our article we will compare the content of LRSMed in the years 1999 [6], 2002 [7] and 2004 (data from November 2004).

2. LRSMed

The LRSMed is a multilingual service that retrieves E-learning modules freely available on the WWW, describes the modules with a metadata standard, stores the metadata in a database and offers a user-interface for retrieval, commenting and authoring. Main target group of LRSMed are medical students, but some material will also be useful for health care professionals as well as for the public. Figures 1 and 2 show screen-shots from the LRSMed. In Figure 1 a search for E-learning modules is specified using the criteria specialism (anatomy), application type (image atlas), and language (English). The result screen is shown in Figure 2. Eleven modules were retrieved from the database and information is presented including the modules' title, specialisms, application types, and languages. The user can call further information or can switch directly to the modules via the title's hyperlink. As part of LRSMed's quality assurance strategy, comments about a module can be entered here. The result set can be transformed into a document in Portable Document Format (PDF) and printed out.

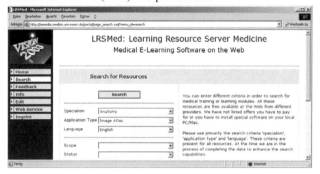

Figure 1 - User interface of the search for E-learning modules

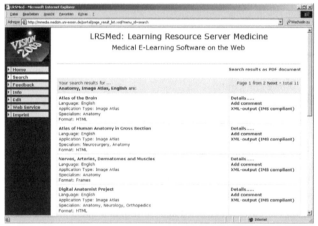

Figure 2 - Result set with further options and hyperlinks to the modules

Key features of LRSMed include the use of Learning Objects Meta-data (LOM) [8] in the implementation of the IMS Learning Resource Meta-data Information Model [9] as metadata-specification, the eXtensible Markup Language (XML) as syntax for interfaces and the Oracle suite for implementation. An application programming interface implemented with the Simple Object Access Protocol (SOAP) enables the integration of LRSMed in other applications as hospital information systems, E-learning platforms, etc.

Learning material has to fulfil several requirements to be accepted for inclusion in the LRSMed: availability (free of charge), technique (standard WWW-browser, only extended by common plug-ins), target group (primarily medical students), language (at the moment German and English), and application type (cf. figure 3).

A critical assessment of the E-learning module's quality is supported in two ways. Firstly, an interested user can read comments of others about that module. The comments are stored within the metadata and comprise free text as well as a simple score. Secondly, LOM had been extended with entities covering information about the module's development process (Was the development based on specific standards for software development?) as well as information about evaluation (Has the module demonstrated its educational impact in a controlled study?).

3. Trends in frequency, specialism and application type

The number of E-Learning modules available in LRSMed has increased dramatically. Having 100 modules in the first quarter of 1999, this number raises linear up to 267 until the second quarter in 2002 and exponential up to 439 the first quarter, 653 the second quarter, and 763 the fourth quarter 2004. The LRSMed offers currently 805 active resources (status 2005-01-07). In comparison KELDAmed provides 1135 resources including 591 eBooks (PDF-files) the same day. The number of resources included in CAL reviews is not published.

Figure 3 shows an overview of the relative frequency of modules categorized according to the application type. Because LRSMed allows multiple classifications of E-learning modules to different application types some modules count twice in Figure 3. Similiar to 1999, simple scripts are most commonly offered in 2004 (30 %). The type info service jumped from a bad position of 2 % in 1999 to position 3 with 12 %. We define info services as enhanced link lists concerning a medical topic. Other application types that received a higher relative frequency in 2004 than in 1999 are textbook, drill and practice, and virtual presentation. On the opposite the relevancy of simulation, image atlas, presentation, and audio database decreased. Video database and questionnaire were introduced later.

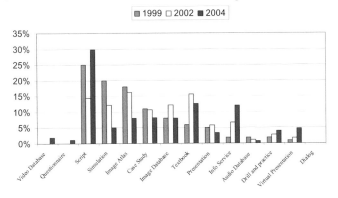

Figure 3 - Relative frequency of E-learning modules in LRSMed 1999 (left column), 2002 (middle column) and fourth quarter in 2004 (right column) categorized according to the application type. From left to right the application types are ordered in descending relative frequency from 1999.

The six most frequent specialities in 1999 are also present in the TOP 10 of 2004: internal medicine divided in its specialities cardiology, hematology and oncology, and gastroenterology; anatomy; neurology; radiology; dermatology; pathology. Medico-theoretical fields as biochemistry, biometry, and epidemiology lost their position in the TOP 10-list. In 2004, number 2 behind anatomy is general medicine, which improved its position from 8 in 2002. Firstly visible in the TOP 10 in 2004 is pediatrics at position 8. Histology (position 4), first aid (position 8), and otolaryngology (position 10) had an intermediate visit in the TOP 10-list 2002. Between 2002 and 2004 internal medicine had been divided into its sub-specialisations due to a high number of respective modules. The most frequent combinations of specialism and application type in 2004 are shown in Table 1.

Table 1 - Combinations of specialism and application type with 10 or more modules in 2004.

Specialism	Application type	Number of modules
Anatomy	Image database	18

General medicine	Info service	17
Microbiology	Script	16
Virology	Script	16
General medicine	Script	15
Cardiology	Textbook	13
Cardiology	Script	13
Radiology	Case study	13
Biochemistry	Script	12
Hematology and Oncology	Script	12
Anatomy	Simulation	11
Gastroenterology	Script	11
Pharmacology	Script	11
Hematology and Oncology	Info service	10

4. Conclusions

On the WWW, the number of freely available E-learning modules in medicine has increased enormously between 1999 and 2004. Some remarkable national and supranational funding programs in the last decade might be one reason for this increase in learning material. For example, the German government funded 180 projects within its program "New Media for Education" between 2000 and 2003 with more than 180 million EURO, from which 16 projects in medicine received 34 million EURO [10]. In addition, the large number of scripts might indicate that many lecturers offer material they have developed for own purposes before. Meanwhile, the coverage of specialities has changed. Image oriented specialities like anatomy, radiology, and pathology dominated in the late 90s as well as medico-theoretical fields like biochemistry. Nowadays clinical fields with a high common relevancy are present in the top-list of E-learning modules. Especially general medicine made its way into the WWW. General surgery is still underrepresented in comparison to its importancy.

The quality of the E-learning modules is difficult to access. Published studies demonstrate a poor reliability in assessing health teaching resources [11]. An impression could be received by the trend in application types. Not the number of complex and sophisticating types had been raised - simple scripts are still the most frequent application type available in 2004. As mentioned in 1999 by Haag et al. [12], modules offering a tutorial dialog are still missing. So the WWW is used mainly for a distribution of classic material. The possibilities of the medium are still not fully exploited.

We do not know whether the situation seen in our LRSMed is representative for the scene. But our analysis demonstrates that a lot of material is available which could be integrated into courses because of its simple structure. Today, lecturers can utilise this material and combine it with face-to-face teaching to establish an ideal synergy of blended learning.

5. Acknowledgements

The development of LRSMed was funded by the German Federal Ministry of Education and Research (BMBF) within the project Vision 2003.

6. References

[1]   The European ODL Liaison Committee. Distance Learning and eLearning in European policy and practice: the vision and the reality. 17 November 2004, available at http://www.odl-liaison.org/, accessed 2004-11-26.

[2]   Jennett B. High technology medicine. Benefits and burdens. Oxford: Oxford University Press, 1986.

[3]   Approbationsordnung für Ärzte vom 27. Juni 2002. Bundesgesetzblatt Teil 1, 2002; pp. 2405-35.

[4]   Gesetz zur Modernisierung der gesetzlichen Krankenversicherung (GKV-Modernisierungsgesetz - GMG). Bundesgesetzblatt Teil 1, 2003; pp. 2190-258.

[5]   Lowe HJ, Lomax EC, Polonkey SE. The World Wide Web: a review of an emerging Internet-based technology for the distribution of biomedical information. *JAMIA* 1996: 3 piii: 1-14.

[6]   Stausberg J, Bündgens D, Prange J. Multimediale medizinische Lehr- und Lernsoftware im World Wide Web: Eine Angebotsanalyse. In Victor N, Blettner M, Edler L, Haux R, Knaup-Gregori P, Pritsch M, Wahrendorf J, Windeler J, Ziegler S, eds. Medical informatics, biostatistics and epidemiology for efficient health care and medical research. München: Urban & Vogel, 1999; pp. 333-6.

[7]   Geueke M, Stausberg J. A meta-data based Learning Resource Server for Medicine. *Computer Methods and Programs in Biomedicine* 2003: 72 piii: 197-208.

[8]   IEEE Learning Technology Standards Committee (LTSC), Learning Object Model 6.1, available at http://ltsc.ieee.org/doc/wg12/LOM_WD6-1_1_without_tracking.pdf, accessed 2002-05-30.

[9]   IMS Global Learning Consortium, IMS Learning Resource Meta-data Information Model Version 1.2. Final Specification. 17 May 2001, available at http://www.imsglobal.org/metadata/index.html, accessed 2002-06-26.

[10] Projektträger Neue Medien in der Bildung + Fachinformation des BMBF in der Fraunhofer Gesellschaft. Förderprogramm Neue Medien in der Bildung. Förderbereich Hochschule. Aktuelle Fördervorhaben aus der Förderbekanntmachung zum Einsatz Neuer Medien in der Hochschullehre. Sankt Augustin Dezember 2002, available at http://www.gmd.de/PT-NMB/Projektdokus/Hochschul_Vorhaben.pdf, accessed 2003-05-05.

[11] Darmoni SJ, le Duff F, Joubert M, le Beux P, Fieschi M, Weber J, Benichou J. A preliminary study to assess a French code of ethics for health teaching resources on the Internet. In Surján G, Engelbrecht R, McNair P, eds. Health data in the information society. Proceedings MIE2002. Amsterdam: IOS, 2002; pp. 621-6.

[12] Haag M, Maylein L, Leven FJ, Tönshoff B, Haux R. Web-based training: a new paradigm in computer-assisted instruction in medicine. *International Journal of Medical Informatics* 1999: 53 piii: 79-90.

Address for correspondence

Priv.-Doz. Dr. med. Jürgen Stausberg, Medical Faculty, University of Duisburg-Essen, Inst. for Medical Informatics, Biometry and Epidemiology, Hufelandstr. 55, D-45122 Essen, Phone: +49 201 723 4512, Fax: +49 201 723 5933, stausberg@uni-essen.de, WWW: http://www.uni-essen.de/imibe/

Connecting Medical Informatics and Bio-Informatics
R. Engelbrecht et al. (Eds.)
IOS Press, 2005

Testing Repeatability of Forces when Using Neurosurgical Spatulas

Lars C Brix, Claus B Madsen, Jens Haase

Aalborg University, Aalborg, Denmark

Abstract

Virtual reality systems seems to be useful for training the use of brain spatulas without damaging brain tissue but the success of such a system is dependant on the human ability to discriminate pressures applied with the spatula. This paper describes an experiment designed to explore some central issues related to this ability: are surgeons better than laypeople, are the abilities in Virtual Reality (VR) and real world (RW) comparable, and will visual feedback enhance the ability. A group of surgeons and a control group of laypeople were tested in VR and RW. The results showed that surgeons performed better than the control group in RW but worse in VR, and that visual feedback improved the surgeons' abilities more than the control group. The results indicated that visual feedback is important for the success of such a virtual training system.

Keywords:
Surgery simulation; Brain spatulas; Haptics ability

1. Introduction

It is believed that surgery simulations will play an important role in surgical training in the future [1]. For the surgeon it is important to perform common and basic elements of the surgical procedure in an effortless and automatic fashion without being consciously aware of the motor performance. The self-regulatory aspect of a motor task must thus be facilitated and the intentional corrective movements must be minimized [2]. Surgical training is therefore basically a training that involves development of automatic skills [1].

In the Virtual Brain Project (VBP) [3] at Aalborg University our main focus is on simulators to train neurosurgical operative procedures. One of the projects in the VBP is the Brain Spatula Simulator Project where our goal is to develop training facilities that minimizes complications from brain spatulas [4].

The function of the brain spatula is to support or retract brain tissue and thereby create a space for the operative procedure. In a Danish thesis Rosenørn [5] showed that brain tissue may become ischemic and eventually infarcted if it is retracted with prolonged, high pressure. Specific training to avoid such complications is not available at present. Our concept is based on the idea of transferring skills trained in a VR setup to the RW operative field.

The ability to discriminate pressure at the tip of an instrument is attached to the ability to discriminate forces exchanged between the fingers and the instrument and the ability to convert these forces to a tip force. According to Dargahi et al. [6] the sensing of the human hand can be somehow compared to a tactile sensor with a sensitivity range of 0.01-10N. Thus it must be assumed that humans actually are able to sense a wide range of forces through an instrument such as a spatula given proper training.

It is hypothesized that neurosurgeons are better than non-surgeons to sense a discriminate pressure difference through an instrument due to their daily practice. It has been found relevant to explore this hypothesis since the goal of the spatula simulator will be to enable the surgery trainees to acquire the skills of an experienced surgeon.

It is furthermore hypothesized that skills and performance in VR are comparable to skills and performance in RW. This may be considered a basic demand for the plausibility of developing a simulator in VR for training skills to be applied in a RW-situation.

A third hypothesis we have is that the skills of sensing forces is enhanced by using visual information as a supplement to the pure haptic information. Since surgeons primarily are visually oriented this seems plausible [7]. This information is furthermore relevant for the design of our training system since it indicates whether the focus should be on pure haptic training or whether visual feedback should be added.

The experimental setup presented in this paper was designed to explore these three hypotheses. The setup is described in section 2 and is followed by a statement of the results in section 3. A discussion of the results are given in section 4 followed by a conclusion in section 5.

2. Materials and Methods

In order to be able to investigate the hypothesis that VR-skills are comparable to RW-skills it was found necessary to use two experimental setups exploring the skills of the test persons:

- A RW-setup where a hanging force meter was attached to a spatula as shown in figure 1 on the left. In this setup the force applied with the tip of the spatula could be read on the scale of the force meter. This setup did not necessarily represent the skills of using a spatula on a brain precisely, but it was a situation where the user was able to use his haptics experiences from the real world.
- A VR-setup based on the ReachIn API^{TM} as shown in figure 1 in the middle. This setup enabled visual feedback in the form of a 3-dimensional projection of objects in front of the user using stereo-glasses and a mirror. It furthermore allowed force feedback through a Phantom^{TM} device with 6 d.o.f. input and 3 d.o.f. output.

It was decided in general to focus on testing the ability to feel forces with three different forces chosen in cooperation with an experienced microsurgeon: 0.2N, 0.5N, and 1.0N. They represent an acceptable force, a force on the limit of what he would use, and a force that the surgeon would never use, respectively.

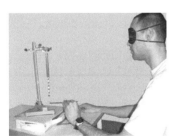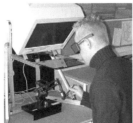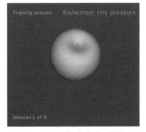

Figure 1 – The two setups used in the experiment and a screenshot from an experiment. On the left the RW-setup is shown and in the middle the VR-setup is shown. On the left is a screenshot from the visual test.

The experiment was divided in three different test types. The first two were focused on the haptic difference between RW and VR and the third on the importance of visual feedback:

1. *RW Force Meter:* The basic ability to sense a force using only haptic feedback tested in the RW-setup. The test persons were blindfolded and were asked to train a specific force and afterward to recreate the trained force 5 times in a row. This was repeated 6 times with the three different forces used twice in randomized order. Training was done with verbal instructions from a test leader guiding the test subject to push with a force within 0.01N from the desired force. During the force recreation the subject verbally indicated to the test leader when he/she felt the force corresponded to the force he/she had trained. The force was then read manually by the test leader.

2. *VR Force Meter:* The *RW Force Meter* test repeated in the VR-setup. The training was here done with guidance from the computer. During the force recreation the subject again verbally indicated to the test leader when the correct was assumed found. In this experiment the actual force was read by the computer when the test leader pushed a button and thus some human nuisance factors in from RW-test were removed. The spatula/hand position was held invisible to the test subject resembling the blindfolding in the RW-test.

3. *Visual Test:* The effect of visual feedback tested in VR. The test person trained a force by pushing a virtual ball that had both visual and haptics feedback as shown in figure 1 on the left. It was visually indicated when the correct force was applied on the ball. After the training the force was recreated three times with three different situations: with both visual and haptic feedback, with only visual feedback, and with only haptic feedback. This was repeated 9 times training each of the three force sizes 3 times in random order.

The experiment was conducted involving a group of 9 surgeons from Århus hospital in Denmark with from 1 to 38 years of surgical experience. The control group was 14 laypeople with various backgrounds but none were surgeons. All test subjects were told to use their preferred hand for the experiment and all were subjected to all three tests.

3. Results

The directly retrieved results from the experiments were the recreated forces. These were converted to an error measure by subtracting them from the force trained. The error measure was thus positive if the force recreated was weaker than the force trained and negative if it was stronger than trained.

In general when a group of errors were investigated the mean value and standard deviation (std) of the data were explored. A mean value of zero would indicate that the test persons were able to recreate the force trained and a mean value different from zero would indicate a systematic error. The standard deviation would show how close the recreated forces in general were to the trained forces and would thus indicate the ability to discriminate forces in the group of results.

Using the assumption that the groups of results were normally distributed two different statistically tests were used for exploring the results. A two-tailed t-test for testing the null-hypothesis that the mean-value of a group of results was zero and a one-tailed F-test for testing the alternative-hypothesis that the standard deviation of a group of results was lower/higher than the standard deviation of another group of results. Visual inspections of histograms and normality plots were used to examine whether the normality assumption seemed valid for the groups of results. In no cases did the assumption seem invalid.

The test results are reported in the following section followed by a discussion in section 4.

Real World Test vs. Virtual Reality Test

As mentioned the RW Force Meter test and the VR Force Meter test were constructed to compare the abilities in RW and VR. It has been found relevant to investigate whether the results are dependant on the size of the force trained.

Table 1 shows the mean and standard deviation of the errors for the two force meter tests dependant on the force trained. Furthermore the p-values are given for the two-tailed t-test of zero mean. The values for which the p-values indicate that the null-hypotheses should be rejected with 95% confidence, i.e. $p < 0.05$, has been marked by a grey background. For these mean-values the given confidence level indicates that the values are not zero, i.e. there is a statistical significant difference between the recreated and trained forces.

Table 1 – Means, stds, and p-values for the force meter tests dependant on trained force.

	RW Force Meter		VR Force Meter	
0.2N	-0.034 (0.074)	$p = 4.9 \cdot 10^{-12}$	-0.0025 (0.16)	$p = 0.81$
0.5N	0.013 (0.11)	$p = 0.067$	0.12 (0.16)	$p < 2.2 \cdot 10^{-16}$
1.0N	0.066 (0.14)	$p = 6.2 \cdot 10^{-12}$	0.13 (0.34)	$p = 1.3 \cdot 10^{-8}$

A general tendency is that the standard deviations get higher with higher forces trained for both tests. This indicates that lower forces can be recreated more precisely than higher forces. When comparing the RW and VR tests it seems obvious that the standard deviations are larger in VR especially for 0.2N and 1.0N.

Table 2 shows a corresponding table of the two force meter tests dependant on which group the test persons belonged to.

The surgeons seem to be better in RW considering the standard deviations than the laypeople (p-value for F-test with alternative-hypothesis that their performances are better is $1.2 \cdot 10^{-7}$) whereas they seem worse in VR (p-value with alternative-hypothesis that they are worse is 0.00012).

Table 2 – Means, stds and p-values for the force meter tests dependant on test person group.

	RW Force Meter		VR Force Meter	
Surgeons	0.00097 (0.097)	$p = 0.86$	0.070 (0.27)	$p = 2.9 \cdot 10^{-5}$
Laypeople	0.023 (0.13)	$p = 0.00024$	0.090 (0.22)	$p = 1.3 \cdot 10^{-15}$

Visual Importance

The visual test was constructed with the purpose of detecting the importance of visual information for the ability to recreate forces. Since the size of a force in this test is coupled to a deformation it has again been considered relevant to investigate the importance of the trained force.

Table 3 shows the results for the three result types dependant on the force trained. As before grey fields indicate that recreated forces are statistically different from trained forces.

Table 3 - Means and stds and p-values for the visual test dependant on trained force.

	Both feedbacks	Only Visual Feedback	Only Haptic Feedback
0.2N	-0.049 (0.11) $p = 0.00036$	-0.11 (0.16) $p = 7.1 \cdot 10^{-8}$	-0.025 (0.13) $p = 0.10$
0.5N	0.025 (0.13) $p = 0.13$	-0.083 (0.17) $p = 0.00013$	0.058 (0.13) $p = 0.011$
1.0N	-0.039 (0.15) $p = 0.038$	-0.066 (0.20) $p = 0.0075$	0.13 (0.21) $p = 1.6 \cdot 10^{-6}$

The standard deviations are generally lower when both feedbacks are present than when only one of the feedbacks is present. It thus seems that the test persons improve their ability to recreate a force when using both feedbacks.

In table 4 the corresponding results for the visual test is shown for each test person group.

Table 4 - Means and stds and p-values for the visual test dependant on test person group.

	Both Feedbacks	Only Visual Feedback	Only Haptic Feedback
Surgeons	-0.030 (0.12) $p = 0.024$	-0.10 (0.15) $p = 8.9 \cdot 10^{-8}$	0.066 (0.21) $p = 0.0054$
Laypeople	-0.015 (0.15) $p = 0.24$	-0.079 (0.19) $p = 7.0 \cdot 10^{-6}$	0.047 (0.17) $p = 0.0026$

The standard deviations indicate that surgeons perform better than laypeople when both feedbacks or when only the visual feedback is present (p-values 0.0087 and 0.027 respectively in F-test with alternative-hypothesis that the surgeons perform better) whereas they actually perform worse when only the haptic feedback is present (p-value is 0.032 in F-test with alternative-hypothesis that they perform worse).

It should be noted that the only-haptic feedback results of the visual test are not directly comparable to the results of the VR Force Meter test due to the different methods in training and recreation of forces

4. Discussion

The two-tailed t-tests of zero mean shows that the mean values in most cases are different from zero with 95% confidence. This means that the test persons in general made systematic errors when recreating the forces trained. That the errors were systematic could indicate that the method of training and the method of recreating forces were experienced differently by the test persons, e.g. that they were forced to move the spatula in an impractical manner during training. This difference does therefore not necessarily mean that people are not able to recreate the same force more than once with high accuracy.

Comparing the RW Force Meter test and the VR Force Meter test it can be seen that the mean error in RW is generally lower than in VR. The difference between training and recreating forces must thus have been larger in VR than in RW. Since the standard deviations of the VR test are also larger in general it must be concluded that some difference must exist between the two situations making it more difficult to recreate forces in the used VR setup than in the used RW setup considering pure haptics.

Whether this would also be the conclusion if the haptics of a surgical simulation was used instead the haptics of a spring-like system is an open question, but we think that the results indicate that the force feedback arm has some properties such as inner friction and position dependency that reduces the precision of the results. That the performance was reduced in the VR setup was supported by the fact that the group of surgeons were significantly better than the laypeople in RW but that their performance were more comparable in VR.

The slightly worse performance of the surgeons in VR could be an indication that the group of laypeople comprised a higher amount of persons experienced in using VR in their everyday live (e.g. through computer games). Proper training in VR could possibly reduce the difference between VR and RW but it would weaken the surgery simulator idea of transferring skills from VR to RW if such a special training was needed.

Another possibility of improving the results in VR is to include visual feedback. The results in the visual test showed that the surgeons again performed worse than the laypeople when only haptic feedback were present but that they on the contrary performed better when the visual feedback was present. This indicates that the visual feedback improved the surgeon's abilities to recreate the forces more than the laypeople's abilities.

It seems that surgeons rely more on their visual sense than on their haptic sense when both are present. This is considered important for the development of VR training systems with the current force feedback technology. Emphasis should be put on the development of the visual feedback in order to enhance the ability of non-experienced persons to transfer knowledge from VR to RW in a manner giving them an intuitive understanding of forces comparable to experienced surgeons.

5. Conclusion

In this paper we investigated the ability to discriminate forces through an instrument in both a RW-setup and a VR-setup. It was found that a difference existed between the haptics ability in the RW-setup and the VR-setup. The ability to recreate forces was superior in RW compared to the ability in VR indicating that the used VR-setup was not able to give a true simulation of the RW haptics.

The difference affected surgeons differently from laypeople. The surgeons were better than the laypeople considering the haptics ability in RW but they were worse in VR. When visual feedback was added in VR it was found that surgeons were able to use it to counteract some of the problems with the lost haptics ability and performed better than the laypeople.

6. Acknowledgements

The authors wish to thank all participants in the experiment. We especially wish to thank Per Bjerre, from Aarhus University Hospital for his help with arranging the experiment.

7. References

[1]   Haase J, Musaeus P, and Boisen E. Virtual reality and habitats for learning microsurgical skills. In: Andersen,P. and Qvortrup,L., eds. Virtual Applications: Applications with Virtual Inhabited 3D Worlds. London: Springer, 2004, pp. 29-48.

[2]   Milton JG, Small SS, and Solodkin A. On the road to Automatic: Dynamic Aspects in the Development of Expertise. *Journal of Clinical Neurophysiology* 2004: 18(3): pp. 134-143

[3]   Larsen OV, Haase J, Østergaard LR, Hansen KV, and Nielsen H. The virtual brain project: development of a neurosurgical simulator. *Proceedings of Medicine Meets Virtual Reality* 2001: 256-262.

[4]   Hansen KV, Brix L, Pedersen CF, Haase JP, and Larsen OV. Modelling of interaction between a spatula and a human brain. *Medical Image Analysis* 2004; 8:23-33.

[5]   Rosenørn J. The risk of ischaemic brain damage during the use of self-retaining brain retractors. *Acta Neurologica Scandinavia* 1989: Supplementum 120 Vol. 79.

[6]   Dargahi J, and Najarian S. Human tactile perception as a standard for artificial tactile sensing – a review. *International Journal of Medical Robotics and Computer Assisted Surgery* 2004: 1(1):23-35.

[7]   Waterhouse JA. Dextrous and Shared Interaction with Medical Data: stereoscopic vision is more important than hand-image collocation. *Proceedings of Medicine Meets Virtual Reality* 2002.

8. Address for correspondence

Lars C. Brix
Aalborg University
Fredrik Bajersvej 7D
DK-9000 Aalborg O, Denmark
brix@hst.aau.dk

Section 5

Handheld and Wireless Computing

Connecting Medical Informatics and Bio-Informatics
R. Engelbrecht et al. (Eds.)
IOS Press, 2005

Exploring Electronic Conversion of Behavioral Instruments for Telehealth

Karen L. Courtney [a], George Demiris [a], Catherine K. Craven [a],
Debra Parker Oliver [a], Davina Porock [b]

[a] University of Missouri-Columbia, Missouri, USA
[b] University of Nottingham, England, UK

Abstract

As research interests in telehealth applications increase, traditional behavioral instruments need to be adapted for use for new mediums in telehealth evaluation. Display and method of presentation changes can affect the reliability and occasionally the validity of the revised instruments. This paper explores critical concerns to be addressed with electronic conversion of psychometric instruments and provides an example of testing methodology and psychometric properties for an instrument measuring quality of life (CQLI) converted in electronic format for use within a telehealth intervention.

Keywords:
Telemedicine; Psychometrics; Quality of Life; Data Collection; Computers, Handheld

1. Introduction

Telehealth seeks to bridge geographic distances between caregivers and clients and enhance the delivery of healthcare through the use of communication technologies. The potential of telehealth applications to address local healthcare infrastructure and spatial access barriers to high quality care is of great interest to health care providers and policy makers. As Finch et al. point out, the production of evidence about the effectiveness of telehealth is vital for its progression, ultimate diffusion and success [1].

The same geographic barriers to healthcare that make telehealth desirable generate challenges for assessment and evaluation of telehealth interventions. Traditional evaluation methods that use focus groups or paper-based behavioral instruments, such as quality of life measures, are difficult to utilize or implement effectively when large geographic distances separate clients from care providers or researchers. In fact, this challenge may contribute to ineffective evaluations of telehealth interventions [2,3].

Due to the growth in Internet use within the last decade and the proliferation of personal computing devices such as handheld computers and smart phones, researchers have begun to explore electronic alternatives to traditional paper-based assessment. Although researchers have developed some new instruments that collect information electronically [4,5,6,7,8,9], most researchers convert traditional paper-based assessment tools to electronic collection versions. Electronic data collection (EDC) methods include use of the Web, e-mail, and desktop and handheld computers for surveys, diaries, behavioral instruments and focus groups. Conversions to EDC can include changes to the display of the instrument, changes to the delivery mechanism or both.

In addition to distance considerations, there are five commonly recognized benefits to electronic collection of data, including: cost savings, time savings, immediacy of results, user preferences and enhanced data integrity. As researchers expand the use of EDC to more diverse populations and include multiple delivery mechanisms, the potential for EDC as a method of telehealth evaluation increases.

Changes in the display or delivery modes or both in the conversion of traditional instruments to electronic versions can produce changes in their reliability, and in some cases, their validity. In order to ascertain that the revised instruments remain adequate evaluation measures, telehealth researchers must also re-evaluate reliability and possibly the validity of the revised tools.

Changes in the display of information can change how a participant perceives a question. Unlike in paper methods, in EDC, font size, font color and the way questions are presented to participants are easily manipulated. Such manipulation could change the psychometric properties of a behavioral instrument. Several researchers have noted, however, that the design flexibility of EDC, which allows for the use of alerts, audio capabilities and dynamic questionnaires, benefits users [11,13,16]. Visual display issues presented problems for other researchers [14], including respondents not following discussion threads [6] or an increased dropout rate in groups assigned complex tables to fill out [23]. Other researchers raised ergonomic issues with the electronic format including confusion over contiguous keys [17] and difficult text entry via keyboards or a stylus [15]. In these studies with display changes, the interaction of the respondents with the new display mode means ergonomics and design are important considerations for the evaluation's effectiveness.

In addition to changes in display, in EDC the delivery mode can change. Self-report instruments can be changed to interview style instruments. Although such changes in tool format can eliminate ergonomic and display challenges for respondents, this change in delivery mode can affect the level of self-revelation in responses. In fact, EDC demonstrates increases in respondents' self-revelation [4,13,24,25]. This is true even in the case of sensitive topics such as intimate partner violence, substance abuse or psychological state [6,7,8,26,27,28,29]. For example, researchers have found that electronic screening can be more effective than face-to-face clinician evaluations of domestic abuse in identifying potential victims and perpetrators [26].

In instruments in which both the display and delivery modes are modified for EDC, further testing is required as demonstrated in the case study described below.

2. Materials and Methods

In order to determine the effect of modification of display and delivery mechanism on instrument reliability, we conducted a case study within the Missouri Telehospice Project [30]. This project uses videophone technology to bridge geographic distance between hospice caregivers and care providers in order to reduce caregiver anxiety and improve their quality of life. One of the instruments used in this project is the Caregiver Quality of Life Index (CQLI) [31].

The CQLI had been used previously in studies of family caregivers of hospice patients. The authors of the CQLI reported adequate reliability and validity testing with our target population. In McMillan's and Mahon's [31] initial CQLI development report, they provided measures of reliability and validity. For measures of reliability, internal consistency, as measured by Cronbach's alpha, were given in addition to the average inter-item correlation. Cronbach's alpha was tested at admission and after four weeks and was 0.76 and 0.88 respectively [31]. The average inter-item correlation was positive and moderate (r = 0.44) [31]. Initial CQLI psychometric testing supported the instrument's reliability.

Similarly, prior psychometric evaluation of the CQLI supported the validity for hospice patient family caregivers. McMillan and Mahon reported both content and construct validity measures [31]. A Content Validity Index (n = 5) was computed for content validity and was 1.0 for the total score and each individual item. Construct validity was measured using known groups of caregivers and non-caregivers. The overall CQLI score was significantly different between the groups as expected with caregivers having lower quality of life scores than non-caregivers (t = 4.36, p<0.001). As expected, the following individual items were also significantly different among the groups: emotional (t = 5.09, p<0.001), social (t = 4.14, p<0.001), and physical (t = 2.9, p<0.005). Caregivers scored lower in quality of life in these three areas than their non-caregiver counterparts. The financial item (t = 1.59, p =ns) was not significantly different between caregivers and non-caregivers although, again, caregivers consistently reported lower quality of life scores than non-caregivers [31].

For the Missouri Telehospice Project, the CQLI instrument was revised to evaluate the quality of life of hospice family caregivers in remote locations. The CQLI was changed from a paper-based, self-report, 100 mm visual analog scale to an interview format, 0-10 rating scale. A research assistant collected responses to the scale via a handheld computer for the reliability testing. This implementation of CQLI-revised allows the evaluation team to assess caregivers' quality of life without having to travel to the remote locations to conduct the assessment. For this case, we changed both the display of the behavioral instrument and the delivery mechanism.

The display changed from a paper, visual analog to an audio, 0-10 scaled, interview assessment which could be conducted via telephone. Because in this study it was the research assistant and not the caregiver who operated the handheld computer, some of the effects of display changes were ameliorated. However, this display change still required appropriate usability testing involving the intervention study data collectors.

The change to an interview format was also a delivery change because the quality-of-life ratings were verbalized to the research assistant, which was a change from the silent, self-reporting of the paper instrument. This change introduced the potential for changes in the level of our caregivers' self-revelation. Thus, these delivery changes necessitated testing the reliability of the CQLI-revised. Because the content of the questions did not change, and the instrument had prior use in the hospice population, validity retesting was unnecessary.

Norbeck [32] suggests that a minimal standard for publication of new behavioral instruments is as follows: one measure of content validity; one measure of construct or criterion validity; test-retest reliability; and internal consistency reliability. However, no universal standards exist for conversions of behavioral instruments for electronic data collection. Based on potential threats to reliability cited in the literature, it seems reasonable that a minimal standard for instrument-conversion testing would include internal consistency, test-retest, and parallel forms reliability. Additionally, further validity testing might be required if the questions or responses change or if the instrument will be used with a different population.

Following IRB approval, we examined the reliability of the revised CQLI instrument in comparison to the original with a convenience sample of 25 adults in an academic medical center setting. CQLI reliability was measured for test-retest stability, internal consistency and stability between versions (parallel forms). The research assistant gave each participant the paper instrument with instructions. Within several minutes of each participant completing the paper CQLI, the research assistant administered the revised, interview version of the CQLI and recorded the responses in the handheld computer. For test-retest reliability, each participant repeated the tandem CQLI testing one hour later. Both paper and interview versions performed well in all three reliability measures.

3. Results

Statistical analysis was performed using SPSS 12.0. Test-retest reliability was comparable for both versions. The paper and electronic versions demonstrated excellent test-retest reliability ($r = 0.944$, $r_s = 0.912$, $p<0.001$ respectively) for the total score. Likewise, the paper and electronic versions exhibited excellent test-retest reliability for the individual items (r ranging between 0.866 and 0.937, $p<0.001$, r_s ranging from 0.811 to 0.955, $p<0.001$ respectively).

Internal consistency of both formats as measured by Cronbach's standardized alpha was acceptable for all sessions. The Cronbach's standardized alpha for the paper version was 0.721 and 0.710 for time 1 and 2 respectively. For the electronic version, Cronbach's standardized alpha was 0.769 and 0.705 for time 1 and 2 respectively.

The paper and electronic versions showed significant positive correlations for both the total score (rs = 0.892, $p<0.001$) and for individual items (rs ranging between 0.684 and 0.897, $p<0.001$) during time 1. Likewise, during time 2, there were significant positive correlations between both versions for total score (rs =0.919, $p<0.001$) and for individual items (rs ranging from 0.848 to 0.957, $p<0.001$). These strong positive correlations indicate that the revised CQLI version is as reliable as the original CQLI instrument.

4. Discussion and Conclusion

Telehealth alters the process of care delivery and introduces new technology and different social mechanisms in the context of a "teleconsultation." When the mode of administering the evaluation tools also utilizes advanced technologies, not only do we need to evaluate the telehealth intervention but also the reliability and validity of our modified evaluation tools.

Instruments that have been modified rarely produce an identical psychometric result; however, the results should be consistent in strength and direction. Of the research completed that has addressed reliability measures, electronic methods have been comparable in internal consistency [8,13,20,21,24,25]. Likewise, researchers who have tested parallel forms also report high reliability between instrument versions [8,10,15, 17,18,19,20,22].

However, the majority of researchers do not report psychometric testing or results for their revised instruments. This lack of reliability and validity testing makes it difficult for evaluators of telehealth research and programs to judge the efficacy of telehealth interventions. Strong positive correlations between parallel forms of psychometric instruments are required to demonstrate the appropriateness of the instrument conversion.

Obtaining similar results for internal consistency for multi-item instruments and test-retest reliability for stable trait measures is necessary as well.

With careful planning, traditional psychometric instruments can be converted for use in evaluating telehealth applications. Current research indicates that converted instruments can be valuable in the assessment of telehealth applications. Without adequate testing and reporting of reliability and validity following conversions, the information retrieved from telehealth intervention evaluations using such conversions could be disregarded by both policy makers and researchers.

4.1 Suggested Guidelines for Psychometric Reporting for Telehealth Evaluation Studies

Just as Norbeck [32] suggested minimal standards for psychometric reports for new instrument development, we suggest that telehealth evaluations using electronically converted behavioral instruments report reliability and when appropriate validity psychometric testing results. At a minimum, we recommend that test-retest reliability and parallel forms reliability be reported for converted behavioral instruments. For scaled instruments, such as the CQLI in the case presented, internal consistency reliability should also be reported. Not every instrument conversion will necessitate further validity testing; however researchers should consider validity testing when the instrument conversion has resulted in a change in either the questions or responses presented to participants.

5. Acknowledgements

This work was supported in part by the National Library of Medicine Biomedical and Health Informatics Research Training Grant T15-LM07089-13 and the Catherine Pouget Research Award of the MAPI Research Institute.

6. References

[1]   Finch T, May C, Mair F, Mort M, and Gask L. Integrating service development with evaluation in telehealthcare: an ethnographic study. *BMJ* 2003: 327: 1205-1209.
[2]   Dillon E, and Loermans J. Telehealth in Western Australia: The challenge of evaluation. *J Telemed Telecare* 2003: 9 (S2): 15-19.
[3]   Grigsby J, Rigby M, Hiemstra A, House M, Olsson S, and Whitten P. The diffusion of telemedicine. *Telemedicine Journal and e-Health* 2002: 8 (1): 79-94.
[4]   Whalen CK, Jamner LD, Henker B, Delfino RJ. Smoking and moods in adolescents with depressive and aggressive dispositions: Evidence from surveys and electronic diaries. *Health Psychol* 2001: 20 (2): 99-111.
[5]   Tsang MW, Mok M, Kam G, Jung M, Tang A, Chan U, et al. Improvement in diabetes control with monitoring. *J Telemed Telecare* 2001: 7 (1): 47-50.
[6]   Moloney MF, Dietrich AS, Strickland O, and Myerburg S. Using Internet discussion boards as virtual focus groups. *Adv Nurs Sci*. 2003: 26 (4): 274-286.
[7]   Formica M, Kabbara K, Clark R, and McAlindon T. Can clinical trials requiring frequent participant contact be conducted over the Internet? Results from an online randomized controlled trial evaluating a topical ointment for Herpes Labialis. *Journal of Medical Internet Research*. 2004: 6 (1): e6.
[8]   Buchanan T, and Smith JL. Using the Internet for psychological research: Personality testing on the World Wide Web. *Brit J Psychol* 1999;90:125-144.
[9]   Stubbs RJ, Hughes DA, Johnstone AM, Rowley E, Reid C, Elia M, et al. The use of visual analogue scales to assess motivation to eat in human subjects: a review of their reliability and validity with an evaluation of new hand-held computerized systems for temporal tracking of appetite ratings. *Brit J Nutr* 2000: 84: 401-415.
[10] Bliven BD, Kaufman SE, and Spertus JA. Electronic collection of health-related quality of life data: validity, time benefits, and patient preference. *Qual Life Res*. 2001: 10 (1): 15-22.

[11] Eysenbach G, and Wyatt J. Using the Internet for surveys and health research. *Journal of Medical Internet Research*. 2002: 4 (2): E13.
[12] Giammattei FP. Implementing a total joint registry using personal digital assistants. A proof of concept. *Orthopaedic Nursing*. 2003: 22 (4): 284-288.
[13] Hanscom B, Lurie JD, Homa K, and Weinstein JN. Computerized questionnaires and the quality of survey data. *Spine*. 2002: 27 (16): 1797-1801.
[14] Schleyer TKL, and Forrest JL. Methods for the design and administration of Web-based surveys. *J Am Med Inform Assn*. 2000: 7: 416-425.
[15] Fletcher LA, Erickson DJ, Toomey TL, and Wagenaar AC. Handheld computers. A feasible alternative to paper forms for field data collection. *Evaluation Rev*. 2003: 27 (2): 165-178.
[16] Selanikio JD, Kemmer TM, Bovill M, and Geisler K. Mobile computing in the humanitarian assistance setting: an introduction and some first steps. *J Med Syst*. 2002: 26 (2): 113-125.
[17] Ryan JM, Corry JR, Attewell R, Smithson MJ. A comparison of an electronic version of the SF-36 General Health Questionnaire to the standard paper version. *Qual Life Res*. 2002: 11 (1): 19-26.
[18] Caro JJ, Sr., Caro I, Caro J, Wouters F, and Juniper EF. Does electronic implementation of questionnaires used in asthma alter responses compared to paper implementation? *Qual Life Res*. 2001: 10 (8): 683-691.
[19] VanDenKerkhof EG, Goldstein DH, Lane J, Rimmer MJ, and Van Dijk JP. Using a personal digital assistant enhances gathering of patient data on an acute pain management service: a pilot study. *Can J Anaesth*. 2003: 50 (4): 368-375.
[20] Jamison RN, Raymond SA, Levine JG, Slawsby EA, Nedeljkovic SS, and Katz NP. Electronic diaries for monitoring pain: 1-year validation study. *Pain* 2001: 91: 277-285.
[21] Chang BL. Internet interventions for community elders: Process and feasibility. *Western J Nur Res* 2004: 26 (4): 461-466.
[22] Cronk BC, and West JL. Personality research on the Internet: a comparison of Web-based and traditional instruments in take-home and in-class settings. *Behavior Research Methods, Instruments, & Computers*. 2002: 34 (2): 177-180.
[23] O'Neil KM, Penrod SD, and Bornstein BH. Web-based research: methodological variables' effects on dropout and sample characteristics. *Behavior Research Methods, Instruments, & Computers*. 2003: 35 (2): 217-226.
[24] Davis RN. Web-based administration of a personality questionnaire: Comparison with traditional methods. *Behav Res Meth Instr C*. 1999: 31 (4): 572-577.
[25] Berthelson CL, and Stilley KR. Automated personal health inventory for dentistry: A pilot study. *J Am Dent Assoc* 2000: 131: 59-66.
[26] Rhodes SD, Bowie DA, and Hergenrather KC. Collecting behavioural data using the world wide web: considerations for researchers. *Journal of Epidemiol Commun H*. 2003: 57 (1): 68-73.
[27] Turner CF, Ku L, Rogers SM, Lindberg LD, Pleck JH, and Sonenstein FL. Adolescent sexual behavior, drug use, and violence: Increased reporting with computer survey technology. *Science* 1998: 280 (5365): 867-873.
[28] Webb PM, Zimet GD, Fortenberry D, and Blythe M. Comparability of a computer assisted versus written method for collecting health behavior information from adolescent patients. *J Adolescent Health* 1999: 24: 383-388.
[29] Weisband S, and Kiesler S. Self disclosure on computer forms: Meta-analysis and implications. In: *CHI:96*; 1996.
[30] Demiris G, Parker Oliver D, Porock D, and Courtney KL. The Missouri telehospice project: Background and next steps. *Home Health Care Technology Report* 2004: 1 (4): 49-55.
[31] McMillan SC, and Mahon M. The impact of hospice services on quality of life of primary caregivers. *Oncology Nursing Forum* 1994: 21 (7): 1189-1195.
[32] Norbeck JS. What constitutes a publishable report of instrument development. *Nurs Res* 1985: 34: 380-382.

Address for correspondence

Karen L. Courtney, RN, MSN
University of Missouri – Columbia
324 Clark Hall
Columbia, MO 65211 USA
CourtneyKL@health.missouri.edu

Pervasive Observation Medicine: The Application of RFID to Improve Patient Safety in Observation Unit of Hospital Emergency Department

Chang-I Chen[a,b], Cheng-Yaw Liu[b], Yu-Chuan Li[a,b], Chia- Cheng Chao [b,c],
Chien-Tsai Liu [a], Chieh-Feng Chen[a,b], Ching-Feng Kuan[d]

[a]*Graduate Institute of Medical Informatics, Taipei Medical University*
[b]*Taipei Medical University, Municipal Wan Fang Hospital*
[c] *National Chen Chi University MIS Graduate School*
[d]*Chungtai Institute of Health Sciences and Technology, Department of Health Care Administration*

Abstract

> Over the past decade, observation medicine has become an important component of
> emergency medicine. There are several settings in which observation medicine has
> been useful and valuable.(1) RFID as the patient identification, not only
> generates the on-line laboratory data and radiology report via hand-held wireless
> PDA, this RFID system help physician stream-line patient admission to acute bed
> or ICU in the emergency department more effectively。

Keywords:
Radio Frequency Identification (RFID); Observation Unit (OU); Patient Safety

1. Background

As part of an interdisciplinary study of patient safety and quality improvement, we implemented the RFID framework in the observation unit of emergency department, defined as a real-time observation utility by medical management, and of the informatics framework enhancement that resulted from patient safety of quality improvement.

METHODS. We are applying RFID technology into emergent medical setting then reviewing 10,000 patients in the observation unit and its records from the emergency department of selected acute care, non-psychiatric hospitals in Taipei, Taiwan in 2004. We then developed wireless web-based RFID framework to implement the real-time safety reminders such as the laboratory and radiology reports to the physician who can make decision promptly to the patients in the observation unit.

RESULTS. The waiting time for physicians to make clinical decision according to laboratory and radiology results is largely reduced within 30 percent due to the RFID system. Observation hours is reasonably decreased by the physician who could actively receiving patient's updated clinical data to make clinical decision via web-based informatics system. **CONCLUSIONS.** We are planning to monitor the effectiveness of pervasive RFID system from these factors, such as length of waiting for acute bed admission, and the potential delayed diagnosis.(2) When these common ER factors can be greatly improved from the adoption of RFID and many practice emergency department quality issues will gain a better result as the application of RFID.

2. Introduction

Emergency medicine in Taiwan is in the face of major change and overcrowding. National Health Insurance (NIH) reimburse emergency department (ED) services as 30% lower pay out-patient basis, as the results, The phrase 'pervasive Observation Medicine' describes the use of pervasive RFID technologies in emergency department of observation unit(OU), including making clinical diagnosis more effectively while patients' diseases on progressing.(3) These observation areas cater for certain categories of patients with surgical, medical, psychosocial and/or medical specialist consulting needs who can be discharged within 24–48 hours. OU has tended to be condition specific need to outpatient follow up or inpatient but tailored to local needs and interests or more often, lack of alternative pathways within the hospital.(3)

RFID technology is already being deployed across the pharmaceutical and many healthcare industries to improve patient identification of patient safety.(4) The focus on this study is the patient care centered, in which the RFID technology will be used to remind in charge physician to track patient's medical instruments as well as patients and hospital personnel. The Joint Commission on Accreditation of Healthcare Organizations (JCAHO) has recently stated new safety goals that should further expedite the process of RFID implementation in this field.(5) It is not difficult to conclude that RFID technology should become a critical success factor for the medical center of the 21st century in terms of both improved patient safety and improved ED clinical decision on the real-time data can be obtained by the physician via wireless PDA.(6)

3. Results

On the monthly ED patients around 5,500, we are applying RFID technology into emergent medical setting then reviewing 5,000 patients in the observation unit on the eight-month period, and its records from the emergency department of selected acute care, non-psychiatric hospitals in Taipei, Taiwan in 2004. We then developed wireless web-based RFID framework to implement the real-time safety reminders such as the laboratory and radiology reports to the physician who can make decision promptly to the patients in the observation unit. Radio frequency identification (RFID), which has focused for its application to inventory control and supply management, can also be implemented in a patient ID wristband system as a substitute in conjunction with, wireless PDA scanner for real-time data collection such as medication administration. (7) The good news is that emerging technologies are available to tap into these potential benefits for improving patient safety.

Using these devices for quick but secure access to essential data can enhance timely clinician decision-making and save lives, improve the flow and ensure security of patient information at the point of care. Wireless technology can provide approach to clinical information further reducing barriers to safe medication delivery.(7) Compared to bar coded bracelets in use at many hospitals today, RFID bracelets are welcomed by patients because they are far less interfering.

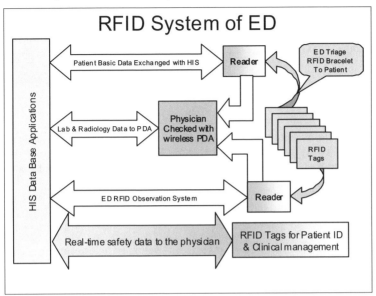

Upon admission, patients receive a paper-thin bracelet embedded with a small RFID chip containing information such as the patient's birth date, ID number, blood type, allergy, doctor's name, medication and other essential medical information.

The application of new technology RFID to improve the patients safety of OU of emergency department had been used from the Sept. 2004.

Table 1 show the 5,010 patients of the length of waiting for acute admission patient used new medical devices RFID from the September, 2004. to the April, 2005 and versus another 3,923 patients not used medical technology RFID from the Jan. 2004 to the Aug. 2004.

Table 1 - Differentiate the used RFID from not used RFID Length of waiting for acute bed admission

Characteristics	Not used RFID	Used RFID
Patient No.	3,923	5,010
Length of waiting (LOW) for acute bed		
Mean	303.6	77.2
SD	225.3	48.8
Not used RFID vs Used RFID	*P Value* = 0.014	

It has been shown that the patients using the medical new device RFID has decreased length of waiting (P=0.014) Medical new technology RFID can make process effectively.

Table 2 shows the 1,096 patients of the length of waiting for ICU used new devices RFID from the Sept. 2004 to April, 2005 which compared with 537 patients not used RFID from the Jan. 2004 to the Aug. 2004.

Table 2 - Differentiate the used RFID from not used RFID Length of waiting for ICU admission

Characteristics	t used RFID	Used RFID
Patient No.	537	1,096
Length of waiting (LOW) for ICU		
Mean	236.7	73.1
SD	166.0	76.9
Not used RFID vs Used RFID *P Value* = 0.026		

It has been shown that the patients using the medical new device RFID has decreased length of waiting for ICU(P=0.026). Medical new technology RFID can make clinical decision process effectively. Physicians or clinician decision can improve patient safety and medical delivery on well-ordered.

4. Discussion

On this study, ED patients who may need short-term observation and /or treatment. There are patients who may not be very reliable in follow-up who might fit into a brief diagnostic work in an observation unit (OU) or get initial therapy in the OU. About 5-7% of all emergency department patients could benefit from an observation unit.(8) The OU may help improve relations with the medical staffs, and improve public relations by improving emergency department(ED) efficiency and turn-around times. The setting of the RFID systems may be used to track patients, doctors and expensive equipment in hospitals. RFID tags can be attached to the ID bracelets of all patients or just patients requiring special attention, or in predictable critical conditions of patients treated in the observation unit of the emergency so their location can be monitored continuously.(9)

Improvements in emergency department patients' safety are the most importance work, and will improve staff training, and depend on a combined access including regular monitoring of practice, a better understanding of the causes of errors, a reduction in the complexity of routine procedures taking advantage of new technology.(10) Further development of the systems is needed to enable staff to carry out bedside caring procedures efficiently and accurately.(11)

A small number of studies using new technology RFID for the patient safety in hospitals have shown promising results in preventing errors. Although the effectiveness of RFID system shown a significant improvement on the basis of length of waiting for acute bed (P=0.014) and ICU (P=0.026) respectively. There are several other factors which may contribute the change such as the High Risk Reminder (HRR) on the critical value of lab. test and radiology report, computerized consulting system, these should perform further study to find out the correlation with RFID.

5. Conclusion

The use of new technology RFID to improve the patients' safety of ER is very promising. (8) Supporter of the RFID system believes RFID tag will improve rapid access to vital medical information on unconscious or uncommunicative patients. RFID will eventually replace bar-code technology at the bedside. But RFID can provide safety in so many ways because it can present so much more information than a bar code.(12) Above all, early studies suggest can cut medical error rates greatly.

With the application of RFID system, emergency department(ED) based observation unit are becoming effectively evaluated for the assessment and treatment of patients whether who may require inpatient or ICU management or monitoring.(13) The RFID based observation unit can be of great value to patient care. Although the concept of the OU is considered good practice especially in minimizing clinical risk, within the framework of RFID, it introduce the concept of wireless medical informatics environment which combined the safety mechanisms of high risk reminder (HRR), pervasive observation management (POM), and there has been significant progress to further develop and improve the quality which is safety centered of OU in ED practice.

6. Reference

[1] Ross, M.A., & Graff, L.G. (2001). Principles of observation medicine. Emergency Medicine Clinics of North America, 19(1), 1–18.

[2] Ross, M.A., & Graff, L.G. (2001). Principles of observation medicine. Emergency

[3] Medicine Clinics of North America, 19(1), 1–18.

[4] Ross, M.A. (1998). Guidelines and clinical pathways. In L.G. Graff (Ed.), Observation units implementation and management strategies (pp. 23–36). Dallas, TX: American College of Emergency Physicians.

[5] Barcode identification for transfusion safety. Current Opinion in Hematology. 11(5):334-338, September 2004. Murphy, M F a,b; Kay, J D.S

[6] Abrahamsen, Cathie RN, MSN Washington taps into healthcare technology [Departments: Tech update] Nursing Management (Springhouse) © 2005 by Lippincott Williams & Wilkins, Inc. Volume 36(3) March 2005 pp 52-55

[7] Poon, E., Blumenthal, D., Jaggi, T., Honour, M., Bates, D., and Kaushal, R.: "Overcoming Barriers to Adopting and Implementing Computerized Order Entry Systems in U.S. Hospitals, "Health Affairs, 23:184–90, 2004.

[8] Sensmeier, Joyce RN, BC, CPHIMS, MS Transform workflow through selective implementation. Nursing Management. 35(12):46-51, December 2004.

[9] Kohn, C and Henderson, C. W. (2004), "RFID-enabled medical equipment management programs to reduce costs," Managed Care Weekly Digest, 5/10/2004, 94-95

[10] Ward, Rod MA Ed, BSc, RGN, RNT NEWS. CIN: Computers, Informatics, Nursing. 23(3):115-118, May/June 2005.

[11] Sensmeier, Joyce RN, BC, CPHIMS, MS Transform workflow through selective implementation. Nursing Management. 35(12):46-51, December 2004.

[12] 2004. Featherly, K.: "Emerging Technologies,"Healthcare Informatics. 21(1): 29–38,

[13] Committee on Quality of Healthcare in America, Institute of Medicine, Crossing the Quality Chasm: A New Health System for the 21st Century, Institute of Medicine National Academy Press, 2001.

[14] Ward, Rod MA Ed, BSc, RGN, RNT NEWS. CIN: Computers, Informatics, Nursing. 23(3):115-118, May/June 2005

Address for correspondence

Yu-Chuan (Jack) Li, M.D., Ph.D.
President, Taiwan Assoc of Medical Informatics
Professor and Chief, Graduate Institute of Med Info
Vice Superintendent, Wan Fang Hospital
Taipei Medical University, Taipei, Taiwan
email: jack@tmu.edu.tw | http://li.tmu.edu.tw/

Connecting Medical Informatics and Bio-Informatics
R. Engelbrecht et al. (Eds.)
IOS Press, 2005

End-to-end Encryption for SMS Messages in the Health Care Domain

Marko Hassinen[a], Pertti Laitinen[b]

[a]*University of Kuopio, Dept. of Computer Science, Kuopio, Finland*
[b]*University of Kuopio, Shiftec, Dept. of Health Policy and Management, Kuopio, Finland*

Abstract

The health care domain has a high level of expectation on security and privacy of patient information. The security, privacy, and confidentiality issues are consistent all over the domain. Technical development and increasing use of mobile phones has led us to a situation in which SMS messages are used in the electronic interactions between health care professionals and patients. We will show that it is possible to send, receive and store text messages securely with a mobile phone with no additional hardware required. More importantly we will show that it is possible to obtain a reliable user authentication in systems using text message communication. Programming language Java is used for realization of our goals. This paper describes the general application structure, while details for the technical implementation and encryption methods are described in the referenced articles. We also propose some crucial areas where the implementation of encrypted SMS can solve previous lack of security.

Keyword:
SMS messages, communication, privacy, confidentiality, mobile phone, information systems

1. Introduction

Number of mobile phone users globally at the end of year 2002 was over 835 million. In Europe the corresponding figure was over 383 million users served by 143 operators over 50 areas. Non-voice traffic, including SMS, is showing remarkable growth with further increase expected. [1,2].

Text messages (SMS messages) are short text based messages usually sent between two mobile phones or by a computer application to a mobile phone [2]. Although gsm traffic is usually encrypted, there is little or no security in cases where the device is lost, stolen or otherwise accessed by an adversary. In such case messages stored in the device can easily be read and misused by the adversary.

We searched electronic databases (Elsevier Sciencedirect, IEEE Electronic Library, Pubmeb Medline) and found that two different ways have been used to utilize SMS messages in the health care domain. Firstly, text messages were used to various remainders. Main point was to improve patients' compliance to the care at the appointed time e.g. arriving to the doctor or to get a vaccination. [3,4]. The other way to utilize SMS was to send information from patients home to the clinical information systems e.g. different kinds of measurements done by a patient with diabetes. [5,6]. How the security issues were dealt with was not mentioned in the articles .

European Union directive on privacy and electronic communications (2002/58/EC) gives regulations on protection of the privacy of individuals. The directive aims to harmonization of regulations in Member States considering protection of fundamental rights and freedom. The directive sets limits on the collection and use of personal data in case of electronic communication. [7]. Same kind of regulations are included in HIPAA (Health Insurance Portability and Accountability Act of 1996) regulations in USA [8]. Each country of Europe has its own, more exact, legislation to handle personal data in the health care domain. Main issue of those regulations is to protect individual's privacy, which is a fundamental base for confidential relationship between health care professionals and patients. We suggest a way to fulfil those requirements in case of using SMS messages in health care.

In chapter 2 we introduce a programming platform based on Java, which we use in a development of an application for encrypted SMS messages in chapter 3. More details of encryption methods are explained in chapter 4. Some proposals for adaptations in the health care domain are explained in chapter 5. Finally in conclusions we will show the benefits of encrypted SMS messages and consider a future development of our work.

2. Mobile Java

J2ME (Java 2 Micro Edition) is a runtime environment specifically designed for devices with very limited resources, such as mobile phones or handheld computers. A program developed for J2ME is called a MIDlet. There is no straight interaction between a MIDlet and the device itself, since MIDlets are run by the Java virtual machine (JVM).

The WMA (Wireless messaging API) is described in specification JSR-120. It provides the means for sending and receiving SMS messages (among other functions) using the GCF (Generic Connection Framework). [9]. A connection for the SMS traffic is created as a MessageConnection object, which has methods for sending and receiving SMS messages.

3. Application

The requirements that were set on the application were the following:

- Encrypt SMS messages, send and store them safely
- Receive encrypted messages, decrypt and store them safely
- Store contacts, including name, phone number and password, safely
- Operate fast enough to provide acceptable service in an environment with very limited processing power
- Be compact enough for use in mobile phone memory space

Because of its portability across different mobile phone vendors, security and existing support for our needs, we chose Java as our development environment.

3.1 Application solution

SafeSMS is an application designed for SMS end-to-end encryption. It can send, receive and store encrypted text messages. Encryption is based on a secret password shared between the sender and the recipient. The encryption key is derived from a password. The application stores the sent and received messages so that they can only be read by a person who knows the relevant password. The application also includes a phone book, which contains the name, phone number and the password for each contact. The phone book can be used by several persons but one can only read contacts created by himself or herself.

The application has been created using the Java programming language. SafeSMS works on phones and PDA's that have Java runtime environment (MIPD 2.0, WMA). In the user manual [10] there is a list of such devices on the market at the moment (30 such devices on 12.10.2004). The application can be tested using an emulator. During the development phase of the software WKT 2.0 (Wireless Toolkit) from Sun Microsystems was used. See [11] for details. An earlier version of this software that runs on the MIDP 1.0 environment was introduced in July 2003. Details can be found in [12].

The application is installed as a Java application and the installation can be done directly from the internet. In order to be able to use the application, both the sending and receiving devices must have the application installed. The messages are sent as binary messages and the device can make a decision whether an incoming message is aimed for SafeSMS or not.

When a new message is initiated, the content of the message is written after which, a number where to send the message is prompted. Finally, a password used to encrypt the message is asked using a dedicated password screen. After receiving a message, the user is notified of a received message and he can read the message from the storage. Unless the message comes from a number listed in the phone book of the current user, the user must provide a decryption password. Figure 1 shows logical function of the application in phone to phone communication. It also shows the function with a server that can be used to send bulk messages.

SafeSMS has five user interface languages, English, Finnish, French, German and Italian. SafeSMS uses the locale selected in the phone to decide which language to use, but the user can select another one of the languages if he so wants. If the locale is anything else than fi (Finland), fr (France), ge (Germany) or it (Italy), the english language is used.

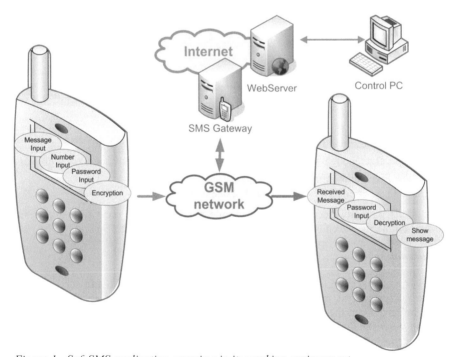

Figure 1 - SafeSMS application overview in its working environment

The Record Store (javax.microedition.rms) is a package containing classes used for permanent storage. Details of how the storage is implemented are left to the device, and the API (Application Programming Interface) provides the programmer means to use the storage without paying attention to details such as file reading and writing. The device is also responsible to guarantee that information on the storage is kept safe during power off's.

SafeSMS stores the received and the sent messages, as well as contacts in the record store. It uses the personal user password to derive an encryption key to encrypt certain values of stored messages as well as contacts. For contacts, all values, hence name, number and password are encrypted. This way contacts can be read only with the correct user password. Also different users can use the same phone book and will only see their own contacts.

The message part of a stored message is already encrypted during transmission. With sent messages also the date and the number of the recipient are encrypted, so that a user sees only messages he has sent. For incoming messages the number is not encrypted, since the user password is not always available when the message is received. This is the case if the application is not running at the time of receiving a message. After reading the message the user may choose to encrypt the message details, after which it can be seen only by that user.

3.2 Push registry

In an earlier MIDP 1.0 version [12] of this software, the application had to be running in order to receive an incoming message. On the Siemens platform this could be solved with a feature called Java SMS caching [9], but a different approach was used in the original version. It was based on archiving the message and reading it from the archive by the application in order to decrypt it.

MIDP 2.0 introduced a construct called Push registry that enables an application to register inbound connections to AMS (Application Management Software). This feature allows AMS to start the application on arrival of a message that is meant for the application. Registering an application to the Push Registry can be done in two ways. SafeSMS uses the static method of describing the Push Registry entry in the application descriptor file (jad), where all SMS messages with port 54321 are registered to be used by SafeSMS. This means that upon arrival of a message on port 54321 the message is directed to SafeSMS. In case the application is not running, it will be launched by AMS.

Sometimes it is necessary to know whether the application was started by the user or by the AMS using Push registry. Whether the application was started by AMS after an incoming connection can be detected using the method listConnections[13].

4. Encryption methods

SafeSMS has two methods for encrypting, Blowfish and Quasigroup. Using the JAD file one can choose which one to use. There are no limitations for adding a new algorithm for encryption.

Blowfish is an iterated block cipher designed by Bruce Schneier. It has gone through an extensive cryptanalytic analysis by the cryptographic community. A description of this method can be found in [14].

The Quasigroup method is based on a mathematical construct called a quasigroup. It is a stream cipher that does multiple rounds of encryption. These encryptions are parameterized by the given password. A description of the algorithm can be found in [12].

5. Conclusions

The ability to encrypt messages opens a wide variety of possibilities in several fields of health care. Our application provides a safe storage for sent and received messages. When the messages include some delicate information such as patient data, it is very important that the messages in the phone cannot be read by outsiders. Currently there are solutions, where text messages are used, but there is no way to avoid a disclosure if the device is lost and the user has not deleted the received messages. Such systems include for example a system for sending assignment messages for emergency response teams, which in Finland often contain patients name and description of the emergency. Clearly this kind of messages should not be disclosed to a third party.

There are various situations where patients or health care professionals would like to elicit a list of the patients' changed medication e.g. patients' appointment to private sector, health care personnel in home care or in emergency situations. In case of asking information from health care providers' databases by SMS, it is essential to authenticate questioner by adequate means.

5.1 Authentication

With our application it is possible to authenticate the counterpart. A mere phone number cannot be considered as a sufficient token of authentication, since in a case of a lost device, the user can be anyone.

Our approach combines the phone number and the secret password to authenticate the user. Even in the case where an adversary can access the phone, he still doesn't have the necessary password. He can use any password, but in that case it is trivial to detect the fraud in the receiving end. In our case, where the EMS staff uses SSN (social security number) to retrieve the list of medication of a patient, the probability that a SSN encrypted with a wrong password decrypts as a valid SSN is extremely small. The sending party (e.g. hospital) will use a password registered between itself and the sender. Upon receiving the list of medications, the adversary is met with a task of decrypting the response. This is as hard as trying all the possible keys of the encryption algorithm, provided that the password is properly selected.

5.2 Customization

Several customizations can be made to the software to make it more suitable for specific purposes. For the use of SMS messages in dispatching EMS crews with SMS messages we propose the following. Current system requires user activity to read the received message. Also the message doesn't differ in any way from a regular message. Our application can be customized so, that the message received from the dispatch is shown on the device immediately and requires no user interaction. Also the sound will differ from any other message, this way drawing the attention of the user.

6. Further work

As stated in section 4, there are no limitations for adding a new algorithm for encryption into our application. We are currently working on an implementation of the AES (Advanced Encryption Standard), which is the follower of DES (Data Encryption Standard) as an approved encryption method for sensitive, but not classified information. Despite the definition it is expected to follow DES as a de facto cryptographic standard for banking, administration and industry [15].

Although many communication needs can be covered using text messages, we see that the adoption of Multimedia messages (MMS) will open a whole new field of possibilities of communication both in health care and emergency response. The ability to transmit images, sound and even video feed has a wide range of new applications e.g. the paramedics can consult a medical specialist from the field with a help of an image. Our current research on how to make this secure already looks promising.

7. Acknowledgments

We would like to thank professors Pekka Kilpeläinen and Martti Penttonen from the Dept. of Computer Science at University of Kuopio for their valuable guidance and advice. Also we would like to thank Pierre-Yves Baumann and Philippe Bolgiani from Switzerland for language translations and for testing the application.

8. References

[1] GSM World. GSM Europe. Facts and figures. (10 Jan 2005.) Available at
    http://www.gsmworld.com/gsmeurope/about/gsm_europe_factsfigures.pdf .

[2] Xu H, Teo H, Wang H. Foundations of SMS Commerce Success: Lessons from SMS Messaging and Co-opetition. Proc. of the 36th Hawaii Int. Conf. on System Sciences, 2003, pp. 90-99(10).

[3] Car J, Sheikh A. Email consultations in health care: 1—scope and effectiveness. *BMJ*. 2004: 329: pp. 435-438 (4).

[4] Vilella A, Bayas J-M, Diaz M-T, Guinovart C, Diez C, Simó D, Muñoz A, Cerezo J. The role of mobile phones in improving vaccination rates in travelers. *Preventive Medicine*. 2004: 38: pp. 503-509(7).

[5] Kwon H-S, Choa J-H, Kima H-S, Lee J-H, Song B-R, Oh J-A, Han J-H, Kim H-S, Cha B-Y, Lee K-W, Son H-Y, Kang S-K, Lee W-C, Yoon K-H. Development of web-based diabetic patient management system using short message service (SMS). *Diabetes Research and Clinical Practice*. 2004: 66 : pp. 133-137(5).

[6] Gómez E, Hernando M, García A, Del Pozo F, Cermeño J, Corcoy R, Brugués E, De Leiva A. Telemedicine as a tool for intensive management of diabetes: the DIABTel experience. *Computer Methods and Programs in Biomedicine*. 2002: 69: pp. 163–177(15).

[7] EU. Directive on privacy and electronic communications 2002/58/EC. (10 Jan 2005.) Available at http://europa.eu.int/eur-lex/pri/en/oj/dat/2002/l_201/l_20120020731en00370047.pdf.

[8] Kibbe D. HIPAA privacy and security regulations. *The Case Manager*. 2001: 12: pp. 34-39(6).

[9] Siemens SMTK Programmer's Reference Manual, Version 4.2 Siemens AG, 10/2004 (3 Jan 2005) Available at http://communication-market.siemens.de/

[10] Hassinen M. SafeSMS 1.0 user manual. October 2004, Department of Computer Science, University of Kuopio. http://www.cs.uku.fi/mhassine/SafeSMS/Manual_en.pdf

[11] Sun Microsystems User Guide, Wireless Toolkit. Version 2.0. Java Platform, Micro Edition (3 Jan 2005) Available at http://java.sun.com/

[12] Hassinen M, Markovski S. SMS encryption using quasigroup encryption and Java SMS API. Proceedings of the Eighth Symposium on Programming Languages and Software Tools.

[13] J2ME API Documentation. Sun Microsystems Inc. (3 Jan 2005) Available at http://java.sun.com/

[14] Schneier B. Applied Cryprography. Protocols, algorithms and source code in C. Joh Wiley and Sons, Inc. 1996.

[15] Daemen J, Rijmen V. The Design of Rinjdael. Springer-Verlag. 2002.

Address for correspondence

Marko Hassinen, University of Kuopio, Department of Computer Science, P.O.B. 1627, Fin-70211 Kuopio, Finland Marko.Hassinen@uku.fi

Connecting Medical Informatics and Bio-Informatics
R. Engelbrecht et al. (Eds.)
IOS Press, 2005

Usability Study on Two Handheld Computers to Retrieve Drug Information

Simon Letellier[a, c], **Klervi Leuraud** [b], **Philippe Arnaud** [c], **Stefan J Darmoni**[a, b]

[a] *L@STICS, PSI laboratory, FRE CNRS 2645, Rouen University, France,*
[b] *Public health department, Rouen University Hospital, France,*
[c] *Pharmacy department, Rouen University Hospital, France.*

Abstract

Objective :Performing a usability study on two handheld computers (personal digital assistant and tablet PC), as tools for retrieving drug information.

Materials and methods: A randomised crossover study was performed: 34 students in pharmacy and medicine used the two handheld tools in a randomised order, to answer a questionnaire containing 12 questions covering all the aspects of a drug database and a qualitative analysis on six different items to measure access to drug information. The availability of the drug information database Vidal on PDA and on tablet PC implied our choice of the database. Three main criteria for evaluation were chosen: success rates, time-on-task, and number of clicks.

Results: There were no significant differences between the two groups neither on age, sex, medical discipline, study years nor previous computer practice. The success rate is significantly higher with the PDA for only one question. The PDA is significantly faster than the tablet PC on 7 of the 12 questions and generates fewer clicks for 3 questions. Compared to the tablet PC, it appears that the PDA is better in terms of clearness, navigability and usefulness for professional practice and it is the only tool which is significantly preferred to all other supports.

Conclusion: In this study with students, the PDA is significantly more effective quantitatively and qualitatively than the tablet PC to retrieve drug information.

Keywords:
Drug therapy, Computer assisted; Computers, Handheld; Ergonomics

1. Introduction

Since the last ten years, the handheld tools are diversified and numerous. Among them, the personal digital assistants (PDA) are already largely integrated into the professional and private life. They are used by the general population as well as the health community. Many physicians and pharmacists have integrated tools into their current bedside practice [1-2]. More recently, the tablet PC is a peculiar and new type of portable microcomputer. It did not reach yet neither all its applicability nor all the popularity which it may hope to reach. However, it already found a place of choice while being used at the bedside of patients in several French hospitals (Hospital European George Pompidou, Rouen University Hospital). The usability studies occupy an increasingly significant place in health informatics and telematics [1-2].

The objective of this study is to determine if there is a significant difference in use between the two handheld tools chosen, namely, the personal digital assistant and the tablet

PC, to retrieve drug information, and to measure, if there is any significant difference in their respective effectiveness.

2. Material and Methods

The Rouen Pharmacy and Medicine Faculty set up an evaluation of two of these handheld tools (PDA and the tablet PC) by a group of voluntary students in medicine and in pharmacy. The usability study was performed on the only French drug knowledge base available on these two tools, namely the Vidal® drug knowledge base. The Vidal accessible on the Tablet PC was the Intranet version of this drug knowledge base. This study was performed during a Master's degree of Medical Informatics (SL) [3].

The model of the study used as a starting point another usability study carried out in Rouen on the Doc'CISMeF search engine [4]. This previous study was a collaboration with the Lille Ev@lab [5], laboratory of ergonomics. The current study also benefits from a 12-year experience in the Rouen University Hospital (RUH) to access electronically the Vidal® drug knowledge base first on a mainframe [6] and later on the RUH Intranet.

This usability study was made on a test user without video recording. All the 34 participants are students in pharmacy and medicine. They were recruited on a voluntary basis. The participants had to fill a questionnaire inspired by another study in progress in the Lille laboratory of ergonomics.

This study has tested the three main aspects of usability : efficiency, effectiveness and satisfaction end-user. The principal criterion to measure the handheld tool efficiency is the success rate for each question of the questionnaire. The success is measured by finding the right answer to the question within a five-minute limit. Two secondary criteria were also selected to estimate the effectiveness of the handheld tool: time in seconds to answer one item of the questionnaire and the number of clicks to answer it. The final qualitative evaluation was used to estimate the user's satisfaction. After a development phase of the study, the evaluation were proceeded on two and half months (from February to April 2004). Thirty four students were included during this time period. Finally, the study was enclosed one month later after statistical analysis of the results.

The study is a prospective, randomised, cross-over study: any student which has participated in this study was his/her own witness. The order attribution of the handheld tools used by the students were chosen according to a randomisation table with two arms. The two arms defined in this study are: the PDA-TPC arm: answers to the questions series are initially required by using first the PDA and next the tablet PC (TPC). And the TPC-PDA arm : the answers to the questions series are initially required by using the tablet PC and secondly the PDA.

This study was an "in vitro" study, which took place in the conference room of the RUH Informatics and Networks Direction because it required a room provided with a wireless network and the handheld tools in the proximity, and furthermore it also needs silence to fill properly the questionnaire. That is why we preferred the choice of an in vitro study vs. an in vivo study in a clinical department, which was already feasible in 2004.

The sessions followed by each participant were carried out by the same trainer and appraiser and lasted each one approximately ninety minutes. The questionnaire of the study includes three parts. The first part checks the profile of the participant: their age, their previous practice in handheld tools use and on drug knowledge bases. The second part of the questionnaire is dedicated to the quantitative evaluation and comprises twelve questions which cover all the main aspects of the drug knowledge base. These questions were elaborated so that each one answers a given set of themes and a possible interrogation in clinical situation (e.g. question 9: Give the list of the drugs, which can be prescribed in case of onchocerciasis or question 5: you wanted to prescribe Nordazepam to a patient, who is intolerant to gluten. Is it possible?). The last part of the questionnaire relates to the qualitative evaluation.

The user's satisfaction of these two handheld tools are appreciated by the participants with five criteria: design, presentation clearness, navigability, and estimated utility of these tools to facilitate the daily professional practice. Each criterion was analysed distinctly by using a 5-point Likert scale: very bad, bad, well, very well and without opinion. Finally, it was requested from the participants to establish a preferential classification of the drug databases available in French among six drug databases: Vidal PDA, Vidal Tablet PC on Intranet, Vidal Intranet via a "regular" microcomputer, Vidal on Internet (URL: www.vidal.fr), Vidal as paper textbook, and finally another drug database Theriaque (URL: www.theriaque.org), mostly used by pharmacists.

The data on the participants profile are compared between the two arms of the study (Wilcoxon nonparametric test for the age, Fisher test or chi-square test for the qualitative variables). A possible influence of evaluated by the Wilcoxon nonparametric test, as well as the possible influence of the preliminary knowledge of the PDA on the number of successes by PDA. The binary criterion of judgement (success/failure) was then evaluated for each of the twelve questions by the methods specific to the cross-over studies: interaction study between the support (PDA or T.PC) and the order (PDA-T.PC arm or T.PC-PDA arm), then study of the support effect. In the absence of interaction, the comparison between the two supports was carried out on the whole of the data by a Mc-Nemar test. In the other case, only the data of the evaluation first period were analyzed by a Fisher test.

The criterion "response time" was analysed by similar methods but specific to the continuous variables (Wilcoxon nonparametric test on the time differences during the two periods of evaluation if there is no interaction, and Wilcoxon test over time during the evaluation first period if there is an interaction). For the students having given up a search before the five-minute limit, time corresponding was fixed at five minutes. The criterion "numbers of clicks" was evaluated by the same methods for the criterion " response time" but for the only questions where all the students answered successfully for the two supports, in order to compare their ease of use. For these three criteria, a Bonferroni procedure was adopted to take account of the repetition of each criterion on the various questions. Was the degree of significance, p, thus regarded as significant for an two-tailed 5% error if $p \leq 0.050$ is divided by the number of questions (twelve for the binary criterion and for the time, i.e. $p < 0.004$).

The qualitative criteria of evaluation (design, presentation clearness, navigability, and estimated utility of these tools to facilitate the daily professional practice) were evaluated by the sign nonparametric test (paired comparisons) and the criterion "preference" was evaluated by the Friedman's nonparametric test. For these criteria, the degree of significance, p, was regarded as significant for a 5 % two-tailed error if $p \leq 0.050$. The whole statistical analyses were carried out using SAS software.

3. Results

The compared analysis of the two arms populations of the study highlights no significant difference on sex, mean age, studied discipline and university level (pharmacy or medicine). No effect of the preliminary knowledge about the tablet PC or VidalCIM® could be highlighted on the successes number. Of the same Tablet PC, no effect of the knowledge of the PDA could not be highlighted on the number of successes by PDA. An effect of the knowledge of VidalPDA® could not be tested: the study counts only two preliminary users of VidalPDA®. The interaction between the order and the support on the twelve questions (Fisher's exact test, significant difference for an 5% error if $p \leq 0.004$) was tested beforehand. No interaction was highlighted. In the absence of interaction, the handheld tools then could be compared with a McNemar's test (significant difference for an 5% error if $p \leq 0.004$) This test is based on the analysis of the unmatched pairs of results. Thus only three questions comprised unmatched pairs and were testable. The order and support interaction was carried out beforehand on the twelve questions (Wilcoxon's test, significant difference for a 5% error if $p=0.004$) about the time criterion. Except for Question 9, for the main criterion of this study "success rate for each question of the questionnaire", there is no significant difference between PDA and Tablet PC. For Question 9, the PDA has a significant better success rate; (Tablet PC success rate (SR) = 18% when randomised first and 18% when randomised second ; PDA success rate (SR) = 71% when randomised first and 100% when randomised second; $p<0.001$ using the Bonferroni procedure).

For the criterion "time in seconds to answer one item of the questionnaire", the PDA was significantly faster than the Tablet PC for 7 out of the 12 items of the questionnaire while Tablet PC were never significantly faster than PDA (e.g. for question 2: average time in seconds for Tablet PC = 54.3 ± 23.29 when randomised first and 40.71 ± 15.93 when randomised second; average time in seconds for PDA = 39.94 ± 31.43 when randomised first and 21,47 ± 5,38 when randomised second; $p<0.0001$ using the Bonferroni procedure).

For the criterion "number of clicks", only 4 items were testable, where all the students answered successfully on the two tools, and are tested in order to compare the ease of use of these tools. The Wilcoxon test highlights significant differences for each one of these questions. A less number of clicks are significantly necessary for three questions with the PDA compared with the tablet PC. For one question, a less number of clicks are significantly necessary with the tablet PC compared with the PDA.

For three out of four qualitative criteria (presentation clearness, navigability and assistance to the daily professional practice), the PDA was significantly better rated (see Table 1). No significant difference was found for the criterion "Design".

Table 1: Good quality of navigability?

	Disagree	More or less disagree	More or less agree	Agree	No opinion
	% (n)	% (n)	% (n)	% (n)	% (n)
PDA	2.9% (1)	2,.% (1)	17.6% (6)	76.5% (26)	0% (0)
Tablet .PC	0% (0)	29.4% (10)	55.9% (19)	14.7% (5)	0% (0)

$p<0,001$, sign test

The Friedman test analyses all the six drug knowledge bases proposed to the thirty four participants (see Table 2). If the test highlights a difference, the tools can then classified according to their mean score. Once classified and according to their classification order, a sign test is applied for a two by two test. The analysis of the user's choice with the sign test highlights a significant difference between Vidal on PDA and Vidal on the tablet PC ($p<0.0001$ using the Bonferroni procedure). Furthermore, Vidal on PDA is significantly preferred by the users vs. the four other bases. For the five others, no significant difference has been found, although there is trend between Vidal on Tablet PC vs. Vidal on "regular" PC using Intranet.

Table 2: Distribution of user preferences among six drug knowledge bases

	First choice	Second choice	Third choice	Fourth choice	Fifth choice	Sixth choice	Mean score
Vidal on PDA	23	8	3	0	0	0	5.82
Vidal on Tablet PC	4	10	10	9	1	0	4.09
Vidal on Intranet	1	7	9	11	6	0	3.65
Vidal on paper	4	6	4	8	7	5	3.32
Theriaque	2	3	6	3	8	12	2.59
Vidal.fr	0	0	2	3	12	17	1.76

$p < 0.001$, test de Friedman

4. Discussion

As far as we know, there is no published usability study on French drug knowledge base. Nonetheless, the Evalab laboratory of ergonomics is already working on another usability study with the Vidal drug knowledge base. Since the end of the study in May 2004, Vidal is not anymore the only drug knowledge base which is available on the handheld tools chosen in this study: the Banque Claude Bernard is now available on Intranet via tablet PC and on PDA. Therefore, a similar study may be performed with this drug knowledge base.

Our current study has nonetheless a serious bias: although we previously checked that the Vidal version on PDA and Tablet PC may give for each item of the questionnaire the right answer, these two drug knowledge bases are nonetheless different, specially in terms of ergonomics. Furthermore, Vidal on PDA seems to have better functionalities, which may explain some of the results (i.e. its start page has a reduced content and is stripped to the essential: the entrance points are specific and without stepping). Moreover, turn back to this page is done with a simple click from any consulted page. Nonetheless, its use remained relatively low in France because of its cost, of its limited content, and its target: PDA users of health professionals. In this direction, critical opinions of users in 2002 [10], were formulated on the cost, the poverty of the content, but also ergonomics, and the dependence of this Vidal® version to Mobipocket Reader®. The result obtained with the tablet PC has to be moderated because of its future possibilities of improvement are significant particularly in weight, autonomy, ergonomics, and support of wireless networks. This tool has already invested the patient bedside in the United States [3] as well as several hospitals in France (George Pompidou European Hospital, Toulouse, Rouen). It makes it possible to transport all the possibilities of the hospital information systems in the health professionals' arms, and to work directly with electronic patient record. It allows also the handling of the heavy electronic documents such as those of the medical imaging and has much less limit of memory, access real time, and storage capacity vs. the PDA capabilities.

This study made it possible to determine the current limits of usability of these two handheld tools to access the Vidal® knowledge bases. The tablet PC, and its drug knowledge base has significant possibilities for improvement. In fact, this knowledge base until now was primarily conceived for a use on a desktop PC. So a tablet PC equipped with Vidal on PDA version would seem more adapted to an effective search but would be deprived of the possibilities of communication and interoperability of this support as well as hospital resources like the therapeutic book. Beyond, a more thorough evaluation could be undertaken to measure the use of Vidal in its integrated version into the hospital information system; this would need an vivo study rather than the in vitro study described here.

Conclusion: In a population of students in pharmacy and medicine, the PDA is a more effective tool on the quantitative and qualitative aspects than the tablet PC to retrieve drug information.

6. References

[1] Cohn WF, Detmer W, Fagan G, Bolick R, Methods for Evaluating Handheld and Wireless Point-of-Care Clinical Reference Tools, Medinfo. 2004;2004(CD):1558.

[2] Kushniruk A, Triola M, Stein B, Borycki E, Kannry J, The relationship of usability to medical error: an evaluation of errors associated with usability problems in the use of a handheld application for prescribing medications. Medinfo. 2004:1073-6.

[3] Letellier S. Usability study on two handheld computers to retrieve drug information: Tablet PC vs. PDA. Master of Medical Informatics, Paris, July 2004 (pp 38).

[4] LeBeux P., Duff F., Fresnel A., Berland Y., Beuscart R., Burgun A., Brunetaud JM., Chatellier G., Darmoni SJ., Duvauferrier R., Fieschi M., Gillois P., Guille F., Kohler F., Pagonis D., Pouliquen B., Soula G., Weber J., The French Virtual Medical University. In: Proceedings of MIE 2000, Sixteenth International Congress of the European Federation for Medical Informatics, Hanover, Germany Stud Health Technol Inform. 2000;77:554-62.

[5] Beuscart MC., Leroy N., Alao O., Darmoni SJ., Usability Study of a Medical Resources Web Site. In: Proceedings of MIE 2002, Seventeenth International Congress of the European Federation for Medical Informatics, Stud Health Technol Inform. 2002;90:133-137.

[6] Darmoni SJ., Massari P., Dufour F., Arnoudts S., Dieu B., Alizon B., Hantute F., Baldenweck M., Consultation du Vidal® Electronique au CHU de Rouen. Télématique et Médecine, Quatrièmes Journées Francophones d'Informatique Médicale, Bruxelles, Belgique, juin 1993. (URL: http://www.chu-rouen.fr/dsii/publi/vidmie.html)

[7] Leroy N., Sites web médicaux spécialisés: VIDAL®, EV@LAB, Octobre 2003 (URL: http://www.univ-lille2.fr/evalab/fp/vidal.htm).

[8] Wilkerson C., Medical Tablet PC, (http://www.medicaltableTPC.com)

[9] SAS/STAT® User's Guide, Version 8, Cary, NC:SAS Institute Inc., 1999 (http://v8doc.sas.com/sashtml)

[10] Thera.info, VidalPDA: revue du produit, 2002 (http://thera.info/archives/dossiers)

Address for correspondence

SJ. Darmoni, MD, PhD
Professor of Medical Informatics, Rouen Medical School
Laboratoire PSI - FRE CNRS 2645
Information & Communication Technologies, Public Health Department,
Rouen University Hospital, 1 rue de Germont, 76031 Rouen Cedex, France
Tel: +33.232.88.88.29; Fax: +33.232.88.88.32
Email: Stefan.Darmoni@chu-rouen.fr
URL: www.chu-rouen.fr/cismef & www.univ-rouen.fr/medecine & www.univ-rouen.fr/psi/

Connecting Medical Informatics and Bio-Informatics
R. Engelbrecht et al. (Eds.)
IOS Press, 2005

The Digital Pen and Paper Technology: Implementation and Use in an Existing Clinical Information System

Christelle Despont-Gros, Christophe Bœuf, Antoine Geissbuhler, Christian Lovis

University Hospitals of Geneva, Service of Medical Informatics, Switzerland

Abstract

Objective: *Evaluation of the technical feasibility of tight integration of the digital pen and paper technology in an existing computerized patient record.*
Technology: *The digital pen is a normal pen able to record all actions of the user and to analyze a micro pattern printed on the paper. The digital paper is a normal paper printed with an almost invisible micro pattern of small dots encoding information such as position and identifiers. We report our experience in the implementation and the use of this technology in an existing large clinical information system for acquiring clinical information.*
Discussion: *It is possible to print uniquely identified forms using the digital paper technology. These forms can be pre-filled with clinical readable information about the patient. When care providers complete these forms using the digital pen, it is possible to acquire the data in a structured computerized patient record. The technology is easy to integrate in a component-based architecture based on Web Services.*
Conclusion: *The digital pen and paper is a cost-effective technology that can be integrated in an existing clinical information system and allows fast and easy bedside clinical information acquisition without the need for an expensive infrastructure based on traditional portable devices or wireless devices.*

Keywords
Digital pen and paper, bedside clinical information acquisition, computerized patient record, human-machine interfaces

1. Introduction

Access to clinical reference information at the point-of-care is a goal that is difficult to achieve by lack of really portable devices. There are many problems that must be addressed when trying to tackle bedside data acquisition, such as global costs, wireless connections, robustness of devices, weight, size, duration of batteries, size of the screen, usability of the acquisition methods (touch pad, keyboard, sensitive screen, …) and cultural acceptance [1], amongst others. By far, the pen and the paper remain the most cost-effective, efficient and easy to use means for acquiring data. The handwriting data acquisition paradigm remains the most adapted in several clinical contexts, mostly because of the mobility of care providers [2]. The transfer of handwritten data into the computerized patient record (CPR) requires digitalizing the paper. This operation can rarely be achieved in real time, and does not provide access to structured data. In addition, it does not allow direct feedback to care providers. Currently, several mobile devices allowing bedside data acquisition are used in clinical settings [3]. They are usually based on PDA's or notebook technologies, including tablet PC's. However, these devices suffer several defaults. The smallest devices are really portable but have very small screens [4] and the larger devices are often heavy. Most of them have short battery life, especially if connected using a wireless network. In addition, these devices are expensive, especially if used in large settings, and are often accompanied with crucial maintenance problems, both for hardware and software.

In Fall 2003, the University Hospitals of Geneva (HUG) had the opportunity to evaluate, in real clinical situation, a beta pre-commercial release of a package, including a digital pen developed by Logitech®, digital paper using a micro pattern of dots developed by Anoto® and a forms and pen management system, the Forms Automation System (FAS), developed by Hewlett Packard®. This technology was tested in two clinical settings with the objectives of evaluating technical integrability, data acquisition reliability and acceptance of users according to both technical aspects and human factors. The assessment of data acquisition reliability and acceptance of users are out of the scope of this paper and are available separately [5]. The objective of this paper is to present our experience in implementing and integrating concretely this new technology in our CPR.

2. Background

The HUG is a consortium of primary, secondary and tertiary care facilities employing 5'000 care providers, with approximately 2'000 beds and managing over 45'000 admissions and 450'000 outpatients encounters each year. The Service of Medical Informatics, in addition to its teaching and research activities, is responsible of the clinical information system (CIS), including the design, development and support of tools and processes for the institutional management of medical knowledge, the computerized patient record and a general medical order entry system. The CIS is a Java based 3-tiers architecture using event-driven processes and interoperability with Web Services. More than 20'000 patient records are open every day in the CIS.

2.1 Clinical context: Post-natal care in Obstetric Anaesthesia (PNC)

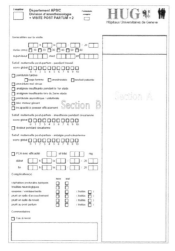

Figure 1: The PNC form

Since July 2001, the anaesthetists evaluated the anaesthetic complications and maternal satisfaction after labour analgesia in the labour room using a paper form. The data collection is performed in two parts corresponding respectively to one of the two columns of the form: a) data about the labour and the delivery, that is pre-printed on the form and comes from the CPR (Figure 1, Section B); b) data relative to the "post partum", which is filled within the next 72 hours of follow up care using the form (Figure 1, Section A).

Since July 2003, a web application allowed acquisition of clinical information pertaining to labour and delivery (Figure 2, PFAnesthesio). This data is usually collected before and during the labour. Normal PC and wireless laptops are available. Within the next 72 hours, the form is printed with this data, and the second part about post-natal care is filled during visits to mothers performed by an anaesthetist, sometimes scattered in several wards. The filled forms are scanned after discharge of the patient to allow data to be transferred in the CPR. When enough forms are entirely filled, an operator collects them and processes a scanning with human-assisted optical character recognition. Only single character fields, such as check-boxes, are reliably recognized. For ambiguous situations, the operator decides which value is correct. This process respects the standards imposed to all CIS in HUG: a secure user authentication and a traceability of the requests and actions performed.

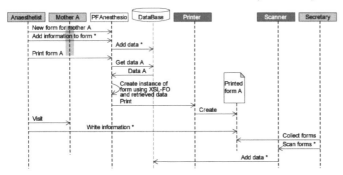

Figure 2: workflow of data acquisition before the DPP trial
"*" means that the request or action can be performed several times

2.2   The DPP technology

The DPP combines mainly three components: a) a HP colour LaserJet Printer with specific drivers; b) a HP software package; c) a Digital Pen with a specific firmware. By the time of the study, all components were in alpha or beta release and not available commercially.

2.2.1   The form: printer drivers, document and the "digital" pattern

When the form is printed, using the dedicated driver, a layer of a slight pattern of black dots is also printed. This layer, using a technology developed by Anoto®, identifies the function of the paper and encodes much information, such as unique ID and 2D position. It allows the pen to record the cursive information, including speed; direction acceleration etc. For the CPR, it is important to ensure an unambiguous association between the pattern, that is the document identification, and the patient whose information has been printed on the document. The pattern allows such kind of unique identification of printed sheets. Only a subset of HP colour LaserJet printers are certified for printing these patterns, which requires extreme precision. In addition to the standard driver of the printer, a digital driver allows to establish a link with a Paper Lookup Server (PLS). This server, which has to be installed first, allows storing the clinical context and the distributed patterns, and ensures the link between clinical contexts and patterns. This is important to be able to reliable link a paper form to a computer clinical session. When a user requests a print of a digital form, the driver sends a request to get an instance of pattern associated to the corresponding clinical form. The PLS stores a) the context received from the CIS, in our case a unique ID identifying the encounter; b) a unique form identifier, and c) the unique ID created for the new pattern to be printed with the form. This pattern is printed with the document and will be recognized by the digital pen. The pattern is made out of very small black dots resulting in a slightly off-white colour. It is almost not visible and gives a slight grey appearance to the paper and can identify categories of paper, such as post-it or notes, or unique documents. The technology developed by Anoto can manage several billion of unique patterns. To increase discrimination of the pen's camera between the pattern and the layout of the form, the black colour is reserved to the pattern. Therefore, layout or any information devoted to human reading on the form has to be printed in another colour, generally blue, but a complete colour palette is provided by HP. The paper used in our study was a standard recycled paper in accordance to HUG requirements, judged as a bad quality paper by experts of HP. However, it is not proved that the paper quality was implied in problems encountered during data acquisition.

2.2.2   The HP software package

In addition to the PLS, several components are required to allow a fine-tuned integration between the existing CPR and the DPP technology. The most important components are a) a plug-in added to Adobe Acrobat® to design forms; b) a toolbox that allows the development of services and the transfer of structured data on the form to web services, and c) several management tools for users and administrators. For care providers, the package includes a tool for validating data transferred and for the identification of users. The tools for administrators allow linking a service with a form, registering and managing users and pens as well as linking specific pens with users. A complete trace is available. The plug-in added to Acrobat allows to design forms. For the form designer, the operation consists to draw an area above each structured field of the form and defines its type, such as Boolean, free text, etc. A unique ID must be assigned to each area, which will be associated with the information recognized by the pens. In addition the pattern area is drawn encompassing all the fields that have to be digitalized. When the form is ready, it must be linked with the corresponding service. The toolbox provided by HP allows to access all information transmitted by pens, but does not process the data nor establishes the link with the existing CPR. In order to get the correct data in its corresponding field in our CPR's database, we had to develop an application service handler (ASH). This has been done using JAVA, but it is not mandatory. The granularity of data recorded by pens allows the access to every single elements corresponding to one sample (see next section), including unique ID of the form, coordinates of the pattern area defined before, timing in millisecond, information from the pressure captor and the ID of the pen used to fill the area. It is also possible to access to consolidated data, where all single points are grouped into strokes, defined as a cursive path performed without pressure interruption. Strokes have a start time (pen down), an end time (pen up), and belong to a field of the form. If a unique form has been filled with several pens, it is possible to reconstitute the consolidated result. The system can be linked to an Intelligent Character Recognition (ICR) system to recognize handwriting.

2.2.3   The Digital Pen

The digital pen contains a standard ink cartridge, a camera, a communication unit, a pressure captor, an image processing unit, a storage unit and a battery. All these components result in a bigger and somewhat bulkier pen than usual. The camera, placed under the ink cartridge, is able to record 50 frames per second. When the pressure captor detects that the ink cartridge is in contact with the paper, the camera samples the position of the pen on the paper using the pattern. Less than 2 square millimetres are needed for the pen to localize its position, whatever the entry place, direction or angle. For each sample, the pen stores at least the pattern, the coordinates, the timing. The pen stores up to 40 handwritten pages between transfers and one full power charge allows writing up to 25 full pages. A led located on its side indicates the battery charge and the status. The activation of the pen is ensuring by the cap which acts as power switch. The pen is able to emit vibrations to provide feedback to users, for example when the pen is unable to recognize the pattern. A digital pen can only interact with patterns groups that are part of its "writing domain", which might be only one form. When docked, the pen will only transmit data if a validation box on the form has been checked. A form will be saved every time that box is checked, allowing multiple save operations. Once docked in its USB cradle, the PLS is called with information of every patterns for which data has to be transmitted. The server retrieves the context and a pointer to the ASH allowing data to be correctly processed. Validated data is automatically transmitted to server. Each pen validates its own data and several pens and users can contribute to a unique given form simultaneously or with time intervals. Data is merged when it is transferred, and at each transfer forms will be consolidated if needed.

2.3   Details of the implementation of the DPP in the CIS

There are two important steps to implement the system: a) installation of all components, required only once and b) development of the ASH for each form to be linked with existing databases. We used the following environments:

For development:
- Windows 2000 Server SP3 or Windows 2000 Advanced Server SP3
- Microsoft SQL Server 2000 SP3, Standard or Enterprise Edition
- Sun Java 2 SDK, Standard Edition 1.4.1_01 or later
- Apache Tomcat 4.1.18 or later

For production:
- Solaris 9
- Oracle 8
- BES or WebObjects application servers

For clients:
- Windows 2000 Professional SP3 or Windows XP Professional SP1
- Microsoft Internet Explorer 5.01 SP2 or 6.0 SP1

As already mentioned, the ASH was developed in JAVA, to meet the production requirements. It has been developed using a Servlet called when a pen requests a transfer. For all simple types, such as lists and checkboxes, the toolbox gives a direct access to the value of the field. For text fields, using the SDK, pen data can easily be transform in two picture formats: BMP and SVG (vector). We used both and stored them.

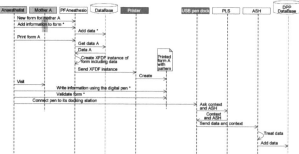

Figure 3: workflow of data acquisition during the DPP study
"*" means that the request or action can be performed several times

Before the DPP study, PDF forms including existing data were generated using XSL-FO

(Figure 2). During the DPP study, the technology requires the registration of the PDF file generated with the plug-in to the PLS. This file is stored on the server and linked with the corresponding ASH. Patient data must then be merged with this file, using XFDF. The printer driver manages directly XFDF files and includes data in the corresponding PDF descriptor file when printing.

2.4 Acquisition quality and satisfaction of users

The scan system has been maintained during the study to compare the reliability of data acquisition (path not represented in Figure 3). The DPP technology proved to be as reliable as OCR using a professional scanner without human intervention. Acquisition errors only occurred for specific fields when the design of the form was badly adapted to the technology. Quality surveys as well as a complete user satisfaction study have been conducted [5]. The DPP appears to be a well accepted technology.

3. Conclusions

The DPP is a promising technology that proved to be easy to integrate with an existing CIS, using new technologies such as JAVA and Web Services. One major inconvenience of the technology is the need to print using colour printers, in order to increase discrimination of the camera of the pen between human-readable information and the pattern devoted to the DPP technology. Structured data originating from single state fields, such as checkboxes and radio buttons, or scales, are immediately addressable to store in a relational databases. Handwriting, for letters and numbers, must be processed with a third-part OCR or ICR.

The data acquisition reliability proved to be similar to a professional scanning system, with the great advantage of mobility and direct acquisition at the bedside. Care providers have been enthusiastic at using this technology, with criticisms towards the ergonomy of the pen that are addressed with new versions of the system.

4. Acknowledgments

This work has been funded by the Swiss National Science Foundation 632-066041 and the Geneva University Hospital, PRD 03-I-05

5. References

[1] Kaplan B. Evaluating informatics applications--some alternative approaches: theory, social interactionism, and call for methodological pluralism. *Int J Med Inf* 2001;64(1):39-56.
[2] Sicotte C, Denis JL, Lehoux P. The computer based patient record: a strategic issue in process innovation. *J Med Syst* 1998;22(6):431-43.
[3] Wilcox RA, La Tella RR. The personal digital assistant, a new medical instrument for the exchange of clinical information at the point of care. *Med J Aust* 2001;175(11-12):659-62.
[4] Lapinsky SE, Wax R, Showalter R, Martinez-Motta JC, Hallett D, Mehta S, et al. Prospective evaluation of an internet-linked handheld computer critical care knowledge access system. *Crit Care* 2004;8(6):R414-21.
[5] Despont-Gros C, Landau R, Rutschmann O, Simon J, Lovis C. The digital pen and paper: evaluation and acceptance of a new data acquisition device in clinical settings. *Methods of Information in Medecine*;Accepted in 2004.

Address for correspondence

Christelle Despont-Gros, Hôpitaux Universitaires de Genève, Service d'Informatique Médicale (SIM), 21, rue Micheli-du-Crest, CH-1211 Genève 4, Switzerland, christelle.despont@sim.hcuge.ch

Connecting Medical Informatics and Bio-Informatics
R. Engelbrecht et al. (Eds.)
IOS Press, 2005

Wireless Transfer of Sensor Data into Electronic Health Records

Ole Anders Walseth[a], Eirik Årsand[a], Torbjørn Sund[b], Eva Skipenes[a]

[a]*Norwegian Centre for Telemedicine, Tromsø, Norway*
[b]*Telenor R&D, Oslo, Norway*

Abstract

The purpose of this study is to explore how wireless transfer of sensor data can be implemented in existing Electronic Health Record (EHR) systems. Blood glucose data from people with diabetes Type 1 has been selected as the case.
As proof of concept, a prototype for sending blood glucose measurements into an EHR system was developed for the DIPS EHR system. For the prototype to be transferable to a general setting, care was taken not to introduce any additional workload for the diabetes nurses or the diabetes Type 1 patients. In the prototype, the transfer of blood glucose data is automatic and invisible to the user, and the data is presented to the nurses within the existing DIPS laboratory module.
To determine whether deployment of such a system would present any risks or hazards to patients (medical or financial), a risk analysis was performed. The analysis indicates that storing blood glucose values in the patient's EHR does not represent any significantly increased risks for the diabetes patient.
The study shows that existing EHR systems are well suited to receive sensor data. The three main EHR systems in Norwegian hospitals are all supported with application programming interfaces (APIs), enabling external vendors to add modules. These APIs are sufficient to implement modules for receiving sensor data. However, none of the systems currently have commercially available modules for receiving such data.

Keywords:
Blood glucose sensor, Diabetes, Diabetes nurse, Diabetes management system, EHR, Electronic health record, Risk analysis

1. Introduction

In the case of a chronic disease such as diabetes, much of the responsibility for managing the disease falls on the patient. When diagnosed, the patient is given a certain amount of initial training and information, but throughout the lifelong course of the illness it is primarily up to the patient to maintain the discipline required to keep blood glucose levels within recommended levels.

Monitoring and control of blood glucose levels are critical in the management of diabetes Type 1 to minimize long-term complications, and people with diabetes Type 1 may need to measure their blood glucose level several times a day [1,2]. Blood glucose measurements are performed by applying a single drop of blood to a measurement strip in a blood glucose monitor.

Norwegian health services put together diabetes teams, combining the skills of different professionals, to help and support patients with diabetes. A diabetes team may include doctors, diabetes nurses, secretaries, dieticians and paediatricians. If patients have poorly controlled diabetes they may require extensive, often continuous, follow-up, while well-regulated patients may require as little as one visit every six to twelve months.

The routines and strategies for storing and maintaining patient information vary between different diabetes teams and health services. The information may be stored on paper health records, in Electronic Health Record (EHR) systems or both. Some hospitals even use special software for storing diabetes health record information. The trend, however, is for health-related information to be collected in fewer and larger systems.

Electronic Health Care Records in Norwegian hospitals

During the last years there has been a considerable increase in the use of EHR systems in Norwegian hospitals. While only 36 % of Norwegian hospitals had implemented EHR systems in 1999, this percentage had reached 84% in 2003 [3].

The Norwegian Centre for Informatics in Health and Social Care (KITH) is responsible for the Norwegian EHR standard. The standard is not mandatory, but the various health sectors may require EHR vendors to comply with certain parts of the standard. The standard is technology independent.

The three main providers of EHR systems for Norwegian hospitals are Siemens (Doculive), DIPS ASA (DIPS) and Tieto Enator (Infomedix). In 2001 the KVALIS project [4] conducted a survey on how Norwegian hospitals use these systems in clinical tasks. This study concludes that "doctors use electronic medical record systems for far fewer tasks than the systems supported" but for the task of "following results of a test or investigation over time" most doctors use the EHR system or other computer software if available.

Hospitals with an EHR system licence often tailor the EHR system to fit the individual hospital's needs. Since smaller hospitals tend to have fewer or less complex needs, such hospitals are often pioneers in taking full advantage of EHR use [4].

This study investigates the feasibility of wireless input and long-term storage in Norwegian EHR systems of routinely collected diabetes data by the patients themselves.

2. Materials and methods

The three main EHR vendors in Norway were asked about the possibility for their systems to receive and use wireless sensor data, and we visited the software division of two of these vendors. We also had contact with external vendors making add-on modules for the EHR systems. Diabetes nurses at four different hospitals were interviewed to provide information on current diabetes practice and how they would prefer diabetes data presented in the EHR system.

The DIPS EHR system was selected to develop and test a prototype for wireless transfer of blood glucose values from patients.

Through collaboration with NR (the Norwegian Computing Centre), we performed a risk analysis. The purpose of this analysis was to investigate whether wireless transfer of blood glucose data from diabetes Type 1 patients into EHR systems is feasible and whether such a system presents any risks or hazards to the patients (medical or financial).

3. Results

The diabetes nurses who were interviewed said they would prefer to have the blood glucose values presented as a list. They said that it was easier to see the actual values when they were presented this way, and that it was faster for them to read a list than to interpret graphs or pie charts since they were used to traditional paper-based lists. However, data presented as pie charts and graphs were also found to be useful. [5]

Wireless transfer of sensor data into Electronic Health Records

The three main EHR systems in Norwegian hospitals are all supported with application programming interfaces (APIs), enabling external vendors to add modules. This makes it possible for smaller or specialised companies to make software that extends or communicates with the EHR. The APIs are openly available for the Infomedix and the DocuLive EHR systems and licensed for the DIPS EHR system. All three EHR APIs contain sufficient functionality to receive and manage the sensor data applied in our prototype.

Chosen EHR system

To develop a prototype for wireless transfer of blood glucose data from diabetes Type 1 patients into an EHR system, we collaborated with DIPS ASA. The company provided access to a DIPS EHR server, complete with a set of fictitious patients, DIPS client software as well as support and technical help. The program for storing blood glucose measurements in DIPS was developed using the DIPS API, which is a COM+ interface. The DIPS API provides functions for creating and updating patient information, lab results, lab requisitions and documents. The interface also includes various search functions.

The prototype

The prototype for wireless transfer of blood glucose data into the DIPS EHR system is a further development of an NST prototype where an in-house developed Bluetooth unit automatically transfers blood glucose values from a OneTouch Ultra blood glucose monitor to a Nokia 7650 mobile phone using a Bluetooth connection [6], and where these data are sent from the mobile phone as an SMS to a preset phone number.

The only part of this process visible to the user is when the diabetes patient measures his/her blood glucose level using the blood glucose monitor.

When the blood glucose monitor is switched off after the measurement, the NST Bluetooth unit is automatically switched on and stays active for 3 minutes. If the Nokia 7650 mobile phone is within Bluetooth range (10 meter) a connection will automatically be established, and the last blood glucose measurement will be transferred. If the Nokia 7650 is not within range (or turned off), the blood glucose measurements taken will be sent the next time the Bluetooth unit is turned on and the phone is within range.

When the Nokia 7650 receives the blood glucose value from the patient, the phone will automatically send the measurement as a SMS to a preset phone number. In this study we have configured the Nokia 7650 to send the measurement data to a PC equipped with a Nokia D211 phone card. The measurement data received at the D211 server contains the blood glucose values together with the date and time of the measurement.

The D211 server runs a small application that accesses an external DIPS server using the DIPS COM+ API over an Internet connection (the Norwegian Health Network in a real setting). The values are stored as lab results in the DIPS EHR laboratory module. Once a measurement is stored in the DIPS server, any DIPS client connected to the server can present it.

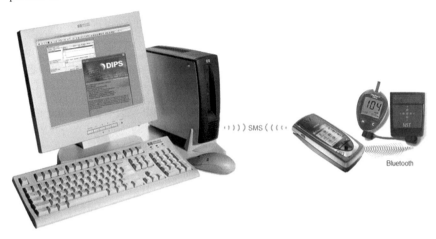

Figure 1 – Transfer of blood glucose measurements into the DIPS EHR system

The DIPS EHR client laboratory module is used to display lab results, and the blood glucose values can be displayed as a list of data or as a time graph.

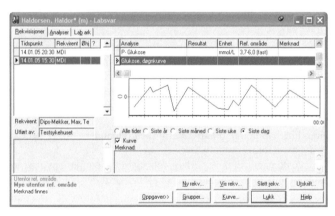

Figure 2 – The DIPS lab module displaying blood glucose values

Risk analysis

In Norway, diabetes patients are not highly stigmatised, and in the case of Type 1 diabetes, the disease is typically not something the patient would hide from his/her surroundings. It is even considered as an extra safety if the surroundings know that a person has Type 1 diabetes, due to the characteristics and consequences of potential low blood glucose values. The OneTouch Ultra blood glucose monitor used in the prototype stores the last 150 values (without any security measures), and the other parts of the prototype are not considered to make the data more accessible for the surroundings. The security for the data once they are stored in the EHR is ensured through the security of the EHR system.

In this context our findings suggest that blood glucose values are not highly sensitive. For the data to be of interest to somebody other than the patient and the hospital, the attacker probably needs to collect data for a certain period of time. The probability of such an attack is small, as would be the consequences.

Blood glucose data as described in the prototype are typically used as a tool for communication between diabetes nurses and patients. Today, the patient brings a handwritten diabetes diary or a computer printout of these values to discuss diabetes management with the diabetes nurse. It is also common for many patients to give an approximate of the values based on memory. Storing the measurements automatically will simplify this process, and should not introduce any new security issues. Loss of data or incorrect measurements may still occur (through hardware or software failure or through intentional manipulation by the user). The average blood glucose level of a patient is also measured through the HBA1c, and this serves as a security mechanism. The measurements provided by the prototype are not by themselves sufficient for providing medical advice.

The Norwegian jurisdiction on confidentiality of personal data is very strict. There are several laws and security requirements that must be followed, addressing issues such as documentation requirements, professional secrecy, privacy protection, disclosure requirements and information requirements. Applicable laws include the Personal Data Act, the Health Personnel Act and the Personal Health Data Filing System Act.

It seems likely that no extra safeguards need to be applied for blood glucose data compared with those necessary for other types of personal data, and security should be satisfied with any solution that complies with Norwegian legislation. Security safeguards include:

- The receiver of the information (blood glucose data) should be able to verify the identity of the sender.
- Sensitive personal data that are transferred electronically via a medium that is beyond the physical control of the responsible institution should be encrypted. SMS messages are encrypted over the radio link from the mobile phone to the GSM base station. The messages are transferred in plain text from the GSM base station through the telecommunication network or the Norwegian Health Network, but tracing these messages in the network is very difficult.
- The data received should be handled in a sufficiently secure manner with respect to confidentiality, integrity, availability and quality.
- In order to be able to make demands with regard to security of the equipment used by the patients, the health care institution should consider whether they should own the equipment.
- Communications (transfer of data) to or from the hospital should be fully controlled by the hospital.
- The blood glucose data should be protected against unauthorised access on the patient's side.

4. Discussion

Norway is approaching complete EHR coverage, and several hospitals are aiming to become totally paperless within the next few years. In order to gain the full benefits of this development, it is important that the EHR systems are not just electronic versions of the old paper-based health records, but take full advantage of the possibilities the new medium presents. EHR systems provide the possibility for automation of data retrieval, data structuring and data presentation. Transfer of sensor data from patients with chronic diseases is one such possibility [7].

In the case of diabetes Type 1, blood glucose data gathered automatically could support health personnel in helping and advising their patients in managing their disease. This function would also spare patients the trouble of keeping handwritten diabetes diaries. For an actual deployment of the system, SMS is probably too expensive. GPRS/3G should therefore be considered as an alternative for data transmission.

The concept can be applied to other settings, such as monitoring patient data at the patient's home and in some cases shortening hospital stays or eliminating the need for hospitalisation.

5. Conclusion

Our study suggests that transfer of sensor data into EHR systems is feasible with the current Norwegian EHR systems. A prototype has been implemented as proof of concept. The risk analysis suggests that the implemented prototype is sufficient for testing in an empirical trial. This is a possible continuation of the project and would help to further understand the usefulness of the concept in diabetes management.

6. Acknowledgments

We would like to thank DIPS ASA and our partners in the Wireless Health and Care project of which this study is a part: Abelia, IBM Norway, Memscap, Norwegian Computing Center, Rikshospitalet University Hospital, Sintef and Telenor R&D.

7. Reference

[1] Prospective Diabetes Study (UKPDS) Group U. Intensive blood-glucose control with sulphonylureas or insulin compared with conventional treatment and risk of complications in patients with type 2 diabetes (UKPDS33). The Lancet 1998;352(9131):837-853

[2] Prospective Diabetes Study (UKPDS) Group U. Effect of intensive blood-glucose control with metformin on complications in overweight patients with type 2 diabetes (UKPDS 34). Lancet North Am Ed. 1998;352(9131):854-865.

[3] Lars Erik Kjekshus. (2004) INTORG - De somatiske sykehusenes interne organisering (STF78 A045005) [online]. Available: http://www.hero.uio.no/publicat/2004/INTORG_Rapport_2004_190304.pdf [2005, January 12]

[4] Hallvard Lærum, Gunnar Ellingsen, Arild Faxvaag. (2001). Doctors' use of electronic medical records systems in hospitals: cross sectional survey. BMJ [Online], 323 (7325), 1344-1348, Available: bmj.bmjjournals.com [2005, January 12]

[5] Årsand E, Walseth OA, Skipenes E. Blood glucose data into Electronic Health Care Records for diabetes management. Øystein Nytrø. In Proceedings of the second HelsIT Conference at the Healthcare Informatics week in Trondheim, Norway, 21-22 September. Trondheim: Norwegian Centre for Electronic Patient Records; 2004;19-23.

[6] Norwegian Centre for Telemedicine. (2004). *Automatic transfer of blood glucose data from children with type 1 diabetes.* [Homepage of Norwegian Centre for Telemedicine], [Online]. Available: http://www.telemed.no/cparticle44523-4357b.html. [2005, January 13].

[7] Ramon Martí, Jaime Delgado. (2003). *Security in a Wireless Mobile Health Care System.* [homepage of TERENA Networking Conference]. [Online]. http://www.terena.nl/conferences/tnc2003/programme/papers/p8d3.pdf. [2003, May 29].

Address for correspondence

Ole Anders Walseth, Norwegian Centre for Telemedicine, University Hospital of North Norway.
E-mail: ole.anders.walseth@telemed.no. Telephone +47 416 68150

Connecting Medical Informatics and Bio-Informatics
R. Engelbrecht et al. (Eds.)
IOS Press, 2005

Integration Architecture of a Mobile Virtual Health Record for Shared Home Care

Maria Hägglund[a], Isabella Scandurra[a], Dennis Moström[b], Sabine Koch[a]

[a]*Uppsala University, Uppsala, Sweden,* [b]*Datavis Sverige AB, Örnsköldsvik, Sweden*

Abstract

The coexistence of different information systems that are unable to communicate with each other is a persistent problem in health care in general, and in shared care in particular. This is especially critical when it comes to information access needed at the point of care, e.g. in the patient's home. The purpose of this paper is to present the technical architecture of a virtual health record (VHR) that both integrates information from different electronic health records (EHRs) and allows for documenting at the point of care using mobile devices. The VHR supports a seamless information and communication flow between different care providers giving them mobile access to selected patient-oriented information. A service oriented system architecture where database functionality and services are separated has been implemented. This guarantees flexibility with regard to changed functional demands and allows third party systems to interact with the platform in a standardised way. Major requirements for the VHR have been documentation support at the point of care, integrated presentation of the information from different feeder systems, and the possibility of offline access to the data on handheld devices. Therefore, publishing was chosen for the integration design. A patient centred XML schema is published as an interface for integration with the information broker. The feeder systems deliver their information in XML.-files that are mapped against the ideal schema and inserted into the mediator database. The paper describes both an online web application and an offline solution that was implemented on personal digital assistants (PDAs). The system has been introduced in a Swedish home care district with an established fiber-optical network infrastructure connecting all the locations forming the study site.

Keywords:
Medical Records Systems, Computerized; Integrated Advanced Information Management Systems; Information Storage and Retrieval; Internet; Home Care Services; Nursing Record

1. Introduction

The coexistence of different information systems that are unable to communicate with each other is a persistent problem in health care. This becomes particularly obvious when the care of a patient is shared between different health care providers. Health care professionals from different organisations will then have to work together in a team-oriented way to provide high quality care for a patient. However, they rarely have access to a common IT-support or even access to basic information from each others systems. If the care is performed in a mobile environment, information access is needed at the point of care. Home care of elderly patients is a typical example [1]. In Sweden a shift in the responsibility for the domestic care of elderly and disabled people from the county councils to the municipalities is increasing shared care and the need for seamless and consistent information and communication flow. The growing number of senior citizens adds pressure to this situation, and tools for increasing the quality of care and supporting coordination and cooperation between the different care providers involved are greatly needed [2].

The electronic health record (EHR) is one of the most important tools of health care professionals, both as a source of information regarding a patient's health, and as a documentation tool [3]. It is however not likely that any single information system could ever cover all the needs of the different care providers [4]. An integrated version of the different EHRs from different care providers is needed to allow for adequate information access and documentation at the point of care. Such a Virtual Health Record (VHR) needs to gather the information needed from the different EHRs, or feeder systems, and to present it to the user in one view [5]. The view might differ depending on which user group is accessing the VHR, but the underlying structure and information source are the same. Moreover, the users' need to be able to document information at the point of care so as to spread the new information. Based on these conditions, the authors have developed a mobile VHR within the research project "Old@Home" [6]. It is the purpose of this paper to discuss the technical architecture of the VHR and its implementation.

2. Materials and methods

Technically, implementation is based on Microsoft .NET, using Biztalk Server 2004 as platform for information handling, SQL Server 2000 and SQL Server CE 2.0 for data storage, Sharepoint Portal Server for handling of Web-portals, and XML as format for data exchange. Microsoft Visual Studio.NET and .NET Compact Framework are used as developer platforms. Microsoft Authorization Manager (AZMAN) is used for handling of access rights.

The test site where the VHR has been implemented, and is currently being tested, has an established fiber optical network infrastructure connecting all the locations forming the study site: two primary care centers, the elderly patients' private homes and one nursing home for the elderly, from where the home care of elderly patients living in their private homes is coordinated. The VHR is used by the three main care provider groups involved in the home care of elderly citizens still residing in private homes: (1) general practitioners (GP) and (2) district nurses (DN), both employed by the county council and (3) home help service personnel (HHS), mainly assistant nurses, employed by the local authority (municipality).

2.1 Integration method

Two different methods for integration were considered when designing the technical platform; indexing and publishing. The major difference between the two methods is the place for storing the information. Indexing implies that the information remains within the data storage of the feeder system, i.e. the EHR, and the role of the integration functionality is to keep track of where the information is stored and how to access it. Each feeder system regularly sends updates of its index information, but the actual information is kept in its original storage. Publishing on the other hand means that there is a separate data storage in form of a mediator database to which the feeder systems publish the information agreed upon on a regular basis. Different types of information can have different timeframes. [7]

When indexing you know whom the information belongs to, and additional benefits are that the information is only stored in one place and that it is relatively easy to add or remove feeder systems. However, indexing requires that all feeder systems are online when the VHR requests information and it is most suitable for so called vertical integration, showing information from one feeder system at a time. The method is mainly used for accessing information, and not for interacting with or updating it. With publishing, issues of ownership and responsibility for the information stored in the mediator database are more complicated to handle. It is also more difficult to add new feeder systems, and a mapping process for each system is needed before the information can be stored in the mediator database. The benefits are that feeder systems need not to be online in order for the VHR-applications to access the information and it is easier to create a horizontal integration, showing information from several different feeder systems in one view. Furthermore, interaction with the feeder systems can be implemented, updated or added information in the VHR can be published back to the respective feeder system. In addition, information which is not available in the feeder systems, such as multimedia information or information used for communication between the different care providers can be stored.

Since major requirements for the VHR have been documentation support at the point of care, integrated presentation of the information from different feeder systems, and the possibility of offline access to the data on handheld devices [8] publishing was chosen for the integration design.

3. Results

We implemented a service oriented system architecture where database functionality and services are separated. This way we guarantee flexibility with regard to changed functional demands and allow third party systems to interact with the platform in a standardised way.

The VHR described here gathers information from three separate feeder systems, used by three different care provider categories. Each feeder system is accessed through a web service. The publishing of information from the feeder systems is triggered by the information broker requesting information about the patients currently listed in the VHR, and the web services deliver the information in an XML-file in a pre-defined format. The format of these XML-files varies depending on the feeder system. The variation in the XML-files structures makes it necessary to map them so the information can be stored in the mediator database. Therefore an ideal XML-schema has been developed within the project. The information broker maps the XML-files from the feeder systems against the ideal schema so that the information regarding each patient is changed to the format of the ideal schema. This information is then sent as input to a web service which inserts it to the mediator database.

Once the information is in the mediator database the health care professionals can access it through their VHR-applications. Each user category (GP, DN and HHS) has a specific view, giving them access only to the information they need and are allowed to read. Two types of applications have been developed; an online web application used by GP and DN, and an offline application for a handheld computer used by the HHS. Each handheld device has a local SQL CE 2.0 database to which the data to and from the mediator database is synchronised using server based filters configured according to the different users' roles. Rule based synchronization is to be implemented, meaning that if synchronization is requested at the point of care and no connection to the Internet is available the client will try GPRS. If the HHS walks into a hotspot area of WLAN the device uses the best performance/lowest cost connection seamlessly, and the device will also drop the connection to the WLAN if it is connected to the fiber optic network.

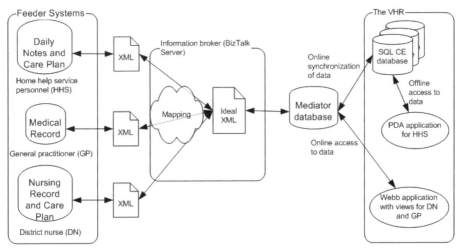

Figure 1: the integration architecture

3.1 Ideal schema

To reach flexibility towards existing feeder systems a patient centred XML schema for information exchange is exposed as a web service for connecting to the information broker. For selected patients, necessary information such as daily notes, prescription lists and care plans are fetched from the respective feeder system and sent to the information broker.

For the mapping between the information from the feeder systems to the ideal schema to be as straight forward as possible it is of course preferable if the XML output from the feeder systems is identical to or closely resembling the ideal schema. The system providers that develop web services in order to communicate with this information broker will be able to adapt to the format of the ideal schema. It is desirable for the ideal schema to be compliant with a standard for information sharing, such as ENV 13606 [9] or HL7 [10]. In Sweden today, no such compliance with the available standards exists. In expectance of national guidelines in this area our ideal schema has been developed taking the ENV 13606 and HL7 into consideration, and can be updated or replaced when a national standard is made available.

3.2 VHR Mediator Database

The publishing integration method requires a mediator database to which the information from the feeder systems can be copied. MS SQL server 2000 is used for the implementation. In this database it is also possible to store information which is not available in the feeder systems, such as certain multimedia information or information used for communication between the different care providers. This type of information is not published back to the feeder systems, but remains in the mediator database, connected to a specific patient. New information of the type that is fetched from the feeder systems can also be added to this database, for example a new daily note written by the HHS, and is subsequently published back to the right feeder system.

When information has been added or updated in the VHR, it is crucial to keep track of this information so that it can be published back to the right feeder system. Therefore a change log structure has been included in the mediator database, and whenever any information is added or changed a new post is created in the change log with information about when the information was changed, which patient it belongs to and where, which table, in the mediator database it is stored.

3.3 Online and offline access

Both an online web application and an offline solution have been developed. The DN and GP access the VHR through a web application, either from the office desk top PC, or from a HP Compaq Tablet PC TC1100, used in mobile work situations such as in the patient's home. Their applications interact directly with the mediator database through a roaming session based virtual private network (VPN). The HHS use handheld devices, HP iPAQ h6340, and on these an offline solution is implemented. The information is synchronised between the mediator database and the local SQL CE databases, and the offline applications interact with the local SQL CE database while the HHS are using it. A filtering functionality ensures that only information about the patients which the current user is allowed to access is transferred to the handheld device when synchronising. Currently the HHS have to return to their office in order to synchronise with the mediator database, but a wireless solution with a roaming session based VPN for wireless applications is to be implemented and tested. This will ensure ubiquitous computing and the possibility to synchronise on the given bandwidth at any given moment.

3.4 Security and access rights

Due to the selection of a publishing and offline application, reliable security mechanisms are vital. Security, authentication and data classification is fundamental to give users, organisations, relatives and patients a feeling of trust and security. On a high level role based access rights enables each different user group (GP, DN and HHS) to only have access to information on the patients they work with, and only to a limited amount of information on each patient. A user needs analysis conducted within the project revealed which information each user group needs to have, the "Information domains". The patients also have the possibility to deny certain user groups access to certain information, although so far no one has chosen this alternative. On a low level all methods in the application have an equivalent operation in AZMAN and each user has one or more roles, all stored in the directory. Every method itself checks if the user has the right to perform that method. Access rights are granted to authenticated users stored in the directory, roles are synchronised to the PDA/SQL CE after a full authentication to the server online. When granted access the data leaving the server is in an encrypted secure channel (SSL or VPN). All data stored is encrypted. To ensure that data in the PDA is read by the right user biometry and certificates can be used. With this security model all security can be managed centrally.

4. Discussion and conclusions

Needing offline access to the VHR in mobile work situations naturally poses certain problems, and a proposed solution to these, is the two level synchronization described above, between the local SQL CE databases and the mediator database, and between the mediator database and the feeder systems.

When giving the health care professionals access to information gathered from several different feeder system one has to take the problem of information overflow into account. If the users are confronted with too much information they will not be able to process it, and therefore a thorough selection of which information each user group should access has been performed and implemented in the VHR. Easy access to the VHR is also crucial in order to facilitate and not hamper the work at the point of care.

The suggested architecture for a VHR, using triggered publishing as integration method, makes mobile and/or offline access to information from different feeder systems and interaction with them possible. This enables a seamless flow of information between the care providers involved in the home care of the elderly patients, ensuring a higher quality of care.

6. Acknowledgements

The project "Old@Home - Technical support for Mobile CloseCare" is supported by VINNOVA – Swedish Agency for Innovation Systems (P23037-1 A) and Trygghetsfonden, as well as by the following clinical and industrial partners: Primary Care Hälsingland, County Council of Gävleborg, Municipality of Hudiksvall, DataVis Sverige AB, Ericsson Network Technologies AB, Bergsjö Data AB and AB Hudiksvallsbostäder.

7. References

[1]   L. Lind, E. Sundvall, D. Karlsson, N. Shashavar, H. Åhlfeldt. Requirements and prototyping of a home health care application based on emerging JAVA technology, *Int. J. Med. Info.* 68 (2002) 129-139.

[2]   A. Andersson, N. Hallberg, T. Timpka, A model for interpreting work and information management in process-oriented healthcare organisations, *Int. J. Med. Info.* 72 (2003) 47-56.

[3]   Blobel B. Comparing Concepts for Electronic Health Record Architectures. In: Surján G et al. (eds): Proceedings of MIE 2002, IOS Press, pp. 209-214.

[4]   Hurlen P, Skifjeld K, Andersen E P. The basic principles of the synapses federated healthcare record server. *Int. J. Med. Info.* 52 (1998) 123-132.

[5]   van der Linden H, Talmon J, Tange H, Boers G, Hasman A. An architecture for a Virtual Electronic Health Record. In: Surján G et al. (eds): Proceedings of MIE 2002, IOS Press, pp. 220-225.

[6]   Koch S, Hägglund M, Scandurra I, Moström D. Towards a virtual health record for mobile home care of elderly citizens. In: Fieschi M, Coiera E, Li J (eds): Proc. MEDINFO 2004 - 11th World Congress on Medical Informatics, San Fransisco, USA, Sept 2004, IOS Press, Amsterdam, pp. 960-963

[7]   Lundmark B, Svedberg H, Westling A. Läroprojekt om IntegrationsPlattform för hälso- och sjukvårdens IT-stöd i Region Skåne (LIPS), Projektrapport, maj 2002, http://www.carelink.se/files/LIPS_Projektrapport.pdf (in Swedish)

[8]   Scandurra I, Hägglund M, Koch S. Integrated Care Plan and Documentation on Handheld Devices in Mobile Home Care. In: Brewster S,Dunlop M (eds.): Proceedings of Mobile Human-Computer-Interaction – Mobile HCI 2004, LNCS 3160, Springer-Verlag, (2004)

[9]   ENV13606 – Health informatics – Electronic Health Record Communication, http://www.centc251.org

[10] Health level 7 – HL7: http://www.hl7.org

Address for correspondence

Maria Hägglund, Maria.Hagglund@medsci.uu.se
Dept. of Medical Sciences, Biomedical informatics and engineering, Uppsala University
University Hospital 82:1, S-75185 Uppsala
http://www.medsci.uu.se/mie/project/closecare/index.htm

The coming pages are blank due to the withdrawal of an article by the editors during the printing process

352

Connecting Medical Informatics and Bio-Informatics
R. Engelbrecht et al. (Eds.)
IOS Press, 2005
© 2005 EFMI – European Federation for Medical Informatics. All rights reserved.

Using Mobile Technology to Improve Healthcare Service Quality

Chia Chen Chao[a,b], Wen Yuan Jen[c], Yu-Chuan Li[d], Y P Chi[a], Chen Chang-I[d], Chen Chjeh Feng[d]

[a]Department of Information Management, Chen Chi University
[b]Department of Health Service Management, Taipei Medical University, Taiwan,
[c]Department of Information Management, National Central University, Overseas Chinese Institute of Commerce Taiwan
[d]Institute of Medical Informatics, Taipei Medical University, Taiwan

Abstract

Improving healthcare service quality for illness of treatment, illness prevention and patient service is difficult for most hospitals because the hospitals are lack adequate resources and labor. In order to provide better healthcare service quality for patients, mobile technology can be used to manage healthcare in a way that provides the optimal healthcare service for patients. Pursuing utilization of mobile technology for better patient service, Taipei Medical University Municipal W. F. Teaching Hospital has implemented a mobile healthcare service (m-HS) system to increase healthcare service quality. The m-HS system improves the quality of medical care as well as healthcare service. The m-HS is a multi-functional healthcare management agent, meets the mobile tendency of the present society. This study seeks to discuss the m-HS architecture and workflow processes. We believe the m-HS does have the potential to improve healthcare service quality. Finally, the conclusions and suggestions for the m-HS are given.

Keywords:
Mobile technology, mobile healthcare service, patient safety, health care

1. Introduction

Due to high cell phone usage, mobile devices have become necessary tools in our daily life, and it is time to make use of mobile for providing patient service. Based on the advantages of mobile technology, this study considers that it is sufficiently reliable and powerful to improve patient service and patient-physician relationships. In order to increase healthcare service quality, Taipei Medical University Municipal W. F. Teaching Hospital has implemented a mobile healthcare service (m-HS) system. The process of the m-HS is conducted by mobile technology, and its primary function is to help physicians and hospital administrators manage individual patients in a systematic fashion. Since cell phones are so popular in Taiwan, it is time to launch mobile healthcare service for patients, physicians and hospital administrators. Better service quality in medical care and health care can be fulfilled by mobile technology.

This paper is organized as follows:

1. To illustrate the features of healthcare and mobile healthcare service application for patient service.
2. To introduce the m-HS architectures.
3. To highlight the functions and workflow processes of the m-HS innovation new services for patient.
4. Two surveys have been conducted for this study. Survey 1 was before the implementation, survey 2 was preceded six months after the implementation of the system.
5. To conclude the mobile contribution ,discussions and implications.

2. Healthcare Literature

The Features of Healthcare

This study summarized the features in three categories: illness treatment, illness prevention and patient service. The detail contents are listed as follows:

1. Illness treatment
   Problems associated with illness of treatment include a number of issues as follows: (1)Long waiting time, extended waits are a waste of valuable time and restrict patients to only brief treatments or consultations with from physicians. (2)Behind schedule appointments by physicians, (3)Appointment reminders, (4)Physician shortage, hospitals need more physicians for some emergency cases to treat large volumes of critical patients. (5)Patient safety, notification of a negative side effect of a drug is possible via a patient and physician-directed alert message. (6)Inpatient ward availability, patients can be notified of pending ward availability as soon as possible.

2. Illness prevention
   Problems also exist from the perspective of illness prevention, three issues are given: (1)Abnormal ancillary test results notification, (2)Ancillary tests procedure reminder, (3)Periodic notifications, for examples, to follow routine check up procedures or schedule their child's vaccinations.

3. Patient service
   Hospitals can foster loyalty in patients by improved relationship management between patients and physicians. Three patient's services provide as follows: (1)Greeting, (2)Lectures for improving health, (3)Appropriate reminder for patients.

Mobile healthcare service

This study proposed to adopt mobile technology to provide better service quality for patients. According to the features of illness treatment, illness prevention and patient service, the solution of the problems or defects of the present health care may lie with the mobile technology of mobile healthcare service.

3. The M-HS-Architecture

The m-HS system proposes a variety of functions to deliver mobile service for dedicated medical processes and patients; hence, six subsystem layers comprise the system (see figure 1).

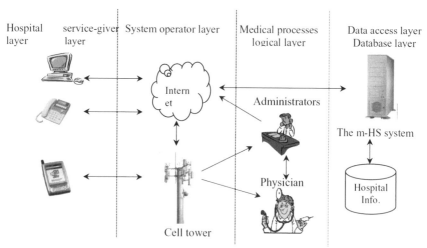

Figure 1 Diagram of the m-HS Architecture

4. Functions and Processes of the M-HS

The m-HS is designed to improve the service quality of illness treatment, illness prevention and patient relationship management. Patients, physicians and hospital administrators are all served.

The M-HS for Patients

The various services for patients are listed below.
1. Appointment number inquiry service, Patient appointment notice,
2. Pre-physical check ups / surgery precaution procedures notification,
3. Patient waiting / inpatient ward notification,
4. Service for patient safety notification,
5. Service for improving patient relationships

The M-HS for Physicians

1. The m-HS emergency physician group notification,
2. Treatment notification,3.Treatment time notification

The M-HS for Administrators

1. The management of physicians and clinics,
2. Performance evaluation

The Workflow Processes of the M-HS

1. 1. The patient session,
2. 2. The examination session,
3. 3 The administrator sessions

5. Survey and Results

Two surveys have been conducted for this study. Survey 1 was conducted by questionnaire before the implementation of the m-HS to survey patient's attitude for 18 functions (Fig 2 & Table 1) while survey 2 was preceded six months after the implementation of the system. Telephone survey was applies by Survey 2 to survey user's satisfaction, willing continuously to use and helpful of m-HS system to aid for service quality.

120 questionnaires were distributed for Survey 1 which 102 questionnaires were completed, reaching 85% high response rate. The reliability of the scales was assessed using Cronbach's alpha. The value of Cronbach's alpha gives an indication of the internal consistency of the items measuring the same construct. The reliability coefficient for the 18 items of our questionnaire was 0.88. As an acceptable range of reliability coefficients for most instruments is over 0.7 [24], the instrument we adopted in analyzing this survey was statistically reliable.Encouraged by the finding of survey 1, the m-HS system was then developed and designed based on user's needs. The m-HS pilot scheme has been implemented in the WanFang Hospital for six months from February to July in 2004. During this period, the mobile message system has delivered around 10,000 service messages to patients. Survey 2 was conducted by telephone survey for receiving feedback from 200 patients after received of the m-HS service. From the result of survey 2, Table 2 shows most patients who adopted m-HS were satisfied with its functions. Many patients expressed willingness to continue using m-HS and agreed that m-HS services enhanced the quality of healthcare. Therefore, it is evident that the finding of survey 2 not only strongly supported the feasibility of applying mobile service in healthcare but also shows such a service reached to the goal of enhancing the quality of service in hospitals. We thus assume that applying a mobile service to improve healthcare service in a hospital is no longer a rhetoric topic, but will be a growing reality in the future.

6. Conclusion

According to the result of survey 1, it shows that items with mean over 4.0 (or domain score over 73%) were related to medical or examination issues. In other words, items participants considered the most are "Medication safety notification", "Pre-surgical operation notification" and "Inpatient wards waiting notification", This indicates participants consider m-HS functions relevant to medical or examination issues are of greater importance. The above-mentioned findings imply that more emphasis should be placed for functions related to patient's personal health management in the future development of m-HS. Mobile healthcare service not only improves the quality of healthcare service, but also improves patient relationships for healthcare providers. If the m-HS enlarges its service domain, it has the potential to be a multi-functional health management agent in the future. We believe that the trend will integrate increasing wire bandwidth, the improvement of mobile technology and health monitor devices, and global positioning software. In short, the practitioners and researchers who want to successfully exploit mobile healthcare should pay attention to various pending issues that have to be addressed.

7. References

[1]   Anantharaman, V. & Han, L.S. (2001). Hospital and emergency ambulance link: using IT to enhance emergency pre-hospital care. *International Journal of Medical Informatics, 61,* 147-161.

[2]   Andrade, R. Wangenheim1, A.V. & Bortoluzzi, M.K. (2003). Wireless and PDA: a novel strategy to access DICOM-compliant medical data on mobile devices. *International Journal of Medical Informatics, 71,* 157-163.

[3]   Banitsas,K. A., Song, Y. H. & Owens, T. J. (2004). OFDM over IEEE 802.11b hardware for telemedical applications. International Journal of Mobile Communications, 2(3), 310 – 327.

[4]   Chau, P.Y.K. & Hu, P.J.H. (2002). Investigating healthcare professionals' decisions to accept telemedicine technology: an empirical test of competing theories. *Information and Management 39 (4),* 297–311.

[5]   Chen, J.C.H., Dolan, M. & Lin, B. (2004), Improve processes on healthcare: current issues and future trends. Internation*al Journal of Electronic Healthcare, 1(2),* 149–164.

[6]   Cocosila, M., Coursaris, C. & Yuan, Y. (2004). M-healthcare for patient self-management: a case for diabetics. *International Journal of Electronic Healthcare, 1(2),* 221–241.

[7]   Côté, M.J. (1999). Patient flow and resource utilization in a patient clinic. *Socio-Economic Planning Sciences, 33(3),* 231–245.

[8]   Ehnfors, M. & Grobe, S. J. (2004). Nursing curriculum and continuing education: future directions. *International Journal of Medical Informatics, 73, 7-8,* 591-598

[9]   Eisenstadt, S. Wagner, M. Hogan, W., Pankaskie, M., Tsui, F.C. & Wilbright, W. (1998). Mobile workers in healthcare and their information needs: are 2-way pagers the answer? in: C. Chute (Ed.), *Proceeding of the AMIA Annual Fall Symposium.* 135–139.

[10] Fishman, S., Prince, J., Herman, J. & Cassem, N. (1996). Pocket-sized electronic clinical referencing, *MD Computer, 13(4),* 310–313.

[11] 11.Gagnon, M.P., Godin, G., Gagne, C., Fortin, J.P., Lamothe, L., Reinharz, D. & Cloutier, A. (2003). An adaptation of the theory of interpersonal behaviour to the study of telemedicine adoption by physicians. *International Journal of Medical Informatics, 71,* 103–115.

[12] Gulur, I. & Muldur, S. (2001). A model approach to sharing electronic medical records between and within the state hospitals in Turkey. Computers in Biology and Medicine, 31, 513–523.

[13] Hameed, K. (2003). The application of mobile computing and technology to health care services. *Telematics and Informatics 20,* 99–106.

[14] Hsu, C.M. (2004). Personal mobile service and wireless application survey. Retrieved October 30, 2004, from http://www.find.org.tw/0105/howmany

[15] Lin, B. & Vassar, J.A. (2004). Mobile healthcare computing devices for enterprise-wide patient data delivery. *International Journal of Mobile Communications, 2(4),* 343– 353.

[16] Lombardo, J.S., McCarty, M. & Wojcik, R.A. (1997). An evaluation of mobile computing for information access at the point of care. *Biomedical Instrument Technology, 31(5),* 465-475.

[17] Michalowskia, W., Rubinb, S., Slowinskic R. & Wilkc, S. (2003). Mobile clinical support system for pediatric emergencies. *Decision Support Systems, 36,* 161–176.

[18] Mylonakis, J. (2004). Can mobile services facilitate commerce? Findings from the Greek telecommunications market. *International Journal of Mobile Communications, 2(2),* 199–198.

[19] Ptochos, D., Panopoulos, D., Metaxiotis, K., Askounis, D. & Psarras, J. (2004). Using internet GIS technology for early warning, response and controlling the quality of the public health sector. *International Journal of Electronic Healthcare, 1(1),* 78–102.

[20] Panagiotakis, S., Koutsopoulou, M., Alonistioti, A., Houssos, N., Gazis, V. & Merakos, L. (2003). An advanced service provision framework for reconfigurable mobile networks. *International Journal of Mobile Communications, 1(4),* 425–438.

[21] Su, S. & Shih, C.L. (2003). Managing a mixed-registration-type appointment system in patient clinics. International Journal of Medical Informatics, 70, 31–40.

[22] Wagner, M., Eisenstadt, S., Hogan, W., & Pankaskie, M. (1998). Preferences of interns and residents for e-mail, paging, or traditional methods for the delivery of different types of clinical information, in: C. Chute (Ed.), *Proceedings of the AMIA Annual Fall Symposium, Hanley and Belfus,* 140–144.

[23] Wee, J. & Gutierrez, J. A. (2005). A framework for effective quality of service over wireless networks. *International Journal of Mobile Communications, 3(2),* 138–149.

[24] Wickramasinghe, N. & Misra, S. K. (2004). A wireless trust model for healthcare. *International Journal of Electronic Healthcare, 1(1),* 60–77.

[25] Wu, C.H. (2004). A survey of mobile service in the 2nd season of 2004. Retrieved October 30, 2004, http://www.find.org.tw/0105/howmany/howmany_disp.asp?id=81.

Address for correspondence

ChiaChen Chao, Doctoral program, Department of Information Management Chen Chi University / Instructor, Department of Health Service Management, Taipei Medical University, Taiwan, vic@wanfang.gov.tw

WenYuan Jen, Doctoral program, Department of Information Management, National Central University / Instructor, Overseas Chinese Institute of Commerce Taiwan, wyjen@mgt.ncu.edu.tw

Dr. Yu-Chuan Li, Graduate Institute of Medical Informatics, Taipei Medical University, Taiwan, jack@tmu.edu.tw

Dr. YP Chi, Department of Information Management Chen Chi University Taiwan, ypchi @nccu.edu.tw

Chen Chang-I, Doctoral program, Graduate Institute of Medical Informatics, Taipei Medical University, Taiwan, danchen@mail2000.com.tw

ChenChjeh Feng, Doctoral program, Graduate Institute of Medical Informatics, Taipei Medical University, Taiwan, clifchen@ms1.hinet.net

Section 6

Healthcare Networks

Connecting Medical Informatics and Bio-Informatics
R. Engelbrecht et al. (Eds.)
IOS Press, 2005

Developing Online Communities with LAMP (Linux, Apache, MySQL, PHP) – the IMIA OSNI and CHIRAD Experiences

Peter J. Murray[a], Karl Øyri[b]

[a]*Centre for Health Informatics Research and Development (CHIRAD), UK*

[b]*Rikshospitalet University Hospital, Norway*

Abstract

Many health informatics organisations do not seem to use, on a practical basis, for the benefit of their activities and interaction with their members, the very technologies that they often promote for use within healthcare environments. In particular, many organisations seem to be slow to take up the benefits of interactive web technologies. This paper presents an introduction to some of the many free/libre and open source (FLOSS) applications currently available and using the LAMP - Linux, Apache, MySQL, PHP architecture - as a way of cheaply deploying reliable, scalable, and secure web applications. The experience of moving to applications using LAMP architecture, in particular that of the Open Source Nursing Informatics (OSNI) Working Group of the Special Interest Group in Nursing Informatics of the International Medical Informatics Association (IMIA-NI), in using PostNuke, a FLOSS Content Management System (CMS) illustrates many of the benefits of such applications. The experiences of the authors in installing and maintaining a large number of websites using FLOSS CMS to develop dynamic, interactive websites that facilitate real engagement with the members of IMIA-NI OSNI, the IMIA Open Source Working Group, and the Centre for Health Informatics Research and Development (CHIRAD), as well as other organisations, is used as the basis for discussing the potential benefits that could be realised by others within the health informatics community.

Keywords:
Nursing informatics; Database management systems; Software design

1. Introduction

One of the key features of many modern health informatics organisations is the need to quickly interact with their members, who are often spread around the world, in order to accomplish their work. However, many health informatics organisations, although they discuss and advocate the appropriate use of technologies, seem to be relatively slow in terms of their own uptake of the technologies to support their day-to-day operations. This seems to be especially the case in respect of the use of web-based technologies for providing information and for interacting with online communities comprising their members and wider constituencies of interest, whether that interaction is sharing resources or knowledge, developing or using tools to support such interaction and dissemination, or seeking to improve benefits to patients and improve health and healthcare.

There are, however, many applications with the multimedia-based [1] modular functionality to enhance organisational information exchange, collaboration and research where knowledge sharing is essential. Many of these are easy-to-use free/libre and open source software (FLOSS) tools that, in addition to carrying the many benefits of FLOSS, are readily available to less developed and wealthy countries, and so can help to fulfil the international commitments of health informatics organisations such as the European Federation of Medical Informatics (EFMI) and the International Medical Informatics Association (IMIA) and their Working Groups and Special Interest Groups. [Note: For the purposes of this paper, we use the term 'open source' or the acronym FLOSS (Free/Libre and Open Source Software) [2] to generically cover open source, free software, and GNU/Linux [3]; other widely used acronyms also exist, e.g. OSS/FS [4]]

The aim of this paper is two-fold: to introduce some of the many FLOSS applications that are available to develop interactive portals and websites and support dynamic online communities as part of the structure of health informatics organisations; and to show how one group in particular, the Open Source Nursing Informatics Working Group (OSNI) of the Special Interest Group in Nursing Informatics of the International Medical Informatics Association (IMIA-NI) is using some of these tools for precisely those purposes on their website, at www.osni.info. The experience of the IMIA Open Source Working Group (OSWG) and of CHIRAD (the Centre for Health Informatics Research and Development) in moving to use these tools also provides supporting evidence for their benefits and ease of use.

The paper will discuss the use of FLOSS applications, and in particular Content Management Systems (CMS) such as PostNuke [5], which has been used by the IMIA-NI OSNI WG to develop an online community to meet the aims of the group. The model that can be derived from this could be of benefit to many other health informatics organisations, especially those in developing countries or other environments where scarce resources limit expenditure on costly proprietary systems.

It is not within the scope of this paper to rehearse the background descriptions of, or perceived benefits of, FLOSS nor to describe some of the common office and productivity open source applications available; these are available in many other papers and sources (for example [6], [7], [8], [9]) and a certain level of knowledge is assumed.

2. Some FLOSS applications for collaboration

2.1 LAMP and e-learning

Many FLOSS applications, especially the kind of Content Management Systems (CMS) we discuss here, use a combination that is often referred to as LAMP - the Linux, Apache, MySQL, PHP (LAMP) architecture - which has become very popular in the industry as a way of cheaply deploying reliable, scalable, and secure web applications. (the 'P' in LAMP can also stand for Perl or Python.) MySQL is a multithreaded, multi-user, SQL (Structured Query Language) relational database server, using the GNU General Public License. The PHP-MySQL combination is also cross-platform, ie will run on Windows as well as Linux servers.

FLOSS applications are gaining widespread use within education sectors, with one example of a widely-used e-learning application being Moodle (www.moodle.org). Moodle is a complete e-learning Course Management System, or Virtual Learning Environment (VLE), with a modular structure designed to help educators create high-quality, multimedia-based online courses. Moodle is translated into more than 30 languages, and handles thematic or topic-based classes and courses. As Moodle is based in social constructivist pedagogy (http://moodle.org/doc/?frame=philosophy.html), it also allows the construction of e-learning materials that are based around discussion and interaction, rather than static content. Such interactive applications are ideal for supporting the learning needs of distributed health informatics organisations. Several OSNI members, working with CHIRAD (the Centre for Health Informatics Research and Development) are developing an open access health informatics repository using Moodle (see http://www.differance-engine.net/hivle/).

2.2 Content Management Systems

There are more than 25 FLOSS Content Management Systems (CMS) designed for developing portals/websites with dynamic, fully searchable content; PostNuke, PHPNuke, and Mambo are among the most commonly used (see http://www.opensourcecms.com/ for a fuller list). A CMS has a flexible, modular framework that separates the content of a web site (the text, images, and other content) from the framework of linking the pages together and controlling how the pages appear. In most cases, this is done to make a site easier to maintain than would be the case if it was built exclusively out of flat HTML pages.

A CMS can be easily administrated and moderated at several levels from an Administration Panel, allowing flexibility of access to make different types of materials available to selected members of an online community, to the whole community, or to the wider world. Registration of members is necessary if different permissions and levels of access are assigned to different types of member, and if registered members of the site upload material direct or submit material for publication to moderators who give approval and publish on the web site. This gives complete control of compliance with the organisation's policy for published material. In addition, the work-load relating to publication of material and overall maintenance of the website can be spread among many members, rather than having only one webspinner, securing frequent updates of content and reducing individual workload, so making likelihood of member participation greater. The initial user registration and redistribution of passwords and access can be carried out automatically by user requests, while assignment to user groups is made manually by the site administrators or moderators.

2.3 Other server-side dynamic applications

In addition, blogs, bulletin boards, discussion forums and other applications such as photograph or picture galleries can be contained within, or linked to a CMS.

Bulletin Board(BB)/Discussion Forums(DF) applications essentially allow users to post and read news items and exchange messages with other users of the systems. From several FLOSS BB/DF applications available, all with good functionality, OSNI has incorporated phpBB (www.phpbb.com) as an external application linked to its OSNI PostNuke CMS web site (http://www.osni.info/phpBB2/index.php). As of mid January 2005, the OSNI BB had 17 registered users from Spain, UK, Norway, USA, India, and Cuba. There are 70 articles, grouped within one open and three closed forums.

The advantage with FLOSS BBS/DF such as phpBB is that the overview of discussions and topics is clear, as the thread of posts in the discussion is displayed and can easily be followed. Some material can be made open in public forums, and other material can be available in closed sections for particular user groups. Iterations of documents and topic based discussions can be handled effectively, directly available to those concerned. Thus the communication becomes much more efficient than communicating via e-mail as it is available to all with user permissions to view. In addition, as the discussions are automatically archived, they and available for later review by new members of an online community, or available as a valuable resources for researchers.

Blogs (weblogs) are open source web applications which contain periodic, reverse chronologically ordered posts on common web pages typically accessible to any Internet user. Their use is being explored to provide reports on health informatics events for those unable to attend, and may be used to provide a form of distant interaction with such events [10]. An example of such a blog is the use of the FLOSS b2evolution software used to provide real-time reporting at medinfo2004 and planned for use to report on HC2005 and MIE2005 (see http://www.differance-engine.net/medinfo2004blog/).

Wikis are web sites that allows users to add and update content on the site using their own web browser, resulting in a site that is collaboratively developed and maintained by its users. [11]

3. IMIA, IMIA-NI and their Open Source Working Groups

IMIA established an Open Source Health Informatics Working Group (OSWG) in October 2002. The OSWG web site began as a series of simple, flat HTML pages. It was quickly realized that this would not meet the needs of the group, and the website was migrated to use PHPNuke, a FLOSS CMS similar to PostNuke, and can be found at: www.chirad.info/imiaoswg

In agreeing to the need to explore nursing-specific issues, IMIA-NI established a Working Group on Open Source Nursing Informatics (OSNI) in June 2003, its purposes to include raising awareness among nurses and exploring the existence or case for nursing-specific components to FLOSS developments and discussions. The IMIA-NI OSNI Working Group developed out of Open Nurse (the nursing open source network) which was initially based around the development of the open-nurse.info website. The network started at the NI2003 conference in Rio de Janeiro resulted in the launch of the OSNI.INFO web-site in March 2004 with the URL; http://www.osni.info/html/index.php, replacing open-nurse.info as the OSNI WG's official website.

The two IMIA groups are complementary and synergistic, and seek to work with other bodies, such as the AMIA OSWG (the Open Source Working Group of AMIA, the American Medical Informatics Association) (http://www.amia.org/working/os/main.html) and other relevant organizations in nursing, healthcare, informatics, education, and other pertinent fields.

At present, the OSNI website aims to develop a comprehensive listing of other online resources. In the longer term, the OSNI network aims to publish a number of papers and other resources outlining for nurses some of the issues around the use of open source and free software within nursing and healthcare. The aim of the OSNI network is to work in a manner akin to that by which open source and free software is developed. We welcome all contributions, and will share all the contributions we receive with anyone who wishes to use them. In the same way that the development of open source software provides for transparency of processes, we wish to provide a transparent process that others can use as they see fit.

4. OSNI.INFO as a model

The decision to move the OSNI website from static html to a CMS was based in a number of issues, including a lack of up-to-date content and the workload on a single webspinner. The osni.info site uses the FLOSS CMS platform PostNuke (http://www.postnuke.com/). The OSNI website has had more than 16,000 page-views between its launch in March 2004 and mid January 2005. It has 14 modules, 74 international members from all over the world, 25 stories published, 5 active topics, 1 special section (member profiles), and 110 web links in 23 categories. The OSNI website has contributed to establishing a new network, where visitors and registered OSNI members can exchange information and news. The number of registered members and site traffic is steadily increasing, indicating a need for this type of virtual organisation and network connecting nurses interested in FLOSS, and nursing informatics in general.

Among the facilities available to members using the website are: the ability to add new articles or news items that appear on the site almost instantaneously, and to add new weblinks are downloadable items; opportunities to contribute to discussion forums and have a complete, reviewable record of discussions; access to member-only areas through access control mechanisms, so as to provide recognizable benefits to members that may not be available to the wider community, and which give potential members a reason to become members.

The benefits that accrue to the group as a whole, and to individual members, are: interaction within a group, many of whose members may rarely meet physically; distribution of workload among members, to providing a feeling of community and interaction for members, and reducing reliance on and workload of a single webspinner; rapid uploading of new materials; and a searchable archive of all materials on the website.

CHIRAD, the Centre for Health Informatics Research and Development, is a virtual health informatics organisation based in the UK, but has members around the world, and is an Academic Institutional member of IMIA. In the past year, it has moved its websites from static HTML pages to FLOSS CMS such as PostNuke and PHPNuke. It has also begun moving its health informatics resources and virtual learning environment to use Moodle.

One author (KØ) is the osni.info webspinner and maintain several other websites using FLOSS CMS. The other author (PJM) is Chair of the IMAI OSWG and of IMIA-NI OSNI, maintaining their websites and the CHIRAD wesbites, in addition to several others. The authors have been involved in the installation and maintenance of over twenty examples of the FLOSS tools such as PostNuke, PHPNuke, Moodle, TikiWiki, Mambo, Moodle, b2evolution and Coppermine described in this paper. Their experience is that many of the tools are relatively easy to install, and with only a short period of exploration and learning how to use them, fully functional dynamic web applications can be developed.

5. Conclusion

The Internet has, in the last decade, played a leading role in facilitating communication across borders, becoming more and more important as a source of communication, education, research and collaboration. Problems with early stage Internet-based communication were related to high costs in developing, maintaining and updating websites as platforms for collaborative organisational work. The Open Source movement is changing all of this and the ways in which the sharing of knowledge and access to new development and refined and enhanced functionality in web-based applications, the healthcare informatics scene has the potential for going through a major change. The structure and functionality of websites has changed a lot from static flat-file html sites with hyperlinks and hypertext, to websites developed on relational databases with completely new dynamic and searchable retrieval of content.

The use of dynamic, FLOSS CMS tools for the development and maintenance of websites such as that used by the OSNI group facilitates the fostering of international links and collaboration among nurses around the world, who need only a simple web browser to access all the functionality of the website. This has particular advantages for developing countries, and activities to support the development of nursing and nursing informatics in such countries, and supports links to the wider global health informatics community. The model developed by OSNI for its website has the potential for easy adoption by other health informatics organisations and associated benefits, including low costs, rapid provision of current, relevant information, and the development of a sense of community.

6. References

[1]   Jakobovits RM, Rosse C, Brinkley JF. WIRM: an open source toolkit for building biomedical web applications. J Am Med Inform Assoc. 2002;9(6):557-70.

[2]   International Institute of Infonomics. Free/Libre and Open Source Software: Survey and Study. [monograph on the Internet]. Maastricht: International Institute of Infonomics, 2002 [cited 2005 Jan 21] Available from: http://www.infonomics.nl/FLOSS/index.htm

[3]   Stallman RM. Linux and the GNU Project.[homepage on the Internet]. Boston (MA): Free Software Foundation; c.1997-2002 [updated 2004 Jul 12; cited 2005 Jan 8 Available from: http://www.gnu.org/gnu/linux-and-gnu.html

[4]   Wheeler DA. Why Open Source Software / Free Software (OSS/FS)? Look at the Numbers! [monograph on the Internet]. 2005 [updated 2005 Jan 15, cited 2005 Jan 21] Available from: http://www.dwheeler.com/oss_fs_why.html

[5]   PN Team. PostNuke -An Open source Content Management System. [homepage on the Internet]. 2005 [cited 2005 Jan 21] Available from: http://news.postnuke.com/Sections-article25-p1.html

[6]   Shaw NT, Pepper DR, Cook T, Houwink P, Jain N, Bainbridge M. Open source and International Health Informatics: Placebo or panacea? Informatics in Primary Care. 2002;10(1):39-44.

[7]   Peeling N, Satchell J. Analysis of the impact of Open Source Software. [monograph on the Internet]. Farnborough: QinetiQ Ltd., 2001. [cited 2005 Jan 21] Available from: http://www.govtalk.gov.uk/documents/QinetiQ_OSS_rep.pdf

[8]   Murray PJ, Wright G. Free/libre/open source software and health informatics: the international priorities. Health Informatics Society of Ireland, 9th Annual Conference & Scientific Symposium. Dublin; 2004.

[9]   Murray PJ. open-nurse.info - building an international community of nurses. Fourth International Congress on Medical Informatics and First International Congress on Nursing Informatics. Havana, Cuba; 2003.

[10] Murray P, Ward R. Engaging in healthcare informatics - let's use the technology. BJHC&IM 2004;21(10):14.

[11] Christensson P. Definition of Wiki. [homepage on the Internet]. Sharpened.net ; c.1999-2004. [cited 2005, Jan 21] Available from: http://www.sharpened.net/glossary/definition.php?wiki

7. Address for correspondence

Dr Peter J. Murray
Chair, IMIA Open Source Working Group; Founding Fellow, CHIRAD,
Coachman's Cottage
Nocton Hall, Nocton
Lincoln LN4 2BA, United KIngdom
Email: peter@open-nurse.info URL: www.peter-murray.net

Connecting Medical Informatics and Bio-Informatics
R. Engelbrecht et al. (Eds.)
IOS Press, 2005
367

Preparing the Electronic Patient Record for Collaborative Environments and eHealth

Petra Knaup[a], Sebastian Garde[b], Reinhold Haux[c]

[a]*University of Heidelberg, Department of Medical Informatics, Heidelberg, Germany*

[b]*Health Informatics Research Group, Faculty of Informatics and Communication, Central Queensland University, Rockhampton, Australia*

[c]*Technical University of Braunschweig, Institute for Medical Informatics,Germany*

Abstract

In the era of eHealth the electronic patient record is increasingly regarded as part of a collaborative environment. To efficiently support the documentary tasks and analyses a cooperative documentation infrastructure which allows multiple use and shared entry of data is necessary. The objective of this paper is to introduce a method for systematically planning such a cooperative documentation environment. It consists of the steps: analyse the prevailing documentation infrastructure, provide terminology, provide documentation management, plan the logical architecture and provide all necessary tools. The steps can be formally specified so that parameters can be automatically controlled and the environment can be updated more easily.

Keywords:
Electronic Health Record, Systematic Planning, Medical Informatics, Clinical Trials, Multipurpose Data

1. Introduction

eHealth is said to be a driving force for nowadays medicine. Although it is recognized as a "general 'buzzword' used to characterize not only 'Internet medicine', but also virtually everything related to computers and medicine, it is an emerging … field in the intersection of medical informatics, public health and business" [1]. The availability of innovative technology will increase the desire to access high quality medical information. According to [2] the major problem of adopting these technologies is the necessity of exchanging the electronic patient record. This is in accordance with the perception of the statement, that "…the meaning of an electronic patient record (EPR), as a representation of documents should be transformed into a collaborative environment that supports workflow, enables new care models, and allows secure access to distributed health data" ([3]). The limits of the 'virtual patient record' [4] can still be seen in data security, data privacy and interoperability, but the medical informatics community is active in handling these problems. Results on data privacy have been published in a recent special issue of the International Journal of Medical Informatics (e.g. [5]) and the use of digital signatures has proven feasible ([6]). With respect to interoperability standardization efforts to better communicate clinical documents ([7]) and electronic patient records respectively parts of them ([8, 9]) are promising.

But when we regard factors for failure or success of electronic patient records ([10, 11]) we are often confronted with additional problems, especially after implementation and introduction of the system. Even if a high quality product is provided and the potential end-users have continuously been involved in the development process, there may be user resistances. The perceived usefulness of a clinical application system is recognized as a key factor for failure or success. According to [12] the perceived usefulness is influenced by a variety of individual attitudes like computer anxiety, satisfaction with the current job situation and the trust in the company to effectively support the management of an EPR system. From a medical informatics point-of-view perceived usefulness can only be reached, when a user presumes a clear benefit of an electronic patient record and this benefit has to become effective immediately after installation of the EPR system. Only if a multiple entry of data can be avoided, a clinical user will be aware of the potential benefit of an EPR system.

The task of medical informatics research is to provide methods to systematically plan the data processing in a collaborative environment. Regarding the fast progress of emerging technologies, these methods should be independent of particular technologies. Likewise, they should not be restricted to a particular architecture. Additionally, legislation and new insight in medical science are continuously placing new demands, so that methodological approaches should be open to integrate new questions of investigation effortlessly.

The objective of this paper is to introduce an approach of systematically planning cooperative documentation environments which is independent of particular architectures and technologies.

2. Methods

Components and procedures are formulated with the help of formal logic. However, for an easier legibility we will present them verbally in this paper. Our approach is in accordance with the systematic planning of clinical documentations ([13]). The terminology we use to describe our approach is in accordance with [14]. As figure 1 illustrates, a cooperative documentation environment is regarded as a coherent group of institutions and documentation systems which cooperate. Nevertheless, data exchange to documentations systems outside the cooperative documentation environment should be supported. We understand documentation systems as a comprehensive concept for application systems which provide attribute types, attribute values and functions that operate on the attributes and which are used for documentation purposes. In this sense, every electronic patient record system is a documentation system.

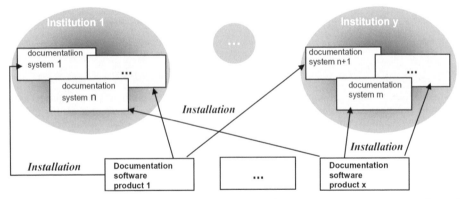

Figure 1: Basic components of a cooperative documentation environment. Several documentation systems are prevailing in the participating institutions. They result from the installation of various documentation software products.

3. Results

Modeling the process of systematically planning cooperative documentation environments involves five steps:

Step 1: Analyses of the prevailing documentation infrastructure

In the first step the participating institutions are identified and existing infrastructure in each participating institution is analyzed. The result of this phase is a set of participating institutions, a set of prevailing documentation systems, a set of prevailing management systems and a set of prevailing data-interfaces between documentation systems, between documentation systems and management systems and for data exchange with external partners.

Management systems provide services for other systems. They are themselves not part of the clinical documentation. Management systems can be administered by technical staff but they are not directly part of documentary tasks in clinical routine. Figure 2 illustrates this concept. Typical examples for management systems are communication or terminology servers.

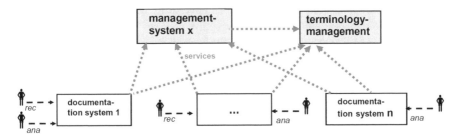

Figure 2: Management systems provide services for clinical documentation systems. With clinical documentation systems data are recorded (rec) and analyzed (ana). Clinical users are not end-users of management systems. A terminology management system is an example.

The aim of the mentioned analyses in the first step is to identify if there is already data which is used multiply and to be able to test in a later phase if the prevailing infrastructure can fulfil several important tasks of the documentation environment.

Step 2: Provision of a terminology management system

In the second step the terminology to be used in the documentation environment is derived. This starts with identifying the questions of investigations of each participating institution. The question of investigation is any clinical or research question a user wants to answer with the help of a documentation system. When we run one or several functions of a documentation system to answer a question of investigation then we perform an analysis.

The aim of the second phase is to build up a terminology management system which comprises all attribute types of the documentation environment and to assign which question of investigation will use which attribute type. According to [15] an attribute type is a "category of attribute values used as a criterion for the establishment of a concept system (cf. ISO 1087)". An attribute value is a "value of an attribute type as observed for a particular object". We call a couple of an attribute type and an attribute value an 'attribute'. For example the attribute value 'brown' of attribute type 'color of hair' leads us to the attribute 'brown hair'.

We suggest adding step by step the attribute types of each documentation system of each participating partner. The challenge is to carefully check whether a new attribute type is identical or overlapping to an already existing attribute value. The degree of multiple usability is highly depending on the quality and consistency of the underlying terminology.

Our methodology suggests algorithms for analyzing the attribute values of documentation systems and questions under investigation, for adding new attribute values and new questions of investigation in the terminology management system and for analyzing the maximum degree of multiple usability of data which can be achieved.

The result of this phase is a terminology management for a multiple use of data.

Step 3: Provision of documentation management system

In this phase a documentation management system has to be planned that 'knows' which attribute values can be documented in which institution with the help of which documentation system and which attribute values are needed in which institution for analysis in which documentation system. In a collaborative documentation environment where data is used multiply and entered by various institutions, the data recorded in an institution is not identical with the data analyzed in this institution.

Our methodology provides an algorithm for building up the documentation management system and controlling its consistency. Additionally, functions to guarantee data privacy and protection should be integrated. The result of this phase is a documentation management system for managing the multiple use and shared entry of data.

Step 4: Planning of the logical architecture

The aim of the fourth phase is to plan the logical architecture of the documentation environment. It has to be decided

- which documentation software and functions have to be developed for providing the documentation systems defined in step 3.
- which modules extend documentation systems for which question of investigation.
- which management systems are necessary.
- which data interfaces are necessary between which documentation systems.
- if there are any data interfaces necessary to exchange data with external institutions.

Modules are non-autonomous documentation systems which can enhance documentation systems. They are added to a particular system and have no own functions. All functions of the documentation system work also on the attribute values of the module. Modules should not contain any attribute types which are already part of the documentation system

The result of this phase is the logical architecture which has to be implemented by the collaborative documentation environment.

Step 5: Provision of tools

The aim of the fifth phase is to prepare all necessary components to establish the cooperative documentation environment. Implementation, adaptation, delivery and introduction of the components can take place according to well-established project management strategies and software engineering methods. Typical decisions are decisions of the physical architecture, the used technologies and standards. Further, it has to be decided if generic tools shall be used to generate a documentation system or a module on the basis of a standard terminology.

The result of this phase should be the final cooperative documentation environment.

4. Additional remarks

The steps have not necessarily to be taken in a sequential order. Depending on the complexity of the documentation systems and the amount of attribute types one may decide to work out step 1 and 2 for each documentation system separately. Even after phase 4 and 5 one may decide to add a new documentation system or a new question of investigation to be answered in the cooperative documentation environment. The procedure is valid as well for building up a new documentation environment as for extending an existing one.

5. Application

The procedure model resulted from our experiences in pediatric oncology (e.g. [16, 17]). In Germany pediatric oncology is realized as a clinical research network. For each diagnose a trial center is established that delivers therapy protocols. Pediatric oncology centers (POC) apply these protocols for treating a patient. Therapy results are recorded and transmitted to the trial centers for further research and eventually optimized therapy protocols. To avoid multiple data entry for clinical routine and research a cooperative documentation environment is desirable.

Step 1: Analyses of the prevailing documentation infrastructure: About 20 POCs are treating the majority of children of pediatric oncology in Germany ([16]). They all are using their local hospital information system. Additionally, they are supported by a best-of-breed system for therapy planning and documentation tailor-made for pediatric oncology. In some POCs interfaces for data exchange with the hospital information system have been implemented. Trial centers run their own trial data base for research data. Data entry takes place manually.

Step 2: Provision of a terminology management system: In Germany a minimum basic data set (MBDS) for pediatric oncology is available ([18]) which represents the data all trials have in common. We adapted the MBDS to make it applicable for multiple use and shared entry ([19]). We built up a terminology management system and entered the adapted MBDS ([20]).

Step 3: Provision of documentation management system: The degree of multiple usability is high since all POC should record the data of the MBDS. Currently, all data are recorded a second time in the trial center.

Step 4: Planning of the logical architecture: We designed a documentation and therapy planning system for pediatric oncology which can be used in the POCs (DOSPO, [21]). We specified data interfaces for data exchange with the trial centers. We designed a generic tool for generating trial specific modules on the basis of attribute types in the terminology management system. Modules can be generated in the trial centers, delivered to the POC and integrated into the local DOSPO system.

Step 5: Provision of tools: We implemented and introduced DOSPO. In some hospitals we established HL7 communication interfaces to the local HIS. We implemented the generic tool so far that trial data bases and electronic case report forms can be generated ([20]).

6. Discussion

The detailed approach comprises formal definitions of the mentioned components and the relations among them. They are used to specify the algorithms provided precisely, so that they can be implemented for various cooperative documentation environments.

The major advantage of our approach is that a multiple entry of data can be avoided and that data can be used for several purposes. This should increase the motivation of the staff involved in data recording. Furthermore, results of clinical and research questions are comparable between all partners. Of course, the approach is only practicable if aspects of data protection and security are carefully regarded. The approach can complement standardization efforts in the field of communication and electronic health record systems. They are integrated in step 4 and 5 of the planning process. If specifications of standards are represented in the terminology management system they can influence the planning process even earlier.

Our suggestions reflect an optimum procedure. In a real setting it may be difficult to analyze every attribute type of every documentation system (phases 1 and 2) in advance. Our example in pediatric oncology demonstrates that the procedure can be adapted to particular documentation environments. The documentation software was installed in 31 hospitals. The main functions in use were therapy planning, report writing, recording diagnosis and procedure codes.

The major restriction of our approach is the claim for a terminology management system. The claim is not new and the maintenance of a terminology system is still a great challenge ([22, 23]). The harmonisation process in pediatric oncology lasted over several years. The new basic data set consists of 262 attribute types. They are organized in a list of items, coding tables and a glossary. For representing integrity constraints 13 disjunct classes of integrity constraints were defined. For the attribute types of the basic data set 1244 particular integrity constraint were specified and entered in the terminology management system. The effectiveness of multiple use and shared entry is highly dependent on the quality and consistency of the underlying terminology.

7. Acknowledgements

The approach results from our 10 year experience in the field of pediatric oncology. We appreciate all contributions from our colleagues in pediatric oncology who have supported the DOSPO-project and its ideas and all contributions from all members of the DOSPO project team over the years. The project was funded by the Germany leukemia research aid and the German Ministry of education and research in the context of the medical research networks.

8. References

[1]   Eysenbach G. What is e-health? *J Med Internet Res*, 2001. 3(2): p. E20.

[2]   ESA, *http://www.esa.int/export/SPECIALS/Telemedicine_Alliance*. last access January 2, 2005.

[3]   Safran C, and Goldberg H. Electronic patient records and the impact of the Internet. *Int J Med Inf*, 2000. 60(2): p. 77-83.

[4]   4.   Costa C, Oliveira JL, Silva A, and Ribeiro VG. A new concept for an integrated Healthcare Access Model. *Stud Health Technol Inform*, 2003. 95: p. 101-6.

[5]   Blobel B. Authorisation and access control for electronic health record systems. *Int J Med Inf*, 2004. 73(3): p. 251-7.

[6]   Brandner R, van der Haak M, Hartmann M, Haux R, and Schmücker P. Electronic Signature for Medical Documents - Integration and Evaluation of a Public Key Infrastructure in Hospitals. *Methods Inf Med*, 2002. 41: p. 321-330.

[7]   Dolin RH, Alschuler L, Beebe C, Biron P, Boyer SL, Essin D, Kimber E, Lincoln T, and Mattison, JE. The HL7 Clinical Document Architecture. *J Am Med Inform Assoc*, 2001. 8(6): p. 552-69.

[8]   Beale T. Archetypes: Constraint-based Domain Models for Future-proof Information Systems, in *OOPSLA 2002 workshop on behavioural semantics*. 2002.

[9]   Bird L., Goodchild A, and Tun Z, Experiences with a Two-Level Modelling Approach to Electronic Health Records. *Journal of Research and Practice in Information Technology*, 2003. 35(2): p. 121-138.

[10]   Beynon-Davies P, and Lloyd-Williams M. When health information systems fail. *Top Health Inf Manage*, 1999. 20(1): p. 66-79.

[11]   Frohwerk, A., Implementing the CPR: a journey. *J Ahima*, 1999. 70(3): p. 32-7; quiz 39-40.

[12]   Dansky, KH, Gamm LD, and Vasey JJ. Electronic medical records: are physicians ready? *J Healthc Manag*, 1999. 44(6): p. 440-454.

[13]   Leiner F, and Haux R. Systematic planning of clinical documentations. *Methods Inf Med*, 1996. 35: p. 25-34.

[14]   Winter A, and Haux R. A Three Level Graph-Based Model for the Management of Hospital Information Systems. *Methods Inf Med*, 1995. 34: p. 378-396.

[15]   Leiner F, Gaus W; Haux R, and Knaup-Gregori P. *Medical Data Management - A Practical Guide*. Health Informatics, ed. K.J. Hannah and M.J. Ball. 2003, New York: Springer.

[16]   Kaatsch P, Spix C; and Michaelis J. *Jahresbericht/Annual Report 1998. German Childhood Cancer Registry*, in Institute for Medical Statistics and Documentation. 1999, University of Mainz: Mainz.

[17]   Kaatsch P, Haaf G, and Michaelis J, Childhood malignancies in Germany - Methods and Results of a Nationwide Registry. *The European Journal of Cancer*, 1995. 31A(6): p. 993-999.

[18]   Sauter S, Kaatsch P, Creutzig U, and Michaelis J. Definition of a Common Data Set for Clinical Trials in Pediatric Oncology. *Klin Paediatr*, 1994. 206: p. 302-312 (in German).

[19]   Merzweiler A, Ehlerding H, Creutzig U, Graf N, Hero B, Kaatsch P, Zimmermann M, Weber R, and Knaup, P. [Standardizing terminology in pediatric oncology--the basic data set]. *Klin Paediatr*, 2002. 214(4): p. 212-7.

[20]   Merzweiler A, Knaup P, Creutzig U, Ehlerding H, Haux R, Mludek V, Schilling FH; Weber R; and Wiedemann, T. Requirements and Design Aspects of a Data Model for a Data Dictionary in Pediatric Oncology, in *Medical Infobahn Europe. Proceedings of MIE2000 and GMDS2000*, A. Hasman, *et al.*, Editors. 2000, IOS: Amsterdam. p. 696-700.

[21]   Wiedemann T, Knaup P, Bachert A, Creutzig U, Haux R, and Schilling. Computer-aided documentation and therapy planning in pediatric oncology. *Medinfo*, 1998. 9 Pt 2: p. 1306-9.

[22]   Rector, AL. Clinical Terminology: Why Is it so Hard? *Methods Inf Med*, 1999. 38: p. 239-252.

[23]   Cimino JJ. Terminology tools: state of the art and practical lessons. *Methods Inf Med*, 2001. 40(4): p. 298-306.

Address for correspondence

Dr. Petra Knaup-Gregori
Department of Medical Informatics
Im Neuenheimer Feld 400
D-69120 Heidelberg
petra_knaup@med.uni-heidelberg.de
Ph +49 6101 85818, Fax +49 6221 564997.

Connecting Medical Informatics and Bio-Informatics
R. Engelbrecht et al. (Eds.)
IOS Press, 2005

Understanding Telecardiology Success and Pitfalls by a Systematic Review

Stefano Bonacina[a,b], Lorenza Draghi[a], Marco Masseroli[a], Francesco Pinciroli[a,b,c]

[a]*Dipartimento di Bioingegneria, Politecnico di Milano, Milano, Italy*
[b]*Multimedica Hospital, Sesto San Giovanni (MI), Italy*
[c]*Istituto di Ingegneria Biomedica, Consiglio Nazionale delle Ricerche, Milano, Italy*

Abstract

Cardiology is the clinical area where death causes are more frequent than in any other clinical area, and it could benefit from telemedicine. At present, assessment about telecardiology application are hard to find, and sometimes can be found in review article about telemedicine, but there is a lack of review on telecardiology application literature. So we reviewed studies regarding telemedicine applications on cardiology specialty.
Sixty-one articles were selected, searching the PubMed database for all years the database were available. All considered articles were published on peer reviewed telemedicine and biomedical journals, from 1992 to 2004. We defined an evaluation grid for the articles in our research result set. Each article was reviewed and catalogued, identifying: 1) Article identification, 2) Content description, 3) Telemedicine manifesto classification, 4) Telemedicine system paradigm, 5) Involved actors.
Most of the analysed literature referred only to feasibility studies, pilot projects and to short-term outcomes, for example only 21 cases reported a project duration greater than one year. The method proposed can be used to analyse literature on others telemedicine specialties.

Keywords:
Telemedicine; Cardiology; Medical Informatics

1. Introduction

The success of a new telemedicine application depends on a large number of sensitive factors, like cost-effectiveness, efficacy, patient satisfaction, doctor-patient communication, and clinical outcomes. In previous systematic reviews these factors were investigated. Whitten et al. [1] addressed the question of whether the existing literature allows any conclusions to be drawn about the cost effectiveness of telemedicine interventions, even though reported studies are often small in scale, methodologically flawed, and reflect pragmatic evaluations rather than controlled trials, making them unsuitable for formal meta-analysis [2]. Whitten et al. [1] found there was no persuasive evidence about whether telemedicine represents a cost effective means of delivering health care.

The study of Hersh et al. [3] focused on the efficacy of telemedicine for diagnostic and management decisions. Authors found that in only a few of analyzed studies the diagnosis and management decisions provided by telemedicine are comparable to those made face to face.

Mair and Whitten [4] highlighted that in the published research methodological deficiencies (e.g. low sample sizes, and study design) affect the validity and generalization of results. Moreover, communication issues can affect the quality of interpersonal relationships based on this medium, and therefore can affect consultation outcomes, although this have still to be fully explored.

The analytical survey of the literature produced by Miller [5] strongly favoured doctor-patient communication via telemedicine, although further research is necessary if nature and content of the communication process are to be fully understood. Miller also proposed a conceptual model [6] that posits telemedicine affects health outcomes through changes in the way doctors and patients communicate. The review of Hailey et al. [7], focusing on studies reporting comparison outcomes with non-telemedicine approaches, shown that there are few good-quality comparative studies of telemedicine, and it may be difficult to generalize findings on a particular application because of significant influence of local circumstances (e.g. case-mix, practice patterns, reimbursement policies, and availability also of other health technologies).

The cited systematic reviews deal with telemedicine literature in general, without focusing on a particular medical specialty. Because of the significantly different ways telemedicine is performed in the specific medical areas, this can lead to disregard important details in favor of general considerations. Therefore, we decided to perform an analytical review of scientific articles regarding the application of telemedicine in a specific medical field. As area of study we chosen telecardiology and telemedicine application in cardiology because cardiology is the clinical area where death causes are more frequent than in any other clinical area, and probably it can benefit from telemedicine. Although at present only a few telemedicine articles regard telecardiology, some interesting review articles exist. For example, the review of Sable [8] that focuses on tele-echocardiography and comparison between the two primary modalities of tele-echocardiography (i.e. "store and forward" and "real time").

To do our analysis, first we designed a literature classification inventory able to orderly store all the relevant attributes characterizing a scientific study on telemedicine applications. Then, we selected and systematically reviewed a set of scientific papers regarding telecardiology and published from January 1992 to October 2004, and populated the inventory with information from the reviewed articles.

Finally, we analyzed the collected data trying to investigate questions like: a) What are the key aspects for telecardiology applications success? b) Which technologies are widely diffused and which others have been abandoned? c) To what extent does Telemedicine benefit from the enhancement of Information and Communication Technology methods and devices?

2. Materials and Methods

2.1 Literature Search and Article Selection

We performed a text based search of title, abstract, and Medical Subject Heading (MeSH) terms in PubMed, the US National Library of Medicine publication database, using Entrez, the National Center for Biotechnology Information (NCBI) search and retrieval system [9]. The terms "telemedicine and cardiology" and "telecardiology" were used for the literature search and the following search string was employed ("telemedicine" [MeSH Terms] OR "telemedicine" [Text Word]) AND ("cardiology" [MeSH Terms] OR "cardiology" [Text Word]) OR ("telecardiology" [All Fields]). Publication date was limited to October 2004.

From the articles retrieved, we selected all publications in English language that were not conference proceedings, editorials, review articles, or historical articles, and we considered for further analyses only those articles published on peer reviewed journals. A value of Impact factor greater than 0,4 was also considered in selecting articles published after 2001.

2.2 Design of Literature Classification Inventory

We developed an for articles in our research result set. Each considered article was reviewed and catalogued according to a specifically developed evaluation grid constituted of the following five groups of characteristics below described and summarized in Table 1: 1) Article identification, 2) Content description, 3) Telemedicine manifesto classification, 4) Telemedicine system paradigm, 5) Involved actors.

2.3.1 Article Identification

This part contains attributes for article identification, such as Author list, Title, Journal, Author affiliation, Type of affiliation (i.e. University, Clinic, Industry, or other), Place of affiliation, PMID (PubMed Identification Number), Year of publication.

2.3.2 Content Description

We used the following attributes to describe article content: Medical specialty, Disease considered, System purposes/objectives, Method description, Aimed Results, Results obtained by applying the described method, Number of patients/cases/sessions evaluated, Project duration, and Comments. In the considered cardiology specialty examples of described diseases are: Congenital/Heart/Vascular/ Diseases (CHD, HD, CVD), Cardiac events (CE), Surgery Candidates (SC), Heart Murmurs (HM), Acute Myocardial Infarct (AMI).

2.3.3 Telemedicine Manifesto Classification

According to the manifesto on telemedicine declared in [10], we classified the telemedicine system presented in an article also by telespecialty, telephase, and teleservice. The first indicates which is the medical specialty the telemedicine system is dedicated (e.g. telephatology, teleradiology, telecardiology). The second, telephase, indicates the medical moment the system is devoted to (e.g. prevention, diagnosis, therapy, treatment). The third, teleservice, refers to the offered healthcare service (e.g. teleconsulting, telemonitoring, telereferral).

2.3.4 Telemedicine System Paradigm

As shown in Figure 1, a telemedicine system can be represented by the four basic block components it is constituted of: Information Sources, Information Users, Tele-services & Tele-specialties, and Connection Technologies. Data are bi-directional exchanged between all these blocks, each of which can be composed of different elements. We considered such blocks and their elements to catalogue a telemedicine system described in an article.

2.3.5 Involved Actors

The different interacting actors involved in a telemedicine system were classified according to their status and characteristics as individual or institutional actors, and service providers or users (Table 1).

Table 1 - Evaluation grid with the attributes considered to catalogue scientific articles on telemedicine applications

Article Attributes	Group
List of Authors	
Article Title	
Journal (Abbreviated Journal Title, Year, Volume #, Issue #, Page #)	
Name of Institution	
Type of Institution (University Department, Industry, Clinic, Laboratory, ...)	Article Identification
Place of Affiliation	
PMID (PubMed Unique Identifier)	
Year	
Medical Specialty	
Disease Considered	
System Purposes/Objectives	
Method Description	
Obtained Results	Content Description
Aimed Results	
Number of Patients/Cases/Sessions	
Project Duration	
Notes	
Tele_Specialty_Type (Telepatology, Teleradiology, Telecardiology)	Telemedicine
Tele_Phase_Type (Diagnosis, Prevention, Therapy, Prognosis, Treatment)	Manifesto
Tele_Service (Teleconsulting, Telemonitoring, Telerefertation, ...)	Classification
Data Sources	
Data Users	
Description of Acquisition System	
Methods of Data Transmission – Hardware	Telemedicine System
Methods of Data Transmission – Software	Paradigm
Type of Transmitted Data	
Methods/Instruments/Technologies of Visualization	
Home Environment Actors (Patients, Relatives, Nursing Personnel)	
Practitioners (General Practitioner, Specialist)	
Points of Care (Hospitals, Medical Centers, Health Centers, Laboratories, ...)	
Local Health Centers	Involved Actors
Health/Clinical Research Organizations	
Universities	
Information & Communication Technology Service Providers	

3. Results

3.1 Retrieved and Evaluated Articles

Our initial literature search yielded 127 references of telemedicine and cardiology scientific articles published till October 2004. Out of these, 61 articles that met the selection criteria described in the method section, were considered for evaluation. More than 59% of these articles (36 out of 61) were published on telemedicine journals: the two peer-reviewed "Journal of Telemedicine and Telecare" and "Telemedicine Journal" (renamed "Telemedicine Journal and e-Health" in 2001), and "Telemedicine Today".

3.2 Analysis of the Classified Articles

By querying the created inventory according to the considered article attributes and analyzing the results obtained for each defined group of attributes, several interesting findings following described were unveiled.

3.2.1 Article identification

The great majority (80.33%) of the considered articles that met the selection criteria were mainly from Europe, 29 (47.54 %), and from the United States, 20 (32.79%). Other 5 (8.20%) were from Canada, 2 from Australia, 2 from Japan, 1 from Azerbaijan Republic, 1 from Israel, and 1 from Mexico.

3.2.2 Content description

As we focused on telecardiology, for all 61 considered articles the "Medical Specialty" attribute was "cardiology", and 20 of the 61 studies were devoted to pediatric cardiology. Of the 61 studies, 41 were specifically addressed to a disease that was CHD, HD, or CVD in 34 cases, HM in 3 cases, SC in 2 cases, and AMI in 2 cases. "System Purposes/Objectives" consisted of early diagnosis and patient screening, evaluation of long distance consultation, and remote interpretation of ECGs or echocardiograms. The most frequent "Methods Description " was about remote transmission of echocardiograms and ECG (32 cases). The "Number of Patients/Cases/Sessions" was specified for 42 studies, and "Project Duration", which was specified in 36 studies, lasted longer than 2 years in 11 cases and longer than 3 years in 2 cases.

3.2.3 Telemedicine manifesto classification

According to the selection criteria, the "Tele_Specialty_Type" attribute was Telecardiology for all the considered articles. However, the "Tele_Phase_Type" was Telediagnosis in 38 cases, Teletherapy in 7 cases, and Telesurgery in 1 case, whereas 15 articles were not addressed to any specific health care moment.

4. Discussion

Previous systematic reviews of telemedicine literature pointed out the following issues: first, there is no evidence about whether telemedicine represents a cost effective mean of delivering health care [1,2]. Second, there are methodological deficiencies that affect the validity and generalization of the results [4]. Third, few good-quality comparative studies of outcomes with non-telemedicine alternatives are available [3,7]. Moreover, a recent systematic review of literature on telecardiology assessment [11], from 1992 to September 2003, found that there is still limited good-quality evidence of telecardiology benefits to health-care.

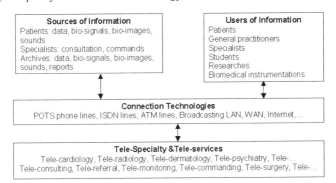

Figure 1- The four basic block components of a telemedicine system, their interactions, and the possible elements within each block

Our study proposes a detailed way of analyzing documents that can contribute to compile clinical or medical guidelines. The attributes used to classify scientific literature, defined in Table 1, can be used together with the data collected to build decision trees, or rules, in order to describe relationships between attributes and to make decisions.

Furthermore, medical professionals can predict the reasonable values of one or more attributes from the known values of others, e.g. to establish the involved actors into a telecardiology system regarding a specific disease.

5. Conclusion

In the present study we developed a method to classify scientific publications and analysed literature on telecardiology from January 1992 to October 2004. If this method would be used to analyse, on large scale, literature about others telemedical specialties like teleradiology, teledermatology, telepathology, telepsychiatry, the differences and similarities among tele-specialties could be deeper addressed.

6. Acknowledgments

This work was supported by the FIRB grant: "Information and Communication Technology for the management of prevention, care and rehabilitation processes", 2003, by the Italian Ministry of the University and Technical Scientific Research - MURST.

7. References

[1]   Whitten PS, Mair FS, Haycox A, May CR, Williams TL, Hellmich S. Systematic review of cost effectiveness studies of telemedicine interventions. *BMJ* 2002;324:1434-7.

[2]   May C, Mort M, Mair FS, Ellis NT,Gask L. Evaluation of new technologies in health care: what's the context? *Health Inform J* 2000;6:64-8.

[3]   Hersh W, Helfand M, Wallace J, Kraemer D, Patterson P, Shapiro S, Greenlick M. A systematic review of the efficacy of telemedicine for making diagnostic and management decisions. *J Telemed Telecare.* 2002;8(4):197-209.

[4]   Mair F, Whitten P. Systematic review of studies of patient satisfaction with telemedicine. *BMJ* 2000;320:1517-20.

[5]   Miller EA. Telemedicine and doctor-patient communication: an analytical survey of the literature. *J Telemed Telecare.* 2001;7:1-17.

[6]   Miller EA. Telemedicine and doctor-patient communication: a theoretical framework for evaluation. *J Telemed Telecare.* 2002;8:311-318.

[7]   Hailey D, Roine R, Ohinmaa A. Systematic review of evidence for the benefits of telemedicine. *J Telemed Telecare.* 2002;8(Suppl.1):S1:1-7.

[8]   Sable C. Telemedicine applications in pediatric cardiology. *Minerva Pediatr.* 2003 Feb;55(1):1-13.

[9]   National Library of Medicine. Entrez-PubMed. Available at: http://www.ncbi.nlm.nih.gov/entrez/query.fcgi. Last access: Jan 12, 2005.

[10] Pinciroli F. A manifesto on telehealth and telemedicine. J Am Med Inform Assoc. 2001 Jul-Aug;8(4):349-50.

[11] Hailey D, Ohinmaa A, Roine R. Published evidence on the success of telecardiology: a mixed record. J Telemed Telecare. 2004;10 Suppl. 1:36-8.

Address for correspondence

Stefano BONACINA
Dipartimento di Bioingegneria
Politecnico di Milano
Piazza Leonardo da Vinci, 32
I-20133 Milano, Italy
E-mail: stefano.bonacina@biomed.polimi.it

Connecting Medical Informatics and Bio-Informatics
R. Engelbrecht et al. (Eds.)
IOS Press, 2005

Architecture Evaluation for the Implementation of a Regional Integrated Electronic Health Record

Daniel Ferreira Polónia, Carlos Costa, José Luis Oliveira

University of Aveiro, DET/ IEETA, 3810-193 Aveiro, Portugal

Abstract

The interconnection between different healthcare information systems is not yet a trivial task. Solid communication infrastructures do exist, solid solutions for Health Information Systems (HIS) are installed, but, unfortunately, too many different solutions hinder the integration of HIS at a regional, national or European level. In this paper we propose a solution and an implementation of an Integrated Electronic Health Record that is a composition of two distinct integration models – centralized and distributed. We exploit this solution against a set of predefined users and institutional requirements, at a regional level in two Portuguese regions. As a conclusion, an evaluation of the cost and inherent benefits is made involving the clinical, economical and organizational perspectives.

Keywords:
Regional Health Planning, Medical Record Linkage, EHR, Health Systems Plans, EPR

1. Introduction

Despite the massive introduction and wide usage of Health Information Systems during the last decade, several problems still exist in these scenarios, most of them related with the lack of integration.

With the evolution of the health information and communication systems, it is now the time for the implementation of systems that allow the unification of the existing Electronic Health Records (EHR). For that, and taking into account the existing architectures, it is necessary to perform an analysis of the architectural possibilities and optimize the mix between them, in order to maximize the benefit from the implementation of such systems.

The analysis scope must include, not only the necessary means required to unify the EHR's, but also the required maintenance and support and, if possible, the creation of an archive that allows the integration of the already existing information, scattered and stored in the systems of the multiple players of the health care provision value chain.

In this paper, we define and describe four main models for the implementation of an Integrated Electronic Health Record (I-EHR), and, in order to perform the implementation analysis of each model, we identify the geographical region where it is to be implemented, identifying and quantifying the number of institutions and involved professionals, as well as the demographic status of the region. It is also presented a methodological evaluation framework that considers the technological, clinical and economic perspectives. Finally it is presented an application of the methodological framework to the proposed architecture and a qualitative cost-benefit analysis is made.

2. Materials

For the definition of concepts, we hereby present the formal definition of Integrated Electronic Health Record (I-EHR) and present four versions of architectures that can be adopted to support its implementation.

According to [1], an I-EHR is a collection of all of an individual's lifetime health data in electronic form, generated during relevant interactions with the healthcare system. In addition to providing support for continuity of care, the I-EHR may prove to be a valuable tool in basic and clinical research, medical decision making, epidemiology, evidence-based medicine, and in formulating public health policy.

Multiple benefits, and associated effort, can arise from the implementation of such a system at a regional or national scale [2, 3]. The benefits can be identified among multiple dimensions, with the most relevant being the clinical and economical, but still with identifiable benefits in the scientific, technological and organizational dimensions.

3. Reference architectures for the implementation of an I-EHR

In what concerns the integration of autonomous and distributed systems, four approaches can be taken. The first, based on a message-based architecture, the second and third one based in the system federation architecture, which are be further subdivided into physically and virtually federated architectures, and finally the fourth one, an evolution of the virtually federated architecture, that is the virtually unique electronic health record (VUEHR) architecture. We briefly present the first three and then make a more detailed analysis of the fourth model in what concerns interoperability, modularity and scalability, migration, stability, management, maintenance, security and, finally, its cost effectiveness.

The message based architecture [4] is characterized by data communication between systems that rely on message communication protocols, with the data structures and message contents following a standardized structure.

The physically federated architecture is based on the existence of a centralized system that gathers all the information from the autonomous distributed systems into a centralized structure, where data is structured, indexed and normalized and further integrated with administrative and medical emergency data [5-8].

The virtually federated architecture is based on the integration of the clinical information components through the use of a set of structured pointers that reference the remote location of the patient data, geographically and physically scattered. This model also demands the existence of a centralized structure, as in the physically federated architecture, that has lower storage and communication requirements. The most simplistic implementation structure can be based in a server unit with a search engine that guarantees the federated structure [9].

Finally, the virtually unique electronic health record (VUEHR) architecture, a model we have developed and proposed in [10, 11] and that has been refined since, provides access to integrated patient information scattered among different systems inside the health provision network. It is based on a smart card containing card-owner information, as well as structured references to its electronic records. The card securely supports the reference structured data set, and the implementation of Public Keys Cryptography and Crypto Smart Cards unequivocally provides a way to securely store, transport and access the card-owner information. It also grants the user full control over the access to its data, through a PIN and/or biometric registration and also allows the card-owner to entitle information access levels to other users such as the healthcare professionals. The main benefits can be characterized by highly scattered geographical storage requirements; a scalable architecture with great flexibility in the addition of new healthcare providers systems to the federation with no impact in the existing systems, guaranteeing an implementation phased approach. It is also a highly reliable model, due to its simplicity and operational and functional independence from any type of centralized unit. The model empowers of patient user, enabling the discretionary access to data, when crossed with the healthcare professional card, and allows open access to the medical emergency data. The system is technology independent and its only requirement is that the institutions provide Web access to patient information and support authentication with digital certificates. The information duplication problem is therefore reduced and the anonymization of data is intrinsic to the system.

4. Methods

We now proceed into describing the region where the I-EHR is to be implemented, in demographic and health care current status, and presenting the users that will be subject to the implementation of such a system. We will them present the evaluation framework that will help us perform the evaluation of the architecture mix that supports implementation.

Region geographical and health care characterization

The region to be analyzed is located in the central sea side of Portugal and is constituted by two NUTS III regions (Baixo Vouga and Entre Douro e Vouga) [12] that are made up of 17 Local Administrative Units (municipalities), scattered by 2.264 square kilometers and comprising 662.536 inhabitants [13].

There are 17 health centers (primary care units), one per municipality, that have 128 local extensions to the small villages. These units employ 1.520 persons, of which 463 are doctors and 314 are nurses.

The region has 8 hospitals (secondary care units) comprising 22 medical and 37 surgical services, 6 intensive care units, 13 clinical pathological services and 19 imaging services [14]. The total staff comprises 3.470 employees, of which, 578 are doctors and 1163 are nurses. It also has 3 privately owned hospitals for which no data is available.

It comprises 169 pharmacies that employ 399 workers, of which 302 are pharmacists.

5. Evaluation framework

The proposed architecture will be a mix of the previously described federated architectures and that will have to comply with the following evaluation framework items [15-17]:

Technical compatibility with other systems and existing legacy systems, including issues such as upgradeability, maintenance, data consistency and adaptability to changing requirements, as well as security and user identification aspects, with these aspects being the fundamental key issues to be considered;

Professional and patient user acceptance, including addressing professional clinical and business needs as well as structural process related impact and impacts in the quality of care provided, aligning these issues with the technical ones but not making them fundamental;

Economical viability of the proposed solution, with calculation of upfront investment and operational costs, as well as cost effectiveness and benefits, thus generating the return on the investment made will be an important aspect of the evaluation, that is heavily related to the technical options made early in the project;

Other aspects such as the social consequences of the implementation of such a system are considered as out of scope from this paper.

6. Results and Discussion

Taking into consideration the previously presented geographical and health specifications of the region under analysis, we now discuss the task of finding the optimal architecture for the system in order to implement the regional I-EHR.

On a top down approach, we would select as the main architecture that would gather all the institutions and participants, the virtually unique electronic health record architecture. It was selected since it provides maximum flexibility in the integration of the different, heterogeneous institutions and at the same time is scalable enough in order to be extensible to other regions that would adopt this architecture with minimum cost. On the down side, it will demand the issuance of new health cards, powerful enough to retain the references created in each interaction with the health institutions, and will demand the integration of the existing software into "institutional data centres".

Analysing the involved institutions, we start with the health centres and its extensions. Since they share similar processes and users, and taking into consideration that they are scattered in relatively small geographical areas, with good coverage of telecommunication services, we propose the interconnection of the health centre to the extensions using the physically federated architecture with the integration and storage of the data to be placed in the main health centre. All the data placed in the data centre, as a result of consultations, prescriptions and other clinical and/or administrative actions, would be referenced to the upper integration level according to the procedures described in the virtually unique electronic health record (VUEHR), with the information stored in the data centre and with a reference placed in the patient health card [18].

The implementation of this option, in what regards the health centers, can be phased over time, starting from the smaller to the bigger ones, with the main requirement being that the health center and its extensions are treated as a single unit and integrated in a one shot basis. Due to the similar nature of the software to be integrated, the experiences and the work performed can be replicated in the subsequent integration efforts, lowering the integration costs and efforts.

In what concerns the hospitals, the architectural option to be taken must allow that the involved services (medical, surgical, intensive care, pathological and imaging) are treated as different units, being able to phase the integration effort of its legacy systems into the main hospital data center according to their own schedule. As in the case of the health centers, it must be noticed that, since the same services, in different hospitals, share the same applications, the integration effort can be replicated among them, thus diminishing the economical integration effort.

The providers of external diagnosis services, that perform clinical exams externally to the hospitals and health centres can, with the implementation of this model, improve their workflow efficiency, with integrated exam scheduling and with online availability of the examinations performed.

The pharmacies that belong to the network only need to access the information regarding the medicines prescribed by the physicians in the health center or the hospital. However, since they all share similar management information systems, there is also the option of integrating this system into the network.

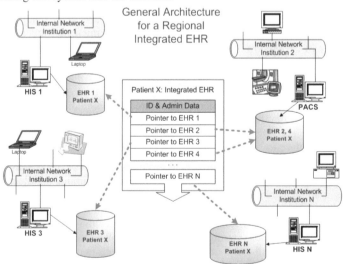

Figure 1 – Main building blocks of the proposed architecture.

7. Conclusion

The results obtained in this study show us that there is no single architecture that can provide all users of the system with maximum results. This objective can only be achieved with the development of a "best of breed" architecture that gathers the best features and adapts them to the local needs and processes. It is shown that some of the units of the system (hospitals and health centres) need to have a preliminary, internal integration using the physically federated architecture in order to gather information from all the underlying units, which then interconnect into a network where the architecture is the virtually unique electronic health record (VUEHR) and that allows the access of all users to all the information, no matter what is the internal architecture adopted by them. The same applies to the remaining institutions where, independently of their size, they can with little integration effort, enter the network and access information provided by all parties.The architecture main components are shown in Figure 1.

Analysing the process in more detail, as mentioned previously, the implementation of this system requires three major activities to be performed concurrently.

First, the implementation of a regional high capacity communications infrastructure that is able to interconnect all the participant institutions.

Secondly, the need to integrate all the existing information systems in health institutions data centers, although it is possible to reuse some of the integration effort since they share similar applications from a reduced universe of sellers.

Thirdly, and the most demanding effort of them all, it is necessary to issue new health cards into the universe of 662.536 inhabitants and 5.389 health professionals employed in the health centers, hospitals and pharmacies of the region.

From a technical point of view, this approach can be implemented with the integration of the existing legacy systems with the new data center structure, thus maximizing the use of the existing software infrastructure and guaranteeing the backwards compatibility of the existing data. The maintenance effort of the central structure is almost inexistent, with the core of the maintenance effort taking place in the institutional health centers. On the security side, it is guaranteed that the clinical data can only be accessed with consent from the patient and, on the other hand, the data physical storage always remains under supervision of the health center. The security tunnelling would also be established automatically between the data center and the access point through the use of digital certificates. The professionals belonging to these institutions would also be able to maximize their requirements, having access to an I-EHR that complies with the requirements previously exposed.

The economical evaluation, at this stage, needs to be performed qualitatively since quantitative data are still not available. However, we can say that the integration effort is probably the main technical and economical difficulty, with the main advantage of having little maintenance requirements of the central system, although there are maintenance costs in the local data centres. This benefit can be annulated by the fact that there is the need to issue new cards for the universe of patients and professionals involved.

In a very preliminary benefit study performed using the TEC methodology developed by NCSU [19], we estimated that the implementation of this architecture could signify a yearly savings of 9,23 € per capita, which could mean a total yearly savings of 6,1 million euros in the region considered.

8. Acknowledgments

The present work has been funded by the European Commission (FP6, IST thematic area) through the INFOBIOMED NoE (IST-507585).

9. References

[1]   Tsiknakis, M., D.G. Katehakis, and S.C. Orphanoudakis, An open, component-based information infrastructure for integrated health information networks. International Journal of Medical Informatics, 2002. 68(1-3): p. 3-26.

[2]   Tsiknakis, M., D. Katehakis, and S.C. Orphanoudakis, A health information infrastructure enabling secure access to the life-long multimedia electronic health record. International Congress Series, 2004. 1268: p. 289-294.

[3]   van Ginneken, A.M., The computerized patient record: balancing effort and benefit. International Journal of Medical Informatics, 2002. 65(2): p. 97-119.

[4]   Katehakis, D.G., et al. An Open, Component-based Information Infrastructure to Support Integrated RegionalHealthcare Networks. in Medinfo 2001. 2001: IOS Press.

[5]   Halamka, J.D., C. Osterland, and C. Safran, CareWeb(TM), a web-based medical record for an integrated health care delivery system. Int. Journal of Medical Informatics, 1999. 54(1): p. 1-8.

[6]   Lenz, R. and K.A. Kuhn, Intranet meets hospital information systems: The solution to the integration problem? Methods of Information in Medicine, 2001. 40(2): p. 99-105.

[7]   Kerkri, E.M., et al., An Approach for Integrating Heterogeneous Information Sources in a Medical Data Warehouse. Journal of Medical Systems, 2001. 25(3): p. 167-176.

[8]   Zucker, A., From computerized patient records to national resource. Stud Health Technol Inform, 2003. 95: p. 892-7.

[9]   Malamateniou, F., G. Vassilacopoulos, and J. Mantas, A search engine for virtual patient records. International Journal of Medical Informatics, 1999. 55(2): p. 103-115.

[10] Costa, C., et al, A Multi-Service Patient Data Card, in Medinfo 2002. 2002. Amsterdam: IOS Press.

[11] Costa, C., et al, A New Concept for an Integrated Healthcare Access Model, in MIE 2003. 2003. St. Malo: IOS Press.

[12] Commission, European, NUTS Statistical Regions of Europe. 2005.

[13] INE, Anuários Estatísticos Regionais (Saúde) - Quadros Nacionais 2003 / Yearly regional statistics for health 2003, Instituto Nacional de Estatística, 2003, Lisboa.

[14] IGIF, Estatistica 2003/Statistics 2003, Health Ministry, 2003, Lisboa.

[15] Ammenwerth, E., et al., Visions and strategies to improve evaluation of health information systems: Reflections and lessons based on the HIS-EVAL workshop in Innsbruck. International Journal of Medical Informatics, 2004. 73(6): p. 479-491.

[16] Stoop, A.P. and M. Berg, Integrating quantitative and qualitative methods in patient care information system evaluation guidance for the organizational decision maker. Methods of Information in Medicine, 2003. 42(4): p. 458-462.

[17] Neame, R. and M.J. Olson, Security issues arising in establishing a regional health information infrastructure. International Journal of Medical Informatics, 2004. 73(3): p. 285-290.

[18] Polónia, D., et al., Um Data Center para a Saúde em Portugal: Análise de Viabilidade Técnico-Económica (Techno economic analysis for the viability of a health data center in Portugal), Instituto de Engenharia Electrónica e Telemática de Aveiro (IEETA), 2003, Aveiro.

[19] Aiman-Smith, L., et al. Real world technology management education: using the TEC algorithm. in Management of Engineering and Technology, 1999. Technology and Innovation Management. PICMET '99. Portland International Conference on. 1999.

Address for correspondence

Daniel Ferreira Polónia
DET /IEETA - Universidade de Aveiro
3810-193 Aveiro, Portugal
dpolonia@ieeta.pt

Connecting Medical Informatics and Bio-Informatics
R. Engelbrecht et al. (Eds.)
IOS Press, 2005

Semantic Integration in Healthcare Networks

Richard Lenz[a], Mario Beyer[a], Klaus A Kuhn[b]

[a]*Philipps-Universität Marburg, Institut für Medizinische Informatik, Marburg, Germany*
[b]*Technische Universität München, Lehrstuhl für Medizinische Informatik, Munich, Germany*

Abstract

A seamless support of information flow for increasingly distributed healthcare processes requires to integrate heterogeneous IT systems into a comprehensive distributed information system. Different standards contribute to ease this integration. In a research project focussing on the development of a reference architecture for inter-institutional health information systems, we identified and categorised concurring integration standards by distinguishing between technical and semantic integration on the one hand, and data and functional integration on the other hand. In addition, standards for semantic integration are roughly categorised according to their scope. By placing standards into a corresponding matrix a "semantic gap" is revealed, which cannot be covered by standards as it contains volatile medical concepts. As a conclusion, it is recommended to conceptually consider the necessity of system evolution in systems architectures and also in future integration standards.

Keywords:
Information Systems, Information Management, HIS

1. Introduction

Healthcare increasingly changes from isolated treatment episodes towards a continuous treatment process involving multiple healthcare professionals and various institutions. This change imposes new demanding requirements for IT. Thereby, IT applications should guide data acquisition in a way that data are ready for reuse in different contexts from the beginning, without the need to manually index or transform the data. To achieve this heterogeneous systems have to be integrated into a comprehensive distributed information system. Integrating autonomously developed applications, however, is a difficult task, as individual applications usually are not designed to cooperate and often based on differing conceptualisations. Powerful integration tools (e.g. application servers, object brokers, different kinds of message-oriented middleware, and workflow management systems [1]) are available to overcome technical and syntactical heterogeneity. Yet, *semantic heterogeneity* remains as a major barrier to seamless integration of autonomously developed software components (cf. [2]). Semantic heterogeneity occurs when there is disagreement about the meaning, interpretation or intended use of the same or related data [3]. It occurs in different contexts, like database schema integration, ontology mapping, or integration of different terminologies. The underlying problems are more or less the same, though they are often complex and still poorly understood. Stonebraker characterises disparate systems as "islands of information" and points out two major factors which aggravate systems integration [4]: (1) Each island (i.e. application) will have its own meaning of enterprise objects.

(2) Each island will have data that overlaps data in other islands. This partial redundancy generates a serious data integrity problem. Based on this statement, data integration can be led back to a mapping problem (semantic mapping of different conceptualisations) and a synchronisation problem (to ensure mutual consistency of redundant data in different data-bases under the control of autonomous applications). The mapping problem has been extensively discussed in the database literature under the term "database schema integration" (e.g. [5-8]). A major perception in this research has been that schema integration cannot be automated in general. Batini et al stated:*"The general problem of schema integration is undecidable."* [9]. Heiler states that *"understanding data and software can never be fully automated"* [10]. Consequently, the process of schema integration always needs a human integrator for semantic decisions. Colomb recognized that there are cases where no consistent interpretation of heterogeneous sources is possible (*"fundamental semantic heterogeneity"*) [11]. In such cases one either has to modify software components or simply accept a low degree of data quality.

Standard ontologies are needed to reduce the effort for semantic integration. Moreover, as medicine is a rapidly evolving domain, concepts for system evolution are needed. Fortunately, far reaching standards for information interchange have already been developed in the medical domain. Yet, healthcare software is still far away from plug and play compatibility. In a research project focused on a reference architecture for comprehensive IS in healthcare networks [12], we have identified concurring and semantically overlapping standards. To get an overview of the standards' characteristics and interrelations, we have arranged them to a system of standards which we find to be helpful for architecture development.

2. Objectives

In this article we try to clarify how different standards contribute to systems integration by distinguishing different aspects and dimensions of integration. The objective of this approach is to identify and characterise the "semantic gap" not covered by standards. Our goal is to derive recommendations for future system architectures and standards development.

3. Methods

At a conceptual level, information systems are designed around three layers: presentation, application logic, and resource management [1]. According to this well known abstract m odel of information systems, we distinguished different aspects of integration: data integration, functional integration and presentation integration:

- *Data integration:* When we characterized semantic heterogeneity as the main cause for high integration efforts, we focused on data integration, because it is the backbone and starting point of each successful integration project. Any process control always requires a meaningful exchange of data, too [13]. The goal of data integration is to create a unique semantic reference for commonly used data and to ensure data consistency. As a basic categorization for such a semantic reference we roughly distinguish three different facets: (1) The *instance level,* referring to the semantics of individual data objects, which corresponds to the meaning of entries in a database. (2) The *type level,* designating the semantic classification of data objects, which roughly corresponds to the database schema. (3) The *context,* which refers to the semantic relationships that associate an object with other objects. To illustrate the difference we may consider a concept "diagnosis" on the type level, and a particular instance, say "Encephalitis", and the context of this instance which is determined by the patient, the physician who made the diagnosis, and other objects that contribute to a particular statement (information).

- *Functional integration* refers to the meaningful cooperation of functions. Uncontrolled data redundancy is often the result of an insufficient functional integration. Autonomously developed systems often provide slightly differing but still overlapping functionality, which aggravates integration even if common ontologies are already used. Data integration is concerned with the consolidation of declarative knowledge, while functional integration is concerned with the consolidation of procedural knowledge on which applications are based. Both aspects have to be considered for *application integration*.
- *Desktop integration or presentation integration* refers to the user interface of a distributed system. Desktop integration is aimed at user transparency, meaning that the user would not know what application was being used or what database was being queried [14]. This requires more than a unified layout and uniform interaction mechanisms. Examples are "single sign-on" and "desktop synchronisation". Desktop synchronisation is needed when a user has multiple windows to different applications on her desktop that share a common context. Synchronisation is required when the context is changed in one of the interlinked applications.

Another orthogonal aspect of integration standards is their *scope*. We can distinguish between technical and semantic integration. By "technical integration" we refer to the technical infrastructure which supports application integration. "Semantic integration", in contrast, refers to the meaning of data and functions. By contrasting the scope with data and functional integration we receive a rough matrix that helps to characterise different integration standards. Table 1 shows how different standards can be positioned into this matrix.

Table 1 – A classification of integration standards

	Technical integration	Semantic integration
Data integration	Syntactic frameworks	Ontology and vocabulary
Functional integration	Middleware	Application frameworks

4. Results

XML and RDF are examples for *syntactic frameworks* supporting data integration. Standards for semantic integration in healthcare are increasingly *based on* XML in order to improve syntactical compatibility with commonly accepted data processing formats.

Middleware standards typically provide a common infrastructure for interconnecting distributed software components. Such standards are primarily intended to provide programming abstractions, which help a programmer to easily bridge different hardware, operating systems, and programming languages. Examples for standardisation efforts in this area are CORBA, .net, EJB, or Web Services.

Ontologies and vocabulary standards support semantic data integration, as they serve as a semantic reference for system programmers and users (cf. [15]). Considering the different facets of data integration we find that well accepted standards like HL7 V2 and DICOM are primarily concerned with organisational issues on a type level. Terminological control is only supported to a limited degree. Yet, numerous standards support terminological control for medical issues at an instance level. Upcoming standards like CDA [16] and DICOM SR cover the interchange of medical contents also on the type and context levels.

Despite well accepted standards for data integration like HL7 V2 and DICOM, healthcare applications are still far from plug and play compatibility. One reason for this is that the existing standards do not address functional integration issues sufficiently. In order to avoid these difficulties common *application frameworks* are required which serve as a reference for programmers to create functionally compatible software components. Requirements for an application framework directed towards open systems in the healthcare domain are described in [17]. In general such a framework must provide clear specifications of interfaces and interaction protocols which are needed for embedding a software component into a system of cooperating components. The best example for such a standard in the healthcare domain is the IHE initiative ("Integrating the Healthcare Enterprise") [18]. IHE does not develop new standards for data interchange but specifies integration profiles on the basis of HL7 and DICOM. Thereby actors and transactions are defined independently from any specific software product. An integration profile specifies how different actors interact via IHE transactions in order to perform a special task. These integration profiles serve as a semantic reference for application programmers, so that they can build software products that can be functionally integrated into an IHE conformant application framework. HL7 V3 will also take a step into this direction, as conformance to HL7 V3 is specified in terms of "application roles" [19]. Like IHE actors, an application role is associated with some dedicated functionality (e.g. "lab order sender") – it comprises a set of trigger events, messages and data elements which are needed to integrate an IT component with this functionality. An IT component will typically fill many such application roles.

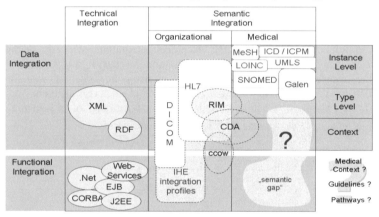

Figure 1 – Contribution of different standards to application integration

Figure 1 shows a rough characterisation of standards according to our classification matrix. The position of HL7 in this diagram refers to HL7 V2. Some improvements that come with HL7 V3 (e.g. RIM, CDA and CCOW [20]) are roughly indicated. The intention of the diagram is not to precisely and comprehensively classify the different standards but to get an idea which aspects of semantic integration are typically covered by such standards. It turns out that there is a gap in the lower right corner where standardised medical processes could have been expected. Medical pathways and guidelines fall into this category. This is essentially medical knowledge which has to be consented by medical experts and which evolves over time. Consented medical knowledge is necessary for cooperative patient treatment, but it is probably unsuitable as a subject of standardisation, as it rapidly evolves.

Despite of many standards for medical terminologies are in place. Yet, a unique and comprehensive ontology of the medical domain is not within sight, and, even worse, all given examples continuously evolve over time – necessarily. Thus, semantic integration of heterogeneous systems in healthcare will have to deal with volatile medical concepts.

5. Discussion and conclusions

Both reference ontologies and application frameworks are needed to support semantic integration. Yet, IT standards should not try to comprehensively map an application domain into a single model, as the domain continuously evolves. Instead, IT systems should be based on generic models and be capable of incorporating the results of ongoing consensus processes among healthcare professionals. The evolution of information systems should be a demand-driven process under the control of healthcare professionals. *Process integration* is concerned with the alignment of IT systems to actual business processes in a concrete setting. This is not addressed by standards, but by appropriate models for demand-driven software development (e.g. [21]). Desiderata for such a demand-driven process are:

- Tools and techniques for *rapid application development* (RAD). These tools should allow reuse of existing data and IT services.
- An IT infrastructure for a healthcare network should provide a *robust and stable basis* for application development. Thus, the framework should be based on generic but stable domain models instead of comprehensive but volatile domain models.
- Modeling of *domain concepts should be separated from IT system implementation.* IT systems should be implemented by IT experts and medical knowledge should be modeled and maintained by domain experts. Yet, this separation is not easy, because algorithms (e.g. reminder systems) typically refer to medical knowledge to fulfill their task. One attempt to support such a separation of concerns, is the "archetype" approach developed in the context of the GEHR project [22].
- To bring application development as close to the end user as possible, a *multi-layered software engineering approach* is proposed. An idealised abstract model for such a multi-level approach for software engineering is shown in Figure 2.
- *Layered ontologies* may serve within this layered software engineering process as semantic references on different levels of software development. The layered approach of the CDA, and the generic HL7 V3 Reference Information Model (RIM) are emerging standards which are already built on this fundamental principle.

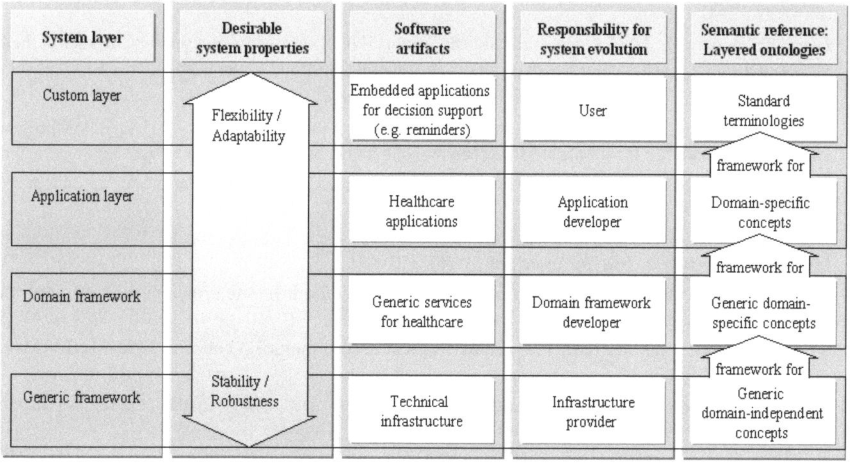

System layer	Desirable system properties	Software artifacts	Responsibility for system evolution	Semantic reference: Layered ontologies
Custom layer	Flexibility / Adaptability	Embedded applications for decision support (e.g. reminders)	User	Standard terminologies
				framework for
Application layer		Healthcare applications	Application developer	Domain-specific concepts
				framework for
Domain framework		Generic services for healthcare	Domain framework developer	Generic domain-specific concepts
				framework for
Generic framework	Stability / Robustness	Technical infrastructure	Infrastructure provider	Generic domain-independent concepts

Figure 2 – A layered approach for system evolution

Layered approaches have proven to be a successful technique for separating concerns and reducing system complexity. Transferring this principle to the development and continuous improvement of information systems in complex application domains is aimed at allowing application developers and end users to build well integrated healthcare applications without the need to do low level coding and debugging. Appropriate tool support is needed at each level of abstraction in order to effectively make use of the lower system layers.

A layered approach, as sketched above, fosters a system evolution process that follows the principle of "deferred systems design" [23]: Volatile concepts are not pre-modelled and hard-coded in software, instead knowledge can be added or modified on demand and at runtime, as the domain evolves.

Our layered model can be used as an abstract reference model for evolutionary information systems. An example for an adaptation of this model to a real world hospital information system on the basis of commercially available system components is given in [21].

References

[1] Alonso G, Casati F, Kuno H, Machiraju V. Web Services - Concepts, Architectures and Applications. Berlin: Springer, 2003.

[2] Pollock JT. The Web Services Scandal - How Data Semantics Have Been Overlooked in Integration Solutions. EAI Journal 2002; 2002(August): 20-23.

[3] Sheth A, Larsen J. Federated Database Systems for Managing Distributed, Heterogeneous, and Autonomous Databases. ACM Computing Surveys 1990; 22(3): 183-235.

[4] Stonebraker M. Integrating islands of information. EAI Journal 1999;(September/October): 1-5.

[5] Elmagarmid A, Rusinkiewicz M, Sheth A (Hrsg.). Management of heterogeneous and autonomous database systems. San Francisco, California: Morgan Kaufmann Publishers, 1999.

[6] Conrad S. Schemaintegration - Integrationskonflikte, Lösungsansätze, aktuelle Herausforderungen. Informatik Forschung und Entwicklung 2002; 2002(17): 101-111.

[7] Bouguettaya A, Benatallah B, Elmagarmid A. Interconnecting Heterogeneous Information Systems. Boston: Kluwer Academic Publishers, 1998.

[8] Rahm E, Bernstein PA. A survey of approaches to automatic schema matching. The VLDB Journal 2001; 2001(10): 334-350.

[9] Batini C, Lenzerini M, Navathe SB. A Comparative Analysis of Methodologies for Database Schema Integration. ACM Computing Surveys 1986; 18(4): 323-364.

[10] Heiler S. Semantic Interoperability. ACM Computing Surveys 1995; 27(2): 271-273.

[11] Colomb RM. Impact of Semantic Heterogeneity on Federating Databases. The Computer Journal 1997; 40(5): 235-244.

[12] Lenz R, Beyer M, Meiler C, Jablonski S, Kuhn KA. Informationsintegration in Gesundheitsversorgungsnetzen - Herausforderungen an die Informatik. Informatik Spektrum 2005; 28(2): 105-119.

[13] Bange C. Von ETL zur Datenintegration. IT Fokus 2004; 3(4): 12-16.

[14] Pille BT, Antczak RK. Application Integration. In: Ball MJ, Douglas JV (Hrsg.). Performance Improvement Through Information Management. New York: Springer, 1999: 144-152.

[15] Lenz R, Kuhn KA. Intranet meets hospital information systems: the solution to the integration problem? Methods Inf Med 2001; 40(2): 99-105.

[16] Dolin RH, Alschuler L, Beebe C, Biron PV, Boyer SL, Essin D et al. The HL7 clinical document architecture. J Am Med Inform Assoc 2001; 8(6): 552-569.

[17] Lenz R, Huff S, Geissbühler A. Report of conference track 2: pathways to open architectures. Int J Med Inf 2003; 69(2-3): 297-299.

[18] Vegoda P. Introducing the IHE (Integrating the Healthcare Enterprise) concept. J Healthc Inf Manag 2002; 16(1): 22-24.

[19] Health Level Seven I. HL7 Version 3 Statement of Principles. Health Level Seven, Inc. URL: http://www.hl7.org/Library/data-model/SOP_980123_final.zip

[20] Seliger R. Overview of HL7's CCOW Standard. Health Level Seven, Inc. URL: http://www.hl7.org/library/committees/sigvi/ccow_overview_2001.doc

[21] Lenz R, Kuhn KA. Towards a continuous evolution and adaptation of information systems in healthcare. Int J Med Inf 2004; 73(1): 75-89.

[22] Beale T. Archetypes: Constraint-based Domain Models for Future-proof Information Systems. In: OOPSLA 2002 workshop on behavioural semantics; 2002

[23] Patel N. Adaptive Evolutionary Information Systems. London: Idea Group Publishing, 2003.

Address for correspondence

Dr. Richard Lenz, Institut für Medizinische Informatik,
Klinikum der Philipps-Universität Marburg
35033 Marburg/Lahn, GERMANY
Tel. +49–6421–28–66298, Fax. +49–6421–28–63599, Email: lenzr@staff.uni-marburg.de

Connecting Medical Informatics and Bio-Informatics
R. Engelbrecht et al. (Eds.)
IOS Press, 2005

A Model-Driven Approach for the German Health Telematics Architectural Framework and the Related Security Infrastructure

Bernd Blobel, Peter Pharow

Fraunhofer Institute for Integrated Circuits IIS, Erlangen, Germany

Abstract

Shared care concepts such as managed care and continuity of care are based on extended communication and co-operation either between different health professionals, or between them and the patient. Health information systems and their components, which are very different in their structure, their behaviour, the respective data, and their semantics as well as regarding implementation details used in different environments for different purposes, have to provide intelligent interoperability. Therefore, flexibility, portability, and future-orientation must be guaranteed using the newest development of model driven architecture. The ongoing work for the German health telematics platform based on an architectural framework and a security infrastructure is described in some detail. This concept of future-proof health information networks with virtual Electronic Health Records as core application starts with multifunctional Electronic Health Cards. It fits into developments currently performed by many other developed countries in Europe and beyond.

Keywords:
Health telematics; Model driven architecture; Electronic health record; Smart cards; Security; Privacy

1. Introduction

Any communication and co-operation between healthcare providers must be supported by intelligently interoperable health information systems (HIS). This challenge needs to be met especially for managed care and continuity of care concepts widely introduced in most of the developed countries with the aim to improve quality and efficiency of patient's care.

Interoperability might be provided at different levels. Those interoperability levels are ranging from simple data exchange and meaningful data exchange with agreed vocabulary to a functional interoperability with agreed communicating applications' behaviour, or finally to a service-oriented interoperability directly invoking applications' services.

Health information systems enabling such advanced co-operation in the managed care context mentioned above are characterised by openness, scalability, portability, distribution at Internet level, service-oriented interoperability, as well as appropriate security and privacy services. Finally, they have to be based on standards [1].

2. The German Health Telematics Platform

As many other countries, Germany has launched a national programme for establishing a health telematics platform supporting seamless care [2, 3]. This platform combines card-enabled communication mediated by the patient with network-based interoperability between all actors involved. For the patient data card called the German Electronic Health Card, a multi-purpose microprocessor card is used. It will serve as a health insurance card for Germany as well as for European purposes, additionally providing an emergency data set, pointers to the patient's Electronic Health Record (EHR) components accessibly distributed on the net, a medication file, provider's reports, patient's receipts, and finally and especially an electronic prescription carrier. An explicitly protected compartment contains information the patient might like to hide from being read by others. The e-prescription was the main motivation for the project aiming to rationalise the process and to improve patient's safety in combination with some of the aforementioned functionalities. For any access to data others than the emergency data set, a Health Professional Card (Electronic Doctor's License) is required. Additionally, the electronic health card provides basic security services based on cryptographic algorithms, such as strong authentication, integrity, accountability, and encoding / decoding services deploying the Qualified Electronic Signature [4] and a related Public Key Infrastructure (PKI). The health card will be rolled out in 2006. It complies with the plan of a corresponding European Health Insurance Card, which will be implemented in all EU Member States until 2008. By that way, the German card will facilitate managed care and quality assurance.

Security services support both communication and application security services for any principals such as users, devices, systems, applications, components, or objects. For supporting trustworthy interoperability between patients and health professionals, the latter group has to use Health Professional Cards (HPC) for adequate security services.

To guarantee future-proof principles for designing and implementing common basic services of the aforementioned health telematics platform, an Architectural Framework and a Security Infrastructure are currently under definition and will be demonstrated as a proof of concept [5]. This architectural framework is characterised by different paradigms such as

- Distribution for openness,

- Component-orientation for scalability and flexibility,

- Interoperability at service level reflecting concepts and knowledge expressed through formal models for enabling conformance agreements,

- Separation of platform-independent and platform-specific modelling separating logic and technologic views on system components as well as

- Installation of reference and domain models.

The latter properties enable openness, portability and future-proof investments for the solutions provided. The approach completely complies with the advanced paradigms including the Model Driven Architecture (MDA) presented in this paper.

3. Modelling Systems

For describing systems and their behaviour in an appropriate way, real systems need to be modelled. A model might hide the internal structural complexity, or might be focused on specific aspects of the system such as form or special functions. Beside this way of a simplification of complex systems by modelling them, grouping elements of a system according to specific commonalities in structure and / or function makes system design, development, and maintenance manageable, realisable, and eligible for financing. The result is a set of components which can be designed, manufactured, and improved separately from other components, however keeping in mind and enabling reasonable interoperation between related components.

To reduce the complexity of a healthcare system consisting of many subsystems following the shared care paradigm, a single unrealistic comprehensive information system covering every thinkable procedure, fact and result will be realised by subsystems constraint to specific tasks, content, etc. In other words, we move from systems to components.

An information system normally reflects processes happening in the real world, by that way on the one hand establishing an information-related model of reality, and on the other hand implementing a real system. Models are systems consisting of components, too. The component paradigm is a basic paradigm which is applicable to real systems but also to models of reality [1]. Therefore, the component paradigm should be shortly examined in the following.

A component is a non-trivial, nearly independent, and replaceable part of a system that fulfils a clear function in the context of a well-defined architecture. A component represents a fundamental building block upon which systems can be designed and composed. A component conforms to, and provides, the physical realisation of a set of interfaces. Due to the underlying recursiveness, the component paradigm is very generic.

In the context of software architecture, components are characterised by attributes, operations, constraints, multi-interfaces and environmental conditions. Attributes are the structural elements of the architectural component, and are usually those relevant to its interface (i.e., observable). The operations themselves are those allowable on the architectural component. The constraints, sequencing requirements and / or interactions are those parts of the architecture description that constrain the usage / interaction and internal composition / state of the component. Properties describing a component's environment are, i.e., reliability, performance, security, safety, and quality which are essential for the acceptance of an application system. Therefore, components can be characterised by:

Component =   attributes + operations + structural constraints + operational constraints +   (1)
              events + multi-interfaces * scenarios + safety + reliability + security + ...

Component-based analysis and development is an interface-focused design approach which is characterised by a clear separation of component specification and its design and implementation. It supports the Plug & Play principle and is architecture-centric. An interface is a collection of operations which are used to specify a component service offered by a component (or a class) that is in turn implemented by a class or a component. The description of a component interface is a black box view of that component. For achieving interoperability, only the service requested by a client component and provided by the server component is of interest, but not the internals of the server's implementation.

4. MDA-Based Architectural Framework and Security Infrastructure

For keeping such complex national project's specification and implementation manageable, the architectural framework including the security infrastructure as its integral part is strictly based on the ISO 10746 Reference Model – Open Distributed Processing (RM-ODP) [6]. This concern all newly developed applications and common services components but also analysis and migration of legacy systems.

The ISO 10746 RM-ODP considers each component in distributed interoperable systems from different viewpoints, thereby abstracting from complex reality to interesting constraints such as concepts, contexts, structure, or behaviour. Thus, a component's purpose (business view, scenario, policy), the information needed to describe content (attributes) and function (operations) of a component (information view), the component's composition and decomposition (computational view), the distribution (engineering view), and the implementation and operation principles (technology view) have been specified.

Components can be composed / decomposed providing different levels of details or granularity. Starting from the granularity level of basic concepts of the corresponding domain, the complexity of aggregated components reflecting the functionality needed may be increased according to the users' needs, evolving over basic services / functions and relations networks up to complex business concepts. By that way, stand-alone applications, distributed applications or even highly complex networks can be implemented. In that context structural and functional complexity has to be considered as well. Components and their level of granularity can be selected according to the users' needs [1, 7].

In the first phase of modelling, the platform-independent specification of the components' properties is performed describing the business, the information, and the computational viewpoint of each component needed. Those models are portable into any environment with specific database models, operating systems' requirements, etc. This specification is transferred into the second phase of platform-specific modelling covering the engineering and the technology viewpoint.

The separation of platform-independent and platform-specific models, distinguishing logic and technologic aspects is the core idea of Object Management Group's Model Driven Architecture (MDA) for component-oriented information systems [8]. The specification of platform-independent models is supported by appropriate tools. The transfer into platform-specific model is automatically performed by the respective tools, too. Both phases describe system components at meta-level using, e.g., the Unified Modeling Language (UML) still abstracting from implementation details. The resulting graphical vocabulary has to be transferred into verbal constraint models using the Extensible Mark-up Language (XML). All the models are developed starting from coarse description up to fine-grained specialisation. Thereby, the models follow the approach of the Generic Component

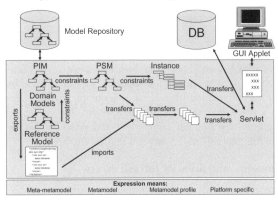

Fig. 1 – Development strategy for semantically interoperable HIS

Model based on the ISO 10746 RM-ODP. For both the model management and the automatic development of running application at runtime, corresponding tools will be deployed. In a model driven architecture, the implementation is automatically performed using tools as demonstrated within the HARP project at the Magdeburg Medical Informatics Department [9]. In the next section, this project will be shortly introduced.

Different views can be described independently by domain experts. Available knowledge can be exploited and specific terminologies can be applied correctly. For example, the concept knowledge of medical doctors or procedural experience of administrators will be expressed in domain models referring to an information reference model established by IT experts. Beside agreed methodologies and tooling, an accepted terminology maintained in a repository is a basic requirement. This terminology and ontology will be reused from SNOMED® with its extensions SNOMED_RT® and SNOMED_CT® as well as from the UMLS® created by the US National Library of Medicine (NLM) and meanwhile internationally maintained with important contributions by the British National Health Service (NHS). The outcome is transferred considering engineering aspects related to, e.g., the specific database model, which can be managed by database experts.

All different development phases from general requirements analysis over domain-specific views up to implementation and maintenance of any HIS can be described by MDA. Therefore, MDA allows also dealing with legacy systems to define interfaces and levels of interoperability. As meta-languages, UML and XML have been introduced as mentioned already. Because of some weaknesses of the approved version UML 1.4, tools supporting the emerging UML version have been used.

5. System Integration and Migration Paths

Having in mind that systems generally consist of either hierarchically built subsystems or capsules, at least three different levels of interoperability can be modelled and implemented as a migration path starting at the highest level of service-oriented collaboration between directly related components down to simple data retrieval.

The next level comprises aggregated services mediated either by super-component interactions or by the exchange of messages via architecture-independent interfaces (e.g. HL7 V2.x) [10].

Eventually, proprietary communication or database import / export functions might be established. The aggregation of components and – implementing them – services is mediated by components, in analogy to CORBA establishing horizontal or vertical services depending on the usability of those services by all domains or by a special one. Platform-specific issues are kept out of scope as long as possible to enable a future proof HIS characterised by the aforementioned properties. For final implementation, they have to be realised, however.

6. Electronic Health Record

Because all facts and items directly or indirectly established during patient's care are needed for its optimised management, shared care information systems and networks have to be based on a comprehensive and lifelong virtual EHR system as the HIS core application. Therefore, the German health telematics platform must be completed by a modern EHR architecture, which is also open, component-based and model-driven, etc.

The EHR architecture deployed in the second phase of the German health telematics project will be based on specifications provided by the revised CEN ENV 13606 "Electronic Health Record Communication" [11] and international projects such as the openEHR Foundation [12]. Accordingly, the German Electronic Health Card provides a tiny EHR extract. Furthermore, it establishes a tool (pointer facilities) for managing future EHR systems in a patient-controlled way.

7. Architecture and Security Infrastructure Implementation

Beside the definition and demonstration of an architectural framework and security infrastructure such as the German Health Telematics Platform, the roll-out of that approach means first to manage the card-enabled environment and second to provide basics and migration path for a future-proof ICT supporting shared care. In that context, the acceptance of the solution by patients and health professionals including the responsible and influencing bodies within the German healthcare and social system is inevitable. For that reason, the creation of acceptance by public relation activities, support of the ministry in creation of positive opinions and resonance is an important work package. Additionally, project management, quality assurance and quality management as well as an appropriate scientific accompaniment of the project are crucial success factors.

8. Conclusion

Modelled as a multi-model approach at the meta-model level, the future-proof secure health information system (HIS) is a virtual and at runtime self-organising architecture consisting of certified components which exchange digitally signed and attributed XML messages. Reference model, constraint models, terminology, and methodology have to comply with international standards or must be standardised.

Following the challenging example of other countries such as Australia, Denmark, Finland, the USA, and certainly some others, Germany launched a programme for establishing a Health Telematics Platform, which has to comply with the advanced paradigm of component-based MDA systems. First feasibility studies have successfully been performed within the European HARP project the author being responsible for the modelling part has been involved in.

9. Acknowledgement

The authors are indebted to thank the German Federal Ministry for Health and Social Security for supporting their activities as well as the partners from GEHR / openEHR and Object Management Group for collegial collaboration.

10. References

[1] Blobel B. *Analysis, Design and Implementation of Secure and Interoperable Distributed Health Information Systems.* Series "Studies in Health Technology and Informatics" Vol. 89. Amsterdam: IOS Press, 2002.

[2] German Federal Republic, Federal Ministry for Health and Social Affairs. http://www.bmgs.bund.de

[3] Aktionsforum Telematik im Gesundheitswesen. http://www.atg.gvg-koeln.de

[4] Council of Europe. Council of Europe 99/93/EC: Directive on Electronic Signatures. Strasbourg, 1999.

[5] German Federal Ministry for Health and Social Affairs. bIT4health.
http://www.bmgs.bund.de/deu/gra/ministerium/ausschreibungen/index.cfm

[6] ISO/IEC 10746 "Information technology – Open Distributed Processing – Reference Model".

[7] Blobel B, Pharow P (Edrs.). *Advanced Health Telematics and Telemedicine. The Magdeburg Expert Summit Textbook.* Series "Studies in Health Technology and Informatics" Vol. 96. Amsterdam: IOS Press, 2003.

[8] Object Management Group, Inc.: CORBA Specifications. http://www.omg.org

[9] HARP Consortium. http://www.ist-harp.org

[10] Health Level 7, Inc. http://www.hl7.org

[11] Comité Européen de Normalisation. http://www.centc251.org

[12] openEHR Foundation. http://www.openehr.org

11. Address for correspondence

PD Dr. Bernd Blobel, Ph.D., Associate Professor
Fraunhofer Institute for Integrated Circuits IIS, Health Telematics Project Group
Am Wolfsmantel 33, D-91058 Erlangen, Germany
Phone: +49-9131 / 776-7350, Fax:+49-9131 / 776-7399
E-mail: bernd.blobel@iis.fraunhofer.de URL:http://www.iis.fraunhofer.de

Connecting Medical Informatics and Bio-Informatics
R. Engelbrecht et al. (Eds.)
IOS Press, 2005

Development of Secured Medical Network with TCP2 for Telemedicine

Kumiko Ohashi, Yuichiro Gomi, Hiroki Nogawa, Hiroshi Mizushima, Hiroshi Tanaka

Tokyo Medical and Dental University, Tokyo, Japan

Abstract

We developed a secure medical image transmission system by using TCP2 which is a new technology that establishes secure communications in transport layer. Two experiments were conducted; TCP2 performance tests, and field tests that transmit real-time digital video image in domestic and international settings by equipping TCP2 with DVTS (Digital Video Transmission System). The results showed DVTS equipped with TCP2 has enough performance to send secure and high quality medical images. It was considered that medical network using TCP2 would contribute as an essential technology to telemedicine.

Keywords:
Medical Network; Telemedicine; Computer security

1. Introduction

As broadband networks have been widely available in ordinary communication, we can transfer a large volume of image data over the Internet without compressing them. As an instance of such enabling technologies, a new type of image communication system named *DVTS (Digital Video Transport System)* [1] has been available to transmit digital video stream over the Internet and it is now widely used for teleconferences [2]. We think DVTS could be used also in the medical field, namely for telemedicine.

However, this system by itself does not have the function for secure communication that is crucial in medical applications. One of the methods to realize secure communication in DVTS is to use TCP2 protocol, which is a new security technology that establishes secure communications in Transport layer. Besides, TCP2 has a retransmission function which sends the packet again if it is lost in the communication. This function would be useful for attaining the high fidelity in image transmission which is another condition required in medical image communication.

Thus, in this study, we developed a new medical image transmission system which we call *"secure DVTS"* by equipping the ordinary DVTS with TCP2.

We conducted two experiments on this new image transmission system, in which we measured performances of TCP2 with loop-back interfaces and those when TCP2 was equipped in DVTS.

Furthermore, we executed an experiment sending colon endoscopic video between University of Hawaii (UH) and our University (TMDU) to examine whether this system can be actually used for telemedicine. We investigated the results of those experiments, and discussed the necessary conditions for secure transmission of medical images.

2. Methods

2.1 DVTS

DVTS is a new network communication technology which enables us to transmit DV stream over the Internet. It has been disclosed as free software on the Internet. Using DVTS, users can transmit real-time video stream with minimum equipments - e.g. notebook PCs and digital video cameras.this system needs 35Mbps bandwidth for sending non-compressing image. But this application itself does not have a secure technology.

2.2. New Secure Protocol"TCP2"

2.2.1 The Feature of TCP2
TCP2 is a new security technology that enables us to encrypt data, exchange keys and execute authentication in the transport layer (OSI fourth layer). TCP2 (developed by TTT Co.) is equipped with TCP, TCPsec, UDP, UDPsec, IP, ICMP and IGMP protocol (Figure 1). TCP2 consists of two emulators, a TCP2 emulator and an UDP emulator. Each emulator provides encryption onto TCP and UDP respectively as well as conventional functions of them. All kinds of encryption algorithms can be implemented. When a sender transmits data with TCP2, only a receiver installed with TCP2 starts an encrypted communication with TCPsec. If a sender transmits data with TCP, the receiver communicates with ordinary TCP or cut off connections. The receiver with TCP2 can avoid illegal accesses by limiting communications of TCPsec packets.

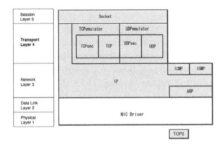

Figure1 – Details of TCP2

2.2.2 Comparison with Other Security Technologies

We compared TCP2 with other security technologies. The details are shown in Table 1. SSL works in the session layer and IPsec works in the network layer. TCP2 works in the transport layer. The SSL works in a layer of higher rank, so that it establishes a security communication at the application level. Therefore it is weak against attacks to lower layers. IPsec cannot be used in the network where IP addresses are dynamically changing. Furthermore, it needs to change firewall settings to pass through IPsec protocol. On the other hand in TCP2 the change of settings is not necessary in all network environments.

Table1 - Comparison with Other Security Technologies
This table shows comparison of IPsec, SSL, and SSL2 with each other.
○: available or possible, ×: unsuitable or impossib □: available or possible only in some cases.

	IPSec	SSL	TCP2
Peer to Peer communication	○	×(The need of a forwarding server)	○
Resistance to DoS attacks to TCP/IP protocol stack	○	×	○
Encryption of UDP	○	×	○
No changing of application settings	○	×(Non-compatibility)	○
Utilization in a network using NAT and IP Masquerade	□(Available using with NAT-T)	○	○
Utilization in ADSL and PPP mobile networks	□(Not available in normal mode)	○	○
In an unstable network environment (Occur many errors-packet losses and physical noises)	×(Reduce throughput by encrypting retransmitted packets)	○	○(Keeping encryption of retransmitting data)
Utilization in a network dynamically changing IP address	□(The need of DHCP server for IPSec)	○	○
Connecting through many carriers	× (Necessity for changing settings of carriers)	○	○

2.2.3 The measurement of TCP2 Throughput

We measured the performance of core protocol stacks of TCP2 comparing with those of the ordinary TCP before mounting TCP2 on DVTS. We prepared a PC installed with TCP2 using AES encryption algorithm (128bit). A loop-back program was mounted on the TCP2 core protocol stacks. This test program transmitted 10220 bytes data and received their replication in the core memory by the loop-back program. These procedures were repeated for 20 seconds and the number of TCP/UDP payload data was counted.

According to Figure 2, performance of TCPsec and UDPsec was about one half of the conventional TCP and UDP respectively. Bandwidth of the network that we used for the telemedicine experiment is ranged from 100Mbps to 156Mbps so that this throughput is enough for transmission images by DVTS. There would be actually no difference if we use broad bandwidth networks.

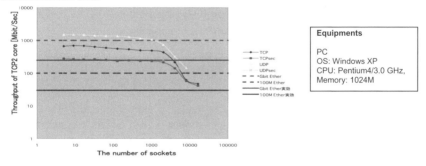

Figure 2 -Throughput of TCP2 core

3. Experiment of Transmitting Endoscopic Video for Telemedicine

3.1 The Experiment in Japan

3.1.1 Method of the Experiment

The network was constructed to examine performances of secure DVTS. The equipment of the experiments are shown in Table 2.The bandwidth was set to 100Mbps. The resolutions of transmitting images were set 780 ×480 pixels and RGB with 32bit.We prepared a videotape cassette of colon-endoscopic examinations and transmitted the video stream from the PC in TMDU to another one located in National Cancer Center (NCC,Tokyo).We measured performance indexes such as a packet loss rate, transmission delays, bandwidth occupied by the streaming, and CPU occupation rate. At first, to measure the throughput, 20000 packets of data were sent by the experimental program. We measured the time that elapsed from receiving the initial packet to receiving the 10000th packet. Then, we counted the number of packet losses while executing another experimental program where 30000 packets were sent at the rate of 4000 packet per second (250μsec) . During this streaming, we also observed qualities of transmitted video and audio data. We examined them under the two conditions – one is normal DVTS, the other is secure DVTS.

Table 2 – Equipments of the Experiment

Equipments	Model	OS	Specifications
Sending client PC in NCC	Mouse Computer	WindowsXP	CPU:Pentium4(3.0Ghz)/Memory:1024MB
Receiving client PC in TMDU	DELL/5150	WindowsXP	CPU:Pentium4(3.06Ghz)/Memory:512MB
Sending client PC in UH	IBM/ M50	WindowsXP	CPU:Pentium4(3.0Ghz)/Memory:512MB
DV camera	SONY/DCR-PC300K		Digital i Link(IEEE1394 compliance)

3.1.2 Result of the Experiment

The results were shown in Table 3. TCP2 throughput was about half in comparison with TCP one. No serious packet loss and the block noise were observed to interrupt communications in both experiments. Moreover packet losses of TCP2 are fewer than TCP ones.

Table 3 – Result of the Experiment (Between TMDU and NCC)

This table summarizes result of the experiment in domestic.
Quality of image: excellent or a few of block noises sometimes appear.

Evaluation of experiments	TCP Throughput average(Mbps)	TCP Packet Loss	DVTS Packet loss (/sec)	DVTS Quality of Image	CPU occupation rate (%)	Delay (sec)
Without TCP2	88.934	0	20~30	Sometimes appear	25~30	0.1~0.2
With TCP2	46.908	0	0~4	Nothing	35~45	No Delay

However, CPU occupation rate of TCP2 is higher than that of TCP. In *secure DVTS*, the quality of DVTS is much better than in the ordinary DVTS. It was found that TCP2 could efficiently encrypt streaming video. Thus, *secure DVTS* provides enough performance for high-quality image transmission.

3.2 Experiments between Japan and Hawaii

3.2.1 Method of the Experiment

We conducted tele-endoscopic experiments with secure DVTS between Hawaii and Japan over APAN (Asia-Pacific Advanced Network)[3]. The bandwidth of APAN is 156Mbps. We transmitted real time endoscopic video from UH to our University. Experimental equipments are showed in Table 2. Audio streams were also simultaneously transmitted over the same network. The Video stream was transmitted without compression at the rate of 30 fames per second. We tracked the route of these packets following by using the Traceroute program.

3.2.2 Result of the Experiment

The number of hops in the network from NCC to UH were 5 hops. Round Trip Time (RTT) was 78 msec. Correspondingly in the domestic network (from TMDU to NCC) they were 9 hops and 11 msec. Table 4 shows the results of this experiment. TCP2 throughput was lower than the former experiment, though it was higher than the bandwidth that DVTS requires for sending non-compression video (35Mbps) in both experiments. Packet losses and the block noise were very few in secure DVTS. Thus, the results show secure DVTS provides enough performance for high-quality image transmission even in large RTT (round trip time) environment. Figure 3 describes equipments used in the experiments, a sample of captured image of the transmitted video.

Table 4 – Result of the Experiment (Between NCC and UH)

This table summarizes result of the experiment in international situation (from Tokyo to Hawaii).

Evaluation of experiments	TCP Throughput Average (Mbps)	TCP Packet Loss	DVTS		CPU occupation rate (%)	Transmission on Delay(sec)
			Packet loss (/sec)	Quality of Image		
Without TCP2	69.593	3.7	1~7	Rarely appear	25~30	Rarely
With TCP2	51.484	0	0	Nothing	35~45	No Delay

4. Discussion

The result means that *secure DVTS* was able to send encrypted video stream efficiently. Furthermore, TCP2 technology was able to ensure the quality of image and audio in DVTS. The transmission experiment over APAN showed that the retransmission function of TCP2 was effective for ensuring high quality images even in the long distance network such as between Hawaii and Japan. Our experiments also showed that, even in UDP protocol that does not have retransmission functions, it was possible to establish secure communications and to ensure the quality of real-time streaming. But it should be noted that CPU occupation rate of *secure DVTS* was high, for it needs high computer power for encryption and decryption. Thus in our experiment, only one-direction experiment was possible due to limit of computer resources available. Our speculation is that, if other application runs during the transmitting images with DVTS, these images would be distorted because of the lack of computer capability.

In the future when the processing speed of computers becomes faster, the *secure DVTS* will be able to transmit images in two directions and to execute multicasting. Our conclusion is that spread of the TCP2 technology would promote the establishment of secure medical network.

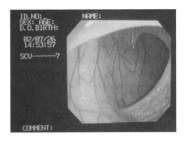 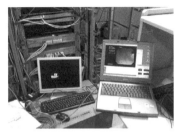

Figure 3–A sample of captured image of the transmitted video and DVTS Equipments.

5. Conclusion

The domestic and international telemedical experiments have shown that *secure DVTS* is available for transmitting encrypted video over Internet. This system has enough security and quality for telemedical applications. Furthermore, it is easy to implement and easy to use. We consider that the secured DV transmission system will be used for other medical application such as intra-hospital network or mobile healthcare communications.

6. Acknowledgments

We would like to express our sincere acknowledgements to Dr. David Lassner and Alan Whinery, University of Hawaii, for their support in our international experiment. We also would like to thank T.T.T Corporation for providing us TCP2 implementation.

7. References

[1]   DVTS: http://www.sfc.wide.ad.jp/DVTS/
[2]   K.Sugiura, T.Sakurada, A.Ogawa, O. Nakamura, S.Nakagawa, J.Murai. DVTS Using Portable Notebook computers.IPSJ SIGNotes Distributed Processing System. 2002;107:139-144
[3]   APAN(Asia Pacific Area Network): http://www.apan.net/

Address for correspondence

Tokyo Medical and Dental University Graduate School.
1-5-45 Yushima Bunkyo- Ku, Tokyo 113-8510 Japan
TEL:+81 35803 5862 FAX: +81 35803 0251
E-mail: ohashi@bioinfo.tmd.ac.jp
URL: http://bioinfo.tmd.ac.jp/~ohashi

Connecting Medical Informatics and Bio-Informatics
R. Engelbrecht et al. (Eds.)
IOS Press, 2005

Security Infrastructure Requirements for Electronic Health Cards Communication

Peter Pharow, Bernd Blobel

Fraunhofer Institute for Integrated Circuits IIS, Erlangen, Germany

Abstract

Communication and co-operation processes in the healthcare and welfare domain require a security infrastructure based on services describing status and relation of communicating principals as well as corresponding keys and attributes. Additional services provide trustworthy information on dynamic issues of communication and co-operation such as time and location of processes, workflow relations, integrity of archives and record systems, and system behaviour. To provide this communication and co-operation in a shared care environment, smart cards are widely used. Serving as storage media and portable application systems, patient data cards enable patient-controlled exchange and use of personal health data bound to specific purposes such as prescription and disease management. Additionally, patient status data such as the emergency data set or immunization may be stored in, and communicated by, patient data cards. Another deployment field of smart cards is their token functionality within a security framework, supporting basic security services such as identification, authentication, integrity, confidentiality, or accountability using cryptographic algorithms. In that context, keys, certificates, and card holder's attributes might be stored in the card as well. As an example, the German activity of introducing patient health cards and health professional cards is presented. Specification and enrolment aspects are on-going processes.

Keywords:
Electronic Health Record, Health Network, Health Cards, Security, Infrastructure, Health Professional Card, Patient Data Cards, Policy

1. Introduction

For the purpose of increasing quality and efficiency, health systems in developed countries throughout the world tend to move towards distributed collaborative and co-ordinated care of patients in the sense of shared care. Additionally, the prevention of citizens comes into the focus of the health care administration and management.

Specialisation and de-centralisation processes in healthcare must be accompanied by comprehensive communication and co-operation in order to meet the challenge of the shared care paradigm. Communication and co-operation may be supported through any kind of networks from a departmental Local Area Network (LAN) up to the Internet. An alternative to networking is the connection of patient's information with the patient's being itself: Acting as data subject and data source but also as carrier of any data collected, the patient can realise the informational self-determination guaranteed by privacy acts and constitutions. In any case, communication and co-operation have to be provided securely.

2. Smart Cards in Healthcare

When an information system, e.g. an Electronic Health Record (EHR) shall be held by a human being, an appropriate media is needed to store data structures and applications providing the required functionality as well as to communicate data items between partners inside or outside the healthcare domain. This generally applies ranging from the use of a simple hardware token for specific functions such as identity-related services up to more or less comprehensive portable information systems carried by the information subject [1].

2.1 Card Technologies and Applications in Healthcare

Over the last 30 years, many technological solutions have been developed and implemented for possessing and using person-related administrative or health information in healthcare. Those technologies can be distinguished according to the medium deployed, according to the purpose the cards are used, or according to the mechanisms and functions provided.

Starting with simple paper cards which can only be written once and read many times, memory cards have been introduced. Providing different storage capacity, magnetic stripe cards, laser written and read optical cards or chip cards have been used to simply store the aforementioned information. Regarding the purpose of use, storage cards can be distinguished from tokens such as access cards, identity cards, authentication cards, signature cards, encoding/decoding cards, etc. Sometimes, cards are also classified by their medical dedication for supporting specific decease's care (e.g. DIABCARD for supporting the care of diabetes patients). Considering both structure and mechanisms applied, programmable processing facilities have been established forming processor cards, sometimes equipped with dedicated co-processors for supporting special complex algorithms. Processor cards are also known as smart cards. The purpose is often combined with special mechanism to provide the functions required. Frequently, several purposes and functions are realised deploying the same physical cards (multi-functional cards).

For electronic health information systems independent of whether it is possessed by patients or additionally network-based, beside the appropriate carrier also an environment must be provided for the authorised use of information in the sense of collecting, storing, processing, and communicating data. Starting in Europe, smart cards, i.e., microprocessor cards, have been used for both purposes mentioned, i.e., as Patient Data Cards (PDC) and Health Professional Cards (HPC) around the world for quite a long time [2, 3].

Generally, it should be mentioned that smart cards could be deployed in two ways. On the one hand, the card could bear all information needed, in the case of PDC, e.g., all relevant medical data as part of an EHR. On the other hand, the card can be used as a pointer providing just references and linkages to the information stored in networked systems. However, even a combination of those two principles could be imaginable.

2.2 Card-Enabled Network Security Infrastructure

In Europe and beyond, smart cards are frequently used for enabling communication and application security services for health networks and records. The basic principle consists of a certified binding of a principle (human user, organisation, device, system, application, component, or even a single object) to its electronic unique identifier or assigned properties, rights and duties, also called attributes of that principal. Communication security services concern the identification and authentication of communicating principals. In an end-to-end secure communication environment (object security), these services are used for authentication and control of access rights of principals communicating as well as integrity, confidentiality, and accountability including non-repudiation of information exchanged. For object security, security aware principals are needed.

On the other hand, integrity and confidentiality of communicated data may also be provided at system level transparent to the application and the user – not requiring the user's specific awareness for those security measures (channel security). Application security services deal with authorisation and access control to data and functions, but also with accountability of principals, audit track and auditing of principals and services ensuring integrity, confidentiality of data and functions. In both concepts, notary's services have to be established. Another important requirement for communication and application security concerns the availability of information and services [4, 5, 6, 7].

3. The German Health Professional Card Specification

Based on results of the European TrustHealth project [3] and the Health Professional Card standard CEN ENV 13729 [2], the German HPC V 2.0 specification has been approved in July 2003 [8]. Its specification had to be linked to decisions setting up the organisational framework such as Trusted Third Party (TTP) services, Public Key Infrastructures (PKI), and related Registration and Certification Authorities (RA, CA). The legal framework for electronic signature processes became a national reality in December 1997 [9, 10, 11].

The main players in German health domain defined the Physicians' ID the first German implementation of a Health Professional Card as it is managed under the authority of the State Medical Associations. The electronic Physicians' ID is intended to completely replace the current paper-based Physicians' ID. For this reason, the Physicians' ID will have a distinctive card cover – similar to the paper-based one.

From a more technical point of view, the HPC is contact a based smart card capable to process Public Key (PK) algorithms. The physical characteristics shall comply with ISO/IEC 7816-1 and related standards. An HPC is a normal size card (ID-001 card). Other card layouts are currently under discussion, e.g. an institutional card (SMC) that could easily be considered a plug-in card (ID-000) for secure devices e.g. in pharmacies.

4. Standard Patient Data Cards and their Data Elements

When intending to generally provide open, interoperable solutions, they must be based on international standards. Regarding patient data cards, series of standards have been specified first at European level (CEN TC 251 "Health Informatics") and after its establishment at ISO TC 215 "Health Informatics" level.

4.1 Standardisation in the Patient Health Cards Domain

Developed under the Vienna Agreement by the ISO TC 215 WG "Health Cards" in collaboration with CEN TC 251, the ISO standard 21549 "Health Informatics – Patient health card data" [12] replaces the European Pre-standard ENV 12018 adopted by CEN back in 1995. ISO 21549 consists of the following parts:

- Part 1: General structure
- Part 2: Common objects
- Part 3: Limited clinical data
- Part 4: Extended clinical data
- Part 5: Identification data

- Part 6: Administrative data
- Part 7: Electronic prescription
- Part 8: Links

Person-related data carried on a data card can be categorised into three types: identification data (of the device itself and the individual to whom the data it caries relates), administrative data, and clinical data. It is important to realise that a given healthcare data card "de facto" has to contain device data and identification data and can in addition contain administrative and clinical data. Furthermore, patient data cards may support the collaboration with network-based systems. For that purpose, any type of link information has been specified. Patient data cards are widely used for a specific communication in patient's care: the electronic prescription. Because of the huge amount of performed transactions, e-prescription is indeed an important health card application, which itself guarantees the return of investment within a short time. Eventually, person-related cards analogue to HPC enable the use of established security infrastructure services.

A data card essentially provides specific answers to definite queries whilst at the same time a need to optimise the use of memory by avoiding redundancies "high level" Object Modelling Technique (OMT) has been applied with respect to the definition of healthcare data card data structures. Using a UML Class Diagram, figure 1 shows the overall structure for patient health card data according to ISO 21549 [12].

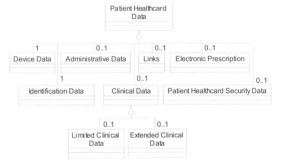

Figure 1 - General Patient Data Health Card Structure

4.2 The bIT4Health Project and the German Electronic Health Card

As many other countries, Germany has launched a national programme for establishing a health telematics platform supporting seamless care [13]. This platform combines card-enabled communication mediated by the patient with network-based interoperability between all actors involved. For the patient data card, called the German Electronic Health Card (elektronische Gesundheitskarte, eGK), a multi-purpose micro-processor card is used. It will serve as a health insurance card, an immunisation and vaccination passport, an electronic prescription carrier, a carrier for pointers to the patient's Electronic Health Record (EHR) components or related information such as drug information distributed on the net, and an information carrier for facilitating managed care and quality assurance [14].

At its backside, the German as well as the future European Electronic Health Card carries the so-called E111 form human readably containing all data needed for care of a citizen from an EU member state to be medically treated in another EU member state. Of course, this data set is also electronically stored on the smart card.

A specifically protected compartment contains information the patient likes to hide from being read by others. For any access to data others than the emergency data set, a Health Professional Card (Heilberufeausweis, HBA) is required. Additionally, the electronic health card provides basic security services based on cryptographic algorithms, such as strong authentication, integrity, accountability, and encoding / decoding services deploying the Qualified Electronic Signature [9, 10, 11] and a related Public Key Infrastructure (PKI).

The German bIT4health project will deploy the patient data card as token in prioritised applications. The priority of applications is defined by the possible savings, improvement of patient's safety as well as basic services for installing a health telematics and telemedicine platform. According to a business analysis, the replacement of the traditional paper-based prescription by electronic means will save about 700 million € a year. Expecting an amount of 1.5 billion € for implementing the health telematics infrastructural services described, the return of investments will be realised within 2 years [13].

Another aspect deals with the loss patient's safety due to medication errors or wrong information provided, which causes about 25.000 death patients a year in Germany. This number corresponds very well with the IOM study performed in the US mentioning 96.000 death patients for the same reasons in the USA. Therefore, e-prescription and medication file are prioritised. The latter may be stored on the health card or kept in a networking environment card-based pointers are referring to. Such solution can smoothly move towards the establishment of an Electronic Health Record (EHR) as the core application of any health telematics or telemedicine environment.

Without ignoring the huge social and societal savings by better patient safety avoiding harm or even death of patients (which is hard to calculate), the optimisation of medication due to the knowledge of the patient's medication applied as well as patient-related specific conditions by using medication files will easily save more than 1 billion € a year. ROI may even be realised within one year. The health card will be rolled out in 2006 replacing the currently used German health insurance card and providing added value services.

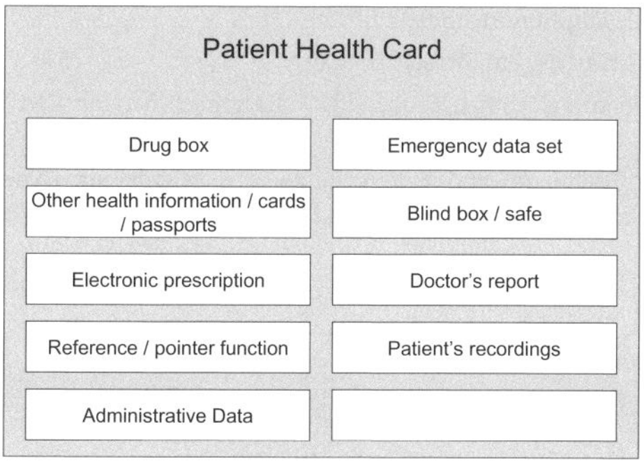

Figure 2 - Functional Blocks of the German eGK

Security services support both communication and application security services for any principals such as users, devices, systems, applications, components, or objects. Supporting trustworthy interoperability between patients and health professionals, the latter deploy Health Professional Cards (HPC) for adequate security services.

Another important aspect of the bIT4health project concerns the acceptance of offered telemedicine solutions by patients and health professionals. Earlier investigations on the acceptance of the DIABCARD demonstrated clearly that more than 95% of patients suffering from chronic diseases (e.g. diabetes) have highly appreciated or appreciated the use of specific patient health cards. For convincing citizens of storing personal health data on patient's health cards, the voluntary choice of specific applications as well as the control functions by patients or at least by trustworthy health professionals is a basic requirement.

5. Conclusions

Shared care solutions all over the world have to be based on trustworthy communication and application security services. Smart cards in general, Patient Identification Cards,

Patient Data Cards, and Health Professional Cards play an important role either as ID token or as health data carrier. Cards have an impact on the related security infrastructure, certification of processes, process interoperability (workflow), and certification of state and relations of principals in longer terms. This is especially true for the upcoming fast development on Electronic Health Record (EHR) architectures, their requirements, their design, their policy details, and their instantiation and implementation strategies.

6. Acknowledgement

The authors are in debt to the European Commission for the funding of several European research projects and especially to the project partners within the "HARP" project as well as all other partners and organisations for their support and their kind co-operation.

7. References

[1] Blobel B. Analysis, Design and Implementation of Secure and Interoperable Distributed Health Information Systems. Series "Studies in Health Technology and Informatics" Vol. 89. IOS Press, Amsterdam 2002.

[2] CEN TC 251 ENV 13729 "Health informatics - Secure user identification – Strong authentication using microprocessor cards (SEC-ID/CARDS)", 1999

[3] TrustHealth: The European TrustHealth Project (1996 – 2000). Project Description and Deliverables. http://www.ehto.org/ht_projects/initial_project_description/trusthealth.html

[4] Object Management Group, Inc.: CORBA Specifications. http://www.omg.org

[5] ISO/IEC 10746-2 "Information technology – Open Distributed Processing – Reference Model: Part 2: Foundations".

[6] Blobel B, Pharow P (Edrs.): Advanced Health Telematics and Telemedicine. The Magdeburg Expert Summit Textbook, pp. 21-28. Series "Studies in Health Technology and Informatics" Vol. 96. IOS Press, Amsterdam 2003

[7] Damianou N, Dulay N, Lupu E, Sloman M. Ponder: A Language for Specifying Security and Management Policies for Distributed Systems. The Language Specification, Version 2.3. Imperial College Research Report DoC 2000/1. 20 October, 2000.

[8] The German Specification for a Health Professional Card v 2.0. PDF Document (English version). http://www.heilberufeausweis.de/

[9] The German Law Governing Framework Conditions for Electronic Signatures and Amending Other Regulations (Gesetz über Rahmenbedingungen für elektronische Signaturen und zur Änderung weiterer Vorschriften – SigG): English version, May 16th, 2001. http://www.iid.de/iukdg/gesetz/engindex.html

[10] The German Electronic Signature Ordinance (Signaturverordnung – SigV): English version, November 2001. http://www.iid.de/iukdg/gesetz/engindex.html

[11] The European Electronic Signature Standardization Initiative (EESSI) – an Industry Initiative in Support of the European Directive on Electronic Signature. http://www.ictsb.org/EESSI_home.htm

[12] ISO standard 21549 "Health Informatics – Patient health card data", 2003

[13] bIT4Health. The German Electronic Health Card Project. Descriptions and Specifications (partly in English). http://www.dimdi.de/de/ehealth/karte/index.htm

[14] The German Specification for an Electronic Health Data Card v 1.1. PDF Document (English version). http://www.dimdi.de/de/ehealth/karte/technik/kartenspezifikation/index.htm

Address for Correspondence

Peter Pharow, Fraunhofer Institute for Integrated Circuits IIS, Image Processing and Medical Engineering Department, Health Telematics Project Group, Am Wolfsmantel 33, D-91058 Erlangen, Germany
Phone: +49-9131 / 776-7350, Fax: +49-9131 / 776-7399, E-mail: peter.pharow@iis.fraunhofer.de
URL: http://www.iis.fraunhofer.de

Connecting Medical Informatics and Bio-Informatics
R. Engelbrecht et al. (Eds.)
IOS Press, 2005

Security Services for the HemaCAM Project

Kjeld Engel, Heiko Kuziela, Bernd Blobel, Peter Pharow

Fraunhofer Institute for Integrated Circuits IIS, Erlangen, Germany

Abstract

Within the HemaCAM project which deals with automated differential white blood cell count by image processing, a security infrastructure has been integrated. The security services for this demonstrator have been derived from the German health network ONCONET that enables a trustworthy framework for both health professionals and patients as well as supports clinical studies. For the solution, services assuring both communication security and application security have to be provided. This task has been realised by the use of the security token Health Professional Card and an appropriate Trusted Third Party infrastructure.

Keywords:
Computer Assisted Microscopy, White Blood Cell Count, Security, Infrastructure, Health Professional Card, Signature

1. Introduction

Shared Care, eHealth as well as regional and national health networks respectively are directions today's healthcare systems are going to. Thereby, supporting information systems have to meet a number of requirements. They have to be distributed, interoperable, and open as well as to comply with sophisticated standards. Normally available applications can fulfil these requirements only partially. Because of the personal and especially of the social impart of personal health information, such data are highly sensitive. Therefore, collection, processing, communication and use of personal health information require enhanced security and privacy services. The integration of security into the application represents the real challenge.

Most of security and privacy services the trustworthy environment needed for healthcare communication and co-operation is based on deploy cryptographic algorithms. At both the European level and the German national level, smartcards for health professionals have been standardised as proper token. These Health Professional Cards (HPC) standards specify three key pairs for authentication, digital signature and encoding / decoding information using a symmetric session key as well as corresponding key-related certificates, but also attribute certificates certifying the card holder's role-defining attributes. The legal, organisational and functional infrastructure framework has been specified by the European Electronic Signature Directive as well as by the European Electronic Signature Standards Initiative [1].

The security infrastructure used within the health network ONCONET has been integrated into a real medical application: HemaCAM (Computer Assisted Microscopy in

Haematology). The ONCONET solution supports secure communication between registered principals enabling the transfer of any file by Secure File Transfer Protocol (SFTP) [2] to exchange patient-related medical data (e.g. physician's letter, diagnostic findings, CT images). Beside the services of mutual strong authentication, non-repudiation of origin and receipt as well as confidentiality and integrity of information communicated, the ONCONET permits secure SQL queries (predefined or freely formulated) using proxy technology to obtain statistical data about patients [3]. The security services mentioned are mainly based on the identity of the principals involved as well as on those principals' properties (attributes), both provable through X.509 v3 certificates issued and managed by a neutral Trusted Third Party (TTP). Smartcard support is realised via Multifunctional Card Terminal and HPC.

2. HemaCAM

A differential white blood cell count (WBCC) test is daily practice in clinical diagnostics and is usually ordered for the majority of patients. This blood cell count may provide first diagnostic indications of various diseases like leukaemia, HIV, bacterial or viral infections or allergic reactions. The generation of such blood cell counts is the most common assignment to clinical laboratories (see figure 1).

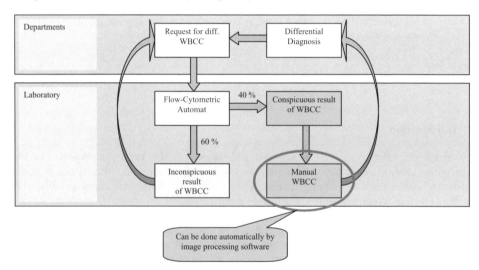

Figure 1 – White blood cell count order and result reporting

As a matter of routine the blood samples are analysed by chemo-physical blood cell count devices. For the majority of blood samples the automated procedures are reliable; abnormal blood samples, however, have to be stained and re-controlled manually under the microscope by trained laboratory operators. The consequences are extra work for the laboratories and extended waiting periods for the physician, the ward staff, and the patient. This costly manual re-examination is necessary for about 40% of all differential blood cell count analyses.

To optimise the performance and to improve the quality of clinical findings, the Fraunhofer Institute for Integrated Circuits IIS in Erlangen has developed an automated classification method: HemaCAM. Novel image processing methods allow for the quick and objective generation of differential blood cell counts – abnormal blood samples included. A method for the automated localisation of leucocytes in digitised blood smear cell counts is being realised at the moment. The project concentrates on the establishment of reference data for the various types of leucocytes. It is complemented by achievements of the Göttingen University (Central Laboratory: specimen selection and preparation, expert classification) as well as Würzburg University (Institute of Biochemistry and Pathobiochemistry: expert classification), and is sponsored by the German Federal Ministry of Education and Research BMBF [4].

The advantages of such an image processing based CAM system are as follows:

- Analysis of 100 cell in approx. three minutes (at medium cell density)
- Various fields of application for hospitals and laboratories
- High-quality reference data
- Intuitive touch screen user interface
- Establishment of a data bank for blood cell counts and proposals for classification ready for download and reproduction
- Quality improvement through operation on standardised data bank
- Shorter waiting periods of ward staff, physicians and patients for clinical findings
- Reduced risk of postural deformities or eye problems for users
- Easy integration into the daily clinical and laboratory routine without major outlay of time or expense

Among others, some of the key features of the HemaCAM system are:

- Fast scanning microscope system
- Adjustable number of WBC's to count
- Automatic detection of the valid scanning area on slide
- Automatic classification of leukocyte, platelets, erythrocytes and artefacts
- Sophisticated segmentation and classification algorithms
- Expert database for differential WBC count
- Manual verification of slide analysis possible

3. The German Health Professional Card Specification

Based on results of the TrustHealth project [5] and the first HPC standard CEN ENV 13729 [6], the German HPC V1.0 specification has been approved in 1999 [7]. The German Physicians' ID card provides a total of five different functions:

1. It's a classic identification card which a physician can use in a number of different settings, e.g. when ordering prescription drugs in a pharmacy where he is not known. For this purpose the card is personalised with name and picture.
2. The first electronic function is that of a certificate providing authentication to any digital device this card is presented to. Here, a fast and simple method for easy identification was realised taking into account that this approach can only be used in an otherwise already secure setting, since there is no special security against theft. This trade-off between security and simplicity will certainly find its use, since it is intended as a direct electronic analogue to the physical presentation of the classic identification card.
3. The second electronic function is that of being carrier of an asymmetric key pair (the private key of the key pair) for the strong authentication in a client/server environment. A public key infrastructure has to be put into place, where virtually

any unit can look up or download the public key of a health professional and can then make use of it to check the private key of the person, presenting his identification in any type of clinical setting. This enables the implementation of strong security in an otherwise untrusted environment.

4. The next major element is another key pair (again, the private key of an asymmetric key is stored on the cards) for the implementation of a hybrid (symmetric/ asymmetric) transport encryption. This is where transportation protocols like S/MIME can come into play by defining how the messages interchanged are to be encrypted.

5. The final element of the HPC is the private key of an asymmetric key pair for the production of a legally binding electronic signature according to the German Signature Law [8, 9]. The specifics of the health professional are contained in a number of attribute certificates which he can append to his signature, specifying his role in medicine [6, 7, 10].

From a more technical point of view, the HPC is a contact-based smartcard capable to process Public Key algorithms. The physical characteristics comply with ISO/IEC 7816-1 and related standards. An HPC is a normal size card (ID-001 card). Other card layouts are still under discussion, e.g. an institutional card (SMC) that could easily be considered a plug-in card (ID-000) for secure devices e.g. in pharmacies. The HPC contains:

- Elementary files (EF) at the master file (MF) level for general data objects and card verifiable (CV) certificates

- HP-related application (HPA) providing services for electronic identification of the health professional, electronic signature creation, client/server authentication, document decipherment, and card-to-card authentication (HPC/eGK and HPC/SMC)

- Cryptographic Information Application providing information for the primary system (e.g. a doctor's office system) to support the communication between the system and an HPC.

The HPC security mechanisms require different types of end user certificates:

- Electronic signature certificates (X.509 v3, type: electronic signature certificates, i.e. public key certificate and attribute certificates)

- Authentication certificate (X.509 v3, type: authentication certificate)

- Key encipherment certificate (X.509 v3, type: key encipherment certificate).

In addition to the aforementioned certificate types all containing a key, additional certificates without a key (so-called attribute certificates) complete the card infrastructure. Attribute certificates in the context of the HPC do rule certain aspects of permission, qualification and privileges.

4. Security services for HemaCAM

Due to the high sensitivity of data there is a need to secure the information exchange between the ordering department, the HemaCAM application and the result reporting laboratories. To integrate security services into the HemaCAM application, the so-called SFTP technology was used - a communication protocol that offers user and system authentication as well as a secure control and data connection. It enables the secure transfer of any type of files ranging from documents up to medical images. The SFTP protocol enables mutual strong authentication, integrity check, confidentiality, accountability including non-repudiation services, and notary's services such as certified time stamps.

The SFTP protocol is a security enhanced version of the fundamental file transfer protocol (FTP) provided in RFC 959 and is based solely on standards (e.g. ISO, NIST FIPS-PUB, ANSI and IETF/IESG RFCs). SFTP has been developed and implemented for TCP/IP-based networks. Following the client/server architecture, SFTP is composed of the SFTP Client (SFTP/C) for the client systems, and the SFTP Daemon (SFTP/D) running on the server. SFTP/C has been developed as a separate component (DLL) that can be integrated into virtually any application. This is the way SFTP was integrated into the HemaCAM application. The software is written in C/C++ using MS Visual C++ 5.0 and is based on Windows platform (9x and higher). Several software packages and some hardware devices are needed for instantiation. Security mechanisms are supplied by the security engine SECUDE (Security Development Environment for Open Systems, developed by SECUDE GmbH Darmstadt) offered through various application programming interfaces (APIs). The smartcard and the card terminal ICT-800 STD are accessed through the CT-API included by SECUDE. All security relevant information of a user (like secret keys, verification keys, certificates etc.) is integrity-protected and confidentiality-protected stored in a so-called Personal Security Environment.

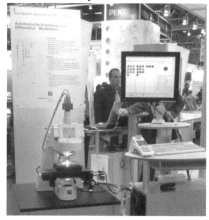

Figure 2 – HemaCAM on MEDICA 2004

For system authentication, a strong mutual three-way challenge-response authentication protocol (applying token identifiers, sequence numbers, timestamps) based on ISO standards has been implemented. The control connection transmitting commands and reply codes is secured by integrity and non-repudiation services using, e.g., token identifiers, sequence numbers and timestamps to enhance the level of security. SFTP offers different cryptographic protocols for the data connection like PKCS#7, Security Multi-parts for MIME (RFC 1847) and S/MIME version 2. It further offers several session key algorithms like IDEA, DES-EDE3-CBC, DES-EDE2-CBC, and DES-EDE2-ECB as well as the hash algorithms MD5, SHA-1, and RipeMD-160. However, any desired cryptographic syntax can be implemented additionally for the data transmission (as PGP/MIME or others). In general, the connection is secured by confidentiality, integrity, and the non-repudiation services.

Figure 2 shows the HemaCAM demonstration at MEDICA Exhibition 2004. Up to now, only the authentication functionality was integrated into the HemaCAM project. But several other possibilities of SFTP allow a much more intensive use in the future.

5. Conclusions

The project's final objective is building up an open and entirely secure application by embedding the fine grained security into the HemaCAM application. Within real three-tier architecture, the solution establishes secure authentication as well as authorisation of principals. The functionality can be enhanced, e.g. by role profiles and security attributes. The solution clearly separates and demarcates security and policy related issues according to the component paradigm.

The solution is strictly based on national and international standards (HPC, IP, CDA, XML, Component Architecture, etc.) and Internet technology. It realises a trustworthy communication with end-to-end security services, offers flexibility, protection of investment, openness for enhancements, and can be expanded on other entities. The solution follows the trend of the reorientation of healthcare information systems on Electronic Health Record basis.

6. Acknowledgement

The authors are in debt to the European Commission for the funding of several European research projects and especially to the HemaCAM project partners as well as the other partners and organisations for their support and their kind co-operation.

7. References

[1]   Blobel, B, Pharow, P, Engel, K. Enhanced Security Services for Enabling Pan-European Healthcare Networks. In: Patel V, Rogers R and Haux R (eds.): MEDINFO 2001. IOS Press, Volume 84 Studies in Health Technology and Informatics.

[2]   Blobel B, Pharow P, Engel K, Spiegel V, and Krohn R. Communication Security in Open Health Care Networks. In: Kokol P, Zupan B, Stare J, Premik M, and Engelbrecht R. eds. Medical Informatics Europe '99. Series in Health Technology and Informatics Vol. 68. IOS Press, Amsterdam 1999; pp. 291-296.

[3]   Blobel B. Onconet: A Secure Infrastructure to Improve Cancer Patients' Care. Eur. J. Med. Res. 2000: 5: 360-368.

[4]   Automated Differential Blood Cell Analysis, Press Release of Fraunhofer Institute for Integrated Circuits IIS, November 15, 2004.

[5]   TrustHealth: The European TrustHealth Project (1996 – 2000). Project Description and Deliverables. http://www.ehto.org/ht_projects/initial_project_description/trusthealth.html

[6]   CEN TC 251 ENV 13729 "Health informatics - Secure user identification – Strong authentication using microprocessor cards (SEC-ID/CARDS)", 1999.

[7]   The German Specification for a Health Professional Card v 1.0. PDF Document (English version). http://www.hcp-protocol.de

[8]   The German Law Governing Framework Conditions for Electronic Signatures and Amending Other Regulations (Gesetz über Rahmenbedingungen für elektronische Signaturen und zur Änderung weiterer Vorschriften – SigG): English version, May 16th, 2001. http://www.iid.de/iukdg/gesetz/engindex.html

[9]   The German Electronic Signature Ordinance (Signaturverordnung – SigV): English version, November 2001. http://www.iid.de/iukdg/gesetz/engindex.html

[10] The German Specification for a Health Professional Card v 2.0. PDF Document (English version). http://www.heilberufeausweis.de

Address for Correspondence

Kjeld Engel, Fraunhofer-Gesellschaft für angewandte Forschung, Institute for Integrated Circuits IIS, Image Processing and Medical Engineering Department, Health Telematics Project Group, Am Wolfsmantel 33 D-91058 Erlangen, Germany, kjeld.engel@iis.fraunhofer.de

Connecting Medical Informatics and Bio-Informatics
R. Engelbrecht et al. (Eds.)
IOS Press, 2005

Purposes of Health Identification Cards in Belgium

Francis H. Roger France[a], Etienne De Clercq[b], Marc Bangels[c]

[a]*Health Services Research, Ecole de Santé Publique de l'Université Catholique de Louvain*
[a]*Unité d'Informatique Médicale*
[b]*Unité de Sociologie et d'Economie de la Santé*
[c]*Service Public Fédéral de la Santé Publique et de l'Environnement, Unité d'Informatique et de Télématique*

Abstract

Although other alternatives might exist, identification cards have been chosen as an acceptable and adequate tool to be used to identify patients and health professionals.
They are planned for a digital signature and for access to electronic health records as well as for health information exchange and for databases querying. Local applications might exist independently, but the Federal State has now developed Be-Health, a platform for health professionals, social security personnel as well as the great public to facilitate a common access to some health data. Security conditions have been defined and are described.

Keywords:
Electronic health record; Standards; Security

1. Specific identification cards in the healthcare sector

After years of discussions in Belgium, there is a consensus at the Federal Public Service for public health to isolate health data from others datasets because of their high sensitivity in nature. It is felt that we should avoid mix administrative data such as fiscal or penal records with health records.

1.1. Patient identifier

At the beginning, it was question of a unique identifier by patient. Now, it is admitted that the patient might have several unique identifiers in relation with various objectives. Three of them have been defined: 1) administrative purpose, 2) health care, 3) studies (research, statistics). These identifiers will be produced by a cryptographic method [1] in order to protect confidentiality and patient's privacy rights. The three defined objectives are processed by different professionals in relation to: 1) financial and administrative applications that should not be mixed with diagnoses, 2) electronic health records that contain diagnoses, treatments and other private information within the care process, 3) statistics and clinical studies that don't have to be linked with health care process, as identification of patients are not needed and could be replaced by pseudonyms allowing to proceed to data checking.

These multiple unique identifiers by patient could be generated from the present "unique" social security number, but by an irreversible crypted method. The social security unique identifier is printed with the citizen authorization on the identification card and inserted on a chip card called SIS for social security information[*]. This number contains, however, identifiable items such as the reversed date of birth, followed by a sequential number of three digits that is even for female and uneven for males, given in the sequential order of arrival at the Federal register when sent by each Commune of the country. This nine-digit number is followed by a check digit of two positions that is a remaining result of a division by 97. The SIS card main purpose is to reduce administrative formalities and to ascertain that the citizen is solvable and covered by the social security.

These identifiers could be read and copied by a human being. They should also take into account international developments, among which the European Directive on data protection [2]. Biological identifiers are not on the agenda in Belgium.

1.2. Health professionals identifier

A unique identifier by health professional is also proposed in Belgium. Before health cards, health professionals as citizens used their handwritten signature to represent themselves with an official symbol that could be verified on an identification card or on a passport. From now, a unique identifier will be obtained by health professional, most likely by using the electronic identification card. It will be associated to some attributes (specialty, time of recognition, ...) certified by specific servers (validated authentic sources).

For healthcare purposes, the professional qualification could be specified and used in the whole country as well as abroad. Each physician in Belgium has a unique number in a comprehensive register. It takes into account requirements from the Physician Council (Ordre des Médecins), the Ministry of Health (diploma authentication) and the INAMI (Institut National d'Assurance contre la Maladie et l'Invalidité), the social security institution allowing reimbursement and recognition of specialty.

There is also "an Order of pharmacists" but no professional Order for nurses. Therefore, a cadaster of nurses is in progress at the Federal Public Service for Public Health. Another cadaster is in building for physiotherapists, dentists and s.o.

The authorization level for access to health data could be attributed by several organisations at a more local level. For example, a physician, recognized to practice medicine in the whole country and to be reimbursed at the level of his specialty, could be recognized as medical director of a hospital only if the institution gives him the rights that belong to his function such as to sign billing data for patient reimbursement. A general practitioner working some days as expert for a health insurance should distinguish his activities when using his identification, by taking the right attribute of his work.

2. The Trusted Third Party (TTP): a key organisation

A main public difficulty was to agree upon an organisation that could be entrusted by all participating parties to healthcare in order to manage unique numbering systems that have to be encrypted [3].

A platform called *Be-Health* [4] for a common access to telematics in the healthcare sector has been financed in order to allow healthcare professionals as well as social security actors and the citizen to deal with the health information they need. On 23 December 2004, the Belgian Government accepted to appoint as technical partner a semi-public organisation called SMALS (société de mécanographie pour l'application des lois sociales), as the TTP

---

[*] Social Security Royal Decree of 16-10-1998

for the health care sector. In order to ensure security, cryptography is used, based on an algorithm that transform clear text to cipher text on the sending site and vice versa on the receiving end. The same algorithm is used in both sides with different keys.

With BeHealth common access, strict identification procedures using the digital identification keys are now in development. A cryptographic key is a string of bits controlling the behaviour of the algorithm. In an assymmetric system, one key is used for encryption, and the other for decryption. The private key is given to the keyholder on the card, while the other key, called public key is made available to all users that wish to share cryptographic functions with the keyholder. We had the opportunity to contribute to the Be-Health project in a working group of experts[*] belonging to the Federal Public Service for Public Health, the INAMI, the National Inter-Mutualist College, the cross-point databank of social security and the Commission Norms for Telematics in Health Care in a project that will be coordinated by the FEDICT (Federal Public Service for information and communication technology).

The objective of *Be-Health* is to allow citizens and patients as well as healthcare and social security partners to have access uniformly to added value services and to information already available in the various organisations in a secure way. Each certification body (Commune, Council of physicians, ...) will communicate to a *Trusted Third Party* (TTP). Authenticated data and the authentic sources of data will be validated both for health professionals and for "patients" (see Figure 1). Authorisations will be specified following their access rights. Security will be also extended to the communication network system.

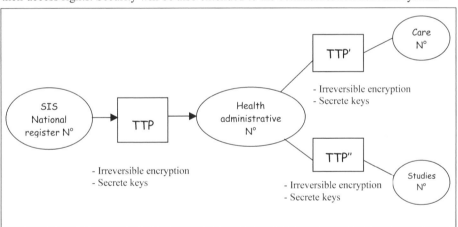

Figure 1 – *A public key infrastructure (PKI) for the healthcare sector in Belgium: Three "unique identification numbers" are proposed by patient, in relation to three different objectives, obtained from the social security identifier (SIS), by a Trusted Third Party (TTP), with two encrypted keys, one public and one private.*

In order to guarantee security and the respect of objectives of *Be-Health*, a sectorial health committee "healthdata" will be included in the commission for the protection of the private life on the basis of Art. 36bis of the Law of 8 December 2002 in relation to the protection of private life. The first budget for this development during the year 2005 is relatively modest, given the philosophy to use all components that exist in order to minimize costs: 1.45 million euros have been accepted by the Government.

---

[*] The Be-Health working group was made of Mr R. De Ridder, R. De Brandt, O. Schneider, J.P. Dercq, D. Cuypers, Th. Gravet, M. Bangels, G. De Moor, F.H. Roger France, J. De Cock, V. Nys, P. Verertbruggen, J. Hermesse, F. Robben and E. Quintin

3. The electronic ID card

The Belgian experiment of the electronic identification card is new and at a scale that has never been encountered. The security level should be higher than for bank cards. In supplement to identifiers printed on the ID card, (name, date of birth,…), encrypted private keys will be available in the chip. Attributes (physician, medical director, …) to be used for specific purposes wo'nt be on the chip but available in specific federal registers that have to be validated.

Its development began with the distribution of the new electronic identification card in ten Belgian communes in 2003. Priorities were given to newborns, new inhabitants as well as the renewal of old ID cards. The whole country should be covered by 2008 and each card will be valid for a period of 5 years. If a card is lost or destroyed a new one could be obtained in a delay of 7 days.

For healthcare purposes, a difficulty might be that all patients won't be covered by this ID card. Among exceptions, let's quote newborns, at least during the first days before their birth is declared to the Commune, foreigners without employment in the country, tourists from another continent. …

4. The use of professional cards for health purposes

Several applications will require health identifiers that could be obtained with the digital ID card:

1) A *signature*: a digital signature [5] is more secure with a electronic ID card than with passwords linked to a local card. Health professional signatures are needed for treatment prescription (drugs, physiotherapy) as well as for requests of diagnostic tests, specialist advice, nursing care and s.o. Physicians sign also medical certificates for disability for work, school absences, … as well as for health insurance, admission prolongation discharge of patients, accident's declaration, refund applications, … A signature is also required to validate medical reports being a discharge letter, an operating room protocol or laboratory results. Minimum Basic Data Set (MBDS) registration should also be certified by a signature. Medical directors of hospitals sign collective hospital inpatients invoices as well as outpatients statement invoices.

2) Another use of professional cards is to enable secure *access* to identifiable electronic health records [6]. The proposed tool might authentify the requester and give access to authorized persons, by category of health professional. It would assure repudiation and should be documented by access journalling.

3) It allows also the *exchange of health information* about identifiable patients [7]. Each patient could be asked to declare to any institution in which he will be treated the identification of health professionals who treat him, especially the name of his general practitioner. Encrypted messages signed by a sender and addressed to a receiver would use the electronic signature. Message authentication could be verified by a hashing mechanism that would disclose whether the message was the same as the one sent.

5. Application in a teaching hospital

In Saint-Luc Hospital at the University of Louvain in Brussels, a large teaching hospital of more than 1000 beds and 350000 outpatient visits a year, the first priorities for electronic signature was drug prescription developed since 1996. The second priority since two years is access right to the electronic health record and the third one concerns the signature to validate discharge letters.

Up to now, only an internal system is used [8], as the Belgian electronic identification card is not yet widely available for all physicians. A local smartcard allows authentication through an electronic warden, a password and an identification number that can be read on ± 1200 PCs. In order to have access to the medical record of the patient, a documentation system called "Medical Explorer" has been developed in JAVA. It allows to reduce the number of paper records and to work more and more with paperless records. It gives access to all clinical reports and technical protocols as well as to laboratory data, imaging reports.

Access rights are given only to authorized health professionals. Physicians and head nurses can consult the whole electronic health record while some secretaries and some nurses cannot have access to everything but only to tables of contents and to the laboratory tests performed, not to results.

Access can be obtained (the *record is open*) if the patient is present or in the file of the appointments to outpatient visits or technical acts (using ultragenda software). The presence of a patient is ascertained when he comes in emergency room or if he is admitted as inpatient or as day-case. The patient record is open 5 days before a planned admission to 15 days after his discharge. *It is closed* otherwise and can only be opened by a physician who has been in charge of the patient. A dialogue for justification is installed and each access is listed on a journal on the opening screen of the session.There is a *security committee* to check the respect of confidentiality for personal health data in the health system. A *security officer* has been appointed halftime. He is a former nurse. As a rule, each physician can always have access to a record but if flags or special security measures have been activated, his access will systematically be examined by the security officer. Furthermore, in order to assure to the personnel of the hospital the respect of the rules, a random selection of persons has been decided. An overview is organised with the security officer and the patient in order to review all accesses made to his record if he wishes to identify abnormalities to be investigated.

It has been decided to ask to each patient to sign a contract where he designates the physician to whom he wishes reports to be sent, like to his general practitioner. But a patient could also forbid some health professionals to have access to his record. In this case, he could rediscuss the matter in case of need of care with this physician. Otherwise, the health professional could limit his responsibility.

6. The federal health network "FLOW"

A prototype has been designed in Belgium supported by the Federal Government to allow links between health records in hospitals and in general practice. Up to now, there is a voluntary participation to the Flow project [1]. The medical record can be opened or closed following the same rules as in St Luc but the access number to the patient is still the SIS number and not yet the ID card encrypted number. In the next future, this identifier should be depersonalised and replaced by an encrypted double key.

In this perspective, the Belgian electronic ID card could play a key role in access to health data as well as for electronic signature and responsibility of health professionals in their practice. There remain some question marks. Among them : will there be sectorial cards, one for healthcare, another one for banking and financing, another for cultural purposes? Each citizen could not carry 100 cards on him for various purposes. Experience will show the way in which such questions could be solved in practice.

Another difficulty that has been mentioned is the exception. The lack of citizenship in the country should not forbid patients to have access to healthcare. Replacement solutions should be prepared. An important aspect that has not been fully appreciated is the *context* in which information is asked. A dialogue has to be planned about objectives of access to identifiable health data. In principle, only the physician who has a contract with the patient, confident in him, can have access to his record, not all physicians in the institution. It would, however, be a disaster if a physician could not obtain access to a record for administrative reasons because he is not well identified as the personal physician of this patient in emergency. Solutions have to be found. An easy one could be to mention the name of the physician who asked an advice or a procedure if the patient did not address himself directly to this physician or to this nurse. Solutions have to be tested and adapted progressively.

7. Conclusion

In conclusion, several major steps have been accomplished recently in Belgium in order to obtain unique identifiers specific to health for citizens as well as health professionals identifiers.

Both are based on the delivery of the Belgian electronic identification card that is currently distributed in the country. Irreversible encryption through a Trusted Third Party (the SMALS) has been planned in 2005 in the framework of a common portal (Be-Health) for access to health data.

Security measures are proposed in order to ensure confidentiality (irreversible encryption, identifiers linked to purposes, taking in account context) of verifiable authenticated requesters and receivers of health data, in function of authorizations. Each access will be documented and there will be a structured organisation to follow security conditions, including a security officer.

8. References

[1]   Roger France FH, Bangels M. Norms for Telematics in Health Care: priorities in Belgium. In: e-Health in Belgium and in the Netherlands, FH Roger France et al, eds. IOS Press, Amsterdam, 2002, 93: 179-183.

[2]   Directive 1999/93/EC of the European Parliament and of the Council of 13 December 1999 on a Community framework for electronic signatures. Official Journal of the European Communities, 19-1-2000.

[3]   De Meyer F, De Moor G, Roger France FH. Electronic signature and certification models in healthcare. In : Medinfo 2001, Proceedings of the 10th World Congress on Medical Informatics, London, 2-5 September 2001 (V. Patel, R. Rogers, R. Haux, Eds), IOS Press, 2001:1252-1256.

[4]   Conseil des Ministres. Séance du 23 décembre 2004. Projet Be-Health. Ref 2004 A707-50-036. Chancellerie du Premier Ministre, 2004.

[5]   De Moor G, Claerhout B, De Meyer F. Implementation framework for digital signatures for electronic data interchange in health care. In: Health Continuum and Data Exchange in Belgium and in the Netherlands, F.H. Roger France et al, eds. IOS Press, Amsterdam, 2004, 110: 90-111.

[6]   Blobel B, Roger France FH. A systematic approach for analysis and design of secure health information systems. Int J Med Informatics, 2001, 62: 51-78.

[7]   Commission "Telematics standards in relation to the health care sector" (Advice n° 4). Recommendations regarding national development of standardized electronic health care messages. In: Health Continuum and Data Exchange in Belgium and in the Netherlands, F.H. Roger France et al, eds. IOS Press, Amsterdam, 2004, 110: 112-117.

[8]   Roger France FH. Security of health care records in Belgium. Application in a University Hospital. Int J Med Informatics, 2004, 73: 235-238.

Websites
     www.belgium.be/fedict, www.smals.be, www.health.fgov .be/telematics, www.saintluc.be

Connecting Medical Informatics and Bio-Informatics
R. Engelbrecht et al. (Eds.)
IOS Press, 2005

The Baltic Health Network – Taking Secure, Internet-based Healthcare Networks to the Next Level

Henning Voss[a], Vigdis Heimly[b], Lotta Holm Sjögren[c]

[a]Danish Centre for Health Telematics, Odense, Denmark
[b]KITH, Trondheim, Norway
[a]Carelink, Stockholm, Sweden

Abstract

*Internet-based health care networks are a step forward compared to first generation health care networks, which has been limited to pushing text-based messages between different systems. An Internet-based network can also "pull" data - and not only text but any digital data – for instance images and video sequences. The Internet-based networks can more effectively fulfil the vision of access to relevant data regardless of time and location. Although far from identical, the health delivery systems of Denmark, Norway and Sweden are similar. They also share a shortage of specialized health personnel – not least radiologists and in some regions obstetricians. Furthermore, over the past ten years they have implemented an IT-strategy to increase efficiency in the delivery of healthcare services. Part of this strategy has been to build three national networks on top of the existing regional, secure and Internet-based healthcare networks. These national networks connect not only all hospitals in the three countries, but also a majority of the other stakeholders in the healthcare sector (GPs, private specialists, laboratories, homecare services etc.). The organizations behind the three networks are now working on creating a trans-national network, the Baltic Health Network (BHN), which will be one of the outcomes of the **Baltic eHealth project** and will not only connect the three national networks but also add two hospital networks from Lithuania and Estonia. The BHN is expected to be operational by June 2005. One of major advantages of the BHN is that the many rural hospitals of the Baltic Sea Area with a few mouse clicks can reach a specialist for second opinion in any of the approximately 200 hospitals connected to the network. For instance the midwives in the rural areas of Västerbottan County, Sweden, are awaiting the establishment of BHN to get access to second opinions from specialists at National Center for Foetal Medicine at the University Hospital of Trondheim, Norway. The BHN will remove a very important technical barrier for collaboration between health professionals and the Baltic eHealth project hopes that this and other project initiatives will facilitate the large-scale usage of second opinion from available health care experts regardless of institutional, regional and even national borders. This will lift the quality of service to patients in the Baltic Sea Region – especially in the rural areas where highly specialized health professionals tend to be geographically far away.*

Keywords:
Internet health care networks; Regional health care networks; Baltic eHealth; Rural health care.

1. Introduction – first generation regional health care networks

Modern healthcare is provided in close co-operation between many different institutions and professional groups – working together and using their specialised expertise in their common effort to deliver the best quality service and the most cost-effective care as possible. Due to this specialisation and division of labour, the need for seamless electronic communication between the parties is still growing. An answer to this need is the development of regional health care networks (RHCN). An ideal RHCN should provide [1]:

- Daily communication of prescriptions, referrals, lab-results etc.
- Secure e-mail for patient related information
- Booking facilities for hospital and diagnostic information
- Shared Medical records
- Emergency and alert systems
- Tele-medicine facilities
- Protocols and guidelines for cross-sector treatment
- Health Information web-sites for professionals, patients and the public
- Administrative cross-sector information and management systems

Such comprehensive RHCN do not exist in Europe today. However, in the last 15 years several less comprehensive first generation RHCNs have been established. The first movers were UK and the Netherlands who already in the late eighties established links to communicate structured messages (based on the EDIFACT[1] standard) between hospitals and GPs. Today EDI-communication is being used in a number of European Regions – not least in Denmark, Norway and Sweden.

The basic idea behind EDI-messages is to send (push) structured electronic text-based messages from one computer to another. This means that data entered once can be re-used elsewhere in the health care sector. EDI-communication is therefore a very effective tool to increase efficiency in communication between GPs and their surroundings (hospitals, pharmacies, specialists, labs etc.) [2] as EDI can save much time in the communication of prescriptions, referrals, lab-results, discharge letters and reimbursement claims [3]. However, EDI-communication has two major shortcomings: First, it is largely text-based and can usually not handle the communication of data like images, ECGs, and video sequences. Second, EDI-messages are "pushed" from a sender to a receiver, which means that both parties have to be involved in the transaction. If a receiver had access to "pull" the data whenever needed, the sender would not have to be actively involved.

2. Next generation Regional Health Care Networks

The Internet technology offers a solution to both shortcomings of the first generation RHCNs, as the Internet technology is capable of meeting a large number of additional communication needs. Some of the most important services are 1) forwarding (push) of e.g. text, pictures, X-rays, sounds, graphics and video sequences, 2) web notices (pull) of EHR-data, X-ray results, laboratory replies, ECGs etc., 3) videoconferences, 4) web-portals that gives access to medical information to relevant health professionals, as well as the individual citizen/patient, 5) appointment making for examinations and treatment, and 6) electronic reporting to quality registries, archives and clinical databases of aggregated and/or anonymized data.

---

[1] UN/EDIFACT = United Nations/Electronic Data Interchange for Administration, Commerce and Trade.

Basically all elements in the above-described ideal RHCN can be handled in a network where the underlying infrastructure is based on the Internet technology. This is not to say, that other technologies could not provide the same features, but the obvious advantage of using the Internet-technology is its rapid spread – the Internet is becoming totally ubiquitous, which means that any IT-department is very familiar with the technology.

Since the late nineties, the above advantages of basing next generation Health Care Networks on Internet technology became obvious to policymakers in the three Nordic countries. The ambition in all three countries was the same: to build not only a regional second generation networks, but to create three national networks, that will be able to meet any communication need any healthcare provider might have.

However, when it comes to security, the Internet leaves something to be desired. Since patient related information is intended to cross borders between sectors, institutions and actors, security became a major concern in all three countries. The only way around these concerns has been to involve all relevant levels, institutions and actors in very difficult consensus processes and to find a common denominator for each country on the security issues. These consensus processes are reflected in the slightly different technical models that where chosen in each country. The three models are described below.

Sweden

In Sweden the National Health Care Network is called Sjunet, which is an IP-based broadband network, connecting all Swedish hospitals, primary care centres and many other health services. Sjunet is built up of nodes connecting the firewalls in all 21 county councils and regions.

The network started as a regional project in 1998, involving only seven counties, where the Sjunet was set up as a virtual private network (VPN) with "tunnels" on the Swedish part of the Internet. The VPN technology guaranteed that information was not accessible from or communicated through the public Internet. The network provider guaranteed that the available bandwidth was sufficient for applications and services. Since 2003 the network is based on VLAN technology with built-in redundancy and is technically separated from the Internet. The separation from the Internet means better availability with regards to bandwidth [4].

The net is being used for many telemedicine services, including the secure transmission of X-rays, patient information, clinical rounds and collaboration between hospitals via videoconference or IP-telephony. The video conferencing service includes a video bridge for multi conferencing, a video number directory, gatekeepers (video switches), and a number of guidelines. Of special interest is the provision on security certificates, following the PKI standard, from a CA-server (Certified Authority) that allows decryption and authentication of messages sent on Sjunet. All hospitals connected to Sjunet can make use of this service [5].

By using Sjunet, local clinics and hospitals are able to consult specialists in neurophysiology from university hospitals for the analysis of EEG and nerve conduction studies. The specialist can access databases with patient information at referring clinics. Once the analysis has been done, the specialist sends the report to the referring physician. A cost-benefit study [6] of this example shows considerable savings - both within health care and for the patients.

Denmark

The Danish network consists of a central hub that connects all existing closed secure networks in the Danish healthcare sector into one large national network. Contrary to the Sjunet, the Danish network does not only use Internet-technology, but is actually running on the Internet. This requires a high degree of security, which is ensured at three levels. To ensure the transmission security, connections to the central hub are established via VPN-tunnels – this is the first level of security. At the second level an electronic "agreement system" controls the incoming and outgoing data flow from the local networks to the central point. When two parties wish to communicate via the central node, they can open a connection between each other in the agreement system. Other parties in the network will not have access to the data communicated between the two parties. The third security level is local user identification and password.

The network structure is established by reusing the existing IP structures. A wide range of public RIPE2 IP addresses are available for the network and the local IP addresses are "translated" into a unique national network address using NAT (Network Address Translation). The use of VPN allows all parties in the network to reuse the existing Internet connections already in use by all organisations [7].

The Danish Internet-based Network has been running since 2003. All hospitals are using the network – not least for the legally required submission of patient data to clinical databases. With regards to GPs, private specialists, and homecare services, they are all connected to the network via their IT-providers, and the usage is increasing but still rather limited. The reason for this is the limited number of services that are offered to this group over the Internet-based network. Most of the communication needs of GPs and private specialists are still covered by the very widespread traditional EDI-based network3. However, several pilots like web-lookup of X-rays on the network indicate a strong demand for a more widespread dissemination. Today a large number of hospitals are getting ready to provide these services to the GPs and specialists in their region. With regards to the homecare sector, the network is being used in a few pilots to strengthen the communication flows between hospitals and homecare units. These pilots also look promising and will hopefully inspire others to initiate similar projects.

Norway

In Norway, healthcare is delivered by the five regional health enterprises. In 1998 the first regional network was established and today all five regions have their own network. The health networks in the region North-Norway and in the region Mid-Norway have had a substantial traffic load for 3 to 4 years, but the development of the regional health networks of the other regions has been slower. This has partly been due to the fact that other types of infrastructure were preferred in these regions, such as county nets and electronic message exchange via a national mail-server. The types of services offered on the networks have also varied between the five regions.

The objective with the Norwegian National Health Network is to contribute to high quality and coherent health and social services, by being a sector network for effective cooperation between the different service sections in the sector. A basic principle of the National Health Network is that one connection point and one joint communication platform shall give access to a broad range of services for electronic exchange of information. Such services will, among other things, be secure e-mail and exchange of electronic messages, telemedicine services, use of common systems on the network and controlled access to the Internet. From one and the same connection point, users shall be able to communicate with all the other actors that are connected to the network.

A special strategy and action plan has been developed for the National Health Network. The network will be operated and further developed in line with this strategy. This involves connecting more actors and offering additional services. So far the main focus has been on

---

[2] RIPE = Réseaux IP Européens.
[3] Messages per year (2004): 32 million. Source: www.medcom.dk.

connecting the hospitals and general practitioners to the network. A municipal programme for electronic interaction shall lead to closer and improved cooperation between primary health services, specialist health services and social services. Connecting the municipalities to the network is therefore also one focus area in the National Health Network strategy.

3. The Baltic Health Network

The three networks described above are very similar but they also differ from each other - especially on two parameters:

- Internet: While the Danish network is based on VPN tunnels over existing Internet connections, the Swedish and to some extent the Norwegian networks are separated from the Internet – but they are still using the Internet-technology.

- Agreement-system: While Denmark has an agreement-system that automates the handling of connections in the network, Norway and Sweden are so far handling the connections manually.

Neither of the two points constitutes a major obstacle for a future connection of the three networks, and the cost of connecting them is estimated to be rather limited.4 The potentials of a cross-national healthcare network are on the other hand very promising – not least because even today, without such a network, several cases of cross-national collaboration in the region can be pointed out.5 The development of a transnational network including the Baltic states, the Baltic Health Network (BHN) is therefore currently ongoing and is expected to be finalized in June 2005, where not only the three Nordic countries will be connected to each other, but also two hospitals in Estonia (East-Tallinn Central Hospital) and Lithuania (Vilnius University Hospital).

The BHN is a significant deliverable in the Baltic eHealth project. The project's goal is to bring about fully developed eHealth solutions that can be directly put into use by health providers throughout the Baltic Sea Area. Any eligible stakeholder in the healthcare sector will be given free and unlimited access to the BHN, which therefore is expected to become a major eHealth facilitator in the Baltic Sea Area, as the establishment of eHealth solutions will become much easier now.

During the three year project period (2004 – 2007), Baltic eHealth will demonstrate the usefulness of the BHN in two clinical pilots. In the eRadiology pilot, specialists from East-Tallinn Central Hospital (Estonia) and Vilnius University Hospital (Lithuania) will assist the doctors at the Funen Hospital (Denmark). In the eUltrasound pilot, specialists from the National Center for Foetal Medicine at the University Hospital of Trondheim (Norway) will assist doctors and midwives at the hospitals in Västerbotten County (Sweden). The primary goal of the pilots is to inspire others to initiate similar eHealth services on the BHN.

The aim of the Baltic eHealth project is that the BHN will be widely used and even expanded in size, as other healthcare networks in the Baltic Sea Area will be encouraged to connect to the BHN. The vision for the BHN in the long run is that it will become a model for other national – and cross-national Internet-based healthcare networks in Europe. This would prove the establishment of a European-wide healthcare network to be a real option.

4. Questions to be answered

The usage of a cross-national network like the BHN brings about a number of critical questions.

---

[4] Approximately 45.000 € for IT equipment.
[5] Examples: Danish and Swedish hospitals collaborate on ultrasound images. Norwegian and Swedish hospitals collaborate on radiology and Norwegian and Swedish hospitals collaborate with a radiology clinic in Barcelona, Spain.

The most frequent are:

1. Is it legal to send patient information between countries?
2. How does a hospital get reimbursed if it delivers a second opinion to another hospital?
3. How do we deal with cultural differences?
4. What if the two collaborating health professionals do not speak the same language?

These questions should be considered carefully before launching a cross-national collaboration. However, the problem is that the answers to the questions are still very unclear and this is a barrier to the full-scale usage of the BHN. Few decision makers will initiate such projects, if for instance the legal basis is unclear.

The Baltic eHealth project will only be successful in persuading decision makers to use the BHN for cross-national communication, if the project can give clear and unambiguous answers to the above questions. For this reason, the project will develop concrete guidelines on how to overcome legal, financial, cultural and linguistic barriers.

5. Conclusion

When operational in June 2005, the BHN will be the only cross-national healthcare network in Europe. At the same time, it will be the largest cross-sector network, as it will connect not only all the 200 hospitals of Denmark, Norway and Sweden, but also thousands of other healthcare stakeholders like GPs, specialist, laboratories, pharmacies and municipalities. The objective of BHN is to remove the technical barrier for collaboration between health professionals. The network and other results from the Baltic eHealth project like best practises from the two pilots and the guidelines on removal of other barriers for eHealth will be made available to decision makers in the Baltic Sea Region and this will hopefully contribute to the large-scale usage of second opinion from available experts regardless of institutional, regional and even national borders. Once the usefulness of the BHN is documented in the Baltic Sea Region, the BHN will be a strong candidate for a universal European model for the next generation health care network.

6. Acknowledgments

Baltic eHealth is funded by the Baltic Sea Region Interreg III B programme. The full list of partners and other information are available at www.baltic-ehealth.org.

7. References

[1] Oates J, Jensen HB. Building Regional Health Care Networks in Europe. *Studies in Health Technology and Informatics, Vol. 67* 2000: 3p.
[2] Jensen HB. The Missing Link. *EC-D6 XIII Health telematics concerted action* 1994: 16.
[3] Cannaby S, Wanscher CE, Pedersen CD, Voss H. The cost-benefit of electronic patient referrals in Denmark. ACCA and MedCom. *European Commission Information Society Directorate – General* (Forthcoming) 2005: 22.
[4] Malmqvist G. Networking in Health Care: An Issue of Conncetion or Co-operation? – The Evolution of Sjunet, The Swedish Health Care Network. *Paper at ICICTH* 2003: 2p.
[5] Norberg H. Health and Social Sectors with an "e". *Nordic Council of Ministers* (forthcoming) 2005: 73.
[6] Dahlgren LE. Öka nyttan av IT inom vården! *Eerlids* 2003: 42p.
[7] CD Pedersen, CE Wanscher. The Story of MedCom. *Picnic* (forthcoming) 2005: 90p.

8. Address for correspondence

hvo@cfst.dk

Connecting Medical Informatics and Bio-Informatics
R. Engelbrecht et al. (Eds.)
IOS Press, 2005

The Israeli Virtual National Health Record: A Robust National Health Information Infrastructure Based on a Firm Foundation of Trust

Esther Saiag

Israeli Ministry of Health, Tel Aviv Sourasky Medical Center, Israel

Abstract

*In many developed countries, a coordinated effort is underway to build national and regional Health Information Infrastructures (HII) for the linking of disparate sites of care, so that an access to a comprehensive Health Record will be feasible when critical medical decisions are made [1]. However, widespread adoption of such national projects is hindered by a series of barriers– regulatory, technical, financial and cultural. Above all, a robust national HII requires a firm foundation of trust: patients must be assured that their confidential health information will not be misused and that there are adequate legal remedies in the event of inappropriate behavior on the part of either authorized or unauthorized parties[2].
The Israeli evolving National HII is an innovative state of the art implementation of a wide-range clinical inter-organizational data exchange, based on a unique concept of virtually temporary sharing of information. A logically connection of multiple caregivers and medical organizations creates a patient-centric virtual repository, without centralization. All information remains in its original format, location, system and ownership. On demand, relevant information is instantly integrated and delivered to the point of care. This system, successfully covering more than half of Israel's population, is currently evolving from a voluntary private-public partnership (dbMOTION and CLALIT HMO) to a formal national reality. The governmental leadership, now taking over the process, is essential to achieve a full potential of the health information technology. All partners of the Israeli health system are coordinated in concert with each other, driven with a shared vision – realizing that a secured, private, confidential health information exchange is assured.*

Keywords:
Health Information Infrastructure; National Health Record; Data confidentiality; Electronic Medical Record

1. Introduction

Nation-wide implementation of health information technology is the only demonstrated method of controlling costs in the long run without decreasing the quality of health care delivered [2][3]. The provision of necessary patient information and medical knowledge in the hands of decision makers at the point of clinical decision making greatly benefits the health care system by significantly reducing errors, avoiding dangerous mistakes, reducing duplicate services and unnecessary hospitalizations and improving clinical decisions.

In Israel, advanced communications and computational infrastructure have made wide adoption of health information feasible. In the ambulatory setting, more than 95% of care givers document medical data almost exclusively into an Electronic Medical Record (EMR), while their colleagues in hospitals use it mainly for clinical admission and discharge. Until recently, the communication between various health care facilities in Israel was often paper-based, rendering the patient to serve as the messenger for data delivery and exchange. During the last 3 years, an outstanding HII project, leaded by Israel's largest HMO (Clalit Health Services) is gradually attracting multiple health care organizations, linking their various information systems through innovative powerful integration engines (the dbMOTION solution).

For 3.5 million citizens, medical encounters are now supported by and based on a comprehensive clinical database, virtually instantly created at the time and place of care and dissipated immediately at the end of the transaction. Transforming this initiative to a national operation involves multiple dilemmas- legal, technical, ethical, financial and practical. One of the leading questions would be, weather to expand the current technology to a nation-wide implementation or to replace it with an alternative solution, one of several available at the moment.

2. Background

A nationalized health system in Israel provides entitlement of every citizen to one of 4 HMO's. Health services are available to all, based on a payment (Health Insurance Tax). However, service provision is not conditioned by payment. The Israeli health system comprises of 4 sectors: the Ministry of Health, 4 HMO's, the private sector (including hospitals, labs etc.) and several Non Profit Organizations. Out of 50 general hospitals,8 belong to the largest HMO (Clalit Health Services), 11 are in governmental ownership, the rest are public or private.

Several times a year may the citizen change his affiliation to a certain HMO. Sick patients may be referred to a secondary care hospital consultant. Generally, healthcare is very collaborative in its nature in Israel, making it easier to understand how such a fascinating extraordinary process, of Information Technology Infrastructure, can take place independently, long before governmental involvements take over.

Israel's current Trans-Institutional -Cooperation

The dbMOTION solution is currently applied for more than half of Israel's population (3.5 million members of the Clalit HMO). All 8 general hospitals, hundreds of primary care clinics, labs and institutes of Clalit Health Services are interconnected through this platform throughout the country. In addition, two largest governmental hospitals, as well as one public hospital, have successfully joined the process, actually serving as a pilot for a possible future expansion of this information-net.

At the point and time of care, be it at the primary care clinic, in one of the above ERs or at the hospital ward, upon demand, relevant information is instantly integrated and delivered, enabling clear decisions. Metadata and maintained indexes assure fast retrieval of data (8 seconds on the average).

3. Methods

As described, step by step, following the Clalit initiative, a growing number of medical organizations in Israel have joined the process voluntarily and with no ministerial drive or support. This partnership speeded the adoption of health information technology and has largely promoted the establishment of the Israeli National Health Record. However, a governmental leadership was essential to achieve formal agreement and full cooperation of all partners of Israel's health system. The goal was to build a national, consistent and comprehensive health care network, for a secure data sharing and exchange. Therefore, a strategy of several steering committees has been worked out.

A Superior Steering Committee

Leaders of all sectors of Israel's health system gathered for the establishment of a conceptual framework for the National Health Record: an integration of medical data from all various origins, and its presentation upon request at all points of care, with no data repository or centralization and with *absolute dissipation of the generated data once the current medical encounter is through.* This unique, innovative approach for the implementation of a national health data communication is by no means the most convincing parameter driving all partners towards the process.

A Technological Committee

The dbMOTION solution, already widely operating, fully addresses the strict demands agreed upon by the superior steering committee, namely the virtual temporary creation of data, followed by its disappearance. Yet, the governmental initiative must involve an impartial analysis of multiple technological solutions, ending up with the most appropriate one for a nation-wide implementation. A Request For Information is been conducted by the committee, asking for proposals for the fulfillment of the agreed strategy.

A 3 layer architecture has been worked out – a basic *connectivity Layer*, to which pre-organized data, originating from multiple local databases, will be imported; An intermediate *Intelligent Layer* to dill with data normalization, conversion and synchronization, data security and authorization, clinical algorithms, alarms and alerts and others; A third *Viewer layer*. Sharing of information is asked to take place between different parties, regardless of the information technology employed by each member. Seeking to address a unified platform for the study and comparison of various technological solutions, a "Testing Lab" is been operated, with the connection of several test-databases installed in a set of servers.

An Advisory Committee for Terminology and Coding

Similarly to other aspects of the national process, moving from an independent initiative to a governmental strategy dictates the need for synchronized and standardized modes of cooperation. Although part of the work is already well underway, this committee will take the appropriate steps for the completion and adoption of standards that will allow medical information sharing electronically.

Originally, the idea of data sharing and exchange relied on the early foundation of a structured minimal set of clinical "items" (*Minimal Data Set*) – several critical diagnoses, allergies, current medications - upon which an agreement would be achieved, regarding the content, format and nomenclature. However, evolving technological solutions, as well as the ambition to link as many (unrelated) members ,as early as possible, have strongly moved us towards the immediate linkage of different databases, long before the completion of a standardized language. Still, exploitation of inter-institutional cooperation will only be fully met by the completion and adoption of a comprehensive medical vocabulary and of health information standards.

A committee for Ethics and Legislation

The Israeli law, through The Patient Rights Act and The People Health Act, permits medical data exchange for the purpose of healthcare provision, regardless of the patient's agreement. The establishment of the nation-wide health information sharing requires strong new legislation activities, carried out through this advisory committee.

The committee will convene task forces to determine ethical and legal means for secure and trusted linking of data, while protecting patient privacy.

The current HII operated by the Clalit, already implements robust standards for authentication and authorization. The system routinely and securely records access to data and is capable of tracking activities in a database. The role of this committee is to determine, on a national level, who will be authorized to what piece of information and how will the patient have control over his clinical data.

4. Discussion

Health Information exchange and interoperability have become an ongoing challenge for the international healthcare community. Examples include "Health Information Infrastructure" in the USA [4], "Healthconnect" in Australia[5], the Canadian "Infoway"[6], The "National Program for IT" in the United Kingdom[7] and others.

Principle questions, by which various national programs might differ from each other, are as follows: Is it going to replace the Medical Record (including intensive data entry), or will it mainly provide a "read only" access to the patients' comprehensive clinical status? Is a Central Database been maintained, populated by aggregative data available at all time (although authorization-dependent), or whether limited relevant data is retrieved upon request, on-line originating from multiple, diverse data repositories? Is it permitted to aggregate identified information or whether statistical unidentifiable data is only available, for the sake of privacy? Is it mandatory to replace all existing information technologies, or whether a powerful integration engine is been used, providing the conservation of current technologies?

The" Centralized Model" is less popular, especially when national involvement is the case, due to privacy violation concern. The "Federation Model", characterized by virtual organization of data "looks and feels" safer, though it doesn't necessarily exclude the existence of stored data- the threat of the "Big Brother".

"The HealthConnect" in Australia is structured for "electronic collection, storage and exchange of consumer health information via a secure network and within strict privacy safeguards" – in Israel we found such declarations insufficient for the achievement of robust consensus and cooperation, as to the willingness of care providers, health organizations and especially the patients to share any piece of data, what so ever. In Israel, therefore, the concept of the National Health Record is pivoted in our real effort to guaranty zero violence of privacy – the virtual clinical data retrieved for temporary use, doe's not exist in its aggregative form in any site in the system. Moreover, there is no way to store the data locally, following its use and before its dissipation.

Standards

Technical and semantic standards are essential for sharing of high quality information across a national health care system. To support better management of shared clinical information, standards are required for privacy and data protection, security and authentication, massaging and communication, data standards and terminology coding and classification systems[8]. Current wide HII in Israel, the dbMOTION-Clalit cooperation, is a self production rather than an open & non proprietary technology.

Transforming from an independent voluntary initiative to a national program, will soon evolve a request for proposals (RFP).. Solutions appropriate for our needs should support various formal terminology systems as Snowmed-CT, ICD-9-CM, CPT-4 and others. Massaging services should be based on the HL7 version 3 massaging standard.

Shifting from a voluntary inter-institutional cooperation, wide and successful as one can be, to a National Health Record, is a revolution of health care. Various characteristics of the Israeli health system have made this revolution feasible.

Paucity of insurers

In Israel, each citizen belongs to one of four HMOs, 55% been affiliated to Clalit, 25% belonging to the second large, leaving the rest to two similar smaller HMOs. In addition, most of the general hospitals belong to one of two owners - the government and the largest HMO.

Current strategy of Israel Ministry of Finance, to establish a unified communicational infrastructure, linking various government ministries to each other and with the citizens (E Government), further augments the homogenous infrastructure of Israel's health system.

Master Patient Index

Personal identification (ID) numbers, like we maintain in Israel, are mandatory for data interchange projects. These nationwide identifiers enable the unambiguously identifying of patients and linking their information from multiple sources within and across clinical enterprises.

Wide Acceptance of IT by Providers

Information technology of all kinds is very popular among care providers in Israel. Wide adoption of various EMRs, knowledge management applications, computerized clinical guidelines and algorithms as well as data warehouse systems, all catalyze the implementation of the national process.

Secondary to the above-mentioned strengths of the Israeli health system "profile", the emergence of the National Health Record was trivial. However, the most powerful strength of our current system is the innovative, unique concept of *virtual data, which is always there when you need it, secured and updated, and at the same time does not really exist anywhere in its integrative manner.* At the current legal atmosphere in Israel, namely the seemingly unlimited permission for medical data exchange among providers, only such robust foundation of trust could make this state of the art cutting edge technology part of our daily reality.

5. References

[1] Patricia Dykes and Susanne Bakken. National and Regional Health Information Infrastructure: Making Use of Information Technology to Promote Access to Evidence. *MEDINFO 2004*;pp.1187-1191

[2] Mark R.Benioff and Edward D.Lasowska. Revolutionizing Health Care Through Information Technology- President's Information Technology Advisory Committee2004

[3] William G.Chismar and Sean M. Thomas. The Economics of Integrated Electronic Medical Record Systems. *MEDINFO 2004*;pp.592-596

[4] A Way Forward for Improving Health Delivery in the USA- a Strategic Framework for change, http://www.medrecinst.com/conferences/seminar/dec04/proceedings/

[5] HealthConnect, A Health Information Network For Australians, www.healthconnect.gov.au

[6] Canada Health infoway, www.infoway-inforoute.ca

[7] National Program for IT IN the NHS, http://www.connectingforhealth.nhs.uk/

[8] Liaw ST,General practice and computing standards, Aust Fam Physician.2002 Jun;31(6):509-14.

Address for correspondence

Esther Saiag, MD,MSc
Tel Aviv Sourasky Medical Center
6, Weizman St.Tel-Aviv64239, ISRAEL
esthers@tasmc.health.gov.il

Section 7

Imaging Informatics

Connecting Medical Informatics and Bio-Informatics
R. Engelbrecht et al. (Eds.)
IOS Press, 2005

435

Myocardium Tissue Analysis Based on Textures in Ultrasound Images

Vytenis Punys[a,b], Jurate Puniene[a], Renaldas Jurkevicius[c], Jonas Punys[a]

[a] *Kaunas University of Technology, Studentu str. 56, Kaunas LT-3031, Lithuania*
[b] *Kaunas Medical University Hospital, Eiveniu str.2, Kaunas LT-3007 Lithuania*
[c] *Kaunas Medical University Hospital, Eiveniu str.2, Kaunas LT-3007 Lithuania*

Abstract

*The heart disease is related to the alterations in the biological tissue of its muscles. The myocardium alterations have been analysed and evaluated on ultrasound images. The statistical parameters of the heart texture on the defined region of interest present information about the state of myocardium. There are hundreds of the texture parameters, which could be used to evaluate the heart tissue structure. The goal was to choose the most informative ones by applying the quantitative analysis technique. The Fisher statistics has been applied for hypothesis testing to define the most informative texture parameters. The quantitative analysis proved that the texture parameters of the myocardium tissue can be estimated significantly, when the sample size of ROI is not less than 900-1000 pixels. The sample cannot be enhanced by combining images on in the diastolic and systolic phases. To evaluate the state of the myocardium the following statistical parameters can be used on **four chamber view images:** the percentiles of order 0.01, 0.1, 0.5, grey level run length non-uniformity (in all directions: horizontally, vertically, 45^0, 135^0), except a lateral wall of the left ventricle, the entropy of the two-dimensional probability distribution, the parameter of the two-dimensional probability distribution, which defines the mean distance between grey levels. On **parasternal images** the informative statistical parameters are: grey level run length non-uniformity (in all directions: horizontally, vertically, 45^0, 135^0), grey level non-uniformity, the entropy of the two-dimensional probability distribution applied to the septum only.*

Keywords:
Echocardiography, Computer-Assisted Image Interpretation

1. Introduction

Echocardiology has been increasing used non-invasive technique for diagnosing heart diseases [1,2]. The ultrasound examination offers opportunity for making anatomical and functional diagnosis by analysing a heart tissue. The use of ultrasound is based on the correlation between the anatomical structure of tissue and its acoustic properties. The reflection and transmission of ultrasound in tissue depends on tissue density, elasticity and acoustic impedance. Changes of these parameters are related to the alterations on an ultrasound image texture [3-5]. The alterations in the biological tissue of its muscles are reflected in echocardiograms. However, the changes of texture are rather imperceptible by the human eye. Even it is more difficult for the human eye to evaluate tissue granularity and direction of fibres. Miocarditis and fibrosis exert influence upon alterations of brightness, heterogeneity and contrast. Image processing techniques may be applied for evaluating these alterations by carrying out quantitative analysis of some regions of a heart image texture.

The goal was to analyse a heart tissue and to evaluate myocardium on the base of statistical parameters of the heart texture alterations. Statistical parameters of the image texture on the defined region of interest can present information about the state of myocardium. In Figure 1 some views of a heart with regions of interest are presented.

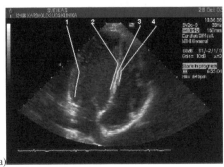 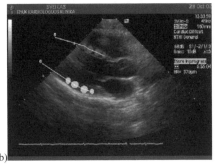

a)   b)

Figure 1- Allotment of the sets of ROIs (region of interest) for the evaluation of myocardium structure in different measurements schemes: (a) four-chamber view (1-the lateral wall of a left ventricle, 2- the right side of septum, 3- the left side of septum, 4- the middle part of septum, where the most intensive echo-signal is detected), (b) parasternal view (5- the septum, 6- the inferior wall of a left ventricle).

2. Materials and methods

Statistical texture parameters enable to extract information about tissue properties and to classify the different regions on an image, which define normal or abnormal tissue fragments of a heart. There are some simple statistical characteristics as a mean, a variation, a histogram, though the higher-order statistics of the texture have to be taken into account [6].

Texture features can be defined by its:

- *Spatial frequency components.* High spatial frequencies dominate for the fine textures, while coarse textures are characterized by low spatial frequencies.

- *Edge per unit area.* Coarse textures have a small number of edges per unit area; fine textures have a high number of them.

- *Grey level spatial dependency*, that means co-occurrence (conditional distribution) of the grey levels and spatial interrelationship of them. The distribution changes slightly for coarse textures and it changes rapidly for fine textures.

- *Grey level run length.* Course textures have many pixels in a run for some grey level and fine textures have only few pixels in it.

- *Auto regression model parameters*, which present relation between the neighbourhood pixels. The parameter values for course textures are similar and for fine textures they have wide variations.

Spatial frequency components are estimated by discrete Fourier transform. It is well known and frequently used technique in image processing.

Textural edgesness can be defined by a gradient for any local area (the sum of absolute value of the differences of neighboring pixels). Gradient techniques are widely applied in a contour estimation.

Co-occurrence defines the spatial distribution and the spatial dependence. Lets analyze this texture feature in more detail. Suppose, that the texture area has N resolution levels in horizontal and vertical directions. The texture is presented by N_g grey levels. The grey level co-occurrence is defined by a matrix of conditional frequencies $P_{i,j}(d,\theta)$, which depends on distance d between neighboring grey levels i and j. The parameter θ defines the angular relationship. For $\theta=0^0$ it is a conditional probability estimation of a left-right transition of grey levels i and j.

Run length of a grey level is a collinear connected set of pixels, which belong to the same grey level. Grey level runs are characterized by the grey level value, the length of the run (a number of pixels in the run) and the run direction. The run length matrix elements $r(i,j)$ define how often a particular grey level value i is met in a particular run length j, $i=1,N_l$, $j=1,N_r$, N_l is the number of grey values, N_r is the run lengths. Usually four matrices $r(i,j)$ are calculated in the directions $\{0^0, 45^0, 90^0, 135^0\}$. Some statistics can be calculated from the matrix $r(i,j)$: short run emphasis, long run emphasis, grey level non-uniformity, run length non-uniformity, fraction of an image in runs.

Short run emphasis
$$\sum_{i=1}^{N_l}\sum_{j=1}^{N_r}\frac{r(i,j)}{j^2} \Big/ \sum_{i=1}^{N_l}\sum_{j=1}^{N_r}r(i,j). \tag{1}$$

Long run emphasis
$$\sum_{i=1}^{N_l}\sum_{j=1}^{N_r}j^2 r(i,j) \Big/ \sum_{i=1}^{N_l}\sum_{j=1}^{N_r}r(i,j). \tag{2}$$

Grey level non-uniformity
$$\sum_{i=1}^{N_l}(\sum_{j=1}^{N_r}r(i,j))^2 \Big/ \sum_{i=1}^{N_l}\sum_{j=1}^{N_r}r(i,j). \tag{3}$$

Run length non-uniformity
$$\sum_{j=1}^{N_r}(\sum_{i=1}^{N_l}r(i,j))^2 \Big/ \sum_{i=1}^{N_l}\sum_{j=1}^{N_r}r(i,j). \tag{4}$$

Fraction of an image in runs
$$\sum_{i=1}^{N_l}\sum_{j=1}^{N_r}r(i,j) \Big/ \sum_{i=1}^{N_l}\sum_{j=1}^{N_r}jr(i,j). \tag{5}$$

Principal component technique has been applied for a covariance matrix to list the statistical parameters in decreasing order according to their informativeness. The next step is to define how many of these statistical parameters should be used for the myocardium state evaluation [7].

There are some test criteria to check the hypothesis about a number of the significant statistical parameters [8,9]. We have carried out the hypothesis testing of the parameter significance on the base of the Fisher test [10].

3. Results

Consequently, we have been solving problems:

- which echocardiographical images (four chamber view or parasternal view, based on native or harmonic imaging techniques) and which myocardium areas to use that the textural parameters were statistically significant and reliable;

- is it possible to improve the reliability of the texture parameters, increasing the sample size by combining images in systolic and diastolic states;
- defining the most significant texture parameters for evaluating the myocardium tissue.

The regions of interest (ROIs), defined by the physician, on the four chamber images and on parasternal images (harmonic and native) were of different size and orientation. These ROIs have been used to evaluate the texture parameters of the myocardium tissue. Experimentally it has been proved that to get statistically significant texture parameters, we need ROIs with at least 900–1000 pixels. The areas of myocardium, limited to this size, have been investigated on (see Figure 1):

- images of four chamber view: the lateral wall [abbrev., LW] of a left ventricle and the septum: right side [abbrev., SR], left side [abbrev., SL] and its middle part [abbrev., SI] (where the most intensive echo-signal is detected);
- parasternal images [abbrev., PS]: the inferior wall [abbrev., IW] of a left ventricle and the septum [abbrev., S].

Table 1 – Statistical characteristics of the set of the images (systolic/diastolic) analysed

	Sound patients	Hypertension patients
Number of patients	152	117
Number of image sequences analysed	2968	2297
Among them:		
Four chamber view, 3 MHz native images	98 / 101	82 / 82
ROIs: lateral wall of a left ventricle	98 / 101	82 / 78
septum, left side	98 / 79	82 / 79
septum, middle (echo-intensive) part	98 / 101	82 / 82
septum, right side	98 / 101	78 / 79
Four chamber view, 4 MHz harmonic images	121 / 117	94 / 94
ROIs: lateral wall of a left ventricle	117 / 113	94 / 94
septum, left side	118 / 102	90 / 91
septum, middle (echo-intensive) part	121 / 117	90 / 94
septum, right side	113 / 116	86 / 90
Parasternal (PS) view, 3 MHz native images	137 / 139	94 / 94
ROIs: septum	137 / 139	94 / 94
inferior wall of a left ventricle	137 / 139	94 / 94
Parasternal (PS) view, 4 MHz harmonic images	137 / 133	91 / 91
ROIs: septum	133 / 133	91 / 91
inferior wall of a left ventricle	137 / 133	91 / 86

To augment the reliability of the texture parameters, the sample size has been increased by combining images of the same patient in systolic and diastolic states. With probability **P=0.8** a hypotheses has been tested if the values of texture parameters of sound patients and ones with hypertension differ significantly in the compound sample. There were only three parameters (Long-run Emphasis at 45^0 direction, Short Run Emphasis at 45^0 direction, Fraction of greyscale series in runs at 45^0 direction), which differ significantly in only two anatomical locations. These texture parameters form 1% of the total amount (280) of the examined parameters. For this reason we gave up the idea of combining systolic and diastolic images.

At the beginning, having limited amount of data, a hypothesis on parameters' significance has been tested with the probability **P=0.7**. Additional to the ordinary statistical characteristics (mean, variance, skewness, kurtosis) some parameters based on two-dimensional probability characteristics, were statistically significant. By having increased the sample size, it was possible to test a hypotheses with the probability **P=0.99**. The amount of significant parameters increased considerably. The significance of texture parameters of the myocardium tissue has been proved on the base of the Fisher criterion [10].

Table 2 – Significant texture features of miocardium tissue, when systolic and diastolic images are combined into a common data set (marked cells indicate discriminative features in corresponding anatomical regions with probability P=0.80)

Imaging technique	Harmonic 4MHz imaging						Native 3 MHz imaging					
Echocardiographic view	4 chamber view				PS view		4 chamber view				PS view	
Anatomical region	LW	SR	SI	SL	IW	S	LW	SR	SI	SL	IW	S
Long run emphasis at 45° (45dgr_LngREmph)		X						X				
Short run emphasis at 45° (45dgr_ShrtREmp)		X						X				
Fraction of an image in runs (45dgr_Fraction)		X						X				

Table 3 – Significant texture features of miocardium tissue (marked cells indicate discriminative features in corresponding anatomical regions with probability P=0.99)

Imaging technique	Harmonic 4MHz imaging						Native 3 MHz imaging					
Echocardiographic view	4 chamber view				PS view		4 chamber view				PS view	
Anatomical region	LW	SR	SI	SL	IW	S	LW	SR	SI	SL	IW	S
Percentiles of histogram:												
(Perc., 1%)	X		X				X		X			
(Perc., 10%)	X		X				X		X			
(Perc., 50%)	X		X				X		X			
Run-length nonuniformity												
(Horzl_RLNonUni)	X				X	X	X				X	X
(Vertl_RLNonUni)	X				X	X	X				X	X
(45dgr_RLNonUni)	X				X	X	X				X	X
(135dr_RLNonUni)	X				X	X	X				X	X
Grey level nonuniformity												
(Horzl_GLevNonU)					X	X					X	X
(Vertl_GLevNonU)					X	X					X	X
(45dgr_GLevNonU)					X	X					X	X
(135dr_GLevNonU)					X	X					X	X
Mean distance between grey levels from co-occurrence matrix (S(,)SumAverg)	X		X				X		X			
Entropy of co-occurrence matrix (S(,)Entropy)	X						X	X				X

4. Conclusions

1. The texture parameters of the myocardium tissue can be estimated significantly, when the sample size of ROI is not less than 900-1000 pixels. For this reason, the septum areas on the four chamber images, except its middle part, are too small to be used for the myocardium tissue analysis.

2. The texture parameters of the myocardium tissue differ in the diastolic and systolic phases. For this reason combining these images into one sample is not acceptable.

3. The significance of texture parameters of the myocardium tissue does not depend on the measurement technique (native or harmonic), though the values of the parameters differ.

4. The significant texture parameters on *four chamber view images* (the lateral wall of the left ventricle and the middle area of the septum) differ between sound patients

and the ones with hypertension. To evaluate the state of the myocardium the following parameters can be used:

- The percentiles of order 0.01, 0.1, 0.5 of the probability distribution;
- Grey level run length non-uniformity (in all directions: horizontally, vertically, 450, 1350). It can only be applied to lateral wall of the left ventricle.
- The entropy of the two-dimensional probability distribution, when the distance between pixels varies from 1 to 5.
- The parameter of the two-dimensional probability distribution, which defines the mean distance between grey levels.

5. The significant texture parameters on parasternal images (the inferior wall of the left ventricle and the septum), which can be used to evaluate the state of the myocardium, are:

- Grey level run length non-uniformity (in all directions: horizontally, vertically, 450, 1350).
- Grey level non-uniformity;
- The entropy of the two-dimensional probability distribution, when the distance between pixels varies from 1 to 5. It can be applied to the septum only.

5. Acknowledgements

This research was supported by the Lithuanian State Science and Studies Foundation (Reg.number 26045) and by the Kaunas University of Technology, Lithuania. We would like to express our gratitude to Dr.Materka and his team for ability to use their package of computer programs MazDa (http://eletel.p.lodz.pl/cost/software.html).

6. References

[1] Feigenbaum H. Echocardiographic tissue diagnosis. *European Heart journal*, 1996, vol.17, pp. 6-7.
[2] Wied G., Bahr G., Bartels P. Automatic analysis of cell images. In: Wied G., Bahr G., eds. *Automated cell identification and cell sorting.* Academic Press, New York, 1970, pp. 195-360.
[3] Bello V., Pedrinelli R., Bianchi M., ect. Ultrasonic Myocardial texture in Hypertensive Mild-to-Moderate Left Ventricular Hypertrophy. A videodensitometric study. *American Journal of Hypertension,* 1998, 11, 155-164.
[4] Lieback E., Hardouin I., Meyer R., Bellach J., R. Hetzer R. Clinical value of echocardiographic tissue characterization in the diagnosis of myocarditis. *European Heart Journal*, 1996, 17, pp. 135-142.
[5] Bhondari A. K., Nanda N.C. Myocardial texture characterization by two dimensional echocardiography. *American Journal of Cardiology*, 1989, 123, pp. 832-840.
[6] Haralick R.M. Statistical and structural approaches to texture.. *Proc. of the fourth International joint conference on Pattern recognition*, Kyoto, Japan, 1978, pp. 45-69.
[7] Materka A. MazDa; Computer program for quantitative analysis of image texture. *Proc. of Int. conference Informatics for health care.* Lithuania, Kaunas University of Technology. 19-20 September, 2002, 1. pp. 39-59.
[8] Rao C. R. *Linear statistical inference and its applications.* John Wiley & Sons Inc., 1965.
[9] Kendall M.G., Stuart A. *The advanced theory of statistics.* Vol.3. Charles Griffin & company limited, London. 1966.
[10] Janko J. *Statisticke tabulky.* (in Russian), GOSTstatizdat, Moscow. 1961.

Address for correspondence:

Vytenis Punys, Image Processing & Analysis Laboratory, Kaunas University of Technology, Studentu str. 56-305, LT-51424 Kaunas, LITHUANIA, E-mail: vytenis.punys@ktu.lt

Connecting Medical Informatics and Bio-Informatics
R. Engelbrecht et al. (Eds.)
IOS Press, 2005

Automatic Measurement of Skin Wheals Provoked by Skin Prick Tests

Michael Prinz[a], Kornelia Vigl[b], Stefan Wöhrl[b]

[a] Core Unit for Medical Statistics and Informatics; Section on Med. Computer Vision
[b] Department of Dermatology; Division of Immunology, Allergy and Infectious Diseases (DIAID)
Medical University of Vienna, Vienna, Austria

Abstract

Skin prick tests (SPT) represent the standard method for the diagnosis of type-1 allergies. The skin wheals provoked by the SPTs are considered positive above certain cut-off diameters, usually 3 mm. At present their size is mostly estimated by measuring the diameter with rulers. Since the shape of wheals usually is not circular, the measurement of diameters leads to imprecise results. Therefore, we developed an algorithm for precisely measuring the wheals' area in mm^2 automatically. The average deviation of the automatic measurement on a test set achieved with the developed algorithm was 6.9 %. Compared to the maximum standard deviation of 6.59 % when measuring the manually redrawn outlines, the automatic method works sufficiently well.

Keywords:
Allergy, urticaria; Skin prick test; Mathematical morphology; Computer-assisted diagnosis; Methodology

1. Introduction

For the diagnosis of type-1 allergies, skin prick tests (SPTs) are applied to the patient's volar forearm. As a preparation, the forearm is marked with a skin-marking pen corresponding to the number of allergens to be applied. After applying the allergens dissolved in aqueous solution onto the skin, each drop is pricked with a standardized, sterile metallic lancet through the drop to provoke a specific dermal reaction described as wheal or hive. The wheal appears as a circumscribed edema of the skin with a characteristic reddened adjacent area. Since it can also be provoked by urticaria stinging, it is also termed an urticarial lesion. After leaving the allergenic solution on the skin for 15 to 20 minutes, the drops are wiped off. The outline of the possibly provoked skin wheals are marked with the skin-marking pen. A standard translucent adhesive tape is sticked onto the marked outline and pulled down again. This way the marker is transferred to the tape. Finally the tape is put on a documentation form.

The wheal size has been demonstrated to correlate with activity of allergic diseases. The measurement of wheal size has therefore been applied in a lot of study settings [1-3]. At present only the wheals' diameter is measured. Some physicians determine the average of the maximum and minimum diameter for estimating the allergic reactions [4].

There has been done some work on determining wheal sizes automatically already [5-7]. These works proved that measuring wheals automatically is an adequate method. We intended to develop an easy-to-use tool for the precise calculation of wheal sizes. The tool should easily integrate into the usual SPT flow of work and should be based on standard computer equipment. Therefore, we decided to use the common skin prick test procedure of outlining the wheals' border with a blue coloured pen and transferring the borders' shape to a form. We implemented an application which scans the documentation form and automatically detects wheals, strokes and empty SPT areas and measures the wheals' area in mm^2.

2. Material and Methods

For the development of the algorithm we used the Khoros Pro 2001 development environment for image analysis applications developed by Khoral Incorporated. Khoros has been installed on a standard 800 MHz Linux PC[1]. The algorithm was based on methods of mathematical morphological image analysis operations [9] and therefore, the MMach-package for Khoros was used [10]. The forms were scanned with a resolution of 200 dpi on a standard HP ScanJet 7400 C.

2.1. Documentation form

For being able to automatically detect the wheals provoked by the various allergens we decided to design a new documentation form onto which all adhesive tape stripes with the transferred wheals' outlines have to be put on (*Figure 1*). Since usually the form is not positioned precisely upright onto the scanner (*Figure 2*) we attached two black dots to the form at the upper left and the lower right corner. These dots are automatically detected by our algorithm after the scanning process. The form is moved and rotated correspondingly to obtain a precisely upright positioned form necessary to for further processing (*Figure 3*). The small boxes at the lower right corners of the SPT-areas are used for marking the clinical relevance of the allergic reaction.

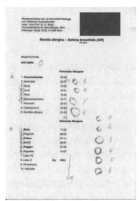 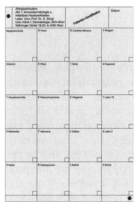

Figure 1 - Old versus newly designed form. The old form shows a "chaotic" order of wheal outlines making it impossible to perform measurements automatically. On the new form the outlines are put on at predefined areas. Two black dots were attached for being able to position the form exactly after the scanning process. The small boxes at the lower right of the SPT areas are used to mark the test's clinical relevance.

---

[1] In the meantime Khoros has been taken over by Accusoft Corporation and has been renamed to VisiQuest [8].

The two black dots at the form's upper left and lower right corner are detected by their shape and size. By eroding and subsequently conditionally dilating the image with a circular structure element all dots larger resp. smaller than the structure element are removed. Only the two marker dots remain visible. The angle between the connection of the detected dots' centres and a vertical line is measured. The form is rotated by the difference between the ideal angle and the measured angle. Afterwards the position of the upper left dot is redetected and the entire form is relocated to the ideal position. As long as both marker dots are visible on the scanned image the algorithm is able to ideally reposition the form.

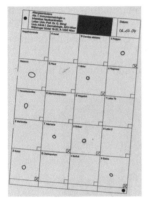 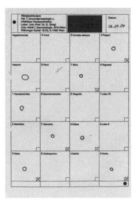

Figure 2 - The form has been put onto the scanner imprecisely.

Figure 3 - By detecting the black dots the algorithm is able to correct the position of the form to obtain a precisely upright positioned form.

Extraction of SPT areas

After positioning the form exactly the individual SPT areas are extracted via their well known coordinates (*Figure 4*). The outlines of the wheals have been marked with a blue coloured marking pen. Thus, by extracting the blue channel of the SPT area images, the black coloured area contours including the small box at the lower right are excluded (*Figure 5*).

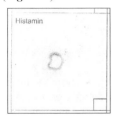 

Figure 4 - An SPT-area has been extracted. The border of the area and the small box at the lower right are still visible.

Figure 5 - The SPT-area's blue colour channel has been extracted. The black borders around the SPT area and the label have disappeared.

Detection and Measurement of wheals

The extracted SPT-areas are inspected one after the other. The area to examine is limited to the wheal's actual extension by detecting the wheal's minimum and maximum coordinates.

These coordinates are extended by a safety margin to be sure not to cut off the wheal's outer border (*Figure 6*). The wheal's border is condensed by a mathematical closing operation. Thus, fine gaps are closed (*Figure 7*). To be able to close larger gaps the border is watersheded to obtain the wheal's middle contour (*Figure 8*). The middle contour is dilated and superimposed on the closed border (*Figure 9*). By applying this procedure large gaps in the wheal's border contour are appropriately reconstructed. A threshold has to be found dynamically to obtain a closed binary border contour. This is achieved by increasing the threshold stepwise starting from a minimum value until a closed border emerges (*Figure 10*). Since the wheal's outer border has been outlined on the patient's arm the inner contour of the border resembles the actual wheal's area. The inner contour is extracted by dilating the border and subtracting the dilated border from the thresholded border. The resulting contour is smoothed to remove peaks which do not resemble manually drawn outlines (*Figure 11*).

The number of pixels inside the extracted contour is measured and converted to mm^2 by considering the scanning resolution.

Figure 6 - The actual area of the wheal (ROI) has been extracted.

Figure 7 - A mathematical closing operation has been applied to the original wheal border.

Figure 8 - The closed wheal border is watersheded to obtain the wheal's middle contour.

Figure 9 - The wheal's dilated middle contour is superimposed on the closed wheal border to fill larger gaps of the wheal border.

Figure 10 - The resulting grey level border is dynamically thresholded to obtain a closed wheal border.

Figure 11 - The inner contour of the border is extracted and smoothed.

When an allergen is not applied to the patient's skin a blue coloured stroke from the lower left to the upper right is manually drawn into the assigned SPT area directly on the form (*Figure 12*). Our algorithm is able to detect these strokes automatically and indicates that the corresponding test has not been applied. The detection of the stroke is started by extracting the stroke's blue coloured pixels. The regression line of these pixels is calculated and the angle between the regression line and the horizontal line is measured. Regression lines with angle values between 10° and 80° meet the requirements for strokes. The length of the stroke has to be at least 300 pixels and the average distance of the stroke's pixels to the regression line has to be less than 5 pixels. If a set of pixels meet these requirements the test is classified as not applied.

Allergens which do not provoke any allergic reactions to the patient's skin are indicated by leaving the corresponding SPT area empty (***Figure 13***). The algorithm also detects empty SPT areas and indicates that there has been no allergic reaction to the allergen.

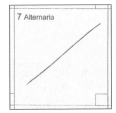

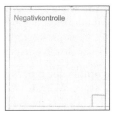

Figure 12 - A manually drawn stroke in a form's SPT area indicates that the corresponding test has not been applied.

Figure 13 - An empty SPT area indicates that there has not been any reaction to the allergen.

3. Results

For evaluating the accuracy of our application we formed a test set of 12 test persons who were treated on both inner forearms with 5 distinct concentrations of histamine ranging from 1:1 to 1:100. Histamine is the main mediator secreted by skin mast cells after activation with allergen and causative for the dermal reaction described as wheal. For each skin prick test, it is used as a positive control to demonstrate skin reactivity that can be hampered by inadvertent intake of drugs with antihistaminic side effects such as antidepressants. We preferred histamine to real allergen for the evaluation of this system, because it produces reproducible wheals also in non-allergic subjects. The overall number of provoked wheals was 111. To obtain the actual wheals' area the outlines were manually redrawn and measured with the image processing software ImageJ [11]. Each wheal was redrawn 3 times by the same physician. The average of the 3 measurement was taken. The standard deviation of the areas derived by the manual outlines was up to 6.59 %. The average deviation of the automatic measurement on the originally scanned forms was 6.9 %. We observed a few runaways with deviations above 20 % which nevertheless resembled the actual outline sufficiently well. Thus, the average deviation of the automatic measurement was only slightly higher than the maximum average deviation of the manual measurement. Similar to [5] we observed higher deviations from the actual size at small wheals < 5 mm^2. We achieved some improvement by enlarging these wheals by a factor of 1.5 to 3.0 for the reconstruction of their border and reducing them again for measuring their size.

The application was also applied to a set of 126 prick tests with allergens in allergic individuals at which the wheal outlines were manually redrawn with a blue coloured pen directly on the form. Only slight parameterizations had to be made to achieve excellent detection and measurement results of these outlines.

The algorithm behaves very stable on varying contrasts and varying intensities of the blue coloured contour on the adhesive tape. By using mathematical morphological operations even larger gaps in the contour are reconstructed very well.

4. Discussion

The accuracy and the stability of our algorithm are very promising and are appropriate for applying it to the routine SPT. The algorithm provides an objective and reproducible method for measuring wheals. So far we have developed a prototype of the application. The processing speed of the wheal detection procedure has to be improved. The overall processing of an entire form with 20 SPT areas takes about 20 minutes on a standard 800 MHz PC.

5. Conclusion

We have presented an algorithm for processing SPTs automatically which works without any interaction by the user. Wheals, strokes and empty SPT-areas are detected automatically. The area of wheals is measured precisely. The algorithm is appropriate for being integrated into the routine process of performing SPTs. The results of the measurement can easily be transferred to medical documentation systems and thus, provides a completion of the patient history concerning treatment of skin allergies.

6. References

[1]   Eigenmann PA, Sampson HA. Interpreting skin prick tests in the evaluation of food allergy in children. Pediatr Allergy Immunol 1998;9(4):186-91.

[2]   Gergen PJ, Turkeltaub PC. The association of allergen skin test reactivity and respiratory disease among whites in the US population. Data from the Second National Health and Nutrition Examination Survey, 1976 to 1980. Arch Intern Med 1991;151(3):487-92.

[3]   Gergen PJ, Turkeltaub PC. The association of individual allergen reactivity with respiratory disease in a national sample: data from the second National Health and Nutrition Examination Survey, 1976-80 (NHANES II). J Allergy Clin Immunol 1992;90(4 Pt 1):579-88.

[4]   Maccario J, Oryszczyn MP, Charpin D, Kauffmann F. Methodologic aspects of the quantification of skin prick test responses: the EGEA study. J Allergy Clin Immunol 2003;111(4):750-6.

[5]   Pijnenborg H, Nilsson L, Dreborg S. Estimation of skin prick test reactions with a scanning program. Allergy. 1996 Nov;51(11):782-8.

[6]   Poulsen LK, Liisberg C, Bindslev-Jensen C, Malling HJ. Precise area determination of skin-prick tests: validation of a scanning device and software for a personal computer. Clin Exp Allergy. 1993 Jan;23(1):61-8.

[7]   Poulsen LK, Bindslev-Jensen C, Rihoux JP. Quantitative determination of skin reactivity by two semiautomatic devices for skin prick test area measurements. Agents Actions. 1994 Jun;41 Spec No:C134-5.

[8]   AccuSoft Corporation. http://www.accusoft.com.

[9]   Serra J. Image Analysis and Mathematical Morphology, volume I. Academic Press, 1982.

[10] Barrera J, Banon JF, Lotufo RA, Hirata R. MMach: a Mathematical Morphology Toolbox for the Khoros System. J of Electronic Imaging 1998; 7(1):174-210.

[11] Rasband W. ImageJ, Image Processing and Analysis in Java, http://rsb.info.nih.gov/ij.

Corresponding author:

Michael Prinz
Core Unit for Medical Statistics and Informatics
Section on Med. Computer Vision
Medical University of Vienna
Spitalgasse 23
1090 Vienna, Austria
tel: (+43)(1) 40400-6655
fax: (+43)(1) 40400-6656
email: Michael.Prinz@meduniwien.ac.at
url: http://www.mbm.meduniwien.ac.at

Connecting Medical Informatics and Bio-Informatics
R. Engelbrecht et al. (Eds.)
IOS Press, 2005

Computed Quality Assessment of MPEG4-compressed DICOM Video Data

Thomas Frankewitsch[a], **Sven Söhnlein**[a], **Marcel Müller**[b], **Hans-Ulrich Prokosch**[a]

[a]*Department of Medical Informatics, University of Erlangen-Nuernberg, Germany*
[b]*Department of Dermatology, University of Freiburg, Freiburg, Germany*

Abstract

Digital Imaging and Communication in Medicine (DICOM) has become one of the most popular standards in medicine. This standard specifies the exact procedures in which digital images are exchanged between devices, either using a network or storage medium. Sources for images vary; therefore there exist definitions for the exchange for CR, CT, NMR, angiography, sonography and so on. With its spreading, with the increasing amount of sources included, data volume is increasing, too. This affects storage and traffic. While for long-time storage data compression is generally not accepted at the moment, there are many situations where data compression is possible: Telemedicine for educational purposes (e.g. students at home using low speed internet connections), presentations with standard-resolution video projectors, or even the supply on wards combined receiving written findings. DICOM comprises compression: for still image there is JPEG, for video MPEG-2 is adopted. Within the last years MPEG-2 has been evolved to MPEG-4, which squeezes data even better, but the risk of significant errors increases, too. Within the last years effects of compression have been analyzed for entertainment movies, but these are not comparable to videos of physical examinations (e.g. echocardiography). In medical videos an individual image plays a more important role. Erroneous single images affect total quality even more. Additionally, the effect of compression can not be generalized from one test series to all videos. The result depends strongly on the source. Some investigations have been presented, where different MPEG-4 algorithms compressed videos have been compared and rated manually. But they describe only the results in an elected testbed. In this paper some methods derived from video rating are presented and discussed for an automatically created quality control for the compression of medical videos, primary stored in DICOM containers.

Keywords:
Computer-Assisted Image Processing, Telemedicine, Coronary Angiography, Quality Control

1. Introduction

Since 1983 Digital Imaging and Communication in Medicine standard (DICOM) has evolved to a widespread and almost best accepted standard in medical image acquisition, transportation, storage and retrieval.[1] Almost every modality is capable to communicate digital data based on DICOM: It is routine usage that computed radiography, nuclear magnetic resonance images, and echocardiography or sonography data are packed within DICOM containers.[2-5] Pathology has adopted this standard for transferring photos of light microscopy, too.[2] Other specialties which document findings in multimedia data are preparing adaptations of DICOM.[6;7]

Additionally, DICOM has proved to be useful in education. Teaching files can be constructed using DICOM information and files.[8-10] Therefore, not only physicians on wards, radiology departments or outpatient practice are interested in such files, students will them use either.

The acceptance of DICOM keeps up with the increasing amount of visual data which are forthcoming on digital devices today. While more multimedia data are available, network transfer and storage capacities have to be enhanced, too, to enable retrieval.

Raw or original data are stored in best quality, because of the fear of loss in medical information. Legal rules force PACS-holding departments to store data in a manner that there is no loss in diagnostic expressiveness.[11;12] Best quality is needed or demanded on diagnostic workstations; hence nobody dares to decide which information can be deleted.

High quality data in image based information systems usually mean high volumes of data. But there are many situations where the amount of data can or even must be reduced: e.g. low-speed connections, low-resolution presentations or printings. In other word, the utilisation of medical images and movies (e.g. a movie of a coronary angiography) is not restricted to diagnostic workstations, they might be behold in situations where the diagnostic report is available and lower resolution is acceptable. Students may want to use teaching files at home, where they are not connected with high-speed backbones to the internet, outpatient practices just want to document a visible and mostly more impressive finding on video or x-ray film together with the written report. In many clinical environments radiology departments discuss results of examinations showing images or video-tapes with a standard video projector.

In multimedia data reduction can be achieved by compression: redundant data can be stored economically, unnecessary data like background noise can be deleted. There are many algorithms on the market, lossy or non lossy, which can be used for image or video compression. Many of them are not very expensive or even freely available and can be integrated in nearly every personal computer system. Non lossy methods usually reduce the amount of data within 50%, lossy ones even spare up to 90%.[13;14] At the moment DICOM accepts lossy and non-lossy JPG compression for still images. Since 2003 MPEG-2 video compression is approved in DICOM standard for videos.[15-18]

While MPEG-2 is standardised in many points, the successor MPEG-4 has got more features: E.g. DIVX which is one of many MPEG-4 realisations, allows not only fixing bit-rate, but also enables psycho-visual enhancements, different variations in sampling and calculations. Therefore results can not be compared on the bit rate only and studies on MPEG-4 usage mostly in cardiology are discordant.

In addition, compression results depend on the input data. Therefore, tools with an enriched set of optimizers will not perform the same way on each individual video sequence. The aim must be to offer the highest quality as possible combined with the lowest amount of data as possible. Manually controlled compressions are feasible, but time and effort are expensive. Consequently manual quality control can only be performed in studies but not in routine usage. Therefore, the urgent need for an automated quality control arises.

Video compression: estimation of loss

There exist two common ways for video compression quality estimation:

On the one hand one compares bytes of non-compressed and compressed frames in pairs. The differences that occur during compression are calculated frame-based and along the whole frameset.

But there are some methical shortcomings: It is important whether a large error occurs in one image of the video stream, where it might affect, hide or create a relevant sign of a disease, or whether there are only slightly modifications that affect all images with or without diagnostic relevance.

Mathematical method – unbiased

Mean square error (MSE)

One way for calculating the error produced is comparing input and output frames pixel by pixel. Different calculation models are available and commonly recommended. E.g. one basic method is the determination of the mean squared error (MSE):[19]

$$(1)\ MSE = \frac{1}{K}\sum_{k=1}^{K}\left\{\frac{1}{N \times M}\sum_{i=0}^{N-1}\sum_{j=0}^{M-1}\left[f_{comp}(i,j,k) - forg(i,j,k)\right]^2\right\}$$

But one has to take into account the display rate of an individual pixel. It is an important factor to compare the error of an image with the amount of bits a pixel is encoded, because an alteration of a 8bit pixel within the distance of one bit must be taken into another focus that the change of a 256bit pixel. The relative alteration is more interesting than the absolute one. The peak signal to noise ratio tries to determine the error in contrast to the maximal value of a pixel:[19]

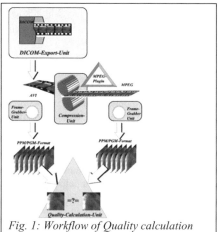

Fig. 1: Workflow of Quality calculation

$$(2)\ PSNR = 10 \cdot \log_{10}\left(\frac{MAX^2}{\frac{1}{N}\sum_{i=1}^{N}MSE_i}\right)[dB]$$

Based on this PSNR the Video Quality Metric has been published by the International telecommunication Union (ITU). [20]

$$(3)\ VQM = \frac{1}{1 + e^{a(PSNR-b)}}$$

The values of a=0.15 and b=19.7818 have been retrieved experimentally. It is recommended that only values of 20≤PSNR≤45 are accepted. The resulting VQM is compared to fuzzy results like "excellent" (VQM<20%) or "good" (VQM<40%).

Human visual system based methods

Shortly the human visual system based methods have to be discussed. While pixel based procedures are machine and human independent in quality estimation of movies the perception of human eye and its weakness in certain circumstances is paid attention. These methods are calculating the 'just notable difference' (JND). While in movies observations depend on the scene displayed, its brightness, its speed and its content, in medical videos there is until now no acceptable proceeding published.

On the other hand conventional movies are compressed using the shortcoming of human eyes. There are many items in a video a human would see, e.g. the movie is to fast to recognize a certain rearrangement of a scene or there is different perceptibility in middle grey and bright parts of an image. Wile medical examinations take count on nearly every detail, such compression methods might not be useful, and therefore the error perception based on such methods might only work on movie based videos.[21]

2. Methods

For evaluation purposes 18 motion video clips were selected, which were representative of typical normal and abnormal findings in coronary angiography. The movies showed different length between 35 and 220 frames. The frames consisted of images with 512x512 pixel resolution. The following procedure performs different steps as shown in figure 1:

1st DICOM-Export-unit

DICOM movies have to be extracted out of their primary container. One problem arises at that peculiar step. Many DICOM videos are stored in 12bit grey scale. Usually compression tools freely available only process 8bit grey scaled images. Therefore the windowing of DICOM frames must be done now to enable a broad usage of MPEG-4 tools, e.g. students usually use standard computers without special decompressing tools. A single windowing option is used for all exports. For first tests a freely available component was integrated in this unit.[22]

2nd Frame-Grabber uncompressed

The resulting video-stream is cut in single frames and each individual image is stored in a system independent PPM/PGM bitmap. These bitmaps served as a reverence for further calculation.

3rd Compression Unit

The compression unit reads the primary video stream and performs a video compression with plugged-in compressor tools. Such tools are easily plugged into Microsoft's windows system environment and commonly available. Most of them offer freely available corresponding decompression units. We used two different version of a MPEG-4 implementation, which is freely available from the DIVX-group: DivX4.12 and DivXPro5.21.[23]

4th Frame-Grabber compressed

The resulting video-stream is again split up into single frames and images are stored PPM/PGM bitmap. At that moment uncompressed and compressed framesets of the DICOM movie are prepared for the calculation unit.

5th Final Calculation

The calculation unit is a constructed as a plug-in to supply further development. In the first version different methods are calculated to evaluate the best indicator for quality estimation in medical

Table 1: Calculated values of PSNR, MSE, VQM related to the in- and output

avg./max. Bitrate	Comp. Ratio (MOVIE)	Comp. (DICOM)	KB	PSNR	MSE	VQM %	Comment	Version
100	348	46	79	33,468	29,257	11,37	foggy and blocks	v04.12
150	328	43	84	33,524	28,886	11,29	foggy and blocks	v04.12
300	199	26	138	34,146	25,029	10,39	foggy and blocks	v04.12
500	123	16	224	34,487	23,143	9,92	min. blocks	v04.12
750	90	12	307	34,524	22,943	9,87	min. blocks	v04.12
1000	87	11	315	34,519	22,971	9,88	min. blocks	v04.12
2000	85	11	325	34,519	22,971	9,88	none	v04.12
4000	85	11	325	34,519	22,971	9,88	none	v04.12
6000	84	11	327	34,541	22,857	9,85	none	v04.12
150/150	562	74	49	39,662	7,0286	4,82	foggy and blocks	v5.21
150/1500	540	71	51	39,769	6,8571	4,75	foggy and blocks	v5.21
500/5000	197	26	140	43,934	2,6286	2,60	foggy	v5.21
750/7500	120	16	229	44,651	2,2286	2,34	foggy	v5.21
2000/2000	73	10	378	45,246	1,9429	2,15	none	v5.21
6000/60000	73	10	379	45,510	1,8286	2,06	none	v5.21

environment. It supports MSE, PSNR and VQM calculation.
For each compressed video file, we noted: DIVX-version, average and maximal bitrate related to compression level (KB/s), file-size of uncompressed video, file-size of compressed movie, compression ratio (uncompressed video file dimension/compressed dimension).

3. Results

Because of limited space only a few typical results can be displayed in this paper. Table 1 shows the results of typical file-compression. The original video-stream of this example is about 27528 KB, while the primary DICOM file shows only 3608 KB.

This difference is a result of video-streaming. Therefore, maximum compression rate can be expected within 1/10 without loosing remarkable quality. Still image compression only achieves a ratio of 1/3.

We did not find any optical differences in bit-rates above 2000 KB/s, but succeeded in high-quality movies in some sources at 500 KB/s.

4. Discussion

As results suggest published tests using one of the most popular video compressors are not unambiguous. [24;25] The compression algorithms proposed and used for real-time movies are acceptable in a greyed environment. Although PSNR and VQM are stated to be markers of quality in movies there is little evidence that in a grey-scale movie both quality estimators will succeed: Within a single file and codec an increasing VQM and increasing PSNR describe really loss of quality. But the absolute values are not transferable to other codecs or files. As shown in table 1 a VQM of 5% (which is usually declared as "excellent") can describe a lowest-quality movie. Additionally the ranges of VQM do not fit into the scheme proposed by the ITU. [20]

Compression without loss of diagnostic information is possible, especially for the distribution on telemedicine or teleteaching, but quality control is surely one of the major tasks.

Further investigation has to be done, to clarify the quality measurement in short-time movies and especially in a grey-scaled environment like CT, angiography or NMR.

5. References

[1]   Bidgood WD, Jr., Horii SC, Prior FW, Van Syckle DE. Understanding and using DICOM, the data interchange standard for biomedical imaging. *J Am Med Inform Assoc* 1997; 4(3): 199-212.

[2]   Balis UJ. Digital imaging standards and system interoperability. *Clin Lab Med* 1997; 17(2): 315-322.

[3]   Andriole KP. Anatomy of picture archiving and Communications systems: nuts and bolts- -image acquisition: getting digital images from imaging modalities. *J Digit Imaging* 1999; 12(2 Suppl 1): 216-217.

[4]   Setti E, Trecate G, Ferrari M, Mainardi L, Musumeci R. Breast magnetic resonance imaging: a computer-based analysis of enhancement curves. *J Digit Imaging* 2001; 14(2 Suppl 1): 226-228.

[5]   Burger R, Kunzel KH, Brenner E. DICOM - a new approach in medical under- and postgraduate education. *Med Educ* 2001; 35(11): 1076-1077.

[6]   Loane M, Wootton R. A review of guidelines and standards for telemedicine. *J Telemed Telecare* 2002; 8(2): 63-71.

[7]   Frommelt PC, Whitstone EN, Frommelt MA. Experience with a DICOM-compatible digital pediatric echocardiography laboratory. *Pediatr Cardiol* 2002; 23(1): 53-57.

[8]   Ernst RD, Baumgartner BR, Tamm EP, Torres WE. Development of a teaching file by using a DICOM database. *Radiographics* 2002; 22(1): 217-221.

[9]   Wu M, Zheng Y, North M, Pisano E. NLM tele-educational application for radiologists to interpret mammography. *Proc AMIA Symp* 2002; 909-913.

[10]   Eng J. Improving the interactivity and functionality of Web-based radiology teaching files with the Java programming language. *Radiographics* 1997; 17(6): 1567-1574.

[11]   (Muster-)Berufsordnung für die deutschen Ärztinnen und Ärzte - MBO-Ä 1997 - geändert durch die Beschlüsse des 103. Deutschen Ärztetages, Köln. 2000.

[12]   Röntgenverordnung. 2005. http://www.laekb.de/40/10aesqr/05Gesetz/Roentgenverordnung.pdf

[13]   Spencer K, Solomon L, Mor-Avi V, Dean K, Weinert L, Gulati M et al. Effects of MPEG compression on the quality and diagnostic accuracy of digital echocardiography studies. *J Am Soc Echocardiogr* 2000; 13(1): 51-57.

[14]   Okura Y, Matsumura Y, Hidaka K, Yokoyama H, Inada H, Harauchi H et al. Evaluation of the effect of varying MPEG-2 compression ratios on digital coronary angiographic assessment of stenosis severity. *J Digit Imaging* 2002; 15(4): 210-215.

[15]   Baker WA, Hearne SE, Spero LA, Morris KG, Harrington RA, Sketch MH, Jr. et al. Lossy (15:1) JPEG compression of digital coronary angiograms does not limit detection of subtle morphological features. *Circulation* 1997; 96(4): 1157-1164.

[16]   Brennecke R, Burgel U, Rippin G, Post F, Rupprecht HJ, Meyer J. Comparison of image compression viability for lossy and lossless JPEG and Wavelet data reduction in coronary angiography. *Int J Cardiovasc Imaging* 2001; 17(1): 1-12.

[17]   Iyriboz TA, Zukoski MJ, Hopper KD, Stagg PL. A comparison of wavelet and Joint Photographic Experts Group lossy compression methods applied to medical images. *J Digit Imaging* 1999; 12(2 Suppl 1): 14-17.

[18]   Kerensky RA, Cusma JT, Kubilis P, Simon R, Bashore TM, Hirshfeld JW, Jr. et al. American College of Cardiology/European Society of Cardiology International Study of Angiographic Data Compression Phase I: The effect of lossy data compression on recognition of diagnostic features in digital coronary angiography. *J Am Coll Cardiol* 2000; 35(5): 1370-1379.

[19]   Final Report from the Video Quality Experts Group on validation of objective models of video quality assessment. http://www.mihandbook.stanford.edu/handbook/home.htm.

[20]   Working Group on Multimedia Communications Coding and Performance: Objective Video Quality Measurement Using a Peak-Signal-to-Noise-Ratio (PSNR). Committee T1 - Telecommunications. T1A1.1/2001-026R7. 2001

[21]   Watson A, Hu J, McGowan J. DVQ: A digital video Quality metric based on human vision. *Journal of Electronic Imaging* 2001; 10(1): 20-29.

[22]   Offis. www.offis.org, 2005.

[23]   DIVX Professional 5.2.1. www.divx.org, 2005.

[24]   Yamakawa T, Toyabe S, Cao P, Akazawa K. Web-based delivery of medical multimedia contents using an MPEG-4 system. *Comput Methods Programs Biomed* 2004; 75(3): 259-264.

[25]   Barbier P, Alimento M, Berna G, Cavoretto D, Celeste F, Muratori M et al. Clinical validation of different echocardiographic motion pictures expert group-4 algorithms and compression levels for telemedicine. *Medinfo* 2004; 2004: 1339-1342.

Address for correspondence

Dr. Thomas Frankewitsch, Krankenhausstr. 12, D-91054 Erlangen.

Connecting Medical Informatics and Bio-Informatics
R. Engelbrecht et al. (Eds.)
IOS Press, 2005

Lung CT Analysis and Retrieval as a Diagnostic Aid

Henning Müller, Samuel Marquis, Gilles Cohen, Christian Lovis, Antoine Geissbuhler

Service of Medical Informatics, University and Hospitals of Geneva

Abstract

Image retrieval is currently a very active research field due to the large amount of visual data being produced in most modern hospitals. Most often, the goal is to aid the diagnostic process. Unfortunately, only very few medical image retrieval systems are currently used in clinical routine. One of the application domains for image retrieval is the analysis and retrieval of lung CTs. A first user study in the United States shows that these systems allow improving the diagnostic quality.
This article describes the approach to an aid for lung CT diagnostics. The analysis incorporates several steps and the goal is to automate the process as much as possible for easy integration into diagnostics. Thus, several automatic steps are proposed from a selection of the most characteristic slices, to an automatic segmentation of the lung tissue and a classification on the segmented area into diagnostic classes. Feedback to the MD will be given in the form of marked regions in the images that appear to be different from the norm of healthy tissue. We are currently working on a small set of training images with marked and annotated regions but a larger set of images for the evaluation of our algorithm is in work. For this reason, the article does currently not contain much quantitative evaluation. For several tasks we use existing open source software such as Weka and itk. This allows an easy reproduction of the search results.

Keywords
Content-based image retrieval; High-resolution lung CT; Diagnostic aid; Classification

1. Introduction

Content-based image retrieval (CBIR) has been an extremely active domain in the fields of computer vision and images processing for more than 20 years [1]. In the medical field, this domain is also starting to become active, as an increasing amount of visual data is being produced in hospitals and made available in digital form [2,3]. General medical image retrieval in PACS-like databases is in this context very different from specialized retrieval in a very focused domain. In the medical field, the main goal is the use as a diagnostic aid and for access to medical teaching files. Current medical use is on the retrieval of tumour shapes [4] as well as on histological images [5], and in other more specific fields (dermatology, pathology). A domain where textures play a very important role in the diagnostic process is the analysis of high-resolution lung CTs [6]. In [7], a user test shows that an image retrieval system can improve the diagnostic quality significantly, especially for less experienced radiologists. Still, most of these systems either rely on much complicated interaction with the user, which makes them hard to introduce into a clinical context, or they are too broad to be used as a diagnostic aid in a specialized domain.

This article details a solution for helping with the interpretation of high-resolution lung CTs, which is a domain where diagnostics are fairly hard especially for non-chest specialists. The diagnostic result strongly depends on the overall texture of the lung tissue, so automatic analysis seems possible. Our project limits the direct interaction with the user and performs as many tasks as possible in an automatic fashion, so a minimum of time is needed to operate the system and get responses for feedback.

2. Steps for a diagnostic aid on lung CT interpretation

This section describes the various steps that are necessary for a complete diagnostic aid system for lung diagnostics and their degree of automation.

2.1 Generation of a test database and acquisition of representative samples

The first and most important part is the creation of a database of thin-section lung CTs. This database needs to include healthy cases as well as pathologic cases. Characteristic regions need to be marked by a radiologist to allow us learning the characteristics of a disease with respect to healthy tissue. Currently, we only have a fairly small database of 10 series containing around 50-60 images per series. 112 regions are marked in the images by a radiologist to represent the following classes of tissue for the further classification step:

- Healthy tissue (52 sample regions);
- Emphysema (21);
- Micro nodules (19);
- Macro nodules (3);
- Interstitial syndrome (5);
- Bronchiectasis (5);
- Ground glass attenuation (1);
- Fibrosis (6).

It is important to note that prototypically healthy regions have to be annotated by the radiologist as well so that a classifier can get a good idea of healthy tissue. Other systems in the literature often use only pathologic classes for the classification but the first step in the diagnostic process is to find out whether the tissue is abnormal or not. We are currently creating a larger database projected to contain at least 100 series of 50-60 images that will allow us a better representation of these classes. In Figure 1 you can see a screenshot of our tool for image annotation. It generates a simple XML file containing the regions of interests as a set of points (outline) and a label for each outline. These files are then fed into the system along with the images at the training step.

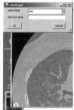

Figure 1 - A screenshot of our utility for the annotation of image regions.

2.2 Analysis of blocks of lung tissue

In Figure 3 you can see the partitioning of the lungs into smaller blocks (size 16x16 pixels in the image) for further detailed texture analysis. A block is taken into account if it is by more than 80% inside of an area marked by the expert or automatically segmented by the system. These lung blocks are stored as references together with the original image. This avoids artefacts of the filters that can occur due to missing border pixels as we can take into account the entire block environment.

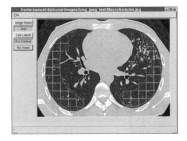

Figure 2 - The partitioning of the lung tissue into small blocks for classification and feature extraction.

The framework is designed to facilitate finding the optimal block size for analysis and classification. From each block we extract and store the following visual features:

- average grey level and standard deviation of the grey levels in the block;
- grey level histogram using 32 grey levels;
- features derived from co-occurrence matrices (four directions, two distances);
- responses of Gabor filters in four directions and at three scales;
- Tamura texture features.

A small number of grey levels in the histogram is sufficient for this kind of classification as has been shown in image retrieval applications, where they often perform better.

2.3 Training

Then, the features together with the region label become a sample in a classification problem [8]. Based on the acquired training data, the weights of the features for classification are calculated. To develop an optimal classification strategy, several classifiers are tested and their performance is evaluated on the currently available data. An open source utility allowing us to compare several classifiers is Weka1, which has also the advantage of being able to connect directly to the feature database (mySQL). We perform cross-validation using various classifiers to get an idea of how discriminant our features are. While Weka is an external tool, we have also included libsvm [9] into, an easy-to-use Support Vector Machine (SVM) classifier. We also plan to integrate torch [10] to discover connections between the various features and the classes of our system. Torch is a fast data-mining tool. In the final version, only the best classifier will be integrated but as for the testing phase we need several to find out the optimal solution.

---

[1] http://www.cs.waikato.ac.nz/~ml/weka/

2.4 Lung segmentation as data preparation for classification

When submitting a new image for analysis and as diagnostic aid, we concentrate on the part of the image that we are interested in, the lung tissue. While manual region selection of the image is still possible (using the tool described in 2.1 – only without a label), automatic segmentation is desired to minimize user interaction in the final diagnostic aid step. To this aim we use an algorithm described in [11] to find an optimal threshold for lung tissue segmentation, which works on DICOM images having a full 12-bit resolution (or more) as well as on the jpeg images from our radiology teaching file. As basis for the segmentation we use itk2. In Figure 2, a lung CT, its segmented version and a view of the outline discovered by the software can be seen.

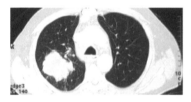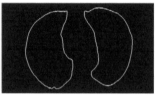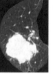

Figure 3 - A lung CT and the tissue of the two lung halves segmented.

For the final texture classification we do not plan to take into account the entire lung tissue but rather the diagnostically interesting part, which is the outside part of the lung with less vessels that can change the texture strongly and introduce noise for the classification. The inside part with the vessels is automatically removed from further analysis.

2.5 Classification of lung blocks

For the classification step of a new lung image, a partitioning of the image into blocks is performed. Then, the features of each block in the (manually or automatically) marked regions corresponding to lung tissue are extracted. The samples are created by the block's features and have no label attached to them, yet. The integrated classifier (currently libsvm) now performs the classification and attaches a label to each block of the lung tissue based on previous learning data. We use the parameters (kernel type, gamma factor, stop criterion, etc.), which performed best at cross-validation (see step 2.3).

2.6 Slice selection from a CT lung volume

This step is currently not implemented and will likely be the last part to be done, as its development is not crucial. Goal is basically to perform the task of the medical doctor to find the slice(s) that best characterize a disease. Once a large database of labelled tissue samples is ready, it will be fairly easy to process the entire volume slice by slice and select those slices with the largest part of the tissue being marked as non-healthy for further inspection. To select several slices, we can give the system a combination of maximum number of slices and a threshold of unhealthy tissue. Selected slices can also be marked in the volume data by highlighting the volume part that contains the most pathologic blocks.

2.7 Result presentation to the medical doctor

The goal of the results presentation is not to make the decision for the radiologist but rather to highlight parts of the lung tissue that were classified as pathologic. A highlighting of the

---

[2] http://www.itk.org/

background in coloured shades is planned instead of the grey scales in the parts of the images that were classified as pathologic. Each colour presents one of the classes that we are detecting in the classification step. Currently, we only present the results in a 2D view and one image at a time, meaning that the slices with the largest pathogenic parts are taken and displayed. It can also be imagined to present the results in 3D, where the entire pathogenic area over several slices can be highlighted within the volume. Retrieval of similar cases from the reference database will enable the MD to verify his diagnosis. This is easily possible through an image retrieval application using features from the currently active case and comparing them thoses stored and labelled for past cases in the database.

3. Results

We currently have a framework in place that allows us to acquire knowledge from the radiologists in the form of marked regions and annotations within images. Our database is still small but a larger number of cases are planned. The acquired data with labels is used to train our classifiers. This means that with a growing number of judged cases from the radiologist, the system is expected to perform better. The lung segmentation phase works reliably and stable as well as the partitioning of the lung tissue into small blocks and the feature extraction. All these steps work in a completely automated fashion. The medical doctor can simply feed a volume of lung CT images into the system. The images are segmented and portioned into smaller blocks automatically. These blocks are then classified and unhealthy tissue is marked in a different colour in the images so the medical doctor has a feedback for regions that he needs to inspect further.

Current results when using the 112 regions and block sizes of 32x32 pixels (corresponding to ~1000 blocks) are 84%, when using cross validation between healthy and non-healthy tissue using SVM classifiers. Nearest neighbours lead to roughly 74% correctly classified. When classifying into the 8 available classes, the nearest neighbour classifier reaches 85.5% correctly classified. Problems occur especially for classes with a very small number of representative blocks. Another problem is that the radiologist marked regions with a margin, leading to several blocks that are actually healthy tissue but close to a pathologic region and labelled as pathologic. This explains part of the errors.

We currently run the framework on a simply desktop computer with a Pentium IV processor with 2,8 GHz and 1 MB of RAM. On this computer, the segmentation takes around 5 seconds per slice and the subsequent cutting into blocks, feature extraction and classification another 2 seconds. Thus the analysis of a single slice is almost interactive whereas an entire volume takes a few minutes before results can be displayed. We still need to experiment with the classification part and also with the features that we extract from the images to obtain an optimal feature set for classification. The current framework is by now a research tool, designed to ease experimentation of features, classifiers, parameters, etc. The final system will probably discard a lot of these options, be much simpler and focus more on the user interface and the results display to the user.

4. Conclusions

This article presents a framework to aid the diagnostic process for lung diseases using lung CTs. The domain has shown its potential in studies and our current cross validations leads to good results. The steps of the diagnostic process are performed in an automatic way. Abnormalities are highlighted in the original images by a change of colour. Once we have a larger database accessible, more quantitative evaluation is needed to evaluate the algorithm quality and show the usefulness of the application in a clinical environment. Many parameters need to be optimized, from the feature extraction phase to the training step and the classifiers employed. We also need to think about optimal block size of lung tissue and whether we should rather take overlapping blocks to avoid misclassifying small parts of the texture and reduce false positives.

Lung CT analysis has shown its usefulness in practice by improving the diagnostic quality especially of non-experts. Now it is important to create large reference databases and evaluate the many visual descriptors and techniques available to create a robust framework for routine use that needs to have as many steps of the process in an automatic way as possible. Several questions still need to be solved before routine use, for example the handling of other available data on the patients. The age can play an important role for the texture of the lung tissue. For the classification we need to integrate all these data into the framework. The possibility to compare the images with annotated cases from the reference databases is expected to further increase acceptance of the technology because the system does not make a decision by itself but rather points out interesting areas of the lung tissue and gives evidence on these areas by supplying similar past cases.

5. References

[1] AWM. Smeulders, M. Worring, S. Santini, A. Gupta and R. Jain, Content-Based Image Retrieval at the End of the Early Years, *IEEE Transactions on Pattern Analysis and Machine Intelligence* **22**(12) pp 1349-1380, 2000.

[2] ·H Müller, N Michoux, D Bandon, A Geissbuhler, A review of content-based image retrieval systems in medicine – clinical benefits and future directions, *International Journal of Medical Informatics*, **73**, pp 1-23, 2004.

[3] TM Lehmann, MO Güld, C Thies, B Fischer, K Spitzer, D Keysers, H Ney, M Kohnen, H Schubert, BB Wein, Content-based image retrieval in medical applications, *Methods of Information in Medicine*,43, pp 354-361, 2004.

[4] P. Korn, N. Sidiropoulos, C. Faloutsos, E. Siegel, Z. Protopapas, Fast and effective retrieval of medical tumor shapes, *IEEE Transactions on Knowledge and Data Engineering*, 10(6) 889—904, 1998.

[5] LHY Tang, R Hanka, HHS Ip, A review of intelligent content-based indexing and browsing of medical images, *Health Informatics Journal* **5**, 40—49, 1998.

[6] C.-R. Shyu, CE Brodley, AC Kak, A Kosaka, AM Aisen, LS Broderick, ASSERT: A physician-in-the-loop content-based retrieval system for HRCT image databases, *Computer Vision and Image Understanding* **75** (1—2), pp. 111—132, 1999.

[7] AM Aisen, LS Broderick, H Winer-Muram, CE Brodley, AC Kak, C Pavlopoulou, J Dy, CR Shyu, A Marchiori, Automated storage and retrieval of thin-section CT images to assist diagnosis: System description and preliminary assessment, *Radiology*, **228**, pp. 265-270, 2003.

[8] A K Jain, R P W Dvi, J Mao, Statistical Pattern Recognition: A Review, IEEE Transactions onf Pattern Analysis and Machine Intelligence, **22** (1) pp. 4-37, 2000.

[9] CC Chang, CJ Lin, libsvm, a library for support vector machines, Technical report, available with software at http://www.csie.ntu.edu.tw/~cjlin/libsvm/

[10] R Collobert, S Bengio, J Mariéthoz. Torch: a modular machine learning software library. *Technical Report* IDIAP-RR 02-46, IDIAP, 2002.

[11] S Hu, EA Hoffman, JM Reinhardt, Automatic lung segmentation for accurate quantitation of volumetric X-ray CT images. *IEEE Transactions on Medical Imaging*, **20**(6), pp. 490-498, 2001.

Address for correspondence

Henning Müller
University and Hospitals of Geneva, Service of Medical Informatics
24, rue Micheli-du-Crest, CH-1211 Geneva 14, Switzerland
henning.mueller@sim.hcuge.ch, http://www.sim.hcuge.ch/medgift/
Tel ++ 41 22 372 6175, Fax ++41 22 372 8680

Connecting Medical Informatics and Bio-Informatics
R. Engelbrecht et al. (Eds.)
IOS Press, 2005

A Generic Concept for the Implementation of Medical Image Retrieval Systems

Mark O Güld, Christian Thies, Benedikt Fischer, Thomas M Lehmann

Department of Medical Informatics, Aachen University of Technology (RWTH), Aachen, Germany

Abstract

This work presents mechanisms to support the development and installation of content-based image retrieval in medical applications (IRMA). A strict separation of feature extraction, feature storage, feature comparison, and the user interfaces is suggested. The concept and implementation of a system following these guidelines is described. The system allows to reuse implemented components in different retrieval algorithms, which improves software quality, shortens the development cycle for applications, and allows to establish standardized end-user interfaces.

Keywords:
Medical Imaging; Medical Image Archive; Content-based Image Retrieval (CBIR); Picture Archiving and Communication Systems (PACS); Digital Imaging and Communication in Medicine (DICOM)

1. Introduction

The growing number of digital image acquisition and storage systems in clinical routine rises demands for new access methods. Still, most picture archiving and communication systems (PACS) only use manually entered textual information to access a patient's image data. Content-based image retrieval (CBIR) depends on automatically extracted content descriptions (features) for each image as well as their storage and comparison upon a query [1].

Considering the implementation of a CBIR system in medical applications, there is currently a gap between monolithic CBIR systems for general-purpose image retrieval, e.g. Blobworld [2], and programming tools for the development of image processing algorithms. Existing general-purpose CBIR systems closely couple feature extraction, feature storage, feature comparison, and the query interface. Since changes often affect all system components, this makes it difficult to extend them. However, existing image processing tools provide a huge number of routines useful for feature extraction and comparison, but they lack support for organising feature storage and easy deployment of algorithms to the end-user, who is not involved in technical details.

Extensibility and flexibility

TAGARE et al. have pointed out the specific demands and challenges of CBIR in the medical domain [3], which significantly differ from demands of general-purpose CBIR [4]. To provide satisfying query results, multiple levels of content abstraction are necessary [5], with each abstraction level using a completely different type of features as well as a rough detection of relevant image regions, e.g. global features for categorization, per-pixel features for local analysis and structural features to express spatial relationships between identified objects. The context in medical queries can also vary, e.g. attention to details of bones or tissue structure. Thus, most medical CBIR implementations focus on a certain domain [1]. Furthermore, medical knowledge continuously evolves and properties or quantifications used in medical language are sometimes difficult to express precisely in computerized methods. To keep the retrieval system extensible, all algorithms must be divisible into reusable computation steps, e.g. pre-processing, feature extraction, and feature comparison, which can be easily parameterised and combined.

Separation of algorithms and interfaces

Standardized guidelines for graphical user interfaces are required to ensure the acceptance by end-users and to minimize required learning time. Although medical retrieval algorithms may carry unique semantics, most image retrieval applications use the query-by-example (QBE) paradigm: the submission of a sample image or image region is answered by the system displaying a list of archived images which are most similar to the sample. Thereafter, query refinement may follow. Decoupling the interface from the application-specific retrieval algorithm allows to compose all interfaces from standardized modules [6].

Development and deployment

Beside the decomposition of the algorithm, each of these steps should optionally be divisible at code level with the development environment hiding as many details of the build process as possible. The major goal is to minimize the amount of information that must be shared between all developers, as this allows them to focus on their primary field of expertise. Especially the implementation of GUIs completely differs from that of image processing algorithms. Thus, the deployment, i.e. the integration of new retrieval algorithms into existing user interfaces for testing and final release, must be as easy as possible.

Efficiency at run-time

The process of automatic image content extraction at various abstraction levels requires considerable amounts of computation time and storage space. The decomposition of algorithms as proposed above can also be exploited for distributed computation at query time. Distributed systems based on standard PC hardware provide a cost effective way to cope with these demands.

2. Materials and Methods

In our approach, a central relational database is used to store all entity definitions and administrative information, while source code and larger feature data are stored separately [7].

Entities of the algorithm model

The system can be extended by adding instances of the following entity types: *feature types*, *methods*, *networks*, i.e. algorithms, and *experiments*, i.e. partly parameterized networks, which are used to generate *queries*. Queries completely parameterize experiments, i.e. they define all input data for the invocation of an algorithm. All entities are defined via the eXtensible Markup Language (XML) and can be imported into the system using the according administration tool. The system provides features as a data container which is transparently stored.

Features carry type information, which defines the semantics of the data inside the container. Consequently, the developer must provide a feature type definition for each newly introduced content description. The system allows symbolic inheritance to express feature type compatibility. For example, a texture feature consisting of a tuple of floating point values should be compatible with a general floating point vector as used by a lot of distance measures:

```
<featuretype name="texture_tamura">
A 3D histogram of texture features proposed by TAMURA:
Directionality, contrast and coarseness.
<isa> vector </isa>
</featuretype>
```

Methods encapsulate a transformation of feature tuples and define the atomic processing steps inside algorithms. To cover all possible transformations, there are three method types: a method can either transform one input tuple into one output tuple (1:1), compress a set of feature tuples into one tuple (T:1, e.g. prototype computations or data set analysis like principal component analysis), or expand one feature tuple into a set of feature tuples (1:T). A method accesses the tuples via its inputs and outputs. Beside the method implementation, the developer must provide the method's feature interface, which defines the expected feature type for each input and the type of the generated feature for each output:

```
<method name="extract_tamura" type="1:1" project="texture_tamura">
<input featuretype="image" keeps_ref="1"> Input image. </input>
<output featuretype="texture_tamura"> Texture feature. </output>
Extracts texture features proposed by TAMURA from an image.
</method>
```

Networks are used to build algorithms by defining the flow of features between methods and their dependencies inside the computation. Consequently, networks also have a feature interface, which is expressed using sources and sinks. Sources are nodes with exactly one output and no input and refer to one feature as part of the algorithm's input. Sinks provide the analogue for the algorithm's output. The network also ensures a consistent parameterisation, e.g. identical parameters for a feature extraction method which is applied to both reference images and a sample image.

Experiments are used to partly parameterise networks. This is done by assigning suitable features to some of the network's source nodes, e.g. empirically determined parameters for feature extraction. Experiments hide fixed parameters from query-relevant parameters, e.g. the selection of a query image. By assigning features to the remaining sources, the end-user provides the complete set of input features.

This triggers a query, which is executed within the backend (see below). Once the backend completes the computations, the user interface can access the features associated with the sink nodes.

Web-based interfaces

All end-user interfaces to the retrieval system are JAVA applications or HTML dialogues implemented in PHP. Therefore, the end-user requires a web browser and a JAVA virtual machine. For interactive applications, a PHP script can initiate a query and blocks until the backend completes the computations. The backend returns the resulting features, i.e. the features propagated at the sinks of the network. For example, this might be a list of images similar to the selected sample. More complex feature types such as hierarchical attributed region-adjacency graphs (HARAGs) [8] demand more sophisticated viewing applications.

Therefore, the PHP script can also generate hyperlinks to a JAVA application responsible for this feature type, which can be integrated into web pages via JAVA WebStart. The JAVA application accesses the demanded feature from the web server via the hypertext transfer protocol (HTTP).

It should be noted that the experiment entity implicitly defines the interface of available algorithms to the end-user. Since each source and sink carries feature type information, it is possible to abstract an algorithm from its interface to the end-user. Thus, it is possible to obtain a functional end-user interface by implementing only a generic one which includes input and output modules for each occurring feature type in the experiment's interface. This is illustrated in Fig. 1.

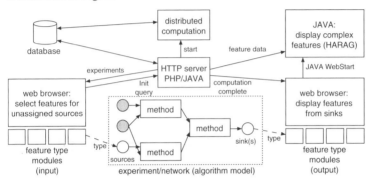

Figure 1 – Schematic view of the system components used for the retrieval process.

Development environment

The development environment organises all implementation parts as *projects*. Projects encapsulate internal functionality, exported functionality, which is visible by other projects, stand-alone programs, and methods. The supported programming languages are C and C++, but all methods must have a C++ interface. The developer provides direct dependencies from other projects and external libraries via the project's configuration file. Known external libraries can be accessed by a project under their symbolic names. The dependencies are automatically unrolled by the build system. Their configuration and integration into the build process is transparent to the developer. The build system is implemented on top of the GNU make utility.

Distributed computing and storage

All entity definitions are stored in a central relational database. For efficiency, small features are directly stored inside the database, while images and complex feature data are stored on file servers and the database only tracks each feature's location.

When a query is issued, a central scheduling service determines the sequence of all necessary method calls using the underlying network definition and the source nodes' features. For each method call, the scheduler picks a suitable host in the network cluster, determines the nearest locations of the involved input features, and allocates the resulting output features. Afterwards, the call is dispatched to a daemon service running on the selected host. The communication between scheduling service and the daemons uses HTTP. Before calling the method, the daemon fetches all input features and provides them as objects, making the features' locations transparent to the method. The database also stores each feature's generation history, so that already computed features can be identified during query processing and the respective computations are skipped.

3. Results

The system was implemented using open standards and free software and currently runs on Intel/Linux and Sparc/Solaris platforms. At this time, the systems holds 13,151 images from the Department of Diagnostic Radiology, Aachen University of Technology and 2,355 dental radiographs obtained from the Department of Oral Maxillofacial Radiology, Göteborg University, Sweden. The contents of these images were encoded by radiologists using a hierarchical coding scheme, which provides the ground truth for query experiments. The system also stores other medical and non-medical image data for evaluation purposes. All important administrative operations like image import, export, and content encoding can be performed using web-based interfaces. The currently available retrieval algorithms use the QBE paradigm and can therefore be used from a single web-based query interface, which also offers a basic relevance feedback/query refinement functionality. An extensive object-oriented and template-based PHP library was developed to support the development of the graphical user interfaces.

The implementation and testing time of methods is significantly decreased, since a number of core projects contain often-required functionality, e.g. image file access and classification-related data structures, and the methods do not need to concern the access to features. Instead, all feature data and parameters are accessible locally via objects. Simple pre-processing steps like image filters can be implemented and deployed within minutes. The feature type concept and the method definition allows it to use a method in arbitrary context compatible with the method's interface. Existing algorithms can be modified without changing the method implementations. For example, additional pre-processing steps can be integrated by modifying the network entity. The parameterisation can be altered by editing the experiment entity. The deployment of new algorithms is done by defining an experiment entity. This mainly consists of setting up algorithm's parameters by assigning parameter features to the respective sources and choosing a set of reference images. If a compatible PHP interface for the algorithm's interaction scheme exists, it is directly available online. So far, several retrieval algorithms were implemented to carry out the experiments for several publications. The retrieval system is accessible from anywhere on the internet via a web browser and a JAVA virtual machine and does not require any maintenance or configuration by the end-user.

The run-time environment can effectively utilize the computation power of a computer cluster. This is also useful during the feature extraction process, which is performed offline. Most content descriptions are computed per image with no dependencies between single images during the extraction process, which is ideal for distributed processing. For this scenario, first experiments with ten identical stations yielded a speedup factor of 8, which is primarily limited by the bandwidth of the file server holding the feature data. Like feature access, the concurrent processing is transparent to the method implementation.

4. Discussion

The more general modelling approach for the retrieval algorithms causes a certain overhead. Thus, the efficiency of optimized monolithic systems cannot be reached. On the other hand, the proposed mechanisms provide several advantages regarding extensibility, maintenance and reusability. The primary benefits result from the strict separation of all system entities, which can be transparently accessed using well-defined interfaces. For each new entity, its creator must provide a proper documentation. Afterwards, the interface documentation is all the co-developers need to use the entity. This very basic concept is employed on all levels. During the implementation, other projects are easily accessible and the build process is configured automatically. At run-time, methods are automatically called and provided with the required feature data, so the developer only has to implement the feature transformation itself. The composition of new algorithms using existing methods can solely rely on the methods' feature interface. A new algorithm for an existing user interaction scheme (e.g. QBE) can be deployed by defining an experiment which fits the scheme. These two steps are manageable without knowing any details about method internals or source code and significantly speed up development and testing cycles. The entity interfaces also help to establish a standardized documentation, which is valuable especially for groups of developers. Based on the concepts proposed in [9], a full integration of the system into the clinical workflow is currently being planned.

5. Conclusion

The proposed concept allows it to effectively support the development and deployment of content-based image retrieval in medical applications. The strict separation of entities at different levels (modelling, implementation, deployment and run-time) allows a maximum transparency for each person involved, both on the developer's and on the physician's side. When fully integrated into clinical routine, content-based access to image data promises a significant impact in the fields of evidence-based medicine, case-based reasoning, and computer-based training.

6. Acknowledgement

This work was performed within the IRMA project, which is funded by the German Research Community (DFG), grant Le 1108/4.

7. References

[1] Müller H, Michoux N, Bandon D, Geissbuhler A: A review of content-based image retrieval systems in medical applications. Clinical benefits and future directions. International Journal of Medical Informatics 2004; 73: 1-23
[2] Carson C, Belongie S, Greenspan H, Malik J: Blobworld – Image segmentation using expectation-maximization and its application to image querying. IEEE Transactions on Pattern Analysis and Machine Intelligence 24(8): 1026–1038, 2002.
[3] Tagare HD, Jaffe CC, Duncan J: Medical image databases – a content-based retrieval approach. Journal of the American Medical Informatics Association 4:184–198, 1997.
[4] Smeulders AWM, Worring M, Santini S, Gupta A, Jain R: Content-based image retrieval at the end of the early years. IEEE Transactions on Pattern Analysis and Machine Intelligence 2000; 22(12): 1349-80
[5] Lehmann TM, Güld MO, Thies C, Fischer B, Spitzer K, Keysers D, Ney H, Kohnen M, Schubert H, Wein BB: Content-based Image Retrieval in Medical Applications. Methods of Information in Medicine 2004; 43(4): 354-361
[6] Lehmann TM, Plodowski B, Spitzer K, Wein BB, Ney H, Seidl T: Extended query refinement for content-based access to large medical image databases. Proceedings SPIE 2004; 5371: 90-98
[7] Güld MO, Thies C, Fischer B, Keysers D, Wein BB, Lehmann TM: A platform for distributed image processing and image retrieval. Procs SPIE 2003; 5150:1109-1120
[8] Thies C, Metzler V, Lehmann TM, Aach T: Extraction of biomedical objects by sub-graph matching in attributed hierarchical region adjacency graphs. Proceedings SPIE 2004; 5370(3): 1498-1508
[9] Lehmann TM, Wein BB, Greenspan H: Integration of Content-based Image Retrieval to Picture Archiving and Communication Systems. Proceedings Medical Informatics Europe (MIE 2003), IOS Press, Amsterdam, ISBN 1 58603 347 6 (CD-ROM only).

8. Address for Correspondence

Mark Oliver Güld, Department of Medical Informatics, Aachen University of Technology (RWTH), Pauwelsstr. 30, D - 52062 Aachen, Germany, Email: mgueld@mi.rwth-aachen.de, Web: irma-project.org

Connecting Medical Informatics and Bio-Informatics
R. Engelbrecht et al. (Eds.)
IOS Press, 2005

Complexity Analysis of the Visual-Motor Cross-Modalities Using the Correlation Dimension Parameter

Monica C Serban, Dan M Dobrea

"Gh. Asachi" Technical University, Iasi, Romania

Abstract

This paper focuses on the tremor signal as a window to observe and analyze the central nervous system's functions and organization. In this idea it is proposed a custom system and some methodologies that reveal the cross-modalities influences, specifically, the increased complexity of the neuro-motor system generating the tremor as a result of photic driving activation method. The correlation dimension is used as a measure of system's complexity change and the behaviour of the physiological system is modelled using the Hindmarsh-Rose neuronal model. The proposed system includes: three neurons and their unidirectional coupling – considered to be a possible way the system changes its complexity –, the dynamical noise and the photic driving action. The correlation dimension (CD) analysis was performed on the real tremor signal and on the output signal of the modelled system. The global behaviour of the CD parameter proved to be similar in both cases. Thus, the results are promoting the idea of a complex and structured system that is accounting for the photing driving induced tremor.

Keywords:
Tremor; Correlation dimension; Central nervous system (CNS)

1. Introduction

In two previously papers it was investigated the dependence between the tremor signals and the visual stimuli [1], [2]. It was proved the existence of a direct relation between basic motor activity and the external visual stimuli. The observed changes in the frequency characteristics of the tremor signal due to visual stimuli demonstrated a significant connection between visual pathways in the central nervous system (CNS) and the regions basically governing tremor [1], [2]. In this context, given a multidimensional dynamical system (CNS – its efferent pathways, the motor units) and its one-dimensional output (a series of scalar observations represented by the tremor signal), it appeared the following question: can it be inferred any characteristics of the original CNS system given only its output? In order to answer this question, the complexity of the system was considered as a key feature to be analysed.

The major theoretical contributions for complexity measurement of one system have been resulted so far from the tools of nonlinear dynamics and those of the information theory. Among these, the methods usually used to assess biological complexity were: correlation dimension [3-5], approximate entropy [6], detrended fluctuation analysis [7], false nearest neighbours [5], recurrence plot analysis [4], [8] and point wise correlation dimension [9-10].

In this paper, in order to characterize the systems involved and to get an insight of the process of visual influence on the tremor movement, the correlation dimension was used. More, the system was modelled using for this the Hindmarsh-Rose neuronal model.

2. Methodology

There were admitted four subjects for this study, three males and one female. All subjects were aged between 26 and 29 years. All subjects were healthy, with no known neurological or endocrine pathology, and no known Ca^{2+} or Mg^{2+} deficiency that could influence the tremor characteristics. In addition, they had been taken no medication in the week previous to the recordings. The experimental protocol was explained to the subjects and they gave written consent regarding the participation in this study. The entire procedure of tremor acquisition was unobtrusive for the subjects, without any physical contact, due to the acquisition system capability [11]. In order to isolate them from the surrounding stray stimuli, other than the stimuli supplied by using a computer display, all the recordings took place in a quiet room without any source of light. Also, they were particularly asked to think at nothing.

It has been made 20 recordings for each subject. Each recording had 98.4 s, but only the first 32.8 s and the last 32.8 s of hand tremor were kept. After the first time segment of 32.8 s a visual stimuli was presented to the subject. The seating subjects were asked to maintain the hand in the same postural position. Moreover, the subject's elbow was fixed in order to avoid the fatigue influence. In the first part of the recording, the display was a uniform black background. The stimuli consisted in a circle of 2 cm radius, placed in the middle of the display, changing its luminosity between a black background and a white flash. The stimuli changes' pattern was a symmetric rectangular wave of 5Hz frequency. The subjects had no visual control of their hand position. The sampling rate was 250 samples per second and they had been 8.200 samples per each acquired segment of a recording.

3. Correlation dimension

Correlation dimension (CD) is a parameter able to describe the global complexity degree of a system based on only one of its outputs [12]. The method proposed by Grassberger and Procaccia [13] was used here to estimate the CD parameter. The CD's algorithm is based on the computation of integral correlation, a parameter that makes no assumption regarding the embedding dimension. In this article, the integral correlation was computed for different embedding dimensions (from 1 up to 10), by using the formula:

$$C(R) = \frac{1}{M(M-1)} \sum_{i=1}^{M} \sum_{i \neq j}^{M} H\left(R - d\left(x_i - x_j\right)\right) \ (1)$$

where: H is the Heaviside function and M is the space dimension; xi and xj are two vectors constructed from the original time series by using the time delay method; R is an arbitrary radius and d is the distance computed by using the Takens norm.

The CD is taken as the average slope of the cumulative curve generated by the integral correlation function obtained for different values of the hyper-dimensional sphere R. Both, the radius R and the integral correlation were plotted in log-log coordinated. When the embedding dimension increases the CD should increase but eventually saturate at the correct value. Due to the variability of the psychological influences in the time series (e.g. the level of subject's concentration) and to the continuous dynamics of the CNS, this kind of behaviour was not confirmed in all time series. Consequently, in order to correctly estimate the CD parameter, the embedding dimension was computed for each time series. The particular value thus obtained was then used for the selection of the correct CD value.

Prior to this, it was established the optimal time delay parameter value needed for the state space reconstruction. It has been used the mutual information function [14], the optimal time delay value being chosen for that point where the average mutual information reached its first minimum. For all tremor series the time delay parameter was within the interval [3÷6]. In Figure 1(a) it can be observed a typical characteristic for average mutual information versus time lag. The mutual information reached its first minimum at a time delay value of 5. This value should be considered, in this particular case, the "optimal" value for the time delay parameter.

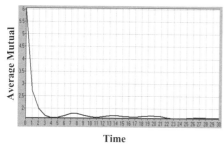 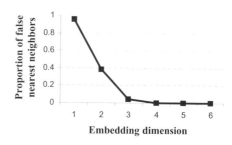

Time   Embedding dimension

Figure 1 – (a) The average mutual information (b) False nearest neighbours calculation for one time series with an embedding time delay of 5 (R_{tol} = 15)

Having the time delay information it is possible to calculate for each one dimensional time tremor series the corresponding minimum embedding dimension. To calculate this last parameter in has been used the false nearest neighbours method [15]. Figure 1(b) presents one of the results obtained for a randomly chosen tremor time series. The proportion of false nearest neighbours drops to 0 when the correct embedding dimension is reached (6, in this case). For almost all time series the obtained embedding dimensions reside within the range from 5 to 8; only for few time series the embedding dimension was greater then 10. The threshold parameter for the embedding criterion (distance tolerance Rtol) was 15 for all determinations [15]. Finally, the CD estimations were calculated for all time series and for all subjects. In the pre-processing step all time series were digitally low-pass pre-filtered, using a cut off frequency of 40 Hz. The aberrant data series were eliminated.

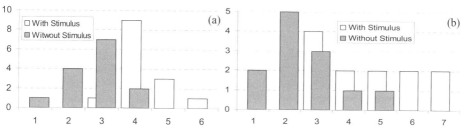

Figure 2 – The histogram distribution for CD parameter based on the time series recorded with and without external visual stimulus for (a) subject 1 and (b) subject 2

In 78.3% of the recordings it was observed an increase of the CD value for the series with stimuli in comparison with the series recorded without any kind of stimuli. For two of the subjects the results are presented in Figure 2. The histogram distributions of the CD parameter for both types of time series (with and, respectively, without stimuli), shown in Figure 2, confirm through their displacement the same global trend. In both graphics the bins' width was 0.275. For subject 2, Figure 2 (b), there are more bins (seven) mainly because the value range of the correlation dimension for this subject was larger. For subject 1 the bins intervals were: [2.4, 2.675), [2.675, 2.95), [2.95, 3.225), [3.225, 3.5), [3.5, 3.775), [3.775, 4.05). For subject 2 the first bin (spanning the range [2.4, 2.675)) had zero elements and the added bins were [4.05, 4.325) and [4.325, 4.6), corresponding to bins 6 and 7.

The correlation dimensions for all time series varied between 2.82 and 4.46. As a consequence, the class of dynamic model that could replicate the complexity of the recorded time series must have at least five independent control variables to account for the system's complexity. The increased complexity of the system, this could be seen as an effect of some underlying structural modifications (new components are added) and/or as an effect of some functional (coupling) changes in the system.

4. Model simulation

As it was shown, data sets analysis reveals that the CD parameter increases from the signals without stimuli to the case with stimuli. Thus, the "measure of complexity" shows that the visual stimulation phase modifies the physiologic system's complexity that becomes a greater one.

It is known that the control of the muscle force can be obtained: (a) by varying the number of recruited motor units (MU) and (b) by varying the activation rate of the motoneurons. In general, MUs fire asynchronously. Moreover, MUs synchrony produces tremor [16]. In our case it was proved [1], [2] that the synchrony was due to external/tuned synchronization that primarily reflects a common driving oscillation, namely the CNS oscillations. The origins for these driving oscillations are still unknown. They could be cortical – even if there is no evidence of sensorimotor induced visual stimuli frequency (this was proved only for primary visual cortical area [17]) –, and/or subcortical (e.g. thalamus, brainstem etc.). Also, from the experimental data there is no evidence for "pure" sensory pathways (dashed line in Figure 3a).

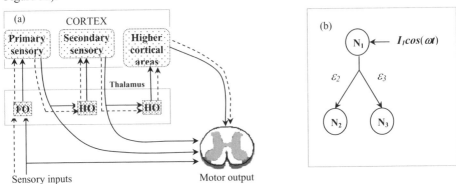

Figure 3 – (a) Sensory processing pathways (b) The proposed model

In [18] it can be found a review on the evidence that many of the afferent sensory inputs reaching the thalamus and then passed on to the cerebral cortex come from axons that branch, sending one branch to the thalamus (namely, to the "first-order" thalamic relays) and the other directly to centres in the brain stem or spinal cord (motor outputs), see Figure 3(a). This pattern is also true for the axons that arise in the layer five of the cortex and pass to "higher-order" thalamic relays (HO). The axons that give off branches to lower motor centres and also innervate the thalamus are crucial for an immediate and completely different behavioural role (e.g. the fast motor actions needed for animal's survival). In terms of complexity this means that the system complexity primes the organism for an adaptive response, making it ready and able to react to sudden physiologic stresses.

Under repetitive visual stimuli the system's complexity can increase at the CNS level as a result of a change in the coupling strength between structural components (cortical/subcortical centre/visual path and, on the other hand, spinal motoneurons) and by recruiting new spinal motoneurons. In order to test these hypotheses a very simple model of the visual influence was proposed and analysed. The proposed system was designed with 3 neurons, all of Hindmarsh-Rose (HR) neuron model type [Figure 3(b)][19]. The HR model, eq. (2), is one with minimal complexity (i.e., three variables only), replicating the main dynamical regimes of regular spiking and chaotic spiking-bursting activity observed in living neurons. One neuron (N1) mimics the central pattern generator; the other two neurons (N2, N3) model two distinct MUs.

$$
\begin{cases}
\dot{x}_i = y_i - x_i^3 + 3x_i^2 - z_i + I_0 + \xi_i + \varepsilon_i(x_i - x_j) \\
\dot{y}_i = 1 - 5x_i^2 - y_i \\
\dot{z}_i = 0.006[4(x_i + 1.6) - z_i]
\end{cases}
\tag{2}
$$

The x variable represents the membrane potential, y is a recovery variable, z is the internal mechanism which regulates the patterns of discharges, ξ represents the background Gaussian white noise (synaptic, dendritic, axonic noise etc.) that is important in the stochastic resonance phenomena (its absolute value ≤ 1.5) and ε is the coupling strength parameter, (i= 1..3, j=1). The I0 parameter denotes the intensity of a constant (tonic) signal that is delivered to the neuron from the external world and its values were chosen as: 14 for N1 and 20 for N2 and N3. Further, we implemented the following four cases: (1) No coupling, $\varepsilon 1 = \varepsilon 2 = \varepsilon 3 = 0$; (2) Light coupling, $\varepsilon 1 = 0$, $\varepsilon 2 = \varepsilon 3 = 0.005$; (3) Strong coupling, $\varepsilon 1 = 0$, $\varepsilon 2 = 0.5$, $\varepsilon 3 = 0.4$; (4) Strong coupling + a forcing term, I1cos(ωt), as input for N1 neuron, $\varepsilon 1 = 0$, $\varepsilon 2 = 0.5$, $\varepsilon 3 = 0.4$, I1 = 22, ω = 5. On successive trials the noise components and the initial state variables were varied for all three neurons, the other parameters of the model being maintained constants. For all cases, there were generated the signals as a sum of N1 and N2 outputs, cut out the first samples corresponding to the transition phase and then, it was applied to them the same CD analysis that was applied to the original tremor data set. The results are summarized in Table1.

Tabel 1: Estimations of the correlation dimension parameter for N_1+ N_2 outputs

	Case 1	Case 2	Case 3	Case 4
N_1+ N_2	3.1954±0.3988	3.13505±0.2917	3.3765±0.2688	3.4402±0.2210

5. Conclusions and further direction

The global complexity of the system increases, fact that is revealed by the tremor signals recorded during a photic driving process. This confirms the emerging coupling strength that appears in the moment of stimuli presentation between the visual CNS pathways and the motor centres generating tremor. With a very simple formal model it has been replicated this behaviour by coupling a HR neuron, modelling the visual CNS input origin, with two other HR neurons that are modelling two independent motor units. The greatest enhancement was observed in case 4, where a new dynamic variable, $I_1 cos(\omega t)$, was introduced. The periodic driving force models the visual repetitive stimuli, also retrieved from the N_1+ N_2 outputs' spectra. The mean growth in the complexity parameter obtained within the model was 0.3052. This represents the difference between strong couplings with driving force and light coupling without any external force. This value is similar with the value obtained for real tremor signals, 0.3717 for subject 1 and 0.5584 for subject 2. This fact shows that, although the proposed model is a very simple one, it still succeeds to capture the main dynamics of the real system. The small increase of only 0.0637 obtained in case 4 compared to case 3 is due to only one new independent dynamic variable $I_1cos(\omega t)$ introduced at N_1's input. The increase of 0.2415 obtained in case 3 compared to case 2 is due to the strength of couplings. These facts can lied to the idea that the greater values achieved with the real data sets (0.3717 and, respectively, 0.5584) beside those achieved with the simulated ones (0.3052) could be explained by a more complex and structured system directly responsible for the photing driving induced tremor. It has to be stressed that these results are only preliminary ones. There is one major drawback in the approach: the length of the real data set is relatively small for this kind of analysis. In order to get sufficient data samples, as a further direction we aim to reshape the acquisition part of our system. Obviously, on the model proposed will be performed further improvements for perfection it.

6. References

[1]   Dobrea DM, Teodorescu HN. Tremor measurements for clarifying the hypothalamic processes and GABA control. *Proc Int Federation for Med and Biol Eng* (IFMBE) 2004: 6

[2]   Serban MC, Dobrea DM, and Teodorescu HN. Evidence for the Central Oscillators in the Physiological Tremor Generation Process. *Proc of 4th European Symp in Biomed Eng*, Patras, Greece, 2004

[3]   Kobayashi T, Misaki K, Nakagawa H, Madokoro S, Ota T, Ihara H, Tsuda K, Umezawa Y, Murayama J, and Isaki K. Correlation dimension of the human sleep electroencephalogram. *Psych Clin Neurosci* 2000: 54 (1): pp. 11-6

[4]   Trzebski A, Smietanowski M, and Zebrowski J. Repetitive apneas reduce nonlinear dynamical complexity of the human cardiovascular control system. *J Physiol Pharm* 2001: 52 (1), pp. 3-19

[5]   May P, Arrouvel C, Revol M, Servant JM, and Vicaut E. Detection of hemodynamic turbulence in experimental stenosis: an in vivo study in the rat carotid artery. *J Vasc Res* 2002: 39 (1), pp. 21 – 29

[6]   Beckers F, Ramaekers D, and Aubert AE. Approximate Entropy of Heart Rate Variability: Validation of Methods and Application in Heart Failure, *An Int J Cardiovasc Eng* 2001: 1 (4): pp. 177-182

[7]   Seely AJ, and Macklem PT. Complex systems and the technology of variability analysis. *Crit Care* 2004: 8 (6): R367-84

[8]   Trzebski A, and Smietanowski M. Non-linear dynamics of cardiovascular system in humans exposed to repetitive apneas modeling obstructive sleep apnea: aggregated time series data analysis. *Auton Neurosci* 2001: 90 (1-2), pp. 106-115

[9]   Kresh JY, and Izrailtyan I. Evolution in functional complexity of heart rate dynamics: a measure of cardiac allograft adaptability. *Am J Physiol* 1998: 275 (3): R720-7

[10]   Dremencov E, Nahshoni E, Levy D, Mintz M, Overstreet DH, Weizman A, and Yadid G. Dimensional complexity of the neuronal activity in a rat model of depression. *NeuroRep* 2004: 15 (12), pp. 1983-1986

[11]   Dobrea DM, and Teodorescu HN, Pattern Classification For Fatigue State Identification. *Fuzzy Syst and Artif Intell* (Reports and Letters) J. 2002: 8 (1-3): pp. 69–84

[12]   Teodorescu HN, and Brezulianu A. Chaos and clustering in fuzzy systems networks. *Int. J of Chaos Theory Appl* 1997: 2 (1), pp. 17-45

[13]   Grassberger P, and Procaccia I. Dimensions and entropies of strange attractors from a fluctuating dynamics approach. *Physica D* 1984: 13, pp. 34-54

[14]   Fraser AM, and Swinney HL. Independent coordinates for strange attractors from mutual information, *Phys Rev A* 1986: 33 (2), pp. 1134-1140

[15]   Kennel MB, Brown R, and Abarbanel HDI. Determining embedding dimension for phase-space reconstruction using a geometric construction, *Phys. Rev. A* 1992: 45, pp. 3403–3411

[16]   McAuley JH, and Marsden CD. Physiological and pathological tremors and rhytmic central motor control. *Brain* 2000: 123, pp. 1545-1567

[17]   Herrmann CS, Human EEG responses to 1–100 Hz flicker: resonance phenomenain visual cortex and their potential correlation to cognitive phenomena, *Exp Brain Res* 2001: 137, pp.346–353

[18]   Guillery RW, and Sherman SM. The talamus as a monitor of motor outputs. *Phil. Trans. R. Soc. Lond. B* 2002: 357, pp. 1809 – 1821

[19]   Baltanás JP, and Casado JM. Noise-induced resonances in the Hindmarsh-Rose neuronal model. *Phys Rev E* 2002: 65, 041915 (1-6)

Address for correspondence

Dan-Marius Dobrea, Faculty of Electronics and Telecommunications, Iasi, Romania, Bd. Carol I, No. 11, Iasi, Postal Code: 700506, mdobrea@etc.tuiasi.ro, http://www.etc.tuiasi.ro/cin/Members/Dan/dan.htm

Connecting Medical Informatics and Bio-Informatics
R. Engelbrecht et al. (Eds.)
IOS Press, 2005

471

Neural Network Screening of Electromyographic Signals as the First Phase to Design Novel Human-Computer Interaction

Pekka-Henrik Niemenlehto[a], Martti Juhola[a], Veikko Surakka[a,b]

[a]Department of Computer Sciences, University of Tampere, Finland
[b]Tampere University Hospital Department of Clinical Neurophysiology
P.O. Box 2000, FIN-33521 Tampere, Finland

Abstract

The present aim was to describe the first phase attempts to recognise voluntarily produced changes in electromyographic signals measured from two facial muscles. Thirty subjects voluntarily activated two facial muscles, corrugator supercilii and zygomaticus major. We designed a neural network based recognition system that screened out muscle activations from the electromyographic signals. When several subjects were tested according to the same test protocol, the neural network system was able to correctly recognise more than 95 % of all muscle activations. This is a promising result and we shall next proceed to modify the system for real-time functioning and then design its utilisation for various multimodal human-computer interaction techniques. The subsequent phase in the future will be the interaction backwards: when a computer program first recognised the use of the facial muscles, it will then follow the instructions given by the user. For instance, by using the facial muscles the subject could select or activate objects on the computer screen. This would be one of the opportunities that we develop to help, e.g., disabled persons, who are unable to use their hands.

Keywords:
Biomedical Signal Analysis; Neural Networks; Electromyographig Signals; Human-Computer Interaction

1. Introduction

Human bioelectrical signals apply to several diagnostic purposes. They are also useful in other contexts. By recording some intentionally controlled phenomena via signal measurements, we are able to extend means for human-computer interaction (HCI) [1]. For example, moving the cursor on the screen by altering the gaze from one point to another seems a reasonable alternative for fast commands. In the present research we developed a method to recognise voluntary muscle activations from electromyographic (EMG) signals, so that it is possible to use facial muscles for HCI. The facial muscles can be used to accomplish various simple and rapid tasks, such as activating a link on the screen. One of the objectives is to help disabled persons to improve their possibilities to use computers. More generally thinking, in the future it might be possible to use multimodal ways to interact with a computer. Let us assume that a head band or eyeglasses would include various sensors to record, e.g., one's facial muscle activity, eye movements (recorded with electro-oculography or small video cameras), heart activity, and brain activity. A computational challenge is then to analyse these signals and search for significant events from them. Our study is the first phase to design an overall HCI system. We tackled the signal analysis of facial EMG signals and the pattern recognition problem of muscular activity variations that appear during subject's voluntary muscle activation.

Some studies were recently published in this field. Barreto et al. [2] studied the use of EMG signals for HCI with motor disabilities. Kübler et al. [3] developed a thought translation device that uses slow cortical potentials of a brain for the simple control influence of a computer. Wolpaw et al. [4] explored the same theme. Surakka et al. [5] studied the multimodal use of facial muscles and eye movements in HCI. We presented the idea to employ neural networks for the analysis of facial EMG signals in [6] and implemented it in [7] for two muscles. Earlier we experimented with a wide set of different multilayer perceptron (MLP) neural networks by varying the topology of the networks (for instance by using different number of hidden nodes), by testing with heavy artificial noise, and by testing various signal conditioning methods, including digital bandpass filters and wavelet denoising. There were only slight differences between various networks, except when we reduced the network to a very small form. Thus, at present we proceeded to use only a few suitable architectures and tested their capacity.

2. Signal Measurements and Recognition

Bipolar surface EMG signals were recorded from healthy 22 males and 8 females. The mean age was 24 years in the range of 20–35 years. The electrodes were placed on the left side of the face above *corrugator supercilii* (activated when frowning) and *zygomaticus major* (activated when smiling) muscle sites. The measurements were conducted according to common procedures described in [8]. The signals were recorded with Grass Model 15 RXi amplifier. The sampling rate was 3 kHz with a passband of 0.1–1.0 kHz. The average signal-to-noise (SNR) ratio was 12.7 dB. Signal examples from the previous muscle sites are shown in Figure 1.

During recordings every subject was seated comfortably and trained to carefully and calmly contract the two muscles, either one of them individually or both at the same time. Naturally, there is some baseline activation all the time in muscles, but its intensity is lower than during contractions that appear as bursts in EMG signals. Four 10 minutes recordings were accomplished for each subject. These tests followed one by one after a short resting period. The first period included the activation of the *corrugator supercilii*, the second period consisted of the activation of the *zygomaticus major*, the third part covered both of the muscles, and finally the last period was pure baseline recording. Due to the large amount of data recorded, we used only a part of it. Rest of the data will be used in our future research.

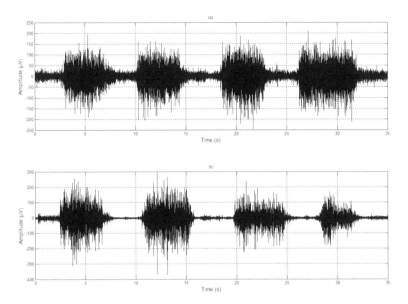

Figure 1 – (a) A 36 s part of a signal recorded from the corrugator supercilii and (b) another from the zygomaticus major.

Our previous work [7] showed that the use of wavelet denoising yielded slightly better classification results than using the more traditional digital bandpass filtering. While applying wavelets, high frequencies are analysed with a relatively effective time resolution, whereas low frequencies are dealt with a good frequency resolution. The transformation was calculated with the pyramidal algorithm [9], in which filters based on the mother wavelet are used. We utilised the Meyer wavelet as the mother wavelet. The principle of the wavelet denoising is as follows. First, a digital signal is transformed with the pyramidal algorithm up to the given level. In our tests the third level generated sufficiently reliable results. Second, the wavelet coefficients of every level are thresholded properly. We applied SURE threshold selection rule and soft thresholding which are described in more detail in [9]. Finally, the thresholded wavelet coefficients and the signal approximation of the last level are inverse transformed into the time domain representation by using the inverse form of the pyramidal algorithm.

To supply training, validation, and test sets, we randomly selected ten groups of three persons from all the subjects for the cross validation procedure [10]. We shared one group at a time to the test set, another to the validation set, and the other eight to the training set. Ten such shares were performed so that each group of three persons was once a test set and once a validation set. Thus we got ten series of sets. This procedure was performed for the data from both muscles. We used the mean square error measure to assess training of the network and checked the behaviour of the validation set to stop the training in time to avoid overtraining.

We randomly extracted 3 times 16 or 48 signal segments from the recording of a subject. Such a part of 16 signal segments corresponded to one of the three output classes applied to the classification: muscle activity onset, muscle activity offset, and plateau segment that contained muscle activity or baseline activity. In other words, there were no significant muscle activity changes in the plateau segments. Consequently, for two muscles of three subjects in a group there were 288 signal segments and 2880 altogether in the whole dataset. The number of 2304 signal segments in a training set was certainly enough for the largest MLP neural network, which consisted of two input nodes, five hidden nodes at two layers, and three output nodes. Thus the largest network contained $2\times5+5\times5+5\times3+13=63$ weights to be trained. Usually, the ratio of at least 10 is recommended between the two preceding figures [10]. Each signal segment was comprised of 1024 successive samples (approximately 0.34 s), which was an appropriate length to the wavelet denoising.

After the prior consideration of several different MLP neural network topologies [7], we restricted ourselves only to the three alternatives here. These were the afore-mentioned 2-5-5-3 network as the one of the maximal topology, a minimal network 2-0-3 (no hidden layer), and an average network 2-5-3. The essential aim was to hold the network size very concise to later apply the network for real-time processing. To gain this, it was important to use a minimal amount of input nodes. Therefore, we shared every signal segment of 1024 samples to halves and calculated a normalised root-mean-square (RMS) value for each. We first computed a RMS value for both

$$RMS = \sqrt{\frac{1}{N}\sum_{i=0}^{N-1}|x(i)|^2} \qquad (1)$$

halves (N=512). One more RMS value was computed for the whole signal segment (N=1024). The ratio of RMS of either half and that of the whole segment is equal to normalised RMS. The normalisation permits the process to be independent of the magnitude of signal segments and the normalised RMS values are mapped to the real interval $[0,2^{1/2}]$. This procedure compressed data considerably, but conserved sufficient information after the wavelet denoising for the recognition process of muscular activity in EMG signals. Either half of a signal segment thus yielded an input value into the network. The normalisation property was useful while scaling the input values to a suitable interval and evolving an invariant feature space with respect to signal amplitudes. The three nodes of the output layer expressed different classes which were mentioned previously: muscle activity onsets, plateau segments from the duration of muscular activity or baseline activity, and muscle activity offsets.

3. Results

When we had a 10-fold cross validation and executed 10 runs for each of them, we obtained a total of 100 runs. We then computed the means and standard deviations of recognition accuracy values (also called sensitivity):

$$a = \frac{tp}{tp+fn}100\,(\%) = \frac{tp}{n}100\,(\%), \qquad (2)$$

where tp and fn are the number of true positive and false negative classifications, respectively, and n is the number of all test cases. In addition to the signals themselves, we also experimented with noisy signals by inserting random white noise to the original signal segments. Two variations were formed by incurring signal-to-noise ratios (SNR) of 5 dB and 1 dB. Table 1 encompasses results of three neural networks tested.

The results in Table 1 show that there were virtually no differences between the three networks. Even the smallest network was able to recognise different types of signal segments very well. It seems that the signal segments were successfully separated in a feature space of two normalised RMS values. Otherwise, such a minimal network could not separate the test cases into the different classes so effectively. We also observed the subtle deterioration in the case of the strongest noise.

Table 1 –Recognition accuracy: means and standard deviations of 100 runs for three neural networks and three signal-to-noise ratios.

Network	Number of iterations	Mean square error of training set	Mean square error of validation set	Recognition accuracy [%]		
				Original signals	Signals with SNR of 5 dB	Signals with SNR of 1 dB
2-0-3	310±20	0.0084±0.0010	0.0089±0.0056	98.3±1.0	97.6±1.7	94.7±2.7
2-5-3	250±28	0.0083±0.0010	0.0086±0.0055	98.3±1.1	97.7±1.8	95.0±2.6
2-5-5-3	225±21	0.0083±0.0010	0.0088±0.0055	98.3±1.1	97.8±1.8	95.1±2.5

The results in Table 2 were computed similarly as those reported in Table 1. In this case the recognition accuracies of different output classes are presented. Only results of the 2-5-3 network are presented, because the variations between the three networks were again slight.

Table 2 –Recognition accuracy: means and standard deviations of 100 runs for 2-5-3 neural network and three signal-to-noise ratios employing three output classes.

Output class	Recognition accuracy [%]		
	Original signals	Signals with SNR of 5 dB	Signals with SNR of 1 dB
Onset segment	99.3±0.7	98.6±1.2	95.4±2.9
Plateau segment	97.7±1.2	99.4±0.7	99.5±0.7
Offset segment	97.9±2.7	95.0±4.3	90.1±5.2

4. Discussion

The developed neural networks functioned properly. On the basis of the current dataset of 30 subjects, it was possible to reliably recognize voluntary muscle activity from the EMG signals measured from *corrugator supercilii* and *zygomaticus major* facial muscle sites. This probably enables us to expand to other (facial) muscles as well. Because the sizes of the networks were very limited, there is an excellent opportunity to construct a real-time neural network based recognition system. To use such a system, a calibration is typically needed. This task could include the training of the network. Even more simply, we might collect a vast dataset of EMG signals from many subjects and rely on it, thus rendering the calibration phase unnecessary. In the future, we shall perform more measurements with more subjects of various ages, build a real-time system, and test some simple human-computer actions, for instance, selection of objects on the computer screen with volitional muscle activations. One practical viewpoint is to diminish difficulties caused by several electrode wires attached to a subject; we shall use wireless electrode recordings to alleviate this practical issue.

Acknowledgments

This research was supported by the Academy of Finland (grants 202185 and 1202183).

References

[1]   Surakka V, Illi M, and Isokoski P. Voluntary Eye Movements in Human-Computer Interactions. In: Hyönä J, Radach R & Deubel H (Eds.) *The Mind's Eyes: Cognitive and Applied Aspects of Oculomotor Research*. Elsevier Science: Oxford, 2003; pp. 473-491.

[2]   Barreto AB, Scargle SD, and Adjouadi M . A practical EMG-based human-computer interface for users with motor disabilities, *Journal of Rehabilitation Research and Development* 2000: 37: 53-63.

[3]   Kübler A, Kotchoubey B, Hinterberger T, Ghanaym N, Perelmouter J, Schauer M, Fritsch C, Taub E, and Birbaumer N. The thought translation device: a neuropsychological approach to communication in total motor paralysis, *Experimental Brain Research* 1999: 124: 223-32.

[4]   Wolpaw RJ, Birbaumer N, Mcfarland DJ, Pfurtscheller G, and Vaughan TM. Brain-computer interfaces for communication and control, *Clinical Neurophysiology* 2002: 113: 767-91.

[5]   Surakka V, Illi M, and Isokoski P. Gazing and Frowning As a New Technique for Human-Computer Interaction, *ACM Transactions on Applied Perception* 2004: 1: 40-56.

[6]   Laakso J, Juhola M, and Surakka V. Neural network recognition of electromyographic signals of two facial muscle sites, In: *Proceedings of Medical Informatics Europe*. Budapest, Hungary, 2002; pp. 83-7.

[7]   Niemenlehto P, Juhola M, and Surakka V. Detection of electromyographic signals from facial muscles with neural networks, submitted manuscript, 2004.

[8]   Fridlund A and Cacioppo J. Guidelines for human electromyographic research, *Psychophysiology* 1986: 5: 567- 89.

[9]   Mallat S. *A Wavelet Tour of Signal Processing*. San Diego, Academic Press, 2001.

[10] Haykin S. *Neural Networks, A Comprehensive Foundation*. New Jersey: Prentice-Hall, 1994.

Address for correspondence

Pekka Niemenlehto, Department of Computer Sciences, 33014 University of Tampere, Finland;
Pekka.Niemenlehto@cs.uta.fi

Connecting Medical Informatics and Bio-Informatics
R. Engelbrecht et al. (Eds.)
IOS Press, 2005

477

Object-Oriented Implementation for the Dual Surface Minimisation Algorithm

Jouni Mykkänen[a], Mikko Itäranta[a], Jussi Tohka[b]

[a]Department of Computer Sciences, University of Tampere, Finland

[b]Laboratory of Neuro Imaging, Department of Neurology,
UCLA Medical School, Los Angeles, CA, USA and Institute of
Signal Processing, Tampere University of Technology,
Finland

Abstract

The automatic surface extraction from volumetric images is important for the medical image analysis. The delineation task is challenging especially with functional imaging where images are noisy and the content of image depends on the study. We have earlier developed a new dual surface minimisation (DSM) algorithm for the optimisation of deformable surfaces and applied it successfully to fully automatic surface extraction from positron emission tomography images. We present a fast object-oriented implementation for the DSM algorithm with a conventional command line interface. The DSM software is a freely available tool for the Internet community at http://www.cs.uta.fi/research/software/. The implementation of the DSM algorithm provides new opportunities to extend experiments, to develop and to study new applications with noisy volumetric images emerging from medical or other applications.

Keywords:
Deformable model; Segmentation, Surface extraction; Object-oriented architecture; Medical images

1. Introduction

Automatic surface delineation methods are required for many applications in medical imaging. The visualisation of the volumetric objects, virtual reality systems and quantitative image analysis are good examples. Deformable models have gained a wide popularity for the surface extraction problems emerging from medical imaging, because their ability to use image independent information about the shape of the surface to be extracted. The underlying idea with deformable models is to optimise a template surface so that the surface is smooth and couples well with salient image features. The largest problem of deformable models is that the optimisation problem is a complex one containing a number of local minima to be avoided. We have developed a new dual surface minimisation (DSM) algorithm for the global optimisation of deformable surfaces [1]. The DSM algorithm is especially dedicated to cope with noisy volumetric images, such as those obtained with positron emission tomography (PET), which is a non-invasive method to measure biochemical processes in living tissue. A substantial amount of noise present in PET images makes the surface segmentation tasks very demanding, and more specifically, local minima related problems with deformable surfaces pressing. We have applied the DSM method to automatically delineate surfaces from fluoro-2-deoxy-glucose (FDG) and Raclopride PET brain images [2] and validated the surface extraction quantitatively with the simulated PET brain data [3]. The software was implemented in Matlab. The DSM method has then been applied to extract the striatum from Raclopride PET brain images and the heart volume from cardiac FDG-PET images [4,5].

In this study, we present a new object-oriented implementation (C++) for the DSM algorithm. Our aim is to clarify the implementation of the DSM algorithm, to make it easy to use and to make it freely available for the Internet community.

2. Dual surface minimisation algorithm

The DSM algorithm is fully presented in [1] and we only give a summary here. We extract surfaces from volumetric images by minimising the energy function of the deformable model. Surfaces are approximated by simplex meshes [6]. The total energy of the surface mesh $\mathbf{W}$ (a set of discrete points $\mathbf{w}_i$, $i = 1, ..., n$, called mexels) is the sum of the internal energy calculated from the mesh and the external energy calculated from the image:

$$E(\mathbf{W}) = \lambda\, E_{int}(\mathbf{W}) + (1 - \lambda)E_{ext}(\mathbf{W}) = 1/n\ \Sigma^n_{i=1}(\lambda\, E_{int}(\mathbf{w}_i) + (1-\lambda)E_{ext}(\mathbf{w}_i)). \quad (1)$$

The regularisation parameter λ is in range $[0,1]$. The external energy E_{ext} couples $\mathbf{W}$ to the salient image features. The internal energy E_{int} regularises the shape of the surface.

The mexel-wise internal energy is defined as

$$E_{int}(\mathbf{w}_i) = ||\mathbf{w}_i - \alpha\, \Sigma^3_{j=1}\mathbf{w}_{i\_j}||^2/A(\mathbf{W}), \quad (2)$$

where $\mathbf{w}_{ij}$ are the neighbouring mexels of $\mathbf{w}_i$ in the mesh, $A(\mathbf{W})$ is the average area of the faces of the mesh, and α is the shape parameter. The shape parameter defines the favoured shape for the internal energy. For example, the thin-plate shape model is defined by setting $\alpha = 1/3$. The thin-plate shape model states that each mexel should be positioned as near as possible to the centre of mass of its neighbouring mexels.

The precise form of the external energy function depends on the applied image content because different image-features characterise surfaces of interest with different type of images. We define the external energy with the help of energy images. An energy image is generated from the image to be processed in such a way that intensity values in the energy image describe salience of voxels for the application and the image content. The external energy at the position $\mathbf{w}$ is

$$E_{ext}(\mathbf{w}) = 1 - B(\mathbf{w}), \quad (3)$$

where B is *the energy image*. The energy image is normalised to have intensity values from 0 to 1.

The energy function (1) is likely to have multiple local minima. Therefore, extracted surfaces obtainable by local energy minimisation would depend highly on the given initialisations. This, within our applications, could cause substantial problems in automating the surface extraction. We proposed a global dual surface minimisation (DSM) algorithm for the deformable mesh optimisation in [1]. The algorithm is global in the sense that it can overcome local minima and hence it reduces the sensitivity of deformable mesh to its initialisation considerably. The algorithm is based on the iterative optimisation of two surface meshes, which approach the surface of interest from different directions.

The standard DSM algorithm begins with two meshes: the outer mesh and the inner mesh. These are created from a given initial mesh preserving its properties, except the size. Their sizes are set in such a way that the surface of the searched structure lies in the space between them. The search is based on the iterative minimisation of the energies of the outer and inner surfaces. One iteration step for a surface is described by the Algorithm 1, which is adapted from [7]. The symbol δ denotes discrete delta function. For the definition of search spaces, see [1]. The whole process is presented in the Algorithm 2.

Algorithm 1 Greedy surface minimisation

Require: W, penalty for current position γ, search spaces S_i for each mexel
for all w_i in **W** do 2:
  set $w_i \leftarrow$ arg $\min_{w \in S_i} E(w) + \gamma\delta(w - w_i)$
end for
return **W**

Algorithm 2 Standard dual surface minimisation	**Algorithm3** Dual surface minimisation - one surface

Require: W$_{outer}$, **W**$_{inner}$
repeat
  if $E(\mathbf{W}_{outer}) < E(\mathbf{W}_{inner})$
    W $\leftarrow$ **W**$_{outer}$
    V $\leftarrow$ **W**$_{inner}$
  else
    W $\leftarrow$ **W**$_{inner}$
    V $\leftarrow$ **W**$_{outer}$
  end if
  $\gamma \leftarrow$ 0
  repeat
    minimise surface **V** by using
      the Algorithm 1 with the penalty γ
    increase γ
  until Change in **V**
  if $E(\mathbf{W}_{outer}) < E(\mathbf{W}_{inner})$
    W$_{inner} \leftarrow$ **V**
  else
    W$_{outer} \leftarrow$ **V**
  end if
until $volme(\mathbf{W}_{outer}) < volume(\mathbf{W}_{inner})$
return **W**
	Require: W, Vol$_{threshold}$
	$E_{min} \leftarrow E(W)$
	W$_{min} \leftarrow$ **W**
	repeat
	  $\gamma \leftarrow$ 0
	  repeat
	    minimise surface **W** to by using
	      the Algorithm 1 with penalty γ
	    increase γ
	  until Change in **W**
	  $E_{cur} \leftarrow E(\mathbf{W})$
	  if $E_{cur} < E_{min}$
	    W$_{min} \leftarrow$ **W**
	  end if
	until $volme(W) <$ Vol$_{threshold}$ (>, if out)
	return **W**$_{min}$

It is favourable approach the surface of interest only from one direction when a level of noise clearly differs between the target and the background. For instance, PET brain images usually contain more noise inside the brain volume than outside of it. The Algorithm 3 presents a DSM-OS (DSM - one surface) version of the DSM algorithm which uses only one surface mesh approaching the target surface, either from inside it or outside it.

3. Object-oriented implementation

We chose an object-oriented approach to achieve clear and flexible program architecture. To obtain the best performance, we selected C++ as an implementation language. The software is divided into image handling, mesh handling, and minimisation modules. The list of the main modules is presented in Table 1.

The mesh module contains classes for mesh handling. Separate mesh loader classes are provided for mesh file I/O. We implemented reading and writing capabilities for Geomview OFF (http://www.geomview.org/) and VRML 1.0 (http://www.web3d.org/) file formats. Whereas the input mesh must be a simplex mesh, the output mesh can be a simplex or triangulated mesh. The triangulated mesh is useful for visualisation purposes. The image module contains classes for accessing image data. The current implementation supports raw image data (dimensions and data type need to be given) and Mayo Analyze 7.5 formats (http://www.mayo.edu/bir/).

Table 1 -Main modules of the implementation of the dual surface minimisation (DSM) algorithm.

Module	Class	description
Mesh	Mesh	Data structures and operations for mesh handling.
	Mesh loaders	Operations for mesh file I/O for various file formats.
Image	Image	Data structures for image data.
	Image loaders	Operations for image file I/O for various file formats.
DSM	DSM	Core algorithm implementation.
	Energy model	Operations for energy calculations.
	Search space	Operations for search space calculations.

The algorithm was implemented so that it is possible to change values for all the parameters of the algorithm without recompiling the source code. However, the default values for the parameters were found reasonable during our software testing. Therefore, the user has to supply only an energy image and an initial mesh. Furthermore, the energy and search space calculations were separated into their own classes, which allows the easy replacement of their implementations.

We implemented a standard command line user interface for the algorithm allowing easy testing and integration to the existing software environment. This is an important feature, since software tools are often heterogeneous with medical imaging. The interface provides access to all parameters of the DSM algorithm. The values can be given in the command line and in a parameter file. The given command line parameters override the default values and the values defined in a parameter file. This provides a convenient and flexible way for controlling the parameter values of the algorithm. The program stores the applied parameter values in the resulting mesh file as a comment. This makes it possible to check the applied parameters afterwards separately for each mesh.

We developed the software under Linux operating system with a 32-bit system architecture. The Gnu 3.2 C++-compiler, the Eclipse 2.1.3. and the Doxygen 1.3. were used for the development. The Blitz++ library was used for vector and matrix operations (http://www.oonumerics.org/blitz/). The new implementation is released under GNU Lesser General Public License (LGPL) (http://www.gnu.org/licenses/lgpl.html). The DSM software   (*Dualsurfacemin*)   package   can   be   found   from http://www.cs.uta.fi/research/software/.

4. Evaluation and results

The new implementation of the DSM algorithm was evaluated to ensure that it works as expected and to find out the practical performance of the software. We used the same image material than with our earlier studies. These include the artificially made meta-sphere images [1], simulated PET brain images [3,8], phantom PET brain image and PET brain images from healthy volunteers [2]. The initial meshes were set with the same parameters than above studies. The evaluation concerns only the automatic surface extraction step with required file I/O, not the image pre-processing. A Linux laptop with the Pentium 4 processor running at 2.6 MHz was used for the experiments. The execution time was measured using the system *time* program. In these experiments, the mesh contained 1280 vertexes. Table 2 summarises the results. The number of iterations are approximated and averaged over several images of the same type. The C++ implementation is about ten times faster than the compiled Matlab version.

Table 2 -Summary of the experiments with dual surface minimisation (DSM) algorithm. Given iteration and time values are approximated.

Material	Image dimensions	Iterations	Time
Meta sphere	64*64*44	1200	18 s
Simulated PET	128*128*63	3850	43 s
Hoffman brain phantom (PET)	128*128*35	3500	35 s
FDG-PET brain	128*128*35	4000	60 s

5. Discussion

We have presented a fast C++ implementation for the DSM algorithm. It is based on an object-oriented architecture which allows flexible integration to the existing software environments. This is very important in medical imaging where often many different software tools must be used together for image analysis. The class structure of the program allows easily adding support for the required image and mesh formats. Modifications to the DSM algorithm are easier to carry out with the object oriented implementation than with the previous procedural implementation. For example, this could be needed for developing a parallel implementation of the DSM algorithm.

We implemented a conventional command line user interface for the algorithm. This way it can be used as any other command line tool program. For example, we could write a shell script to extract surfaces from a set of energy images. The software were found fast and very convenient to use. Compared to our earlier procedural Matlab implementation, we got from eight to ten times speed up, which is a significant improvement. Due to the object-oriented design, the command line interface can be easily replaced by a graphical user interface (GUI). It will be the next step in the development. The plan is to implement GUI using some external scripting languages (e.g. TK/TCL).

The C++ implementation of the DSM algorithm provides new opportunities to extend evaluations to large high resolution images and meshes with tens of thousands vertexes included. This is important when applying the DSM algorithm for the other imaging problems where the image dimensions and surfaces to be extracted are larger and more complex. The implementation was developed in the Linux i586 platform with 32-bit architecture. We also tested the implementation on the Ultra SPARC 2 running 32-bit Solaris operating system.

In summary, we presented a fast object-oriented implementation of the DSM method and released it freely available under GNU LGPL. For the Internet community, this software provides a new tool for automatically extracting surfaces from noisy volumetric images and this way it could help to develop new analysis methods for medical images.

6. Acknowledgements

Thanks to Turku PET Centre, Finland, for providing the image material. J. Tohka's work was supported by the Academy of Finland (grants 204782 and 104834) and by the NIH/NCRR grant P41 RR013642, additional support was provided by the NIH Roadmap Initiative for Bioinformatics and Computational Biology U54 RR021813 funded by the NCRR, NCBC, and NIGMS.

7. References

[1]   J. Tohka and J.M. Mykkänen. Deformable mesh for automated surface extraction from noisy images. International Journal of Image and Graphics, 4:405-432, 2004.

[2]   J. Mykkänen, J. Tohka, and U. Ruotsalainen. Delineation of brain structures from positron emission tomography images using deformable models. In R. Baud, M. Fieschi, P. Le Beaux, and P. Ruch, editors, The new navigators: from professionals to patients, stud. health technol. Inform. volume 95, pages 33-38. IOS Press, 2003.

[3]   J. Tohka, A. Kivimäki, A. Reilhac, J. Mykkänen, and U. Ruotsalainen. Assessment of brain surface extraction from pet images using monte carlo simulations. IEEE Transactions in Nuclear Science, 51(5) 2641-2648, 2004.

[4]   A. Kivimäki, J. Tohka, M. Anttila, and U. Ruotsalainen. Automatic extraction of the heart volumes from dynamic FDG PET emission images for movement corrections. 2004. European Journal of Nuclear Medicine and Molecular Imaging, pp. S406, Volume 31, Supplement 2 (Abstracts, Annual Congress of The EANM, Helsinki 2004).

[5]   J. Tohka, E. Wallius, J. Hirvonen, J. Hietala, and U. Ruotsalainen. Improved reproducibility in dopamine D2-receptor studies with automatic segmentation of striatum from PET images. 2004. In Proc. of IEEE Medical Imaging Conference (MIC2004), Rome, Italy, October 2004 (In press, 5 pages).

[6]   H. Delingette. General object reconstruction based on simplex meshes. International Journal of Computer Vision, 32:111-142, 1999.

[7]   D.J. Williams and M. Shah. A fast algorithm for active contours and curvature estimation. CVGIP: Image Understanding, 55(1):14-26, 1992.

[8]   A. Reilhac, C. Lartizien, N. Costes, S. Sans, C. Comtat, R.N. Gunn, and A.C. Evans. PET-SORTEO: A Monte Carlo-based simulator with high count rate capabilities. IEEE Transactions on Nuclear Science, 51:46-52, 2004.

8. Address for correspondence

Jouni Mykkänen, Department of Computer Science, Kanslerinrinne 1,
FIN-33014 University of Tampere, Finland.
E-mail: Jouni.Mykkanen@cs.uta.fi. Homepage: http://www.cs.uta.fi/~jm/

Connecting Medical Informatics and Bio-Informatics
R. Engelbrecht et al. (Eds.)
IOS Press, 2005

Analyzing Sub-Classifications of Glaucoma via SOM Based Clustering of Optic Nerve Images

Sanjun Yan[a], Syed Sibte Raza Abidi[a], Paul Habib Artes[b]

[a]Health Informatics Lab, Faculty of Computer Science, Dalhousie University, Halifax, Canada
[b]Department of Ophthalmology and Visual Sciences, Dalhousie University, Halifax, Canada

Abstract

We present a data mining framework to cluster optic nerve images obtained by Confocal Scanning Laser Tomography (CSLT) in normal subjects and patients with glaucoma. We use self-organizing maps and expectation maximization methods to partition the data into clusters that provide insights into potential sub-classification of glaucoma based on morphological features. We conclude that our approach provides a first step towards a better understanding of morphological features in optic nerve images obtained from glaucoma patients and healthy controls.

Keywords:
Glaucoma; Optic Discs, Confocal Scanning Laser Tomography, Neural Networks, Self-Organizing Maps, Classification

1. Introduction

Glaucoma is an eye disease that is characterized by damage to the optic nerve and corresponding losses in the field of vision [1, 2]. The prevalence of the disease increases strongly with age, making the disease the second most important cause of blindness in North America and Europe. At present, neither the cause nor the natural course of the disease is well understood. However, novel eye imaging technologies such as confocal scanning laser tomography now allow for accurate and reproducible structural measurements of the optic nerve and surrounding retina, thought to be the key site of damage in glaucoma [3]. Over the last decade, imaging technologies have become more widely used clinically, mainly with the objective of improving the accuracy of diagnostic decisions in the care of glaucoma patients.

The data from imaging devices are not, as yet, as well understood as those from older technologies [4]. Also, our understanding of the multi-factorial nature of the disease itself is evolving rapidly. An important theme in glaucoma research is the large variation in the appearance of the optic nerve, both within groups of healthy subjects and in patients with glaucoma [5], and the sub-classification of glaucoma patients according to morphological features is likely to be an important task in the future. It is now thought that patients with certain patterns of nerve damage may behave differently during the course of the disease [6], making it more important clinically to recognise and differentiate between such patterns. One principal problem with the sub-classification of patterns of optic nerve damage is that it is a subjective task, giving rise to considerable levels of disagreement even between highly trained experts.

Previous work in this area has largely focused on diagnostic accuracy, i.e. the distinction of diseased from healthy optic nerves. Artificial Neural Networks have been used for diagnostic decision-making with Confocal Scanning Laser Tomography (CSLT) images. This work suggested that machine classifiers can lead to small though significant gains in diagnostic accuracy over more traditional classifiers such as linear discriminant analyses [7].

The equally important task of supporting the differentiation between different subtypes of healthy and glaucomatous optic nerves has not previously been attempted. Since there may not be any clear boundaries, we posit that unsupervised clustering of imaging data might be a way forward to identify different subtypes of healthy and glaucomatous optic nerves. Given the apparent lack of an objective characterization of optic disk images, our initial aim here is to propose an objective and automated method to characterize optic disk images into multiple sub-types. Our approach is not to pursue *hard* partitioning of the images into explicit sub-classes (that can be related to existing studies and evidence), rather seek a data-driven characterization of the optic disk images so as to acquire a *smooth* partitioning of the images into potential sub-classes (as inherent within the data) with flexible boundaries. The rationale here is that by analyzing the morphological features leading to these smooth partitioning we may be able to better understand their role and can relate them to other variables that might even be able to provide insights into the progression of the disease.

Taking a data-driven approach and using machine learning algorithms, in particular self-organizing unsupervised neural networks, we learn and abstract from the glaucoma (and normal) image data the inherent class and sub-class structures. We posit that intra-cluster analysis may highlight the similarities between patients and give us an understanding of the role of the different morphological features in determining similarities at this level, whereas inter-cluster analysis may lead to objective, data-driven characterization of the disease in terms of broad classes and sub-classes of the disease patterns.

In this paper we present a data mining framework that uses a mix of data clustering techniques to partition the optic disk data (of both normal subjects and glaucoma patients) into meaningful clusters. In particular we demonstrate the use of Self-Organizing Maps (SOM) [8] for the analysis of CSLT data with the objective of increasing the understanding of the data. We apply multiple test readings taken at intervals—i.e. multiple CSLT images obtained from the same subject —to analyze the dispersion of the test results within and across clusters. We present our results and conclude that our approach provides intuitive insight into the inherent relationships between the morphological features provided by CSLT imaging. We conclude that further study of the emergent clusters may enhance our understanding of optic nerve damage in glaucoma and may ultimately lead to more informed clinical care of patients with this disease.

2. Clustering of CSLT Images: Methodology and Methods

To meet the above-objectives we have designed a CSLT Images Clustering System, that firstly conducts a broad clustering of the data-set to partition the data into distinct clusters, and secondly draw soft boundaries around the prevalent clusters using EM algorithm [9]. There are three benefits of using SOM as the first abstraction level in the clustering [10]. First, the computational cost is reduced. Even with a relatively small number of samples, many clustering algorithms become intractably heavy. Second, data noise is significantly reduced because the prototypes are local average of the data and hence less sensitive to random variations than the original data. Third, the two dimensional SOM map allows a topological representation of the data and provides visualization of the clusters. The sequence of operations is as follows:

2.1 Step 1: Data and its Pre-Processing

The CSLT data-set comprises 3479 optic disc images of 100 glaucoma patients and 63 healthy controls, obtained in intervals of 6 months over a period of up to 9 years. Using the software of the Heidelberg Retina Tomograph [11], 17 morphological features were extracted from these images using a surface-fitting algorithm [12]. The features have continuous values and hence required some pre-processing. Since the SOM algorithm uses Euclidian metric to measure distances between data vectors, scaling of variables was deemed to be an important step and we normalized the variance of all variables to unity, and their means to zero.

2.2. Step 2: Data Clustering Using SOM

SOM is based on a competitive learning algorithm which leads to the formation of a topographic map of the input patterns in which the spatial locations (e.g., coordinates) of the units in the lattice are indicative of intrinsic statistical features contained in the input patterns. The principal goal of the SOM is to transform an incoming signal pattern of arbitrary dimension into a two-dimensional discrete map, and to perform this transformation adaptively in a topologically ordered fashion. The SOM learning algorithm involves three main processes—i.e. competition, cooperation, and synaptic adaptation—that constitute two phases of topological ordering of the data—in the first phase broad clustering is done to demarcate the data into potentially broad clusters, and then in the next phase fine-grained clustering is achieved by fine-tuning the emergent clusters and even breaking larger clusters into more meaningful and compact clusters.

In our experiments, the topology of the SOM is a hexagonal lattice. The number of units is set to 5*sqrt (N), where N is number of input data vectors. Given the number of data vectors, we set the SOM to comprise 300 units arranged as 20 rows and 15 columns. The units were linearly initialized by first calculating the eigen-values and eigenvectors of the given data. Then, the map weight vectors are initialized along the two greatest eigenvectors of the covariance matrix of the training data. The SOM was trained using the sequential training algorithm in two phases: a rough training phase comprising 100 epochs starting with a large neighbourhood radius of 12 linearly reduced to 3 with learning rate 0.5. Then second fine-tuning phase runs for 1000 epochs with a small initial neighbourhood radius 3 that is reduced to 1 with learning rate 0.1. In both cases the neighbourhood function is Gaussian and the learning rate function is inversely proportional to time in order to ensure that all input samples have approximately equal influence on the training result. The resultant is a learnt SOM map that manifests clusters of similar data vectors, shown in Figure 1. Next, the projection of trained map is investigated by applying a principle component projection on the trained SOM (as shown in Figure 2). A U-matrix representation of the learnt SOM is used to observe the cluster structure of SOM. It shows distances between neighbouring map units: high values of the U-matrix indicate a cluster border, uniform areas of low values indicate clusters themselves. The U-matrix is achieved by spreading a colour map on the projection in figure 2. Based on the visualization offered by the SOM (figures 1-3), one can notice the presence of data clusters, hence the need to identify the cluster boundaries for a clearer view of the data.

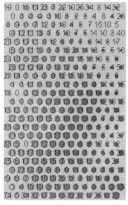 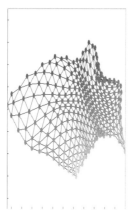 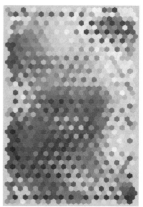

Figure 1: Topological ordering of the data point on the SOM. Also shown is the number of hits each units receives for the entire data-set.

Figure 2: Projection of the learnt SOM depicting the dispersion of the clusters.

Figure 3: U-Matrix representation of the learnt SOM in figure 1. The representation does not exact indicate cluster boundaries.

2.3. Step 3: Fine-Grained Clustering by Defining the Cluster Boundaries

In this step, we attempt to objectively determine cluster boundaries, given our assumption that the distribution of the clusters within the trained SOM is Gaussian. Clustering using finite mixture models is a popular method. In this approach, the input data is generated from a mixture of component density functions where each component density function represents a component. The probability distribution function is given by:

$$f(X_i \mid \Phi) = \sum_{j=1}^{k} \pi_j P(X_i \mid \theta_j)$$

$f_j(Xi\theta j)$ is the probability density function for cluster j, πj is the proportion weight of cluster j, k is the number of clusters, Xi is a input data vector, θj is the set of parameters for cluster j, $\Phi = (\pi; \theta)$ is the set of all parameters and $f(Xi\mid\Phi)$ is the probability density function of our observed data vector Xi given the parameters Φ. There is one method to estimate Φ by calculating Φ which maximizes the log-likelihood, $\log f(Xi\Phi) = \sum_{i=1}^{N} \log f(Xi\Phi)$. In order to get $f(Xi\mid\Phi)$, we find the assignments of all data points to the finite mixtures.

The Expectation Maximization (EM) algorithm [9] is suitable to find distinct components in the case of Gaussian mixtures, it initiates with an estimate of the number of components and an initial guess of the component parameters. In general, the following steps were observed:

Expectation step: This is the E step in which we determine the posterior probability for each component (cluster).

$$E[z_{ij}]^{(t)} = p(z_{ij} = 1 \mid X, \Phi^{(t)}) = \frac{f_j(X_i \mid \theta_j^{(t)}) \pi_j^{(t)}}{\sum_{d=1}^{k} f_d(X_i \mid \theta_d^{(t)}) \pi_d^{(t)}}$$

Maximization step: This is the M step that involves updating the component proportion coefficients, the cluster means and the covariance matrices in each iteration. The proportion coefficient is updated using:

$$\pi_j^{(t+1)} = \frac{1}{N} \sum_{i=1}^{N} E[z_{ij}]^{(t)};$$

In our work we maximize the likelihood of the optic disc image data in distinct clusters given the parameters and our model—a maximum likelihood (ML) measure indicates how well the Gaussian mixtures fit the data into clusters. We use a Bayesian Information Criterion [9], where the best estimate (e.g., number of clusters, parameter estimates) is chosen based on the estimate that gives the highest value of BIC, such that BIC $\equiv$ log $(f(X|\Phi)) - 0.5*P*$log (N), where log (f(X|Φ)) is the log-likelihood of the observed data X given the parameters Φ. P is the number of free parameters in Φ, and N is the number of input data vectors.

We initialize the EM using 10 random re-starts method, and then select a parameter setting to maximize the log-likelihood of our initial clusters. We run the EM clustering with different number of clusters. Table.1 illustrates the number of tested clusters K accompanied with their corresponding BIC values. Note that the BIC is 7953.1 when there are only 2 clusters, and it increases with increase in K such that when K = 5 we get the maximum value of 8799.5 for all reasonable values of K. Hence, we are able to determine that given the trained SOM there are 5 clusters in it that best fit our data (shown in Table 1).

Table 1 - Number of clusters (K) vs. BIC values

# of Clusters (K)	2	3	4	5	6	7	8
BIC value	7953.1	8384.6	8733.5	**8799.5**	8697.1	8616.9	8608.9

To finalize the cluster boundaries for the 5 clusters determined earlier, we calculate the assignment probabilities of each data point to all the cluster labels, the cluster label with the highest probability value is assigned to the data point. Figure 4 shows the SOM with the emergent clusters, the clusters are colour coded for visualization purposes.

3. Evaluation and Concluding Remarks

The partitioned SOM, as shown in figure 4, is evaluated in terms of its efficacy in representing the optic disc images for individual subjects. This method serves two purposes: (1) estimation of the compactness—a measure of cluster goodness—of the emergent clusters vindicating the efficiency of the SOM method; and (2) visualizing the dispersion of multiple observations from any individual subject.

In figures 5 (a&b) we applied multiple optic disk images for two *healthy control* subjects to the learnt SOM. The images were obtained over a time period of 3 and 5 years, respectively, in intervals of 6 months. It may be noted that the data maps in close proximity to each other, and is confined to a small topological area on the map. Moreover, most repeated images activate the same map units, demonstrating little variability within the measurement series of these subjects.

Next, we mapped the data from the *glaucoma patients* to the learnt SOM. For each patient, multiple images were available, obtained at intervals of 6 months. Figure 6(a, b & c) show the results for three glaucoma patients. The results indicate that the data of each of these three patients cluster into different regions of the map. Some dispersion is evident which lead to crossing of the cluster boundaries. This dispersion may be due to several factors, primarily random variability in the measurements as well as systematic changes in optic disc topography over time (disease progression). Based on the evaluation, one can assume that the top-left region represents data from normal subjects, while the emergence of 4 other regions is tantamount to the presence of four morphological patterns of glaucomatous optic discs within the data.

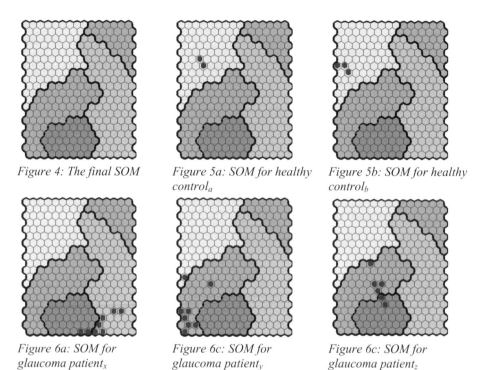

Figure 4: The final SOM   Figure 5a: SOM for healthy   Figure 5b: SOM for healthy
                                 control$_a$ control$_b$

Figure 6a: SOM for   Figure 6c: SOM for   Figure 6c: SOM for
glaucoma patient$_x$ glaucoma patient$_y$ glaucoma patient$_z$

In conclusion, the data-driven clustering approach presented in this paper is the first step towards automated characterization of morphological patterns in optic disc data from healthy subjects and patients with glaucoma.

4. References

[1] Hoskins H, Kass M. Primary open-angle glaucoma, *Becker-Shaffer's Diagnosis and Therapy of the Glaucomas.*, The C.V. Mosby Company, St.Louis, 1989, pp. 277-307.

[2] Epstein D. Primary open-angle glaucoma, *Chandler and Grant's Glaucoma.*, Lee and Febinger, Philadelphia, 2004, pp. 183-231.

[3] Zinser G, Wijnaendts-van-Resand RW, Dreher AW. Confocal laser tomographic scanning of the eye, *Proc SPIE*, vol. 1161, 1989 pp. 337-344.

[4] Ford BA, Artes PH, McCormick TA, Nicolela MT, Leblanc RP, Chauhan BC. Comparison of data analysis tools for detection of glaucoma with the Heidelberg Retina Tomograph. *Ophthalmology* 110 (6):2003, pp. 1145-1150.

[5] Broadway DC, Nicolela MT, Drance SM. Optic disc morphology on presentation of chronic glaucoma. *Eye* 17 (6), 2003, pp. 798-799.

[6] Nicolela MT, McCormick TA, Drance SM, Ferrier SN, Leblanc RP, Chauhan BC. Visual field and optic disc progression in patients with different types of optic disc damage: A longitudinal prospective study. *Ophthalmology* 110 (11), 2003, pp. 2178-2184.

[7] Zangwill LM, Chan K, Bowd C, Hao J, Lee TW, Weinreb RN, Sejnowski TJ, Goldbaum MH. Heidelberg retina tomograph measurements of the optic disc and parapapillary retina for detecting glaucoma analyzed by machine learning classifiers. *Invest Ophthalmol.Vis.Sci.* 45 (9), 2004, pp. 3144-3151.

[8] Haykin S. *Neural Network: A Comprehensive Foundation*. Second Edition. New Jersey: Prentice Hall, 1999

[9] Schwarz G. Estimating the dimension of a model. *The Annals of Statistics*, 6(2), 1978, pp. 461–464.

[10] Vesanto J, Alhoniemi E. Clustering of the Self–Organizing Map, *IEEE Transactions on Neural Networks*, Vol.11(3), 2000, pp.586-600.

[11] http://www.heidelbergengineering.com/

[12] Swindale NV, Stjepanovic G, Chin A and Mikelberg FS. Automated Analysis of Normal and Glaucomatous Optic Nerve Head Topography Images. *Invest Ophthalmol.Vis.Sci.* 2000; 41:1730–1742.

Section 8

Implementation & Evaluation of Clinical Systems

Connecting Medical Informatics and Bio-Informatics
R. Engelbrecht et al. (Eds.)
IOS Press, 2005

3LGM²-Modelling to Support Management of Health Information Systems

Alfred Winter[a], Birgit Brigl[a], Gert Funkat[a], Anke Häber[b], Oliver Heller[a], Thomas Wendt[a]

[a] *Leipzig University, Department for Medical Informatics, Statistics and Epidemiology, Leipzig, Germany*
[b] *University of Applied Science Zwickau, Department of Informatics, Zwickau, Germany*

Abstract

Both regional health information systems and hospital information systems need systematic information management. Due to their complexity information management needs a thorough description or model of the managed HIS. The three layer graph based meta model (3LGM²) and the 3LGM² tool provide means for effectively modeling HIS. The 3LGM² tool has been used to build a model of the health information system of the German federal state Saxony. The model is not only used to support the further development of the Saxonian health information system but also for supporting strategic information management planning in the medical center of Leipzig University. Acceptance of the method depends strictly on its integration in management structures on the institutional, regional, national or even European level.

Keywords:
Hospital Information Systems, Health Information Systems, Information Management, Systems Integration, Organizational Models, 3LGM², Information Systems Modeling

1. Introduction

The driving force for health care has recently been the trend towards a better coordination of care. The focus has been changed from isolated procedures in a single health care institution (e.g. a hospital or a general practice) to the patient-oriented care process spreading over institutional boundaries. Health care providers and health care professionals in a region - and in many cases even worldwide – have to cooperate in order to achieve health for the patient. [1]

The hospital's system for communicating and processing information, i.e. the hospital information system (HIS), is that socio-technical subsystem of a hospital which presents information at the right time, in the right place to the right people [2, 3]. Consequently the heterogeneity of a hospital is reflected by its information system. It has to be actively designed and constructed like a (complex of) building(s) out of different and usually heterogeneous bricks and components.

Widening the scope to the health care region and the necessity for regional cooperation of health care professionals and institutions, we have to claim for the respective cooperation of institutional information systems, e.g. hospital information systems or information systems of practitioners. They shall form again an integrated information system, i.e. the regional health information system (rHIS). Since the complexity of an rHIS is something like the product of the complexity of the information systems included, there is an even stronger demand for systematic information management in the region [1].

Like an architect each hospital's information manager needs a blueprint or model for the information system architecture respectively the enterprise architecture [4-6]. Obviously this holds, a fortiori, for the manager of an rHIS.

The aim of the paper is to illustrate, how models for (r)HIS can be constructed and used for information management tasks. We therefore will shortly introduce the meta-model 3LGM² and the 3LGM² tool for modeling information systems, present a 3LGM² model of parts of the rHIS of the German federal state Saxony, and illustrate some benefits of the model for further development of digital image communication in Saxony and for strategic information management planning in the Leipzig University Medical Center.

2. Method: The Three Layer Graph Based Meta-Model 3LGM² and the 3LGM2 tool

In [7] we proposed the three layer graph-based meta model ($3LGM^2$) as a meta model for modeling HIS. $3LGM^2$ has been designed to support the hospital information management in its enterprise architecture planning (EAP) (see e.g. [6, 8]) activities. Accordingly, it distinguishes three layers of information systems, which especially provide a framework for describing both information processes at the domain layer and communication paths between application components and their interdependencies. $3LGM^2$ is defined using the Unified Modeling Language (UML).

The *domain layer* of $3LGM^2$ describes a hospital independently of its implementation by its enterprise functions. Enterprise functions need information of a certain type about physical or virtual things of the hospital. These types of information are represented as *entity types*. The access of an enterprise function to an entity type can be in a using or an updating manner. The *logical tool layer* concentrates on *application components* supporting enterprise functions. Application components are responsible for the processing, storage and transportation of data representing entity types. *Component interfaces* ensure the communication among application components. The *physical tool layer* consists of physical data processing components (like personal computers, servers, switches, routers, etc), which are physically connected via data transmission connections (e.g. data wires). They carry the application components.

The meta model has been supplemented by the 3LGM² tool [9]. Using 3LGM² as the ontological basis this tool enables information managers to graphically design even complex HIS (Figure 1). It assists information managers similarly to computer aided design tools (CAD) supporting architects. The tool provides means for analyzing an (r)HIS model and thus for assessing the (r)HIS's quality. On the modeling canvas, which dominates the main window of the tool, an information system can be modeled and displayed on three layers as explained before. The three different layers can be viewed and edited separately but also in a multi-layer view. Models especially of rHIS tend to be rather complex. Depending on the complexity and the required level of detail the model diagram may easily get unclear and confusing. The 3LGM² tool includes functionality to extract subsets of models into submodels. It provides a set of predefined analysis functions, which are designed to answer specific questions arising in information management business.

3. Results

3.1 A 3LGM² model of the rHIS of the German federal state of Saxony

Applying the 3LGM² tool we constructed a 3LGM² model comprising a detailed description of the current state of the Leipzig University Medical Center's HIS (UKL-KIS) ("KIS

Universitätsklinikum Leipzig") and important elements of the rHIS of Saxony. The rHIS of Saxony has been further developed by the SAXTELEMED project, funded by the Saxonian ministry of social affairs [10]. The project focused mainly on the exchange of radiological images and intended to improve integration of ambulatory and inpatient care.

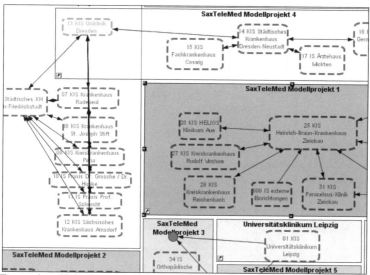

Figure 1 – 3LGM² model of the Saxonian rHIS: Cutout of the overview at the logical tool layer (Names in German since figure is taken from the original model)

Figure 1 gives an overview of the model (SAX-rHIS model) at the logical tool layer. At a low level of granularity it shows the hospital information systems and the information systems of practitioners involved as application components. Frames and respective headers (in German, e.g. "SaxTeleMed Modellprojekt 4") indicate sub projects of SAXTELEMED. Sub projects had been defined at seven medical centers to realize an infrastructure for exchanging radiological images between these centers and healthcare institutions in the neighborhood. Now the ministry's focus is on connecting these 'islands'. One of the frames contains the UKL-KIS. Each frame is linked to the related, more detailed submodel of the respective information system and their components. The 3LGM² tool thereby provides comfortable means for switching between different levels of granularity.

3.2 Supporting further development of the Saxonian rHIS

Investments in Saxonian hospitals – especially those for information technology – are funded by the ministry of social affairs. Respective proposals are reviewed by experts in this field.

The SAX-rHIS model is the only central repository for information concerning the rHIS infrastructure in Saxony. Using this model and the analysis tools provided by the 3LGM² tool, officers in the ministry, reviewers, and applicants among others gain the following advantages:

- If e.g. application components at different sites support the same enterprise function (e.g. report writing), they are linked to the same model element representing the function. In general same real world entities (e.g. communication standards, message types, software products and brands etc.) are represented by the same modelling concepts and elements. So the different information systems' architectures are described in a coherent way, which overcomes the very individual methods usually used in different proposals. Thus the model supports the stakeholders mentioned above in understanding

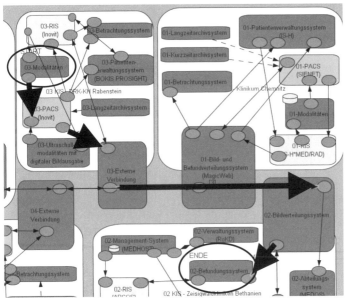

Figure 2 – calculated communication path in the Saxonian rHIS: Images can be sent from the application component "03-Modalitäten" (a modality in the hospital of Rabenstein City) to the component "02-Befundungssystem" (component for supporting writing of radiological findings in the hospital of Bethanien City). (Names in German since figure is taken from the original model)

and comparing different solutions.

• Given, hospital A wants to introduce an application component for radiological imaging, i.e. a radiological modality. In order to avoid unnecessary investments it should be questioned, whether there is already a similar modality in another hospital B and whether it would be possible to transport images from hospital B to A. Appropriate modalities can be found by selecting the function "radiological imaging" at the domain layer; the analysis tool will then highlight the components used for imaging at their different sites. Communication paths on which images could be transported can be found by using a shortest path algorithm implemented in the 3LGM² tool [11]. Figure 2 shows a calculated communication path, if for B the hospital of Rabenstein City and for A the hospital of Bethanien City is taken. The algorithm finds, that images from the modalities in Rabenstein can be sent to the diagnosing system in Bethanien.

3.3 Preparing a strategic information management plan (SIM plan) for the Leipzig University Medical Center

We are now completing the third issue of the SIM-plan for the Leipzig University Medical Center which is valid for 2005 – 2007. Its structure is close to the recommendations in [3]. So, description and analysis of the current state of the UKL-KIS form an important part of the plan.

The sub model of the UKL-KIS in the SAX-rHIS model can be seen as the central repository for information about the UKL-KIS. For example it delivers detailed information concerning interfaces between application systems and the communication server as well as descriptions about redundant storage and communication of patient data. Similar as illustrated in figure 2 it can be derived, what communication links might be used to transport pathological findings to the application systems used at the ward.

For preparing the strategic plan rather simple features of the 3LGM² turned out to be very helpful. Besides features for exporting graphical illustrations like figure 2 we used the reporting facilities of the 3LGM² tool to generate tables describing what application systems are used for particular enterprise functions in different organizational units. As an example figure 3 shows, that for admission of outpatients four different software products are used and that one product (MCS IKA) has been installed as two different and separated application systems. Additionally it can be seen, that in department STRA1 (Radiation Therapy and Radiation Oncology) two different application systems are in duty for the same function. So the table clearly shows a heterogeneity, which is worth to be discussed very seriously.

Even those things, which can not be found in the model turned out to be of mayor

enterprise function	organizational unit	application system (software product)
...	...	...
Admission (outpatient)	KCHA1, GYNA4, IN4A4, HUG, IN1A2, IN1A3, HNOA1, GYNA8, IN1A5, GYNA5, CHZA, AUG, NCHA1, ...	Patient management system (SAP IS-H)
	NET	Outpatient management system NET (MediTec)
	PSYA1	Outpatient management system PSY (MCS IKA)
	RADA1	RIS Radiology information system RAD (MEDOS)
	STRA1	Patient management system (SAP IS-H)
		Outpatient management system STR (MCS IKA)

Figure 3 - Excerpt from the table of enterprise functions, organizational units and application components, generated automatically by the 3LGM² tool

importance for the strategic plan: The lack of powerful interfaces to other health care institutions in the region lead to the clear statement, to concentrate on better integration into the rHIS of Saxony within the next three years.

4. Discussion

Information management in health care regions should be and can be supported by dedicated modeling methods and tools coming from hospital information management. The 3LGM² tool with its means for analysing information processes and related communication paths is suitable to support documentation and planning an (r)HIS and to illustrate its capabilities.

Experiences in Saxony show, that the application of our approach only makes sense, if there is an institution in the region, which feels responsible for information management from a regional perspective. This institution could be a ministry for health, another health care body or even a health care enterprise. Without such an institution a systematic planning and development of an rHIS is impossible – and our approach is not needed.

Experiences at the Leipzig University Medical Center additionally show, that the model can be maintained if (and only if) tactical and strategic information management [12] are closely connected. As a consequence the model has been implemented as the central documentation device for information systems components in the Leipzig University Medical Center. Project managers are obliged to document the information system components created or updated during their projects in the 3LGM² model.

As a conclusion we found, that a systematic organization of information management in health care institutions and regions is the prerequisite for 3LGM² modeling; but modeling and thorough documenting (r)HIS, e.g. using 3LGM², is the basis for systematic information management in health care (regions). This also holds for a nationwide or European perspective.

6. Acknowledgments

This work is part of the research project 'Integrative modeling of structures and processes in hospital information systems' supported by the Deutsche Forschungsgemeinschaft (DFG), grant no. WI 1605/2-1.

7. References

[1]   Winter A. Health Information Systems. In: Yearbook of Medical Informatics. Stuttgart: Schattauer; 2004. p. 359-8.

[2]   Berg M. Medical Work and the Computer-Based Patient Record: A Sociological Perspective. Methods of Information in Medicine 1998: 37 294-301.

[3]   Brigl B, Ammenwerth E, Dujat C, Gräber S, Große A, Häber A, Jostes C, and Winter A. Preparing strategic information management plans for hospitals: a practical guideline. International Journal of Medical Informatics 2005: 74 (1) 51-65.

[4]   Chief Information Officer Council. A Practical Guide to Federal Enterprise Architecture. Boston: Chief Information Officer Council c/o Rob C. Thomas, U.S. Customs Service 7681 Boston Boulevard Springfield, VA 22153; 2001 February 2001. Report No.: http://www.cio.gov.

[5]   Martin J. Information Engineering, Book II: Planning & Analysis. Englewood Cliffs: Prentice Hall; 1990.

[6]   Spewak SH, and Hill SC. Enterprise Architecture Planning: Developing a blueprint for Data, Applications and Technology. New York: John Wiley & Sons; 1992.

[7]   Winter A, Brigl B, and Wendt T. Modeling Hospital Information Systems (Part 1): The Revised Three-Layer Graph-Based Meta Model 3LGM2. Methods Inf Med 2003: 43 544-51.

[8]   Zachman JA. A framework for information systems architecture. IBM Systems Journal 1987: 26 (3).

[9]   Wendt T, Häber A, Brigl B, and Winter A. Modeling Hospital Information Systems (Part 2): Hospital Information Systems (Part 2): Using the 3LGM2 Tool for Modeling Patient Record Management. Methods Inf Med 2004: 43 (3) 256-67.

[10]   Saxonian Ministry for Social Affairs. Saxtelemed [Website]. www.saxtelemed.de; 2003

[11]   Brigl B, Wendt T, and Winter A. Modeling interdependencies between information processes and communication paths in hospitals. Methods of Information in Medicine 2005: in press.

[12]   Winter AF, Ammenwerth E, Bott OJ, Brigl B, Buchauer A, Gräber S, Grant A, Häber A, Hasselbring W, Haux R, Heinrich A, Janssen H, Kock I, Penger O-S, Prokosch H-U, Terstappen A, and Winter A. Strategic Information Management Plans: The Basis for systematic Information Management in Hospitals. In: Yearbook of Medical Informatics. Stuttgart: Schattauer; 2003. p. 431-441.

[13]   Gunasekaran S, and Garets DE. Business value of IT: the strategic planning process. J Healthc Inf Manag 2003: 17 (1) 31-6.

[14]   Thomas M, and Vaughan G. Preparing for the Joint Commission Survey: The Information Systems Perspective. HIMSS Proceedings 1998: 3 369-382.

[15]   Gartner Group. Three Documents for Healthcare IT Planning. Gartner Group's Healthcare Executive and Management Strategies Research Note; 1998. Report No.: KA-03-5074.

[16]   Ward J, and Griffiths P. Strategic Planning for Information Systems. Chichester: John Wiley & Sons; 1996.

Address for correspondence

Prof. Dr. Alfred Winter, Department for Medical Informatics, Statistics, and Epidemiology, Leipzig University, Haertelstr. 16-18, D-04107 Leipzig, Germany, alfred.winter@imise.uni-leipzig.de, www.3lgm2.de

Connecting Medical Informatics and Bio-Informatics
R. Engelbrecht et al. (Eds.)
IOS Press, 2005

497

Specification of a Reference Model for the Domain Layer of a Hospital Information System

Gudrun Hübner-Bloder[a], **Elske Ammenwerth**[a], **Birgit Brigl**[b], **Alfred Winter**[b]

[a] *Institute for Health Information Systems, UMIT – University for Health Sciences, Medical Informatics and Technology, Hall in Tyrol, Austria*
[b] *Institute for Medical Informatics, Statistics and Epidemiology, University of Leipzig, Germany*

Abstract

Objectives: One of the tasks of information management is systematic planning of a Hospital Information System (HIS). However, the description and the analysis of the current state of a HIS typically create high costs and are not well supported. The aim of this paper is therefore to report about the specification of a reference model for the domain layer of a Hospital Information System. Methods: We developed a reference model for the domain layer of a Hospital Information System based on the requirements index for information processing in hospitals for describing the enterprise functions, and based on the object types from the Health Level 7 Reference Information Model (HL7-RIM) for describing the entity types. Result: The developed reference model is a comprehensive hierarchic model of the enterprise functions of hospital information systems. The central enterprise function "patient treatment" for example is described with 35 enterprise functions and 38 entity types on a three-level hierarchy. Discussion: Reference models provide a kind of modelling patterns that can easily be used and adapted to a respective Information System. The availability of reference models should therefore provide a highly valuable contribution to keep the costs for modelling Hospital Information Systems low. We will start to evaluate the reference model by using it in the description of the information systems of a University Clinic of the Tiroler Landeskrankenanstalten GmbH (TILAK), Austria. If this pre-test is positive, it is planned to extend the use of the reference model to the overall Hospital Information System of the TILAK.

Keywords:
Reference models, Hospital Information Systems, Information Management

1. Introduction

Information Systems, especially Hospital Information Systems (HIS), have the task to support patient care, hospital administration and economic business management within hospitals. As a result of the increasing importance of efficient information processing, systematic information management is typically seen as a central management task. The complex processes in health care, which are highly informative and communicative, have to be analysed, controlled and continuously adapted [1]. Hospital Information Systems play a significant role in providing quality health care services [2]. In such a dynamic environment, information and communication technologies (ICT) are taking a leading role and are currently significantly impacting the practice of health care at all levels. The catalyst for change in the health care sector, based on the use of ICT, is the improved quality of health care services and the containment of related costs, as reported in [3].

A HIS is defined in [4] as a sociotechnical subsystem of a hospital, which comprises all information processing as well as the associated human or technical actors in their respective information processing roles. In [5], the central importance of socio-technical and organizational issues for information systems are further discussed. The main objective of information management is described in [6] as the systematic continuous development of the information system as well as the reliable and high-quality operation of the information system. The main tasks of strategic information management in a hospital are "planning", "directing" and "monitoring" of the HIS. The strategic information management is responsible for the overall planning of the whole information system and for the initiation of corresponding projects. A strategic information management plan plays an important role in guiding the deployment of applications and technologies for management service organizations. The IT strategy provides the framework, or "road map", for the chief information officer (CIO) making critical decisions about the deployment of ICT [7].

Before any planning can begin, the HIS's current state must be thoroughly described. This description and the assessment of the current state is the basis for identifying those functions of the hospital that are well supported, and those functions that are not (yet) well supported. Thus application components as well as existing information and communication technology have to be described, including how they contribute to the support of the hospital's functions [4]. However, describing and modelling the Information System from scratch is often found rather labour costly [8-10]. Reference models for a HIS may be very useful here, as they can be used as model patterns. One further advantage of reference models is that they help to standardise HIS terminology between various institutions. This problem of using different terminologies may also be avoided [11].

There are various reference models for hospital information systems as the common basic specification of the British National Health Services (NHS), which is a functional reference model. The framework of the European "Réseau d'Information et de Communication Hospitalier Européen (RICHE) [12] is a process reference model for the activities in hospitals. There exist a lot of reference models for typical processes of a hospital, but functional reference models are hardly available.

The aim of this paper is:

- to report about the development of a reference model for the domain layer of Hospital Information Systems.
- to investigate, based on case studies whether this reference model is in fact useful for the information management of a hospital

2. Materials and Methods

Reference Model of the Domain Layer of a HIS

Reference models can be defined as models that present a kind of pattern for a certain class of aspects. On the one hand these model patterns can help to derive more specific models through modifications, limitations, or add-ons (generic reference models). On the other hand, these model patterns can be used to directly compare models concerning their completeness (nongeneric reference models) [4]. Reference models evolve inductive from consolidation of know how of existing models, documentation of applications, concepts of experts etc., or deductive from theoretical findings [13].

For planning the reference model we used the process model based on Rosemann and Schütte [14], which consists of five phases:

- phase 1: Definition of the problem
- phase 2: Construction of a framework for the reference model
- phase 3: Construction of the structure of the reference model
- phase 4: Completion of the reference model
- phase 5: Application of the reference model

Phase 1:

The basic problem is the great amount of effort needed when modelling hospital information systems. This is both supported by the literature as well as by own experiences in various HIS analysis and modelling projects. The definition of enterprise functions and related entity types especially takes a lot of time. Therefore, we decided to develop a reference model of the domain layer of a HIS.

Phase 2:

We decided to use the three-level graph-based meta-model ($3LGM^2$) for modelling the reference model because it has been approved in some projects in the University Hospital of Innsbruck and in the University Hospital of Leipzig for the static view of a HIS [15, 16]. This meta-model can be used to model HIS on three layers, thus offering more than one point of view on the information model. The domain layer of this meta-model describes the hospital enterprise functions (e.g. patient administration) and the entity types. The entity types present the information on physical or virtual objects in the hospital (e.g. patient, clinical finding). There are two different instances of association between the enterprise functions and the entity types. Enterprise functions either *use* or *create* information about entities of a given entity type.

Phase 3 and phase 4:

We use the $3LGM^2$-meta-model and the respective tool for describing a reference model of the domain layer of a HIS.

Enterprise functions: We decided to take the Heidelberg requirements index for information processing in hospitals [6] as a basis for describing the enterprise functions. The requirement index is separated into two main parts, the "functional requirements" and the "function-independent requirements". The advantage to other comparable work is that these requirements are formulated independent of information processing tools or of information system architectures.

The major enterprise functions are: Treatment of patient, handling of patient records, scheduling and resource allocation, hospital management and research and education. Each major enterprise function consists of several sub-functions, for example, the sub-functions of patient treatment are: patient admission, planning and organisation of patient treatment, order entry, execution of diagnostic or therapeutic procedures, administrative documentation, billing, clinical documentation, discharge and referral to other institutions.

Entity Types: We settle for describing the entity types based on the object types as defined in the Health Level 7 Reference Information Model (HL7-RIM) Version 2.04 [17]. The RIM is the cornerstone of the HL7 version 3 development processes. The HL7 RIM is an object model created as a part of the HL7 version 3 methodology. The RIM intends to provide a coherent shared information model that contains all data content relevant to HL7 messages. The elements of the domain layer of the reference model of a HIS were also adjusted with other resources like HISA [18] and the German Frame architecture for Telematics in Health Care [19].

To check completeness and comprehensibility of the reference model, we organised workshops with employees of the strategic information management of hospitals, with care professionals, with employees of business consultancy for health care institutions and also with medical informaticians.

Phase 5:

For the continuous development of the reference model it is important to consider the whole cycle from the construction to the application of the model. We will start to evaluate the reference model by using it in the description of the information systems of the University Clinic of Radiodiagnostics - Radiology II in Innsbruck, Austria. After the first practical application, an adaptation of the reference is necessary which we will add to the reference model. If this pre-test is positive, it is planned to extend the use of the reference model to the overall Hospital Information System of the Tiroler Landeskrankenanstalten GmbH (TILAK).

3. Results

Our resulting reference model of Hospital Information Systems is hierarchically structured and consists in its actual state of one primary model with the central enterprise function "patient treatment" and the four cross-sectional enterprise functions "handling of patient records", "scheduling and resource allocation", "hospital management" and "research and education". This primary model is then subdivided into 21 submodels that describe the sub-functions according to their refinements. For example, the enterprise function "patient treatment" is subdivided into 8 sub-functions. Four of these sub-functions are associated with further sub-functions.

Figure 1 shows for example a section of the submodels of the enterprise function "patient treatment". According to the 3LGM² tool rectangles denote an instance of the class "enterprise function". Ovals denote an instance of class "entity type". Arrows from rectangles to ovals describe if the enterprise functions use or create information about entities of that entity type.

The hierarchical structure enables a modeller to create a model of the HIS in that degree of refinement that he finds necessary. The modeller can decide, depending on his or her analysis question, to take over the whole or a part of the reference model. He will then only have to adapt and/or refine the elements to his respective information system. Of course; it is also possible to add elements to the model if necessary. The hierarchical structure of the reference model also helps to keep an overview of HIS, and to only show those details that are found necessary in a given situation.

This reference model is available for the modeller in the 3LGM2-Tool.

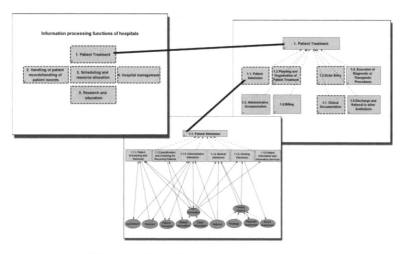

Figure 1 - Section of the submodels of the central enterprise function "patient treatment"

4. Discussion and Conclusion

We developed a reference model for the domain layer of a HIS. We expect that the availability of a reference model will provide a highly valuable contribution to keep the costs for the creation of HIS models low - the modeller can decide, depending on his or her analysis question, to take over the whole or a part of the reference model. He will then only have to adapt the elements to the respective information system.

While creating the reference model, we incorporated available experiences and know how from different domains and from existing models such as HL7-RIM, and we included future users in the development process. This procedure is recommended by [14]; it advises validation through a potential user. We also want to adjust our reference model for the domain layer of a HIS with other approaches like the Reference Model of Open Distributed Processing (RM-ODP) [20].

Using the reference model should not only make modelling easier, but it will also present a kind of central repository of terms of hospital information systems, i.e. a standardised HIS terminology, at least on the domain level (not yet on the tool levels). This standardised terminology will help to make HIS models more comparable.

In the next weeks we will start to evaluate the reference model by using it in the description of the HIS of the University Clinic of Radiodiagnostics - Radiology II in Innsbruck, Austria. If this pre-test is positive, it is planned to extend the use of the reference model to the overall Hospital Information System of the Tiroler Landeskrankenanstalten GmbH (TILAK). The TILAK is a publicly owned holding company established in Tyrol, Austria. The TILAK manages six hospitals, with a total of approximately 2,300 beds, with more than 6,000 staff members, including more than 1,000 physicians [21]. So we have the opportunity to evaluate the reference model by modelling both a whole hospital information system as well as a departmental information system.

We will report on first results during MIE 2005 in Geneva.

5. Acknowledgements

We thank our partners at Information Technology for Healthcare (ITH) in Innsbruck for their fruitful discussion about the reference model. This project is being supported by the Austrian Ministry for Economy and Labour.

6. References

[1]   Brigl B, Ammenwerth E, Dujat C, Gräber S, Große A, Häber A, et al. Preparing strategic information management plans for hospitals: a practical guideline. Int J Med Inf 2005(75 (1)):51-65.

[2]   Ribiére V, LaSalle AJ, Khorramshahgol R, Gousty Y. Hospital Information Systems Quality: A Customer Satisfaction Assessment Tool. Proceedings of the 32nd Hawaii International Conference on System Sciences 1999.

[3]   Tsiknakis M, Katehakis DG, Orphanoudakis SC. An open, component-based information infrastructure for integrated health information networks. Int J Med Inf 2002;68(1-3):3-26.

[4]   Haux R, Winter A, Ammenwerth E, Brigl B. Strategic Information Management in Hospitals. An Introduction to Hospital information Systems. New York, USA: Springer; 2004.

[5]   Kuhn KA, Giuse DA. From hospital information systems to health information systems. Methods Inf Med 2001;40(4):275-87.

[6]   Ammenwerth E, Buchauer A, Haux R. A requirements index for information processing in hospitals. Methods Inf Med 2002;41(4):282-8.

[7]   Lubinski D. Information Strategies for Management Services Organizations. In: Ball M, Douglas JV, Garets DE, editors. Strategies and Technologies for Healthcare Information. New York, United States of America: Springer; 1999.

[8]   Blick KE. Reference Information Model for Clinical Laboratories. RILA as a Laboratory Management Toolbox. Henk M.J. Golschmidt, ed. Clinical Chemistry 1999(45):912a-913a.

[9]   Ten Hoppen AJ, Van der Maas AAF, Helder JC. Modeling of health Care for Information Systems Development. In: H. VBJ, Musen MA, editors. Handbook of Medical Informatics. Heidelberg, Germany: Springer; 1997.

[10] Winter A, Winter A, Becker K, Bott OJ, Brigl B, Gräber S, et al. Referenzmodelle für die Unterstützung des Managements von Krankenhausinformationssystemen (Reference Models to support the Management of Hospital Information Systems). Informatik, Biometrie und Epidemiologie in Medizin und Biologie 1999(30 (4)):173-189.

[11] Fettke P, Loos P. Referenzmodellierungsforschung. Wirtschaftsinformatik 2004;331-340(46).

[12] Réseau d'Information et de Communication Hospitalier Européen (RICHE-2221). Available at: http://www.newcastle.research.ec.org/esp-syn/text/2221.html.Last acces: December 10, 2004.

[13] Schwegmann A, Laske M. Istmodellierung und Istanalyse. In: Becker J, Kugeler M, Rosemann M, editors. Prozessmanagement. 4 ed. Berlin, Germany: Springer Verlag; 2002.

[14] Rosemann M, Schütte R. Multiperspektivische Referenzmodellierung. In: Becker J, Rosemann M, Schütte R, editors. Referenzmodellierung. Heidelberg, Germany: Physica-Verlag; 1999. p. 22-44.

[15] Winter A, Brigl B, Wendt T. Modeling hospital information systems. Part 1: The revised three-layer graph-based meta model 3LGM2. Methods Inf Med 2003;42(5):544-51.

[16] Wendt T, Haber A, Brigl B, Winter A. Modeling Hospital Information Systems (Part 2): using the 3LGM2 tool for modeling patient record management. Methods Inf Med 2004;43(3):256-67.

[17] Health Level 7. HL7 Reference Information Model V01-20; Available at: http://www.hl7.org. Last access: August 10, 2004.

[18] CEN TC251. N-97-024, Healthcare Information System Architecture Part 1 (HISA) Healthcare Middleware Layer - draft. Report no. PrENV12967-1 1997E. Brussels: European Commitee for Standardisation. Available at: http://centc251.org. Last access: August 10, 2004.

[19] German Institut for Medical Documentation and Information (DIMDI) Available at: http://www.dimdi.de/dynamic/de/ehealth/projekte/index.htm. Last access: August 10, 2004.

[20] Tanaka A, Nagase Y, Kiryu Y, Nakai K. Applying ODP Enterprise Viewpoint Language to Hospital Informationsystems. In: Enterprise Distributed Object Computing Conference; 2001. EDOC '01. Proceedings. Fifth IEE International. p. 188-192.

[21] Lechleitner G, Pfeiffer KP, Wilhelmy I, Ball M. Cerner Millenium: The Innsbruck Experience. Methods Inf Med 2003; 42(1):8-15.

[22] Address of correspondence:

Dr. Gudrun Hübner-Bloder, MSc., Institute for Health Information Systems, Eduard Wallnöfer-Zentrum I, 6060 Hall in Tyrol, Austria, Fon: ++43/ (0)508648-3814, Fax: ++43/ (0)508648-3850, Email: gudrun.huebner-bloder@umit.at

Connecting Medical Informatics and Bio-Informatics
R. Engelbrecht et al. (Eds.)
IOS Press, 2005

503

Analysis and Specification of Telemedical Systems Using Modelling and Simulation: the MOSAIK-M Approach

O J Bott[a], J. Bergmann[a], I Hoffmann[a],
T Vering[b], E J Gomez[c], M E Hernando[c], D P Pretschner[a]

[a]Institute for Medical Informatics, Technical University of Braunschweig, Germany
[b]Disetronic Medical Systems AG (Roche Group), Burgdorf, Switzerland
[c]Bioengineering and Telemedicine Group, Universidad Politécnica de Madrid, Spain

Abstract

Background and motivation: INCA (Intelligent Control Assistant for Diabetes) is a project funded by the EU with the objective to improve diabetes therapy by creating a personal control loop interacting with telemedical remote control. Development of telemedical systems generally is a complex task especially in international projects where engineering and user groups with different social and cultural background have to be included into the system development process.

Objectives: To explore if and how sophisticated information system modelling and simulation techniques can improve the development of telemedical systems.

Methods: For system analysis and design the MOSAIK-M approach was chosen. MOSAIK-M means "Modelling, simulation, and animation of information and communication systems in medicine". It includes a generic process scheme, a meta model and a tool environment. The generic process scheme guides modelling projects to produce models of high quality in terms of correctness, completeness and validity. The meta model defines the modelling language.

In INCA MOSAIK-M is used for analysis of the problem domain, specification of the telemedical system and cost/benefit-analysis.

Results: The MOSAIK-M approach was used to create two models: an "As Is"-model of the problem domain and a "To Be"-model of the INCA system. The "As Is"-model of conventional insulin pump based diabetes care comprises submodels of diabetes management, ambulatory and clinical care. The "To Be"-model describes a patient's diabetes management using a smart phone that controls an insulin pump based on continuously measured interstitial glucose. It also describes telemedical care of a patient by diabetologists and a call centre. Both models can be simulated enhanced by visualisation capabilities to explore specific cases or scenarios. This feature proved valuable for the evaluation of both models through domain experts. The "To Be" model is used to guide the implementation of the system. Both models are being augmented by cost structures to support cost/benefit-analysis.

Conclusions: Even a complex telemedical system like the INCA system can be successfully specified using sophisticated modelling and simulation based approaches like MOSAIK-M. The resulting specification is a result of its own and ensures a lasting effect of the definitions and specifications produced during the project. International cooperation and evaluation of the system design prior to its implementation profit from simulation and visualisation capabilities of MOSAIK-M.

Keywords:
Information Systems; Systems Analysis; Model; Simulation; Evaluation; Telemedicine; Diabetes Mellitus

1. Introduction

The combination of insulin pumps for continuous insulin application with devices for continuous blood glucose measurement to achieve a *closed loop* is object of current international research and development [1]. The intended automation of medication raises the question of how to provide the diabetic with professional help in case of technical or medical problems. Goal of the European research project INCA (Intelligent Control Assistant for Diabetes; www.ist-inca.org) is the development of a *closed loop* for type 1 diabetics integrated in a system for telemedical care. INCA is subsequent to the projects M²DM (Multi-access services for telematic Management of Diabetes Mellitus [2]) and ADICOL (Advanced Insulin Infusion using a Control Loop, [3]).

Development of telemedical systems like INCA is a complex task. It requires a professional software development process incorporating identification of requirements as well as a formal specification in preparation of its implementation. Both requirements analysis and system specification profit from the involvement of users and a thorough analysis of the organisational environment of the planned system. This task gets even more complicated in international projects like INCA: different engineering and user groups with different social and cultural background need to be considered as well as national differences in organisational structures and care processes. The successful use of sophisticated information system modelling and simulation techniques in projects concerned with the analysis, design and management of medical information systems in smaller projects (e.g. [4][5]) raises the question if these techniques are suitable to guide the system development process in an effective and efficient way.

2. Materials and Methods

For analysis and design of complex medical information systems (IS) like telemedical systems methods and tools are needed which combine process and organisation modelling with information and application modelling. For the INCA project MOSAIK-M was selected to support system analysis and design.

MOSAIK-M

MOSAIK-M was developed at the Institute of Medical Informatics at the University of Hildesheim and the Technical University of Braunschweig [6] and has been successfully used in several projects since 1995 (e.g. [4][5]). MOSAIK-M is a *methodical framework* and *tool environment* which support modelling, simulation, and animation of information and communication systems in medicine. The methodical framework consists of a *generic process scheme* and an IS *meta model*.

The meta model of MOSAIK-M (Fig. 1) defines the modelling language for creating IS models and is based on the IS definition similar to [6][7]: *An IS is the partial system of an organisation that comprises all information processes and all of the human and technical resources that are involved in these processes in their information processing roles.* The concept of human and technical resources in their information processing roles is formalised by the meta model components *actor* and *actor role*. An actor role is assigned to a *functional unit*. A functional unit itself can contain other functional units or actors. Further organisational structures and interdependencies can be modelled such as representation, delegation, etc.

The behaviour of an actor or a functional unit is described through *processes*. Processes are modelled using a specific Petri-net syntax [8] and can be structured both in a partitive (part-of-relation) and a specialisation (is-a-relation) manner. The MOSAIK-M tool simulates an IS model through stepwise execution of processes by actors. A process execution is initiated by corresponding *events*. While executing a single step of a process, the manipulation of objects or applications by an actor is also simulated, eventually triggering further events. All relevant object structures of the information system, i.e. real world objects and application objects are modelled using the Unified Modelling Language (UML; [9]) that is partly integrated into MOSAIK-M.

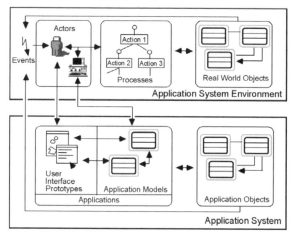

Fig. 1: MOSAIK-M's meta model of medical information systems

To emphasise importance of the computer supported part of IS, the meta model is divided into two parts: the *application system environment* and the *application system* (Fig. 1). Actors, functional units, dynamical behaviour, events and real world objects are parts of the *application system environment*, i.e. all components of the IS except any software-components. Software-components are described within the *application system* submodel. The application system itself is divided into *application objects* and *applications*, which work with them. Applications are structured into *application models* and *user interface prototypes*. Application models as well as application objects are modelled using UML. An application model defines its functionality independent of its implementation and the application objects it works with. It describes the content of any user or system interaction with the application, but does not describe the interaction design. To ease the communication about an application, application models can be exemplified by user interface prototypes that can be incorporated into the simulation of the model.

The MOSAIK-M generic process scheme (Fig. 2) has been developed to guide modelling projects in producing IS models of high quality in terms of correctness, completeness and validity with respect to the objectives of the modelling project. The process scheme, that has to be adapted for specific modelling projects, starts with the *definition of the problem domain*. Objective of this phase is to explicitly define the modelling project's objectives and the boundaries of the relevant subsystems of the IS. The subsequent *analysis* of the problem domain (an existing IS, an organisation for which an IS has to be developed, etc.) using suitable analysis techniques like interviews, observation, etc. should reveal the information needed to construct the IS model. The latter is done in a subsequent *modelling* phase using suitable modelling and simulation tools. This need not to be the MOSAIK-M tool environment. The MOSAIK-M generic process scheme is on principle independent of any specific IS modelling environment.

To ensure correctness, completeness, and validity of the constructed model the project process scheme includes an evaluation phase. The evaluation should be done by members of the analysed organisation and/or domain experts. The perspicuity of the model plays an important role for the expressiveness of the evaluation and its results and can be enhanced by using simulation and visualisation techniques [4][5]. In case the model fails this evaluation the process scheme demands backtracking to former steps of analysis and modelling. If the evaluation is passed, the modelling project is usually finished and the model can be utilised for the objectives of the project.

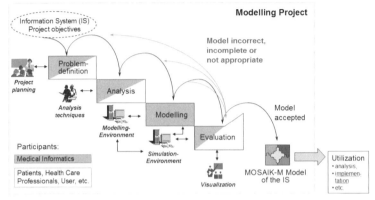

Fig. 2: MOSAIK-M's generic process scheme

INCA and MOSAIK-M

IS models can be used for several purposes like IS analysis, IS design, business process (re)engineering and IS management. MOSAIK-M supports this broad spectrum of IS related projects. In INCA MOSAIK-M is used for IS analysis and design purposes. Therefore the generic process scheme of MOSAIK-M is instantiated three times (Fig. 3): for the project phases "Identification of user needs", "Analysis and system design" and "Deployment and exploitation".

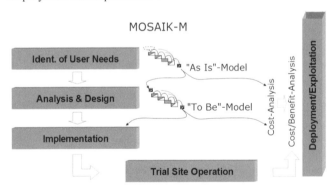

Fig. 3: MOSAIK-M and the INCA-Project

The first iteration of the MOSAIK-M process scheme in the INCA work package "Identification of User Needs" resulted in the so called "As Is"-model that identifies the users of the system, the basic processes and care-flows to support, and the definition and sources of medical data, i.e. the problem domain. The "As Is"-model has been verified by experts of the application field (diabetologists and diabetics).

The "As-Is"-model defines the starting point for stepwise generating a model of a telemedical system (the so called "To Be"-model) that supports the activities within the considered IS of diabetes management. This second instantiation of the generic process model in the INCA project phase "Analysis and Design" leads to a model that includes the system specification useful for the implementation phase. The "To Be"-model has been validated by experts of the application field (diabetologists and diabetics).

The third iteration of the generic process scheme in the INCA project phase "Deployment and exploitation" prepares the cost/benefit analysis of the INCA-system. Both the "As Is"- and the "To Be"-model can be parameterised with current cost factors to determine the total costs of the systems based on the simulation of their models.

3. Results

The "As Is"-model of conventional care for diabetics of the focus group comprises sub-models of diabetes management and insulin pump training. It is divided into an object model with 75 class descriptions, a model of organisational structures (8 institutions and 25 role descriptions) and 156 process descriptions. After setting up a patient description and a blood glucose profile the model allows simulating an episode in the life of a diabetic under conventional insulin pump therapy with outpatient or inpatient treatment if needed.

The "To Be"-model includes 193 class descriptions, a submodel of organisational structures, 341 processes and software-models (358 application models and 112 application objects). It describes the personal diabetes management of a patient using a personal digital assistant (PDA) with mobile phone capabilities, an insulin pump and continuous and discrete blood glucose measurement within a closed loop scenario. Additionally it describes the telemedical care of the patient by diabetologists and a call centre. Modelling and simulation of the INCA-system allow a deeper analysis of the INCA system characteristics and provide possibilities to simulate different control strategies and scenarios.

The required systematic involvement of potential users already in the design process of such a complex system could be realised. Scenarios which describe the *anticipated* way of care and treatment could be effectively discussed with diabetics, physicians and technical partners before implementing the system. Organisational as well as technical problems could be recognised and eliminated in preliminary stages of the implementation. In an international context linguistic differences can be a source of error in system design and particularly in user interface design. The integration of user interface prototypes into the simulation based evaluation of the system helped to identify and resolve these problems. Additionally MOSAIK-M eased project documentation. Communication about intermediate results within the INCA consortium and between the consortium and project reviewers succeeded well based on automatically generated system documentations.

4. Discussion and conclusion

Other methods and tools for IS modelling and/or simulation (e.g. [9]-[12]) are comparable with the MOSAIK-M approach. UML [9] is the de facto standard for modelling object systems. But caused by its generic nature UML does not explicitly support the modelling of MIS consistent to their definition. Comparability of MIS models would depend on agreements beyond UML. Additionally UML does not directly support simulation of UML models and user interfaces. The 3LGM^2 tool [10] allows to model hospital information systems (HIS) from a rather static point of view mainly for HIS-management purposes. For design purposes the approach lacks of process modelling and simulation capabilities. MedModel (see e.g. [11]) focuses on simulation and optimisation of dynamic systems and has a sophisticated animation and visualisation component, but lacks of convenient means to model complex processes and object structures. The ARIS approach [12] is very comprehensive and allows modelling complex organisational structures and processes as well as UML based object and application modelling. The simulation and animation capabilities are rather restricted but can be enhanced by third party tools. Advantages of the MOSAIK-M approach are its sophisticated process modelling and simulation capabilities combined with UML-based object oriented modelling. Moreover functional user interface prototypes can directly be modelled in the MOSAIK-M environment. The MOSAIK-M tool still is a research prototype and not commercially available. Further work is needed to improve the user interfaces of the tool environment. Additionally interfaces to other modelling tools would enhance the exchangeability of modelling results.

The INCA project demonstrates that even a complex telemedical system like INCA can be successfully specified using a sophisticated modelling and simulation based approach like MOSAIK-M. A high degree of user participation within system analysis and design can be realised before implementing the system. The resulting specification is a result of its own and ensures a lasting effect of the definitions and specifications done during the project. Especially in the international context of system development modelling and simulation techniques proved valuable to discuss national differences.

5. Acknowledgments

The project is funded by the EU 5th FWP (IST). We thank our clinical partners O. Schnell and T. Kaupper from the Diabetes Research Institute in Munich (Germany), M. Rigla, E. Brugués and A. de Leiva from the Fundacio Diabem in Barcelona (Spain), and the diabetics and diabetologists which supported our work.

6. References

[1]   Steil GM, Pantaleon AE, Rebrin K: Closed-loop insulin delivery – the path to physiological control. Advanced Drug Delivery Reviews 2004; 56(2): 125-44.

[2]   Bellazzi R, Arcelloni M, Bensa G et al: Design, Methods, and Evaluation Directions of a Multi-Access Service for the Management of Diabetes Mellitus Patients. Diabetes Technology & Therapeutics 2003; 5(4): 621-29

[3]   Hovorka R, Chassin lJ, Wilinska ME, et al.: Closing the Loop: The Adicol Experience. In: Diabetes Technology & Therapeutics 2004; 6(3): 307–18

[4]   Dresing K, Bott OJ, Sturmer KM, Bergmann J, Pretschner DP: Rationalizing the organization and structure of a trauma surgery clinic based on rationing of personal and financial resources--analysis, simulation and conversion using modern data processing techniques, Langenbecks Arch Chir Suppl Kongressbd. 1997;114: 812-4. German

[5]   Lang E, Bott OJ, Pretschner DP: Specification of an Information System for Ophthalmology using Modelling and Simulation Techniques. In: Greens, R.A. et al.: MEDINFO '95 Proceedings, IMIA 1995: 1092

[6]   Rading M: An approach to explorative modelling of computer-based medical information systems (Ein Ansatz zur explorativen Modellierung rechnergestützter Medizinischer Informationssysteme). Dissertation, University of Hildesheim, 1993. German

[7]   Winter A, Haux R: A three-level graph-based model for the management of hospital information systems. Methods Inf Med. 1995; 34(4):378-96.

[8]   Jensen K: High-level Petri nets: theory and application. Berlin a.o.: Springer, 1991.

[9]   Rumbaugh J, Jacobson I, Booch G: The Unified Modeling Language Reference Manual. Addison-Wesley, 2004

[10] Winter A, Brigl B, Wendt T: Modeling Hospital Information Systems (Par 1): The Revised Three-layer Graph-based Meta Model 3LGM2. International Journal of Medical Informatics 2003; 42(5): 544-51.

[11] Groothuis S, van Merode GG, Hasman A: Simulation as decision tool for capacity planning. Comput Methods Programs Biomed. 2001; 66(2-3):139-51.

[12] Scheer A-W: ARIS-Business Process Modeling. Berlin a.o.: Springer, 2. ed., 1999.

Address for correspondence

Dr.-Ing. Dipl.-Inform. Oliver J. Bott, Technical University of Braunschweig, Inst. for Medical Informatics, Muehlenpfordtstr. 23, D-38106 Braunschweig, +49(0)531/391-9505, o.bott@mi.tu-bs.de, www.mi.tu-bs.de

Connecting Medical Informatics and Bio-Informatics
R. Engelbrecht et al. (Eds.)
IOS Press, 2005

Realizing a Realtime Shared Patient Chart using a Universal Message Forwarding Architecture

Achim Michel-Backofen[a], Robert Demming[a], Rainer Röhrig[b], Matthias Benson[b],
Kurt Marquardt[a], Gunter Hempelmann[b]

[a]Department of Medical and Administrative Data Processing, University of Gießen, Gießen, Germany
[b]Department of Anesthesiology and Intensive Care Medicine, University of Gießen., Gießen, Germany

Abstract

The goal of this paper is to describe the clinical needs and the informational methodology which led to the realization of a realtime shared patient chart. It is an integral part of the communications infrastructure of the Patient Data Management System (PDMS) ICUData which is in routine use at the intensive care unit (ICU) of the Department for Anesthesiology and Intensive Care Medicine at the University Hospital of Giessen, Germany, since February 1999. ICUData utilizes a four tier system architecture consisting of modular clients, message forwarders, application servers and a relational database management system. All layers communicate with health level seven messages. The innovative aspect of this architecture consists of the interposition of a message forwarder layer which allows for instant exchange of patient data between the clients without delays caused by database access. This works even in situations with high workload as in patient monitoring. Therefore a system with many workstations acts a blackboard for patient data allowing shared access under realtime conditions. Realized first as an experimental feature, it has been embraced by the clinical users and served well during the documentation of more than 18000 patient stays.

Keywords:
Intensive care, computerized patient record, patient data management systems, networking, Health Level 7

1. Introduction

In 1998 the head of the Department for Anesthesiology and Intensive Care Medicine at the university hospital of Giessen, Germany decided to replace it's running PDMS with a new one that was more adapted to the informational needs of a German hospital especially in the fields of statistical data analysis. The system which is described here is called ICUData and has been developed by a small local company (IMESO Gmbh, Hüttenberg) in close cooperation with the Department of Anesthesiology and Intensive Care Medicine. The goal of the ICUData project was to develop a cost efficient and highly modular PDMS for intensive care units in both large and small hospitals based on today's standard technologies. From the start of the project it has been very clear that ICUData should allow for the integration of all relevant patient data within its clinical database to support detailed online statistical analysis and medical decision making using clinical reminders. With regard to this concept ICUData stands in the tradition of some well known HIS like

HELP [1,2], Regentreat [3,4] and Columbia University [5,6].

2. Materials and Methods

Clinical medicine as a whole and especially intensive care medicine is a highly cooperative tasks which requires the coordinated and shared work of multiple persons of different medical specialties. These persons are often working at different locations within a hospital. The patients continuous treatment requires decisions that should be based on accurate, complete and actual information. It is one of the most important benefits of an electronic patient record that it allows for simultaneous access by many interested users independent of their different physical locations. Nevertheless conventional forms oriented clinical information systems limit the scope of this data access to a relative small number of data items. Also traditional user interface programs need to poll against the database if they want to get the actual state of its data content. This continuous polling can result in serious performance degradation of the clinical database. It becomes especially difficult in the complex monitoring environment of intensive care medicine with it's massive amount of rapidly changing data. Due to the fact that the quality of clinical decisions lives from both the amount and actuality of visible data it was a central goal of ICUData to overcome the limits of form based data display and continuous database polling. ICUData's graphical data chart is designed for a simultaneous display and access to all clinical data groups and instant propagation of all changes in the patients data pool to all interested medical staff.

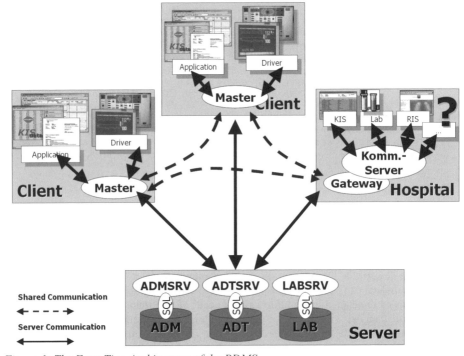

Figure 1: The Four-Tier-Architecture of the PDMS

The basic architecture of ICUData (Figure 1) is a message based four layer client server architecture with message forwarders and application servers interposed between the user interface clients and the relational database management system (RDBMS). ICUData currently utilizes an Oracle RDBMS [7] running on Windows-Server 2003 for its permanent data storage. All message flow between the ICUData components is accomplished using TCP/IP as transport layer and HL7 [8] as a presentation layer. ICUData uses three different logical databases which may also be physically separated over different computers; patient administrative data (ADT), system administration data (ADM) and patient clinical data (LAB). Each application server accesses only one logical database and resides normally on the same computer as the physical database to optimize data throughput. The client layer is also modularized consisting of the authorization and patient management module (ICULogin), the graphical patient chart module (ICUFiles) and a couple of medical device interface processes (MDIP). The basic task of these MDIP's is to transform the vendor dependent content of the medical device data which is received over serial communication interfaces to standard HL7 laboratory messages which could be handled by the ICUData application servers. It's a basic characteristic of ICUData's overall design philosophy that the database design especially for clinical patient data is rather trivial. It currently consists of only two tables which closely resemble the structure of a HL7 laboratory message consisting of header and detail data segments [9]. Also the application servers are rather primitive because their only task is to insert the received HL7 messages into the database or execute HL7 query's. All relevant work regarding to data organization, data manipulation and data presentation is handled within ICUData's object oriented client modules. This has the great benefit of being able to take full advantage of both the logical power of object oriented program design and the computing power of modern workstations. As a result of this strategy, every client module and particularly the graphical patient chart module (ICUFiles) contains always a complete picture of all patient data for its particular domain and a defined timeframe. It is loaded during the startup phase of the program. After the initialization has completed the ICUFiles module has only two ways to expand its actual data set:

- if the user enters new data or manipulates existing data values
- if it receives patient specific data from another data source (e.g. second ICUFiles module which has the same patient open or MDIP receiving monitoring data Mean aterial pressure (MAP) and heart rate

To accomplish data updates from other sources without actually polling the database the ICUData architecture introduces a fourth level of communication between the client modules and the application servers. It's called the ICUMaster communicator. The ICUMaster communicator realized as a Windows service without a user interface. It acts as a universal message forwarding instance. No client server communication can take place without passing an ICUMaster communicator process. The ICUMaster communicator actually gets it´s knowledge about the location of specific clinical database services (which are work units within a specific application server) from a configuration process called ICUMapper. Requests to the ICUMapper are realized as UDP broadcasts. Therefore multiple copies of the ICUMapper could coexist within a network as long as they are sharing a coherent view of system resources. This allows for dynamic relocation of database services without any visible interruption.

The interposition of the ICUMaster communicator into every message flow also opens the way for the most important side effect of this architecture; the realtime shared patient chart. The key to this feature is the introduction of the logical concept of a patient master communicator and related "enter shared communication" messages. The patient master communicator is the ICUMaster communicator which resides on the bedside machine of a patient. Within the overall ICUData communication architecture the patient master communicator takes the role of a centralized forwarder for all data messages related to this specific patient. Any patient chart module residing on another machine at the network can register itself at the patient master communicator by sending an "enter shared communication" message to it. After this registration any message which flows through the patient master communicator (e.g. vital signs monitoring data, user entered data) is also passed to the client module which issued the "enter shared communication" message. The message must be renewed every minute to detect client modules that might have crashed. If the client module on another machine has finished it's activity, it normally terminates the communication with the patient master communicator by sending a "leave shared communication" message. Using this messaging technology the data image of all open patient chart modules could be easily synchronized in realtime. This means that any monitoring data that arrives at the patients master communicator is immediately displayed on all client machines that share the virtual chart. Also if any user drags a data item over the patient chart at one machine the dragging is visualized at all registered machines within the virtual data pipeline in realtime without any polling to the database servers. As a result multiple users may share the same virtual patient chart throughout machines at different locations in the hospital using it as a blackboard for the communication of their patient related decisions.

3. Results

The initial release of ICUData system has been introduced at the surgical ICU unit in February 1999 after one year of development. This short development time was only feasible because all members of the team had some years of experience in developing either hospital information systems [10, 11] or anesthesiology information systems. Since that time more than 18.000 patient stays have been fully documented using ICUData. Most of the strategic data for patient treatment could be moved to the electronic patient record so the need for paper based documentation could have nearly been eliminated. This was only possible through the tight integration of other major HIS resources like central laboratory, microbiology and radiology and even the close coupling to the anesthesiology information system which guarantees an uninterrupted data flow during the surgical treatment of a patient [12]. Especially the data integration benefits from ICUData's strong communication oriented basic architecture. Until now ICUData has also been introduced into the other 5 ICU (interneal medicine, pediatric and neonytology, neurology, neurosurgery, cardiac surgery). Also a intermediate care unit for internal medicine, a ward for pain treatment and two outpatient clinic have been equipped. Throughout all this installations ICUData's ability for realtime sharing of the electronic patient chart (EPR) has been welcomed by the users. The main reason for that may be that the informational model of ICUData is based on an order-performer approach which is strongly supported by the realtime communications aspects of the EPR. Also the basic task of overlooking the data of all patients through the attending physician is simplified because it's possible to put multiple patient charts on a single machine and watch for all the incoming data in realtime. With regard to this aspects the ability for realtime sharing of the electronic patient chart has become an indispensable feature of ICUData in the minds of most users.

4. Discussion

Until now we have detected lots of triggers within the overall systems state that are not directly related to a single patient and therefore not handled with our current forwarding mechanism. These are events like patient bed swaps, patient admissions etc.. We plan to forwarded them by introducing the new instance of a ward and even departmental master communicator. Handling the propagation of these events using a message forwarding architecture could dramatically reduce the frequency of related database requests by simultaneously increasing the correctness of data on all machine's.

5. Conclusion

Whereas the implementation of the ICUData master communicator was an integral part of the ICUData communications architecture to allow for multiple client modules, the project of a shared patient chart has been considered at the first glance as somewhat exotic and experimental for the initial release of ICUData. Surprisingly this exotic feature became very rapidly a central part of the end users daily work exposing some reliability and performance problems of the software. Once accepting the strategic role of this feature the problems could be fixed within the next two months of practical use. Since June 1999 the shared patient chart works rather well and has been established as an integral part of the daily work.

6. Acknowledgements

The authors thank the members of the IcuData developer team of the IMESO company for there support and critical review during the preparation of this article.

7. References

[1] Gardner, RM, Pryor TA, and Warner HR. The HELP hospital information system: update 1998. Int.J.Med.Inf. 54:169-182.

[2] Stanley M.Huff, Peter J.Haug, Lane E.Stevens, Robert C.Dupont, T.Allan Pryor. HELP The Next Generation: A new Client-Server Architecture. Judy G.Ozbolt, editor. Transforming Information, Changing Health Care. Eighteenth Annual Symposium on Computer Applications in Medical Care 18, 271-275. 5-11-1994. Washington, Hanley & Belfus.

[3] McDonald C, Overhage JM, Dexter PR, Tierney WM, Suico JG, Zafar A, Schadow G, Blevins, J. Warvel, J. Meeks-Johnson, L. Lemmon, T. Glazener, A. Belsito, D. Lindbergh, B. Williams, P. Cassidy, D. Xu, M. Tucker, M. Edwards, C. Wodniak, B. Smith, and T. Hogan. 1999. The Regenstrief Medical Record System 1999: Sharing Data Between Hospitals. Proc.AMIA.Symp.1212.

[4] Clement J.McDonald, J.Marc Overhage, William M.Tierney, Paul Dexter, Greg Abernathy, Lisa Harris et al. The Regenstrief Medical Record System (RMRS): Physician use for input and output and Web browser based computing. James J.Cimino, editor. Beyond the Superhighway: Exploiting the Internet with Medical Informatics. 1996 AMIA ANNUAL FALL SYMPOSIUM 20, 989. 26-10-1996. Washington, Hanley & Belfus.

[5] Stephen B.Johnson, George Hripcsak, Joan Chen, Paul Clayton. Accessing The Columbia Clinical Repository. Judy G.Ozbolt, editor. Transforming Information, Changing Health Care. Eighteenth Annual Symposium on Computer Applications in Medical Care 18, 281-285. 5-11-1994. Washington, Hanley & Belfus.

[6] James J.Cimino, Socrates A.Socratous, Paul D.Clayton. Internet as Clinical Information System: Application Development Using the World Wide Web. Journal of the American Medical Informatics Association 2[5], 273-284. 1995.

[7] Oracle9, Release 9.1.0.2 Documentation, Oracle Corporation, 500 Oracle Parkway, Redwood City, CA 94065, USA

[8] Health Level Seven, Inc. The Standard for Electronic Data Exchange in Health Care, Version 2.2 © 1994, 3300 Washtenaw Ave., Sweet 227, Ann Arbor, MI 48104-4250, USA

[9] Renske K.Los, Astrid M.van Ginneken, Marcel de Wilde, Johan van der Lei. OpenSDE: Row Modeling Applied to Generic Structured Data Entry. Journal of the American Medical Informatics Association 11[2], 162-165. 2004

[10] Michel A, Zörb L, Dudeck J: Designing a Low Cost Bedside Workstation for Intensive Care Units: in Proceedings of the 20th. Symposium on Computer Applications in Medical Care, Washington 1996

[11] Prokosch HU, Dudeck J, Junghans G, Marquardt K, Sebald, Michel A: WING - Entering a New Phase of Electronic Data Processing at the Gießen University Hospital. Methods of Information in Medicine 1991, 30:289-298

[12] Fuchs C, Benson M, Michel A, Junger A, Brammen D,Marquardt K, Hempelmann G: Anbindung eines Anästhesie-Informations-Management-Systems an das Patienten-Daten-Management-System einer Intensivstation. Medical Infobahn for Europe. Proceedings of MIE2000 and GMDS2000. eds. Arie Hasman, Bernd Blobel, Joachim Dudeck, Rolf Engelbrecht, Günther Gell, Hans-Ullrich Prokosch, IOS Press 2000, Amsterdam

8. Address for correspondence

Dr. Rainer Röhrig, Dept. of Anaesthesiology, Intensive Care Medicine and Pain Therapy, University Hospital of Giessen, Rudolf-Buchheim-Str.7, D-35392 Giessen, E-Mail: rainer.roehrig@chiru.med.uni-giessen.de

Connecting Medical Informatics and Bio-Informatics
R. Engelbrecht et al. (Eds.)
IOS Press, 2005

Designing Web Services in Health Information Systems: From Process to Application Level

Juha Mykkänen[a], **Annamari Riekkinen**[a], **Pertti Laitinen**[b],
Harri Karhunen[c], **Marko Sormunen**[a]

[a]University of Kuopio, HIS R & D Unit, IT Service Centre, Kuopio, Finland
[b]University of Kuopio, Shiftec, Dept. of Health Policy and Management, Kuopio, Finland
[c]University of Kuopio, Dept. of Computer Science, Kuopio, Finland

Abstract

Service-oriented architectures (SOA) and web service technologies have been proposed to respond to some central interoperability challenges of heterogeneous health information systems (HIS). We propose a model, which we are using to define services and solutions for healthcare applications from the requirements in the healthcare processes. Focusing on the transition from the process level of the model to the application level, we also present some central design considerations, which can be used to guide the design of service-based interoperability and illustrate these aspects with examples from our current work in service-enabled HIS.

Keywords:
Health information systems, Services, Integration, Interoperability, Interfaces

1. Introduction: Service-oriented architectures for HIS?

Central challenges for Health Information Systems (HIS) include lack of reuse, redundant data and functionality and heterogeneous technologies. Adaptation to new requirements and multiple medical cultures and integration with existing systems is difficult in constantly changing health environment. [1,2]. There are also growing demands to coordinate or automate various processes, and to find common description and ways to execute them via electronic transactions to support seamless and quality care to the patients [3-6].

Service-oriented architectures (SOA) have been suggested as a design and technology strategy of complex enterprise application environments [7,8]. SOA includes practices and frameworks that enable application functionality and information to be provided and consumed as services [8-10]. From technical viewpoint SOA is essentially a collection of software services that communicate with each other over network to pass data or to coordinate some activity. Services can be implemented using different technologies, and can encapsulate functionality and information from existing applications, thus allowing the reuse of the existing IT investments. [10,11,7]. Thus, the main expected benefits of SOA seem to support well the requirements of heterogeneous IS domains such as healthcare.

We argue that a SOA-based approach must support different *interoperability needs*, *different degrees of integration*, different *messaging patterns*, and different phases of the *development process.* In this paper we propose a model for design considerations that should be perceived in service-based application development and integration for HIS.

2. Methods: Web services and service design approach

Web services are software components or applications which interact with one another using XML-based Internet technologies [12,5,13]. They offer a platform-neutral interfacing and communication mechanism, have wide infrastructure support and have significantly increased the interest in SOAs [7]. However, two distinct approaches to web services can be identified [14]. The *procedural* approach focuses on bottom-up application integration. It is based on the architecture of the existing remote procedure call (RPC) middleware, and current SOAP, WSDL and UDDI specifications. The *document-oriented* approach focuses on top-down business exchanges, and tries to describe the elements of (commercial) exchange, including the technology solutions. It is based on electronic commerce, documents and loosely-coupled messaging, and includes e.g. ebXML specifications.

We are using a high-level service-oriented approach to analyse healthcare processes and requirements and to define services and solutions, which support the needs of health professionals and patients (see Figure 1). We have adapted the viewpoints from Gartner's four-platform model [9]. The *producer platform* includes tools and technologies for Web services. The *provider platform* hosts services in the enterprise. The *management platform* contains solutions for managing the infrastructure for Web services. The *consumer platform* consists of techniques by which the services are used. The four-platform framework, however, focuses mainly on technical issues and does not represent the way the organizations really use Web services [15]. In comparison to [9], the solutions require a broader approach in which the requirements of the processes and the applications drive technical solutions. We examine the design considerations on three levels – *process, application and platform*, from the four viewpoints – provider, consumer, production and management. On each level the viewpoints require different kinds of considerations. The process level is the most relevant to the healthcare domain. While moving from the process level to the application level and to the platform level, the design considerations become more independent from the healthcare domain and more technology-oriented.

The viewpoints on the *platform level* have been presented above. On the *application level,*

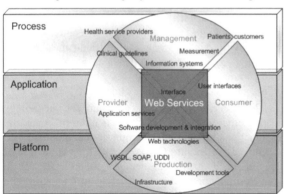

Figure 1. Service-oriented analysis and design approach on Process, Application and Platform levels and some example considerations on these levels.

software services are providers, and applications that use services are consumers. Management is the control and maintenance of the applications and the services, and production refers to the tools, technologies and methods used in the development on the platform level.

On the *process level* the service providers are personnel who provide health services to their customers, including patients. The management of the processes, and services themselves are supported by different conventions and especially information systems, which links process level to the application level. The process level must drive all the application design decisions: its requirements must be addressed in the design of the solutions and services on the application level using the tools and technologies on the platform level. On each level, consumer, provider, management and production issues must be addressed to consider the needed aspects of a given solution.

3. Results: Design considerations for healthcare software services

In this paper, we consider the linkage of process level to the application level design. We present several questions, whose answers guide the design of different types of service-oriented solutions. To define basic solutions for service specifications, we apply the integration specification process in [16]. In particular, we focus on the phase where the main design decisions are made. This phase has the following steps:

1. Select the set of *requirements* to be included in the services, and the basic *integration model*.
2. Evaluate and select the content *standards* and other specifications to be utilised. These standards may have explicit or implicit consequences to the further design.
3. Link the *information and functions in the participating systems* to the requirements.
4. Identify and name the *participating components* (e.g. providers and consumers).
5. Map the selected requirements to the *responsibilities* of the identified components.
6. *Refine the interaction solution*, for example the deployment and interaction style.
7. Identify *integration points* in the architecture of the participating systems. Refine the responsibilities of the components, identify possible extension needs.
8. Specify *interaction sequences*, which may also contain user interaction.
9. Specify service *interfaces*. Information contents and semantics are specified as e.g. document definitions in document style, and as parameter definitions in procedural style, and functional needs as e.g. operation names or document/message types.
10. Define features as either *required, optional* or *extensible* from all implementations.
11. Refine the *requirements* for implementations or further technical specifications.

We propose the following questions to guide the solution specification, especially in steps 1 and 6. The design implications of different options are also discussed briefly. The list in non-exhaustive, but according to our experiences, it covers the main considerations to guide the design of services.

a. What is the main *integration model*? Integration models can be *information-oriented, service-oriented, user-driven or process-oriented* (adapted from [17]). If the main requirements are focused on information sharing or transfer, document approach with declarative messages or documents is often selected. If the main requirements are computationally oriented, e.g. shared functionality, a service (or API) interface with imperative operations is a natural fit. If the main requirements focus on usability or a consistent view to information or several applications, it should be considered whether to use services or other approach, although service-oriented context management interfaces or visually-oriented services such as WSRP (Web Services for Remote Portals) [18] can also be used. If the main requirements are focused on processes, a breakdown of the steps of the process into smaller (information or service) interactions, and the use of process-oriented specifications such as BPEL (Business Process Execution Language) should be considered.

b. What is the required level of *adaptability*? Changes can occur in the information contents, the context of the system, or the system itself. In the procedural style, exact parameters for operations are defined. This results in precise standard interface, and can be supported by automated tools. In the document style, there are more chances for adaptation. To support maximum flexibility, a two-level approach with e.g. (meta) reference model and constraining archetypes can be selected [2], but this type of solution may impose difficulties for existing systems due to the changes in the development approach. Requirement may also be to encapsulate changes, e.g. to support legacy migration, or to provide content-neutral operations, which may carry different information (e.g. templates) in different settings.

c. Is the goal to use a *shared/unified* model, or *federation/mediation* between the participants? In information-oriented integration, a shared document repository and message-based document transfer using messaging broker to copy information from one system to another are examples of unified and federated solutions, respectively. Common service interfaces such as those of OMG Healthcare DTF [4] are examples of shared service-oriented model.

d. What is the required level of *granularity*? For rapid and repeated interaction, e.g. related to the atomic user actions, small procedure calls are suitable as parts of a larger service. For batch-oriented or cross-organizational transactions, with large amounts of diverse information, document-oriented messaging can provide benefits.

e. How *tight integration* is aimed at? Typically in a shared service, only an identification or a reference to a given entity is given, whereas in loose integration (e.g. between organizations), all the relevant information is transferred between the systems. Tight integration often requires guaranteed availability of the invoked service, whereas in document style messaging, guaranteed delivery is aimed at. Also bidirectional invocations and strict data typing tighten the integration solutions.

f. What is the *number of consumers and providers*? In RPC/API style, point-to-point request/response model is usually used between the consumer and the provider, and registries are used for addressing. In document style, mediating brokers or buses can route and copy the messages to several consumers or providers. This requires additional addressing and routing specifications and infrastructure.

g. What is the *message exchange pattern,* e.g. is a response needed and should it be immediate? While RPC is inherently designed for user-driven call-reply with quick response, this can also be implemented with document-oriented services.

h. Does the provider need to maintain consumer-specific *state, context* or *session* between invocations? Common design recommendation for services is to avoid stateful services to ensure performance. However, state management may be an explicit requirement for a service (e.g. user-specific context repository, authorized session management or to maintain state in lengthy processes).

To efficiently solve design problems, answers should be specified for each of these questions. After this it is relatively straightforward to select technologies and tools capable of supporting the needed solutions, or to select another approach instead of services.

4. Discussion: Examples of different types of service specifications

In Table 1, we have compared three solutions for software services from the HIS projects we have been involved in, using the approach above. DRG classification services are used for assessment of resource utilisation in healthcare facilities for billing or care assessment. EPR archive interfaces support the storing of clinical documents in archives. Context repository interfaces are used to provide single sign-on and application synchronization to improve the usability of various clinical and administrative applications.

As seen in Table 1, the answers to the specified questions point the designs for different cases towards different types of services: in DRG and Context interfaces, API/RPC approach is used, whereas documents and integration platforms are utilised for EPR archiving. Procedural services are useful in interactive requirements and e.g. within one organization, whereas document-oriented interfaces are often used in situations where the integration is more loose and flexible, and the infrastructure or applications are controlled by different organizations. For stabile functional and computational requirements where the participants are well-known, API-style invocations are used, where automated tools hide many technical aspects. For cross-organizational, federated, or one-to-many solutions, document style and messaging platforms are needed, typically along with additional work. Such solutions include Enterprise Service Bus (ESB) approach [3], which includes also SOA and web services. In any selected integration model, standards ease the implementation and improve the tool support.

Table 1. Comparison of three service scenarios.

Scenario	DRG classifier interfaces	EPR archive interfaces	Context repository interfaces
Requirement	Produce information based on diagnosis and other information for the assessment and comparison of resource consumption	Provide a common interface for archiving different types of clinical documents related to a patient (e.g. referrals, prescriptions)	Maintain user-specific context information for several applications (user, patient, encounter etc.)
Integration model	service	information	user
Adaptability	static, parameters well-known	dynamic, different types of documents, support for local variation	static interface, extensible subject definitions
Unified or federated	unified model (common service)	unified model (common archive) and federated model (may need local content translations)	unified model (common service)
Granularity	fine-grained operations and parameters	large-grained documents	fine-grained operations and parameters
Tight/loose	tight, common service must be available	loose, archive may be queued, notification	tight, but applications work also without the service
Consumers / providers	many consumers use one provider	many consumers use one provider, variations exist	many consumers use one provider
Message exch. pattern	immediate response needed	no immediate response needed, guaranteed delivery needed	immediate response
State	stateless	stateless	stateful
Additional conside-rations	can be used in interactive and/or batch-oriented way	clinical documents, simple transfer/ archiving interface, additional digital signatures	low implementation threshold for participating applications, no bi-directional invocation

5. Conclusions and future work

We presented an approach and a set of considerations for analysing and designing software services in healthcare applications. We illustrated the approach with examples of different types of solutions. Our model considers essential differences in service designs to support different requirements in the healthcare domain. This model alone does not cover the requirements elicitation on the process level, or the most technical platform considerations. We are using the presented approach to define several healthcare-specific solutions, and also participating in the standardization of service interfaces and specification approaches.

6. Acknowledgements

This work is part of the SerAPI and SOSE projects, funded by the National Technology Agency of Finland TEKES grants no. 40437/04 and 70070/04 together with a consortium of software companies and hospitals.

7. References

[1]   Van de Velde R. Framework for a clinical information system. Int J Med Inf 57 (2000) 57-72.

[2]   Beale T. Archetypes: Constraint-based Domain Models for Future-proof Information Systems. OOPSLA 2002 workshop of behavioural semantics, 2002.

[3]   Chappell D. Enterprise Service Bus. O'Reilly, 2004.

[4]   OMG Healthcare Domain Task Force. CORBAmed Roadmap, Version 2.0 (draft). OMG Document CORBAmed/2000-05-01; 2000.

[5]   Wangler B,   Åhlfeldt R-M, Perjons E. Process Oriented Information Systems Architectures in Healthcare. Health   Informatics Journal 2003: 4: pp. 253-265(13).

[6]   Ryynänen O-P, Kinnunen J, Myllykangas M, Lammintakanen J, Kuusi O. Suomen terveydenhuollon tulevaisuudet. Skenaariot ja strategiat palvelujärjestelmän turvaamiseksi. Esiselvitys. Eduskunnan kanslian julkaisu 8/2004. In Finnish. (The Future of Finnish Health Care - Strategies and scenarios to secure health care services in Finland in the future).

[7]   Natis YV. Service-Oriented Architecture Scenario. Gartner group, 2003. (28 Dec 2004.) Available at http://www4.gartner.com/DisplayDocument?ref=g_search&id=391595.

[8]   Champion K. SOA: the new architecture that leverages the old. Developers.net, 2004 (28 Dec 2004.) Available at http://www.developers.net/node/view/106.

[9]   Smith D. Web Services Architecture: A Four-Platform Framework. TopView, 16 May 2002. Gartner group, 2002.

[10]   Plummer D. A Closer Look at Service-Oriented Architecture. Bea dev2dev, Bea Systems, 2003. (3 Jan 2005) Available at http://dev2dev.bea.com/trainingevents/webinars/Gartner_02_14.jsp.

[11]   Sprott   D.   Moving   to   SOA.   Cbdi   forum,   2003.   (3   Jan   2005)   Available   at http://roadmap.cbdiforum.com/reports/soa/ index.php.

[12]   Aissi S, Malu P, Srinivasan. E-Business Process Modeling: The Next Big Step. IEEE Computer 2002:35(5):55-62.

[13]   Turner M, Zhu F, Kotsiopoulos I, Russel M, Budgen D, Bennet K, Brereton P, Keane J, Layzell P, Rigby M. Using Web Service Technologies to create an Information Broker: An Experience Report. Proc. of the 26th Int. Conf. on Software Engineering, IEEE, 2004, pp. 552-561.

[14]   Alonso G, Casati F, Kuno H, Machiraju V. Web Services Concepts, Architectures and Applications. Springer, 2004.

[15]   Schmelzer R.& Bloomberg J. Retiring the Four-Platform Framework for Web Services. Zapthink, 2003. (28 Dec 2004.) Available at http://www.zapthink.com/report.html?id=ZAPFLASH-12032003.

[16]   Mykkänen J., Porrasmaa J., Rannanheimo J, Korpela M. A process for specifying integration for multi-tier applications in healthcare. Int J Med Inf 2003:70(2-3):173-182.

[17]   Linthicum D. Leveraging the heritage – Approaches to Integrating Established Information Systems. Intelligent EAI, April 15, 2003. CMP Media LLC, 2003.

[18]   Reshef E. Building Interactive Web Services with WSIA & WSRP.Web Services Journal 2002:12(2):2-6.

7. Address for correspondence

Juha Mykkänen, University of Kuopio, HIS R & D Unit, P.O.B. 1627, Fin-70211 Kuopio, Finland, Juha.Mykkanen@uku.fi

Connecting Medical Informatics and Bio-Informatics
R. Engelbrecht et al. (Eds.)
IOS Press, 2005

521

Medflow – Improving Modelling and Assessment of Clinical Processes

Samrend Saboor[a], Elske Ammenwerth[a], Manfred Wurz[b], Joanna Chimiak-Opoka[c]

[a] *Institute for Health Information Systems, UMIT - University for Health Sciences, Medical Informatics and Technology, Hall in Tyrol, Austria*

[b] *Department for Information & Software Engineering, UMIT, Hall in Tyrol, Austria*

[c] *Institute of Computer Science -University of Innsbruck, Austria*

Abstract:

Introduction: Clinical processes are meant to restore the patient's health but often show weaknesses regarding their efficiency (e.g. ineffective task distribution for clinicians, long waiting times for patients). In order to improve these processes an assessment of their quality is needed. This assessment is based on adequate process models and proper systematic assessment procedures. Both seem not sufficiently present in the Activity Diagrams of the Unified Modeling Language (UML) or ARIS Event-driven Process Chains (EPC). *Objectives:* The aim of this paper is to develop and test a process modelling method which explicitly includes all details of clinical processes necessary for a systematic and even semiautomatic quality assessment. *Methods:* We propose a model which is separated into process model, tool model, organisation model and information model. Its visualisation is based on the extended UML Activity Diagrams. *Results:* After being defined formally the graphical elements of the proposed model were implemented into a commonly used modelling software. As a first validation step, various versions of the process of ordering a radiological examination were modelled. *Discussion:* The advantage of our modelling approach is the combination of different aspects (i.e. description of processes, used tools, information objects and actor roles) into an integrated model so that details important for a systematic process assessment are now more explicitly included than in Activity Diagrams or EPC. Further evaluations will help to improve the model and to develop strategies for the semi-automatic analysis.

Keywords:
Process Assessment (Health Care), Process measure, Public Health Informatics, Information System

1. Introduction

Clinical processes, as a specialisation of the classic service processes, are meant to restore the patient's health or at least allay his/her disease. But in practice, the achievement of this aim is aggravated by the nature of healthcare institutions.

A main characteristic of health care is that several healthcare providers (e.g. hospital departments) are involved in the treatment of an individual patient. Each department has its own workflow, role definitions, objectives and fiscal interests [1]. This interdepartemental and interprofessional separation of tasks is seen as one main reason why clinical processes often show weaknesses, e.g. with regard to their efficiency [2] [3] [4]. The only person involved in all areas of the clinical process is the patient himself [1] – making the clinical process unique, as every patient and his or her situation and therefore diagnostic and therapy is unique. Therefore, comprehensive planning of an individual clinical process is often difficult.

These and further characteristics must be taken into account, in order to be able to improve the clinical processes. A basic step of a process improvement is an adequate and systematic process assessment and optimisation which is also known as business process reengineering (BPR). The BPR uses detailed process models (business process models - BPM) which are analysed systematically for weaknesses within the modelled processes in order to develop solutions for them [5]. In healthcare, the systematic analysis of the modelled processes is still missing [6]. Also the modelling methods show deficiencies when applied on processes in healthcare. Established process modelling methods like Activity Diagrams of the Unified Modeling Language (UML) or ARIS Event-driven Process Chains (EPC) claim to be generally applicable – however, important details for process assessment are either disregarded or included just implicitly. For example, it is important to mark clearly the beginning and end of alternative process segments, in order to be able to compare them and to find the best one. For instance, some details could certainly be modelled with the other diagrams of UML, but then the necessary details would be scattered on several models.

Models based on the common Activity Diagrams or EPC notation seem not optimal for the development of systematic assessment procedures. As an important precondition an adequate modelling method must be developed or rather existing modelling methods must be improved.

Aim of this paper

The aim of this paper is to develop and test a process modelling method that includes details of clinical processes necessary to describe and evaluate their quality in a systematic and partly semi-automatic way.

2. Material and methods

As a first step we searched systematically for essential process attributes in literature from fields like process and quality management. The main question we asked was: "Which details are necessary to model processes in health care properly?" Further, we interviewed healthcare professionals and reviewed reports of process analysis in hospitals to find out characteristics of clinical processes. Finally we compared our results with the abilities of UML Activity Diagrams (in version 2.0) and the ARIS EPC – both are often used in health care and versatile modelling software for them is available. We also took several extensions for those methods into account: for the Activity Diagrams the Eriksson-Penker Extensions (EPE) [7], for the EPC the extended EPC (eEPC) and the object-orientated EPC (oEPC) [8] [9].

We found that none of those available process modelling methods seemed suited for our task of a systematic and semi-automatic assessment of clinical processes. The following list shows the main deficiencies we found:

1. Both, Activity Diagrams and EPC, just *model* processes. There are no additional information or special views on models that explicitly support the *assessment* of the quality of the process.
2. The way the information processing tools are described is often rather simplistic – for example, various kinds of tools are described in the same way (e.g. workstations, software tools, paper-based folders, servers, modalities etc.). A differentiation in e.g. hardware and software is often not done (e.g. EPC), however we found this necessary to be able to detect weaknesses such as use of heterogeneous software, or necessary change of hardware tools during one activity. For instance in UML, Deployment Diagrams must be used in addition to Activity Diagrams to model this as-

pect. In order to assess the quality of a treatment process, models of these two kinds must be compared. Further, Deployment Diagrams just focus on the relationship between software components and the hardware they are implemented on – paper-based tools (e.g. folders) are not considered.

3. It is not possible to show clearly that several actors synchronously take part in a single activity , e.g. two people negotiating a meeting. If one of these actors is missing, the process may stuck - it must therefore be possible to express their strong connection. Activity diagrams for instance only have parallel transitions (fork and join) where all parallel control flows are totally independent.

4. Generally exceptions in clinical processes (e.g. patient does not appear for examination) can cause mistakes. Therefore, exceptions as well as their handling have to be included into a process model. Their visualisation is important to be able to improve the exception management, which EPC do not provide.

5. There is no possibility to represent the hierarchy of the actors in hospital, their responsibilities and what each is allowed to do (e.g. data access permissions, competences). This seems, however, necessary to be able to describe exceptions in the task handling properly (e.g. the effects when an actor with high responsibilities is missing).

6. Activity Diagrams and EPC have no possibilities to point out the beginning and end of alternative process segments clearly – which can also consist of several complete XOR- or AND-branches. It is important to be able to compare alternatives and find their weaknesses in order to finally determine the best alternative.

7. In this context there is also no standardised possibility to indicate the probability of each alternative. These probabilities are important for the comparison of the alternatives – because they have to be examined more closely.

8. There is no possibility to model a clear data flow, i.e. creation, usage and eventual destruction of information objects. This is important to be able to find weaknesses in the information handling (e.g. redundancies, information objects get lost).

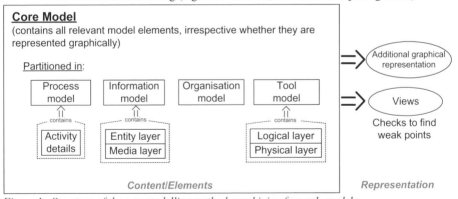

Figure 1 - Structure of the new modelling method, combining four sub-models.

The described requirements for an extended process modelling method can be sorted into four groups: those related to the process itself (1, 3, 4, 6, 7 - process model), those of the organisation of actors (5 - organization model), those of the used tools (2 - tool model) and information objects (8 - information model). Thus our new developed process model (figure 1) consists in fact of four integrated sub-models - each concentrating on the aspects of just one of the groups. The sub-models contain the relevant information irrespective whether these are later being visualised in a process modelling tool by graphical elements or not (separation of content and representation). A central meta model formally expresses the linking of the elements of the four sub-models.

Also the graphical representation is based on the elements of the Activity Diagram. It is extended by selected elements of each sub-model (table 1 - related models in parentheses):

Table 1 – Some new added graphical model elements

	Element	Meaning
tool model	Software tool / PC	A *tool* – represents an IT- or paper-based application system (e.g. software tool) and the implementing physical system (e.g. PC). Besides it can store the information about the location of the physical system.
information model	Picture / digital	An *information object* – is an abstraction of a real-world entity. It can represent a patient record or a picture etc. The lower layer tells how the information object is stored/ transmitted (digital, paper or verbal)
process model	◇	*Alternative process flow* – it marks the beginning and end of a process segment which has several possible alternatives.
	Note	*Alternative process actors* – it represents those alternatives which only differ in the actors who perform the highlighted activities. All affected activities are grouped in the frame. The note contains information about the alternative actors.
	Actor 1 Actor 2 / Activity 1 Activity 1	*Shared activity* – represents an activity which is performed simultaneously by several actors. Thus the affected activity is split into activity parts. The synchronisation bars show that these parts are performed in parallel.

The tool model is based on the Three Layer Graph-Based Meta-Model (3LGM) that distinguishes the logical tool layer (e.g. software tools, conventional application systems) and physical tool layer (e.g. computer systems on which the software is installed, paper-based forms that are used for conventional information processing) [11].

In order to asses the quality of a process, the details from two of the sub-models can be combined to find out weaknesses (generating views). Table 2 shows an example for such a view: information model and tool model are combined to find redundantly stored information objects. In the example the clinical finding is stored in a computer-based clinical information system (CIS) but also in the paper-based patient record (grey background colour).

Table 2 – Example view: Combination of an information model with the tool model

Information object \ Logical tool	Picture Archiving and Communication System	Patient record (digital)	Patient record (paper-based)	...
Picture	X			
Ordering		X	X	
...				

5. Results

The elements of the described four sub-models have already been defined formally (explicit semantic). Further, the new graphical elements were implemented into a commonly used modelling software tool. In order to evaluate the new modelling method a typical and sufficient complex clinical process was selected – the ordering of radiological examinations, and the communication of the related findings. Those processes were described based on a systems analysis performed at the University Hospitals of Innsbruck, Austria. By now, two processes were modelled – the stationary and the ambulatory ordering. Because both models are too detailed to be included into this article, the following example will describe some advantages of the new method:

The left hand side of figure 2 shows how an ordering request would be modeled with the traditional UML Activity Diagram: the activity *ordering of records* adds new information to the object *Ordering* and changes its *state* to *manipulated*. An important weakness here is that information about used logical tools (e.g. Clinical information system [CIS] workstation) are only included textually using notes. This information are therefore not part of the model and not usable for (semi-automatic) assessments.

In contrast, the new modelling method represents the logical tools (and with them the used hardware) explicitly with an own element (here: CIS workstation and PC-1, see table 1). Further the new model highlights that the ordering is recorded twice (both in the digital and the paper-based patient record)! This is a possible weakness that can now be better detected than in the traditional Activity Diagram.

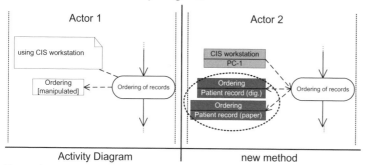

Figure 2 – Example: shows an extraction of an UML Activity Diagram model of the request ordering (left) in comparison to the new modelling method (right).

The new modelling method seems to meet our collected requirements on modelling methods for processes in health care so far. However, its elements (e.g. their semantic) and their implementation have to be tested and to be improved using the selected ordering process. The method and further results will be presented in more detail on the MIE conference 2005.

3. Discussion and Conclusion

The new modelling method supports the assessment of the quality of processes in healthcare. We decided to support this quality assessment by an extended modelling method that supports not only the description of clinical processes, but also the semi-automatic assessment of their quality. Some extensions have been developed and tested based on a typical clinical process, the radiological ordering. Further necessary extensions are still under development.

There are still quite a few open questions to be answered in this project:

- Possible weaknesses of clinical processes: Our core model should be able to describe as many possible weaknesses of clinical processes as possible. We developed a list of typical weaknesses based on an intensive literature search (e.g.[1]). However, at the moment, we are not able to describe all possible weaknesses in our process model. For example, we still have to decide how alternatives which are definitely needed to handle exceptions are represented.
- Complexity of the process model: The graphical representation we chose is mainly based on the elements of UML Activity Diagram. By extending this with new ele-

ments, graphical models may tend to get confusing and difficult to understand, especially in those cases when they are used not only by informaticians, but also by healthcare professionals. We must therefore be careful when selecting and extending the already available elements.

- Semi-automatic assessment: the extensions highlight *possible* weaknesses which have to be examined further. For example, when same information objects (e.g. order forms) are handled at different departments this *could* indicate unnecessary redundancies which could cause mistakes. We still have to decide how this tool should analyse a given model and how it should present its results.

The advantage of our modelling approach is the combination of different aspects (i.e. description of processes, used tools, information objects and actor roles). Each aspect is an integrated part of the model. Details which are important for a proper (semi-automatic) quality assessment are included explicitly. Extracted views help to compare different alternatives and to build reference processes more explicitly. Because UML Activity Diagrams and EPC claim to be generally applicable they fail to represent some important information needed for process assessment as clear and explicit as our method intends to do. The assessment of the models is not primarily taken into account. Further steps in our project will be the evaluation and improvement of the current model elements and the development of strategies for the semi-automatic analysis.

4. Acknowledgements

This project is being supported by the Austrian Ministry for Economy and Labour. It is being realised in close cooperation with the Institute of Computer Science (University of Innsbruck), the Department for Information & Software Engineering (UMIT) and the Information Technologies for Healthcare GmbH.

5. References

[1] Mosley C. Coordination of care in disease management: opportunities and financial issues. Semin Dial 2000;13(6):346-50.
[2] Ammenwerth E, Ehlers F, Kutscha U, Kutscha A, Eichstädter R, Resch F. Supporting patient care by using innovative information technology - A case study from clinical psychiatry. Disease Management & Health Outcome 2002;10(8):479-87.
[3] Bhasale L, Miller G, Reid S, Britt H. Analysing potential harm in Australian general practice: an incident-monitoring study. The Medical journal of Australia 1998;169(2):73-6.
[4] Coiera E. When conversation is better than computation. JAMIA 2000;7(3):277-286.
[5] Luo W, Tung Y. A framework for selecting business process modeling methods. Industrial Management & Data Systems 1999;99/7:312-319.
[6] Ehlers F, Ammenwerth E, Haux R. Process-Potential-Screening: An Instrument to Improve Business Processes in Hospital. Methods of Information in Medicine 2005;Paper accepted for publication.
[7] Brücher H, Endl R. Erweiterung von UML zur geschäftsregelorientierten Prozessmodellierung. Heidelberg, Germany: Physica-Verlag; 2002.
[8] Scheer AW, Nüttgens M, Zimmermann V. Objektorientierte Ereignisgesteuerte Prozeßkette (oEPK) - Methode und Anwendung. Veröffentlichungen des Instituts für Wirtschaftsinformatik 1997;141:1-25. (Available on: http://www.iwi.uni-sb.de/frameset/frameset.php?menu=3. Accessed at: January 30, 2005)
[9] Loos P, Allweyer T. Process Orientation and Object Orientation - An Approach for Integrating UML and Event-Driven Process Chains (EPC). Veröffentlichungen des Instituts für Wirtschaftsinformatik 1998;144:1-17.
[10] OMG. UML Ressource Page. 2005; Available on http://www.uml.org/#uml2.0. Accessed at: January 14, 2005;
[11] Winter A, Brigl B, T W. Modeling hospital information systems. Part 1: The revised three-layer graph-based meta model 3LGM2. Methods Inf Med. 2003;42 (5):544-51.

Address of correspondence:

Institute for Health Information Systems, UMIT – University for Health Sciences, Medical Informatics and Technology, Eduard Wallnöfer-Zentrum 1, A-6060 Hall in Tyrol, Contact: Samrend.Saboor@umit.at

Connecting Medical Informatics and Bio-Informatics
R. Engelbrecht et al. (Eds.)
IOS Press, 2005

527

SomWeb – Towards an Infrastructure for Knowledge Sharing in Oral Medicine[1]

Göran Falkman[a], Olof Torgersson[b], Mats Jontell[c], Marie Gustafsson[a]

[a]*School of Humanities and Informatics, University of Skövde, Skövde, Sweden*
[b]*Department of Computer Science and Engineering, Chalmers University of Technology, Göteborg, Sweden*
[c]*Clinic of Oral Medicine, Faculty of Odontology, The Sahlgrenska Academy, Göteborg, Sweden*

Abstract:

In a net-based society, clinicians can come together for cooperative work and distance learning around a common medical material. This requires suitable techniques for cooperative knowledge management and user interfaces that are adapted to both the group as a whole and to individuals. To support distributed management and sharing of clinical knowledge, we propose the development of an intelligent web community for clinicians within oral medicine. This virtual meeting place will support the ongoing work on developing a digital knowledge base, providing a foundation for a more evidence-based oral medicine. The presented system is founded on the use and development of web services and standards for knowledge modelling and knowledge-based systems. The work is conducted within the frame of a well-established cooperation between oral medicine and computer science.

Keywords:
Integrated Advanced Information Management Systems; Evidence-Based Medicine; Oral Medicine; Software Design; Internet; Community Networks

1. Introduction

It has been argued that optimal health care should be evidence-based [1]. To practice evidence-based medicine (EBM) implies the integration of the expertise of individual clinicians with the best clinical evidence obtainable from external sources [2].

A net-based society provides the necessary foundation for developing computerised tools that support EBM. Equipped with the right IT tools, clinicians can come together and help each other in the collection, analysis, validation, dissemination and harmonisation of clinical knowledge that are prerequisites of EBM.

SomWeb is a project for managing clinical knowledge, with the intention to provide a foundation for evidence-based oral medicine. To create a sufficiently large base of clinical data, nation-wide collaboration is required, which in turn requires an instrument for multiparametric data analysis based on a large number of cases. The purpose of SomWeb is to develop the necessary infrastructure for such an instrument, based on the following:

- Techniques and standards in component-based program development and web services should be used to obtain a more transparent system with better support for reuse and global access to components and services [3].

---

[1] The work presented in this paper was supported by the Swedish Agency for Innovation Systems (VINNOVA).

- Knowledge management services should to as large extent as possible be generic, using standards for knowledge modelling and implementation of knowledge-based systems. This should facilitate knowledge dissemination, use of external knowledge sources and communication with other information systems [4].

- To increase IT-maturity, proposed methods and applications should be user-centric, and should be developed in close collaboration with end-users [5].

- The use of web-based tools for computer-supported collaborative work (CSCW) in the analysis and validation of data and harmonisation of knowledge carried out by clinical experts as part of EBM, and as a source of information and remote consultation for other interested parties, e.g., care providers and care receivers [6].

- Proposed methods and tools should be tested and evaluated in daily clinical work [7].

1.1. MedView

SomWeb is based on a medical information system called MedView [8]. MedView already contains the basis of SomWeb, in the form of elaborated content when it comes to services for knowledge management, together with a well-established user community.

To provide rapid prototyping and deployment of applications in daily clinical work, and to support the harmonisation of clinical processes and knowledge within oral medicine, Med-View has been developed in close collaboration between experts within the Swedish Oral Medicine Network (SOMNet) and experts in computer science.

MedView consists of a suite of applications for the formalisation, acquisition and sharing of knowledge, and for visualisation and analysis of data. So far, data and digital images from more than 8,000 clinical examinations have been collected into a large database.

1.2. Overview

First, the overall aim and objectives of the project are stated, followed by an outline of the general methods used. The next three sections introduce the three major parts of SomWeb. Then, initial results are presented. A discussion that further motivates the SomWeb approach then follows. Finally, the paper is summarised by some concluding remarks.

2. Aim and Objectives

The overall aim of SomWeb is to obtain further knowledge about how interactive, user-centred knowledge-based systems supporting evidence-based oral medicine should be designed, implemented and introduced in the daily clinical work.

The work on achieving the above aim is divided into three partially overlapping objectives: (1) The formalisation of clinical processes and knowledge, (2) the development of web services for oral medicine and (3) the construction of an intelligent web community for oral medicine. These three objectives are described in more detail below.

3. Methods

SomWeb is being developed in collaboration with the clinicians of SOMNet, which together represent approximately 100,000 patients with problems related to oral medicine. These patients will generate relevant clinical data, providing a foundation for analysis and evaluation of models, methods and applications developed in the project. Only anonymous patient data will be used.

Through the work within MedView, a close cooperation between experts within oral medicine, experts in computer science and end-users has been established. A basic principle is that the development of computerised tools supporting clinical activities should be carried out in parallel with the daily clinical use of these tools. Thus, applications are developed using a user-centred and activity-based approach.

SOMWeb is based on the use of public and open standards, open-source and platform-independent tools (e.g., Java), and modern methods for object-oriented software development and design according to well-established design patterns.

4. Formalisation of Clinical Concepts and Processes

In order to conform to modern approaches to the construction of knowledge-based systems (KBS), proposed standards in knowledge modelling and KBS will be analysed and used for re-modelling and re-implementing clinical concepts and processes in oral medicine.

4.1. Ontology for Oral Medicine

Knowledge-based systems can be described as a number of knowledge bases (KBs), which are instances of ontologies, to which a collection of problem solving methods (PSMs) are applied [9]. Recently, both the Resource Description Framework (RDF) and the Web Ontology Language (OWL) have become World Wide Web Consortium recommendations for representing information, exchanging knowledge and for publishing and sharing ontologies.

With the knowledge model in MedView as a starting point, proposed standards for the generic description and implementation of ontologies, primarily RDF/OWL, will be used to construct an ontology for oral medicine.

4.2. Reusable Knowledge Components for Oral Medicine

The construction of KBS is largely based on re-usable 'knowledge components'. Applied to the medical domain, this means that medical KBSs should be constructed from re-usable and clinically validated components [10]. The Unified Problem solving Method develop-

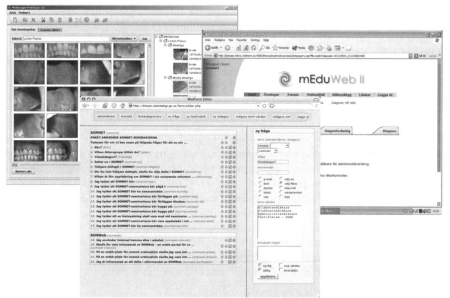

Figure 1 – SOMWeb components: MedImager, mForm and mEduWeb II

ment Language (UPML) [11] has been put forward as a future standard for modelling PSMs and for developing the kind of 'knowledge fusion' and cooperative knowledge management services that are the focus of SOMWeb.

Starting at the developed ontology for oral medicine, useful knowledge components in current MedView applications will be identified and then implemented in UPML.

5. Web-Services for Oral Medicine

The new net-based society has provided the possibility to let KBSs be accessible over the Internet. Another consequence is that, to an increasingly larger extent, a KBS can be based on data from multiple and heterogenous sources of data.

MedView is locally installed, and, with few exceptions, neither the applications nor the databases are externally accessible. To increase IT-maturity within oral medicine and to increase the possibility of information sharing, thereby further the development of evidence-based oral medicine, MedView will be made accessible over the Internet.

Starting with the developed knowledge components, standards and techniques in web services [12] will be studied and used for the development and publication of web services for oral medicine.

6. An Intelligent Web Community for Oral Medicine

Based on the developed knowledge and service models, a web community for oral medicine will be designed, implemented and brought into clinical use. The services offered will include the functionality provided by current MedView applications.

The first step is to analyse forms of collaboration within SOMNet. Then, a first community providing support for the activities of SOMNet will be constructed. This community will include the possibility of structured input of clinical cases and multi-modal presentation of cases using natural language generation over the Internet. Finally, a community with a more complete support for cooperation between different types of users will be developed. User modelling and approaches within intelligent user-interfaces and CSCW will be used to enable individually adapted interfaces. Other possible functionality include some form of recommender system, e.g., in the form of social navigation [13].

7. Results

In order to realise the plans of the SOMWeb project, parallel development along several paths has been initiated.

7.1. Ontology for Oral Medicine

Initial work on knowledge representation has identified some general requirements on an ontology for oral medicine, and has shown how these can be alleviated by using RDF and OWL. Most work so far has been in representing basic clinical concepts, e.g., clinical terms, values, examination templates and language support. There are also some results in the area of representing data types of elements and using meta-data. We have also begun identifying external ontologies of interest for reuse. During this initial work, it has become apparent that RDF and OWL are very applicable in fulfilling the identified requirements.

This work will be continued with further modelling of examinations and related concepts. Other future aspects include supporting different conceptual views, modelling interactions between entities, representing pictorial data and using ontologies for user modelling.

7.2. Computer-Supported Collaborative Work within SOMNet

Increasing the IT-maturity of involved clinicians is of utmost importance for successful medical IT-systems. Within SOMNet, the previous method used for tele-conferencing was that all attendants sent e-mail to each other with case presentations. This practice has been replaced by the use of a central web-based case repository. During tele-conferences, the attendants view the cases from our web-server. Furthermore, cases are kept and thus a common repository of difficult cases is starting to develop.

7.3. Adaptable User Interfaces

To develop suitable techniques for adapting the user interface to the IT-maturity of the individual participant, we intend to deploy the principles of multi-layered user interfaces [14]. In a multi-layered user interface, the user can start using an application without needing to worry about more than the most basic features. As the user matures, he or she can select to add more functionality in a principled manner. As a case study, MedImager for viewing images of the oral mucosa has been developed (see the left picture in Figure 1 above).

7.4. Web-Based Clinical Trials and E-Learning

The focus of the mForm system is to build a tool that enables collection of data from clinical trials over the web that can be handled by any reasonably mature IT-user without special training (see the middle picture in Figure 1).

The mEduWeb system supports learning in oral medicine by providing access to the material collected within MedView and SOMNet. Diagnostic tests and exercises can be included and the student can perform these tasks through the Internet. Lectures, edited cases and other relevant course information can be added as well (right picture in Figure 1).

8. Discussion

It has been noted that the lack of multi-disciplinary teams, who can tackle and solve complex research problems, limits the exploitation of modern information technology within public health care [15]. In this case, SOMWeb has a great advantage through the long and continuous discussion within MedView, which has resulted in that highly specialised care providers and experts in computer science have developed a necessary common ground for communication. Even though the fundamental issues in SOMWeb have previously been studied within the scope of medical informatics, the field of dental informatics is less explored [15]. Therefore, SOMWeb has all the requirements to become a precursor in its field.

As different types of users should have access to one common system, it is important to provide 'intelligent' interfaces with the capability to adapt itself to each user. Although much research has been carried out in this area, there are still many unsolved problems, both in terms of methodology and in terms of concrete solutions. An advantage of SOMWeb is that it requires application to a real clinical environment, with real end-users. This provides a good foundation for subsequent evaluation of obtained results.

9. Conclusions

- The use of standards for knowledge modelling, KBS, web services and web communities forms the basis for the development of a medical information system supporting a more evidence-based oral medicine. Through the application to a large and realistic case, SOMWeb contributes to the work on standardisation in these areas.

- Widely accepted recommendations such as RDF/OWL and UPML will be used to facilitate the development of re-usable and clinically validated knowledge components, i.e., ontologies and PSMs.

- Techniques in web services will enable the development and publication of knowledge services over the Internet, thereby increasing the possibility for knowledge sharing and re-use.

- The creation of a virtual meeting place for oral medicine will provide a forum in which the collected knowledge of a large number of expert users can be accessed. This will in turn promote both the validation of information and the harmonisation of knowledge within the field.

- The use of developed methods and tools in daily clinical work strengthens the basis for EBM in oral medicine, in that users become more accustomed to IT and in that the continuous collection of basic clinical data is a prerequisite for obtaining new medical knowledge.

10. Acknowledgements

The MedImager application is the work of Linn Gustavsson Christiernin and Fredrik Lindahl, Chalmers University of Technology. The mForm application was developed by David Breneman, Chalmers University of Technology.

11. References

[1] Rosenberg WMC and Donald A. Evidence based medicine: An approach to clinical problem solving. Brit. Med. J. 1995: 310(6987), 1122–1126.

[2] Sackett DL, Rosenberg WMC, Gray JAM, Haynes RB, and Richardson WS. Evidence based medicine: What it is and what it isn't. Brit. Med. J. 1996: 312(7023), 71–72.

[3] Aarts J. On articulation and localization – some sociotechnical issues of design, implementation, and evaluation of knowledge based systems. In: Quaglini S, Barahona P, and Andreassen S, eds. Artificial Intelligence in Medicine in Europe. Proc. AIME 2001. Springer, 2001; pp 16–19.

[4] Mendonça EA, Cimino JJ, Johnson SB, and Seol YH. Accessing heterogeneous sources of evidence to answer clinical questions. J. Biomed. Inform. 2001: 34(2), 85–98.

[5] Wetter T. Lessons learnt from bringing knowledge-based systems into routine use. Artif. Intell. Med. 2002: 24(3), 195–203.

[6] Mendonça EA. Clinical decision support systems: Perspectives in dentistry. J. Dent. Edu. 2004: 68, 589–597.

[7] Zeng Q and Cimino JJ. A knowledge-based, concept-oriented view generation system for clinical data. J. Biomed. Inform. 2001: 34(2), 112–128.

[8] JontellM, Mattsson U, and Torgersson O. MedView: An instrument for clinical research and education in oral medicine. Oral Surg. Oral Med. Oral Pathol. Oral Radiol. Endod. 2005: 99, 55–63.

[9] Musen MA. Modern architectures for intelligent systems: Reusable ontologies and problem-solving methods. In: Chute CG, ed. Proc. 1998 AMIA Annual Symposium. 1998; pp 46–52.

[10] Musen MA and Schreiber AT. Architectures for intelligent systems based on reusable components. Artif. Intell. Med. 1995: 7, 189–199.

[11] Fensel D, Benjamins VR, Motta E, and Wielinga B. UPML: A framework for knowledge system reuse. In: Proc. International Joint Conference on AI (IJCAI-99). 1999.

[12] McIlraith S, Son TC, and Zeng H. Semantic web services. IEEE Intell. Syst. 2001: 16(2), 46–53.

[13] Svensson M, Höök K, Laaksolahti J, and Waern A. Social navigation of food recipes. In: Proc. SIGCHI Conference on Human Factors in Computing Systems. ACM Press, 2001; pp 341–348.

[14] Shneiderman B. Promoting universal usability with multi-layer interface design. In: Proc. Conference on Universal Usability, CUU'03. ACM Press, 2003; pp 1–8.

[15] Schleyer T and Spallek H. Dental informatics: A cornerstone of dental practice. J. Am. Dent. Assoc. 2001: 132, 605–613.

Address for Correspondence

Göran Falkman, School of Humanities and Informatics, University of Skövde, PO Box 408, SE-541 28 Skövde, Sweden. Email: goran.falkman@his.se

Connecting Medical Informatics and Bio-Informatics
R. Engelbrecht et al. (Eds.)
IOS Press, 2005

Measuring the Impact of Online Evidence Retrieval Systems using Critical Incidents & Journey Mapping

Johanna I Westbrook[a], Enrico W Coiera[a], Jeffrey Braithwaite[b]

[a]Centre for Health Informatics,
[b]Centre for Clinical Governance Research in Health, University of New South Wales, Australia

Abstract

Online evidence retrieval systems are one potential tool in supporting evidence-based practice. We have undertaken a program of research to investigate how hospital-based clinicians (doctors, nurses and allied health professionals) use these systems, factors influencing use and their impact on decision-making and health care delivery. A central component of this work has been the development and testing of a broad range of evaluation techniques. This paper provides an overview of the results obtained from three stages of this evaluation and details the results derived from the final stage which sought to test two methods for assessing the integration of an online evidence system and its impact on decision making and patient care. The critical incident and journey mapping techniques were applied. Semi-structured interviews were conducted with 29 clinicians who were experienced users of the online evidence system. Clinicians were asked to described recent instances in which the information obtained using the online evidence system was especially helpful with their work. A grounded approach to data analysis was taken producing three categories of impact. The journey mapping technique was adapted as a method to describe and quantify clinicians' integration of CIAP into their practice and the impact of this on patient care. The analogy of a journey is used to capture the many stages in this integration process, from introduction to the system to full integration into everyday clinical practice with measurable outcomes. Transcribed interview accounts of system use were mapped against the journey stages and scored. Clinicians generated 85 critical incidents and one quarter of these provided specific examples of system use leading to improvements in patient care. The journey mapping technique proved to be a useful method for providing a quantification of the ways and extent to which clincians had integrated system use into practice, and insights into how information systems can influence organisational culture. Further work is required on this technique to assess its value as an evaluation method. The study demonstrates the strength of a triangulated evidence approach to assessing the use and impact of online clinical evidence systems.

Keywords:
Information retrieval; Evaluation; Medical informatics; Journey mapping, Evidence-based medicine

1. Introduction

Provision of online evidence systems to support clinical work at the point-of-care has been adopted as a strategy to support evidence-based practice in the UK, USA and Australia.[1-3]. Few evaluations of their effectiveness have been reported. Most studies have focused on assessing frequency of use.[4] Measuring the impact of an information system on clinical practice is problematic. There are many potentially confounding variables for which it is often not possible to control. Thus establishing the relationship between online evidence use and changes in clinical practice and patient outcomes is difficult. There are few studies that have attempted this task. The state of New South Wales, Australia implemented the Clinical Information Access Program (www.ciap.health.nsw.gov.au) a website providing around 55,000 clinicians' (doctors, nurses and allied health professionals) with 24 hour access to evidence at the point-of-care in public health care facilities. A two year evaluation was undertaken to assess the extent to which the system was used, supports clinical decision-making and results in improvements to patient care. A triangulated research program consisted of four stages of data collection. Results from the first three stages have been reported elsewhere and are summarised below.

Stage one - Web log analysis: An analysis of 7 months of CIAP web-logs of the 55,000 clinicians who have access allowed a quantification of the rates of use by geographical Area Health Services, hospitals and professional groups. Considerable variation in the rates of use for individual hospitals and professional groups was found.[5] Medical staff used CIAP at double the rate of nursing staff. Results showed that use of CIAP was related to patient care decisions. For example, searching activity was highly positively correlated with patient admissions at individual hospitals. The wide variation in use required further investigation to understand factors related to high and low use organizations. Stage two sought to address these issues.

Stage two - Case Studies: In-depth case studies investigated the influence of professional and organisational factors on health professionals' use of CIAP. Results from focus groups, interviews and surveys from clinical groups within three case study sites identified a range of cultural, organisational and team factors which were important in explaining variations in CIAP use within and between professional groups and hospitals.[6] Positive promotion of CIAP, and support and encouragement to use it were major factors influencing use. Nurses and allied health staff reported needing most support in the effective retrieval of information. CIAP was used by all three professional groups. Doctors were the highest users and most likely to use CIAP for patient care. Nurses' awareness of CIAP was the lowest of the three groups.

Technical issues were also highlighted but were found not to be the central factor influencing CIAP use. Investigation of the association between clinical team functioning and use of CIAP to improve patient care produced interesting results, demonstrating that well-functioning teams were more likely to report effective use of CIAP. However clinical team functioning was not associated with greater awareness of CIAP.[7]

Stage three - State-wide survey: A statewide survey of 5,511 clinicians (doctors, nurses and allied health professionals) from a random selection of 65 hospitals was undertaken to determine awareness and use of CIAP, how and why clinicians use, or do not use, online evidence, technical issues related to use of CIAP, and clinicians' perceptions of its impact on clinical care.

The survey showed that 63% of clinicians had heard of CIAP and of those who had, 75% had used it. Colleagues were the primary channel via which clinicians heard about CIAP. The survey results reinforced the key findings of the log analysis and in-depth cases study findings. For example, clinicians' actual and reported use of CIAP was consistent in terms of types of resources used. Clinicians' views about the importance of organisational factors in supporting an evidence-based approach to care and the integrated use of CIAP, reported during the focus groups in stage two, were reflected in the survey responses from the respondents. The survey identified high levels of satisfaction with the technical features of CIAP, such as ease of use and search speed. Analysis of the log data indicated that use was related to direct patient care decisions and the survey results reinforced this with, for example, 55% of doctors reporting that they had had direct experience of CIAP use resulting in improved patient care. There were significant differences between professional groups[8] and also between senior and junior clinicians[9] within the same profession. For example, senior and specialist nurses had more positive attitudes to use, perceived more support and legitimation for its use, and reported more frequent use than did junior nurses. [10]

The results from stages 1-3 provided the context and direction for the last stage of the evaluation which sought to pilot two techniques, critical incident[11] and journey mapping[12], to assess integration of the use of CIAP and impact on clinical decision-making and patient care. These methods create a narrative of change from the perspective of system users allowing an examination of professional and organisational cultural changes and how users experience these changes. Few studies have attempted to assess the impact of online evidence systems on clinicians' practice and outcomes of care. The largest was conducted by Lindberg et al[13], who applied the critical incident technique to survey 552 US physicians about their use of MEDLINE. Physicians reported using MEDLINE for a range of clinical tasks, from choosing diagnostic tests to developing treatment plans. In 2% of instances of MEDLINE use physicians reported finding essential information that led to saving patients' lives or sparing limbs and organs.

Two US studies used surveys to examine clinician satisfaction with hospital library services and the reported impact of the information provided on patient care.[14, 15] King [15] surveyed a random sample of physicians, nurses and other health providers in eight hospitals. Doctors reported using the library more than nurses and other health professionals. All groups reported that over 90% of the information obtained was of clinical value and influenced their clinical decisions, contributing to increased quality of care. The second study surveyed physicians in one hospital, who reported a positive response to the hospital library service.[14] In 80% of reported cases, information obtained from the library changed or influenced clinical decisions. However, both studies had low response rates, limiting interpretation of the results.

The introduction of MEDLINE into clinical settings in a US hospital was evaluated through interviews with a random sample of physicians who participated in MEDLINE training. Physicians reported that 47% of searches influenced their clinical decisions, most frequently through confirmation of a decision[16]. Another study found that length of stay was shorter for patients for whom a MEDLINE search had been conducted earlier in their hospitalisation. A causal relationship could not be established and a number of confounding factors such as the severity of patients' conditions limited interpretation of the findings.[17] There have been no reported studies of the clinical impact of access to an electronic resource such as CIAP, where multiple databases are accessible at the point of care.

2. Methods

Sixteen Clinical Nurse Specialists (CNS) and 13 hospital-based specialist physicians were selected who were experienced and regular CIAP users. A three-part semi-structured interview schedule was used. The first two parts were designed to obtain information about critical incidents. First, clinicians were asked to recall examples of when CIAP had been helpful in their clinical work. For each, a series of questions was asked about the type of information sought, databases used, impact of having the information and outcome of the clinical situation. Second, clinicians were asked to recall any searches that had been unsatisfactory.

A grounded approach was taken to coding the interviews.[18, 19] Initially, two researchers coded each critical incident independently. Subsequently in several meetings, coding was clarified and

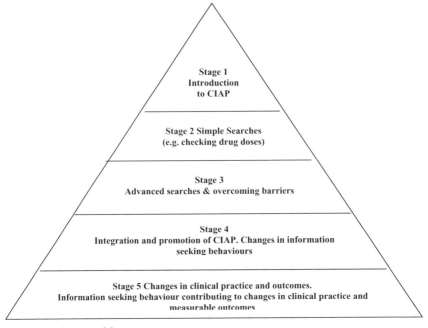

Figure 1 - Journey Mapping stages

refined until agreement was reached on coding and the definition of each category. In this way, categories of the types of impacts were developed. The third part of the interview illicited information about clinician's CIAP Journey. Transcribed interview accounts were then mapped against the journey stages and levels and scored (Figure 1). The journey mapping technique was adapted[12] as a method to describe and quantify clinicians' integration of CIAP into their practice and the impact of this on patient care. The analogy of a journey is used to capture the many stages in this integration process. A journey must commence with an introduction to CIAP (stage 1) and each subsequent stage in the journey represents a greater level of integration of CIAP into clinical practice ending at stage 5 (changes in clinical practice and patient outcomes). Scores are assigned to different levels and stages in the journey. The higher the journey score the further a clinician has integrated the use of CIAP into his/her clinical practice.

3. Results

In total, 85 incidents were described by 29 clinicians interviewed. The average was 3 per clinician (range 1-5). Three categories of impact were derived: micro clinical impacts (a positive clinical impact, but no specific outcomes could be identified; eg 31% of incidents involved a policy change); macro impacts (a positive impact with some objective

---

Box 1 Example of CIAP use changing clinician behaviour
CNs (peri-operative care): "[CIAP] has helped us make it more evidence based and make it more grounded in good information and not just the ritual"

Box 3 Example of CIAP use improving patient health
Specialist (renal): "a patient who had peritonitis which he'd got from a bug he'd picked up in Central Australia....I found the epidemiology, which antibiotics to use, the formula for treatment...We were able to treat the patient successfully"

Box2 Example of CIAP use for a differential diagnosis
Specialist (anaesthetics): "a patient had had an unusual metabolic acidosis after major surgery in the recovery room. In the recovery room here we have access to CIAP and we looked through Harrison's for a differential diagnosis for metabolic acidosis and that helped us solve the problem."

---

measurement of the outcomes reported; and impacts on the clinicians (Box 1); eg 45% of clinicians reported that use of CIAP improved confidence in their decisions. One quarter of all incidents relating to CIAP use, resulted in measurable improvements in patient outcomes. These included improvements in medication use, improved management of complications, differential diagnosis, and identification of effective treatment for drug interactions (Box 2 & 3 for examples of reported incidents).

The journey mapping technique was found to be a useful measure for quantifying changes in clinicians' actions, behaviours, and clinical practice, which occurred in association with CIAP use. The results demonstrated that among this sample of active users all had reached stage 5.

Total scores for the CNSs and doctors did not differ significantly. Thus among active CIAP users CNCs and doctors appear equally likely to achieve optimal benefits. Individuals did however report very different CIAP journeys. For example, one CNS had contributed to the promotion of CIAP across her organisation, but described no macro clinical impacts. The emergency department CNS described major changes to her information-seeking behaviour and had overcome some barriers to using CIAP. The ICU physician specialist reported that his information-seeking behaivour had changed through the availability of CIAP, but he had not been active in promoting CIAP locally or in any broader context. In contrast, the anaesthetist described instances where information gained via CIAP contributed to improvements in clinical practice, but CIAP availability had not changed his information-seeking behaviour to the same degree as his colleagues.

4. Discussion

The data from the critical incidents provided an enhanced understanding of how the online evidence system was being used in clinical practice and reinforced the information gained from other stages of the evaluation. These narratives of system use are an important ingredient in beginning to understand how real-world culture change occurs. Clinicians were able to relate clear narratives of how CIAP use had impacted on patient care. The journey mapping technique proved to be a useful method for quantifying changes in clinicians' actions, behaviours and clinical practice which occurred in association with CIAP use and demonstrated how integration of such technologies is rarely a linear process. Clinicians had individual stories about how use had influenced their practice and the care of their patients. The sample was highly selective and it is likely that a random sample would reveal clinicians who were content with integrating CIAP at lower levels and who may never proceed to stage 5. For an organisation journey mapping may provide a useful measure for assessing the level of integration beyond rates or frequency of use. However further testing using larger, more hetergeneous samples would be beneficial.

More broadly, studies of these type realise accounts of situated practice which may be part of a longitudinal trend of new cultures of information use. Ultimately, new information systems must positively influence clincial practice and organisational culture, otherwise claims of their benefits are unlikely to be sustained.

5. Acknowledgements

We would like to acknowledge Dr Sophie Gosling's contribution to the original study design and data collection while at the Centre for Health Informatics.

6. References

[1]   Gray, J., *National electronic Library for Health (NeLH)*. BMJ, 1999. 319: p. 1476-1479.

[2]   Hersh, W., *Information retrieval. A health care perspective*. Computers and Medicine. 1996, New York: Springer. 320.

[3]   Ayres, D. and M. Wensley, *The clinical information access project*. Med J Aus, 1999. 171: p. 544-546.

[4]   Hersh, W., *Information retrieval: A health and biomedical perspective*. 2nd ed. Health Informatics Series, ed. K. Hannah and M. Ball. 2003, New York: Spinger-Verlag. 517.

[5]   Westbrook, J., A. Gosling, and E. Coiera, *Do clinicians use online evidence to support patient care? A study of 55,000 clinicians*. J Am Med Inform Ass, 2004. 11(2): p. 113-120.

[6]   Gosling, A., J. Westbrook, and E. Coiera, *Variation in the use of online clinical evidence: a qualitative analysis*. Int J Med Inform, 2003. 69: p. 1-16.

[7]   Gosling, A., J. Westbrook, and J. Braithwaite, *Clinical team functioning and IT innovation: A study of the diffusion of a point-of-care online evidence system*. J Am Med Inform Ass, 2003. 10: p. 246-253.

[8]   Gosling, A. and J. Westbrook, *Allied health professionals' use of online evidence: A survey of 790 staff working in the Australian public hospital system*. Int J Med Inform, 2004. 73: p. 391-401.

[9]   Westbrook, J., A. Gosling, and M. Westbrook, *Use of point-of-care online clinical evidence retrieval systems by junior and senior doctors in NSW public hospitals*. Intern Med J, 2005. 35 (6): in press

[10] Gosling, A., J. Westbrook, and R. Spencer, *Nurses' use of online clinical evidence*. J Ad Nurs, 2004. 47(2): p. 201-211.

[11] Flanagan, J., *The critical incident technique*. Psych Bull, 1954. 51(4): p. 327-358.

[12] Kibel, B., *Success stories as hard data: An introduction to Results Mapping*. Prevention in Practice Library, ed. T. Gullotta. 1999, New York: Kluwer Academic/Plenum Publishers.

[13] Lindberg, D., et al., *Use of MEDLINE by physicians for clinical problem solving*. JAMA, 1993. 269(24): p. 3124-3129.

[14] Marshall, J., *The impact of the hospital library on clinical decision-making: the Rochester study*. Bull Med Lib Assoc, 1992. 80: p. 169-178.

[15] King, D., *The contribution of hospital library information services to clinical care: a study of eight hospitals*. Bull Med Lib Assoc, 1987. 75: p. 291-301.

[16] Haynes, R., et al., *Online access to MEDLINE in clinical settings. A study of use and usefulness*. Ann Intern Med, 1990. 112(1): p. 78-84.

[17] Klein, M., et al., *Effect of online literature searching on length of stay and patient care costs*. Acad Med, 1994. 69(6): p. 489-495.

[18] Glaser, B., *Basics of Grounded Theory Analysis*. 1992, California: Sociology Press.

[19] Glaser, B. and A. Strauss, *The Discovery Of Grounded Theory*. 1967, New York: Aldine Publishing Company.

Connecting Medical Informatics and Bio-Informatics
R. Engelbrecht et al. (Eds.)
IOS Press, 2005

Design and Implementation of an ICU Incident Registry

Sabine van der Veer[a], Ronald Cornet[b], Evert de Jonge[c]

[a]*Clinical Engineering Department,* [b]*Department of Medical Informatics,* [c] *ntensive Care Adults,*

Academic Medical Centre (AMC) - Universiteit van Amsterdam, Amsterdam, the Netherlands

Abstract

Due to its complexity intensive care is vulnerable to errors. On the ICU Adults of the AMC (Amsterdam, the Netherlands) the available registries used for error reporting did not give insight in the occurrence of unwanted events, and did not lead to preventive measures. Therefore, a new registry has been developed on the basis of a literature study on the various terms and definitions that refer to unintended events, and on the methods to register and monitor them. As this registry intends to provide an overall insight into errors, a neutral term ('incident') –which does not imply guilt or blame- has been sought together with a broad definition. The attributes of an incident further describe the unwanted event, but they should not form an impediment for the ICU nurses and physicians to report. The properties of a registry that contribute to making it accessible and user friendly have been determined. This has resulted in an electronic registry where incidents can be reported rapidly, voluntarily, anonymously and free of legal consequences. Evaluation is required to see if the new registry indeed provides the ICU management with the intended information on the current situation on incidents. For further refinement of the design, additional development and adjustments are required. However, we expect that the awareness of errors of the ICU personnel has already improved, forming the first step to increased patient safety.

Keywords
Medical errors, Registries, Quality assurance, Intensive Care

1. Introduction

Medical errors and adverse events occur frequently and are thought to result in up to 98.000 unnecessary deaths in the United States each year [1]. The likelihood of adverse events and errors increases with the intensity of care, the severity of illness and the complexity of the care-providing system. Especially in the intensive care setting the risk of clinical errors increases due to the complexity of patients' problems and the frequency of (invasive) interventions. Furthermore intensive care medicine has become increasingly fragmented involving multiple transitions between different health care providers. This leads to failures of communication, which are involved in 37% of the human errors committed in the ICU, resulting in increased patient harm, length of stay and resource use [2]. In most high risk industries, learning from accidents and near misses is a long-established practice and a cornerstone of safety analysis and improvement [3]. Surprisingly, however, this susceptibility to errors is not universally acknowledged by ICU staff [4].

At the ICU of the AMC three methods co-existed to report complications, accidents and (near) misses. Besides causing ambiguity about what, where and when should be reported, the three registries failed to give complete insight in the situation regarding incidents. Explanations for this are the used medium (one registry consisted of a paper form), the tendency to report only severe events or the fact that one registry did not explicitly focus on reporting incidents. Therefore we designed a new ICU incident registry. By registering incidents, the awareness is expected to increase, which will change clinician behaviour and therefore improve patient safety.

2. Material and Methods

In order to come to a clear definition of a reportable event, a literature study was performed resul-ting in a list of terms and definitions, all related to undesired events. Together with the ICU management we determined the intended goal of the registry and selected a matching definition. For the collection of possible events to be reported, a list of complications from one of the three existing registries was adopted as a starting point, assuming it concerned the main part of the ICU interventions. After discussing it with several ICU physicians and nurses, observing their daily practice and comparing it to other similar registries, the final list was attained.

Cases found in medical journals describing incidents and medical errors in the intensive care en-vironment were analyzed to determine the attributes for an undesired event and then discussed with the staff physician, closely involved in designing the new registry, and a head nurse and senior nurse, both taking part in the committee for Reporting Incidents in Patient Care (Meldingen Incidenten Patiëntenzorg). This led to a selection of attributes, forming the items to be registered for every reported event. To gain further insight into the design of an incident registry, another literature study was performed on methods by which incidents are reported, re-sulting in a list of properties of such registries. By discussing them with the same group of people and comparing the number of reported events of the different methods, the specific requirements for each property were set. The resulting incident registry was implemented and integrated as an add-in in the currently used Patient Data Management System (PDMS) of the ICU of the AMC. As an evaluation, a pilot version of the software was presented to a group of nurses and physi-cians using predefined test cases. The results were noted before implementing the final version.

3. Results

Defining an incident

From the literature study it appeared that there are many taxonomies for undesired events [1,5]. Different terms are used, varying from 'complication' [6] to 'adverse event' [7] and from 'human error' [8] to 'critical incident' [9], each with a specific definition and context. Before being able to determine the most applicable one, we defined the main goal of the registry as 'to estimate and detect patterns in the occurrence and severity of undesired events': data that might lead to effective interventions. An expected side effect of implementing the registry is the increased awareness of ICU personnel for patient safety. In order to gain insight in the overall situation regarding unwanted events, a broad definition is required having no strict limitation as to what to report. Therefore, we finally opted for the term *incident*, defined by the Australian Incident Monitoring System in Intensive Care (AIMS-ICU) as *any event or outcome which could have reduced, or did reduce the safety margin for the patient. It may or may not have been preventable and may or may not have involved an error on the part of the healthcare team* [10]. Considering that according to this definition a planned, preventive operation –causing a significant increase of the risk on complications, hence reducing the safety margin for the patient- would also be an incident, we extended the first part of the definition to *any undesired or unintended event or outcome* [6].

Collection of incidents

The new list of incidents consisted of 110 events in 14 categories. In the process of composing this list of reportable events the main focus was on including the major part of the incidents that might occur on the ICU. An existing list of complications forms the basis of this collection, containing events related to frequently performed medical actions, such as 'pneumothorax' in the category 'Central-/Arterial lines'. We adapted it's classification by excluding interventions that are less common on the ICU nowadays and including new categories like 'device related'. Within each category the events have been reviewed, i.e. deleted or added in order to tune them to the ICU domain. Others have been renamed to bring them into line with the attributes to be reported for every incident, e.g. 'severe decubitus' has become 'decubitus' with the severity separately registered as the outcome for the patient (see *figure 1*, item 5) .

Attributes of reported events

To enable focused research on how to decrease the occurrence of certain incidents, a set of attributes has been determined. For each event they form the background information on possible influencing factors and patient outcome. While selecting which attributes to include as items in the registry, we have tried to find a balance between obtaining sufficiently detailed information on one hand and on the other limiting the effort and time required for users to report. Finally, six attributes have been selected. Together with a description of the event in free text (item 6) and the question if the user wants to create a form for the hospital's mandatory registration (item 7), they constitute the items that should be reported for each incident.

One of the selected attributes is 'factors that have contributed to the occurrence of the incident' (item 3), which consists of six predefined contributing factors –such as 'device deficiency'- and the option to enter any other factor under 'Other, namely'. In similar registries the list of possible factors might be much more extensive, but to keep it acceptable for the users, we choose to keep it limited. The selected factors all represent an important field of attention within the ICU policy, such as the use of protocols or the training and supervision of new ICU physicians and nurses.

Another attribute that will be discussed here is 'patient outcome' (item 5), indicating the severity of the incident. The scale of the harm score as described by Kivlahan et al [5], has been used. It consists of six levels: '0' signifying the reported event has no negative outcome for the patient, (e.g. in case of a near miss) and '5' representing 'death'. The description for each level contains information on the patient outcome and in most cases on the interventions that were required as a result of the event. Where needed the description of the levels has been adapted to the ICU domain.

Properties of the registry

After analyzing the design of other incident registries, a list of properties of such registries has been composed. When setting the value for each property, the focus was on maximizing the accessibility. Therefore we have chosen not to identify the reporter of the incident and to use the results of the registry only for internal quality purposes. The patient can be identified by MR number, in order to be able to retrospectively analyze patient related factors. Although it would be possible to track the responsible physician or nurse combining the MR number with the registered shift (item 4a/b), it is emphasized that the results from the registry will not be used for (legal) prosecution. We expect that the anonymous and voluntary character of the registry will decrease the fear of blame and guilt, hence making it less troublesome for ICU personnel to report incidents.

Software

The emphasis during software development has been on accessibility and user friendliness. For each reported incident all items are displayed on one form, creating a scopic view of which data should be entered. To limit the time needed to report, two pull-down lists –one containing the incident categories and one presenting the reportable events within the selected category (items 1a/b)- can be used to select an incident. Another option is using the provided search functionality. Where possible, check boxes and radio buttons are used and free text fields are avoided.

Some incidents should also be reported to the paper, mandatory hospital's registry of Errors, Accidents and Near-misses (FOBO: Fouten, Ongevallen, Bijna-Ongevallen). To avoid double registration, it is possible to create a printable FOBO form, using the previously entered information.

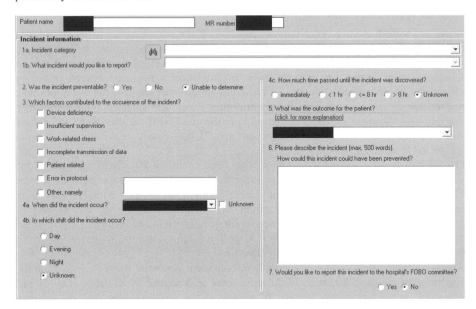

Figure 1- Incident Registry Form

To facilitate easy access, the software is integrated as an add-in in the ICU PDMS, already available on many point-of-care workstations on the wards. Presenting the pilot version to a group of physicians and nurses has not resulted in adjustments in the designed software. It has, however, led to additional instructions regarding to what should be reported as an incident.

4. Discussion

As the aim of the registry is to provide insight in the occurrence of incidents at the ICU, it is essential to know the extent to which incidents are actually registered, and whether they are registered correctly. The first months after implementing the registry it appeared that the number of reported FOBO-events increased, indicating a reduction of underreporting rather than an actual increase of events. The proportion of incidents that does get reported remains to be determined. We will discuss some barriers that can lead to underregistration. Furthermore, we will examine the classification of incidents as it is currently defined, in order to estimate the correctness of the registered incidents.

Barriers towards complete registration

Many reasons exist why incidents are not recorded. An incident must be noticed, recognized as such and the person noticing it must be aware of the possibility of registering and must be willing and able to do so. This requires instructing ICU nurses and physicians on which events are regarded as incidents and how they are registered. To reach a high level of registration, the costs must be minimal and benefits apparent. Costs do not only involve the time spent, but also "mental costs", e.g. fear of being blamed. The broad definition of an incident might not fit the experiences of physicians and nurses as they consider many incidents as 'expectable' and 'unpreventable', not triggering them to report. This indicates that the objective of the registry –i.e. gaining insight into the occurrence of undesired events- needs to be very clearly propagated. The pilot shows that especially physicians should be stimulated to report. This emphasizes the importance of providing feedback, which is crucial to increasing the completeness and correctness of registration. A committee of two physicians and two nurses is established to analyze and report to the ICU the registry's results on a regular basis.

Classification of incidents

Minimum variability within the reporting of events is essential. This means it must be obvious what constitutes an incident and how it should be recorded. An incident however, is often part of a chain of events, in which different linked elements can be determined: errors or other factors can lead to an induced patient condition, which can have a certain outcome [11].

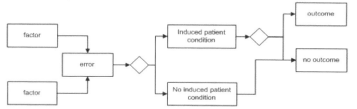

Figure 2: Chain of Events

Attempts to classify incidents according to 'root causes' are complicated by the fact that often several interlocking factors contribute to an error or a series of errors that in turn result in an incident (see *figure 2*). Thus an unambiguous instruction is needed, which clarifies which element of the chain ought to be reported as the incident. Therefore we instruct physicians and nurses to report the induced patient condition. Contributing factors and outcome can be recorded as items, the errors that have led to the incident can be mentioned in the free text description. In case of a near miss –i.e. no induced patient condition exists- the error itself becomes the incident, recording level '0' as the outcome.

5. Conclusion

Medical errors and adverse events occur frequently, but the susceptibility to these is not always admitted by ICU staff. Due to lack of insight into the situation regarding unwanted events at the ICU of the AMC, a new registry has been developed, which should make it possible to estimate the occurrence and severity of undesired events and detect patterns, in order to come to effective interventions. To achieve this we have created an approachable and accessible registry. Within this frame of reference we opted for a neutral term ('incident'), together with a broad definition, including all undesired and unintended events. The collection of reportable incidents is expected to contain the major part of undesired events occurring on the ICU. For the selection of attributes of an incident, a balance is sought between obtaining enough background information to enable focused research on preventive interventions and at the same time limiting the effort and time required to report. ICU personnel can use the registry anonymously and voluntarily, without having to worry about blame, guilt or legal consequences. The developed software is made available electronically as an add-in in the existing PDMS, presenting all items for each reported incident in one form, creating an overview of which data need to be entered.

During the first eight months after implementation 286 incidents have been reported. Analyzing these results will only give a rough idea of the unwanted events that actually took place on the ICU. It is essential to keep track of exactly which incidents get reported and also if they are reported correctly. This emphasizes the importance of providing feedback to increase the completeness and correctness of registration. Furthermore, we can theoretically assume that by implementing the new registry clinicians' awareness and attitude towards errors and near-misses has changed positively, yet further development and adjustments are required to come to a systematic method of incident monitoring, that can contribute to an actual patient safety increase.

6. Acknowledgments

We greatly acknowledge Andrew Jong, who graduated on this subject in November 2004. He has put a lot of time and effort into designing and developing this ICU incident registry. His thesis for Medical Information Sciences has been of significant value for writing this paper.

7. References

[1]	Kohn LT, Corrigan JM, Donaldson MS. *To err is human: building a safter health system*. Washington: National Academy Press, 2000.

[2]	Bracco D, Favre JB, Bissonnette B, et al. Human errors in a multidisciplinary Intensive Care Unit: a 1-year prospective study. *Intensive Care Medicine* 2001; 27: 137-45.

[3]	Willems, R. Either Hier werk je veilig, of je werkt hier niet. Final report Shell Holland, November 2004.

[4]	Sexton JB, Thomas EJ, Helmrich RL. Error, stress, and teamwork in medicine and aviation: cross sectional surveys. *British Medical Journal* 2000; 320: pp. 745-9.

[5]	Kivlahan C, Sangster W, Nelson K, Buddenbaum J, Lobenstein K. Developing a comprehensive electronic adverse event, reporting system in an academic health center. *Joint Commission Journal on Quality Improvement.* 2002; 28: 583-94.

[6]	Stevens CT, Simons MP, Vahl AC. Complicatieregistratie. *Nederlands Tijdschrift Heelkunde*. 2000; 9: 57-60.

[7]	Beckmann U, Bohringer C, Carless R, Gillies DM, et al. Evaluation of two methods for quality improvement in intensive care: facilitated incident monitoring and retrospective medical chart review [comment]. *Critical Care Medicine*. 2003; 31: 1006-11.

[8]	Flaatten H, Hevroy O. Errors in the intensive care unit (ICU). Experiences with an anonymous registration. *Acta Anaesthesiologica Scandinavica*. 1999; 43: 614-7.

[9]	Frey B, Kehrer B, Losa M, Braun H, Berweger L, et al. Comprehensive critical incident monitoring in a neonatal-pediatric intensive care unit: experience with the system approach [comment]. *Intensive Care Medicine*. 2000; 26: 69-74.

[10]	Beckmann U, West LF, Groombridge GJ, Baldwin I, Hart GK, et al. The Australian Incident Monitoring Study in Intensive Care: AIMS-ICU. The development and evaluation of an incident reporting system in intensive care [comment]. *Anaesthesia & Intensive Care*. 1996; 24: 314-9.

[11]	Helmreich RL, Musson DM. Threath and error management model: components and examples. (http://bmj.bmjjournals.com/misc/bmj.320.7237.781/sld001.htm)

Address for correspondence

Sabine van der Veer, Academic Medical Centre, room R01-438, PO box 22700
1100 DE Amsterdam, phone: + 31 20 566 6927, e-mail: s.n.vanderveer@amc.uva.nl

Connecting Medical Informatics and Bio-Informatics
R. Engelbrecht et al. (Eds.)
IOS Press, 2005

Applicability of Textual Clinical Practice Guidelines: Impact of Physician Interpretation

Jean-Charles Dufour[a], Roch Giorgi[a], Jean-Robert Harlé[b], Dominique Fieschi[a],
Françoise Volot[a], Marius Fieschi[a]

[a] Laboratoire d'Enseignement et de Recherche sur le Traitement de l'Information Médicale, Faculté de Médecine, Université de la Méditerranée, Marseille, France.
[b] Service de Médecine Interne, Hôpital de la Conception, Assistance Publique des Hôpitaux de Marseille, France

Abstract

OBJECTIVES: 1) Determine whether textual Clinical Practice Guidelines (CPGs) are interpreted accurately and unequivocally by targeted physicians. 2) Specify audience and perception of the CPGs.
METHOD: Comparative analysis of answers given by a panel of general practitioners to a series of questions and clinical case studies related to three textual CPGs produced and published by the French National Agency for Accreditation and Evaluation in Health (ANAES).
RESULTS: 68 to 96% of physicians are aware of the existence of the CPGs studied. Less than 50% state having read them. On average, 38% of physician interpretations of CPGs are incorrect (i.e., not in agreement with expert interpretation). Furthermore, there is disagreement among physicians responses.
CONCLUSION: This study credits the argument of disparities in practice which derive from inaccurate and discordant CPGs' interpretations. The results should prompt those responsible for producing such decision-making support to design documents that are better structured, less ambiguous, and more precise. In a model which facilitates their computerisation the expression of CPGs provides a solution that should be included upstream in the publication process.

Keywords
Guideline Adherence; Practice Guidelines; Physician's Practice Patterns; Decision Support Systems, Clinical

1. Introduction

Clinical Practice Guidelines (CPGs) are designed to compile the best recognised medical knowledge in order to provide physicians with a practical decisional aid. Their main objective is to improve the quality and effectiveness of medical care. Also they aim at reducing unjustified disparities in medical practice by providing physicians with consensual and reliable referential documents on which physicians can base their practice. To achieve such objectives, CPGs must be accessible, correctly interpreted and properly applied by the physicians for whom they are designed.

Currently, CPGs are expressed in essentially text format. They are published in various medical journals and/or published on the Internet to guarantee a wide dissemination and a relative accessibility [1]. This mode of dissemination cannot in itself impact medical practice sufficiently and modify habits in an appropriate and lasting way. For greater effectiveness, physicians should be regularly reminded of CPG content during their everyday clinical practice [2]. A way to achieve this objective is to provide computerized CPGs which can be readily and easily consulted in day-to-day practice and integrated within the care process [3]. We have being developing such computerized CPGs [4]. The first stage in computerizing CPGs is based on the analysis and interpretation of textual documents published by medical professional societies or specialised organisations like ANAES (the French National Agency for Accreditation and Evaluation in Health). The aim is to identify, within the textual document, the criteria and conditions that should influence a diagnosis or a therapeutic approach during medical consultation [6]. This analysis allows us to structure a CPG in the form of a decision tree and to implement it. As a result, we produce a computerized version which provides quick and direct access to the recommendations adapted to the patient profile. Structuring CPGs from an initial textual document often is difficult because of text ambiguities and incompleteness. For example, concepts contained within the initial CPG can be imprecise; certain notions implicitly rely on specialized expert knowledge; the narrative structure of a document does not always indicate an unequivocal care pathway; there are "knowledge gaps" which are not explicitly mentioned; etc [7]. Consequently, there is a real risk of partial or even erroneous interpretation in the development of the computerized version.

These considerations lead us to further question the editorial content of CPGs. We observe from experience that the latter is ill-adapted to the computerisation of CPGs. Further, do they properly reflect their original objectives (recommend an optimal care pathway, reduce disparities in practice) when used by physicians in appropriate conditions? In other words, are the difficulties of computerising textual CPGs specifically due to the change in formalisation, or rather do they reveal that the CPGs should be improved before distribution to physicians?

The main objective of this work is to determine whether the textual CPGs studied are interpreted accurately and unequivocally by the physicians for whom they are intended. The secondary objective is to further define physician audience and perception.

2. Material and Method

We choose to study three textual CPGs[1] published by ANAES and entitled:

1. « *Health care management for type 2 diabetic patients without complication, march 2000* »

2. « *Diagnosis, health care management and treatment of chronic lumbago patients, december 2000* »

3. « *Health care management for adult patients with primary high blood pressure, april 2000* »

Our study is based on an analysis of answers given by general practitioners (GPs) or residents (Rs) in response to a series of questions and clinical cases developed by the internist co-investigator of this study and related to these three CPGs. Participants were required to adhere strictly to the recommendations given by the CPGs when responding to the clinical cases. A sample of participating physicians was pulled at random from the GPs and the Rs in contact with our research laboratory. All physicians who agreed to take part in the study were included. The physicians were remunerated for their participation.

---

[1] These three CPG were mainly chosen as we had prior knowledge of their computerisation

A general questionnaire and two clinical cases were designed for each of the three CPGs:

- The general questionnaire was composed of four questions as follows: 1) Were you aware of the existence of the CPG? 2) Had you read it before? 3) How long did it take you to read it? 4) How do you rank the clarity of the CPG?

- Each clinical case was composed of 3 to 5 open-ended and focused questions such as « What treatment would you prescribe? », « When do you plan to see the patient again? » etc. Each of these questions addresses one of the following four medical tasks categories: diagnosis assessment, patient's medical follow-up, therapeutic options, and disease check-up. Further, physicians had the option of expressing any comments or problems concerning the description of the clinical case.

The answers were recorded directly by the physicians via an on-line questionnaire. Physicians were systematically reminded to consult and strictly observe the CPG recommendations when discussing the clinical cases. The original PDF documents of the CPGs published by the ANAES were instantly available and could be downloaded from the questionnaire interface.

Each physician possessed a username and a password which allowed him to add to or modify their answers while consulting the study website. Participants could not be identified from their login. No time limit was imposed for answering the questions.

For each clinical case, we asked the internist expert to provide his answer while strictly adhering to the CPG recommendations. The expert's answers supplied served as the "gold standard" in evaluating the physicians' answers to the same CPG. Each physician's answer was compared to the expert's answer by two medical observers who worked independently. An answer-score with two values (0 = physician's answer disagrees with expert's answer; 1 = physician's answer agrees with expert's answer) was defined. In the event of scoring disagreement between the first two medical observers, a third was called upon to give a definitive answer-score. The two values answer-score enabled us to calculate the percentage of answers in agreement with the expert's answers for each CPG.

The degree of agreement between the two medical observers was measured by the Kappa coefficient.

The degree of agreement between the participant physicians was measured by the intraclass coefficient correlation of the answers-scores. This coefficient allowed us to appreciate the degree of discordance concerning answers to the clinical cases within the physicians group.

3. Results

Twenty seven physicians took part in this study: 14 GPs (52%) and 13 Rs (48%).

The study questionnaire, primarily composed of clinical cases, contained 26 questions which the medical observers had given a score to. A total of 629 answers were given a score [26 * 27 - (73 missing data)]. The first two observers agreed for 549 answers (94.4%) and disagreed for 35 answers (6.4%). There was a good degree of agreement between the two observers (Kappa coefficient of 0.88, $p < 0.0001$).

3.1. CPG audience and perception

Table 1 records the percentage of physicians aware of the existence of each CPG and the percentage of physicians who had previously read each CPG. In general, we observed that whereas physicians are relatively well aware of the existence of the CPGs studied (68% to 96% according to the CPG), less than 50% of physicians stated that they had read them beforehand. The lumbago CPG attracted the lowest audience. It was also considered the least clear: more than 66% of physicians considered it "not clear at all" or "moderately clear". While 46.2% and 23.8% thought likewise about the CPGs on diabetes and HBP respectively.

Table 1: CPG audience and perception

	Diabetes	Lumbago	HBP
Aware of the existence	92%	68%	96%
Previously read	48%	36%	50%
Perfectly clear	53.8%	33.3%	76.2%
Moderately clear	23.1%	33.3%	19%
Not clear at all	23.1%	33.3%	4.8%
Average reading time (standard deviation)	27 mn (15)	42 mn (39)	27 mn (16)
Number of A4 pages	21	95	17

3.2. Concordance with the « gold standard »

The overall percentage of answers in concordance with the expert is only 62% (standard deviation, sd = 11%). Only 54% (sd = 18%) of answers were tallied with this reference for the lumbago CPG, 63% (sd = 14%) for HBP and 65% (sd = 15%) for diabetes (non-significant statistical difference). Table 2 shows a synthesis of the results for each physician group (GPs or Rs). We did not find any significant statistical difference in score distribution by CPG between the GPs and Rs groups, except for the CPG for HBP (p = 0.02).

Tableau 2 -Percentage of agreements with the 'gold standard' reference depending on CPG and physician group

	Diabetes	Lombago	HBP
GPs + Rs	65%	54%	63%
GPs	65%	49%	57%
Rs	64%	61%	70%

Table 3 shows the percentage of agreements with the reference, depending on the CPG and on the category of medical task addressed by clinical case questions. Whatever the CPG, the agreement with the expert was significantly stronger for questions focused on diagnosis assessment (p<0.01 when 'diagnosis assessment' was compared with every other category).

Table 3 - Percentage of agreements with the 'gold standard' reference depending on CPG and question category

	Diabetes	Lombago	HBP	Overall CPGs
Diagnosis assessment	98.2% (sd=9.6%)	69.6% (sd=36.1%)	87% (sd=22.4%)	86.4% (sd=15.4%)
Patient's medical follow-up	59.3% (sd=29.7%)	Not Applicable	58.7% (sd=35.8%)	58.5% (sd=24.1%)
Therapeutic options	72.2% (sd=32%)	52.2% (sd=51.1%)	54.4% (sd=23.4%)	62.7% (sd=24.9%)
Disease check-up	29.6% (sd=28.6%)	44.9% (sd=25.8%)	Not Applicable	37.2% (sd=27.4%)

If we consider the overall CPGs, the lower agreement was for questions on 'disease check-up' and the percentage of agreement between each question category is statistically significant (p<0.01), except for the comparison between 'Patient's medical follow-up' and 'Therapeutic options'.

3.3. Concordance between physician answers

Whichever CPG was considered, the calculation of the intraclass coefficient correlation (ICC) revealed a low rate of answer agreement between physicians (ICC Diabetes = 0.43, confidence interval at 95% (CI95%) 0.23-0.77; ICC Lombago = 0.13, CI95% 0.03-0.53; ICC HBP = 0.39, CI95% 0.19-0.77; $p<10-6$ in every case). This variability in answers to the clinical cases suggested divergence in understanding and interpreting CPGs. Indeed, we can consider that problem in understanding the clinical cases themselves can be excluded since no criticism was made by the physicians concerning the description of these cases.

4. Discussion

The objective of this study was to determine if the CPGs studied helped physicians respond correctly to a given clinical problem and if they gave rise to divergences in interpretation and/or in understanding. The results obtained showed that on average, in 38% of cases, physician interpretation of the CPGs was incorrect (did not match the expert interpretation). Above all, our results revealed the disparities between the physicians' answers themselves, a fact that minimizes the potential bias due to the choice of a "gold standard". Although the difference was not significant, the rate of incorrect answers was higher for the CPG concerning chronic lumbago. It is worth pointing out, that this particular CPG presented the most difficulties during its computerisation stage (a stage carried out prior and independently of this study). Its editorial content did not lend itself easily to structuring as a refined decision tree. The other two CPGs (diabetes and HBP) were more easily structured in this form, but were not exempt from imprecision and ambiguity.

A frequent observation about the textual and static format of CPGs is that they are difficult to use in daily practice. Partly this might explain why physicians hardly followed the recommendations given by CPGs in their daily care activity. Thus it was implicitly felt that the observed divergence between practice and CPGs was mainly due to the fact that, for various reasons, such as inadequate format, physicians did not use CPGs and consequently did not follow their proposed recommendations. Although the physicians used and followed the CPGs, in our study we observed disparate interpretations brought to light by divergent answers to the clinical cases. Therefore our findings tend to argue that some of the disparity in practice is derived from inaccurate and unequal interpretation of CPGs, even though used by physicians. This hypothesis should be backed up by further in-depth studies involving a greater number of physicians and an increased diversity of CPGs.

In our study, there were open-ended questions in the clinical cases so as to avoid influencing physician answers (even if more easily used statistically, close-ended questions do not correspond to the reality of clinical practice). The scoring of the answers by the medical observers, indispensable for statistical result analysis, showed a certain stability (the Kappa coefficient measuring agreement between the two medical observers was 0.88).

5. Conclusion

In their classical editorial format, CPGs are not adapted to computerisation [8]. The same difficulties encountered in developing a computerised CPG from a text version are also experienced by physicians themselves when they translate a CPG into operational behaviours within a clinical context. The results of our study tend to support the argument that Cpgs are a source of incorrect and different interpretations among physicians for whom they were specifically designed. These results should encourage those responsible for producing such decision-making supports to provide documents which are better structured, less ambiguous and more precise to ensure correct and unequivocal interpretation. The computerisation of CPGs which requires explicit knowledge clarification and rigorous content structuring is a means to detect potential stumbling-blocks upstream. The advantage of computerisation is not just to provide a support which is easier to use and more readily available than a textual document. It also imposes the need to organize and structure information in a more comprehensive, coherent and consistent way so as to guarantee a better and unequivocal understanding. The development of CPGs according to a computerisable model should precede the publication stage of classical textual CPGs. Computerisation itself gives advance warning of weaknesses that must be addressed upstream of the publication stage so as to benefit both the computer solution and the physicians who actually use the textual version.

6. Acknowledgments

We thank Dr. Omar Bouhaddou for his helpful proofreading and comments.

7. References

[1]   Zielstorff RD. *Online practice guidelines: issues, obstacles, and future prospects.* J Am Med Inform Assoc 1998; 5 (3):227-36.

[2]   Durieux P, Ravaud P, Dosquet P, Durocher A. [Effectiveness of clinical guideline implementation strategies: systematic review of systematic reviews] fr. Gastroenterol Clin Biol 2000; 24(11):1018-25.

[3]   Ciccarese P, Caffi E, Boiocchi L, Quaglini S, Stefanelli M. *A guideline management system.* Medinfo 2004; 2004:28-32.

[4]   Dufour JC, Fieschi M, Fieschi D, Giorgi R, Gouvernet J. *A platform to develop and to improve effectiveness of online computable guidelines.* Stud Health Technol Inform 2003; 95:800-5.

[5]   Agence Nationale d'Accréditation et d'Evaluation en Santé [Web Page]. Available at http://www.anaes.fr. (Accessed January 2005).

[6]   Dufour JC, Fieschi D, Fieschi M. *Coupling computer-interpretable guidelines with a drug-database through a web-based system--The PRESGUID project.* BMC Med Inform Decis Mak 2004; 4(1):2.

[7]   Patel VL, Arocha JF, Diermeier M, Greenes RA, Shortliffe EH. *Methods of cognitive analysis to support the design and evaluation of biomedical systems: the case of clinical practice guidelines.* J Biomed Inform. 2001; 34 (1):52-66.

[8]   Riou C, Dréau H, Séroussi B, Bouaud J, Venot A. *Recommandations de rédactions des guides de bonnes pratiques en vue de leur implémentation dans un système d'aide à la décision.* Proc Technologies de l'information et de la communication pour les pratiques médicales. Eds: Harmel A, Hajromdhane R, Fieschi M. Informatique et Santé, Springer 16, 2004: 267-76.

Address for correspondence

Dr Jean-Charles Dufour.
LERTIM, Faculté de Médecine, 27 boulevard Jean Moulin, 13385 Marseille Cedex 05.
Email : jean-charles.dufour@medecine.univ-mrs.fr / URL : http://cybertim.timone.univ-mrs.fr

Connecting Medical Informatics and Bio-Informatics
R. Engelbrecht et al. (Eds.)
IOS Press, 2005
551

Semantic Challenges in Database Federation: Lessons Learned

Thomas Ganslandt[a], Udo Kunzmann[b], Katharina Diesch[a], Péter Pálffy[c],
Hans-Ulrich Prokosch[a,c]

[a] *Department of Medical Informatics, University of Erlangen, Germany*
[b] *DRG Coordination Unit, Erlangen University Hospital, Germany*
[c] *Center for Medical Information and Communication, Erlangen University Hospital, Germany*

Abstract

In this project an integrated analysis of data from disparate surgery and anaesthesiology departmental information systems was carried out. Due to the lack of shared primary keys, a multi-stage "soft" matching method was implemented. Results of the matching steps are described in detail. Inconsistencies were shown to exist for identifying data, semantic definition of documentation content and documented data itself. Minimum requirements for interdisciplinary documentation in autonomous systems should include shared semantic definitions of documentation content as well as robust and regularly validated interfaces for identifying data.

Keywords:
Hospital Information Systems, Analysis, Database Federation

1. Introduction

Clinical IT infrastructure has traditionally been very heterogeneous[1]. In many cases, adoption of IT systems started with departmental applications like laboratory automation which were later supplemented with enterprise-wide hospital information systems (HIS). Even though the case for integrated enterprise-wide information systems has been convincingly made[1;2], ancillary systems continue to be implemented, driven by the needs of individual clinical disciplines. The proliferation of departmental systems in areas of interdisciplinary cooperation can lead to situations where aspects of the same process are being documented in several systems concurrently. Semantic differences in the definition of documentation items and primary keys result in contradicting reports generated from such systems and raise barriers towards the successful implementation of an enterprise-wide unified reporting infrastructure[1;3].

In this paper we describe the results of a federated reporting project consolidating the input from four separate documentation systems. The project was initiated to provide the foundations for the introduction of time-based service charges between the anaesthesiology and surgical departments at a German university hospital. The project focused on the comparison of time-spans relevant to surgery process measures (e.g. entering/leaving the operating room (OR), cut/suture-time) separately documented in all systems.

2. Materials and Methods

Four documentation systems were included into the study:

- an administrative system which generates the enterprise-wide patient and case IDs and manages admission/discharge/transfer data (ADT) as well as billing information
- an ancillary system for anaesthesiology documentation
- an ancillary system for the documentation of surgical procedures used by all surgical departments except cardio- and neuro-surgery
- a separate ancillary system for the documentation of cardio-surgery procedures

All systems are supposed to share the enterprise-wide patient and case IDs as common identifiers, which are transferred from the administrative system to the ancillary systems by means of a central HL7-based communication server. Each ancillary system uses self-generated primary keys for anaesthesias and surgical procedures. There is no shared key linking them between systems, so it was necessary to identify surrogate fields suitable for matching records during the course of the study. Operating room-IDs were not consistently documented between systems (the cardio-surgery system allowed free-text entry), so it was decided to identify a timestamp field suitable for matching.

Data warehouse tools (Cognos DecisionStream^{TM}) were used to import data from all systems into a central database (Oracle 9i^{TM}). The administrative and surgical ancillary systems were accessed using a direct SQL-based interface to the respective system databases. The anaesthesiology data was imported using flat files (CSV format). The observation period was set to the 2nd and 3rd quarter of 2004.

The following processing steps were carried out (see fig. 1):

1. After importing data into a staging area, all case IDs were compared to the case ID table of the administrative system. Records containing invalid, cancelled or missing case IDs were excluded from further processing.

2. A matching of records from the surgical systems to the anaesthesiology system was performed using the shared case IDs. The distribution of non-matched records among the surgical departments was analysed.

3. The time-spans documented in the remaining records were extracted and their exact definitions gathered from the administrators of the respective systems. Time-spans with identical or similar definitions were identified and the percentage of fully documented records was calculated for each time-span in each system.

4. A field suitable for further matching of surgery and anaesthesiology records within each case ID was selected and matching performed.

5. A sample of non-matching records were visualized using the Pathifier workflow visualization tool[4] to identify possible mismatch causes.

6. For the remaining records the duration of identically or similarly defined time-spans was calculated and the differences were compared.

3. Results

A total of 10026 records were imported from the anaesthesiology (AN) system, 14926 and 679 records were imported from the general surgery (GS) and cardio-surgery (CS) systems, respectively. Figure 1 shows the matching process and the records matched or rejected at each step:

1. Case ID validation: From the AN dataset 614 records (6.2%) were rejected because of invalid (527) or cancelled (79) case IDs or case IDs referring to previously closed hospital visits (8). The GS dataset contained 272 records (1.9%) with invalid (254), cancelled (10) or previously closed (8) case IDs. The CS dataset contained 5 records (0.7%) with invalid (4) or cancelled (1) case IDs.

2. Case ID matching of the remaining data: 928 records (9.3%) of the AN dataset could not be matched to either surgical dataset based on case IDs. 6225 records (41.7%) of the GS and 53 records (7.8%) of the CS datasets could not be matched to the AN records. Further analysis shows that the majority of unmatched GS records come from departments which typically carry out procedures where general anaesthesia is not necessary (e.g. ophthalmology (23%), ambulatory general surgery (20%), dermatology (14%)). The majority of the 928 non-matched AN records (72%) were related to the neurosurgery department, which started production use of the GS system only after the study period.

3. A total of 6 semantically distinct time-spans was found in all datasets (Figure 2). The 3 time-spans from the surgical datasets were identically defined, with 1 time-span being differently named. Of the 4 time-spans from the AN dataset only one matched the surgical time-spans (cut/suture). The definition of the "suture" timestamp, however, differed in that the surgical departments documented the end whereas the anaesthesiology department documented the beginning of suturing.

4. The "cut" timestamp was chosen for the second matching stage as it was identically defined in all datasets and was present in >98.9% of the remaining records of all datasets. At this stage records were joined both on case ID and "cut"-timestamp with a variable time window to allow for slight differences between documented timestamps. Figure 3a shows the percentage of matched records plotted against the size of the time window. Large time windows allowed multiple matching of 2 or more distinct procedures and anaesthesias within the window. Figure 3b show the number of multiply used primary keys plotted against time window size.

5. A match time window of ±2 hours was selected, resulting in successful matches for 6458 (43.3%) records of the GS and 541 (79.7%) of the CS datasets as well as 6447 (69.6%) records from the AN dataset. A remainder of 1876 (12.6%) records from GS, 80 (11.8%) records from CS and 1461 (14.6%) records from AN could not be matched on the "cut"-timestamp even though a case ID match existed. A random sample of the cases was visualized with the Pathifier tool to determine mismatch causes. Excerpts showing typical configurations are displayed in Figure 4.

6. For all 6985 matched procedure/anaesthesia pairs, the durations of the cut/suture time-spans documented both by the surgical and anaesthesiology departments were determined and their differences calculated. Figure 5 shows the distribution of differences.

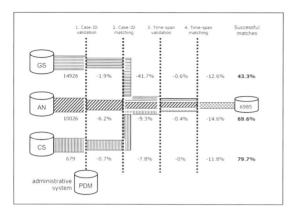

Figure 1: Filtering and matching process with percentages of records from general surgery (GS), anaesthesiology (AN) and cardio-surgery (CS) datasets rejected at each step and the percentage of records successfully matched for each data source.

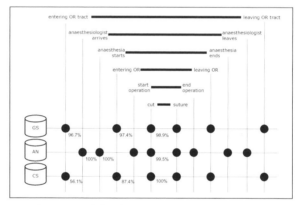

Figure 2: Time-spans documented the datasets. Dots show the presence of timestamps in each system. The percentage of records containing the time-span is displayed to the right of each dot.

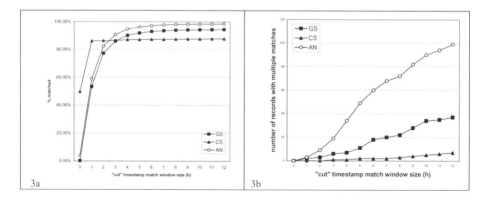

Figure 3: (a) percentage of records from each dataset matched with case ID and "cut"-timestamp plotted against match window size (b) number of primary keys from each data set present in multiple matches.

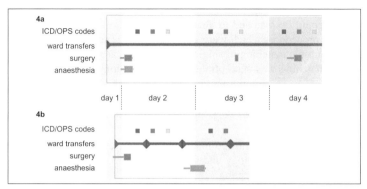

Figure 4: Visualization of 2 typical cases. (a) 3 surgical procedures were documented, only 1 of which is accompanied by a documented anaesthesia, with the patient being on an intensive care unit (ICU). (b) an operation and anaesthesia are documented, but exactly 24hrs apart.

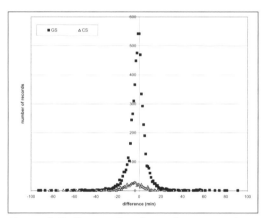

Figure 5: Difference distribution between cut/suture-durations documented by surgery and anaesthesiology departments

4. Discussion

In [1] Lenz et al argue that the coexistence of autonomous departmental information systems entails semantic heterogeneity and inconsistencies of data replicated between systems. Our findings are in many aspects consistent with these statements. While most records contained valid case IDs imported from the administrative system, a relevant percentage (6.2%) of the AN dataset could not be processed because of invalid or cancelled IDs. Procedures for the correct processing of cancellation messages and automatic or manual revision of manually entered case IDs (e.g. in emergency situations) appear to be insufficient. Without a shared primary key for surgical procedures and anaesthesias, a "soft" matching method based on case IDs and documented timestamps had to be devised.

The matching was further complicated by differing semantic definitions of the one timestamp present in all three systems. Non-matches of case IDs could largely be explained by surgical procedures carried out without general anaesthesia and anaesthesias performed for a surgical department not yet taking part in electronic documentation during the study period. Even with a relatively lax match time-window of ±2 hours only 77-86% of the remaining surgical records could be matched to anaesthesias based on case ID and "cut" timestamp. Interdisciplinary procedures which were documented as separate records in the GS and CS systems led to multiple matching of single corresponding anaesthesia records in several cases. Time-based matching was susceptible to documentation errors (cf. Figure 4b).

Case visualization proved to be a valuable tool for identifying prototypical scenarios behind the remaining non-matched records (e.g. operations on an ICU (Figure 4a) or documentation errors (Figure 4b)).

The majority of cut/suture-durations within the matched records were documented with only slight deviations between anaesthesiology and surgery (±20min), but there were also records which differed up to ±2 hours in duration.

5. Conclusions

Integrated analysis of data from 4 administrative and departmental systems in this study showed inconsistencies of identifying data and semantic definitions of documentation content as well as documented data itself. Use of a shared enterprise-wide documentation system would have eliminated many of these problems as well as the need for "soft" matching methods. A time-motion-study could be carried out to gather workflow data independently from the existing departmental documentation systems.

A minimum requirement for documentation in autonomous departmental systems should be shared semantic definitions of documentation content. Interfaces for exchange of case IDs between administrative and departmental systems should robustly handle update and cancellation messages and be validated on a regular basis.

6. References

[1] Lenz R, Kuhn KA. Intranet meets hospital information systems: the solution to the integration problem? Methods Inf Med 2001; 40(2):99-105.

[2] Stead WW. Systems for the year 2000: the case for an integrated database. MD Comput 1991; 8(2):103-110.

[3] Xu Y, Sauquet D, Zapletal E, Lemaitre D, Degoulet P. Integration of medical applications: the 'mediator service' of the SynEx platform. Int J Med Inform 2000; 58-59:157-166.

[4] Ganslandt T, Frankewitsch T, Mueller ML, Kunze U, Buerkle T, Krieglstein CF et al. Visualization of clinical workflows merging data from multiple information systems. Medinfo 2004; 2004(CD):1606.

7. Address for Correspondence

Dr. Thomas Ganslandt
Department of Medical Informatics
FAU Erlangen
Krankenhausstr. 12
D-91052 Erlangen
Germany
Email: thomas.ganslandt@imi.med.uni-erlangen.de

Connecting Medical Informatics and Bio-Informatics
R. Engelbrecht et al. (Eds.)
IOS Press, 2005

557

Mobidis: Toward a Patient Centric Healthcare Information System

Fabrizio L Ricci[a], Luca D Serbanati[b]

[a] IRPPS-CNR, Via Nizza, 128, 00198 Rome, Italy
[b] Politehnica University, Spl. Independentei, 313, 060032 Bucharest, Romania

Abstract

The paper presents some results of the MobiDis project. MobiDis is an information system that includes healthcare consumers and providers in a unique, virtual organisation aimed at promoting a patient centric paradigm in healthcare. It allows logons from desktop or laptop computers, as well as wireless PDAs or tablet PCs connected to Internet. In MobiDis the clinical data of each consumer are stored in the consumer's virtual healthcare record (VHR), a highly structured entity that exists on the network and is simultaneously updated with information from multiple locations. The MobiDis architecture creates an environment for VHRs by providing them with a large variety of services. In order to prove that our proposed architectural solution meets the project goals a prototype was developed. The paper describes the MobiDis architecture and the VHR services, and briefly presents the prototype.

Keywords:
Electronic medical record; Continuity of care; Web services-oriented architecture; Location-based services

1. Introduction

Healthcare is an important area for applications based on new ITC infrastructures. With the arrival of location-based services and increased mobility the range of applications used in the provision of healthcare is expected to enhance the quality of life of citizens in terms of prevention and treatment.

The MobiDis system is designed to provide a fast, secure access to healthcare processes in a location-independent fashion. The infrastructure uses the new technologies available in order to provide a robust, platform-independent usage and location-transparent environment.

The paper emphasis is on the system architecture. After a presentation of the system, the Section 3 introduces the Virtual Healthcare record which is the central, structuring concept of the system. We describe the prototype in Section 4.

2. General Presentation

The MobiDis project aims to study and propose an information system architecture necessary to support the healthcare process including healthcare consumers (HCCs) and providers (HCPs) in a unique, virtual organisation by promoting a patient centric paradigm in healthcare. MobiDis federates different healthcare organizations and individuals in one virtual structure able to guarantee the continuity of the cure. In such an organization the role of hospitals is to treat only patients which need complex therapies. In order to improve the quality of life of the patients, MobiDis promotes home healthcare delivery making use of telemedicine and wireless communications.

Many nations are planning the introduction of electronic medical record systems in order to allow integration of healthcare between the individual care providers and hospitals, and increase the efficiency due to the reduction of the time necessary to gather existing patient's medical data.

Actually similar projects are carried out at both European and national level. Both the Good European Health Record project and the projects carried out in Great Britain, Canada, New Zeeland, and Australia [1] [2] [3] [4] are studying how to implement an electronic medical record-based national system using recent progress in software technology and research results on complex systems.

The MobiDis architecture emphasises:

1. the care consumer-centric solution for the system architecture: the care consumer's VHR is central in this architecture and integrates the most relevant information regarding the consumer's health, medical data as well as local jurisdictions;

2. the national/regional-wide distribution of services, many of them based on legacy systems or services;

3. the ubiquitous access to information regarding the care consumers' health and medical data;

4. the use of wireless devices in the healthcare systems;

5. the flexibility of taking future design decisions and adaptability to environment changes.

In MobiDis the clinical data of each consumer are stored in the consumer's virtual healthcare record (VHR), a highly structured entity that exists on the network and is simultaneously supplied from multiple locations with updated information. The VHR can be viewed as an information container but often this information is distributed in remote databases or systems and the VHR uses only references to it.

VHR is an electronic healthcare records (EHR) too, but it is shared by all potential health care providers and contains all data about the care consumer's significant health episodes. VHR provides medical professionals and organizations with services for accessing clinical data of the healthcare consumers. Sharing EHRs between several care providers gives the opportunities to support coordinated care consumer assessment, facilitate the identification of health risks as well as contributors to health. It also supplies healthcare providers with information they need to plan and allocate resources appropriately and efficiently. The VHR can facilitate the referral process by allowing for the interoperability of information between points of care and ensuring levels of speed, information ubiquity, accuracy, completeness, reliability and clarity. Finally, the EHR can enable decision support (not decision making) by applying validated healthcare guidelines to patient/person information.

In order to better illustrate the VHR, in the followings we present the VHR main features.

3. Virtual Healthcare Record

Accessing VHR

Interaction with the MobiDis system is performed only by registered users and external systems that comply with a certain profile. Every user (medical professional or simple citizen) has an account which gives her/him the possibility to access the system. Their registration is performed by system administrators and controlled by careful designed registration procedures. The system provides tools for the development of new VHRs. Thus, a subgroup of HCPs has the rights to create new VHRs for new-born babies or for people that do not possess a VHR yet. In such a situation the system queries the National Social Register for confirmation and for data initialization.

In MobiDis' approach VHR is a multifaceted [10], reactive entity, which offers to each stakeholder a customised view and acts as an event-driven mediator between other systems and users in the environment.

Medical Events

A cornerstone of the MobiDis system is the medical event (ME). VHR structures the contained information in a chronological order as a list of MEs of that care consumer.

An ME is a complex object that contains information related to a noteworthy healthcare episode (or closely connected series of episodes) in the life of a HCC. Information includes: event type, referral purpose, insert time, event time, duration, and place, identity of the referring care provider (including her/his signature), support used for taking the decision: observations, measurements, diagnostic tests, additional documents that provide evidence (analysis results, x-rays with both text interpretation and image scan, etc), diagnostic, referral report, therapy supplied, and so on.

Each ME may be associated with a schedule (in fact a workflow) of future activities to be executed by certain agents (HCC or HCP) as a consequence of the ME occurrence. These activities will be queued and traced by the system and their completion confirmation will be accounted.

Information Updating

The MobiDis system environment consists not only of users but also of other information systems. In order to connect VHRs with external systems, messages regarding MEs are exchanged with these systems. The clinical data in VHRs may be automatically updated with electronic clinical annotations obtained from electronic patient records (EPR) or EHR which are located at primary health care organisations and different hospital departments, and respectively at GP practices. Conversely, when changes in the VHR of a care consumer occur, every EPR or EHR related with that consumer is notified and it can request VHR exporting services for updating.

The clinical data may be modified by the HCP that created it only by giving/providing a new version: previous versions of the HCE are not overwritten, but archived.

Electronic Personal Medical Record Booklet (EPMRB)

Care consumers retain a degree of control over their own medical information. A GP, for instance, may release information available to other care providers only with the consent of the patient or her/his relatives. A HCC can access her/his own VHR any time, but only partially: her/his view. This view translates specialized terms or explains the difficult-to-understand-by-novices information in simple understandable phrases.

One of the most valuable views on the VHR is the *electronic personal medical record booklet*. ModiDis provides appropriate services for such views. With these services the care consumers are managed with care programmes usually home-based. The booklet can be used by chronic illness patients or children' parents. A need for accurate, up-to-date information on patients' respectively children's current problems is of vital importance. In these cases constant interventions with an upgradable treatment record as well as relatives information and councils are compulsory. It enables them with a constant transfer of information between involved medical practitioners, nurses or hospital staff, and care consumers. The transfer is bidirectional so that the booklet becomes a multimedia intermediary between involved care providers and consumers. In MobiDis the booklet is directly derived from the virtual medical record of the child or of the chronic illness patient.

Of course, such a booklet may be considered useful for any citizen. It might used/him during his/her entire life.

Heterogeneous Platforms

MobiDis allows logons from desktop or laptop computers, as well as wireless PDAs or tablet PCs connected to Internet. The access to the requested critical information is in real-time and as safe as possible. So, the system allows the use of various client platforms. The data sent by the system differs within these platforms, corresponding to the resources of each platform. Each platform would use a client application to connect to a VHR system. At the first connection, client application will access a server which provides the identification needed by the client in order to gain the desired services. The system analyses the client queries and dispatches the services to the client according to the desired service types and platform. If the client system doesn't have all resources needed to process the requested information, the system must adapt the information to the available resources on the client. Some options are: a) the elimination of oversized tags; b) removal of high-resolution images whose resize isn't an option or it is not necessary because they won't be correctly interpreted; c) exclusion of less significant tags; d) style modification (font decrease, spaces removal); and e) splitting data into pages and sending them one by one.

Service-Orientation

From an architectural point of view, MobiDis is a web services-oriented, multi-level distributed system (Figure 1), which is aligned with the service-oriented architecture (SOA) principles. The MobiDis architecture creates a rich environment for a VHR by providing it with a large diversity of services, mainly web-services, that is entities located somewhere

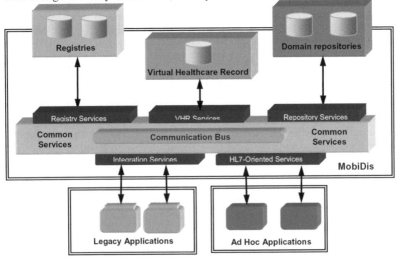

Figure 1 - Services in MobiDis

on the Internet, with a well-defined interface and associated semantics, which can be discovered or directly accessed by authorized clients. We chose the web services paradigm for the MobisDis architecture because this model facilitates integration of legacy applications and platform interoperability.

A client for MobiDis services is any system, application or service which is authorized to approach the medical data supplied by MobiDis. The users of these clients are doctors, patients, medical and sanitary staff, organisations, and authorities. The clients can access specialized, ubiquitously reachable services in order to obtain information stored in VHRs or request transactional activities. For such clients the MobiDis services are only access points.

Such a client may previously know the service or may dynamically discover it using the service's associated semantics and a discovery service included in MobiDis. A new service may also be dynamically composed from some existing services by defining the service semantics as a workflow which integrates these services.

4. MobiDis Prototype

The MobiDis prototype implements some of the previous requirements and uses the J2EE technologies in order to create a distributed, robust, VHR-based system. The prototype consists of four applications, tied together by the architecture presented in Figure 2. Each of them is a complete, modular, independent entity which implements a number of services regarding the tier functionality.

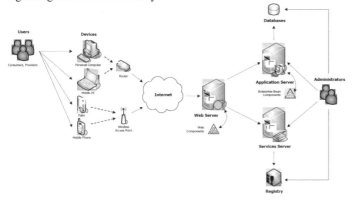

Figure 2 - Architecture of the MobiDis prototype

1. Client Application implements four platform-oriented types of graphical interfaces (Java window- and applet-based interfaces running on PDA and PC platforms) allowing users to experience, interact with, and perceive the MobiDis system. It is a friendly, simple way to benefit from full functionality, without having to be familiar with IT technologies and entities implied in the MobiDis architecture. A hint about presentation of healthcare events in a PDA-based graphical interface is presented in *Figure 3*.

2. Web Application implements the functionality of the server-side presentation tier. It consists from a layer of JSP and servlet components. Servlets are responsible for the dialogue with the user: logon, access device identification, request processing, and session monitoring. JSPs generate the Web pages sent to the Client Application.

3. Service Server implements a specialized naming and directory service. It can be viewed as a "Yellow Pages" of services available in MobiDis. The client can access different services by only making remote calls to the lookup services of the Service Server. All the services that can be accessed in MobiDis have their locations on remote, usually-unknown-by-clients platforms. In order to access them MobiDis uses a flexible lookup mechanism which de-couples the physical address of the service implementation of the service client. The mechanism is implemented by a UDDI-Registry server.

4. Application Server is the core of the MobiDis prototype. It provides data access to the clients, manages user roles security and provides persistence to the business objects. The relevant data is stored in the database and encapsulated in the entity beans. Some of the entity beans behave as web service by exposing service endpoint interfaces which are accessed by web components and client applications.

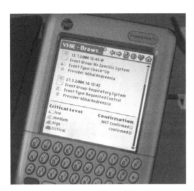

Figure 3 - The HCEs list in a PDA graphical interface

5. Conclusions

The cooperation among HCPs and HCCs for promoting better quality and reducing of costs requires IC&T support, distributed computing in conditions of location transparency and clients' mobility, semantic interoperability among applications, and service composition functions. The MobiDis project investigated an architectural solution of a such distributed, service-oriented system. In the paper some results of this research were presented. Much remains to do in the field of semantic interoperability, semantic annotation of services, and service composition. Other projects with this aim were already started.

6. Acknowledgments

The authors wish to acknowledge and thank their partners in the MobiDis project, the valuable contribution of the "Gang of Four" who implemented the MobiDis prototype at the University "Politehnica" of Bucharest (Cristi Radu, Razvan Lucrateanu, Catalin Barcau, Ovidiu Manolache), and Daniela Luzi for the support she gave us in the paper writing.

7. References

[1]   Blobel B, et al (eds.) *Contribution of medical informatics to health*. IOS Press, 2004
[2]   Canada Health Infoway, *EHRS Blueprint, an Interoperable HER framework*, July 2003.
[3]   www.health.gov.au, *HealthConnect Business Architecture Overview*, March 2002
[4]   Department of Health, Delivering 21st Century IT Support for the NHS. *National Specification for Integrated Care Records Service*, July .
[5]   Ferrara FM, Grimson W, Sottile PA. The holistic architectural approach to integrating the healthcare record in the overall information system, Proceedings of MIE 1999
[6]   Ferri F, Pisanelli DM, Ricci FL, Consorti F, Piermattei A. Toward a general model for the description of multimedia clinical data. In: Methods of Information in Medicine 1998, Vol: 37(3)
[7]   Iakovidis I. From electronic medical record to personal health records: present situation and trends in European Union in the area of electronic healthcare records. Medinfo 1998;9 Pt 1:suppl 18-22
[8]   Peterson H, Ljungkvist G, Appelqvist O. *User Requirements on Electronic Health Care Record*, Springer Verlag, Stockholm 1996
[9]   Ricci FL, Rossi Mori A, Consorti F. Purposive views in patient records: influence on reuse of clinical information and interoperability. In: *Proceedings of the International Working Conference "Electronic Patient Records in Medical Practice"*, 1998
[10] Serbanati L.D. *Integrating Tools for Software Development*. Yourdon Press Computing Series, Prentice Hall, Englewood Cliffs, New Jersey (1992).
[11] Thought Leaders. *Connected Health*. Ed. K. Dean, Premium Publishing, 2003

Address for correspondence

Fabrizio L. Ricci, IRPPS-CNR, Via Nizza, 128, 00198 Rome, Italy, *f.ricci@irpps.cnr.it*

Connecting Medical Informatics and Bio-Informatics
R. Engelbrecht et al. (Eds.)
IOS Press, 2005

Obstacles to Implementing an Execution Engine for Clinical Guidelines Formalized in GLIF

Petr Kolesa, Josef Špidlen, Jana Zvárová

EuroMISE Centre, Institute of Computer Science AS CR, Department of the Medical Informatics, Prague, Czech Republic

Abstract

This article is on obstacles we faced when developing an executable representation of guidelines formalized the Guideline Interchange Format (GLIF). The GLIF does not fully specify the representation of guidelines at the implementation level as it is focused mainly on the description of guideline's logical structure. Our effort was to develop an executable representation of guidelines formalized in GLIF and to implement a pilot engine, which will be able to process such guidelines. The engine has been designed as a component of the MUltimedia Distributed Record system version 2 (MUDR^2). When developing executable representation of guidelines we paid special attention to utilisation of existing technologies to achieve the highest reusability.

Main implementation areas, which are not fully covered by GLIF, are a data model and an execution language. Concerning the data model we have decided to use MUDR^2's native data model for this moment and to keep watching the standardisation of a virtual medical record to implement it in execution engine in the near future. When developing the execution language, first of all we have specified necessities, which the execution language ought to meet. Then we have considered some of the most suitable candidates: Guideline Execution Language (GEL), GELLO, Java and Python. Finally we have chosen GELLO although it does not completely cover all required areas. The main GELLO's advantage is that it is a proposed HL7 standard. In this paper we show some of the most important disadvantages of GELLO as an executable language and how we have solved them.

Keywords:
Guidelines, Clinical Decision Support Systems, GLIF.

1. Introduction

One of the main research projects running at EuroMISE Centre is the development of clinical decision support systems. The aim of this effort is to develop tools that will reduce routine activities performed by the physician as well as allow standardisation and improving of given care, which implies substantial financials savings. Many projects focused on formalization of the knowledge contained in clinical guidelines were recently running at EuroMISE Centre.

It is known that only a small number of physicians uses clinical paper-based guidelines during diagnosing and treatment. This problem is caused by the existence of a large amount of relevant guidelines, which are frequently updated in addition[1]. It is very time-consuming to monitor all relevant guidelines.

We have experience formalizing clinical guidelines using the Guideline Interchange Format (GLIF) [1]. Guidelines formalized in such a way have been used mainly for education of medical students, but a tool for automatic execution of formalized guidelines [2, 3] did not exist.

Another important project recently realized at EuroMISE Centre was the development of a new system for structured electronic health record called MUltimedia Distributed Record version 2 (MUDR[2]) [4]. One of the MUDR[2]'s most valued features is that it allows to change the data model dynamically and on-fly [5]. In addition, it supports versioning of the data model, so the access to the data is possible not only by the current date, but also at an arbitrary point in the past. This feature is important for checking whether a treatment conforms to the guidelines.

2. Materials and Methods

We have decided to join outputs from both these projects to create a *guideline based decision support system*. We have created an execution engine that is able to process formalized guidelines and added it to MUDR[2] system. MUDR[2] already contained some decision support system tools. These tools could be extended by plugins, but the knowledge gained from guidelines was required to be hardwired in the program code of plugins. This approach was not convenient, since it was difficult and expensive to change a plug-in, when a certain guideline had been updated. The utilisation of GLIF-formalized guidelines solves this problem. As the GLIF does not specify the guideline's implementation level, we have developed our own executable representation of the GLIF model.

When developing an executable representation of guidelines we paid special attention to utilisation of existing technologies and tools wherever possible. We have already converted some guidelines to the GLIF model in Protègè 2000 [6]. These guidelines are transferred to an executable representation in XML. It is also possible to export a formalized guideline from Protègè to the Resource Description Framework [7] (RDF) format. This export depicts static structure very well, but there are few possibilities to represent a dynamic behaviour like data manipulation. Therefore we have developed our own representation, which is based on XML and has all features missing in the Protègè RDF export.

From the point of implementation, two areas of executable representation are important: the data that are processed (*data model*) and the program that works with these data (*execution language*). In the next sections we will describe them in greater details.

3. Results

3.1   The Data Model

The data model must define following three topics: *which data it provides, a data naming convention* and *a structure of these data*. An obvious choice of the data model for clinical guidelines is a virtual medical record (VMR) [8]. As the standard of the VMR is still being developed, we have decided for now to use the native data model of MUDR[2] and keep watching the standardisation process to be able to implement the VMR in the future.

---

[1] Approximately 2000 pages of new or updated guidelines are distributed to physicians in the Czech Republic annualy.

3.1.1   Which Data It Provides

As the $MUDR^2$ allows to represent arbitrary data in its data model, it does not fully specify which kind of data it contains. For the purposes of guidelines we can use the *minimal data model* (MDM), which is specified for certain medical specialties. The MDM for a medical specialisation is an agreement made by specialists on the minimal data set, which is necessary to know about a patient in the medical specialisation, for instance *Minimal Data Model for Cardiology* [9].

3.1.2   The Naming Convention

The naming convention specifies the name of certain data. The naming convention of the $MUDR^2$ data model has its origin in the logical representation of this model [6]. Data are represented as an oriented tree, where each node has a name. A certain piece of data is addressed by its full name, which is build of nodes' names on the path from the root to the given node.

3.1.3   The Structure of Provided Data

The data structure specifies which information is carried by a data item (a node in $MUDR^2$). A data item in $MUDR^2$ contains a value and a unit of measurement. Further, it contains some administrative information about when the item was created, by whom it was created, how long it will be valid, etc.

3.2   The Execution Language

The execution language is another important issue of the executable representation of guidelines. All expressions contained in a formalized guideline are written using this language. An execution language consists of four sublanguages with different roles.

- The *arithmetic expression sublanguage* is a language for algebraic formulae and for the control of the program flow.
- The *query sublanguage* is probably the most important part of the execution language. Its role is to retrieve the requested data from an underlying data model. It must meet two conflicting requirements: sufficient language's power and performance. SQL, for instance, is a good example of a suitable query sublanguage.
- The *data manipulation sublanguage* contains constructs for non-trivial data transformations like manipulation with strings, converting data from one format to another (e.g. sorting of a sequence by a given attribute), etc.
- The *date related functions*. Although it is not a real sublanguage, we mention it separately, because it is very important for medical guidelines. It must be possible to write expressions like *three month ago* or to count a difference between two dates, and to represent this difference in arbitrary time units (days, months, etc.). These operations must conform to the common sense, e.g. a month is from 28 to 31 days long depending on the context.

When choosing the execution language, we considered four languages: GEL, GELLO, Python and Java. They are shortly described below and theirs pros and cons are mentioned.

- GEL is an execution language defined in the GLIF specification version 3.5 [1]. GEL is not object-oriented and it does not contain a query sublanguage. The data manipulation language is in some aspects very limited (e.g., it is impossible to order sequences according to other attributes then time.). At this state of development, GEL is not suitable to be an execution language.

- GELLO [10] is an object-oriented successor of GEL. It contains a query language, which is semantically very similar to SQL. The data manipulation language is more powerful than in GEL, but it still lacks some important features, e.g. working with strings. Furthermore, GELLO does not contain any date related functions, which have to be provided by the underlying layers. A great advantage of GELLO is that it is proposed to be an HL7 standard.

- Java is an all-purpose modern programming language. The advantage is that Java is a widespread language and it contains all sublanguages mentioned above. It is easily extendable through packages. In addition, many compilers and interpreters are available. Moreover, there is an embeddable interpreter called BeanShell [11]. Beside this, Java's standard packages java.util.Date and java.util.Calendar meet all requirements on data and time processing. A disadvantage is that Java is too general and it is more complicated to use it in guidelines than any specialised language.

- Python has an advantage over Java – though it is a procedural language, it has many functional features. That is useful in the knowledge representation. But compared to Java, there is a major disadvantage: datetime, a build-in module for working with time and date, does not fully comply with the above stated requirements (the months in datetime module have always 30 days, etc.) Other pros and cons are the same as in Java.

Although GELLO does not meet all requirements, we have finally chosen it as the execution language, mainly because it is a proposed HL7 standard. Then we solved how to cope with the features it lacks. Specification of GELLO left all things that GELLO does not solve to the technologies or languages in the sublayers. In this case a programmer formalizing clinical guidelines would have to master another formal language in addition to GELLO and GLIF. We have decided not to solve missing features by another language, which would appear in GELLO´s expressions, and we have introduced all necessary extensions directly into GELLO. The extensions are described in the rest of this section.

First, GELLO does not contain constructs that make the code maintenance significantly easier and that are usually present in modern programming languages. These missing constructs are for instance the *typedef* and the *function* (or similar) construct. We have added both of them to the execution language.

Second, neither GLIF nor GELLO specify the scope of variables. There exist three logical scopes in formalized guidelines: an *entire guideline*, a *subgraph* and a *step*. By adding the *function* construct there is another scope: a *body of the function*. There is no need to have a variable with scope of the entire guideline, since each guideline consists of one or more subgraphs and GLIF specifies that subgraphs interact only through the *in*, *out* and *inout* variables. It is useful to distinguish among the remaining three scopes. To do so we have added three keywords that are to be used when defining a new variable with either the function scope, the step scope, or the graph scope.

Finally, we faced the problem of missing date functions. GELLO does not define any date or time functions. This functionality it is left to the underlying facilities. We have added all the necessary time constructs that were defined in GEL.

3.3   Encoded Guidelines

To verify that the described representation is suitable for clinical guidelines formalized in the GLIF model, we have converted six guidelines to the executable representation: European Guidelines on Cardiovascular Disease Prevention in Clinical Practice [12], Guidelines for Diagnosis and Treatment of Ventricular Fibrillation [13], 1999 WHO/ISH Hypertension Guidelines [14], 2003 ESH/ESC Guidelines for the Management of Arterial Hypertension [15], Guidelines for Diagnosis and Treatment of Unstable Angina Pectoris 2002 [16], Guidelines for Lung Arterial Hypertension Diagnosis and Treatment [17].

4. Discussion

There are some projects concerning the issues of computer-interpretable guidelines. The best known are Asbru [18] language and SAGE project [19].

Asbru has been developed at the University of Vienna as a part of the Asgaard project. The Asbru represents clinical guidelines as time-oriented skeletal plans. This is a very different approach compared to the GLIF's flowchart-based point of view. We believe that the flowchart-oriented approach is more natural to physicians than the Asbru's one. Thus we assume that flowchart-oriented decision support systems will be more acceptable for them.

The SAGE project is built up on GLIF's experience, but it uses the opposite approach to formalizing of guidelines (GLIF's *top-down* approach versus the *from-the-bottom* approach in SAGE). Unlike GLIF, SAGE specifies the implementation level of guidelines, but it gives up the aspiration of shareable guideline representation. As SAGE is still in the testing stage, it remains debatable which approach is more advantageous. Thus we have decided to utilise the guidelines that had been formalized in GLIF and we have converted them into the described execution language.

5. Conclusion

When developing an executable representation of guidelines formalized in the GLIF model, we realised that GLIF version 3.5 meets the needs of formalized guidelines very well.

During the conversion of formalized guidelines into the executable representation we have found out that the execution language GEL (a part of the GLIF 3.5 specification) lacks important features. Further, we have found out that GELLO, the successor of GEL, made considerable progress in bridging these gaps. However, GELLO still does not address some important features like date-related functions. Also the constructs that simplify maintenance of the code are still missing. We have added these features as an extension to the GELLO language. Further, we have developed a component that can process an executable representation of a guideline. This component is a part of the MUDR2 system, which allows guidelines to use the data from structured health records stored in MUDR2. Finally, we have converted six guidelines to the executable representation and verified that this representation is suitable for clinical guidelines formalized in the GLIF model.

6. Acknowledgments

The work was partly supported by the project no. 1ET200300413 of the Academy of Sciences of the Czech Republic and by the Institutional Research Plan no. AV0Z10300504.

7. References

[1] Mor P, Aziz B, Samson T, Dongwen W, Omolola O, Quing Z. Guideline Interchange Format 3.5 Technical Spec. http://smi-web.stanford.edu/projects/intermed-web/guidelines/GLIF_TECH_SPEC.pdf, InterMed Collaboratory, 2002.

[2] Ram P, Berg D, Tu S, Mansfield G, Ye Q, Abarbanel R, Beard N. Executing Clinical Practice Guidelines Using the SAGE Execution Engine. In: MEDINFO 2004 Proceedings, Amsterdam 2004, pp. 251-5.

[3] Wang D, Shortliffe EH. GLEE – a model-driven execution system for computer-based implementation of clinical practice guidelines. In: *Proceedings AMIA Annual Fall Symposium,* 2002, pp. 855-9.

[4] Hanzlíček P, Špidlen J, Nagy M. Universal Electronic Health Record MUDR. In: Duplaga M, et al. eds. Transformation of Healthcare with Information Technologies, Amsterdam: IOS Press, 2004, pp. 190-201.

[5] Špidlen J, Hanzlíček P, Říha A, Zvárová J. Flexible Information Storage in MUDR2 EHR. In: Zvárová J et al. eds. International Joint Meeting EuroMISE 2004 Proceedings. Prague: EuroMISE Ltd., 2004, p. 58.

[6] Stanford Medical Informatics. Protègè 2000. http://protege.stanford.edu/.

[7] World Wide Web Consortium. Resource Description Framework. http://www.w3.org/RDF/

[8] Johnson PD, Tu SW, Musen MA, Purves IN. A Virtual Medical Records for Guideline-based Decision Support. In: Proceedings AMIA Annual Fall Symposium, 2001, pp. 294-8.

[9] Mareš R, Tomečková M, Peleška J, Hanzlíček P, Zvárová J. User Interfaces of Patient's Database Systems – a Demonstration of an Application Designed for Data Collecting in Scope of Minimal Data Model for a Cardiologic Patient. In Cor et Vasa Brno, 2002:44, No. 4, p 76. (in Czech).

[10] Sordo M, Ogunyemi O, Boxwala AA, Greenes RA. GELLO: An Object-oriented Query and Expression Language for Clinical Decision Support. In: Proceedings AMIA Annual Fall Symposium, 2003, pp. 1012-5.

[11] Been Shell. Lightweight Scripting for Java. http://www.beanshell.org/.

[12] Backer GD, et al. European Guidelines on Cardiovascular Disease Prevention in Clinical Practice. In: European Journal of Cardiovascular Prevention and Rehabilitation, 2003: 10: S1-S78 : 2003.

[13] Čihák R, Heinc P. Guidelines for Diagnosis and Treatment of Ventricular Fibrillation. http://www.kardio.cz/index.php?&desktop=clanky&action=view&id=83. (in Czech: Doporučení pro léčbu pacientů s fibrilací síní).

[14] 1999 World Health Organisation – International Society of Hypertension Guidelines for the Management of Hypertension. In: Journal of Hypertension, 1999, pp. 151-83.

[15] 2003 European Society of Hypertension – European Society of Cardiology Guidelines for the Management of Arterial Hypertension. In: Journal of Hypertension, Vol 21, 2003, No. 6, pp. 1011-53.

[16] Aschermann M. Guidelines for Diagnosis and Treatement of Unstable Angina Pectoris. http://www.kardio.cz/index.php?&desktop=clanky&action=view&id=86. (in Czech: Doporučení k diagnostice a léčbě nestabilní anginy pectoris)

[17] Jansa P, Aschermann M, Riedel M, Pafko P, Susa Z. Guidelines for Diagnosis and Treatement of Lung Arterial Hypertension. http://www.kardio.cz/resources/upload/data/2_030_guidelines.pdf. (in Czech: Doporučení pro diagnostiku a léčbu plicní arteriální hypertenze v ČR).

[18] Shahar Y, Miksch S, Johnson P. An Intention-based Language for Representing Clinical Guidelines. In: Proceedings AMIA Annual Fall Symposium, 1996, pp. 592-6.

[19] Tu SW, Musen MA, Shankar R, Campbell J, Hrabak K, McClay J, Huff SM, McClure R, Parker C, Rocha R, Abarbanel R, Beard N, Glasgow J, Mansfield G, Ram P, Ye Q, Mays E, Weida T, Chute CG, McDonald K, Molu D, Nyman MA, Scheitel S, Solbrig H, Zill DA, Goldstein MK. Modeling Guidelines for Integration into Clinical Workflow. In: MEDINFO 2004 Proceedings, Amsterdam 2004, pp. 174-8.

Address for correspondence:

Petr Kolesa
Institute of Computer Science AS CR, EuroMISE Centre
Pod Vodárenskou věží 2,
182 07 Prague 8,
Czech Republic
email: kolesa@euromise.cz

Connecting Medical Informatics and Bio-Informatics
R. Engelbrecht et al. (Eds.)
IOS Press, 2005

569

Implementing a New ADT Based on the HL-7 Version 3 RIM

Stéphane Spahni[a], **Christian Lovis**[a], **Richard Mercille**[b], **Hervé Verdel**[b], **Michel Cotten**[b]
Antoine Geissbühler[a]

[a] *SIM, Radiology and Medical Informatics Dpt, University Hospitals of Geneva, Geneva, Switzerland*
[b] *Computing Services, University Hospitals of Geneva, Geneva, Switzerland*

Abstract

> The University Hospitals of Geneva (HUG) are the result of the merge of six hospitals into one single organization. While a true fusion of the management has been effectively done, it was not the case five years after for several databases, and in particular the ADT (Admission, Discharge, Transfer). In order to truly realize the fusion, a new ADT service has been built using state of the art technology and standards in order to replace the existing seven services. This paper presents the results of the redesign and development of the new ADT service. The data model, based on HL-7 RIM, is described and the technologies selected are presented. Finally, a status after a few months of production is presented.

Keywords:
Hospital Information Systems (HIS), ADT, HL7, Databases migration

1. Introduction

The administrative system of the HUG was based on two different architectures: Diogène [1] for the primary care hospital and Philos [2] for 5 other sites (psychiatric, geriatric and long term care hospitals). Diogène was in place since the seventies, and already went through a migration when the mainframe-based system was progressively replaced by a fully distributed system.

At the end of the nineties, the six hospitals were merged to form one single organization – the University Hospitals of Geneva. However it was not possible to immediately merge the IT infrastructures – for political as well as technical reasons. Each hospital continued therefore to operate its own ADT, with few relations with the others.

The deployment of common applications and the need to have a global view of all information about patients being treated in more than one of the six hospitals [3] introduced the need for linking the various identities in order to be able to retrieve all information about one person, wherever he/she was treated.

A Master Patient Index – MPI was therefore built for storing links between the various identities of the same person in the up to six databases. However such a solution had its limits and several important points were left aside:

- patients still had several active identities, and databases in each entity stored information associated to the "local" identity;

- there were often differences between the various identities of the same person, and changes made on one identity were not reported to the other identities of the same person but in different sites;
- the semantic of the trajectory elements was not exactly the same in all databases, making the job of applications deployed in all institutions harder than necessary.

2. Materials and Methods

Problem to be addressed

The true merge of the databases having failed for several years, a completely new ADT has been built in order to finalize the merge of the institutions in the domain of the administrative patient management and to suppress the differences in the handling of patients identities and trajectories in the various entities of the HUG. The new application, called "SIL" for "Service d'Identification et de Localisation" fully replaces the existing ones, all existing data being migrated into the SIL thus merging all trajectories and identities into one single database with a single data representation.

Constraints

When designing the solution to implement, several constraints had to be taken into account. The most important ones were:

- Migration of all existing data into the new system (i.e. almost 30 years of history!);
- Transparent migration for existing applications: medical as well as non-medical applications like laboratory systems, management applications etc.;
- The new system should have performances at least at the same level than the existing ones, without being penalized by the increased volume of data and the potentially higher complexity of the model;
- The new ADT has to be compliant to the JAVA-based architecture being progressively implemented for the new applications.

  Some additional constraints were also given, in order to take into account the evolution of other elements of the HIS:

- The administrative management of the patients as well as the billing system had to be replaced at the same time the SIL started. Existing data had therefore to be migrated into two different databases: the SIL for clinic-related data and the DPA ("Dossier Patient Administratif") for administration-related data. This introduced a strong constraint in terms of planning, as the two projects had to be ready at the same time!
- The migration of the six hospitals towards the new system for patient management and billing had to be implemented over several months, enabling a migration site by site in order to distribute the teaching over time and to limit the number of persons required for supporting the users during the first days of the move.

Methodology

In order not to loose time reinventing the wheel by designing our own solution for the ADT, we decided to use existing work done in this area and selected the HL7 Reference Information Model version 1.24 (RIM) [4]. This quite complex information model aims in particular at offering a structure for representing persons, things and organizations as well as patient encounters, acts, etc. The potential disadvantage of this model is that aiming at being as exhaustive as possible makes it quite complex to grasp: a substantial amount of time was therefore required in order to understand the reasons behind the choices made in the RIM.

In parallel with the study of the RIM ran the task of making the inventory of the data existing in the various databases (of course not everything is clearly described with its reason for being there…) as well as the list of interfaces made available over the time, sorting out which ones were still in use and which ones were obsolete. Here again we were confronted with the usual lack of documentation, the existing interfaces being well described in terms of fields returned but the algorithm behind the selection of the entries in the databases being often not formalized (e.g. at what time do you notify planned events like pre-admission or planned exit?).

It was only when both phases were advanced enough that it was possible to think at our implementation of the RIM. Indeed the model represents far more than the data managed by the ADT: it potentially describes every act concerning a patient or performed by an actor as well as the messages exchanged between application modules. Choices have therefore been made in order to select the relevant parts of the model and to link the RIM concepts with the local concepts – a task necessary for being able to respect the constraint of transparent migration of existing applications. This resulted in what is called in HL7 a D-MIM or Domain Message Information Model. However it has to be noted that our implementation is only using the data model of the HL7 standard and not the messaging part itself, although this could be a future extension of our implementation. We therefore did not define our Refined Message Information Model – or R-MIM. One reason behind this restriction is the level of compatibility that has to be supported for existing application, another one being the resources available for implementing the new ADT.

Implementation choices

Implementation choices had to be made at different levels: e.g. software environment and components, information model, data model.

Software environment

The software environment was quite well defined for new developments: JAVA / J2EE for programming environment, Borland Enterprise Server as application server and Oracle as DBMS. No object-oriented DBMS is currently supported for production applications.

Information model

The choice of the components of the RIM that had to be implemented was driven by the data that had to be migrated into the SIL. As we implemented ADT functions only, we selected four basic classes from the model:

- Entities, covering the notions of persons (patients as well as clinicians, nurses, etc) and of entities like wards, medical services, care units, rooms etc.;
- Acts, representing admissions, transfers and discharges of patients.
- Roles played by entities (e.g. a person can be a patient as well as a clinician);
- The relations between roles played by entities and acts are implemented using two additional classes of the model: participations which link acts to actors (roles played by entities during a certain time); act relationships representing the relations between acts (several types of relationships do exist; their use will be discussed later).

3. Results

The project started in spring 2003 with the study of the HL7 version 1.24 model and the inventory of existing services. The implementation itself started mid 2003, while the work on the migration of existing data started in autumn 2003. A too optimistic planning expected a production phase by mid-2004: various factors explained in the discussion delayed the switch to the new infrastructure for a few months, the true production having started effectively on the 1st of November 2004 for the first two hospitals, and on the 2nd of January 2005 for the next two (all four representing at the end more that 95% of the activity and of the users). The last two small hospitals migrated beginning of March 2005.

Information model

The figure below presents the data model of the SIL version 1. It is effectively a subset of the RIM, presenting the data that is being handled by the SIL itself. The interfaces are not presented in the diagram: they are either proprietary (SOAP interfaces) or simply based on the classes of our D-MIM.

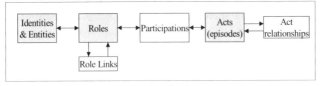

Figure 1: Subset of the RIM for the SIL project

One can see in this picture from left to right the identities of persons (i.e. every person needed to be known) and entities (e.g. ward units, rooms, divisions, etc.), the roles played at a certain time by these entities, then participations which provide the relations between one act and the various actors implied (patient, clinician(s), wards, locations, etc.). We are already planning to integrate non-living objects our D-MIM in order to take into account non-persons (e.g. organs, substances to be analyzed, etc.). These kind of "objects" are manipulated by laboratories and are often non living things. Act relationships are used in particular to represent information migrated from existing systems:

- Relations between episodes, like the relation between the episodes of the mother and her baby (the mother's episode being the one during which she gave birth);

- In the previous system, all ambulatory visits concerning the same problem were grouped into one episode or "outpatient treatment": the act relationships enable us to link all visits (each being an episode) to one "master" episode that represents the same concept as the former "outpatient treatment". While we can find now papers about modeling such situations (e.g. [5]), it has to be noted that at the time we started our work (mid 2003), there was no "white paper" about this subject.

- Other uses are already planned, like e.g. for implementing the notion of "case". As such extensions of our implementation are not yet designed, an in-depth review of the latest version of the model as well as of the literature will have to be made in time.

Architecture

The software architecture of the services implemented to access the SIL data has been partially driven by the needs of the clients. We basically had to support two types of clients:

- New clients, implemented in JAVA and using a global and unified development framework. These clients are using Enterprise Java Beans technology [5] to interact with the SIL. The new administrative application for the management of the patients ("DPA", the client side of the ADT) is the first application using this technology.

- Existing applications, using CORBA services to retrieve data from the ADT. In order to facilitate the transparent migration of these applications, generally without requiring a recompilation of the modules, we decided to use a Web Services approach and selected the AXIS [6] Web Services technology from Apache for implementing all existing services.

Data Migration

One crucial step of the deployment of the SIL was the migration of the almost 30 years of data. This phase proved to be far more complex than expected, and is one major reason for the delayed start up of the SIL. Indeed, the quality of the data was not has high as expected, and many theoretically impossible situations were effectively found in the databases. Typical incoherencies found in the databases were:

- Patients in care units at a time the care unit was not existing (i.e. stay outside the period of validity of the administrative structure);
- When the admission of a patient was delayed, the period between the planned admission and the true admission was considered as a vacation before the start of the episode of care;
- Some patients left the hospital several times the same day, without coming back (i.e. several fugue departures, no return).

Moreover, the true merge of the six databases into one single database with one single active identity per patient made pre-existing incoherencies visible, asking for immediate correction of the links between the identities.

The task was also highly complicated by the progressive replacement of the system across all hospitals: during several months, the two systems had to run in parallel, the new DPA being deployed in some hospitals and the old ADTs being still running in others. While this could have been easily managed in completely separate sites, it required a permanent synchronization of the ADT databases, as close as possible to the real time, for the applications that were already running in all sites.

4. Discussion

Three months after the start of the production phase we are quite satisfied of the performance of the system – in terms of functionality as well as performance.

The HL7 RIM model was very attractive and powerful. Nevertheless this power had a cost as it was sometimes not trivial to grab the reasons behind the choices that were made for the RIM. However we found the investment worthwhile for the future of the system.

We were often tempted to "enhance" the RIM in order to be able to keep the existing concepts or the existing representation of data into the RIM-based SIL, assuming that "this case has not been taken into account, therefore we have to add this or that". While this would have greatly simplified the implementation of the compatible interfaces, we tried not to pollute the data model at the risk of having limited and well documented discrepancies with the existing services. In addition, we found during the comparison of the behavior of existing and new services that the same service did not perform exactly the same way when the data came from one of the initial architectures or the other. It was therefore easier to justify these differences as a full backward compatibility was not reachable anyway.

The data migration was a crucial phase for the project. A few temporary extensions in the data model helped us during the migration period for keeping the synchronization with the non-migrated sites. These extensions will be progressively removed. While we were aware of the importance of the migration of the data, its complexity was certainly underestimated resulting in delays for the start of the new service. However we decided to keep the higher quality of migrated data, at the cost of a delayed start.

The AXIS development environment for the Web Services proved to be a very good choice: the services developed using this technology are performing very well, and we never had stability problems whatever the load on this part had been. It uses only a very small amount of processing power, and supports quite well hot deploy – which is valuable when you completely rebuild your architecture and set of services.

We were unfortunately not as happy with the EJB-based services, or its implementation in the application server. Indeed we had to make several compromises either due to the restrictions imposed by the framework or to the availability of well-performing key components. We e.g. had to abandon two-phases commit due to bugs in the JDBC driver for Oracle. We also encounter problems in the communication between EJBs deployed in separate partitions of the application server. We were nevertheless finally able to reach a situation as stable as the Web Services one also for the EJB-based part of the infrastructure.

5. Conclusion

The SIL project is a major project at the HUG, aiming at truly merging six ADT systems into a single one for the whole institution. The project cumulated several challenges, which ranges from the migration of six databases into a single one to cultural changes by introducing new concepts for representing the objects managed by the ADT.

The choice of the HL7 version 3 Reference Information Model was a challenge: it is considered as having been successfully taken up.

Three months after the first hospital moved towards the new infrastructure, and with now the whole activity performed directly on the new system, we can say that the migration is a success. Of course everything is not solved yet, and some functionality is still missing. Some deficiencies also appeared in the application server, and ask for a rapid solution from the provider of the software. However the system runs already quite fine, and enters now its fine tuning phase.

6. References

[1]   Scherrer JR, Lovis C, Baud R, Borst F, Spahni S. Integrated computerized patient records: the DIOGENE 2 distributed architecture paradigm with special emphasis on its middleware design. Stud Health Technol Inform. 1998;56:15-31.
[2]   Assimacopoulos A. The computer in a health system. Rev Med Suisse Romande. 1990 Oct;110(10):841-4.
[3]   Lovis C., Spahni S., Geissbühler A. Sharing clinical documents in a national care provider network to support community based- medicine. Mednet 2003 Proceedings, Geneva, Switzerland.
[4]   HL7 Reference Information Model: http://www.hl7.org/
[5]   Russler D, Rowed D, Warren JJ, Frankel H, Goossen W, Gabriel D, Frean, I, Chu S, Jongeneel-de Haas I, Nurse D, Patitucci A, (2005). Domain Care Provision in the HL7 v3 standard Ballot 10. Ann Arbor, HL7.
[6]   Monson-Haefel R. Enterprise Java Beans. O'Reilly, 1999.
[7]   AXIS: Apache Web Services project: http://ws.apache.org/axis/
[8]   Spahni S., Lovis C., Mercille R., Trolliard P., Verdel H., Geissbuhler A. Building a new ADT Based on HL-7 Version 3 RIM. Medinfo. 2004;2004(CD):1869.

Address for correspondence

Stéphane Spahni, Medical Informatics Service, Radiology and Medical Informatics Department, University Hospitals of Geneva, 24 rue Micheli-du-Crest, CH-1211 Geneva 14, Stephane.Spahni@hcuge.ch

Connecting Medical Informatics and Bio-Informatics
R. Engelbrecht et al. (Eds.)
IOS Press, 2005

Design and Development of a Monitoring System to Assess the Quality of Hospital Information Systems: Concept and Structure

Frauke Ehlers[a], **Elske Ammenwerth**[a], **Bernhard Hirsch**[b]

[a] *Institute for Health Information Systems, UMIT - University for Health Sciences, Medical Informatics and Technology,*
Hall in Tyrol, Austria
[b] *ITH – Information Technology for Healthcare GmbH, Innsbruck, Austria*

Abstract

Hospital information systems (HIS) are a substantial quality and cost factor in health care. Systematic monitoring of HIS quality is an important task for information management; however, this task is often seen to be insufficiently supported by available methods and tools. The aim of this research project is to develop a comprehensive monitoring system to assess the quality of hospital information systems, taking into account both computer-based and paper-based information processing.
The structure of the developed monitoring system consists of a matrix, crossing HIS quality criteria on one axis (e.g., accessibility of information, or correctness and completeness of information) with a list of process steps within patient care on the other axis (e.g., patient admission, order entry, or clinical documentation). Relevant fields in this matrix ,being defined by one quality criterion and one process step, contain detailed questions, that access the HIS quality with regard to the given criterion in a given process step.
Based on the matrix, a questionnaire with around 140 questions has been developed, consisting of specific questions for physicians, nurses and other professional groups. The ongoing international evaluation will verify completeness, reliability, validity, and feasibility of this HIS quality monitoring system. First evaluation steps point to a high acceptance of this approach among IT staff and clinical staff.

Keywords:
Information management; hospital information systems; monitoring; evaluation; quality

1. Introduction

Hospital Information Systems (HIS) can be understood as the complete information processing and information storing subsystem of a hospital. HIS are becoming an important quality and cost factor for health care. An important task of HIS management is to analyse and regularly supervise HIS quality in order to promptly recognize weaknesses and improve information processing.

While planning and directing of information systems are well understood and supported (e.g. [1]), monitoring of information systems is often seen as insufficiently supported. In most hospitals, regular HIS monitoring activities with quantified assessments of HIS quality are missing both on the strategic and tactical management level. One reason could be that standardized methods and tools for monitoring are missing. For example, hospital quality programmes such as JCAHO [2] or KTQ [3] only comprise very few aspects of HIS quality. Other approaches such as software ergonomic standards (e.g. ISO 9241) focus only on computer-based tools and ignore the significance of paper-based tools in a hospital.

Therefore, the aim of this research project is to develop and validate a comprehensive monitoring system to assess the quality of a hospital information system in a quantitative form.

2. Material and Methods

2.1. General concept of the HIS monitoring system

We reviewed the available literature on HIS quality, analysed our own experiences in the area of HIS assessment, and conducted informal interviews with representatives of IT departments on the requirements with regard to a HIS monitoring system. Based on those activities, we finally decided on the following concept:

- Quality can typically be split into quality of structure, quality of processes, and outcome quality (according to Donabedian, [4]). We decided to focus on outcome-oriented quality criteria, because aspects of structural quality of HIS (e.g. how many computers are used) in our opinion seem not sufficiently informative to describe HIS quality.
- The outcome of information processing is to make available the right information and knowledge at the right time and place in the right form to the right people. This definition describes in our opinion the most important criteria for outcome quality of HIS.
- Clinical working processes are best supported when all information processing tools collaborate in an optimal way. This means that we must address both computer-supported and paper-based information processing in the same way.
- HIS quality should be assessed with direct connection to the various steps of the treatment process of a patient. Thus, the main process steps of patient care should be part of the monitoring system, to allow a context-dependent assessment (e.g. "how is the availability of data during patient admission?").
- HIS quality, defined as the fulfilment of certain criteria in given process steps, can be best assessed by asking those people who are involved in the process step. Thus, clinical and administrative staff members are the real experts of HIS quality.

2.2 Structure of the HIS monitoring system

Based on the general concept of the HIS monitoring system, and after an intensive literature analysis from various fields such as medical informatics (e.g. [5]), business informatics (e.g. COBIT), information management theory, quality management and organizational science (e.g. [6]) as well as accreditation programmes on the issue of HIS quality, we developed a generic matrix-oriented structure for our monitoring system, combining two axes: quality criteria and process steps (see Figure 1).

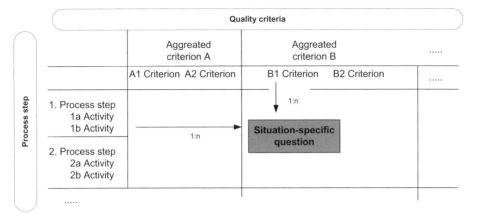

Figure 1- General structure of the monitoring system for HIS quality. Each field within the matrix of quality criteria and process steps contains one or more situation-specific questions on the quality of information processing.

The overall **HIS quality criteria** are described on the x-axis:

- Q1 Availability of information (e.g. "is the patient record available when needed?").
- Q2 Correctness and completeness of information (e.g. "Is the nursing care plan complete?").
- Q3 Readability and clarity of information (e.g. "Is the x-ray order readable?").
- Q4 Usability of information (e.g. "Can statistical analysis be performed?").
- Q5 Fulfilment of legal regulations (e.g. "Is data security guaranteed?").
- Q6 Time needed for information processing (e.g. "Is multiple data entry avoided?").

These quality criteria are put into relation with the **process steps of patient care** that are described on the y-axis. Its structure is based on [7]:

- P1 Patient admission (e.g. administrative and clinical admission);
- P2 Decision-making, planning and organisation of treatment (e.g. care planning);
- P3 Order entry and communication of findings;
- P4 Execution and documentation of diagnostic and therapeutic tasks;
- P5 Patient discharge and transfer to other institutions.

2.3. Contents of the HIS monitoring system

The matrix (Figure 1) presents the overall structure of the HIS monitoring system. By crossing the process steps with the general quality criteria, concrete questions can be defined for assessing HIS quality. For example, the availability of information (Q1) during the process step communication of findings (P3) is assessed in the field Q1 x P3 by one question: "How easily can an overview on new lab findings be obtained during a ward round?".

As already discussed, those specific questions will be answered by staff members who take part in the various process steps. HIS quality will thus be assessed based on a comprehensive, standardized questioning of a representative sample of various stakeholder groups (e.g. physicians, nurses, and administrative staff). The valid answers for each question are described on a standardized 4-point Likert scale. This allows aggregation of answers in the sense of a HIS benchmarking as well as the derivation of an overall HIS total quality score.

3. Preliminary Results and Evaluation

The first German version of the questionnaire (available on request from the authors) contained about 165 questions that were reduced to 140 relevant questions during the first evaluation steps (see below). Not all questions have to be answered by all groups – for example, physicians have to answer around 110 questions and nurses around 100 questions. Figure 2 shows an excerpt of the questionnaire.

		Type of tools used	bad/ seldom/ not adequate			good/ frequently/ adequate
P1.2.1	How easy is it for you to find out whether the patient who is to be admitted has already been treated in your organization before? *(process step P1: patient admission; quality criterion Q1: availability of information)*	O more paper O more IT	– –	–	+	+ +
P2.1.11	How easy can you access relevant clinical information on a patient during the ward round? *(process step P2: decision-making, planning and organization of treatment; quality criterion Q1: availability of information)*	O more paper O more IT	– –	–	+	+ +
P2.2.2	How often does it happen to you that patient-based nursing care plans are not readable? *(process step P2: decision-making, planning and organization of treatment; quality criterion Q3: readability and clarity of information)*	O more paper O more IT	– –	–	+	+ +
P3.19	How adequate do you consider the time effort to search, fill-in and sign forms for order entry (e.g. radiology)? *(process step P3: order entry and result reporting; quality criterion Q6: effort and time needed for information processing)*	O more paper O more IT	– –	–	+	+ +
P4.2.6	How adequate do you consider the time effort for documenting nursing care? *(process step P4: execution and documentation of diagnostic and therapeutic tasks; quality criterion Q6: effort and time needed for information processing)*	O more paper O more IT	– –	–	+	+ +
P5.1.5	During patient's discharge, how well do you feel supported to discover incomplete documentation (e.g. a missing diagnosis)? *(process step P5: patient discharge; quality criterion Q2: correctness and completeness of information)*	O more paper O more IT	– –	–	+	+ +

Figure 2: Example of questions from the HIS monitoring system.

The questionnaire is organized according to the process steps, starting with questions on patient admission, and then following patient treatment until patient discharge. Each process step is first introduced with a short scenario, helping the questioned person to imagine a specific clinical situation (not indicated in Figure 2).

The evaluation concept for the monitoring system is based on the fact that it is intended to be a standardized measurement instrument. We will evaluate the following aspects:

1. Relevance and completeness of the questions, by interviewing representatives from information management (e.g. CIOs) and from various clinical user groups.
2. Relevance and comprehensibility of the questions, by conducting test interviews with selected clinical staff members.

3. Applicability and feasibility of the monitoring system, by pre-tests in various settings.
4. Reliability of the monitoring system, by checking e.g. split-half reliability.
5. Validity of the monitoring system, e.g. by checking criterion validity.
6. Usefulness of results, by focus group interviews with CIOs and hospital managers.

The evaluation concept will be followed one step after the other. The first two evaluation steps are just under way; step 3 is just being prepared in two Austrian and German hospitals.

4. Discussion

The results of the monitoring system shall help to assess 'wellness' or 'illness' of a hospital information system. The monitoring system is meant to be a kind of screening or benchmarking instrument. It will not show in detail the reasons for good or bad information processing, but rather indicate whether information logistics is good or bad.

Our list of quality criteria on the x-axis was based on an extensive literature review. The main difference between our approach and major accreditation programmes lies in the fact that our monitoring system focuses outcome-oriented aspects, while accreditation programmes use a mix of structural-, process- and outcome-oriented aspects.

We based the assessment of HIS quality on a standardized questioning of various involved user groups. In our opinion, the only experts on the question how much the HIS supports their tasks are the users themselves ("customer voices", [8]). There are several examples where hospital staff rejected new tools [9], stressing the importance of the point of view of the staff.

There are other authors who tried to provide methodologies to assess HIS quality. For example, Ribière [18] presents a lot of questions which are comparable to our monitoring system. However, most of them are formulated in a rather general way. What is missing here is the clinical context, i.e. the description of a specific process step, as the availability of information will depend on the situation where it is used. That is why we added the process steps to the monitoring system.

One of the greatest challenges when trying to assess HIS quality is to separate HIS quality from the quality of process organization in the hospital. For example, the number of days needed to complete a discharge letter does not only depend on the tools used, but also e.g. on the workload of the secretaries. Therefore, we decided to focus only on those parts of patient care where information processing and the corresponding tools play a major part – fully aware of the fact that patient care does also depend on organizational factors, motivation of staff etc.

It is sometimes argued that only "objective" HIS evaluation (meaning quantitative measurements) creates new knowledge; however, there are various arguments against this. First, to measure characteristic numbers (e.g. time needed until lab results are available on a ward) is not always helpful, as the assessment of this number will depend on the context, e.g. the type of unit (e.g. psychiatric versus emergency unit). This context-dependence can only be taken into consideration when asking involved people, as we do. Second, measurements of numbers can be quite time-intensive. It will be just impossible to broadly analyse several quality criteria in several process steps as would be necessary for a global HIS monitoring. Anyway, the measuring of characteristic numbers of information processing in itself is just a description of a situation, not an assessment of HIS quality. Which time effort for the discharge letter will be acceptable, which not? To achieve an evaluation we need an assessment scale that attributes the pure numbers with the value "good" or "bad". Third, from a more constructivist point of view, there may not be something as an "objective reality". The "truth" is constructed by people and does not exist in itself, and facts and values cannot be separated [10]. As Ribière [8] puts it "A 'good' information system, perceived by its users as a 'poor' system, is a poor system" (underlining by us, indicating that reality depends on subjective constructions).

5. Conclusion

The quality scores which we plan to aggregate from the questionnaire shall help to find weaknesses in the own HIS, to describe long-term developments of HIS quality, to compare own HIS with other HIS, and to compare quality of information logistics in one department with other departments. Whether our approach leads to an objective, reliable, valid and feasible measurement instrument for the quality of a hospital information system has to be evaluated in the ongoing evaluation studies in different hospitals in various countries.

6. Acknowledgments

This work is supported by the Austrian Ministry for Economy and Labour.

7. References

[1]   Gartner Group. Gartner Group's Healthcare Executive and Management Strategies Research Notes: Gartner Group; 1998.

[2]   JCAHO. Joint commission for accreditation for healthcare organizations (JCAHO).   2002   Available from: http://www.jcaho.org

[3]   Deutsche Krankenhausgesellschaft. Kooperation für Transparenz und Qualität im Krankenhaus: KTQ-Katalog 4.0: Deutsche Krankenhausgesellschaft; 2002.

[4]   Donabedian A. The Definition of Quality and Approaches to its Assessment. Ann Arbor: Health Administration Press; 1980.

[5]   Krobock JR. A taxonomy: hospital information systems evaluation methodologies. J Med Syst 1984;8(5):419-29.

[6]   National Institute of Standards and Technology. Baldrige National Quality Program.   2004. Available from: http://www.baldrige.org

[7]   Ammenwerth E, Buchauer A, Haux R. A Requirements Index for Information Processing in Hospitals. Methods of Information in Medicine 2002;41(4):282-8.

[8]   Ribière V, LaSalle A, Khorramshahgool R, Gousty Y. Hospital Information Systems Quality: A Customer Satisfaction Assessment Tool. In: El-Rewini H, editor. Proc 32nd Hawaii International Conference on System Sciences (HICSS-32), Maui, Hawaii, January 5-8, 1999: IEEE Computer Society Press; 1999.

[9]   Beynon-Davies P, Lloyd-Williams M. When health information systems fail. Topics in Health Information Management 1999;20(1):66-79.

[10]   Guba E, Lincoln Y. 4th Generation Evaluation. Newbury Park London New Delhi: Sage Publications; 1989.

8. Address for correspondence

Univ.-Prof. Dr. Elske Ammenwerth
Institute for Health Information System
UMIT – University for Health Sciences, Medical Informatics and Technology, Hall in Tyrol, Austria
E-Mail: elske.ammenwerth@umit.at
Phone: +43 50 8648 3809

Connecting Medical Informatics and Bio-Informatics
R. Engelbrecht et al. (Eds.)
IOS Press, 2005

Trends in Evaluation Research 1982 – 2002: A Study on how the Quality of IT Evaluation Studies Develop

Nicolette de Keizer[a] , Elske Ammenwerth[b]

[a]*Department of Medical Informatics, Academic Medical Center, Amsterdam, The Netherlands*
[b]*Institute for Health Information Systems, UMIT - University for Health Sciences, Medical Informatics and Technology, Hall in Tyrol, Austria*

Abstract

During the last years the significance of evaluation studies as well as the interest in adequate methods and approaches for evaluation has grown in medical informatics. In order to put this discussion into historical perspective of evaluation research, we conducted a systematic review on trends in evaluation research of information technology in health care from 1982 to 2002. The inventory is based on a systematic literature search in PubMed.

In the first step of our inventory, we concentrated on describing long-term developments in questions, approaches, setting, methods and criteria of IT evaluation studies as described in the abstracts of the identified 1.035 publications. We found some signs of a maturation of evaluation research in medical informatics. However, these findings are only based on study abstracts that do not give sufficient information to assess the quality of studies in more detail.

In a second step of our inventory, we are now looking at the quality of IT evaluation studies in health care, describing in more detail study design and assessing 10 quality indicators. For this second step, we analyse a randomized sample of 105 evaluation full papers in more detail. Besides more descriptive details on study design, the results will show whether IT evaluation studies are credible, and how their quality changed in the last 20 years. An interim analysis of the first 64 papers shows a stable quality of IT evaluation studies over the last 20 years.

Keywords:
Information management; Hospital information systems; Evaluation studies; Quality of studies; Study design

1. Introduction

During the last years the significance of evaluation studies has grown in medical informatics. Evaluation can be defined as the act of measuring or exploring some property of a system, the result of which informs a decision concerning that system in a specific context [1]. Discussion in medical informatics addresses best evaluation methods and approaches and the need for an evaluation framework. The quality of evaluation studies often seemed insufficient [2], [3], [4]. This discussion went on for some years now. In order to put this discussion into historical perspectives of evaluation research, we conducted a review of evaluation research of information technology (IT) in health care from 1982 to 2002. The aim of this review was to identify trends of evaluation research in this area in the last 20 years. The inventory is based on a systematic literature search in PubMed.

1.1 First part of inventory: Description of evaluation studies 1982 – 2002

In the first part of this study, we were interested in the dynamics of studies in recent years, as a reflection of interest in evaluation of information systems. Overall, we identified 1.035 abstracts of evaluation papers in PubMed from 1982 to 2002. Each of the identified abstracts was then classified according to a multi-axial classification developed for this inventory purpose, to allow for a systematic historical analysis on the various aspects we were interested in. We wanted to learn what countries or journals dominate in evaluation research publications, supporting a focused search for evaluation studies. We were then interested to learn which type of information systems (e.g. CPOE) are predominantly evaluated, and whether there are shifts in recent years. Our inventory then emphasizes the focus of a study (e.g. software quality, effect on outcome quality) and the methods applied (e.g. qualitative versus quantitative methods), as methodological discussions have been going on for some years now in medical informatics (compare e.g. [5]). Overall, this first part was an analysis based on the abstracts of the found PubMed studies.

Summarizing, we found interesting developments in evaluation research in the last 20 years. For example, there has been a shift from medical or other journals to medical informatics journals. Also, the number of systematic reviews is steadily rising. In addition, the evaluation of expert systems decreased in prevalence, while that of telemedical systems increased, reflecting rising interest towards cooperative, shared care.

On the other hand, we also identified rather stable trends. For example, explanatory research and quantitative methods dominated evaluation studies in the last 20 years which does not yet reflect the rising awareness of the benefits of qualitative methods. How much those findings are biased due to publication bias cannot be analyzed based on the available data.

Detailed results have been reported elsewhere ([6], [7]) and are available online in our database at http://evaldb.umit.at.

1.2 Second part of inventory: Quality of evaluation studies 1982 - 2002

In the first part of this study, we focused on a rather broad description of evaluation studies in the last 20 years, based only on the abstracts of the selected papers. Since we were also interested into more study details, we now also analysed randomly selected full IT evaluation papers. Here, we were interested in:

- details on the type of research design conducted in evaluation studies;
- the quality of evaluation studies in the last 20 years;
- the effect of IT on the quality of the care process and on the outcome of the care process.

The question of developments of quality of studies is of high importance. Research in medicine must provide sound data that clinicians can rely on in making decisions about patients. Similarly, evaluation research in medical informatics must provide sound data to make decisions about the value of information technology interventions in health care. The question is therefore: How believable are the results of published evaluation studies? In medicine, several authors have analysed the quality of medical studies (e.g. [8] or [9]). They often point to rather weak research designs and a lot of methodological weaknesses. We were interested to analyse this for medical informatics evaluation studies.

The quality of an evaluation study primarily depends on the quality of the study design. There have been some attempts to describe levels of evidence of studies (e.g. [10]). However, the study design itself can only be judged in relation to the study question. While, e.g., a randomized controlled trial (RCT) provides best evidence when analysing the effects of an intervention on patient outcome, a randomization is not necessary when a study does not focus on proving the effect of an intervention, but e.g. on the long-term description of workflow changes or user satisfaction etc.

Finally, we were interested in the outcome of the IT evaluation studies with regard to the effects of IT on health care.

The aim of this paper is to present the design of this second part of our inventory, together with a preliminary analysis of the first results.

2. Methods

Overall, we decided to analyse 105 papers in detail for this second part of the inventory. We chose the papers as a random sample from the 1.035 abstracts found in the first part of our study. To be able to analyse trends, we divided the period 1982-2002 in 7 periods of 3 years. For each 3-year period we randomly selected 15 papers.

The primary aim of this study is to describe the quality of IT evaluation studies. As a start, the research design used has to be described in more detail than we did in the first part of our inventory. To describe the **research design**, we focus on the following aspects:

- Single or multi-center
- Cross-sectional or longitudinal
- Prospective or retrospective
- Case study, Case control study, Cohort study, or clinical trial
- In case of clinical trials: Uncontrolled, non-randomized controlled, randomized controlled
- Data acquisition methods: Questionnaire, Interviews, Observation, Chart review, Automated Logging, or Worksampling

Then, quality indicators are analysed to judge the overall **quality of the study**. Our list of quality indicators is based on earlier work, e.g. on Verhagen et al. [11], Greenhalgh and Taylor [12], CONSORT [13] and the quality criteria of the IMIA Yearbook of Medical Informatics [14]. It was important to find quality indicators that were applicable not only to randomized quantitative trials, but to all kinds of studies (e.g. qualitative case studies, longitudinal descriptive studies, uncontrolled clinical trials, etc.). Finally, we decided on the following indicators:

1. Motivation, problem and study questions are clear.
2. Type, number, and sampling of involved study population are clear.
3. Setting and population seems justified to answer study question.
4. Evaluated information system, or intervention, is described in sufficient detail.
5. Methods for collecting data are sufficient clear.
6. Methods for analysing data are sufficient clear.
7. Methods seem adequate to answer study question.
8. Any comparison that is done between groups is fair.
9. All results are credible and seem valid.
10. All conclusions seem justified by the results.

For each selected study, 0 – 2 points (0=not fulfilled, 1=partly fulfilled, 2=fully fulfilled) could be assigned for each indicator. A maximum of 20 points could be obtained as an overall quality score. All papers have been independently analysed by the two authors, different judgement has been discussed and solved. To calculate interrater variability, 9 randomly selected papers were analysed in a pre-test.

To describe the **results of the studies**, we analysed for each of the applied evaluation criteria, whether the study found negative, positive, no or mixed effects of the investigated IT system.

3. Preliminary results

The sampling of the study papers was done in December 2004, their analysis started in January 2005 and is still ongoing. We will now report on the results of the interim analysis of the first 64 papers (of overall 105 papers).

Figure 1 shows the outcome of the studies. Most studies evaluated the aspect "appropriateness of care". It is also this aspect for which the most positive effect can be measured. The second and third often measured aspects are "efficiency of working process (time)" and "cost of care". Among these two aspects only about 50% of the studies showed positive effects. Most studies evaluated more than one aspect.

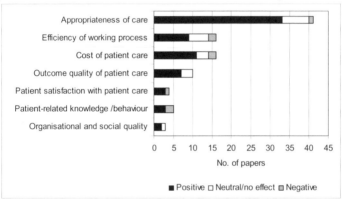

Figure 1 - Results of evaluated aspects on process or outcome of patient care 1982-2002 (n=64 studies; one study can cover more than one aspect).

The majority (89%) of the evaluation studies evaluated an IT intervention using a clinical trial design. Of these clinical trials 21.9% did not use any controls, 37.5% used non-random controls and 29.7% used random controls. In our random sample of evaluation studies, case studies did not appear since the second half of the nineties.

The quality of each study was calculated as sum of the 10 quality indicators of the evaluation studies in time, leading to a minimum score of 0 and a maximum of 20 points for each study. The results show that the quality of the evaluation studies is rather stable over time, being around 15 points (out of 20) for the last 20 years.

Of the ten quality indicators, the indicators "detail in which the IT intervention is described", "the methods of data collection", "the methods of analyses" and "fair comparison between groups" had the lowest scores. The mean total quality score for RCTs (17.7) was significantly higher than for non-RCTs (14.8). No significant differences could be detected between single and multicentre studies, cross-sectional and longitudinal studies, prospective and retrospective studies.

4. Discussion

The idea to describe the quality of research papers is not new. However, to our knowledge, most of comparable work focussed on the quality of controlled trials, borrowing quality indicators for clinical trials from the medical sciences.

For example, van der Loo [15] described a taxonomy of evaluation studies of automated information systems including an axis on study design. However, this taxonomy is restricted to quantitative evaluation studies. He also calculated a quality score, containing 18 quality attributes, focussing on the quality of clinical trials, such as: specify alpha and beta level; use blinding; describe treatment and control; or provide test statistic. In a comparable way, Johnston [16] analysed 28 controlled trials on clinical decision support systems. While these studies both used established quality indicators for quantitative clinical trials, they are not appropriate for most of IT evaluation studies, which are often explorative studies or which do not use a controlled trial to assess an IT system.

We chose a different approach from all those studies. As we learnt from our first part of the inventory, not all IT evaluation studies want to prove an effect of IT on health care outcome and consequently use controlled trials. Other studies are explorative or descriptive in their methods. We were thus forced to generalize the quality indicators from clinical trials to be usable for all kinds of studies. For example, blinding of participants is a typical technique that aims at increasing credibility of results. Instead asking for blinding in our study, we tried to assess the credibility of results.

In a pre-test, the interrater variability of our quality score was good, indicating that our quality score was useful for objectively assessing studies on evaluation of IT interventions in health care.

We are aware that our quality score is more general than detailed lists such as [13]. One weakness of our method might be that due to the general level of the 10 quality indicators we can not distinguish between quality of the study and quality of the paper. However we expect these to be highly correlated.

RCTs in evaluation studies on IT interventions had significant higher quality scores than non-RCT studies. Since our 10 quality indicators are generalized for all kind of study designs, we conclude that papers on RCTs do have a higher quality.

In contrast to others [8], [15] we found a rather stable quality of evaluation studies of IT interventions in health care between 1982 and 2002. The analysis of the remaining papers will show whether this trend continues.

5. Conclusion

Progress in health informatics depends to one part in the scientific credibility of IT evaluation studies. We want to contribute to this topic by analysing the quality of IT evaluation studies in the last twenty years.

6. References

[1] Ammenwerth E, Brender J, Nykänen P, Prokosch H-U, Rigby M, Talmon J. Visions and strategies to improve evaluation of health information systems - reflections and lessons based on the HIS-EVAL workshop in Innsbruck. Int J Med Inf 2004;73(6):479-91.

[2] Heathfield H, Buchan I. Current evaluations of information technology in health care are often inadequate. BMJ 1996;313(7063):1008.

[3] Kaplan B. Evaluating informatics applications - some alternative approaches: theory, social interactionism, and call for methodological pluralism. International Journal of Medical Informatics 2001;64:39-56.

[4]   Tierney W, Overhage J, McDonald C. A Plea for Controlled Trials in Medical Informatics. Journal of the American Medical Informatics Association 1994;1(4):353-5.

[5]   Moehr JR. Evaluation: salvation or nemesis of medical informatics? Comput Biol Med 2002;32(3):113-25.

[6]   Ammenwerth E, de Keizer N. An inventory of evaluation studies of information technology in health care: Trends in evaluation research 1982 - 2002. In: Fieschi M, Coiera E, Jack LI Y-C, editors. Proceedings of the IIth World Congress on Medical Informatics (Medinfo 2004); 7 - 11 September 2004, San Francisco; 2004. p. 1289-1294.

[7]   Ammenwerth E, de Keizer N. An inventory of evaluation studies of information technology in health care: Trends in evaluation research 1982 - 2002. Methods Inf Med 2005;44:44-56.

[8]   Fletcher RH, Fletcher SW. Clinical research in general medical journals: a 30-year perspective. N Engl J Med 1979;301(4):180-3.

[9]   Mihan L, Windeler J. Methodological quality of controlled studies in the "Medizinische Klinik" journal. Analysis of contributions appearing between 1979 and 1996 (in German). Med Klin 1999;94(1):1-8.

[10] CEBM. Levels of Evidence. 2004 . Available from: http://www.cebm.net/levels_of_evidence.asp

[11] Verhagen A, de Vet H, de Bie R, Kessels A, Boers M, Bouter L, et al. The Delphi list; a criteria list for quality assessment of Randomized Clinical Trials for conducting systematic reviews developed by Delphi consensus. J Clin Epid 1998(51):1235-41.

[12] Greenhalgh T, Taylor R. How to read a paper: Papers that go beyond numbers (qualitative research). BMJ 1997;315:740-743.

[13] Moher D. The CONSORT Statement: Revised Recommendations for Improving the Quality of Reports of Parallel-Group Randomized Trials. Annals of Internal Medicine 2001;134(8):657-662.

[14] Ammenwerth E, Wolff A, Knaup P, Ulmer H, Skonetzki S, van Bemmel J, et al. Developing and evaluating criteria to help reviewers of biomedical informatics manuscripts. J Am Med Inform Assoc 2003;10(5):512-4.

[15] van der Loo R. Overview of Published Assessment and Evaluation Studies. In: van Gennip EMSJ, Talmon JS, editors. Assessment and evaluation of information technologies. Amsterdam: IOS Press; 1995. p. 261-82.

[16] Johnston M, Langton K, Haynes R, Mathieu A. Effects of Computer-based Clinical Decision Support Systems on Clinician Performance and Patient Outcome - A Critical Appraisal of Research. Annuals of Internal Medicine 1994;120:135-42.

7. Address for correspondence

Dr. Nicolette de Keizer, Dept. of Med. Informatics, Academic Medical Center (AMC), Amsterdam, The Netherlands,E-Mail: n.f.keizer@amc.uva.nl, Phone: ++31 20 566 5205

Connecting Medical Informatics and Bio-Informatics
R. Engelbrecht et al. (Eds.)
IOS Press, 2005

Interfacing Clinical Practice and Error Prevention

Carola Hullin[a, b, c], Sioban Nelson[a], John Dalrymple[b], Graeme Hart[c]

[a]*School of Nursing, The University of Melbourne. Australia*
[b]*Centre for Management Quality Research, RMIT University. Australia*
[c]*Department of Information Technology, Austin Health, Australia*

Abstract

Medication error is a major source of preventable harm to patients in hospitals and is an area in which, it is suggested, information technology will have a positive impact. This paper presents findings from part of a study that examined current information utilisation patterns during nursing medication rounds. Nursing working patterns in medication administration are poorly understood despite being one of the most likely sources of medication error. Methods used were drawn from principles of Human Computer Interaction (HCI), using a semi-structured observational tool for analysing system requirements and data elements. Results from this study indicated that clinical and contextual factors impact on nursing patterns of information handling in many ways, including documentation quality, location of information sources and current patterns of computer utilization. Numerous extraneous interruptions also impact on the ability of nurses to assimilate and use clinical information effectively. These results were used to develop a conceptual framework for interfacing error prevention in clinical practice. These insights into the human factors that are the reality of clinical practice allow us to design and develop effective information technology systems to help prevent nursing medication administration errors.

Keywords:
Nursing practice; Errors; Mobile computing; Safety

1. Introduction

Medication error is a major source of preventable harm to patients in hospitals and these errors can be prevented by using the right information and information technologies(1, 2). According to the report "Crossing the Quality Chasm: A New Health System for the 21st Century", "*Health care today harms too frequently and routinely fails to deliver its potential benefits*" (p.1)(3). One of the potential benefits for healthcare provision is the appropriate utilisation of information technologies at the patient's bedside for acquiring clinical information(4). Furthermore, the healthcare industry is one of the slowest sectors to adopt and implement information technologies(3, 5).

An area in which information technology has been proposed as having a positive impact is medication error reduction by using electronic medication management systems(6, 7). Leape et al.(1995) argued that medication administration is one of the most likely sources of preventable medication errors and ranks beside prescribing (8). Nurses are often the healthcare professionals administering medication to patients in hospitals. They work in a complex and dynamic environment and the manner that they access, gather, process and store clinical information impacts on patient care. Factors that remain unexplored relate to the current quality of paper-based documents for medication administration. Systems that incorporate electronic prescribing as part of medication management have been shown to be effective in handling clinical information for medication management and preventing errors in practice (6, 7) . However, medication administration is rarely incorporated in those systems and nursing working patterns in medication administration are poorly understood. This paper presents findings from the initial phase of a study that examined current information utilisation patterns during nursing medication rounds for use in designing information systems.

2. Material and Methods

Methods used in this study were drawn from the principles of Human Computer Interaction (HCI). Research methods used in HCI provide several approaches to investigate the human factors for analysing, designing and developing information systems. The major aim of Information System (IS) design is to collect, store, retrieve, communicate and utilise data as a symbolic concept for the development of computerised systems (9, 10). The most appropriate research method for the purpose of this part of the overall study was an ethnographic inquiry and a semi-structured observational tool adapted from Kendall (11). Participants were ninety (n=90) registered nurses from three clinical settings (A, B & C) providing inpatient and outpatient oncology services. The inclusion criterion consisted of nurses that administer medication to patients as part of their daily work. Nursing personnel that did not actively conduct this clinical task were excluded from the study. Ethics approval was obtained from the hospital and university Human Ethics Committees prior to the commencement of the overall study, which was part of a doctoral program conducted by the principal investigator (C.H).

3. Results

The results from this initial phase of the overall study show that some clinical and contextual factors impact on nursing patterns of information handling in many ways, including documentation quality, location of information sources and current patterns of computer utilisation. The instrument used for observable elements was adapted from an existing research tool (Kendall, 1999) (11). For the scope of this paper three out seven observable elements found during this initial phase will be reported on in the next section.

Documentation quality

The quality of the paper- based documentation was audited for each clinical setting. One hundred medication charts for A, B & C sites were obtained by photocopying randomly each time the researcher conducted field visits (as part of the ethnographic inquiry). A typical example of documentation used by nurses for medication administrations is shown in Figure 1.

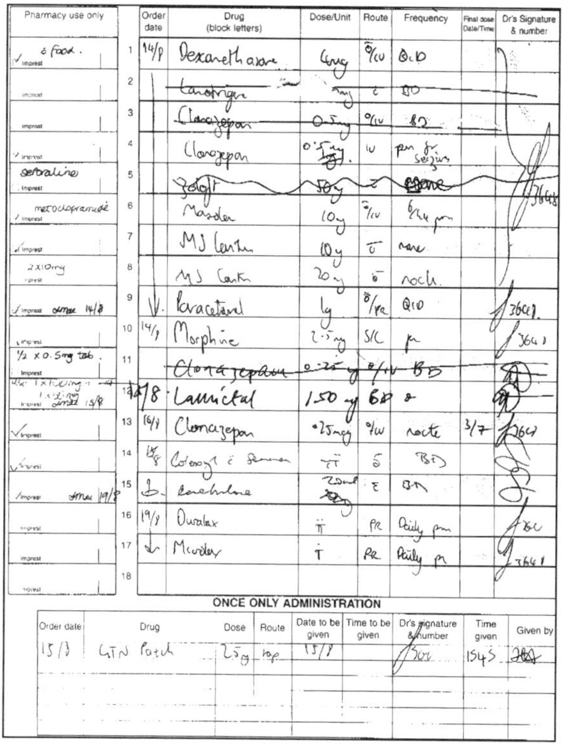

Pharmacy use only		Order date	Drug (block letters)	Dose/Unit	Route	Frequency	Final dose Date/Time	Dr's Signature & number
ē food. Imprest	1	14/8	Dexamethasone	4mg	O/IV	QID		
Imprest	2		Lamotrigine			BD		
Imprest	3		Clonazepam	0.5mg	O/IV	BD		
Imprest	4		Clonazepam	0.5mg	IV	prn for seizures		
sertraline Imprest	5		Zoloft	50mg		mane		3644
metoclopramide Imprest	6		Maxolon	10mg	O/IV	6/24 prn		
Imprest	7		MS Contin	10mg	O	mane		
2 x 10mg Imprest	8		MS Contin	20mg	O	nocte		
Imprest	9		Paracetamol	1g	O/PR	QID		3644
Imprest	10	14/8	Morphine	2.5mg	S/C	prn		3644
½ x 0.5mg tab. Imprest	11		Clonazepam	0.25mg	O/IV	BD		
Imprest	12	18	Lamictal	150mg				
Imprest	13	16/8	Clonazepam	.25mg	O/IV	nocte	3/7	3644
Imprest	14	18/8	Coloxyl ē Senna	ii	O	BD		
Imprest	15			20ml	O			
Imprest	16	19/8	Duralax	ii	PR	Daily prn		
Imprest	17		Microlax	i	PR	Daily prn		3641
Imprest	18							

ONCE ONLY ADMINISTRATION

Order date	Drug	Dose	Route	Date to be given	Time to be given	Dr's signature & number	Time given	Given by
15/8	GTN Patch	25mg	top	15/8			1545	

Figure1- An example of paper-based document

Figure 1 presents some of the elements found during the auditing of the paper documentation used by nurses. The medication chart displayed above was selected randomly for illustration purposes. The descriptive analysis of these documents displayed some common elements. For instance for the 'Pharmacy use only' section, written instructions were not always consistent and the clarity of the data was poor. Identification of the pharmacist providing the professional advice became cumbersome for users of the medication chart. In the case of the 'Order Date' section, the results indicated that users attempt to complete the data required for an order entry which is the date of the medication order but if there was more than one order at the time of admission all the fields required to be filled out were not always completed. This data element becomes relevant for nurses when reviewing the patient's response to the medication treatment, since nurses rely on this factual information to evaluate patient care. Results for 'Name of Drug (Block letters)' examination showed that most of the drug prescriptions are handwritten and block letters are not always used by the provider. Clarity of the medication orders was not always achieved, and this becomes evident for medication treatment with more than one page. Findings for the 'Dose/Unit' section of the medication chart were the most concerning of the data elements. Entries were not clearin several cases and the prescribed dosage was open to misinterpretation when the handwritten value was not clear. In the case of the 'Route' column, the major finding during the analysis was that multiple route options were placed in the same medication order. This element does not meet Australian legislated standard for medication management. An example of this finding is the order for paracetamol (analgesic) where it is prescribed for pain when necessary (PRN order) and the route is written as oral (O) and/or per rectum (PR). This is a situation open to misinterpretation by the nurses administering the drugs. Results for the 'Frequency' column indicated some discrepancies in the manner that frequency is presented in the medication chart. The most common findings during the analysis of this data element was the prescription of daily (once a day) medication but another frequency term would be placed next to it, such as PRN (when necessary). The Dose data element found in the examination of medication charts strongly indicated that this data is not effectively completed and the symbolic manner health professionals used for finalising medication treatment is by placing a line across the order. In the case of 'Date/Time' information required for indicating the termination of medication administration, this is rarely completed and for those medication charts that were completed the identification of the healthcare professional that performed the cessation is not recorded formally in the medication chart.

Location of information sources

This element consisted of the observation of the location of information sources used by nurses while administering medication. The medication charts were the main source of information used by nurses while conducting the clinical task under investigation. The data presented in this paper documents for healthcare delivery was complex in nature (See figure 1). The most frequent location of the medication chart was at the end of the patient's bed for clinical settings A & B. The medication chart was placed inside a folder that hooked onto the end of the patient's bed. In the case of clinical setting C, the outpatient unit, medication charts were located on the working bench where nurses prepared the medication for administration. Patients were seated on armchairs rather than bed for receiving treatment. The location of information was a tray placed next to the medication (pharmacy dispensing box).

Current patterns of computer utilisation

This element consisted of the assessment of the frequency nurses use computerised information for medication administration Ninety nurses participated in this initial phase of the overall study that examined current information utilisation patterns during nursing medication rounds. The results showed a poor level of usage of computerised information while conducting this clinical task. Nurses had computerised information available at their point of work including protocols, medication references and Australian medicines guidelines, during this study. Findings demonstrated that only two nurses out of ninety participants actively used computerised information while administering medication. The factor the influenced nurses during this investigation in not using the computerised information was the lack of computers at their point of work.

Extraneous interruptions

Numerous extraneous interruptions also impacted on the ability of nurses to assimilate and effectively use clinical information for medication administration. For the scope of this paper a summary of the findings from this initial investigation is provided next.

The number of interruptions nurses experienced while accessing information for medication administration averaged six per observational episode (X=6). As demonstrated in Figure 2, clinical setting A averaged two interruptions per observation, while clinical setting B showed slightly more with four interruptions per observation. Clinical setting C experienced frequent interruptions while handling information, with an averaged of eight interruptions per observation. These findings are critical when designing information systems for clinical practice, since nursing care is heavily dependent upon access to clinical information.

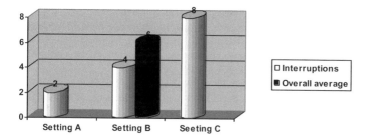

Figure2- Interruptions per Observational episode

Figure 2 shows an overview of the average number of interruptions per clinical setting. The complexity of clinical care was highlighted by analysing the source of these interruptions.

4. Discussion

The results from this part of the study were actively used in developing a conceptual framework for interfacing error prevention in clinical practice. The findings of this initial investigation are critical in effectively introducing and managing information technologies for preventing errors in clinical care. It is essential that newly designed information systems do not produce more interruptions for the already complex healthcare environment. Nurses are the largest group of healthcare professionals in any modern health system and their information utilisation patterns are poorly understood. These insights into the human factors reality of clinical practice allow us to design and develop effective information technology systems to help prevent nursing medication administration errors.

5. Conclusion

This paper presented some of the results from a study that examined current information utilisation patterns during medication nursing rounds. The results of the overall study were used for designing and developing effective information technologies (in this case mobile computing) to help accessibility and prevention of potential medication administration errors. Some of the system requirements need to include the complexities found in this study.

6. Acknowledgements

This study was sponsored by the Information Technology of the hospital where this study took place. Also, The University of Melbourne scholarship was awarded as part of the principal investigator doctoral program. Lastly, the research team is grateful to all participants of this study.

7. References

[1] 1. Borenstein SH, Choi M, Langer JC. Error and adverse outcomes on a surgical service: what is the role of the resident? Journal of Surgical Research 2003;114(2):296.

[2]   2. Borenstein SH, Choi M, Gerstle JT, Langer JC. Errors and adverse outcomes on a surgical service: What is the role of residents? Journal of Surgical Research 2004;122(2):162-166.

[3]   3. Institute, of, Medicine. Crossing the Quality Chasm: A New Health System for the 21st Century. Washington, D.C.: National Academy Press; 2001.

[4]   4. England I, Stewart D, Walker S. Information Technology Adoption in Health Care: When Organisations and technology collide. Australian Health Review 2000;23(3).

[5]   5. Medicine Io. To err is human: building a safer health system. Washington, D.C.; 2000.

[6]   6. Bates DW, Cullen DJ, Laird N, Petersen LA, Small SD, Servi D, et al. Incidence of Adverse Drug Events And Potential Adverse Drug Events: Implications for Prevention. [Article]. JAMA Jul 1995;274(1):29-34.

[7]   7. Bates DWMDM, Spell NMD, Cullen DJMDM, Burdick EMS, Laird NP, Petersen LAMDM, et al. The Costs of Adverse Drug Events in Hospitalized Patients. [Article]. JAMA January 1997;22(29):307-311.

[8]   8. Leape LL, Bates DW, Cullen DJ, Cooper J, Demonaco HJ, Gallivan T, et al. Systems Analysis of Adverse Drug Events. Journal of American Medical Association 1995;274(1):35-43.

[9]   9. Staggers N. Human Computer Interaction in Health Care Organization. In: Englebardt S, Nelson R, editors. Health Care Informatics: An Interdisciplinary Approach. Sydney: Mosby; 2002.

[10] 10. Preece J, Rogers I, Sharp H, Benyon D, Carey T. Human-Computer Interaction. England-Menlo Park-New York-Ontorio-Sydney-Madrid-Mexico City: Addison-Wesley; 1994.

[11] 11. Kendall K, Kendall J. System Analysis and Design. Fourth ed. New Jersey: Prentice Hall; 1999.

Address for Correspondence

Carola Hullin
Level 1, 723 Swanton Street Carlton. Victoria 3053. Australia. Phone: +61 3 83440800

Connecting Medical Informatics and Bio-Informatics
R. Engelbrecht et al. (Eds.)
IOS Press, 2005

Using Feedback to Raise the Quality of Primary Care Computer Data: a Literature Review

Simon de Lusignan

St. George's – University of London, UK

Abstract

Background: Primary care is recognised as a medical specialty and its unique information needs justify the existence of its own health informatics sub-specialty: primary care informatics (PCI). A challenge for PCI is how to raise the standard of computerised medical records so that meaningful conclusions can be drawn from them. In the UK the Primary Care Data Quality (PCDQ) programme has eight years experience of using feedback in an educational context to improve data quality.
Objective: This literature review set out to define the characteristics of a feedback process most likely to achieve change; the principles of which could be applied to PCDQ or to other data quality initiatives.
Method: A literature review of the major medical bibliographical databases, and the websites and working groups of the international medical informatics associations.
Results: There are generalisable lessons for primary care derived from the literature about implementing best evidence, feedback and the theory of diffusion of innovation. The principles identified are: (1) Engage and support local innovators – i.e. those most likely to adopt change, demonstrate the evidence-base for the intervention and the form of feedback most acceptable to them (2) Model the clinical context in which quality improvement is required; (3) Develop an understanding of the health system, its culture and management system; and, (4) Identify and address technical issues relating to computer use and coding.
Conclusions: Feedback is most effective when: clinically relevant, educationally orientated, given by peers, and sensitive to the socio-technical context.

Keywords:
Primary health care; Review, literature; Family practice; Medical Informatics; Computers; Feedback, Diffusion of Innovation

1. Introduction

Primary care was recognised internationally in the World Health Organization's Alma-Ata declaration of 1978 [1] which stated that primary care was key to attaining "health for all". Definitions of primary care focus on the types of patients, their problems, and that they are seeing specially trained primary care professionals [2]. Many countries have comprehensive primary care computer systems; all are quite distinct from those used in secondary care.

De facto primary care informatics (PCI) has evolved as a subspecialty of health informatics. PCI has its own journal [3], and within many national and international informatics organisations has its own working groups [4,5,6,7,] that help promulgate best practice in PCI. Medical informatics is a science: studying how data, information and knowledge can promote health and improve medical care [8]. PCI is also defined as a science (Box 1) The development of a high quality computerised medical record is a core part of the discipline [9,10].

The scientific study of data, information and knowledge, and how they can be modelled, processed or harnessed to promote health and develop patient-centred primary medical care.

Its methods reflect the biopsychosocial model of primary healthcare and the longitudinal relationships between patients and professionals.

Its context is one in which patients present with unstructured problems to specially trained primary care professionals who adopt a heuristic approach to decision making within the consultation."

Box1 - Definition of Primary Care Informatics

The author has over eight year's experience of using an educational intervention (Primary Care Data Quality Programme – PCDQ) to improve data quality [11]. Whilst the use of feedback is not new [12], as yet, there has been no published review of the literature about how to most effectively deliver feedback to improve data quality in primary care. This literature review seeks to fill this gap and suggest principles that can be used to critically appraise the PCDQ programme or other data quality initiatives.

2. Method

There were four components of the literature review:

1. Literature searches. : A standard approach to literature searching was used [13,14]. This approach inevitably only finds retrospective material so in a fast moving field like informatics needs to be supplemented.
2. Searches of health and medical informatics association websites, and their associated primary care informatics working groups [4,5,6,7,], journals and conference proceedings.
3. Using standard internet search tools; e.g. Google.
4. e-mail contact with useful individuals identified from searches 1 to 3 above.

3. Results

General findings about appropriate change strategies

A systematic review of the strategies likely to achieve change, conducted in the context of implementing evidence based practice, summarised the evidence as follows [15]:

5. Interventions based on exploration of the barriers are more likely to succeed.
6. Multi-faceted interventions targeting the different barriers are more likely to be effective.
7. Educational outreach, in the USA, changes prescribing behaviour
8. Reminder systems are generally effective
9. Audit and feedback have mixed results
10. Most interventions work under certain circumstances, none is effective under all.
11. Passive dissemination is unlikely to result in behaviour change.

How to use feedback effectively

Feedback has been used in a number of contexts in primary care, and been shown to change behaviour [16]. Providing feedback about the use of laboratory tests has been shown to reduce the number of tests ordered [17] and to reduce inadequate cervical smear rates [18]. It has also been shown to modify the choice of medication prescribed [19,20], adherence to prescribing guidelines [21], and to help control the costs of prescriptions [22]. Feedback can also improve data quality [23].

The effectiveness of feedback is reported internationally. The studies above are reported from: Australia, Netherlands, New Zealand, United Kingdom, Norway, United States and Denmark.

Who provides the feedback may be important. Feedback by peers achieved a greater quality improvement than that achieved by non-physician observers [24] though practices reported preferring quality improvement visits by non-physicians [25]. An educational intervention to control antibiotic prescribing had proved successful with its effectiveness lasting after six years [26].

Not all studies show benefit from feedback. One study, counter to what is reported above, found no effect from feedback on test ordering [27]. In some disease areas feedback does not seem to alter morbidity. Where there is scepticism about the reliability of the data about referral rates then no such benefit could be found [28].

There may be some features of feedback which makes it more likely to be successful. Hickey et al., suggest that keeping feedback brief, and pragmatic are important if it is to be successful [29]. Watkins et al., recommend that if an educational intervention is to be successful it needs: a credible facilitator, protected time for learning, and explicit links to everyday practice [30].

The theory of diffusion of innovation

The theory of diffusion of innovations (DOI) became well known as the result of Rogers' work [31]. He created a very precise definition of diffusion:

> *Diffusion is the process by which an innovation is communicated through certain channels over time among the members of a social system.*

Rogers assigned all the key words in this definition a precise meaning, which are described below:

The *communication channels* that he concluded were important were with the peer group. Rogers believed that most people adopt changes based on what their peer group says rather than the basis of scientific evidence.

The *time* taken to adopt a change is dependant on the duration of the innovation-decision process; something that varies between individuals and subject matter. The first to adopt a change are the *innovators* (first 2.5%), next the *early adopters* (next 13.5%), then the *early majority* (next 34%), followed by the *late majority* (next 34%), and finally the *laggards* (last 16%).

The *social system* is critical in determining whether a change is adopted. A social system is defined as a set of interrelated units that are engaged in joint problem-solving to accomplish a common goal. Within such a system the role of *opinion leaders* and *change agents* (individuals who attempt to speed others innovation decisions) are critical. Encouraging, rewarding, and making change agents, innovators, and early adopters work more visible will help the innovation gain *critical mass:* the point at which that change becomes self sustaining. Because of their relatively high prevalence getting the early adopters on board is judged to be critical in this regard.

Rogers' model of the diffusion of innovation has been given recent impetus by Berwick [32] who has reviewed the diffusion of innovations in some detail – from a medical perspective. Berwick proposed that "evidence" (based medicine) represents innovation – which even if implemented in one location does not necessarily diffuse to others. He suggests that application of the theory of DOI to implementing evidence concentrating on three areas of influence:

- The perception of innovation
- The characteristics of individuals who adopt change
- Contextual and managerial factors within the organisation

Many of the concepts in DOI are compatible with the sociotechnical school [33], soft-systems modelling [34] and systems thinking [35]. An important difference is that the DOI models is more prescriptive with much more fixed roles for individuals – and maybe over-exact proportions of individuals who adopt those roles.

The experiential learning from data quality projects in the UK

PRIMIS is a national data quality initiative in the UK. Its process is one of non-judgmental adult learning, supported by a national comparative service so that practices can compare their data quality with others [36]. PCDQ is an educational intervention with quality initiatives focusing on one disease area at a time [11]. The directors of these two large UK data quality projects (the author and the PRIMIS Director), have published features of what they consider to be an effective data quality programme [37], Table 1.

Table 1:   Characteristics of an effective data quality programme.

1. Motivation of professionals to have a positive attitude of their structured computer data	
2. Working with lead clinicians receptive to evidence-based quality improvement initiatives	
3. Respect for the "clinical judgement" (phronesis) of experienced clinicians	
4. Using informatics as an enabler of quality improvement*	*Best provided by an academic partner with the appropriate skill set.
5. Using education as an appropriate change agent*	
6. Data quality feedback using parameters with a positive predictive value and high sensitivity	
7. Personally provided feedback, by a skilled facilitator, within the workplace	
8. Professionally led programmes, supporting local clinical champions	
9. Alignment with national, evidence-based, quality improvement programme	
10. Financially incentivised	

We recognised that experienced clinicians tend not to blindly follow rules that they don't see as important. This may represent what Aristotle called "phronesis" – wisdom born of practical experience [38] – with clinicians not prepared to blindly record data for no apparent benefit [39]. This issue was also recognised, although rationalised in a different way, by Suchman [40] in her appraisal of why deciasion support tools are often not adopted; and, appears to fits with the theory of DOI which states that it is individuals not evidence that influences individuals to adopt an innovation. There are also many parallels with Soumerai and Avron's work on *academic detailing*, which also stressed the importance of understanding motivation, focussing on opinion leaders, working in an unbiased concise educational mode [41].

4. Discussion

Four themes emerge from this literature review, which provides a framework for giving feedback about data quality in primary care. .

Firstly, clinician engagement is essential. If GPs and nurses fail to get involved in the feedback process the risks of failure are high. It helps if there is an achievable clinical objective with a sound evidence-base. Ideally the feedback document should be brief. The theory of DOI suggests *innovators* should be engaged first. Feedback should be given in an educational context and be given by peers.

Secondly: understand context in which clinical coding takes place. This is best achieved by modelling the scenario within which data recording takes place. Usually, this will be during or after the clinical consultation, though sometimes by clerical staff.

Thirdly, recognise that culture is important. When designing a feedback strategy recognise the cultural norms within practices, clinics, localities, and health care system within which the initiative is operating. Be sensitive to pre-existing initiatives and perverse incentives that might exist.

Finally, look at technical issues. For example: the human computer interface, the coding system used, may influence a practitioner's abilities to use the computer system.

5. Conclusions

Feedback is a useful tool which can be used to raise the quality of computerised medical records in primary care. This literature review suggests that feedback is more likely to be effective where: it is clinically relevant with a strong evidence-base; is piloted among innovators; is feedback in an educational context within a peer group; and, is sensitive to the socio-technical context.

6. Acknowledgments

The PCDQ programme has been supported though an unconditional educational grant by MSD, and participating primary care organisations.

7. References

[1] Pan American Health Organization. Primary Health Care – 25 years of the Alma-Ata declaration. www.paho.org/English/DD/PIN/alma-ata_declaration.htm

[2] Starfield B. *Primary care: concept, evaluation, and policy.* New York: Oxford University Press, 1992

[3] Informatics in Primary Care. www.radcliffe-oxford.com/ipc

[4] American Medical Informatics Association Primary Care Informatics Working Group (AMIA PCIWG). www.amia.org/working/pci/main.html

[5] European Federation for Primary Care Informatics (EFMI) Primary Care Working Group. www.efmi.org/efmi/wg.asp?page=groups2&wgid=6

[6] International Medical Informatics Association (IMIA). Working Group No 5: Primary Care. www.imia.org/

[7] World Organisation of Family Doctors (Wonca) Informatics Working Party. www.globalfamilydoctor.com/aboutWonca/working_groups/index.htm

[8] Musen MA, van Bemmel JH. Challenges for medical informatics as an academic discipline. Methods of Information in Medicine 2002; 41:1–3

[9] Sullivan F. What is health informatics? *Journal of Health Services Research Policy* 2001; 6(4):251–254

[10] de Lusignan S. What is Primary Care Informatics? *J Am Med Inform Assoc* 2003; 10:304–309

[11] de Lusignan S, Hague N, Brown A, Majeed A. An educational intervention to improve data recording in the management of ischaemic heart disease in primary care. *J Public Health (Oxf)*. 2004 Mar;26(1):34-7.

[12] van der Lei J, Musen MA, van der Does E, Man in 't Veld AJ, van Bemmel JH. Comparison of computer-aided and human review of general practitioners' management of hypertension. Lancet. 1991;338(8781):1504-8.

[13] D. L. Hunt, R. Jaeschke, K. A. McKibbon, and for the Evidence-Based Medicine Working Group. Users' Guides to the Medical Literature: XXI. Using Electronic Health Information Resources in Evidence-Based Practice *JAMA,* 2000;283(14):1875 - 1879.

[14] Greenhalgh T. How to read a paper. The Medline database. *BMJ.* 1997;315(7101):180-3.

[15] NHS Centre for Reviews and Dissemination, University of York. Getting evidence into practice. *Effective Healthcare* 1999, 5(1). URL: http://www.york.ac.uk/inst/crd/ehc51.pdf

[16]   Buntinx F, Winkens R, Grol R, Knottnerus JA. Influencing diagnostic and preventive performance in ambulatory care by feedback and reminders. A review. *Fam Pract.* 1993;10(2):219-28.

[17]   Pop P, Winkens RA. A diagnostic centre for general practitioners: results of individual feedback on diagnostic actions. *J R Coll Gen Pract.* 1989;39(329):507-8.

[18]   Buntinx F, Knottnerus JA, Crebolder HF, Seegers T, Essed GG, Schouten H. Does feedback improve the quality of cervical smears? A randomized controlled trial. *Br J Gen Pract.* 1993;43(370):194-8.

[19]   Ferguson RI, Maling TJ. The Nelson general practice prescribing project. Part II: Prescribing reports for self audit. *N Z Med J.* 1990;103(902):560-2.

[20]   Fraser RC, Farooqi A, Sorrie R. Use of vitamin B-12 in Leicestershire practices: a single topic audit led by a medical audit advisory group. *BMJ.* 1995;311(6996):28-30.

[21]   Rokstad K, Straand J, Fugelli P. Can drug treatment be improved by feedback on prescribing profiles combined with therapeutic recommendations? A prospective, controlled trial in general practice. *J Clin Epidemiol.* 1995;48(8):1061-8.

[22]   Lassen LC, Kristensen FB. Peer comparison feedback to achieve rational and economical drug therapy in general practice: a controlled intervention study. *Scand J Prim Health Care.* 1992;10(1):76-80.

[23]   Porcheret M, Hughes R, Evans D, Jordan K, Whitehurst T, Ogden H, Croft P; North Staffordshire General Practice Research Network. Data quality of general practice electronic health records: the impact of a program of assessments, feedback, and training. *J Am Med Inform Assoc.* 2004;11(1):78-86.

[24]   van den Hombergh P, Grol R, van den Hoogen HJ, van den Bosch WJ. Practice visits as a tool in quality improvement: mutual visits and feedback by peers compared with visits and feedback by non-physician observers. *Qual Health Care.* 1999;8(3):161-6.

[25]   van den Hombergh P, Grol R, van den Hoogen HJ, van den Bosch WJ. Practice visits as a tool in quality improvement: acceptance and feasibility. *Qual Health Care.* 1999;8(3):167-71.

[26]   Zwar N, Henderson J, Britt H, McGeechan K, Yeo G. Influencing antibiotic prescribing by prescriber feedback and management guidelines: a 5-year follow-up. *Fam Pract.* 2002;19(1):12-7.

[27]   Baker R, Falconer Smith J, Lambert PC. Randomised controlled trial of the effectiveness of feedback in improving test ordering in general practice. *Scand J Prim Health Care.* 2003;21(4):219-23.

[28]   de Marco P, Dain C, Lockwood T, Roland M. How valuable is feedback of information on hospital referral patterns? *BMJ.* 1993;307(6917):1465-6.

[29]   Hickey A, Scott I, Denaro C, Stewart N, Bennett C, Theile T. Using clinical indicators in a quality improvement programme targeting cardiac care. *Int J Qual Health Care.* 2004;16 Suppl 1:i11-25.

[30]   Watkins C, Timm A, Gooberman-Hill R, Harvey I, Haines A, Donovan J. Factors affecting feasibility and acceptability of a practice-based educational intervention to support evidence-based prescribing: a qualitative study. *Fam Pract.* 2004;21(6):661-9.

[31]   Rogers E. *Diffusion of Innovations,* 4th ed. New York, Free Press, 1995.

[32]   Berwick DM. Disseminating innovations in health care. *JAMA.* 2003;289(15):1969-75.

[33]   Berg M. *Rationalizing medical work.* Massachusetts: MIT Press, 1997.

[34]   Checkland P, Scholes J. *Soft Systems methodology in action.* Chichester: Wiley, 1999.

[35]   Chapman J. A systems perspective on computing in the NHS. *Informatics in Primary Care* 2002;10:197-9.

[36]   Teasdale S, Bainbridge M. Improving information management in family practice: testing an adult learning model. Proc AMIA Annu Fall Symp. 1997; 19:687–692.

[37]   de Lusignan S, Teasdale S. The features of an effective primary care data quality programme. . In, Ed. Bryant JR. *Perspective in Healthcare Computing.* Proceedings of HC2004. Swindon: British Computer Society,2004.

[38]   Fugelli   P.   Clinical   practice: between   Aristotle   and   Cochrane. *Schweiz   Med Wochenschr*1998;128(6):184-8.

[39]   Suchman L. *Plans and situated actions.* Cambridge: Cambridge University Press, 1987.

[40]   de Lusignan S, Wells SE, Hague NJ, Thiru K. Managers see the problems associated with coding clinical data as a technical issue whilst clinicians also see cultural barriers. Methods Inf Med. 2003;42(4):416-22.

[41]   Soumerai SB, Avorn J. Principles of educational outreach ('academic detailing') to improve clinical decision making. .*JAMA.* 1990 Jan 26;263(4):549-56.

Address for correspondence

Dr Simon de Lusignan, Primary Care Informatics, Division of Community Health Sciences, St. George's – University of London, London SW17 0RE email: slusigna@sgul.ac.uk

Connecting Medical Informatics and Bio-Informatics
R. Engelbrecht et al. (Eds.)
IOS Press, 2005

Usability Evaluation of a Laboratory Order Entry System: Cognitive Walkthrough and Think Aloud Combined

Linda W P Peute, Monique M W Jaspers

Department of Medical Informatics
Academic Medical Center- Universiteit van Amsterdam

Abstract

Though designing physician order entry (POE) systems has been a highly discussed research topic in the last decade, it seems that engineering POE systems that truly optimise the quality and efficiency of ordering is still a challenge. This study addresses a usability evaluation of an emerging POE for the electronically ordering of laboratory tests. By applying two complementary cognitive approaches, specifically the cognitive walkthrough and think aloud method with seven potential end users of the system, we analyzed usability problems in the prototype system and their potential effect on the quality of orders in terms of efficiency and errors in ordering. The cognitive walkthrough provided a coding scheme that was used to analyse in more detail usability errors encountered during the think aloud tests with the seven end users. The analyses revealed a total of 33 usability problems, which indeed led to inefficiency, omissions in ordering and even to cancelled orders. Most of these usability problems referred to incomprehensiveness of required actions by the user and incomprehensiveness of text used in the system. Next to the discussion of the reasons for these usability problems, the surplus value of the think aloud method as supplementary to the cognitive walkthrough in evaluating physician order entry systems is outlined in this paper.

Keywords:
Physician Order Entry Systems; Usability Evaluation; Information Systems

1. Introduction

A Laboratory Physician Order Entry system (LPOE) is a medical computer application, designed to support and to advance the process of laboratory test ordering by physicians. Physician Order Entry systems (POE) are known to offer numerous benefits among which increased quality of written communication and decreased variation in orders due to order sets based on standard practice protocols [1]. Yet, the lessons learned from implementations that failed show that the complexity of POE implementation involves the adoption of the system in clinical practice [2]. Based on these negative experiences with POE implementations it has been emphasized that it is highly important that these systems can be effectively integrated into daily working routines and provide sufficient benefit to the user to offset the burden of system use [3]. To increase the success of a POE implementation, among other things, asks for better understanding of how physicians are to interact with the POE system and whether this interaction supports their working routines.

In 2004 we were asked to evaluate the emerging system prototype of a LPOE system, OMLab, before this system would be implemented in a pilot phase at the outpatient neurology department. The project team was particularly interested in evaluating whether the prototype, based on a 6-step model, which was to be used for ordering laboratory tests, would easily integrate into the working routines of the physicians and whether specific usability problems would lead to errors in orders. If required the prototype system would be optimized before the pilot implementation would proceed. To gain insight into potential usability and learnability problems we applied both the Cognitive Walkthrough inspection method (CW) and the Think Aloud (TA) method for the evaluation of the OMLab system prototype to get insight in usability problems with the OMLab order entry system. More specifically, we investigated whether the TA method had a surplus value to the CW in revealing underlying causes of these usability problems and in revealing more categories of usability problems.

2. Methods

Two researchers from the field of medical informatics conducted a CW on the OMLab order entry system. CW is a usability inspection method, developed to offer system designers a tool to evaluate how easily a system can be used through exploration with the aim to improve the systems design before implementing it in daily practice [4]. CW focuses on the identification of goals and of subsequent actions to complete tasks within the system, thereby analysing whether the users' background knowledge would enable completion of these tasks. In this way evaluators consider the behaviour of the interface and its effect on the user, with the aim to identify those actions that would be difficult to perform in the system. In this study the CW was used to define a framework of sub-goals and related action-sequences per sub-goal. The researchers used this framework to identify potential usability problems in the action-sequences to be executed in the OMLab system. Each of these potential usability problems was then coded according to 'Norman's theory of action' into 'goal problems' (the user tries to accomplish the wrong thing) or 'action problems' (the user would like to perform the correct action but does not know how) [5]. Thereafter seven potential end users of the OMLab order entry system were asked to perform four simulated laboratory-ordering tasks supported by the OMLab system. In accordance with the TA method, the users were instructed to verbalize their thoughts in performing tasks [6]. These tasks were based on four real life clinical scenarios, which were reviewed by an expert clinician to prevent interpretation problems. The scenarios were designed so that together they would cover all usability problems identified by the CW. Standard practice laboratory protocols were used as input for three of the four scenarios. The potential end users differed in age, computer experience and in their experience with paper-based laboratory ordering. None of the end users had prior experience with a system for ordering laboratory tests and all worked with the same paper forms to request laboratory tests. Sessions took place in the clinical environment of the potential end users and lasted 40 to 50 minutes. Sessions were videotaped; screen sequences of the OMLab system were captured for subsequent analysis. The coded usability problems predefined by the CW, were used to interpret the video recordings and to analyze the problems the physicians actually encountered during the TA tests. The verbal protocols of end users were transcribed and physicians' utterances were linked to the occurrence of usability problems encountered in the TA testing sessions. As such the TA method was to characterize both the problems of potential end user physicians in interaction with the OMLab system, and the ways in which these problems could negatively influence the quality of laboratory orders.

3. Results

The CW identified six subtasks and 29 associated actions that needed to be executed by a user in order to enter and send an order. The six subtasks included: (1) Check name and phone number of requester, (2) Select a protocol, (3) Select laboratory tests, (4) Enter patient clinical data, (5) Enter reason for ordering laboratory tests, and (6) Send the order to the outpatient clinical laboratory. These subtasks represent the six states of the 6-step model of the OMLab system (see Figure 1). For example, an action associated to the subtask of selecting laboratory tests is: click on the drop down menu 'material'. For a relative simple order, ordering one laboratory test with the help of the system, only four of these six subtasks are to be performed and 13 actions. In executing a relatively complex order all six subtasks of the system need to be performed and all 29 associated actions, of which some are to be performed several times. The in-depth CW analysis of the OMLab user interface revealed a total of 25 potential usability problems associated with actions to be performed in executing the 6-step model.

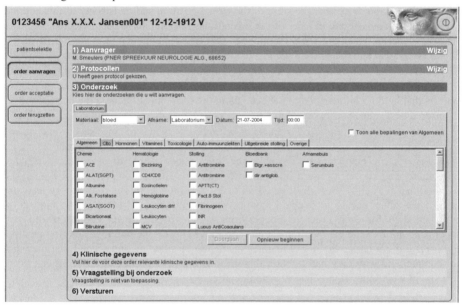

Figure 1- Example of an OMLab screen, activated in step three- the general sheet

In the next section, examples of the most severe or most frequently encountered usability problems, revealed by the CW and TA analyses, will be given per subtask.

Subtask two 'Select a protocol'

Inflexibility of protocol selection: This usability problem referred to the inflexibility of selecting a protocol in the system. Once an end user had selected a protocol the selection was not reversible. It was likewise not possible for a user to select more than one protocol in the system, though in practice this situation frequently occurs. The TA usability test showed that two end users choose a wrong protocol and after discovering their mistake were not able to change their selection. Instead of restarting the system, one end user deselected all of the system's protocol based pre-selected set of 16 laboratory tests, before selecting the set of laboratory tests he had decided on.

Subtask three 'select laboratory tests'

Inability to navigate to laboratory tests in the system: To select a laboratory test, end users first searched the general sheet by clicking on the scrollbar (see Figure 1). In performing the four scenarios, the seven end users clicked the scrollbar 298 times. Because searching of tests with use of the scrollbar arrows took additional time, all end users were dissatisfied and complained about system performance. Though all tests were alphabetically organized the users on average still needed two and a half minutes to find the test they were searching for. Five of the seven users verbalized more than once, while searching for a test in the OMlab system, that the laboratory tests in the program were not organized as they were used to with the paper ordering forms. They all expressed the need for a search function by which they could find tests by entering the first letter of a test or a test synonym.

Incomprehension of button texts: For ordering infrequently ordered laboratory tests a button 'extra tests' needs to be selected in the system. After selecting this button additional laboratory tests appear on the OMLab screen. End users experienced severe difficulties in ordering these laboratory tests, because of the wrong position and invisibility of this button. The button was only found in three of the seven times it should have been selected conform the task scenario. Most end users complained that many laboratory tests were difficult to find in the system and that selecting a test required too many actions by the user.

Appearance and information content of error messages in the system: In 14 of the in total 28 scenarios that were to be performed by the users, system error messages were presented to users that held no information to the user about the cause and effects of the occurrence of the error. The TA analysis revealed that no user understood these error messages.

Understandability of required sequence of actions: None of the seven end users understood nor executed the required sequence of actions in the system to order tests cito (tests that require results fast). To make the 'cito' sheet visible to users, the designers deliberately had chosen to use a different color for this sheet. However, the TA analysis revealed that the 'cito' sheet disoriented all users, resulting in missing laboratory tests on each of the seven occasions it could have occurred. Furthermore, users had to indicate a time and date for each order to be performed. Five of the seven end users did not understand nor execute the required actions correctly. The TA method revealed first that the end users did not notice that these features needed to be filled in, and second that they did not comprehend why they had to enter this information in step three already, instead of in step six, in which they finally had to send the order.

Subtask 4 'Enter clinical patient data'

Self-descriptiveness of tasks in the system: In the TA analysis all seven end users verbalized that they did not understand the necessity of filling in clinical patient information in a laboratory order, as only they themselves would review the order results. Since physicians did not want to enter this extra information, they started searching for different routes in the system to send the order. This led to inefficiency of ordering. Five of the seven users were dissatisfied and uttered complaints. The CW analysis did not identify this as a user interaction problem, because the CW mainly focuses on the ease with which tasks in the system can be executed. The TA analysis gave us, next to the occurrences of usability problems, additional insight into the working practices of the physicians in ordering tests and whether the system supported efficient ordering. However the necessity to enter clinical patient data in step four of the OMLab system originated from the requirement analyses of the OMLab system. Since the end users of the OMLab system in daily practice do not supply patient clinical information on the paper order forms, they were not willing to fill in any such information.

A different problem revealed by the TA analysis was the fact that users missed the possibility in the system to supply additional information concerning a specific test, like a patient's weight or length. As they missed this feature in the OMLab system end users supplied this information only in step four 'patient clinical information', though this information was not visible for the laboratory personnel.

Subtask 5 'Enter reason for ordering laboratory tests'

Understandability of required sequence of actions/ User workload: Five of the seven users were disoriented about the correct sequence of actions they needed to execute in entering a reason for ordering a specific laboratory test in the OMLab system. The laboratory personnel needed this information in order to perform a more specific analysis on the ordered tests. Users ineffectively tried to skip this step to accomplish sending the order. After on average executing the wrong action three times, most end users finished this subtask correctly. However it seemed that this system feature was not easily learned, for an end user performed the same "ineffective" action several times in different task scenarios.

Redundancy of information: In evaluating the manner in which users executed the steps in the system, the TA usability test revealed a specific usability problem referred to as 'redundancy of information given by end users'. Users, after having selected a specific protocol in step two of the system, were forced to add information for individually ordered test concerning the reason for ordering a particular laboratory test, whereas they felt that they had supplied this information in step two by selecting a protocol.

Table 1- An example of a usability problem revealed by the TA analysis

CW Code	Interaction problem	# encounters	Verbalizations
No Code TA [5]	Physicians did not enter appropriate clinical patient information in step 4 or a research question in step 5, though the system required this information.	Encountered 18/21	"I don't need to give additional information; I have already selected a protocol. That seems enough information to me" [10], "This is silly, I will enter both in step 4 and 5 that I already selected a protocol" [5]

During the TA test eight additional usability issues arose which were not identified by the CW. These issues were concerned with overall system understandability, information content of the OMLab system, redundancy of information in the system, and comprehension of texts on buttons. Moreover, these problems were all revealed in the context of actions to be performed in the system that did not directly link to the standard paper ordering routines, thereby forcing the user to change them. For example, end users did not comprehend the button 'start new order' in step three of the system in relation to their goal for completing the order. Two end users clicked this button with the goal to send the order. The system provided no feedback on the fact that the order was cancelled. So they had ended the previous order before sending the order to the laboratory. In real practice the physician would have to enter the entire order again.

4. Discussion and conclusions

In this study we performed a usability evaluation of the OMLab system by means of a CW, performed by two experts in the field of medical informatics, combined with the TA method with seven potential end users of the system. The CW framework could be adequately applied for the analysis of the OMLab interaction problems encountered during the TA tests. Sixteen of the in total 25 usability problems identified by the CW, actually occurred and indeed resulted in inefficiency of ordering, omissions and factual errors in ordering tests and even in cancellation of orders. For example, seven of the usability problems introduced a potential source of inefficiency in completing orders with the OMLab system. Furthermore, the incomprehensiveness of texts in the OMLab system in subtask three, and the non-descriptiveness of subtask five resulted in factual errors in ordering. The CW however did not reveal all usability problems encountered by end users in interaction with the OMLab system. The TA analysis revealed eight more OMLab usability problems. These perceived usability problems influenced the way physicians behaved in interaction with the system. Despite the strength of the CW in discovering potential usability problems, it seems that the CW only revealed about 76% of the usability problems the end users actually encountered in interaction with the OMLab system. Though these results indicate that the CW method does not predict all usability problems we still abide that applying the CW in evaluating the design of a system is an effective and relative easy way to find potential user-interaction problems based on which the system might be improved. The surplus value of the TA analysis to the CW analysis was in providing us with a deeper understanding of the underlying causes of usability problems the physicians encountered in interaction with the system and the ways in which these problems might be tackled in adjusting the system's user interface. By combining these methods in the evaluation of the OMLab system, specific recommendations for enhancement of the system could be communicated to the developers of the system.

Computerized physician order entry is an inherently complex process, but the way in which the system is designed can either increase or minimize its complexity. The 6-step model of the OMLab system is a tool to minimize the complexity of ordering laboratory tests in a computer system by visualizing the steps the end user needs to perform to order laboratory tests. The question is, however, whether the 6-step model guides the physician through the ordering process in an efficient and usable way; thereby supporting ordering laboratory tests of high quality. From the analysis of the TA results the conclusion can be drawn that to order tests the 6-step model of the OMLab system is easy to follow. Yet, the manner in which actions were to be executed within each of the six steps caused severe usability problems. Although the prototype OMLab system missed a lot of features and still is at an early stage of development, knowing whether the redesigned system will support good quality of ordering in clinical practice is ever more important.

5. Acknowledgements

The authors thank M. Smeulers, J. de Gans, P. F. Mooijweer- Groen, T.L.F. Urbanus and P. J. M. Bakker for their cooperation in conducting this study.

6. References

[1] Sittig DF, Stead W. Computer-based physician order entry; The state of the art. *J Am med Inform Assoc* 1994:1: 108-123.
[2] Horsky J, Kaufman DR, Patel VL. The cognitive complexity of a provider order entry interface. *Proc. AMIA Annu. Fall Symp.* 2003: 294-298.
[3] Horsky J, Kaufman DR, Patel VL. Computer-based drug ordering: evaluation of interaction with a decision-support system. *Proc. Medinfo* 2004.
[4] Polson PG, Lewis CH, Rieman J, Wharton C. Cognitive walkthroughs: A method for theory-based evaluation of user interfaces. *International Journal of Man-Machine Studies* 1992: 36:741-773.
[5] Norman DA. Things that make us smart: defending human attributes in the age of the machine. Reading, MA: Addison Wesley; 1993.
[6] M.T. Boren, J. Ramey, Thinking aloud: reconciling theory and practice. IEEE Transactions on Professional Communication 43 (2000) 261-278.

Address for correspondence

L.W.P. Peute, M.W.M. Jaspers, Dept. of Medical Informatics, Academic Medical Centre, Room J1b-115-1, P.O.Box 22700, 1100 DE Amsterdam, The Netherlands, E-mail: L.W. Peute@amc.uva.nl, M.W.Jaspers@amc.uva.nl

Connecting Medical Informatics and Bio-Informatics
R. Engelbrecht et al. (Eds.)
IOS Press, 2005

605

Operation Management System Evaluation in the Central Finland Health Care District -

End Users' View of System Implementation

Kaisa Lemmetty[a], Eija Häyrinen[b]

[a,b] Central Finland Health Care District, Information Management, Finland, http://www.ksshp.fi
[a] University of Kuopio, Department of Health Policy and Management, Social and Health Informatics,
http://www.uku.fi,kaisa.lemmetty@ksshp.fi, eija.hayrinen@ksshp.fi

Abstract

In this paper we evaluate the implementation of the operation management system in the Central Finland Health Care District. The implementation of the operation management system changed the practice of operation management for the surgical clinic and concerned 500 personnel in total. A survey was carried out to investigate the end users' views on the system's usefulness, usability and the training and user support provided. The users' possibilities to accomplish their tasks and the kind of obstacles they face in operation management were explored. The assessment revealed that more end support is needed after the system implementation, even though a generally positive attitude towards the system was manifested among the staff.

Keywords:
HIS implementation, evaluation, usability

1. Introduction

The evaluation of healthcare information systems is challenging: system evaluation in itself is complex, there are technical and human aspects to consider, as well as the complexity of reorganizing clinical practice. [1] Evaluation studies concerning information systems are useful as they help to perceive relations and may change current practice. Acquired evaluation results cannot be generalized on the basis of statistical argumentation only, but have to be substantiated stepwise, taking into account the specificity of the object and context of each evaluation. [2, 3, 4] Systems usability is more than mere usefulness and utility. When combining the concepts of usefulness and utility copability emerges. No system is complete before it encounters practice. [5, 6, 7]

The surgical clinic in the Central Finland Health Care District performs approximately 15 000 procedures a year in altogether 22 operating rooms. Within the last year a complete operation management system was implemented in the surgical clinic and healthcare professionals were urged to rearrange their work practice concerning operation planning and following the operating room activity. In Central Finland the operation system was integrated into the hospital information system to enable the retrieval of administrative data, the patient registers and the national coding system for diagnosis and medical procedures. The specific needs and processes of the hospitals were configured into the system. The application includes a complete program for operating room and surgery management. The system of planning, scheduling and analysis of operations permits the following of the entire preoperative process, starting from the surgery request and the waiting list to the final operation schedule. All the staff members have access to information about the operation activity and get a general view of the status of patients in operation.

2. Material and Methods

The surgical staff's (doctors, nurses and secretaries) facilities for and attitudes towards the use of the operation management system were studied in the survey. The questionnaire included 48 arguments and the alternatives were from one to five on the Likert-scale. The questionnaire was sent as an e-form to 180 users for data collection. The answers were statistically analyzed and a qualitative analysis was conducted with the open answers. Responses were received from 110 participants (61%). The participants consisted of nurses 64%, doctors 15% and secretaries 21%.

3. Results

In the analysis, average values (1 poor-5 good) were calculated for usability, utility and copability. A comparison was also made between different occupations, age, training model and clinical background.

Table 1 End users' view of system usability, utility and copability

Participants (N=110)	Usability	Utility	Copability
Doctors (15%)	3,49	3,10	3,15
Nurses (64%)	2,83	2,88	3,09
Secretaries (21%)	3,23	3,24	3,14

The average value for system usability varied from 2, 83 to 3, 49. Doctors were the most content with the system usability, while nurses expressed lower satisfaction. The system utility average values were from 2, 88 up to 3, 10. Concerning utility, secretaries revealed the highest value at 3, 24 and nurses the lowest at 2, 88. The system copability value varied the least between different occupations. The only statistically significant topic was that doctors were more pleased with the system's data accuracy and data retrieval than secretaries.

The survey revealed that the staff requires further training and user support. For the efficient use and utility of the operation management system it is important to take into account how the users relate to the real life use of the system. It seems that support and the implementation training should be targeted to different professions dissimilarly. Operation management is a process and the team consists of doctors, nurses and secretaries who all have specific demands. They have profession-based tasks and need different skills and competence when using an information system. System copability may be the fact that requires further addressing.

The evaluation of the operation management system provided us with information about the users' views on usability, utility and copability. End user assessment reveals how the system meets practice in operation management after the implementation. Both organizational and educational issues were addressed in the survey. The evaluation of the system helps us to comprehend the necessity of dialogue and educational support given to users not only during the implementation phase but also in the routine use of the system.

End users' satisfaction with the system may directly reflect organizational efficiency [8]. Better utility of operation resources permits users to focus on high priority cases and the most urgent care. The system offers good opportunities for the further development of surgical care and accessibility to operations.

In this evaluation study we found that implementation training had no significant impact in promoting the end users' satisfaction with the system's utility, usability and copability. For further studies, more relevant data of the system implementation, training and user satisfaction is required to achieve a better understanding of the complexity of change in clinical practice.

4. Acknowledgments

This work was supported by the Central Finland Health Care District, Research Unit.

5. References

[1]   Ammenwerth E. Iller C. & Mansmann U. 2003. Can evaluation studies benefit from triangulation? A case study. *International Journal of Medical Informatics* (2003) 70, 237.

[2]   Friedman C. Wyatt J.C. 1997. Evaluation Methods in Medical Informatics, Springer, New York.

[3]   Brender J. 1998. Trends in assessment of IT-based solutions in healthcare and recommendations for the future. *International Journal of Medical Informatics.* 52 (1 -/ 3) (1998) 217/ 227.

[4]   Kaplan B. 2001 Evaluating informatics applications. Alternative approaches: theory, social interactionism, and call for methodological pluralism, *International Journal of Medical Informatics.* 64. (2001)

[5]   Boisen E. & Bygholm A. & Hejlesen O K. 2001: Activity Theory and Medical Informatics: Usability, Utility and Copability. Patel V.-L.; Rogers R. Haux R. MEDINFO-2001.604-8 vol.1. IOS Press, Amsterdam, Netherlands.

[6]   Boisen E. & Bygholm A. Cavan A & Hejlesen OK. 2003. Copability, coping, and learning as focal concepts in the evaluation of computerised diabetes disease management. *International Journal of Medical Informatics* (2003) 70, 353. / 363.

[7]   Engeström Y. 1990: Learning, working and imagining. Twelve studies in activity theory. Orienta konsultit Oy. Helsinki.

[8]   Vimarlund V. Timpka T. & Hallberg N. 1999. Healthcare professional's demand for knowledge in informatics. *International Journal of Medical Informatics* 53 (1999) 107–114.

Address for correspondence:

Kaisa Lemmetty, RN, Clinical nurse specialist, M.Sc. student, kaisa.lemmetty@ksshp.fi
Central Finland Health Care District,
Information Management, Jyväskylä, Finland, http://www.ksshp.fi

Connecting Medical Informatics and Bio-Informatics
R. Engelbrecht et al. (Eds.)
IOS Press, 2005

Comparisons of Physicians' and Nurses' Attitudes towards Computers

Gordana Brumini, Ivor Ković[a], Dejvid Zombori[b], Ileana Lulić[a], Lidija-Bilic-Zulle, Mladen Petrovečki

Department of Computer Science, Rijeka University School of Medicine, Rijeka,
[a]*Student of Rijeka University school of Medicine,*
[b]*Student of Rijeka University School of Philosophy, Department of Psychology*

Abstract

Before starting the implementation of integrated hospital information systems, the physicians' and nurses' attitudes towards computers were measured by means of a questionnaire. The study was conducted in Dubrava University Hospital, Zagreb in Croatia. Out of 194 respondents, 141 were nurses and 53 physicians, randomly selected. They surveyed by an anonymous questionnaire consisting of 8 closed questions about demographic data, computer science education and computer usage, and 30 statements on attitudes towards computers. The statements were adapted to a Likert type scale. Differences in attitudes towards computers between groups were compared using Kruskal-Wallis and Mann Whitney test for post-hoc analysis. The total score presented attitudes toward computers. Physicians' total score was 130 (97-144), while nurses' total score was 123 (88-141). It points that the average answer to all statements was between "agree" and "strongly agree", and these high total scores indicated their positive attitudes. Age, computer science education and computer usage were important factors witch enhances the total score. Younger physicians and nurses with computer science education and with previous computer experience had more positive attitudes towards computers than others. Our results are important for planning and implementation of integrated hospital information systems in Croatia.

Keywords:
Attitudes; Computers; Education; Nurses; Physicians; Questionnaire

1. Introduction

The rapid progress of information technology influences to the major political resolves and it's the reason for many necessary changes in all segments of the activity in medicine. So that, most 'healthcare reform' plans includes the development of a reliable and competent healthcare information system. The part of these reforms is the implementation of integrated hospital information systems (IHIS). During 2003, Croatian Ministry of Health and Social Welfare announced informatics projects in health care system. Pilot projects of IHIS implementation were tested in four Croatian hospitals: Dubrava University Hospital and "Holly Spirit" General Hospital in Zagreb, and Rijeka and Split University Hospital Centers [1].

One of the key issues, constantly present during arrangements for IHIS implementation, was to find the adequate way of transition from standard "paper and pen" environment to the one based on modern and more effective information technology (IT) [, 3]. IHIS can dramatically improve performance, reduce costs, provide more time for direct patient care, and ensure a better connection with patients, suppliers and physicians [4-6]. The implementation included three major components: the brand-new hardware and software technology, and all medical or nomedical employers in the hospital. In our study we concentrated to the end users of IHIS, physicians and nurses. The experiences from some other countries point that the positive users' attitudes towards computers are the necessary prerequisite for successful implementation of IHIS [6,7].

We had already examined the nurses' attitude towards computers in two Croatian's hospital: Dubrava University Hospital, Zagreb and Rijeka University Hospital Center, Rijeka and our results were recently published in Croatian Medical Journal [8]. Also, in the Medix journal, were published all the results of the first phase of healthcare information system in Croatia [9,10]. The aim of this study was to estimate and compare physicians' and nurses' attitudes towards computers in Dubrava University Hospital. Gathered information will be helpful in meeting the needs and demands of physicians and nurses during IHIS implementation in Croatia.

2. Subjects and Methods

Subjects

The study was conducted during November 2003 in Dubrava Clinical Hospital, Zagreb. Head nurses distributed questionnaires during usual daily meetings of nursing staff to randomly selected one quarter of nurses. Out of all employed physicians we surveyed one third, major of them as chiefs of hospital units. Before questionnaire distribution, respondents were informed about the subject of the study and confidentiality of responses was ensured. Out of 210 respondents surveyed, 194 returned and properly filled in the questionnaire: 141 nurses and 53 physicians (response rate 92%).

Questionnaire

The well-known Nurses' Attitudes towards Computers (NATC) instrument [11] was modified, supplemented with new items and used in this study. Final questionnaire consisted of 8 closed questions about demographic data, computer science education and computer usage, and 30 statements on attitudes towards computers. The statements measured the respondents' attitudes towards computers. The answers were defined by Likert one to five response scale, where "1" indicated strongly disagree, "2" disagree, "3" undecided, "4" agree, and "5" strongly agree with a particular statement. Respondents were advised to give their first reaction to the statements after reading.

Statistics

Factor analysis was performed on all statements [12]. According obtained one factor solution ($\alpha = 0.91$), it was decided to form one measure of attitudes. Thirty answers were summarized and the total score for each respondent was computed. Total score range was 30 to 150. The results are shown with median and range presented with 5th-95th percentile boundaries. Non-parametric tests, Mann-Whitney test and Kruskal-Wallis test, were used to compare average total score between groups.

All statistical values were considered significant with p<0.05. Statistics was done using Statistica for Windows (release 6.1, StatSoft. Inc., Tulsa, OK, USA) and MedCalc (release 7.5, MedCalc, Maraikerke, Belgium).

3. Results

The total score presented attitudes toward computers (Table 1). Physicians' total score was 130 (97-144), while nurses' total score was 123 (88-141). It points that the average answer to all statements was between "agree" and "strongly agree". Therefore, the total score value of 123 and a higher was assumed to be the indicator for positive attitude in this study.

Although, the physicians and nurses showed positive attitudes towards computers, physicians had a significant higher score than nurses (130 vs. 123, p=0.008). There was no difference among men and women in their total score in both groups (women vs. men, physicians: 127 vs. 130, p=0.584; nurses: 123 vs. 126, p=0.496). The total score according to age showed the significantly difference, so physicians younger than 50 had a higher total score compared to elderly (133 vs. 121, p=0.048). There was significant difference between nurses younger than 50 and elderly in their total score (125 vs. 119, p=0.048).

We also examined if the computer science education, frequency, and purpose of computer usage had the influence on the scores on the attitudes towards computer (Table 1). Computer science education was related to the achievement of significant higher nurses' positive attitudes. Nurses who attended classes of medical informatics during their formal education obtained significantly higher total score than others (127 vs. 121, p=0.012). Also, the physicians with computer science education have more positive attitudes than they without it; difference in total score is significant (133 vs. 120, p=0.018). The analysis also revealed that computer usage had a significant influence on the total score. Nurses and physicians who did not use computers at all had lower score compared to all others, irrespective location using of computers at home, at work or at home and at work (Kruskal-Wallis test, p<0.001). But, there is no difference in the total score among physicians and nurses (physicians vs. nurses, at work: 126 vs. 125, p=0.125; at home: 136 vs. 126, p=0.088; at home and at work: 137 vs. 130, p=0.486).

The frequency of computer usage enhances total score in both groups, but no significantly (Kruskal-Wallis test, physicians: p=0.459; nurses: p=0.164). Finally, we analyzed and compared difference in attitudes towards computers between four main purposes of computer usage: using computers at work, for education, in communication with others, and for pleasure. For all these purposes, there was no significant difference between physicians and nurses. Comparisons the total score obtained between using computers for any of these purposes or for all of them and no using computers at all showed significant differences. The physicians and nurse who used computers have more positive attitudes than nonusers (Kruskal-Wallis test, physicians and nurses: p<0.001).

Table 1. Physicians' and nurses' total score according to gender, age, computer science education, computer usage, and frequency of computer usage.

	Physicians		Nurses		Statistics
	N	Total score[*] Median (5th-95th)	N	Total score[*] Median (5th-95th)	p
Gender					
Women	23	127 (88-144)	141	123 (88-141)	0.584
Men	30	130 (111-145)	10	126 (89-146)	0.496
p		0.584		0.496	
Age (years)					
< 50	29	133 (103-144)	108	125 (88-142)	0.004
≥ 50	24	121 (88-144)	33	119 (88-140)	0.049
p		0.048		0.048	
Computer science education					
No	23	120 (88-144)	102	121 (88-141)	0.486
Yes	30	133 (103-144)	39	127 (104-145)	0.110
p		0.018		0.012	
Computer usage – where?					
Nowhere	6	117 (88-122)	50	108 (82-133)	0.340
Work	8	126 (87-139)	24	125 (89-140)	0.125
Home	12	136 (107-145)	33	126 (108-142)	0.088
Work & home	27	137 (112-144)	34	130 (109-145)	0.468
p	0.004[†]		<0.001[†]		
Computer usage – hours per week					
< 1	8	119 (77-143)	24	124 (97-142)	0.516
1-5	16	129 (97-145)	26	125 (105-141)	0.670
>5	25	136 (112-144)	41	132 (104-142)	0.234
p	0.061[‡]		0.164[‡]		
Purpose of computer usage					
Work	28	131 (103-144)	63	130 (103-142)	0.840
Education	34	133 (107-145)	25	127 (109-142)	0.132
Communication	30	133 (115-145)	30	133 (108-142)	0.745
Pleasure	18	133 (112-144)	47	130 (108-142)	0.538
All	10	136 (115-144)	11	136 (128-142)	0.715
No use	6	117 (88-122)	50	108 (82-133)	0.340
p	<0.001[ʃ]		<0.001[ʃ]		
All	10	130 (111-145)	141	123 (88-141)	0.008

[*]Total score indicates summarized score of all items (higher score represents more positive attitudes towards computers)
[†]Mann-Whitney test reveals significant difference between group nowhere and the rest three groups
[‡] Mann-Whitney test reveals no significant difference between all groups
[ʃ]Mann-Whitney test reveals significant difference between group no use and all others groups

4. Discussion

There are no previous reports on physicians' and nurses' attitudes towards computers in Croatian hospitals. Successful implementation of IHIS is highly influenced by the acceptance of its end users [6,7]. We hoped that gathered information would be helpful in all aspects of IHIS implementation, from designing the system to the training the staff and customer support.

In our study, the physicians and nurses showed a high total score that indicates positive attitudes towards computer. Age, education and computer usage had statistically significant influence on the attitudes. The total score according to age showed the difference, so physicians and nurses younger than 50 had a significantly higher total score compared to elderly, that is consistent with other published studies [13, 14]. It might be due to their awareness of information technology and of benefits introduced by IHIS as well as their willingness to change and adapt to IHIS. Elderly users in general may be less amenable to the introduction of information technology in their daily practice. Furthermore, for the last six years, courses of basic computer science are mandatory in all Croatian nursing schools and that could explain why younger nurses had a higher total score compared to elderly ones who mainly lack computer science education. Physicians younger than 50 have more positive attitudes compared to nurses the same age group. The reason is probably also connected with computer science education, because for the last 30 years physicians had to attend classes of Medical Informatics during their studies and acquired knowledge and skills of computer usage as well as the importance IT use in healthcare. Additionally, Littlejohns and authors consider that one of major reasons for the failure of IHIS implementation in Limpopo province (South Africa) lied in not recognizing the education of users as an essential precursor [7].

Computer usage increased total score in both groups. Physicians and nurses using computers were already familiar with computer usage and aware of its benefit. Our data are consistent with studies by other authors who have found that physicians and nurses with computer experience are convinced in abilities of IHIS [4, 15, 16]. We noticed that the purpose of computer use was no important. However, our data revealed that physicians and nurses using computers for any purpose showed more positive attitudes towards than those who no used it.

Our findings suggest that computer science education and computer usage are the most important parameters that particularly contribute to development of positive attitudes towards computers. Therefore, it is important to assess and develop adequate computer science education program for users, which will provide successful implementation of IHIS.

5. References

[1] Ministry of Health of the Republic of Croatia. Evaluation of Bidders' Trial Software Installation in Tender for Integrated Hospital Information System, project "IHIS – Trial Installation". [original in Croatian], dated April 14, 2003.

[2] Newbold SK, Kuperman GJ, Bakken S, Brennan PF, Mendonca EA, Park H, Radenovic A. Information tehnology as an infrastructure for patient safety: nursing research needs. *IJMI* 2004;73:657-662.

[3] Carvalho PM, Carvalho VCL, Menita RHG. Introducing Health Informatics for Active Learners in an Innovative Nursing Curriculum: a Four Years Experience at Marilia Medical School. Proceeding of the 8ht International Congress in Nursing Informatics, 2003, Jan 20-25; Rio de Janeiro, Brasil. [cited 2004 Aug 29]; [3 screens]. Available from URL: http://www.famema.br/disc/is/ni2003_1.pdf.

[4] Meijden MJ, Tange H, Troost J, Hasman A. Development and implementation of an EPR: how to encourage the user. *Int J Med Inform.* 2001;64:173-85.

[5] Menke JA, Broner CW, Campbell DY, McKissick MY, Edwards-Beckett JA. Computerized clinical documentation system in the pediatric intensive care unit. *BMC Med Inform Decis Mak.* 2001;1:3.

[6] Fraenkel DJ, Cowie M, Daley P. Quality benefits of an intensive care clinical information system. *CritCareMed* 2003;31:120-5.

[7] Littlejohns P, Wyatt JC, Garvican L. Evaluating computerized health information systems: hard lessons still to be learnt. *British Med J* 2003;326:860-3.

[8] Brumini G, Kovic I, Zombori D, Lulic I, Petrovecki M. Nurses' Attitudes Towards Computers. *CMJ* [accepted 2005 Jan 7].

[9] Vukovic D. Implementation of Integrated Hospital Information Systems. Medix 2004;54/55:104-6.

[10] Brumini G, Bilic-Zulle L, Bišćan J. Physicians and Nurses' Attitudes towards Computers in Healthcare. Medix; 54/55:113-4.

[11] Stronge JH, Brodt A. Assessment of Nurses' Attitudes Toward Computerization. *Computers in Nursing* 1985;3:154-8.

[12] Stricklin MV, Bierer SB, Struk C. Home Care Nurses' Attitudes Toward Computers:A Confirmatory Factor Analysis of the Stronge and Brodt Instrument. *Computers in Nursing* 2003;21:103-11.

[13] Marasovic C, Kenny C, Elliott D, Sindhusake D. Attitudes of Australian Nurses Toward the Implementation of a Clinical Information System. *Computers in Nursing* 1997;15:91-8.

[14] Simpson G, Kenrick M. Nurses' attitudes toward Computerization in Clinical Practice in a British General Hospital. *Computers in Nursing* 1997;15:37-42.

[15] Burkes M. Identifying and Relating Nurses' Attitudes toward Computer Use. *Computers in Nursing* 1991;9:190-8.

[16] Curtis E,Hicks P,Redmond R. Nursing students experience and attitudes to computers: A survey of a cohort of students on a Bachelor in Nursing Studies course. *Information Tehnology in Nursing* 2002;14:7-17.

Correspondence to:

Gordana Brumini
Department of Computer Science
Rijeka University School of Medicine
Braće Branchetta 20, 51000 Rijeka
E-mail: bgord@medri.hr
Tel: 385 051-651-255

Section 9

Terminologies, Ontologies, Standards and Knowledge Engineering

Connecting Medical Informatics and Bio-Informatics
R. Engelbrecht et al. (Eds.)
IOS Press, 2005

617

Nursing Outcome Documentation in Nursing Notes of Cardiac-Surgery Patients

Yun Jeong Kim[a], Hyeoun-Ae Park[b]

[a]*Asan Medical Center, Seoul, Korea*
[b]*College of Nursing, Seoul National University, Seoul, Korea*

Abstract

This study analyzed what nurses wrote in narrative nursing notes for nursing outcome of cardiac-surgery patients. The nursing notes of 46 patients were decomposed into phrases and analyzed based on the nursing process. Eight patterns were extracted according to different combinations of nursing-process components, of which 29.2% have nursing outcome phrases. The content of the nursing notes was also classified into 15 categories, of which nursing outcomes were recorded more frequently in nursing care driven mainly by physician's order, such as disease-related symptom management, insomnia care, respiratory care, and pain control, than in independent nursing care such as education and emotional care. A survey on the attitudes of nurses toward the nursing record revealed that they do not document nursing outcomes as much as they think they do. The main reasons for this discrepancy were insufficient time for recording and lack of knowledge about why, how, and what to evaluate. Even though there is room for improvement, nursing notes represent a useful resource for determining nursing contributions to patient outcomes.

Keywords:
Nursing documentation; Nursing notes; Nursing Outcome; ICNP; Outcomes research; Cardiac surgery

1. Introduction

The continuing increase in demands for health services and the associated healthcare costs have led both healthcare professionals and consumers to focus on the outcomes such as the effectiveness and efficiency of healthcare. At the same time, as evidence-based practice is emerging as an important method for clinical decision making, healthcare providers are required to demonstrate that their services are effective both clinically and financially [1].

The effectiveness and efficiency of nursing can be evaluated by assessing how patient outcomes are affected by nursing practice. Nursing sensitive outcomes refer to observable and measurable changes in the health status or behaviours of patients as a result of nursing actions [2]. Interest in nursing-sensitive outcomes was stimulated by nurses' beginning to assert themselves as an autonomous profession rather than having a subservient relationship to physicians [3]. By demonstrating that nurses contribute positively to patient outcomes, a nursing component of care can be identified, a body of knowledge unique to nursing can be accumulated, and the foundation of their professional status can be developed.

Though nursing undoubtedly contributes to the curing of diseases and recovery of health, the effect of nursing cannot be proven unless it is documented. Thus, the nursing record can represent a significant body of evidence supporting the effectiveness of nursing care. To establish the effectiveness of nursing, nurses should specify nursing inputs (who gives what care, where, and when, and how care is provided) and patient outcomes that are sensitive to and can be attributed to these inputs, since patients are in an increasingly interdisciplinary milieu in a variety of settings and their responses to treatment or care are affected by several healthcare professionals [3, 4]. For this purpose, nursing diagnoses, interventions, and outcomes should be recorded according to the nursing process. However, not all of these factors are included in the nursing record; instead, patient assessments have mainly been emphasized due to the problem-oriented recording [5].

Therefore, the aim of this study was to identify the current status of nursing outcome documentation through an analysis of the nursing record in clinical settings, and to present ways of ameliorating problems with nursing outcome documentation by conducting a survey of nurses who documented the nursing records analyzed.

2. Materials and methods

This study was undertaken in two parts. The first part involved an analysis of narrative nursing notes to identify the current status of nursing outcome documentation. The second part involved a survey of nurses to explore problems with the recording of nursing outcomes.

2.1. Current status of nursing records

The notes related to 518 days of nursing 46 patients who were hospitalized and underwent cardiac surgery from November 1 to November 30, 2002, in a tertiary hospital in Korea were collected. The narrative nursing notes were decomposed into phrases that were divided into three groups according to their content: (i) nursing-phenomenon-related phrases describing problems, signs, and symptoms of the patients and the nursing diagnosis, (ii) nursing-action-related phrases describing the nursing care provided to patients, and (iii) other phrases that could not be classified into either nursing phenomena or nursing actions and were used to describe contextual information, for example, a phrase quoting the statements of a patient or the treatment plan of a physician.

Nursing-phenomenon-related phrases were divided into nursing assessments, diagnoses, and outcomes according to the definitions of the International Classification for Nursing Practice (ICNP) [6]. A nursing assessment is a definitive phrase that is not influenced by the judgment of the nurse (e.g., "BST 60 mg/dl, patient is in a cold sweat"), whereas a nursing diagnosis is influenced by judgment (e.g., "Patient shows hypoglycemia symptoms"). A nursing outcome is the measure of the status of a nursing diagnosis at some time point after a nursing intervention.

Nursing-action-related phrases were divided into nursing actions and interventions, which refer to nursing-action-related phrases with no prior and with prior nursing-phenomenon-related phrases, respectively. A clinical nurse specializing in cardiac surgery and an ICNP expert verified this work.

The nursing notes were classified into eight patterns according to the combinations of nursing assessment, diagnosis, action, intervention, and outcome. Then, the frequencies of each pattern were tabulated and the characteristics of each pattern were explored. Eight patterns were classified into 15 cardiac-surgery patient care categories to determine differences in the eight patterns.

2.2. Survey of nurse attitudes toward nursing outcome documentation

To study the attitude of nurses toward nursing records and problems with nursing-outcome evaluation and documentation, 30 nurses who had documented the nursing records analyzed for this study were surveyed using questionnaires from April 10 to April 14, 2004, of which

27 returned the questionnaires. The survey questionnaire was developed through interviews with a clinical nurse specialist in cardiac surgery and nurses working in the ward, and consists of items asking priorities in 15 nursing-care categories and how often they perform and record each component of the nursing process: nursing assessment, intervention, and outcome. They were also asked to provide reasons for poor outcome recording and ways of improving nursing-outcome documentation. The survey results were compared with the results of our analysis of the actual nursing records.

3. Results

3.1. Characteristics of subjects

The nursing records of a total 46 patients who underwent cardiac surgery were analyzed. Over two-thirds (69.6%) of the patients had coronary heart disease and received a coronary artery bypass graft. The mean hospital stay was 11.3 days (SD=3.4 days), and ranged from 3 to 19 days.

According to the demographic data of the nurse who participated in the survey, two-thirds (66.7%) of the nurses had more than 2 years of work experience in nursing and 85.1% had worked for more than 1 year in cardiac surgery. Twenty nurses (74.1%) had a baccalaureate.

3.2. Analysis of nursing notes according to the nursing process

The narrative notes related to 518 days of nursing the 46 patients were decomposed into 5,099 phrases, which were divided into three group: 3,448 nursing-phenomenon-related phrases (67.6%), 1,403 nursing-action-related phrases (27.5%), and 248 other phrases (4.9%) (Table 1). The removal of phrases with redundant meanings resulted in 466 unique nursing-phenomenon phrases, 288 unique nursing-action phrases, and 42 unique other phrases. Each unique nursing-phenomenon phrase appeared a mean of 7.4 times, each nursing-action phrase appeared 4.9 times, and other phrases appeared 4.2 times. Out of 466 unique nursing-phenomenon phrases, 25 phrases appeared more than 83 times, representing 60.8% of all nursing- phenomenon-related phrases, and 37 unique nursing-action-related phrases appeared more than 22 times, representing 60.2% of all nursing-action-related phrases.

Table 1 - Classification of nursing phrases, categorized by nursing phenomena and actions

	Total no. of phrases	No. of unique phrases	Mean redundancy
Nursing phenomena	3,448 (67.6%)	466 (58.5%)	7.4
Nursing actions	1,403 (27.5%)	288 (36.2%)	4.9
Others	248 (4.9%)	42 (5.3%)	4.2
Total	5,099 (100%)	796 (100%)	5.5

The phrases in nursing notes were classified into nursing assessments, diagnoses, actions, interventions, and outcomes. These phrases were categorized into eight patterns depending on the different combinations of nursing process components (Table 2). In this process, the 248 phrases that did not relate to nursing phenomena or nursing actions were extracted. The nursing-assessment-only pattern (which was the most frequent) accounted for 45.8% of the 4,851 phrases. Further examination of these eight patterns revealed that phrases containing only nursing assessments or nursing diagnoses represented 48.3% of the total, phrases containing nursing interventions with nursing assessments or nursing diagnoses represented 8.2%, and phrases containing nursing outcomes represented 29.2%.

These eight patterns were classified into 15 categories according to their content in order to explore differences in patterns by category. Nursing outcomes were recorded more often in the areas of pain control, disease-related symptom management, insomnia care, respiratory care, medication, and vital-sign-related care. However, nursing outcomes were documented less in the preparation for surgery, examination-related care, education, and neurological care.

Table 2 - Frequency of nursing phrases according to nursing-record pattern and category

Category	A*	B	C	D	E	F	G	H	Total
Disease-related symptom management	429	6	12	2	16	25	131	2	623
Vital-sign-related care	353	6	22	53	10	160	68	0	672
Examination-related care	60	2	117	77	15	126	21	48	466
Insomnia care	219	13	1	8	9	34	60	0	344
Preparation for Surgery	22	2	103	0	7	0	0	37	171
Emotional care	1	1	0	0	6	0	10	0	18
Education	4	0	76	7	0	0	3	5	95
Nutrition and elimination	33	6	65	22	40	42	85	10	303
Medication	14	0	37	2	5	31	31	14	134
Respiratory care	143	4	89	5	11	41	69	43	405
Pain control	98	50	5	5	33	28	215	2	436
Wound care	575	21	25	5	19	7	42	0	694
Drainage care	51	6	7	0	0	0	3	0	67
Neurological care	23	3	0	3	2	0	0	0	31
Bedsore care	4	0	0	9	7	5	15	0	40
Others	193	0	132	7	16	4	0	0	352
Total	2222	120	691	205	196	503	753	161	4851
Percentage	45.8	2.5	14.3	4.2	4.0	10.4	15.5	3.3	100

* A: Nursing assessment only
  B: Nursing diagnosis only
  C: Nursing action only
  D: Nursing assessment + nursing intervention
  E: Nursing diagnosis + nursing intervention
  F: Nursing assessment + nursing intervention + nursing outcome
  G: Nursing diagnosis + nursing intervention + nursing outcome
  H: Nursing intervention + nursing outcome

3.3. Survey of nurse attitudes toward nursing outcome documentation

The nurses reported that they documented the effectiveness or the patient's response to nursing actions in more than 78% of nursing-outcome evaluations: pain control, vital-sign-related care, and drainage care in more than 87%, and emotional care and education in less than 65%.

We asked the nurses to provide reasons for nursing outcomes being documented so poorly in actual nursing notes. The reasons provided differed by category, with a lack of time provided as the principal reason for all most categories except for emotional care, respiratory care, and bedsore care. For emotional care, nurses reported insufficient knowledge about how and when to evaluate as a major factor preventing adequate nursing-outcome documentation. Nurses also pointed out that the correct evaluation time for bedsore care and respiratory care was ambiguous.

The largest proportion of nurses commented that they needed more time to make a quality recording in order to improve nursing-outcome recording (42.9%), which was followed by increasing nurses' awareness of the need for nursing-outcome evaluation (20.0%), education about the evaluation method (17.1%), and nursing-outcome recording in general (17.1%).

4. Discussion

The categorization of nursing notes into eight patterns revealed that the frequency of the nursing-assessment-only pattern was the highest and that the frequency of nursing outcomes with nursing assessments or diagnoses and nursing-intervention patterns were very low. Of the 15 nursing-care categories for cardiac-surgery patients, nurses documented nursing outcomes in the areas of pain control, disease-related symptom management, vital-sign-related care, insomnia, and medication more than the other areas. These areas involve nursing care that is driven mainly by the order of physicians. However, for independent nursing involving aspects such as education, neurological care, and emotional care, nurses documented neither nursing outcomes nor nursing assessments and actions. This has also been revealed by other studies. Davis et al. reported that nursing assessments emphasized biomedical rather than psychosocial concerns [7]. Kim's study of nursing audits indicated that information on oxygen supply, nutrition, fluid balance, and skin care was well documented, but that on educating patients about health maintenance and illness prevention was hard to find [5].

There is another problem in nursing-outcome documentation. Nurses do not use standard outcome indicators or tools to measure objective changes in nursing outcomes. Even in nursing notes about pain control, which exhibit a high frequency of nursing-outcome recording, the criteria of nursing outcomes are not clear because nurses documented nursing outcomes using their own rephrasing of patients' self-reporting to describe their response to nursing actions, such as "pain relieved", "a little bit reduced", "somewhat reduced", and "a lot reduced". This results in a communication problem between not only nurses but also with other healthcare professionals. Therefore, outcome indicators or tools should be developed to facilitate the objective evaluation of nursing outcomes.

When surveyed, there was a prominent discrepancy in the nursing-outcome documentation. The frequency of nursing-outcome documentation was 37.0%, and rest of the total nursing-action-related phrases did not contain nursing-outcome phrases. However, nurses reported that they evaluated and documented nursing outcomes in 78.7% of evaluations. The survey revealed that nurses were unaware of their poor outcome documentation and that they considered themselves as good at evaluation and recording the responses of patients to nursing actions that they provided. On the other hand, nurses agreed that they documented nursing assessments, actions, and outcomes in education and emotional care poorly, even though they considered these areas important. The study by Hale et al. produced similar results, in that there were no discrepancies between what nurses said they did and what was recorded in nursing notes on the pain management of patients with myocardial infarction [8], whereas on anxiety, nutrition, and health education, the intervention nurses reported that they provided to patients was not well documented in the nursing notes. They concluded that nursing documentation did not provide a comprehensive data source for nursing interventions provided to patients or their effectiveness.

Several studies have shown that nurses have significant influence over patient outcomes in areas where nurses play the dominant role, and nursing outcomes can be measured in these areas [9,10]. In the study by Carr-Hill et al. [9], these areas included patient hygiene, nutrition and hydration, pressure sores and skin integrity, intravenous therapy, discharge planning, pain control, education and rehabilitation, and elimination. Cullum [10] showed that nurses contribute to patient outcomes in the following areas: patient education, health promotion, cardiac rehabilitation, postoperative and preoperative care, anxiety prevention and reduction, and pain management. These two studies and the 15 categories of our study have the following areas in common: pain control, nutrition, elimination, bedsore care, education, and emotional care. Out of these areas, nurses documented nursing outcomes well in pain control. Thus, the nursing record can be useful in demonstrating the nursing contribution to patient outcomes in pain control.

However, nursing outcome was barely documented in other areas. According to our survey, the major barrier to the evaluation and documentation of nursing outcomes was a lack of time. To improve accuracy and reduce recording time, new charting formats such as computerization of the nursing record need to be developed, especially given that this barrier has been described many times in previous studies [11, 12]. The main reason for poor recording in education and emotional care was insufficient knowledge about how and when to evaluate. Therefore, comprehensive education on nursing outcomes including when and how to measure the results of nursing actions should be provided to improve nursing-outcome recording.

5. Conclusion

This study reveals that present nursing outcome documentation has many shortcomings. To solve these problems, education and training should be provided on the importance of nursing records based upon the nursing process, and regulations and guidelines should be provided for nursing outcome documentation. Moreover, outcome indicators and tools need to be developed for the objective measurement of nursing outcomes and to facilitate communication between healthcare professionals. To improve nursing-outcome recording, nurses should be provided with continuous feedback based on systematic and regular evaluations and audits. The development of electronic nursing records that take these problems into consideration would further improve nursing records and make them a useful source for information on patient outcomes.

6. References

[1]   Jennings BM, Loan LA. Misconceptions among nurses about evidence-based practice. *J. Nurs. Scholarsh.* 2001: 33(2) pp. 121–7.

[2]   Harris MR. Clinical and financial outcomes in patient care in a home health care agency. *J. Nurs. Qual. Assur.* 1991: 5(2) pp. 41–9.

[3]   Bond S, Thomas LH. Issues in measuring outcomes of nursing. *J. Adv. Nurs.* 1991: 16(12) pp. 1492–502.

[4]   Spilsbury K, J. Meyer J. Defining the nursing contribution to patient outcome: lessons from a review of the literature examining nursing outcomes, skill mix and changing roles. *J. Clin. Nurs.* 2001: 10(1) pp. 3–14.

[5]   Kim YS. A study on nursing care process approach to quality of nursing care through nursing audit. *J. Inst. Health Environ. Sci.* 1992: 2(2) pp. 153–60.

[6]   International Council of Nurses, International Classification for Nursing Practice Web Document, Geneva (2002). Available from: www.icn.ch/icmpupdate.htm.

[7]   Davis BD, Billings JR, Ryland RK, Evaluation of nursing process documentation. *J. Adv. Nurs.* 1994: 19(5) pp. 960–8.

[8]   Hale CA, Thomas LH, Bond S, Todd C. The nursing record as a research tool to identify nursing interventions. *J. Clin. Nurs.* 1997: 6(3) pp. 207–14.

[9]   Carr-Hill R, Dixon P, Griffiths M, Higgins M, McCaughan D, Wright K. *Skill mix the effectiveness of nursing care.* New York: Centre for Health Economics, University of York, 1992.

[10] Cullum N. Identification and analysis of randomised controlled trials in nursing: a preliminary study. *Qual. Health Care.* 1997: 6(1) pp. 2–6.

[11] Moloney R. Maggs C. A systematic review of the relationships between written manual nursing care planning, record keeping and patient outcomes, *J. Adv. Nurs.* 1999: 30(1) pp. 51–7.

[12] Brooks JT. An analysis of nursing documentation as a reflection of actual nurse work, Medsurg. Nurs. 1998: 7(4) pp. 189–98.

Address for correspondence

Hyouen-Ae Park, Professor, College of nursing, Seoul National University,28 Yongon-dong Chongno-gu, Seoul, 110-799, Korea, hapark@snu.ac.kr

Connecting Medical Informatics and Bio-Informatics
R. Engelbrecht et al. (Eds.)
IOS Press, 2005

623

Icpcview: visualizing the International Classification of Primary Care

Pierre P Lévy[a,b], Laetitia Duché[a], Laszlo Darago[c], Yves Dorléans[b], Laurent Toubiana[b], Jean-François Vibert[b], Antoine Flahault[a,b]

[a] *Hôpital Tenon(Assistance Publique Hôpitaux de Paris), France*
[b] *INSERM U707, Paris, France*
[c] *University of Debrecen, Hungary*

Abstract

This paper proposes a method to visualize the semantic content of data bases where the medical information is coded with the International Classification of Primary Care. The main idea is the identification of a pixel with a code and the conversion of all the data associated with these into an image the ICPCview. The method proceeds in two step, defining the reference frame and using this reference frame to visualize data. The reference frame is built by using a sign/diagnosis binary criterion, a seventeen category nosological criterion and an age ordinal criterion .The results are visualization of the signs and diagnosis of the ICPC according to gender, age and time period of the year. A limitation of the method lies in the fact that the result depends on the chosen reference frame. Further work has to be done with various reference frames and data. However the main point is that, when both the reference set of the image and of the mind of the user are built, the method is powerful at extracting the hidden content of a very large amount of data.

Keywords:
ICPCview, Caseview; Information visualization; International Classification of Primary Care, General practitioner, Code. French Sentinelles network

1. Introduction - Context

A current problem in medicine and biology is the existing of huge data banks whose semantic content is difficult to grasp. A solution was proposed for the Diagnosis Related Group (DRG) data base used in the context of hospital tarrifing. This solution was the caseview method proposed as a generic method applicable to all DRG classifications in the world [1,2,3,4,5].

In the present paper a new step is taken: the method is generalised and applied to the International Classification of Primary Care (ICPC). The ICPC [6] is a classification originating from the International Classification of Diseases (ICD) . It was defined to account for the specific activity of general practitioners. Each contact of a practitioner with a patient is described with a chain of codes corresponding to the implied signs, diagnoses and processes. The codes are classified according to three axes: signs, diagnoses and processes. These three axes are used to browse seventeen socio-nosological categories (social, haematology, metabolic…).

In the present study, this coding was applied to the data transmitted by 1200 general practitioners belonging to the French Sentinelles[©] network [7,8,9].

The point of this paper is to show the various insights offered by the generalised caseview method applied to this huge ICPC coded medical data bank

2. Material and Methods

The main idea of the generalised caseview is to assimilate an informational entity to a pixel. Then the method proceeds in two steps. The first step is to define a reference frame by ordering these pseudo-pixels according to three criteria. Using this reference frame and defining a colour scale, the second step allows the visualization of the associated with these informational entities data.

The three criteria are a binary criterion which allows splitting of the reference frame into two parts, a nominal criterion which allows the definition of columns where the entities share a common property and an ordinal criterion which allows the arranging of pseudo-pixels symmetrically for the two parts inside each column.

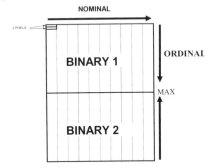

Figure 1- The three criteria of the generalized caseview method

Since August 1997 the data base was built applying a coding algorithm to the transmitted by the practitioners' data. These data correspond to the in-hospital set of their patients. A program converted these referrals into three codes which were allocated to three specific fields of the central data base. Indeed, this automatic coding represents a unique real time system allowing to monitor health at the national level [7,8].

3. Results

3.1 Defining the reference frame

The informational entities used are the diagnosis and signs of the ICPC. The processes are not included because the small number of data.

The binary criterion was signs versus diagnoses: the diagnoses are in the upper part of the reference frame and the signs are in the lower part.

The nominal criterion was the 17 categories of the ICPC: each column of the reference set corresponds to a category (Table 1).

Table 1 –Title of the columns of the reference frame

SOCIAL	HEMATO	METAB, ENDOC	GENERAL	SKIN	MUSCULO-SKELETAL
NEURO	MENTAL	RESPI	CARDIO	DIGESTIVE	KIDNEY
PREGNANCY	FEMALE SYST.	MALE SYST.	EYE	EAR	

The ordinal criterion was the ordering of the codes according to the average age associated with them in the data base.

The reference frame is shown on figure 2. In this figure each "pixel" contains the average age associated with the corresponding "pixel" code. Dark colour corresponds to "old" code (patient older than 65 years old) whereas very light grey corresponds to children (younger than fifteen years old).

The first result appears after analysing the reference frame: the proportion of codes concerned by the study is rather large. This pattern of codes is approximately symmetric, with a larger proportion of diagnoses compared to the signs. Moreover the area where the age is older than sixty five is asymmetric in that there are more "old" diagnoses than "old" signs. This is particularly prominent for the "circulatory" column.

The paediatric diagnoses and signs are marginal.

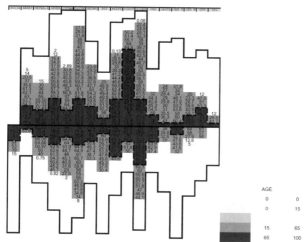

Figure 2 - The Reference frame: each pixel contains the average age associated with the code

3.2 Using the reference set to visualize data

Figure 3 shows in-patient counts corresponding to the three fields of the data base.

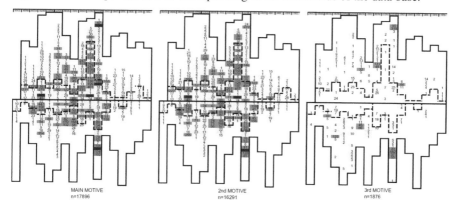

Figure 3 – In-patient count of the three motives

The image on the left is the main in-patient motive: there are many diagnoses for the circulatory, digestive and respiratory systems. The three motives have show similar patterns: only the total number of diagnoses decreases from the left to the right.

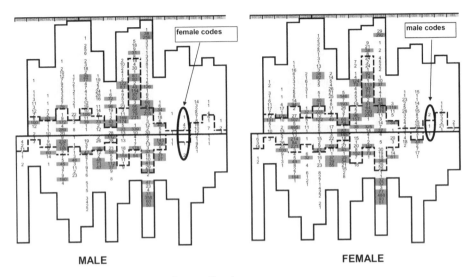

MALE   FEMALE

Figure 4 –in-patient count according to Gender

Figure 4 shows that the male and female patterns seem similar. However there are coding errors as it shown on the figure.

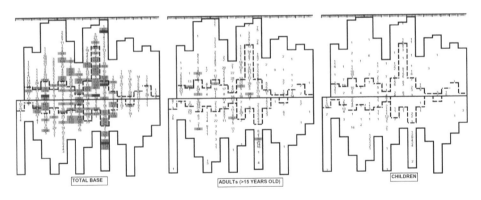

Figure 5 –in-patient count according to age.

Figure 5 shows that in general, the patterns of the total data base are similar to those corresponding to the "adult". The pattern corresponding to children presents a low number of cases at the nucleus level.

To analyse the temporal data, the year was split into two semesters: a cold semester – October to March- and a hot one – April to September.

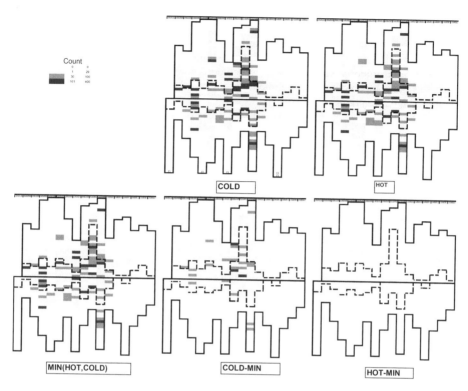

Figure 6 –In-patient count according to the time period of the year.

On the top of figure 6 we can see that the two periods seem similar. The intersection of the two images is shown on the lower left corner. The two images on the lower right show a higher number of diseases (respiratory, circulatory and general) for the "old" diagnoses of the cold period.

4. Discussion

The first benefit of the method lies in its capability to give a first look at the enclosed inside the data base information. However the nature of this information is limited to the point of view "window", in other words, the reference frame. In this way, the data base is viewed from the point of view of the sign/diagnosis, nosological and age triple axis. Only the meaning paned by these axes is visible. More precisely it is important to keep in mind that the ordinal age criterion corresponds to the codes of the first field used to encode pathology. This was visible in figure 2 . The information outside the set of codes present in the first field, is lacking. To summarise, the "window" is restricted to the first field and to the set of information existing in the actual data base. This is the limitation of the method. Other ordinal criteria have to be tested to improve the reference frame.

However the main point is that, when both the reference set of the image and of the mind of the user are built, the method is powerful at extracting the hidden content of a very large amount of data. [10].

5. Conclusion

The main benefit of the method is its capability to allow quick insight on the data. Furthermore it has to be used in combination with other methods.

Moreover, it is important to note that this method is not static: the images can be processed and compared by simple computing (intersection difference…) leading to new results and interpretations.

6. Acknowledgments

We are grateful to the GPs from the French Sentinelles system for transmitting their hospital referral reports.

Moreover, we are grateful to Ann Rocheford for correction of the English version of the paper.

7. References

[1]   Lévy PP. Le case view une methode de visualisation du case mix. *Journal d'économie médicale mars 2002*; 20(2), 118-127.

[2]   Lévy PP The case view a generic method of visualization of the case mix. *International journal of Medical Informatics 2004, 73*, 713-718.

[3]   www.b3e.jussieu.fr/caseview/drgview

[4]   www.medinfo.hu/darago/caseview.php

[5]   László Daragó: Caseview_HUN: easy DRG overview. *Studies in health Technology and Informatics.* Volume 105. Transformation of Healthcare with information technologies. IOS Press. Editors: Marius Duplaga, Krzysztof Zielinski, David Ingram.pp182-189, 2004

[6]   World organization of National Collges, Academies and Academic Associations of General Practitioners/Family Physicians (WONCA). *ICPC-2 International Classidication of primary Care; Second Edition.* Oxford University Press, 1998

[7]   Letrilliart L, Viboud C, Boelle PY, Flahault A. Automatic coding of reasons for hospital referral from general medicine free-text reports. *Proc AMIA Symp.* 2000; 487-91.

[8]   www.sentiweb.org

[9]   Valleron AJ, P Garnerin (1992). "Computer networking as a tool for public health surveillance: the French experiment." *MMWR Morb Mortal Wkly Rep 41 Suppl*: 101-10, 1992.

[10]   Lévy PP. Caseview: building the reference set. In: *Studies in Health Technology and Informatics.* Volume 105. Transformation of Healthcare with information technologies. IOS Press. Editors: Marius Duplaga, Krzysztof Zielinski, David Ingram.pp172-181, 2004.

Address for correspondence

Pierre Lévy
Hôpital Tenon, Unité de Biostatistique et informatique Médicale
4, rue de la chine, 75970 Paris cedex 20, France
Email: pierre.levy@tnn.aphp.fr

Connecting Medical Informatics and Bio-Informatics
R. Engelbrecht et al. (Eds.)
IOS Press, 2005

Common Nursing Terminology for Clinical Information Systems

Yardena Kol, Patricia Zimmerman, Zipora Sadeh

Clalit Health Service (CHS), Israel

Abstract

The lack of professional agreement upon chosen terminology in nursing detracts from the role of Clinical Information Systems (CIS) as central repositories of patient health records. The purposes of this paper are: (1) Identification of common terminology for clinical nursing information in CHS according to the following stages: patient history of health and illnesses; nursing assessment; nursing interventions and outcomes. (2) Implementation of the common terminology into computerized applications in several nursing settings. The sample included 224 nurses divided into four groups. Each group was asked to identify the common initial data for patient history and nursing interventions, based on professional experience, expertise, clinical standards and organizational / legal policy. The identification of nursing assessments and outcomes was done according to evidenced-based Clinical Guide-Lines (CGL) for each nursing setting. The CGL were chosen as a source for assessment and outcome classification for two main reasons. First, the CGL include criteria of the clinical state by the degree of severity base, which are acceptable and comprehensible to other disciplines within the healthcare system. Second, the lack of evidence-based researches related to clinical nursing outcomes. Results: Standard patient history of health and illnesses (admission and discharge) was developed for all departments in the hospital with flexibility to add any specific clinical data upon requirement. A total of 62 nursing assessments / outcomes were identified from the CGL in the four chosen nursing settings. 43 (70%) nursing assessments / outcomes were common both for nursing practice in hospitals and community clinics. 30 (40%) were implemented in the community clinics CIS application, 19 (31%) in the oncology CIS application, and 16 (26%) in the delivery CIS application. The groups identified a total of 70 nursing interventions. 49 (70%) nursing interventions were common both for nursing practice in hospitals and community clinics. 59 (84%) were implemented in the community clinics CIS application, 18 (26%) in the oncology CIS application, and 29 (41%) in the delivery CIS application. For summary, the definition process, including computerization, spread across four years. The community CIS application serves about 1500 clinics in CHS Israel (which employs about 2500 nurses). The admission and discharge CIS application serves 7 general hospitals, and is currently implemented in the internal and surgical departments (about 30 departments, 35 average beds each). The oncology CIS application is implemented in two oncology centers, and the delivery CIS application will soon be implemented in 8 hospitals.

Keywords:
Terminology; Clinical Health System; Patient Records; Nursing; Guideline; Application

1. Introduction

In recent years, Clinical Information Systems (CIS) have been developed progressively as a "collection of various information technology applications that provides a centralized repository of information related to patient care across distributed locations." [6 pp 63]. The CIS include clinical documents recorded by various healthcare agents such as physicians and nurses. The main advantage of CIS is the capability to share and exchange essential information between different healthcare providers in a safe and secure manner. Today, hospitals and community health services (e.g., Clalit Health Services - CHS) are forced to rely upon various applications customized for different areas of clinical expertise. Needless to say, each application has its own approach for structuring health records.

To enable a productive exchange of clinical information between caregivers in every clinical setup, it is essential to adopt a common terminology. Several studies addressed this issue in medicine and nursing [1, 2, 3, 4, 5]. Common terminology is important for medico–legal, quality management, education, research, policy development, health service management and finance management.

There are more than five different applications in our health organization - CHS (that includes 14 hospitals and more than 1600 community clinics). The lack of standardization led us into developing a common nursing terminology.

The purpose of this paper is twofold:

1. Identification of common terminology for clinical nursing information in CHS Israel according to the following stages: patient history of health and illnesses; nursing assessment; nursing interventions and outcomes.
2. Implementation of the common terminology into computerized applications in several nursing settings.

2. Materials and methods

The development process for a common nursing terminology initiated in four nursing settings: hospital admission and discharge, delivery unit, oncology unit and community health clinics.

In order to identify the terminology related to *patient history of health and illnesses, and nursing interventions,* registered nurses from 50 community clinics (only clinics responsible for over 7,000 insured residents) and 14 hospitals were included in our sample. Overall - a total of 224 nurses working in selected clinical fields: 100 from community clinics and 124 from hospitals (admission and discharge=64, delivery=22, internal medicine=28, oncology=10). A demographic breakdown of participant nurses showed 100% full time employees; 87% were female. The average age was 40 years (s.d.= 9.7); average tenure in the required clinic / department was 10.6 years (s.d.= 8.3). 75% had a B.A. degree or higher.

Four groups of nurses in the above clinical fields were formed. Each group of participants was asked to identify the common initial data for patient history and nursing interventions. The identification was based on professional experience, expertise, clinical standards, and organizational / legal policy.

The identification of nursing assessments and outcomes was done according to evidenced-based Clinical Guide-Lines (CGL) for each nursing setting. The CGL were chosen as a source for assessment and outcome classification for two main reasons. First, the CGL include criteria of the clinical state by the degree of severity based on objective scales, which are acceptable and comprehensible to other disciplines within the healthcare system.

Second, the lack of evidence-based researches related to clinical nursing outcomes. We've used the same criteria for assessment and outcomes under the assumption that comparison of health status before and after intervention should be done by similar indicators (reassessment). Furthermore, reassessment by itself reflects the outcomes - improvement or retreat in health condition.

3. Results

Standard nursing record related to patient history of health and illnesses (admission and discharge) was developed for all departments in the hospital with flexibility to add any specific clinical data upon requirement. The following screenshot demonstrates a menu for patient history health record.

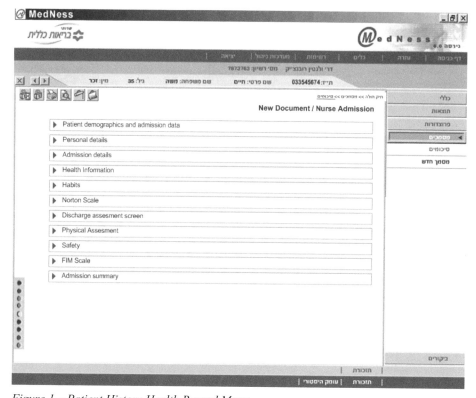

Figure 1 – Patient History Health Record Menu

Assessment and Outcome Classification

A total of 62 nursing assessments / outcomes were identified from the CGL for the CIS applications in the four chosen nursing settings. 43 (70%) nursing assessments / outcomes were common both for nursing practice in hospitals and community clinics. 30 (40%) were implemented in the community clinics CIS application, 19 (31%) in the oncology CIS application (10 common and 9 specific), and 16 (26%) in the delivery CIS application (10 common and 6 specific).

The next two screenshots demonstrate an example of one specific nursing assessment / outcome and one common.

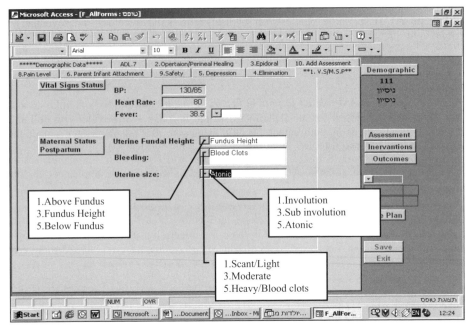

Figure 2 - Specific Example of Nursing Assessment / Outcome - Nursing Delivery

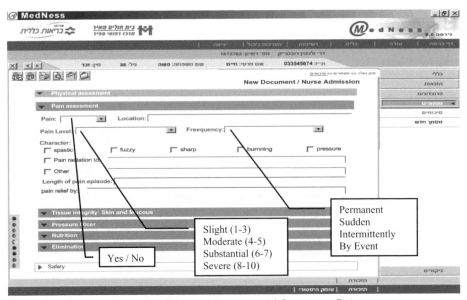

Figure 3 – Common Example of Nursing Assessment / Outcome – Pain

Nursing intervention classifications

The groups for the CIS applications in the four chosen nursing settings identified a total of 70 nursing interventions. 49 (70%) nursing interventions were common both for nursing practice in hospitals and community clinics. 59 (84%) were implemented in the community clinics CIS application, 18 (26%) in the oncology CIS application (13 common and 5 specific), and 29 (41%) in the delivery CIS application (18 common and 11 specific).

Implementation

The community CIS application serves about 1500 clinics in CHS Israel (which employs about 2500 nurses). The admission and discharge CIS application serves 7 general hospitals, and is currently implemented in the internal and surgical departments (about 30 departments, average of 35 beds each). The oncology CIS application is implemented in two oncology centers, and the delivery CIS application will soon be implemented in 8 hospitals.

There are 5 different software infrastructures in CHS Israel hosting clinical applications. Computerized implementation of the joined terminology has been achieved through a cross-infrastructure communication system able to collect clinical information from each application and present it in a unified form. This interface enables caregivers to share and exchange patient data regardless of patient location.

4. Conclusion

The definition process, including computerization, spread across four years. Nurses report very high satisfaction of the application, mainly derived from the common terminology allowing them to share and exchange information related to the same patients between different departments of hospitals and clinics.

In spite of numerous publications of common nursing terminology in the literature, still, there is no acceptable version of international language in nursing. Each country makes the effort to develop a terminology customized for its own requirements. Notably, there is a wide similarity between the different developments, which can be explained by the global likeness of health problems, health needs and interventions, also seen in the mass acceptance of the international CGL for these issues.

The progress of technology is highly rapid, and the nursing profession found itself unprepared by professional conceptualization.

Nevertheless, it is impotent to continue such trials, for hope that in the future, it will be a wide spectrum of trials that will cover all nursing fields. After gathering sources and proper examination, a true base of common terminology in nursing could be established.

5. References

[1]   Bakken S, Cimino JJ. Haskell R, Matsumoto C, Chan GK, and Huff SM. Evaluation of the Clinical LOINC (Logical Observation Identifiers, Names and Codes) Semantic Structure as a Terminology Model for Standardized Assessment Measures. *J Am Med Inform Assoc. 2000: 7 (6)* pp. 529-538.

[2]   Campbell JR, Carpenter P, Sneiderman C, Cohn C, Chute CG, and Warren J, CPRI Work Group on Codes and Structures. Phase II Evaluation of Clinical Coding Schemes: Completeness, Taxonomy, Mapping, Definitions, and Clarity. *J Am Med Inform Assoc 1997: 4 (3)* pp. 238-251.

[3]   Maas JM, and Moorhead S (Eds.). *Nursing Outcomes Classification (NOC) 2nd ed.* St Louis: C.V. Mosby, 2000.

[4]   Martin KS, and Scheet NJ. The Omaha System: Applications for community health nursing. Philadelphia: WB Saunders, 1992.

[5]   Matney S, Bakken S, and Huff SM. Representing Nursing Assessment in Clinical Information Systems Using the Logical Observation Identifiers, Names, and Codes (LOINC) Database. *J Biomed Inform 2003: 36* (4-5) pp. 287-293.

[6]   Sitting DF, Hazlehurst BL, Hsu J, Jimison H, and Hornbrook MC. A Clinical Information System Research Landscape, *Perm J 2002: 6 (2)* PP. 62-68. http://xnet.kp.org/permanentejournal/

6. Address for correspondence

Yardena Kol, RN, Ph.D.
Manager of Research and Professional Development Dept.
Clalit Health Service, Chief Nurse Office
101 Arlozorov St., Tel Aviv, 62098
PO Box 16250, Israel
Tel: 972-3-6923048   Fax: 972-3-6923547   Email: yardenako@clalit.org.il

Connecting Medical Informatics and Bio-Informatics
R. Engelbrecht et al. (Eds.)
IOS Press, 2005

An Ontology for Carcinoma Classification for Clinical Bioinformatics

Anand Kumar[a], Yum Lina Yip[b], Barry Smith[a,c], Dirk Marwede[a,d], Daniel Novotny[a,c]

[a]IFOMIS, University of Saarland, Saarbruecken, Germany
[b]Swiss Institute of Bioinformatics, Geneva, Switzerland
[c]Department of Philosophy, University at Buffalo, Buffalo, New York, USA
[d]Department of Diagnostic Radiology, University of Leipzig, Leipzig, Germany

Abstract

There are a plenty of existing classifications and staging schemes for carcinomas, one of the most frequently used being the TNM classification. Such classifications involve entities which exist at various anatomical levels of granularity and in order to apply such classifications to the Electronic Health Care Records, one needs to build ontologies which are not only based on the formal principles but also take into consideration the diversity of the domains which are involved in clinical bioinformatics. Here we outline a formal theory for addressing these issues in a way that inferences drawn upon the ontologies would be helpful in interpreting and inferring on the entities which exist at different anatomical levels of granularity. Our case study is on the colon carcinoma, one of the commonest carcinomas prevalent within the European population.

Keywords:
Clinical bioinformatics, Ontology, Oncology

1. Introduction

Over 40 carcinomas have been analyzed in terms of the Tumor, Node and Metastasis (TNM) classification, which classifies a carcinoma on the basis of the extent of their spread, lymph node involvement and metastasis and which is used for staging of providing guidelines for the management of the patient who bear them.[1,2] An automated ontology-based system designed to establish for each specific pathology the appropriate TNM class would first need to register the anatomical structures (colon, lung, prostate, etc.) involved. Unfortunately, however, the Electronic Healthcare Records (EHCRs) often use anatomical terms different from those in the TNM classification. Thus the systems need to provide a methodology by which different anatomical terms can be related to the corresponding TNM anatomical entity. In addition to anatomy, however, the system would need to take account also of pathologies, cellular characteristics, and other salient features. For an efficient integration with EHCRs, the ontology system would need to represent such features explicitly and in such a way that it supports inferences drawing not only on EHCR data but also on biological databases dealing with the mutations and protein variants which are involved in the different stages of carcinoma development.

Clinical bioinformatics is a field bases on integration and interpretation of life-sciences data at many levels of granularity, from the coarser (clinical) levels of signs, symptoms, radiological findings, to the finer levels of genotype-phenotype expression and associated molecular pathways. To achieve this end, an ontological theory is required that is able to deal with such a diversity among the entities involved. Here, we present a theory of the needed sort, which is designed to do justice to the fact that the anatomical entities present within FMA can be used to support the drawing of inferences relating to the anatomical and pathological data present within the EHCRs of individual patients. We use the example of colon carcinoma as a case study and present an extension to our previous work where we integrated terms in Gene Ontology[1] with our own ontology for relations, together with the mutant database present within Swissprot[2]. [3,4,5]

2. Formalization

Classes and individuals

The Foundational Model of Anatomy (FMA)[3] is a representation of *canonical* anatomy. [6] Thus *colon* as it appears within the FMA represents a *normal colon* – where in the present context of course we need to deal also with the *abnormal* colon. Nonetheless the FMA is designed as a reference ontology that can serve as a basis also for *non-canonical* anatomy, and in our treatment, the entity colon within FMA stands for a normal colon. Thus,

> *abnormal colon is_a colon*
> *normal colon is_a colon*

can still be accepted is true from the perspective of this extended FMA.

We distinguish between colon carcinoma disease and the pathological structure. Thus,

> *colon carcinoma pathological structure is_a carcinomatous pathological structure*

and:

> *colon carcinoma pathological structure **part_of** abnormal colon*

and since is_a relations are transitive:

> *colon carcinoma pathological structure **part_of** colon*

though it should be stressed that the latter holds only on the reading of *part_of* preferred in [7] and adopted by us here, according to which *A part_of B* means that every instance of *A* is an instance-level part of *some* instance of *B*, rather than on the reading of *part_of* (as meaning something like 'integral part') that is normally adopted in the FMA, where *A part_of B* requires also that every instance of *B* is such that there is some instance of *A* which stands to it in the instance-level part relation. Every colon carcinoma is part of some colon, but not every colon has some colon carcinoma as part. We also have

> *abnormal colon transformation_of normal colon*

where *A transformation of B* holds where for any instance *a* of *A* and any time *t*, there is some earlier time t_1, at which *c* is the instance of the distinct class *B*. (Some abnormalilities are abnormal from the start when they are present abnormally within the fetus.). [7]

> *carcinomatous colon is_a abnormal colon*
> *carcinomatous colon **transformation_of** normal colon*

Parthood and location relations

The FMA integratal parthood relations among anatomical entities include for example:

> *ascending colon part_of colon*
> *mucosa of colon **part_of** wall of colon **part_of** colon*

The parthood relation implies a location relation. [8]

> *region of ascending colon located_in region of colon*
> *region of mucosa of colon part_of region of wall of colon part_of region of colon*

---

[1] www.geneontology.org
[2] http://au.expasy.org/sprot/
[3] http://sig.biostr.washington.edu/projects/fm/AboutFM.html

Bearer relation

A carcinomatous pathological process demands in every case some anatomical entity as its bearer. Thus

> carcinomatous pathological function in ascending colon born_by ascending colon
> T1 stage carcinomatous pathological function in ascending colon born_by mucosa of ascending colon

The bearer relation implies location relation. Thus,

> carcinomatous pathological process in ascending colon **has_participant** ascending colon
> T1 stage carcinomatous pathological processin ascending colon **has_participant** mucosa of ascending colon

Creation relation between process and anatomical entity

We have dealt with relations between process and anatomical entities elsewhere. [9] One of them is the creation relationship. A process creates a substance when the substance did not exist before the initiation of the process and exists after the process has been concluded. It is not necessary that a single process brings a substance into being by itself. It is also not necessary that each process brings a substance into being. However, in case of carcinoma of colon, the pathology leads to a pathological structure, though not always. Thus,

> carcinomatous pathological process in ascending colon **creates** carcinomatous structure in ascending colon
> T1 stage carcinomatous pathological process in ascending colon creates T1 stage carcinomatous structure in ascending colon

The pathological structure is part of the organ affected by the pathology. There is also a parthood relation between a pathological structure and the pathological organ. Thus,

> carcinomatous structure in ascending colon part_of carcinomatous ascending colon
> region of carcinomatous structure in ascending colon part_of region of carcinomatous ascending colon
> > T1 stage carcinomatous structure in ascending colon **part_of** carcinomatous mucosa of ascending colon

Anatomical levels of granularity

We have dealt in greater detail elsewhere with the levels of granularity in anatomy. Every anatomical entity in the FMA has a default level of granularity. For example, *colon* has an *organ* level of granularity; *ascending colon* has an *organ part* level of granularity. This characteristic of an anatomical entity is present within each of its instances and is implied with each of the instances and also at the class level. We then have a mapping gran from FMA terms to levels of granularity, such that for example:

> gran(*colon*) = *organ*

and

> gran(*ascending colon*) = *organ part*

Finer levels of granularity – of atoms, molecules and subcellular organelles – are also needed for our carcinoma ontology in order that we can represent processes at the cellular level, markers like p53 and the various mutant proteins associated with colon carcinoma and represented in the modSNP database of Swissprot.

TNM Classification

TNM classification classifies carcinomas on the basis of the extent of tumor spread, lymph nodes involved and metastasis. There are certain levels of granularity in anatomy which apply to each of the TNM classes. We have dealt with in more details in [10] and here we apply it on the entities which are involved in a specific T, N or M class. However anatomy is not the only partitions which exist within TNM classes. Other partitions, for example pathogenesis and number of lymph nodes involved are also taken into consideration. Our formalism represents the levels of granularity and mentions the other partitions involved.

Table 1. Anatomical levels of granularity for TNM classification

TNM	Explanation as stated in the TNM Classification by the respective Cancer Societies	Level of Granularity	Other partitions
TX	Primary tumor cannot be assessed	--	
T0	No evidence of primary tumor	--	
Tis	Carcinoma in situ: intraepithelial or invasion of the lamina propria	Intraepithelial cell (C); Epithelium & lamina propria (ORP/MPOT)	
T1	Tumor invades submucosa	Submucosa of colon (ORP/MPOT)	
T2	Tumor invades muscularis propria	Muscularis mucosa of colon (ORP/MPOT)	
T3	Tumor invades through the muscularis propria into the subserosa, or into nonperitonealized pericolic or perirectal tissues	Subserosa of colon (ORP/MPOT), nonperitonealized pericolic or perirectal tissues (ORP/MPOT-E)	path of invasion (pathogenesis)
T4	Tumor directly invades other organs or structures, and/or perforates visceral peritoneum	organs (OR-E), visceral peritoneum (ORP)	path of invasion (pathogenesis)
NX	Regional nodes cannot be assessed	--	
N0	No regional lymph node metastasis	--	
N1	Metastasis in 1 to 3 regional lymph nodes	lymph node (ORP), collection of lymph nodes (ORP-C)	number
N2	Metastasis in 4 or more regional lymph nodes	lymph node (ORP), collection of lymph nodes (ORP-C)	number
MX	Distant metastasis cannot be assessed	--	
M0	No distant metastasis	--	
M1	Distant metastasis	ORG	

ORG = Organism; OR = Organ; OR-E = Organ (external to the original organ); ORP = Organ Part; MPOT = Maximal Portion of Tissue (equivalent to organ part but in a different partition); C = Cell; SC = Subcellular

TNM Classification and Staging

Various cancer societies have proposed different staging criteria for carcinomas, which apply at two different levels. Among those carcinomas for which a TNM classification exists, stages are not classified further than by means of the relevant TNM classes. The corresponding management guidelines are then based on these classes, so that for example there is a specific management protocol for T1N2M0 class of bladder carcinomas. However, in case of some carcinomas, including colon, an additional grouping is imposed upon the TNM classification by the American Joint Committee on Cancer (AJCC). For example, stage IIIa of colon carcinoma includes T1N1M0 and T2N1M0. The management protocols applicable to these TNM classes are similar and thus are usually specified in terms of stage IIIa. This means that the ontological representation of carcinomas like colon is incomplete if the Stages clustered over the TNM classes are not included, and therefore, we provide those representations in our ontology also.

Other staging systems

There are other staging systems for colon carcinoma, for example, the Modified Asler-Coller (MAC), Duke's and so on. These take into consideration entities similar to the ones for TNM, for example, invasion of mucosa or submucosa and so on. , and they will not be considered here. According to the kinds of cells predominantly present within the pathology, the different classes are adenomatous, mucinous, signet-ring, scirrhous and neuroendocrine. This classification involves entities are cellular and organ part levels.

Table 2: Definitions for AJCC staging for colon carcinoma

Stage	Clinical definition	Logical definition
0	Tis, N0, M0	Tis & N0 & M0
I	T1, N0, M0; T2, N0, M0	(T1 or T2) & N0 & M0
IIa	T3, N0, M0	T3 & N0 & M0
IIb	T3, N0, M0	T4 & N0 & M0
IIIa	T1, N1, M0; T2, N1, M0	(T1 or T2) & N1 & M0
IIIb	T3, N1, M0; T4, N1, M0	(T3 or T4) & N1 & M0
IIIc	Any T, N2, M0	N2 & M0
IV	Any T, Any N, M1	M1

Pathologic features

In addition to the features taken account of in the TNM classification, there are also several other features which are important in order to understand the prognostic factors and treatment planning for carcinomas. They are primarily related to finer levels of granularity.

Table 3: Pathologic features, their involvement in processes and their anatomical levels of granularity

Pathologic features	Process involved	Level of granularity
vascular endothelial growth factor	angiogenesis	M
reverse transcriptase	lymph node micrometastasis	M
radial margins of carcinomatous structure	carcinoma penetration	OR
degree of tumor differentiation	carcinoma penetration and metastasis	SC, C
mucin producing cancer cells	peritoneal seeding	SC, C
aneuploidy	karyotypic and phenotypic heterogeneity	SC
proliferation index (the sum of the percentage of cells in S phase plus those in G(2)/M phase)	karyotypic and phenotypic heterogeneity	C

Clinical Genomics Model in HL7 v3

Health Level 7 (HL7)[4] provides standards for the exchange, management and integration of data that supports clinical patient care. There are various domains represented within HL7 and each of those has a Domain Message Information Model (DMIM), based on which various Refined Message Information Models (RMIMs) are built.

The purpose of the clinical genomics domain of HL7 is to provide the facility to communicate genomic data within disparate organizations in a uniform way. It encapsulates various types of genomic data relating to a pair of alleles (a locus-genotype) including sequencing, expression and proteomics data. It also incorporates emerging standard formats like BSML[5] (Bioinformatic Sequence Markup Language) and MAGE-ML[6] (Microarray and Gene Expression Markup Language).

The main classes within the clinical genomics Genotype DMIM include genotype attributes, gene associated observation, Individual allele, sequence (recursive class), sequence variation property and expression. These classes represent entities present at the subcellular and molecular levels of granularities and are parts of the cell where they are present.

There are many pathological features which are present at these finer levels of granularity and usage of clinical genomics model would help connect to patient data at those levels of

---

[4] www.hl7.org
[5] http://www.bsml.org/
[6] http://www.mged.org/Workgroups/MAGE/mage-ml.html

granularity for the purposes of inferences to be drawn on EHRs for carcinoma classifications.

3. Conclusion

The main advantages of assigning levels of granularity and dependence relations are:

a. Entities within clinical bioinformatics are present at different levels of granularity and various annotations related to genotypes and their expression as phenotypes are associated with them. The interpretation of those annotations are relevant only at the respective granular levels.

b. Inferences derived upon the entities and their annotations depend on their granularity levels. For example, a mutation at subcellular level within a collection of cells is not enough to be diagnosed as a carcinoma. The TNM classes clearly distinguish on the basis of anatomical entities existing at various granularity levels.

c. The formalism provides a basis of relations that exist between substances, functions, processes and their attributes. These are further elaborated in [10].

These advantages outweigh the disadvantages of this approach which include initial complexities and constraints of the representation and training of personnel in order to apply these formalisms. This formalism has been applied in the case of Colon carcinoma representing entities at coarser levels of granularity applicable principally for medical informatics and representing entities at finer levels of granularity applicable principally for bioinformatics. [3, 4] This formalism is a step towards bridging the gaps in representing entities for clinical bioinformatics especially in the domain of oncology.

4. Acknowledgements

This paper was written under the auspices of the Wolfgang Paul Program of the Alexander von Humboldt Foundation, the European Union Network of Excellence on Medical Informatics and Semantic Data Mining, and the Volkswagen Foundation under the auspices of the project "Forms of Life".

5. References

[1]   Colon and rectum. In: American Joint Committee on Cancer: AJCC Cancer Staging Manual. 6th ed. New York, NY: Springer, 2002, pp 113-124.

[2]   V.T. DeVita, S. Hellman and S.A. Rosenberg. Cancer: Principles and Practice of Oncology, 6th Edition, Lippincott Williams & Wilkins (2001).

[3]   Kumar A, Yip L, Smith B, Grenon P. Bridging the Gap between Medical and Bioinformatics Using Formal Ontological Principles. Computers in Biology and Medicine. (submitted)

[4]   Kumar A, Yip L, Jaremek M, Scheib H. Ontological Model for Colon Carcinoma: A Case Study for Knowledge Representation in Clinical Bioinformatics. GMDS 2004. 29 Sept. Innsbruck, Austria: 196-198.

[5]   Kumar A, Smith B, Borgelt C. Dependence Relationships between Gene Ontology Terms based on TIGR Gene Product Annotations. CompuTerm Aug 29, 2004: 3rd International Workshop on Computational Terminology: 31-38.

[6]   Rosse C, Mejino JL Jr. A reference ontology for biomedical informatics: the Foundational Model of Anatomy. J Biomed Inform. 2003 Dec;36(6):478-500.

[7]   Smith B, Ceusters W, Koehler J, Kumar A, Lomax J, Mungall C, Neuhaus F, Rector A, Rosse C. Relations in Biological Ontologies. (submitted) http://ontology.buffalo.edu/bio/OBORelations.doc

[8]   Donnelly M. On parts and holes: the spatial structure of the human body. Medinfo. 2004;2004:351-5.

[9]   Smith B, Grenon P. The Cornucopia of Formal-Ontological Relations, Dialectica, 58:3 (2004), 279-296.

[10] Kumar A, Smith B, Novotny DD. Biomedical Informatics and Granularity. Comparative and Functional Genomics. (In Press)

Address for Correspondence

Anand Kumar, IFOMIS, Universität des Saarlandes, Postfach 151150, D-66041 Saarbrücken, Germany. Phone: +49-172-8984640. Email: akumar@ifomis.uni-saarland.de, URL: http://www.uni-leipzig.de/~akumar/

Connecting Medical Informatics and Bio-Informatics
R. Engelbrecht et al. (Eds.)
IOS Press, 2005

Integration of Multiple Ontologies in Breast Cancer Pathology

David Ouagne, Christel Le Bozec, Eric Zapletal, Maxime Thieu, Marie-Christine Jaulent

INSERM, U729, Paris, F-75006 France

Abstract

The diagnostic variability in pathology, widely reported in the literature, is partly due to the use of different classification systems by pathologists. The descriptions of morphological characteristics on the same image within different classification systems can be considered as different points of view of pathologists. Our aim is to represent the points of view of the experts in pathology during image interpretation and to propose a methodological and technical solution in order to implement interoperability between these points of view. According to the hybrid ontology approach, we developed a system in three stages consisting in 1) the representation of the various points of view in local ontologies 2) the realization of a shared vocabulary and the development of a mapping tool used to allow the matching of local ontologies and shared vocabulary 3) the development of a transcoding algorithm for the translation of a case description from one point of view to another. A first evaluation of the transcoding algorithm was conducted for 33 cases of breast pathology. Our results show that the pathologists generally produce descriptions of the cases which do not follow rigorously the interpretation rules corresponding to the point of view they assert to adopt. While most of the concepts of local ontologies can be transcoded from a local ontology to another one (varying from 62.5 % to 100% according to the local ontology), the transcoding of a description which is valid according to a certain point of view, often results in a description which is not rigorously in accordance with the new point of view. These results underline the differences of interpretation rules existing in the different points of view.

Keywords:
Knowledge representation; Ontologies integration; Semantic interoperability; Medical imaging; Breast pathology

1. Introduction

Pathologists establish diagnosis and/or give prognostic indications on microscopic lesions observed in images of tissues and cells. Diagnostic variability in pathology is widely reported in the literature [1]. To reduce the variability, pathologists apply rules allowing to establish a diagnostic from morphological characteristics observed on images, and these rules are published within the framework of classification systems. However, at the moment there are many systems evolving quickly. Thus, identical cases can have different diagnostic conclusions according to the pathologist point of view, that is the system of classification he/she used [2].

Our aim is to represent the knowledge contained in the pathologists' various points of view within local ontologies in order to be able to compare and make interoperable conclusions supplied by various pathologists.

A point of view is characterized by an "angle of view" related to a type of individual (profession, age, level of training, etc.) and "a point of focalization" corresponding to a specific usage. Indexing the knowledge, according to points of view, make it accessible and reusable. Ribière [3] proposes models and methods allowing the representation of multiple points of view. Other papers propose solutions for knowledge integration based on ontologies in order to compare different points of view [4-7]. An ontology clarifies a set of the concepts of a domain – e.g. entities, attributes, and processes – their definitions and their interrelations [8-10].

According to Wache [4], there are three main approaches for the integration of diverse knowledge which are generally distinguished. The single ontology approach uses a global ontology providing a shared vocabulary for the specification of the different sources (referenced here as the classification systems) [7]. In the multiple ontologies approach, each source is described by its own ontology and an additional formalism of representation defining the inter-mapping ontology is provided [11]; finally the hybrid approach combines the two previous ones. Each source is described by its own ontology built upon one global shared vocabulary. The main point is how the terms of the source ontologies are described by the primitives of the shared vocabulary [5].

There are developed technical solutions allowing to manage multiple ontologies. These solutions can be classified according to the operations they can handle (mapping, transformation, version management etc.) [7]. One of the difficulties of the multiple ontologies and the "hybrid" ontology approches is the definition of the mapping. There are several environments making the operations of mappings based upon translator agents (KRAFT [12]), description logics (OBSERVER [11]), statistic models allowing the mapping between expressions in natural language (GLUE [13], Lab ISI/USC [14]), lexical techniques (co-occurrences of terms in corpuses) (ONION [15]). The environment to be used must be chosen according to the task envisaged (merging, difference, mapping, transformation, etc.) and depending on the local ontologies which one has to deal with. In our case we chose to use the PROMPT suite, an Open Source software, which allows, among others, to compare and to merge ontologies [16].

We proceeded in three stages consisting in 1) the representation of the various points of view within local ontologies, 2) the realization of a shared vocabulary and the development of an environment of mapping, which allows to match local ontologies and shared vocabulary 3) an algorithm of transcoding allowing to translate the description of a case according to a point of view to a different point of view. A first evaluation was conducted for 33 cases described according to two different classification systems.

2. Material and methods

2.1 The constitution of the local ontologies

In the field of the breast cancer pathology, we considered three classifications of ductal carcinoma in situ (DCIS) - Holland, Van Nuys and Lagios [2] – expressing the rules of interpretation of the cases of DCIS according to different points of view. Each of these classifications supports pathologists to make a structured report of a case of DCIS whose grade (high, intermediate or low) is inferred from given morphological characteristics observed in images. To build the local ontology corresponding to each of these classifications, we extracted the morphological characteristics of the classification and organized them according to a taxonomic hierarchy (" is a ") by anatomy (for example nucleus, cell, canal, etc.) and then by type of morphological characteristic (for example size, forms, etc.). Furthermore, we added a relation called "is inferred from" which allows to represent the rules of diagnostic interpretation of the considered classification. We used

Protégé environment for the construction of local ontologies [17].

2.2   *The mapping between the shared vocabulary and the local ontologies*

We chose a hybrid approach to compare and make interoperable the various points of view of the pathologists. In this way, we developed an environment allowing the definition of a shared vocabulary and the creation of relations - solutions of matching and transformation - between this shared vocabulary and the local ontologies. Every concept of the shared vocabulary is explicitly matched with a concept of every local ontology in order to make possible a transcoding.

We chose to adapt an existing management tool for multiple ontologies, the PROMPT suite, which is particularly adapted when local ontologies have no instances but many relations between concepts [7].

We modified the merging tool of PROMPT to realize a mapping between local ontologies. The mapping tool is based on the algorithms used by the merging tool which suggests what should be merged. As an input for the process of mapping, we have two concepts which are suggested to be merged but, contrary to the merging process, as an output we do not obtain a new concept. Indeed, we want to be able not only to choose the concept to be placed in the shared vocabulary but also to create a relation between this favorite concept and the corresponding concepts in each local ontology. The relation could be either simple or complex. At the moment, there are three different situations (identical, similar or synonym concept) coming along with an explanatory sentence. A relation is defined by four properties: *toClass* (indicate the name of the concept of destination for a relation), *code-value* (clarify the semantic type of the relation – identical, similar or synonym –), *coding-scheme-designator* (clarify the name of the ontology source) and *code-meaning* (sentence of justification of the relation).

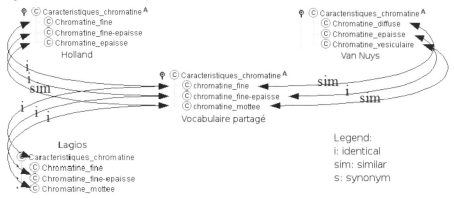

Figure 1 Example of relations between the shared vocabulary and the local ontologies

2.3   *The transcoding*

The transcoding algorithm transforms the description of a case in a given classification system into a new description based on a different point of view. In addition, the resulting description has to be validated against this new point of view.

For each concept to be transcoded, the algorithm takes three parameters in input (concept to be expressed, ontology source, target ontology) and then returns the matched concept of the target ontology if it exists.

2.4   Material and experiment

Each concept of each local ontology was transcoded in the two other local ontologies in order to estimate, for each local ontology, the rate of concepts that can be transcoded. Besides, thirty three cases were described according to Holland's classifications and Van Nuys using the description module of a computerized platform, IDEM, dedicated to on-line inter-pathologists consensus [17]. This platform allows pathologists to produce XML files corresponding to structured reports according to a given point of view. Each XML file of a case description was transcoded according to the two other points of view.

The preservation of the validity of the cases after transcoding was one indicator to evaluate the transcoding procedure. A case description is valid, according to a given point of view, if it conforms to the interpretation rules expressed in the local ontology corresponding to the point of view. An algorithm was developed based on rules embedded in the classifications in order to validate case descriptions according to a given point of view. This algorithm uses the syntactic validation of an XML file (the case description) with regard to an XML schema containing the rules expressed in the given local ontology. Agreement of the validity of cases, before/after transcoding, was estimated thanks to the Kappa coefficient.

3.   Results

3.1   Local ontologies

Local ontologies built in Protégé corresponding to Holland, Lagios and Van Nuys classifications contain respectively 27, 24 and 18 concepts. These concepts are either diagnosis of breast pathology or morphological characteristics observed on images. Relations "is a" and "inferred from" were defined in the local ontologies.

3.2   The matching between the shared vocabulary and the local ontologies

New heuristics of the merging tool of PROMPT were added to build the shared vocabulary from local ontologies. This new plug-in allowed to build a shared vocabulary of 30 "favorite" concepts. The rules for transcoding were extracted from the shared vocabulary.

3.3   Transcoding and experiment

3.3.1   Transcoding the local ontologies

The results of the transcoding of each of the three local ontologies to the two others are given in table 1:

Table 1 : Ratio of « transcodable» concepts for each local ontology

	Tot. nb. of conce pts	« Transcodable » concepts (%)		
		VN	HL	LA
VN	18		100	83,3
HL	27	66,6		66,6
LA	24	62,5	75	

3.3.2   The conservation of the validity of cases during the transcoding

Thirty three cases were described according to Holland's and Van Nuys's classifications. Concerning Van Nuys's classification, 11 cases on 33 (that is 33 %) are exactly conform to the rules of Van Nuys's classification (embedded in the Van Nuys's XML schema extracted from the local ontology). Concerning, Holland's classification, none of the thirty three cases is rigorously in accordance with the classification. In other words, none of the descriptions is prototypical of one of the three DCIS grade. When cases don't conform to the rules of a classification, they generate an error message (resp. 2 error messages or more) in 39 % of cases (resp. 61 % of cases) for Van Nuys's classification. For Holland's classification, when cases don't conform to the rules of a classification, they generate only an error message (resp. 2 error messages or more) in 67 % of cases (resp. 33 % of cases).

We compared the validity of a case to the diagnostic rules from the point of view, in which it was described, with its validity after transcoding in the new point of view. The obtained agreement is bad (Kappa=0 whether it is for transcoding from Van Nuys towards Holland or the contrary).

4. Discussion

The main objective of this work was to represent different points of view of pathologists during image interpretation and to propose a methodological and technical solution for the interoperability of points of view. We implemented the "hybrid" ontology approach described by Wache and experimented by Buccella consisting in representing the different points of view within the local ontologies, in building a shared vocabulary and in defining the mapping between concepts of local ontologies and those of the shared vocabulary. Then, this mapping allowed developing a transcoding module able to translate structured reports expressed according to a local ontology towards another local ontology. Finally, we evaluated the transcoding process.

We showed in our experiment that the pathologists produce generally descriptions of DCIS cases which do not correspond rigorously to prototypical descriptions according to the classification systems. We developed a validation module, which allows the pathologists to become aware of this gap between their practice and the rules expressed in the classification system that they use when interpreting images.

Results show that most of the concepts can be transcoded from a local ontology to another one. On the other hand, we noticed that the transcoding of the case descriptions did not necessarily keep the validity of these cases according to the new point of view. So, the transcoding of a valid description according to a classification often gives as result a description which is not any more rigorously in accordance with the rules of interpretation of the new reference classification. This point highlights the impact of relying on different interpretation rules coming from different points of view.

Short-term improvements consist in defining more specific diagnostic relations of inference at the level of local ontologies. Indeed, apart the "is a" relation, we used only the relation "inferred from". The pathologists also use more specific relations of that type like "is a necessary and sufficient diagnostic criterion of" or "is an optional diagnostic criterion of". It would allow better to take into account the semantic of the interpretation rules of the classifications. Concerning the transcoding, we aim to enrich the merging algorithm PROMPT to improve the quality of suggestions of the system during the constitution of the shared vocabulary.

As long–term improvements, an interesting perspective consists in integrating the tools we have developed in the IDEM collaborative platform, dedicated to virtual slides interpretation. As pathologists using IDEM, do not necessarily use the same classifications to determine their diagnoses, the transcoding process would allow to quantify the part of the diagnostic variability related to the use of different interpretation rules compared to the variability in recognizing morphological characteristics in images.

5. Acknowledgments

The authors wish to thank the IDEM team for their continuous help during the development of this work, all the primary care practitioners for their patience and enthusiasm and Alexandra and Iulian Alecu for their comments on this paper.

6. References

[1]   Fleming KA, Evidence-Based Pathology, *J Pathol*, 179(2); pp. 127-8; 1996.

[2]   Wells WA, Carney PA, Eliassen MS, Grove MR, Tosteson AN. Pathologists' Agreement With Experts and Reproducibility of Breast Ductal Carcinoma-in-Situ Classification Schemes, *Am J Surg Pathol*; 5(24); 2000; pp. 651-670.

[3]   Ribière M. Représentation et gestion de multiples points de vues dans le formalisme des graphes conceptuels, *Thèse de l'université de Sophia-Antipolis*; 1999.

[4]   Wache, H., V ogele, T., Visser, U., Stuckenschmidt, H., Schuster, G., Neumann, H., and Hubnet, S. Ontology-based integration of information - a survey of existing approaches. In Stuckenschmidt, H, *IJCAI-01 Workshop: Ontologies and Information Sharing*, 2001, pp. 108-117.

[5]   Buccella A, Ceclich A. An Ontology Approach to Data Integration, *JCS&T*; 3(2), 2003; pp 62-68.

[6]   Cui Z, Jones D, O'Brien P. Issues in Ontology-based Information Integration. In: (A. Gomez-Perez, M. Gruninger, H. et al.) *Proceedings of the IJCAI-01 Workshop on Ontologies and Information Sharing*, Seattle, USA, August 4-5, 2001; pp 141-146.

[7]   Noy N. Tools for Mapping and Merging Ontologies, Handbook on Ontologies, *S.Staab and R. Studer editors*, pp. 365-384. Springer-Verlag, 2003.

[8]   Bachimont B. Engagement sémantique et engagement ontologique : conception et réalisation d'ontologie en ingénierie des connaissances, Eyrolles, pp. 305-23, 2000.

[9]   Grüber T, *A* Translation Approach to Portable Ontology Specifications, *Knowledge Acquisition 5*, pp. 199–220, 1993.

[10] Uschold M, Grüninger M. *Ontologies:* Principles, Methods and Applications, *Knowledge Engineering Review*, 11(2), pp. 93-155, 1996.

[11] Mena E, Illarramendi A, Kashyap V, Sheth A.P. OBSERVER: An approach for query processing in global information systems based on interoperation across pre-existing ontologies. *Distributed and Parallel Databases*, 8(2); pp. 223-271, 2000.

[12] Preece A, Hui K, Gray A, Marti P, Bench-Capon T, Jones D, and Cui Z. The KRAFT Architecture for Knowledge Fusion and Transformation, in M Bramer, A Macintosh & F Coenen (eds), *Research and Development in Intelligent Systems XVI* (Proc ES99), Springer, New York, 1999, pp.23-38.

[13] Doan A, Madhavan J, Domingos P, Halevy A. Learning to map between ontologies on the semantic web. *In Proceedings of the eleventh international conference on World Wide Web*, pp. 662-673. ACM Press, 2002.

[14] Hovy EH. Combining and Standardizing Large-Scale, Practical Ontologies for Machine Translation and Other Uses, Proc. *1st Int'l Conf. Language Resources and Evaluation* (LREC), European Language Resources Assoc., Paris, 1998, pp. 535-542.

[15] Mitra P, Wiederhold G, Kersten ML. A Graph-Oriented Model for Articulation of Ontology Interdependencies. *In Intl. Conference on Extending Database Technology* (EDBT), pp. 86-100, 2000.

[16] Noy N, Musen MA. *The* prompt suite: Interactive tools for ontology merging and mapping. *Journal of Human-Computer Studies*, 59(6); pp. 983-1024, 2003.

[17] Zapletal E, Le Bozec C, Degoulet P, Guinebretiere J.M, Jaulent MC. Specifications and implementation of a new exchange format to support computerized consensus in pathology. *Medinfo*. 2004; pp. 693-700.

Address for correspondence

15, rue de l'école de Médecine 75006 PARIS, David.Ouagne@spim.jussieu.fr

Wüsteria

Barry Smith[a], Werner Ceusters[b], Rita Temmerman[c]

[a] IFOMIS (Institute for Formal Ontology and Medical Information Science), Saarland University, Germany and
Department of Philosophy, University at Buffalo, NY, USA
[b] ECOR (European Centre for Ontological Research), Saarland University, Germany
[c] CVC (Centre for Terminology and Communication), Erasmushogeschool, Brussels

Abstract

The last two decades have seen considerable efforts directed towards making electronic health records interoperable through improvements in medical ontologies, terminologies and coding systems. Unfortunately, these efforts have been hampered by a number of influential ideas inherited from the work of Eugen Wüster, the father of terminology standardization and the founder of ISO TC 37. We here survey Wüster's ideas – which see terminology work as being focused on the classification of concepts in people's minds – and we argue that they serve still as the basis for a series of influential confusions. We argue further that an ontology based unambiguously, not on concepts, but on the classification of entities in reality can, by removing these confusions, make a vital contribution to ensuring the interoperability of coding systems and healthcare records in the future.

1. Introduction

The goal of an electronic health record (EHR) is to achieve faithful clinical data entry in such a way as to meet the requirements of communicability for both human and machine. [1] To this end much emphasis has been placed on clinical coding, with the rationale that it is codes that will make it possible to associate with the terms used by humans in expressing patient data the sorts of uniform syntax and precise meanings that can be interpreted by software. Code-based terminologies now exist in many different flavours. The Unified Medical Language System contains in its MetaThesaurus over 100 such systems, which are said to comprehend in all some 3 million medical "concepts" [2].

On the EHR front, too, progress is being made. CEN/TC251 has brought Europe-wide acceptance of the need for a comprehensive, communicable and secure EHR as a prerequisite for the delivery of high-quality healthcare, and this European vision has gained international acceptance, leading to the establishment of new standards at the ISO level [3]. As we shall show, however, the realization of this vision is stymied by the fact that the new standards inherit from the earlier work of ISO Technical Committee (TC) 37 a fundamental incoherence.

ISO TC 37 was founded in 1951, largely through the efforts of a certain Eugen Wüster (1898–1977), an Austrian businessman, saw-manufacturer, professor of woodworking machinery, and devotee of Esperanto, who ran the secretariat of TC 37 for the first decades of its existence. [4] Wüster was principal author of almost all the seminal documents on terminology standardization and thus responsible for very many of the ideas which, because of ISO's rules governing re-use of prior standards, have been propagated in ever widening circles ever since. Given this astonishing influence, it is worth spending some time to convey the flavour of Wüster's thinking.

First, we need to note that four distinct views of concepts can be distinguished in the literature. On the psychological view concepts are *mental entities*, analogous to ideas or beliefs; on the linguistic view concepts are the (somehow regimented) *meanings of general terms*; on the epistemological view concepts are *units of knowledge* (as this term is used in phrases such as 'knowledge representation'); and finally, on what some might call the 'ontological' view, concepts are *abstractions of kinds, attributes or properties* (i.e. of general invariant patterns on the side of entities in the world). Sadly, elements of all four views are found mixed up together in almost all terminology-focused work in informatics today. [5]

Wüster himself is a proponent of the psychological view. Our knowledge of concepts, he tells us [6], is rooted in the experiences of the new-born infant, which finds itself "constantly amidst a panoply of diverse sensory impressions". The child begins thereupon to mentally sub-divide this sensory mosaic into individual objects (and Wüster stresses repeatedly in this connection that objects in reality are *constructed* by human beings, and that there is a high degree of arbitrariness and variability to such construction). The child can thereafter also *remember* objects, such memories constituting what Wüster calls "individual concepts". Examples are: "'Napoleon' or the concept of my fountain pen." [6]

If, as Wüster would have it, "a speaker wishes to draw the attention of an interlocutor to a particular individual object, which is visible to both parties or which he carries with him, he only has to point to it". Otherwise, however, "the only thing available is the individual concept of the object, provided that it is readily accessible in the heads of both persons." (Those engaged in communication about, say, Napoleon, are thus somehow required to gain access to the interiors of each other's heads.)

In the course of time, the child notices that some individual objects – e.g. apples, or bricks, or cans of paint – are "interchangeably alike" and are given the same name by older speakers of the language. "The child learns to blend the individual concepts of such objects in its thinking" and thus arrives at *general concepts*, which are, like individual concepts "thought (= mental) objects. They exist only in the heads of people." As individual concepts can be grouped together into general concepts, so general concepts can be grouped together into concepts of higher degrees of abstraction, as when we move from the general concept *apple* to the superordinate concept *fruit*. The formation of concepts at these higher levels, too, Wüster thinks, is "highly dependent on human discretion."

Terminology work is designed to provide clear delineations in this "realm" of concepts via definitions [7], and Wüster thinks that *terms* can be assigned to concepts only when such definitions have been formulated. (How else, after all, are we to gain access to the denizens of this strangely ethereal realm?)

2. Concepts and Characteristics

Wüster's account of concept learning and his insistence on the arbitrariness of concept-formation have long since been called into question by cognitive scientists. Even very small children manifest in surprisingly uniform ways an ability to apprehend objects in their surroundings as instances of natural kinds – in ways which go far beyond what they apprehend in sensory experience. There is now much evidence (e.g. in [8]) to the effect that, for objects in the biological realm, this ability rests on a shared innate capacity to apprehend the surrounding world in terms of underlying structures or powers. The latter are invisible to the child, but adults may learn to recognize them as structures of a molecular sort.

Wüster's idea according to which, before we can assign a term to a concept, we must first "delineate" the concept, is also open to serious objections. To delineate means: to list the totality of "characteristics" which form a concept's *content* or *intension*. Unfortunately Wüster provides conflicting elucidations of what such "characteristics" might be [7], conceiving them sometimes as if they were themselves *concepts* (so that, like other concepts, they would exist in the heads of people), and at other times as *properties of objects* existing in the world. (This is in keeping with the general failure to discriminate clearly between objects and concepts which runs through all of Wüster's thinking.)

Some recent terminology work is clearer in this respect [9]. Unfortunately, however, even in more recent ISO documents [10] the problems still linger, since the relevant communities have still to find a coherent means by which concepts and their characteristics should somehow span the divide between concepts as creatures of the mind and as properties of objects in the world. This lingering incoherence, which spreads also independently of ISO's influence [11], explains why so many terminologies contain certain characteristic families of errors in coding and documentation which flow from the fact that those involved in their authoring and maintenance are unsure as to whether their task is the representation of *ideas in people's heads, meanings of words, consensus knowledge of experts in a discipline* or *types of entities in the world* [5]. Consider for example the definition of *disorder* that we find in SNOMED: "Disorders are concepts [!] in which there is an explicit or implicit pathological process causing a state of disease which tends to exist for a significant length of time under ordinary circumstances." [12, p. 23]. Taken together with SNOMED's definition of concepts as "unique units of thought" [12, p. 11], this would seem to imply that all disorders are imagined.

3. Wüsterian Medicine

Wüster's assumption to the effect that concepts are formed through the application of human discretion to perceived similarities may have led some to suppose that his ideas are well-suited to the area of medical terminology, which is after all subject to the constant coinage of novel terms. Unfortunately, however, there is one prominent feature of medical reality which makes Wüster's approach here inapposite. For in medicine we often have to deal with families of entities in reality in relation to which we are able to grasp few characteristics "identifiable in encounters of similars", and certainly too few to allow definitions of the corresponding concepts. (It is in part for this reason that some 85% of SNOMED-CT's concepts remain in its July 2003 version [12] undefined.)

Consider, for example, a tumour. This starts out as initially undetectable mutations in a small number of cells and then becomes transformed by degrees into a full-fledged object on the scale of coarse anatomy. For very many types of pathogenic process it seems at best simplistic to suppose that we could isolate in perception certain "essential properties" which could be identified in definitions as the "characteristics" of corresponding general concepts. That the detection, classification and diagnosis of such processes involves to such a high degree the application of statistical techniques is already a sign of the fact that we are dealing here with patterns in reality which go beyond the realm of concepts as this is conceived, in Wüsterian fashion, in terms of lists of necessary and sufficient conditions.

The reason for this miscalibration turns on the fact that the Wüsterian notion of concept *has nothing to do with medicine (or biology) at all*. Wüster and his early TC 37 colleagues were concerned primarily with standardisation in the domain of *commercial artefacts*, and especially of *manufactured products*. Wüster himself was the author of a multivolume work entitled *The Machine Tool. An Interlingual Dictionary of Basic Concepts* (London 1976). Machine tools truly are such as to manifest characteristics identifiable in encounters of similars – because they have been manufactured as such. Vocabulary itself is treated by Wüster and his TC 37 followers "as if it could be standardised in the same way as types of paint and varnish or aircraft and space vehicles" [13, p. 12].

Certainly, there are also non-artefactual objects in the Wüsterian universe. As ISO/IEC JTC1 SC36 N0579 (for example) puts it:

> *an object is defined as anything perceived or conceived. Some objects, concrete objects such as a machine, a diamond, or a river, shall be considered material; other objects are to be considered immaterial or abstract, such as each manifestation of financial planning, gravity, flowability, or a conversion ratio; still others are to be considered purely imagined, for example, a unicorn, a philosopher's stone or a literary character. [14]*

Unfortunately such elucidations are so vague as to leave the putative user of the corresponding standards in the dark. Are *processes* objects? Are they concrete or abstract? Are *characteristics* objects? Are *concepts* objects? Are dispositions, functions, limbs, body cavities, blood flow, apoptosis, or types of pus, objects? Are they concrete or abstract? Material or immaterial? Real or imagined? The ISO literature still leaves us with no coherent means to provide answers to such questions, and this in spite of the fact that the task of creating a principled framework in which such answers could be given is of increasing importance to the future of medical coding and of the EHR. In the document just cited, however, in which real objects such as rivers are placed on the same level as imagined objects such as unicorns, ISO makes it clear what it thinks of the importance of this task for the future of terminology research:

> *In the course of producing a terminology, philosophical discussions on whether an object actually exists in reality ... are to be avoided. Objects are assumed to exist and attention is to be focused on how one deals with objects for the purposes of communication. [14, emphasis added]*

As we have argued at length elsewhere, however [5], it is precisely such philosophical discussions which are required if we are to undo the sore effects of Wüster's influence.

4. How Medical Terms Are Introduced

The typical scenario for the introduction of new terms into medical language is as follows. A new disease or virus is encountered in reality, and the communities involved recognize that they need some way to refer to the newly discovered kind as they encounter its successive instances. Agreement is then reached in these and those languages that these and those terms should be used henceforth to refer to *instances of this kind of entity*.

In terminology circles, however, the demand is now raised to add in addition some third thing: the corresponding *concept*. Because concepts themselves are ethereal in nature, they require the support of something else – namely *definitions* – to enable terminology users and associated software applications to gain access to them. At the same time the definitions thus created serve henceforth to restrict the sorts of entities that can be admitted as falling under the corresponding concepts.

In areas like manufacturing or commerce the purpose of standardization is precisely to bring about a situation in which entities in reality (such as machine parts, or contracts) are indeed *required* to conform to certain agreed-upon standards. Such a requirement is however alien to the world of medicine, where it is the entities in reality which must serve in every case as benchmark. Even in medicine, however, terminologists have been encouraged to focus on concepts and definitions rather than on the corresponding entities in reality.

We can now understand more precisely why so many of the medical 'concepts' in terminologies like SNOMED-CT remain undefined. The reason turns on the way in which medical terms are introduced into our language. Such terms reflect entities in reality for which we characteristically have access to only a small fraction of the relevant biological or clinical features. Almost all disorder terms are introduced, not because we already have a clear definition reflecting known characteristics, but because we have a *pool of cases*.

This means that many medical terms are introduced before their users have any 'conceptual' understanding of what they *mean*. These users are however able to grasp what they *designate in reality*: they can see the relevant entities before them in the lab or clinic.

5. An Ontological Basis for Coding Systems and the EHR

There are many who hold that it will suffice to establish communication standards for the EHR if we can only establish a way to refer unambiguously to "concepts" as units of knowledge agreed upon by domain experts and defined in formal ways. As we hope to have shown in the foregoing, this detour through "concepts" – at least as realized in the domain of biomedicine – represents rather an alien accretion of what we can only call *International Standard Bad Philosophy*. It is time, we believe, to pursue new means of conceiving the relation of terms to medical reality in which the detour through concepts is abandoned and in which we draw instead on the best theories and tools which contemporary philosophy has to offer – and this means above all the right sort of ontology, an ontology that is able explicitly and unambiguously to relate to the universal types or kinds in reality as well as to the individual tokens (such as you and me) which are their instances.

The principal task of medical terminology systems is to represent such universal types or kinds, and the principal task of the EHR is to represent the corresponding instances. Our proposal, then, is to develop an ontology in which these two kinds of representations are tied together from the start, without the detour through the realm of concepts.

Note that we are not hereby claiming that to establish the ontology of the world of biomedical universals and instances will be a simple task. There is, as is clear, no single unified perspective on which all reasonable persons must agree if they would only open their eyes. Hence the popularity of T. S. Kuhn's ideas on conflicting paradigms, and hence the influence of Wüster's own ideas on what he sees as the human-induced arbitrariness involved in the "construction" of both objects and concepts. Against both Kuhn and Wüster, however, we see these matters precisely in terms of the existence of a plurality of different perspectives *on one and the same world* – perspectives corresponding, for example, to the different life science disciplines and to different biomedical terminologies. It is because of the immense complexity of this one world that it is accessible to us only in terms of a wide variety of such different perspectives.

On our view, however, some terminologies are to be preferred to others because they project onto the world beyond in a way which enjoys a higher level of correctness or adequacy to the universals or kinds in reality. On the view of Wüster and his followers, in contrast, there is no independent benchmark in relation to which concept-systems could be established as correct, and thus also no independent fulcrum in terms of which concept-systems could be integrated together in robust fashion. On our view such integration can be attained precisely because perspectives are projected onto this common independent reality, which embraces entities at all levels of granularity, from the molecule to population [15].

Our approach does not, be it noted, ignore the psychological and linguistic dimensions of the application of medical terms. Indeed, it takes great pains to ensure that its categories apply to the world itself in all salient dimensions, including beliefs and observations, utterances and terms. It is thus in a position to make it crystal clear, in relation to all the clinical data registered in EHRs, whether entities in the associated coding systems refer to *diseases*, or to *statements made about diseases*, or to *acts on the part of physicians*, or to *documents in which such acts are recorded*, or to *observations of such acts*, or to *statements about such observations.* In this respect, too, it is opposed to the established approaches to the construction of coding systems for use in the EHR in recent years.

6. Conclusion

The application of a sound realist ontology to the domain of healthcare can make coding systems both logically more coherent and also more closely compatible with our commonsensical intuitions about the medically salient objects and processes in reality. It can thus not only help in detecting errors in existing coding systems but also, by allowing the formulation of intuitive principles for the creation and maintenance of such systems, help in avoiding similar errors in the future [16].

To achieve the requisite coding systems and the associated EHR architecture will of course require a huge effort, since the relevant standards need to be overhauled from the ground up by experts who are cognizant of the need for clarity and familiar with the methods of sound ontology. Even before that stage is reached, however, there is the problem of making all constituent parties – including patients, healthcare providers, system developers and decision makers – aware of how deep-seated the existing problems are.

7. Acknowledgements:

Work on this paper was carried out under the auspices of the Alexander von Humboldt Foundation, the EU Network of Excellence in Medical Informatics and Semantic Data Mining, and the Project "Forms of Life" sponsored by the Volkswagen Foundation. Thanks for helpful comments are due also to Gerhard Budin and Gunnar Klein, who however bear no responsibility for the positions here adopted.

8. References

[1]   Redondo JR, Ceusters W, González JM, Iakovidis I. European electronic healthcare records towards the future. *Health in the New Communications Age*, 671-675, IOS Press 1995.
[2]   National Library of Medicine; UMLS Fact Sheet, updated 7 May 2004.
[3]   ISO 18308: Health informatics – Requirements for an electronic health record architecture. 2002 (http://www.iso.ch/iso/en/CatalogueDetailPage.CatalogueDetail?CSNUMBER=33397).
[4]   Oeser E, Galinski C. Eugen Wüster (1898–1977). Leben und Werk, Vienna: Infoterm, 1998.
[5]   Smith B. Beyond concepts, or: Ontology as reality representation, *Formal Ontology and Information Systems* (FOIS), Amsterdam: IOS Press, 2004;:73–84.
[6]   Wüster E. The wording of the world presented graphically and terminologically (selected and translated by JC Sager), *Terminology*, 2003;9(2):269-297.
[7]   Wüster E. *Einführung in die Allgemeine Terminologielehre und Terminologische Lexikographie*, Vienna/New York: Spring, 1979.
[8]   Gelman SA, Wellman HM. Insides and essences: Early understandings of the non-obvious. *Cognition*, 1991;38:213-244.
[9]   Wright SL, Budin G (eds.): *Handbook of terminology management*. Amsterdam: Benjamins 1997.
[10]   ISO-1087:1990 and ISO-1087-1:2000 *Vocabulary of terminology* (versions of 1990 and 2000).
[11]   See for example: http://www.w3.org/2004/02/skos/core/spec/2005-05-04
[12]   College of American Pathologists. *SNOMED Clinical Terms® User Guide*. January 2003 Release.
[13]   Temmerman R. *Towards new ways of terminology description*. Amsterdam: Benjamins, 2000.
[14]   ISO/IEC JTC1 SC36 N0579:1999. Text for FDIS 704. Terminology work: Principles and methods.
[15]   Smith B, et al. Relations in biomedical ontologies, *Genome Biology*, 2005; 6(5): R46.
[16]   Ceusters W, Smith B, Kumar A, Dhaen C. Mistakes in medical ontologies. *Ontologies in Medicine. Proceedings of the Workshop on Medical Ontologies*, Amsterdam: IOS Press, 2004:145-63.

Address for correspondence:

Barry Smith, IFOMIS, Saarland University, Postfach 151150, D-66041 Saarbrücken. phismith@buffalo.edu.
Internet: http://ifomis.org.

Connecting Medical Informatics and Bio-Informatics
R. Engelbrecht et al. (Eds.)
IOS Press, 2005

Desiderata for Representing Anatomical Knowledge

Robert H Baud, Christian Lovis, Paul Fabry, Antoine Geissbuhler

Medical Informatics Division. University Hospitals of Geneva, Switzerland

Abstract:

> The general problem of knowledge representation for gross anatomy supporting both computers and human is rarely globally solved. Partial solutions are flourishing, but the actual and potential users are left with a lack of satisfaction and uncomfortable feeling of incompleteness. Moreover, these solutions are not ready for a sound evolution and are at risk to disappear at any moment by default of adequate maintenance. In addition, the problem is complicated by the fact that any solutions should be relevant for Natural Language Processing applications in a multilingual environment.
>
> This paper tackles with this problem and defines the basic steps for a proper knowledge representation scheme. Taking the subdomain of gross anatomy, it shows how each step has been solved and what performances and benefits are expected by such a solution. A discussion is done on the way to interface from a common source for both computers and humans.

Keywords:
Knowledge representation, Natural Language Processing, ontology, anatomy

1. Desiderata

Considering a medical subdomain like gross human anatomy, one is faced to the global problem of knowledge representation of all relevant objects. The objective is a proper usage of this knowledge by computer programs as well as adequate understanding by human beings and their pedagogical support. The main desiderata consist in a formal model of this domain of anatomy, organizing all the objects and encompassing their relationships. The model should be accessible by computer programs as well as supporting intelligent browsers of anatomy atlases [1].

Two aspects are superposed to this first drawing of the situation: first, the model shall support reasoning on objects of the domain with global coherence and satisfying the needs of sound formal logics. Second, the model shall be extended for NLP processing in multiple languages. Any solution shall maintain the uniqueness of the source (therefore its coherence) when facing so many different needs.

All these prerequisites are rarely found altogether in any implementation, but hopefully the situation of gross anatomy is privileged and tends to this satisfactory solution. This paper aims at introducing and discussing all aspects of this situation and will enhance the expected advantages and benefits. Moreover, it traces the way of an exemplary solution, having the potential of being reproduced in another domain.

2. Methods: the basic modelling steps

In a companion paper, the first author has developed with some details what are the minimal procedural steps for acquiring and developing a model covering a specific domain [2] and only a short presentation is given here. The basic steps for a successful development of a model of a domain are the following:

- **Enumeration of the valid terms**: this initial task is basically the making of an inventory. At this stage, any object may be represented by multiple words or terms: this is part of the next step of detecting the synonyms.

- **Unique identification**: the task is to provide one identifier for any single object, and only one. The difficulty is that the very same object may be recognized by more than one term. In other words, there are less identifiers than terms.

- **Taxonomic organization**: A taxonomic hierarchy is by definition based on *isa* links. It is the backbone of any consistent model, because this type of links preserves the inheritance of properties and attributes. If the father object has a specific attribute value, the child object, which is of the same kind as the father, necessarily has this attribute value.

- **Other hierarchies (like meronomy)**: taxonomy is fundamental, but it is not necessarily natural or convivial. For this reason, other hierarchies like a meronomy based on the part_of attribute of any object are important to define and to make explicit in a model.

- **Horizontal links**: if a hierarchy is usually associated to the vertical direction, horizontal links are the expression of relationships between objects in different branches. Such relationships are as essential in a model as the hierarchical links.

- **Definitions**: when modelling objects of a domain and when each object has been given a unique identifier, the need to be very precise about this object is present. When communicating about an object, one wants to be sure to be understood! This raises the problem of definition of the objects[1].

- **Evolution and maintenance**: This point is related to the methodology used for modelling and its repercussions on evolution and maintenance of the model, where numerous pitfalls are awaiting the newcomers.

3. The modelling of gross anatomy

In this section, the most relevant above steps will be reviewed when applied to the domain of gross anatomy. It will be shown that the convergence of actions from several groups working independently brings an excellent solution to the scientific community. Of course, the process of final integration remains to be done, but this paper wants to emphasize a possible realistic solution not so far from being concrete.

Each step as given in the preceding section should be developed in turn. In all cases, the following aspects of the model shall be considered: adequacy for computer programmes, including the multilingual constraints, adequacy for human beings, logical soundness and coherence and uniqueness of the source. In order to concentrate on the major aspects, the points on meronomy, horizontal links and evolution will be skipped. They will certainly be developed in another paper.

---

[1] Not everybody is really sure of what is meant by the TA term A02.6.02.010: hidden part of duodenum!

Naming the objects of the domain

For centuries now, human beings have compiled list of terms relevant for the description of the human body. Facing a plethoric vocabulary emerging from uncontrolled sources, the Federative Committee on Anatomical Terminology edited in 1998 the first version of the TA [3], which has the statutes of a universal agreement. For a predefined degree of detail, this compilation is representative with more than 7400 different entries of the whole body.

In addition, there are thousands of alternative terms naming the same objects, either from historical sources, national variations and eponyms[2]. Whatever the recommendation for their usage, all these alternate terms do exist and do occur elsewhere in the patient medical record if not in the scientific literature. Therefore, the proper naming of this domain requires an extension of the TA naming by existing sources. This task is partially language dependent; hopefully large similarities between languages exist. The authors are preparing now a database for French, Latin and English starting from the original TA and compiling several lexicons [4] and atlases. Currently more than two terms per object and per language are present as a mean value for the TA.

This effort is only partially adequate for computer applications, because of the versatility of languages: there are tens of different ways to speak about the same objects, as it has been demonstrated in a recent article [5]. The current list of anatomical terms is representative but it is not exhaustive. This means that some intelligent processing should take place elsewhere for a close to perfect recognition of body parts entities spread into free texts. On the contrary, this effort is satisfactory for human beings: the reader usually retrieves more names for a specified object than he knows and he is able to solve more or less trivially the language variations.

Logical soundness is a major difficulty when naming anatomical objects, because there is always a need or a temptation to document this object at the same time: what is the formally sound name for *deltoid tubercle of spine of posterior surface of scapula* or anything shorter? There is certainly a need to make a term self explanatory when seen outside of its context, but this need should not spill out the naming task (a quite common error). The solution to this problem, as implemented by the author [6], is to perform automatically the expansion of a term and to store only the minimal distinctive part (*deltoid tubercle* only). A few specific database attributes are driving the expansion on an individual term and language basis. Basic terms as well as their expansion are later available for display or for other programs. The minimal distinctive part sometimes generates polysemies, but the expansion is here for solving this problem.

The existence in a single database of all variants in multiple languages and the fact that this database may be updated with new terms at any time is part of a guaranty that no other source is necessary. This reference database may de facto act as a unique source, saving the underlying principle.

Identification or code

The main quality of an identifier is its uniqueness: one object of the domain gets one and only one identifier. Setting a unique identifier is often complicated by the fact that one is embarrassed by taxonomy considerations: it is certainly a quite common error to mix identification and hierarchy representation[3]. Nothing is better than a sequential number.

---

[2] Eponyms concern the usage of Proper names when naming body parts (like Meckel's diverticule).
[3] This is the case for ICD10, where the code represents the chapter and the category, with a huge embarrass when more than 10 subdivisions happen, because they are not accepted!

Anyway, there are several situations where the position in the hierarchy is reflected in the identifier or what is often called a code.

The former naming task provides in general more than one term for each existing object. In the domain of anatomy, it is not rare to have five or more terms in one language for a single object. The goal of the identification task is to assign an identifier to each set of terms pointing to the same object. As a consequence each synonym in the set is linked to the same identifier.

The difficulty is due to the fact that it may not be known precisely what is the meaning of a given term. In addition, it will be seen below that the problem of definitions is not yet fully resolved. In these conditions there is always a risk of attributing a term to the wrong object.

The easiest solution is the attribution of a code systematically by program, often using sequential numbers not reusable after deletion. The solution is totally adequate for computer usage, but not convivial nor error prone for human beings, who are not good when handling long numbers. The anonymous aspect of such an identifier makes it logically sound. The computer generation of identifier guaranty the uniqueness of the identifiers.

In the case of anatomy, the design of the taxonomy is realized under the form of the FMA model as shown in the next subsection. This system implemented as a computer application generates sequential numbers having the necessary qualities. Moreover, such an internal identifier is substituted to the TA code, this later becoming simply an attribute of each object. This is the way to escape numerous difficulties arising from the badly shaped TA code [7].

Taxonomy

Building the taxonomy of objects in a domain is the princept part of any knowledge representation schema. For a domain as complex as the gross anatomy, this task should be counted in months if not in years of work. Hopefully, the work has already been done by Cornelius Rosse and his team at University of Washington, giving birth to the Foundational Model of Anatomy, and incorporating the objects of the TA [8]. This project is a long-term development and has not yet reach a full coverage of all attributes of the objects of the domain, but its 80'000 existing objects including totally the TA is a solid ground. Copy of the model is available from the developer for free if the goal is research and development.

The taxonomy has been developed on a sound logical basis, without compromise, by a team competent in anatomy and with solid background on knowledge representation with computers, knowing the last refinements of the science of ontology. The isa taxonomy is pure from top to bottom including all objects. A Protégé implementation is an easy way to play with this model and to understand its intricacies and goodies. In addition, the model allows seeing the objects in several side hierarchies like a part-of hierarchy, but nowhere the different hierarchies are intermixed. The original TA hierarchy is ignored in this model; only the TA objects are considered and matched to the FMA.

A computer program based on this model receives the benefit of the sound isa hierarchy: inheritance of properties and possibility to generalize through the hierarchy. This last feature is typically necessary to match a query against a factual data when they are not given at the exact same level of detail.

However, such taxonomy is not really convivial for human beings: it lacks the natural feeling of the more traditional organization by system for example. The answer to this criticism is coming from the possibility to browse several hierarchies in parallel. Typically, a meronomy (part-of links) is more natural when teaching anatomy than the given taxonomy: a *renal papilla* is part of the *inner zone*, which is part of the *renal medulla*, which is part of the *kidney*, which is part of the *urinary system*. Being built on formal basis, the model is perfectly coherent and satisfactory to this point of view.

The uniqueness of this model is guaranteed for at least three reasons: the model is good; to develop another model is too expensive and necessitates a large know-how; this model is adequately available to any interested scientific user.

Definitions

In a companion paper [6], the author has made the distinction between 5 approaches to the problem of definition on the basis of a research on actual publications in this matter. The 5 solutions are the following: encyclopedic definitions, formal taxonomic definitions, other hierarchical solutions (meronomy), multimedia definition and semantic stemming. It soon appears that any solution is either favorable to human beings or to computers, but generally not to both of them.

The encyclopedic definitions are the kind of definitions we find in a regular dictionary. They are made of natural language and therefore, despite they are very useful for human beings, computers rarely use them. A number of good dictionaries are made available in electronic format.

Formal definitions are built on the basis of a recognized taxonomy, by application of the principle of *genus et differentia*. Other hierarchical definitions may be constructed following links like *part_of* or *branch_of*. In theory, when appending successive extracted sentences through several consecutive levels in the hierarchy, a concrete definition is prepared. With the help of a few syntactic clues, it is possible to arrange such definition to something acceptable for a human reader. But the final result is somewhat artificial for human beings. Work in this direction is to be mentioned [9].

Multimedia definitions may be important and significant in several domains, in particular anatomy: an image with a pointer may act as an extremely precise definition[4].

Semantic stemming allows extracting the meaning of compound words on the basis of known rules validated for a specific language. A recent development on automatic extraction of definitions [10] based on morphosemantic decomposition technique is valid for neoclassical compound words quite frequent in the medical domain. An example is *achloropsy*, which automatically extracted meaning is *pathology characterized by the lack of vision of green*.

Computer programs are satisfied either by the formal definition, the hierarchical solutions or partly by the semantic stemming solution. NLP applications may take advantage of these definitions, but to the expense of delicate supplementary processing: it is indeed not easy to take advantage of a formal definition to disambiguate a term.

Human beings will be happy with the encyclopedic solution, the hierarchical solution and the multimedia definition. The best intersection between the two modes is the hierarchical solution. This means that a particular effort should be agreed with good priority on this topic.

A typical and prevalent example of hierarchical definition is the meronomy or *part_of* hierarchy. It is pleasant to human because it is natural and has been adopted for decades by the teachers of anatomy: it is direct to sketch an anatomical site with all its parts and subparts in a unique drawing. But the same technique of presentation is also convenient for programs if it is issued automatically from a formal model. This is actually the case with

---

[4] The *carpal bones* are usually presented in a vertical view of the hand, but the *carpal tunnel* is invisible there and a transverse view is necessary, in order to act as a definition.

the FMA. It comes with the logical soundness of the model. It is particularly effective in the subdomain of anatomy. The uniqueness of source is preserved with this solution.

4. Discussion and conclusion

Is the coverage of the FMA model sufficient for NLP applications? This implies that besides the structure of the model, each object should have attached several attributes relevant for linguistic processing. The authors of the FMA know about this aspect. Second the author of this paper is preparing new terms with more extensive coverage in English and in French to be possibly made available with some future version of the FMA. Extension to other languages is expected to take place in the future.

We have shown on all the developed points above that the FMA is a satisfactory if not an excellent solution. This is also true for the other points, which have been skipped. This is enough to conclude that anatomy is a favoured terrain, because such a complete solution is generally not available in other subdomain of medicine. This is due to the fact that anatomy is one of the oldest basic medical sciences and that it has been extensively documented for centuries now. But this also means that current formal representations and state of the art for knowledge representation using extensively computer programs have reach a productive status. Last but not least, it indicates that knowledge representation techniques have to be married with NLP techniques in order to reach such a degree of satisfaction. In the future, it will be difficult to trust a totally ontological perspective as well as a purely terminological approach: only mixed solutions have a chance to convince the potential users.

5. Acknowledgements

This work has been partly funded by the Swiss National Science Foundation (SNF 632-066041).

References

[1] C Rosse. Anatomy atlases. Clin. Anat. 1999; 12(4):293-9.

[2] R Baud. Natural Language as an Ontology: Who is Teaching to Whom? EFMI Special Topics Conference 2005, Athens. To be published in Int J Med Inform.

[3] Federative Committee on Anatomical Terminology. Terminologia Anatomica: International Anatomical Terminology. Thieme Ed. 1998.

[4] Dorland WAN. Dorland's Illustrated Medical Dictionary. 30rd ed. Philadelphia. Saunders; 2003.

[5] Baud RH, Ruch P, Gaudinat A, Fabry P, Lovis C, Geissbuhler A. Coping with the variability of medical terms. Medinfo. 2004;2004:322-6.

[6] Baud RH, Fabry P, Namer F, Griesser V, Ruch P, Lovis C, Geissbuhler A. Version francophone de la Terminologia Anatomica. Journées francophones d'informatique médicale, Lille France, May 2005.

[7] Rosse C. Terminologia anatomica: considered from the perspective of next-generation knowledge sources. Clin Anat 2001;14(2):120-33

[8] Rosse C, Mejino JL. A reference Ontology for Biomedical Informatics: the Fundational Model of Anatomy. J Biomed Inform 2003 ;36(6) :478-500.

[9] Michael J, Mejino JL Jr, Rosse C. The role of definitions in biomedical concept representation. Proc AMIA Symp. 2001;:463-7.

[10] Namer F, Baud R. Guessing lexical relations between biomedical terms: towards a multilingual morphosemantics-based system. Proceedings of MIE2005, Geneva Aug 2005, this conference.

Connecting Medical Informatics and Bio-Informatics
R. Engelbrecht et al. (Eds.)
IOS Press, 2005

659

Building Medical Ontologies Based on Terminology Extraction from Texts: an Experimentation in Pneumology

Audrey Baneyx[a], Jean Charlet[a,b], Marie-Christine Jaulent[a]

[a]*INSERM U729, Paris, F-75006, France;*
[b]*STIM DSI/AP-HP, Paris, F-75014, France;*

Abstract

Pathologies and acts are classified in thesauri to help physicians to code their activity. In practice, the use of thesauri is not sufficient to reduce variability in coding and thesauri do not fit computer processing. We think the automation of the coding task requires a conceptual modelling of medical items: an ontology. Our objective is to help pneumologists code acts and diagnoses with a software that represents medical knowledge by an ontology of the concerned specialty. The main research hypothesis is to apply natural language processing tools to corpora to develop the resources needed to build the ontology. In this paper, our objective is twofold: we have to build the ontology of pneumology and we want to develop a methodology for the knowledge engineer to build various types of medical ontologies based on terminology extraction from texts.

Keywords:
Ontology, Terminology Extraction, Knowledge Engineering, Differential Semantics, Natural Language Processing, Pneumology.

1. Introduction

In many medical specialities, pathologies and acts are classified in thesauri to help physicians to code their activity. It has become obvious that the use of such thesauri is not sufficient to reduce variability in coding. Indeed, wording of thesauri is ambiguous (for instance as several pathologies apply to a unique code) and non-exhaustive; the chosen classification method is difficult to use; lastly, maintaining either consistency or coherence of thesauri is impossible. Moreover, the interpretation of wording of medical terminologies depends on the human reader, and as such are not adapted to computer processing. We think that the automation of the coding task requires a conceptual modelling (an ontology non-contextual and unambiguous) of medical items whose meaning would be written inside the model's structure itself. Such modelling is called "ontology" [1]. The word "ontology" used in philosophy has been reused since the beginning of the 1990's mainly in artificial intelligence, knowledge engineering and knowledge representation. Nowadays, its scope is growing and it becomes a common item in the field of information-system modelling [2]. An ontology is a formal system whose objective is to represent a specific domain knowledge by means of basic elements, the concepts, that are defined and organised each one in relation to the others [3]. Ontology insures to maintain axioms' coherence and system's integrity as well as extensibility of the structure without modifying it. The main difficulty is to identify and classify the items of a given domain. Since classification criteria depend on purposes and are not universal, we do not seek to build a universal ontology, but merely a specific ontology of pneumology. This work is part of the PERTOMed[1] research project whose objective is to develop an internet platform offering a range of methods and tools to produce and use terminological and ontological resources in the medical field. Specific medical ontologies are created in close partnership with user groups, who will participate in the evaluation processes of these resources in their real use environment. Our task in the project is to help pneumologists code acts and diagnoses with a software that represents medical knowledge by an ontology of the concerned specialty. The main research hypothesis of PERTOMed is to apply natural language processing (NLP) tools to corpora to develop the resources needed to build the ontology. Thus, an important task is to create textual corpora necessary for NLP tools.

In this paper, the objective is twofold. On the one hand, we have to build the ontology of pneumology and, on the other hand, we want to contrive a methodology for the knowledge engineer to build various types of medical ontologies based on the differential semantics theory [4].

Section 2 presents the material and tools used for the experimentation. Section 3 details the different steps of the methodology. Section 4 presents the results we obtained and last, in section 5, we conclude this paper by discussing perspectives expected from this work.

2. Material

Presentation of the two corpora

In order to cover the whole area of pneumology, we have gathered patient discharge summaries (PDS) in six hospitals of the Assistance Publique-Hôpitaux de Paris. We ended up with a total of 1 038 PDS. In a previous work about a different domain, it has been showed that 350 000 words seems to be a good indicator [5]. In the pneumology case, the first corpus [PDS] has about 417 000 words which is a good base for the experimentation. We added a teaching book to that first corpus, which permitted to refine and control the hierarchical structure of the ontology during the development. That second corpus [BOOK] has about 823 000 words.

Available tools

We use SYNTEX-UPERY as an NLP tool. SYNTEX is a syntax analyser module allowing us to get a network of syntactic dependencies between terms - or terminological network - whose elements are the candidate terms that will be used for the building of the ontology. UPERY is a distributional analyser module computing distributional proximities between candidate terms on the basis of shared syntaxical contexts. It exploits all the network data to cluster needed terms. We obtain a network of candidate terms, their contextual associations and their links to the corpus. The differential ontology editor DOE[2] allows us to build our ontology according to the differential semantics theory proposed in [4].

3. Method

The Bachimont's methodology used to design differential ontologies allows us to describe variations of the words' meaning in context. It stresses the importance of the textual corpus [6], since that corpus is the best source to characterize notions useful for the ontological modelling and the semantic content that is associated with them. We distinguish four successive steps: 1) the constitution of the corpus of knowledge and its analysis by NLP

---

[1] http://www.spim.jussieu.fr/Pertomed
[2] http://opales.ina.fr/public/

tools, 2) the semantic normalization of the set of terms through the application of differential principles, 3) the ontological engagement to formalize defined concepts, 4) the finalization of the process in a language, based on description logics, understandable by the computer [4]. Our experimentation in the pneumology specialty brings both precision and adapts the first two steps of the methodology to the knowledge engineer which is a contribution of our second objective.

Processing of basic resources

The two [PDS] and [BOOK] corpora resources are first processed in order to obtain an anonymous [PDS] corpus, and a didactical [BOOK] corpus, both in XML format. They are processed by SYNTEX-UPERY. The result of the analysis of candidate terms in the [PDS] corpus allows us to build the basic elements – i.e. primitives – of the ontology. A candidate term is a noun phrase (NP) composed by a head and an expansion. For instance, in the NP *Opacity in the left lung*, the term *Opacity* is the head and *in the left lung* is its expansion. The results of the analysis of the [BOOK] corpus are processed themselves to identify hyperonymy links between candidate terms [6], using lexico-syntactic patterns. Those links help us to structure the hierarchy of primitive concepts.

Building of the ontology, stage 1: choice of the candidate terms

Candidate terms representative of pneumology are chosen within the results provided by SYNTEX-UPERY from the [PDS] corpus in two steps:

1) We scan all the results provided by the syntaxical analysis and choose to first study the NP that appear in the corpus more than 12 times (2% of the corpus). From then, we spot the major conceptual axes that are typical of the corpus and the medical field. To each candidate term, we associate a validity criterion that matches one of those axes, on a 1 to 6 scale: 1 (non pertinent terms, axis: other), 2 (reserved for terms which are modellised in the ontology), 3 (axis: symptoms), 4 (axis: pathologies), 5 (axis: treatments) and 6 (axis: examinations). For instance, we associate the validity criterion 6 with all candidate terms on that axis – e.g. *echography, doppler, ultrasonography*, and so on… At the beginning of the method, all the candidate terms have a validity criterion equal to 1 and at the end they are all classified on the axis 2 (which means they have been completely defined in the ontology). Validity criteria 3, 4, 5 and 6 are used temporarily during the building phase (stage 2). This gathering allows the beginning of a first stage of work on the connection by context and the selection by validity criteria leaves 35% of candidate terms on which we can work out the heart of our ontology.

2) The distributional analysis connects terms sharing the same contexts (descendants in head and descendants in expansion). It also connects the contexts according to the terms they share (neighbours in head and neighbours in expansion). On the example (Cf. Table 1), *effusion* is the head of the NP *effusion of pleura* and *of pleura* is its expansion. Descendants in head yield information on what could be child-concepts or defined concepts. Descendants in expansion provide information about the concept's position in the hierarchy. Neighbours in head and in expansion allow us to constitute the groupings of candidate terms semantically close to the one under study, *effusion of pleura*. Groupings are a great help for the development of the hierarchical structure of the ontology, for both horizontal and vertical axes. The example below shows a first possible connection: we can link group A *{effusion, lesion, infection, uncompensation}* with *{symptoms}*. The candidate terms of group A share the same semantical context. Our first hypothesis will be to consider the candidate terms of group A as sibling-concepts and *symptoms* as the parent-concept.

Table 1 – Sample results of the contextual connections for the NP "Effusion of pleura"

Descendants in head	Descendants in expansion	Neighbours in head	Neighbours in expansion
Effusion of the right part of pleura	Tapping of pleural effusion	Lesions	Liquid
Effusion of liquid	Recurrence of pleural effusion	Infections	Infiltration
Effusion of the pleural cavity	Link between dyspnoea and pleural effusion	Symptoms	Uncompensation

Building of the ontology, stage 2: application of differential principles

In order to work the hierarchy out, the candidate terms chosen in stage 1 are organised by refining the differential principles that define them. We have to express in natural language the similarities and differences of each concept with respect to its parent-concept and its sibling-concepts. For instance, the concept of *Ultrasonography* and the concept of *IsotopicExamination* are sibling-concepts whose parent-concept is *RayImaging*. The principle of similarities with the parent-concept is the projection or the injection of an artificial substance in order to take measures. The principle of similarities between sibling-concepts is related to the injection medium. The differencial principle between sibling-concepts is related to the kind of artificial medium used: an isotope in the case of an isotopic examination and ultrasounds in the case of ultrasonography. The 4 axes (3, 4, 5, and 6) are refined that way. In addition, we use the results of the processing of the [BOOK] corpus to help us in applying the differential principles according to the method described in [4].

During the building process, the knowledge engineer must distinguish between primitive and defined concepts. A primitive concept is essential to the representation of the specialty. A defined concept is built from one or more primitive concepts and one or more relationships. The NP *left thoracic pain* is modellised by the following defined concept: [pain] (at the) [thorax] (located on) [left][3].

At the end of this stage, we have a semantic normalization of the set of terms of the specialty and we have represented the hierarchy of primitive concepts and relationships with DOE.

4. Results

Primitive concepts and their organisation

After using SYNTEX process, the [PDS] corpus gives 36 881 NP and the [BOOK] corpus gives 17 666 NP. According to the results of the syntaxical and distributional analyses, the NP *Chemotherapy of <noun>* has the most neighbours in head, 28, and has 90 appearances in the corpus. The NP *<noun> of chemotherapy* has the most neighbours in expansion, 52, and has the highest appearance rate, 454. We can check the pertinence of the connections by group of candidate terms whose appearance contexts are semantically close. For instance, *course of chemotherapy* has *{Hospitalization, Examination, Navelbine, Cisplatine, Taxotere, Carboplatine}* as its neighbours in head and has *{Treatment, Check-up, Antibiotherapy, Injection, Radiotherapy}* as its neighbours in expansion. These results are examined and then transformed into ontological form, using DOE. We build the following hierarchy: *MedicalAction/Treatment/DrugTreatment/Chemotherapy*. Chemotherapy being considered as a drug treatment, we find the following medicinal principles classified under *Medicine/.../MedicinalPrinciple/Navelbine,   Cisplatine,   Doxorubicine,   Taxotere,*

---

[3] The square brackets indicate a primitive concept and the brackets indicate a relationship. In our methodology, relationships are processed in the same way as concepts.

Carboplatine. The candidate terms *Antibiotherapy* and *Radiotherapy* are also located under *Treatment.* This method for regrouping yields an ontology and makes the task much easier for a knowledge engineer who would not be a specialist in the modellised medical specialty. Our ontology includes today 750 primitive concepts stemming from the first study of the candidate terms. Given that the building stages 1 and 2 are iterative, we will rapidly increase the hierarchy by examining the candidate terms which appear less than 12 times in the [PDS] corpus.

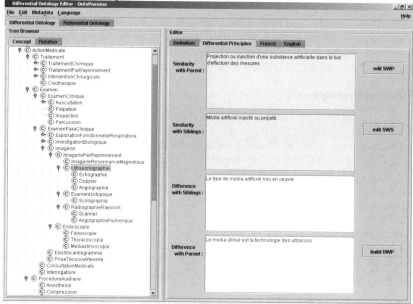

– *An extract of the ontology of the pneumology viewed with DOE*

Preliminary method of validation

The ontology is to be evaluated in terms of both quality and coverage. The conceptual hierarchy must be corrected and validated by pneumologists from the French Pneumology Society with whom we collaborate. The evaluation will also test the completeness of the ontology compared to the specialty thesaurus. To estimate that completeness, we will check the possibility of building a conceptual representation of medical knowledge by combining the primitive concepts and the relationships in the ontology. Today, we are able to build some phrases, for instance the phrase *Chemotherapy intra-pleural*, which is in the Pleura chapter in the thesaurus.

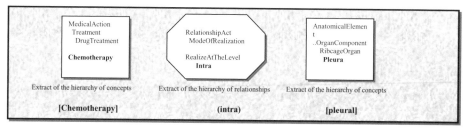

5. Discussion and conclusion

An important issue of this work is to show that our methodology allows a knowledge engineer, a non-specialist in the modellised field, to build ontology from texts, using NLP tools. As a new experimentation, we have tried to work out an organisation of the pneumology concepts, both coherent and stable, based on the practical application of the principles of differential semantics. The initial results of our research coupled with a recent work on surgical intensive care gives us reasons to think we are moving in the right direction [5]. We also forecast an extension of the ontology by analysing the terms specific to pneumology in the ICD-10[4] and CCAM[5] thesauri. We plan to complete this ontology by connecting it to the head (conceptual high level) of the Ménélas project ontology[6] [7]. We assume we will rapidly get an ontology of pneumology of approximately 1 200 concepts. The validation of the ontology can only be done through its use in concrete applications. It must be made available for the medical profession through an environment for helping the coding of acts and diagnoses and the representation of medical knowledge, as part of the terminological platform of the PERTOMed project.

6. Thanks and acknowledgments

We would like to particularly thank Pr Thomas Similowski for his help, Mr Didier Bourigault for making available SYNTEX-UPERY, Mrs Raphaël Troncy and Antoine Isaac who helped us in the use of DOE. We also wish to thank Pr Bruno Housset (Service de Pneumologie, Centre Hospitalier InterCommunal de Créteil, et Société de Pneumologie de Langue Française), Pr Bernard Maitre (Unité de Pneumologie, CHU Henri-Mondor, Créteil), Dr François-Xavier Blanc (Unité de Pneumologie, Service de Médecine Interne, CHU du Kremlin-Bicêtre, le Kremlin-Bicêtre), Dr Nicolas Roche (Service de Pneumologie, Hôtel-Dieu, Paris), Pr Christos Chouaid (Service de Pneumologie, Hôpital St-Antoine, Paris), Pr Jacques Cadranel (Service de Pneumologie, Hôpital Tenon, Paris), Pr Marc Humbert (Service de Pneumologie, Hôpital Antoine Béclère, Clamart), and Dr Alexandre Duguet (Unité de Réanimation du Service de Pneumologie, Groupe Hospitalier Pitié-Salpêtrière, Paris) for having taken time to collect the resources necessary for our work.

7. References

[1]   Staab S and Studer R. *Handbook on Ontologies.* 1st ed. Berlin: Springer, Handbooks in Information Systems, 2003.

[2]   Gomez-Pérez A, Fernandez-Lopez M, and Corcho O, eds. *Ontological Engineering.* 2nd ed. Madrid: Springer, Advanced Information and Knowledge Processing, 2004.

[3]   Rector A. L. Thesauri and Formal Classifications: Terminologies for People and Machines. *Methods of Information in Medicine, 1998.* 37: 501-9.

[4]   Bachimont B, Isaac A, and Troncy R. Semantic Commitment for Designing Ontologies: A Proposal. In Gomez-Pérez A and Richard Benjamins V, eds. *EKAW'2002.*

[5]   Le Moigno S, Charlet J, Bourigault D, Degoulet P, and Jaulent M-C. Terminology extraction from text to build an ontology in surgical intensive care. *AMIA, 2002.* 9-13.

[6]   Malaisé V, Zweigenbaum P, and Bachimont B. Mining defining contexts to help structuring differential ontologies. In Ibekwe-San Juan F, Condamines A and Cabré T, eds. Terminology, 2005. 11(1).To appear

[7]   Zweigenbaum P, Bouaud J, Bachimont B, Charlet J, Séroussi B, and Boisvieux J-F. From text to knowledge: a unifying document-oriented view of analyzed medical language. Methods of Information in Medicine, 1998. 384-393.

Address for correspondence

Audrey BANEYX, INSERM U729 - Laboratoire SPIM, Faculté de Médecine Broussais-Hôtel-Dieu
15 rue de l'Ecole de médecine, 75006 Paris – France, Email: audrey.baneyx@spim.jussieu.fr, Mobile: 06 62 77 59 85

---

[4] The ICD-10 thesaurus is a medical and economic code for patients and allows analysing the activity of hospitals via diagnostic related groups.
[5] The French CCAM thesaurus is a complete and new classification of medical acts.
[6] http://www.biomath.jussieu.fr/Menelas/Ontologie/html/

Connecting Medical Informatics and Bio-Informatics
R. Engelbrecht et al. (Eds.)
IOS Press, 2005

Towards a Multilingual Version of Terminologia Anatomica

Paul Fabry, Robert Baud, Christian Lovis

Service d'Informatique Médicale, Hôpital Universitaire de Genève, Suisse

Abstract:

Objective: Terminologia Anatomica (TA) is the new standard in anatomical terminology. This terminology is available only in Latin and English and its worldwide adoption is subdued to the addition of terms from others languages. On the other hand Nomina Anatomica (NA), the previous standard, has been widely translated. Aim of this work was to append foreign terms to TA by using similarity matching algorithm between its Latin terms and those from NA.
Methods: A semi-automatic matching of Latin terms from TA with those of NA was performed using a string-to-string distance algorithm and manual assessment. We used a French – Latin version of NA together with TA and we suggested French terms for TA. Coverage was evaluated by the number of exact and approximate matches. A target of 80% was set due to the superior number of terms in TA compared to NA. Relevance was estimated by manually comparing the meanings of the English and French terms related to the same Latin term. The question was whether they refer to the same anatomical structure.
Results: Exact or approximate matches were found for 5,982 terms (76.5%) of TA. Our results outlined that more than 75% of the terms from TA came from NA, most of them were left unchanged and all were used with the same meaning.
Conclusion: This method produces relevant results, reaching our 80% target. The method is based only on Latin terms and can be used for other languages and for others terminologies including Latin terms.

Keywords:
Anatomy, Terminologia Anatomica, Nomina Anatomica, Terminology mapping, French language

1. Introduction

The advancement of human anatomy took centuries and occurred in many countries, each using its own language. It was estimated that there were some 50,000 anatomical terms in use at the end of the 19th century but they applied only to some 5,000 to 6,000 structures [1]. Not only several terms were related to the same structure (synonyms) but one term could be used to name different structures (homonyms) depending on its author. In addition, many of these terms were eponyms, i.e. terms including a proper noun.

In order to overcome this obstacle, the International Federation of Associations of Anatomists (IFAA) led to the publication of the first international terminology of anatomy, the *Nomina Anatomica*, (NA, [2]) in 1955. NA included a list of 5,640 Latin terms related to the macroscopic anatomy, to be translated into existing languages.

From 1955 to 1989, NA had six editions with additions in embryology (Nomina Embryologica) and histology (Nomina Histologica) but with only minor modifications in anatomy compared to the original version. Meanwhile, the advances in medicine, particularly in surgical procedures and neurosciences, led to the individualization of new anatomical structures and therefore, to the creation of new anatomical terms, especially in regard to the central nervous system.

In order to provide standardization for these new terms, a new terminology, the Terminologia Anatomica (TA, [3]), was published in 1998. TA provides a list of some 7,500 structures considering the macroscopic anatomy. In addition to Latin terms, TA includes their English counterparts in current usage and the most frequent eponyms, and indexes all the terms using alphanumerical codes.

TA is now considered as the new international standard in anatomical terminology [4]. However, to support its diffusion in non English-speaking countries, an important work is needed to translate its terms and to match them with the multiple synonyms and eponyms present in the anatomical language. On the other hand, NA is still widely used as a reference throughout the world and its Latin terms are associated with terms in other language such as French, Spanish, etc.

An approach for easing the translation of TA is to use a bilingual version of NA and match its Latin terms with those of TA. In this article, we present a methodology using a string-to-string distance algorithm to perform a semi-automatic matching of Latin terms from TA with those of NA. The method was evaluated by using a French – Latin version of NA together with TA in order to suggest French terms for TA.

2. Materials and methods

2.1 Nomina Anatomica and Terminologia Anatomica

Nomina Anatomica (NA) provides a list of approximately 6,000 Latin terms without definition (Figure 1). The order of terms follows a classification by functions and regions into nine chapters. In addition, text indentations and styles of headings are used to represent relationships between the terms but without explicating the type of the relationship (*is a, part of, branch of,* etc.).

NOMINA ANATOMICA	TERMINOLOGIA ANATOMICA		
Arteria auricularis posterior	A12.2.05.037	**Arteria auricularis posterior**	**Posterior auricular artery**
A. stylomastoidea	A12.2.05.038	A. stylomastoidea	Stylomastoid artery
A. tympanica posterior	A12.2.05.039	A. tympanica posterior	Posterior tympanic artery
Rami mastoidei	A12.2.05.040	Rr. mastoidei	Mastoid branch
†(Ramus stapedialis)	A12.2.05.041	†(R. stapedius)	(Stapedial branch)
Ramus auricularis	A12.2.05.042	R. auricularis	Auricular branch
Ramus occipitalis	A12.2.05.043	R. occipitalis	Occipital branch
	A12.2.05.044	R. parotideus	Parotid branch

†*The terms in brackets refer to inconstant anatomical structures.*

Figure 1: The Posterior auricular artery and its branches in Nomina Anatomica, 5th edition (left) and in Terminologia Anatomica (right). A new structure, Ramus parotideus (parotid branch) has been individualized in Terminologia Anatomica.

In order to limit its size, a compositional approach was adopted. For example, in Figure 1, text indentations designate the term *Rami mastoidei* (mastoid branches) as a child (or hyponym) of *A. tympanica posterior* (posterior tympanic artery). The term *Rami mastoidei* alone is not relevant and the user has to infer that the proper term is *Rami mastoidei arteriae tympanicae posterioris* (mastoid branches of the posterior tympanic artery).

There is no bilingual version of NA directly available but its terms are usually found associated with terms in other languages in various anatomy textbooks.

Terminologia Anatomica (TA) is departing from the fifth edition of NA and keeps the compositional approach (Figure 1). TA also uses a classification by function and regions, though more precise as it includes sixteen chapters. TA maintains the use of Latin and includes the terms of NA with minor differences (*stapedialis* in NA vs. *stapedius* in TA in Figure 1), but adds English terms and eponyms. TA has a richer structure: each anatomical structure is represented by a code, which is used to index all the related terms.

Both terminologies make use of abbreviations such as A. for arteria, R. for Ramus, etc.

2.2 Methodology

NA and TA were considered as raw lists of terms, letting apart all the knowledge implied by the position of a term in the list and its relationships with adjacent terms.

The methodology was designed in three main steps:
- Creation of electronic sources for TA and NA.
- Semi-automatic mapping of Latin terms.
- Evaluation of the coverage and the relevance of the results.

2.2.1 Creation of electronic sources

For NA, we used the index of French anatomy textbook and a dictionary [5, 6]. We chose these sources instead of the original NA hardcopy for two reasons: first, they provide French terms related to those of NA, second, they do not have a compositional approach and the Latin terms are fully extended. These sources were processed with an optical character recognition (OCR) software. We manually corrected the errors generated by the OCR and created a list including couples Latin term – French term.

The task was easier for TA as its codes and Latin terms (extended) are present in the Foundational Model of Anatomy (FMA, [7]). Nevertheless, we also processed the hardcopy of TA with OCR software to generate our own version and combined it with the one present in the FMA to be as exhaustive as possible.

2.2.2 String matching

An algorithm was developed using edit distance for matching approximate strings. Prior to the distance computation, all terms were pre-processed for normalization: conversion to all lower case, removal of punctuation signs and brackets, expansion of abbreviations and alphabetical sorting of the words in each term. All the pre-processing steps were performed automatically; the abbreviations present in our corpuses were unambiguous and easily expandable. Then, for each normalized term of TA, the edit distance was measured with all the normalized terms from NA.

Edit distance defines a set of edit operations on characters, such as deletion, insertion or substitution, together with a cost for each operation. Given two strings x and y, the distance between them is the minimum number of edit operations required to transform x into y. We used a rather simple edit distance known as the Levenshtein-Damereau [8, 9] distance, which assigns the same cost for each edit operation.

Three cases were considered for string matching: 1) the strings are equal: there is an exact match; 2) all the strings from NA have a distance superior to 0. Then the five closest strings are provided for manual validation. If one of these strings is validated: there is an approximate match; 3) if none of the five closest strings is validated: there is no match.

2.2.3 Evaluation

The former steps resulted in the generation of a list of quadruplets including a TA code, the corresponding Latin and English terms, and a French term. An evaluation of the coverage was given by the number of TA codes found in the list. However, as there are approximately 1,500 more anatomical structures in TA than in NA, the expected coverage could not exceed 80%. Then, the meanings of English and French terms related to the same code were manually compared. The question was whether they refer to the same anatomical structure.

3. Results

For NA, a list of 8,885 couples Latin term – French term was generated[1]. Regarding TA, we found 7,415 different codes related to 8,449 Latin terms and 9,201 English terms.

Exact and approximate matches were found respectively for 4,863 and 1,119 terms of TA. The large majority of Latin terms from NA present in TA have been left unchanged.

The methodology provided a French term for 5,671 (76.5%) codes of TA. An excerpt of the results is given in Table 1. The overall coverage is satisfactory taken into account the limit of 80% due to the superior number of terms in TA.

Table 1: Results for the Posterior auricular artery and its branches.
The "?" indicates that no match have been found. [†]All terms are extended.

TA Code	[†]English Term	[†]French Term
A12.2.05.037	Posterior auricular artery	Artère auriculaire postérieure
A12.2.05.038	Stylomastoid artery	Artère stylo-mastoïdienne
A12.2.05.039	Posterior tympanic artery	Artère tympanique postérieure
A12.2.05.040	Mastoid branch of posterior tympanic artery	Branche mastoïdienne de l'artère tympanique postérieure
A12.2.05.041	Stapedial branch of posterior tympanic artery	?
A12.2.05.042	Auricular branch of posterior auricular artery	Branche auriculaire de l'artère auriculaire postérieure
A12.2.05.043	Occipital branch of posterior auricular artery	Branche occipitale de l'artère auriculaire postérieure
A12.2.05.044	Parotid branch of posterior auricular artery	?

More than 75% of the matching strings were the strings with the smallest distance. On the other hand, there was no correlation between the distance value and the rank.

No approximate match due to an OCR error was found. The main cause of approximate matches was the term extension. Because of the compositional approach taken by both NA and TA, the terms require to be extended and variants may appear during this process. For example, three different extensions were found in our sources for the term *Lamina horizontalis* (Horizontal plate) and its hypernym *Os palatinum* (Palatine bone): *Lamina horizontalis (Os palatinum)*, *Lamina horizontalis ossis palatini*, and *Lamina horizontalis palatini*. English and French terms also showed these kinds of modifications.

---

[1] The number of Latin terms obtained in our corpus (8,885) is surprisingly large compared to the size of NA (about 6,000 terms). This is due to the presence of variants among the Latin terms and to the fact that the used sources included also Latin terms from Nomina Histologica and Nomina Embryologica.

The relevance of the results was evaluated by comparing the meanings of French and English terms related to the same TA code. This comparison was done manually by a physician with the help of medical dictionaries and anatomical atlases. No difference was found and the terms from NA present in TA are used with the same meaning.

4. Discussion

Our goal was to propose a practical method to append terms in others languages to the anatomical structures enumerated in TA. Several approaches have already been explored to align anatomical terminologies [10-12]. However, the problems we faced were distinct from those works, in that one of our sources existed only in hard copy with no explicit relationship between the terms. Using structural methods to map the two terminologies would have required to manually rebuild their semantic structures.

TA had a conservative approach towards the terms of NA despite the evolution of the structure. Our results outlined that more than 75% of the terms from TA came from NA, most of them were left unchanged and all were used with the same meaning.

We used a rather basic string-to-string edit distance, compared to the numerous distances which have been developed [9]. On the other hand, the Levenshtein-Damerau distance do not need prior knowledge about the terms and has relevant results on relatively small strings. In addition, this distance has already been used with significant results for spell-checking in medical texts [13].

Evaluation shows good result with an overall coverage reaching the 80% limit. However, an important limitation of this work was the lack of validated source in an electronic format. These sources had to be created and we have no assurance of exhaustiveness. For example, we identified 7,418 codes, 8,450 Latin terms and 9,204 English terms in Terminologia but the textbook includes no references about the total number of codes or terms and we can not be sure to have created an exhaustive version.

More important is the compositional approach taken by both terminologies. The variation in terms due to their different extensions was the main cause of approximate matches and led us to use a widely manual evaluation.

French terms were used as it is the native language of the authors. Yet, this work's strength is that only the Latin terms were involved in the matching process. Therefore, the method is suitable for any other languages, to the condition that they have their own version of NA. The IFAA confirmed the Latin as the language of the definitive terminology [4] because of its neutrality and international character. In addition to this role of "depository" of the anatomical knowledge, we suggest that Latin may be of some interest in the creation of multilingual terminologies. For example, the method described in this paper may be used with Terminologia Histologica and Nomina Histologica which include Latin terms.

The knowledge implied in the semantic structure of TA is accessible for humans but this structure lacks the requirement to be relevantly processed by computer programs [14]. Ontology, by providing a formal definition of the concepts of a given domain and by representing all the relationships between these concepts, is a recognized method for expressing biomedical knowledge in a computer accessible format. The reference ontology in Anatomy is the FMA. As it includes terms and codes from TA, a multilingual version of TA could be used to add terms from other languages to the FMA.

5. Conclusion

In this work, we tested a method using the similarity between Latin terms from NA and TA to expand the latter with French terms. This method allows minimizing human resources with relevant results, reaching a specified target of 80% due to the fact that TA includes 1,500 more terms than NA. In addition, as the method is based only on Latin terms, it could be used for other language as well. However, further work requiring sanction of anatomists is yet to be done to produce a validated and comprehensive translation of TA. Finally, we consider this work as a starting point for adding terms to other anatomical knowledge sources such as the FMA.

Acknowledgements

This work has been funded by the Swiss National Science Foundation (SNF 632-066041). The authors wish to thank Dr. Henning Müller for his help.

References

[1]   Rosse C, Gaddum-Rosse P, Hollinshead WH. Hollinshead's textbook of anatomy. 5th ed. Philadelphia, PA: Lippincott-Raven Publishers; 1997.

[2]   International Anatomical Nomenclature Committee. Nomina anatomica : fifth edition, approved by the eleventh International Congress of Anatomists at Mexico City, 1980, together with Nomina histologica, second edition, and Nomina embryologica, second edition. Baltimore, Md.: Williams & Wilkins; 1983.

[3]   Federative Committee on Anatomical Terminology. Terminologia anatomica : international anatomical terminology. Stuttgart ; New York: Thieme; 1998.

[4]   Whitmore I. Terminologia anatomica: new terminology for the new anatomist. Anat Rec 1999;257(2):50-3.

[5]   Rouvière H. Anatomie humaine, descriptive, topographique et fonctionnelle. 14e éd. revisée ed. Paris: Masson; 1997.

[6]   Kamina P. Petit dictionnaire d'anatomie, d'embryologie et d'histologie (nomina anatomica). Paris: Maloine; 1990.

[7]   Rosse C, Mejino JL, Jr. A reference ontology for biomedical informatics: the Foundational Model of Anatomy. J Biomed Inform 2003;36(6):478-500.

[8]   Damereau F. A Technique for Computer Detection and Correction of Spelling Errors. Communications of the ACM 1964;7(3):171-6.

[9]   Manning CD, Schütze H. Foundations of statistical natural language processing. Cambridge, Mass.: MIT Press; 1999.

[10] Mork P, Pottinger R, Bernstein PA. Challenges in precisely aligning models of human anatomy using generic schema matching. Medinfo 2004;2004:401-5.

[11] Rickard KL, Mejino Jr JL, Martin RF, Agoncillo AV, Rosse C. Problems and solutions with integrating terminologies into evolving knowledge bases. Medinfo 2004;2004:420-4.

[12] Zhang S, Bodenreider O. Aligning representations of anatomy using lexical and structural methods. AMIA Annu Symp Proc 2003:753-7.

[13] Ruch P, Baud R, Geissbuhler A. Using lexical disambiguation and named-entity recognition to improve spelling correction in the electronic patient record. Artif Intell Med 2003;29(1-2):169-84.

[14] Rosse C. Terminologia anatomica: considered from the perspective of next-generation knowledge sources. Clin Anat 2001;14(2):120-33.

Address for correspondence

Paul Fabry <paul.fabry@usherbrooke.ca> CRED – Centre Hospitalier Universitaire de Sherbrooke, 3001, 12ème Avenue Nord, J1H 5N4 Sherbrooke, Québec, CANADA

Connecting Medical Informatics and Bio-Informatics
R. Engelbrecht et al. (Eds.)
IOS Press, 2005

Toward a Unified Representation of Findings in Clinical Radiology

Valérie Bertaud[a], Jérémy Lasbleiz[ab], Fleur Mougin[a], Franck Marin[a], Anita Burgun[a],
Régis Duvauferrier[ab]

[a]EA 3888, LIM, Faculty of Medicine, University of Rennes1, Rennes, France
[b]Département de Radiologie et Imagerie Médicale , CHU de Rennes, France

Abstract

The representations of findings in clinical radiology are heterogeneous. Motivations for developing a unified representation include the semantic integration of medical reports based on DICOM-SR(Digital Image Communication in Medicine Structured Reporting), bibliographic databases in the context of evidence-based medicine, and teaching resources. In this work, we propose a unified representation integrating the representations of findings in the UMLS, the GAMUTS in Radiology and the DICOM-SR. We analyse the UMLS and the DCMR (DICOM Content Mapping Resource) of DICOM SR to figure out their own representation of findings. Then we set up a syntax between the UMLS concepts using DICOM-SR relations in order to rewrite the GAMUTS sentences. The translation of the whole GAMUTS using the UMLS concepts and the DICOM SR syntax could be a method to create or supplement the DCMR TIDs (Template ID : Identifier of a Template) and CIDs (Context ID : Identifier of a Context Group) in the field of description of findings in medical imaging. This method could also enable to give an ontologic dimension to the DICOM SR representation system of information. The meaning of the CIDs would then be enhanced far beyond the simple use of the SNOMED vocabulary.

Keywords:
Diagnosis [Subheading], Radiology, Unified Medical Language System, Medical Informatics

1. Introduction

The representations of findings in clinical radiology are heterogeneous : medical reports (DICOM SR), bibliographic databases (MEDLINE), teaching resources. A unified representation would enable to create a bridge between clinical activity, evidence based medicine and teaching. This concern has already been the subject of some works (e.g. [1,2]). But a unique representation of findings that would fit to all these kinds of resources was missing in those works. Our work could make it possible to provide the basis which will be necessary for the "semantic Web" [3] and for the "just in time" in clinical activity [4].

The Unified Medical Language System (UMLS®) [5] already unifies the main medical classifications and nomenclatures in its Metathesaurus [6]. The DCMR (DICOM Content Mapping Resource) is used by DICOM SR (Digital Image Communication in Medicine Structured Reporting) [7] to carry out standardized imaging reports. We have to consider this representation of medical information as a reference insofar as it is integrated in HL7 v3 (Health Layer 7). This representation of radiological information has already admitted the importance of a rigorous terminology since it largely integrates the SNOMED (Systematized NOmenclature of MEDicine).Description of radiological findings are proposed in books of ranges of diagnosis based on descriptions of findings[8,9,10]. These books are numerous. Most of them have been edited a lot of times and some have been translated into several languages [11]. We can notice that the descriptions of findings remain unchanged (in vocabulary and in structure) in various books from various authors and in various editions[12].

The aim of this work is to propose a unified representation integrating the representations of findings in the UMLS®, the GAMUTS in Radiology from Reeder and Felson [8] and the DICOM-SR.

2. Materials and methods

First, we analyse how findings are represented in the ULMS®. The UMLS® has been developed and maintained by the U.S. National Library of Medicine since 1990. It comprises two major inter-related components: the Metathesaurus®, a huge repository of concepts, and the Semantic Network, a limited network of 135 Semantic Types, and 54 Relations. The latter is a high-level representation of the biomedical domain based on Semantic Types under which all the Metathesaurus concepts are categorized, and which is intended to provide a basic ontology for the biomedical domain. In order to analyse the representation of findings in the UMLS®, we start from the 500 sentences of osteo-articular semiology of the Gamuts 2003. Some examples are given in the table 1. We use the Metamap program[13] to discover UMLS® Metathesaurus concepts in the Gamuts phrases.

Table 1 - Example of findings descriptions (GAMUT in Radiology 2003)

Code	Phrase
D-126	Hypoplastic (spindle-shaped or stubby) terminal phalanges
D-127-1	Acro-osteolysis (erosion or destruction of multiple terminal phalangeal tufts)
D-127-2	Acquired acro-osteolysis confined to one digit
D-127-3	Band-like destruction or erosion of the midportion of a terminal phalanx
D-128	Acro-osteosclerosis (terminal phalangeal sclerosis)
D-129-1	Amputation or absence of a phalanx, digit, hand, or foot – acquired
D-129-2	Amputation or absence of a phalanx, digit, hand, or foot – congenital
D-129-3	Self-mutilation of digits
D-130	Gangrene of a finger or toe
D-131	Lytic lesion(s) in a phalanx (often cyst-like)

Then, we analyse the DICOM-SR, and particularly the Part 16 [14] and the supplement 23 [15], to identify the architecture of findings held in this model. Part 16 of DICOM has been created in 2001. It gathers all the coding and terminology elements which appear in the DICOM objects (images, structured reports, physiological signals…). Thus it is considered as the DICOM Content Mapping Ressource (DCMR). This document contains all the terms sorted by applicative domains (Context groups ID: CIDs). Data templates (TIDs) are built from these resources. The structured report is based on the TIDs.

Lastly, we set up a syntax between the UMLS® concepts using DICOM-SR relations in order to rewrite the GAMUTS sentences.

3. Results

Findings in radiology according to the UMLS®

MetaMap makes it possible to discover UMLS® Metathesaurus concepts in the Gamuts phrases (500 phrases, 3780 words, 476 different words). It also indicates for each UMLS®

concept (1271 different concepts, 1149 different CUIs), the corresponding Semantic Types (Table 2).

Table 2 - The Metamap results for the most frequent Semantic Types: number of words in Gamuts phrases, number of UMLS® different concepts, number of different CUIs (Concept Unique Identifier).

Semantic Types	Words	Concepts	CUI
1. Entity			
1.1. Anatomical structure	26	4	4
1.1.1. Anatomical abnormality	78	19	15
1.1.1.1. Congenital abnormality	195	50	42
1.1.1.2. Acquired abnormality	82	18	16
1.1.2. Fully formed anatomical structure	186	3	1
1.1.2.1. Body part, organ, or organ component	855	118	99
	323	24	19
1.1.2.2. Tissue	243	33	33
1.2. Temporal concept	721	97	91
1.3. Qualitative concept	370	44	41
1.4. Quantitative concept	949	123	117
1.5. Functional concept	842	146	137
1.6. Spatial concept	101	15	13
1.6.1. Body space or junction	246	63	49
1.6.2. Body location or region	232	64	59
1.7. Finding	241	93	21
1.8. Sign or symptom			
2. Event	297	39	34
2.1. Pathologic function	464	100	89
2.1.1. Disease or syndrome	174	33	21
2.1.1.1. Neoplastic process	67	21	17
2.2. Injury or poisoning			

First, we can identify the part of the Semantic Network regarding the findings. Among the UMLS® Semantic Types, those which are the most frequently assigned to findings in clinical radiology and the relations that hold between these Semantics Types are presented in figure 1.

Secondly, a great amount of Gamuts phrases are combinations of simple UMLS® concepts. The composed concepts need to use a syntax to be represented (Fig. 2). On this point, we notice that :

- Quantitative concepts", "qualitative concepts" and "functional concepts" can be attributes that make "spatial concepts" and "anatomical structures" pathologic.

- "Finding", "sign or symptom", "disease or syndrome", "pathologic function", "anatomical abnormality", are either self supporting to express pathologies or they can be, like previously, attributes that make "spatial concepts" and "anatomical structures" pathologic.

Beyond these syntactical considerations, some terms of Gamuts cannot be found in the UMLS®. The coverage of the UMLS® is not complete in particular for the description of the images characteristics. Thus, the following concepts are missing in the UMLS® : radiopaque ; high attenuation ; low attenuation ; hypodense ; isodense ; hyperdense ; hypoechoic ; isoechoic ; hyperechoic ; Enhancing ; intravenous contrast ; homogeneous ; heterogenous... Some proper nouns are also missing (e.g. Magdelung deformity), some metaphoric expressions (e.g. salt and pepper demineralization), some anatomic localizations (e.g. parosteal) and various findings (e.g. cupping).

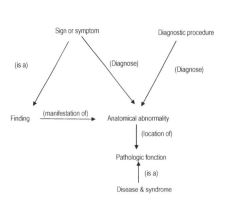

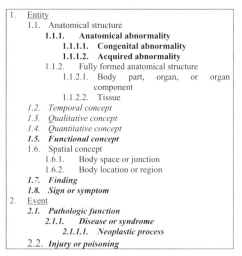

Figure 1 – The semantic network representing findings in the UMLS®

Figure 2 - In this semantic network, in bold the semantic types which are self-supporting, in normal writing the semantic types of the nouns that need an adjective, in italic writing the semantic types of adjective

Findings in radiology according to DICOM SR

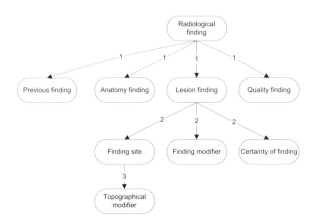

Figure 3 – Representation of findings in DICOM SR. The main relations are : 1 - CONTAINS, 2 - HAS PROPERTIES, 3 - HAS CONC MOD

In the DCMR, the "Findings" are found in multiple CIDs (Fig.3). They are for example: "Previous findings" (former results), "Clinical findings" (clinical elements) coming within the scope of the patient's history or the procedure reason. They can also be the "anatomy findings" (anatomical elements observed) and the "finding site" (site of lesion) possibly specified by "topographical modifiers" (for example the "former part" for the mitral valve). But they are especially the "lesion findings" (lesion element or anomaly) possibly specified by a "finding modifier" (modifier related to a visual anomaly) which states, for example, that the radiological line is a liquid level. It is necessary to add the "quality finding" (quality standards) which includes the artefacts like the CID 6041 (Mammography image quality Finding) or the CID 6135 (Chest image quality finding). The "certainty of finding" means the level of certainty expressed by a percentage of the result. This wealth makes it possible to describe the radiological lesions with a high level of accuracy.

The relations used between CIDs and TIDs to express the findings in DICOM SR are: CONTAINS, HAS CONCEPT MOD (has concept modifier), and HAS PROPERTIES.

Rewriting the GAMUTS phrases using the UMLS® and DICOM SR

Although the coverage of the UMLS® is not complete, it is possible to represent a great amount of the GAMUTS phrases by combining the UMLS® concepts with boolean operators, brackets and the DICOM SR relations regarding the findings (HAS CONCEPT MOD: has concept modifier, HAS PROPERTIES) (Fig. 4).

- D-126 *Hypoplastic (spindle-shaped or stubby) terminal phalanges* : **Hypoplastic**; Functional Concept; C0543481; **HAS PROPERTIES**; **Terminal phalanx**; Body Part, Organ, or Organ Component; C0576464

- D-127-1 *Acro-osteolysis (erosion or destruction of multiple terminal phalangeal tufts)* : **Acro-Osteolysis**; Disease or Syndrome; C0917990 / **Terminal phalanx**; Body Part, Organ, or Organ Component; C0576464; HAS **CONCEPT MOD**; **Multiple**; Quantitative Concept; C0205294; **HAS PROPERTIES**; **Erosion**; Acquired Abnormality; C0333307

- D-127-2 *Acquired acro-osteolysis confined to one digit* : **Acro-Osteolysis**; Disease or Syndrome; C0917990; **HAS CONCEPT MOD**; **Acquired**; Temporal Concept; C0439661; **HAS PROPERTIES**; **Digit**, NOS; Body Part, Organ, or Organ Component; C0278455; **HAS CONCEPT MOD**; **One** Quantitative Concept; C0205447

- D-127-3 *Band-like destruction or erosion of the midportion of a terminal phalanx* : **Erosion**; Acquired Abnormality; C0333307; **HAS PROPERTIES** ; **Band**; Spatial Concept; C0439645; **HAS PROPERTIES**; **Terminal phalanx**; Body Part, Organ, or Organ Component; C0576464

- D-128 *Acro-osteosclerosis (terminal phalangeal sclerosis)* : **Osteosclerosis**; Disease or Syndrome; C0029464 / **Sclerosis**; Finding; C0036429; **HAS PROPERTIES** ; **Terminal phalanx**; Body Part, Organ, or Organ Component; C0576464

- D-129-1 *Amputation or absence of a phalanx, digit, hand, or foot – acquired* : (**Amputation**; Therapeutic or Preventive Procedure; C0002688; **OR**; **Absences**; Finding; C0424530); **HAS CONCEPT MOD**; **Acquired**; Temporal Concept; C0439661; **HAS PROPERTIES**; (**Phalanx**, NOS; Body Part, Organ, or Organ Component; C0222682; **OR**; **Digit**, NOS; Body Part, Organ, or Organ Component; C0278455; **OR**; **hand** <2>; Body Part, Organ, or Organ Component; C0018563; **OR**; **Foot** <2>; Body Location or Region; C0016504)

- D-129-2 *Amputation or absence of a phalanx, digit, hand, or foot – congenital* : Congenital n'est pas reconnu en UMLS mais en fait il s'agit de congenital abnormality

- D-129-3 *Self-mutilation of digits* : **Self Mutilation**; Injury or Poisoning; C0036601; **HAS PROPERTIES**; **Digit**, NOS; Body Part, Organ, or Organ Component; C0278455

- D-130 *Gangrene of a finger or toe* : **Gangrene**; Disease or Syndrome; C0017086; **HAS PROPERTIES**; (**Finger**; Body Location or Region; C0016129; **OR**; **Toe**; Body Location or Region; C0040357)

- D-131 *Lytic lesion(s) in a phalanx (often cyst-like)* : (**Lytic lesion**; Disease or Syndrome; C0221204;**OR** ; **Cyst**; Neoplastic Process; C0010709); **HAS PROPERTIES**; **Phalanx**, NOS; Body Part, Organ, or Organ Component; C0222682;

Figure 4 – GAMUTS phrases translation using the UMLS® concepts and the DICOM SR syntax. In italic writing, the GAMUTS phrases, in bold the UMLS® concepts, in bold and upper case letters the DICOM relations and boolean operators, in normal writing the UMLS® semantic types and their CUI (Concept Unique Identifier).

4. Discussion

In this work, after analysing the structure and the content of the UMLS® and DICOM SR concerning the representation of findings, we demonstrate that it is possible to represent the findings using the UMLS® terminology and the DICOM SR syntax.

Nevertheless, some essential findings in radiology remain missing in the UMLS® like in particular the terms regarding the images characteristics. From this point of view, the UMLS® needs to be supplemented.

Our unified representation enables to connect the medical report (DICOM SR) to the bibliographic databases (MEDLINE) and reference books used for students. We envision potential applications in evidence based medicine, or in information retrieval in the framework of the semantic web for example.

5. Conclusion

The translation of the whole GAMUTS using the UMLS® concepts and the DICOM SR syntax could be a method to create or supplement the DCMR TIDs and CIDs in the field of the description of imaging findings. This method could enable to give an ontologic dimension to DICOM SR system of information representation. The meaning of the CIDs would then be enhanced far beyond the simple use of SNOMED vocabulary.

6. References

[1]   Sneiderman CA Rindflesch TC, Aronson AR. Finding the findings: identification of findings in medical literature using restricted natural language processing. *Proc AMIA Annu Fall Symp.* 1996;:239-43.
[2]   Hersh W, Mailhot M, Arnott-Smith C, Lowe H. Selective automated indexing of findings and diagnoses in radiology reports. *J Biomed Inform.* 2001 Aug;34(4):262-73.
[3]   Berners-Lee T., Hendler J., Lassila O. The Semantic Web. *Scientific American*, May 2001
[4]   Chueh H, Barnett GO. "Just-in-time" clinical information. *Acad Med.* 1997 Jun;72(6):512-7.
[5]   UMLS Knowledge Source Server Version 4.2.3 available at :
      http://umlsks.nlm.nih.gov/kss/servlet/Turbine/template/admin,user,KSS_login.vm
[6]   Burgun A, Bodenreider O. Mapping the UMLS Semantic Network into general ontologies. *Proc AMIA Symp.* 2001;:81-5
[7]   Hussein R, Engelmann U, Schroeter A, Meinzer HP. DICOM structured reporting: Part 1. Overview and characteristics. *Radiographics.* 2004 May-Jun;24(3):891-6.
[8]   MM Reeder, B Felson. *Gamuts in Radiology Comprehensive lists of roentgen differential diagnosis.* Springer – fourth edition 2003.
[9]   R.L. Eisenberg. *Clinical Imaging. An atlas of differential diagnosis.* Aspen publishers, 1988.
[10] S. Chapman, R. Nakielny. *Aids to radiological diagnosis.* Third edition. Saunders, 1995.
[11] S. Chapman, R. Nakielny. *Guide du diagnostic différentiel en radiologie.* Traduit par G. Coche de l'édition 1984. Vigot, 1989.
[12] MM Reeder, B Felson. *Gamuts in Radiology Comprehensive lists of roentgen differential diagnosis.* Audiovisual Radiology of Cincinnati, inc. 1975.
[13] Aronson AR. Effective mapping of biomedical text to the UMLS Metathesaurus: the MetaMap program. *Proc AMIA Symp.* 2001;:17-21.
[14] National Electrical Manufacturers Association. *Digital Imaging and Communication in Medicine (DICOM), part 16 : Content Mapping Ressource.* Rosslyn, Va : NEMA, 2001.Available at : http://medical.nema.org/dicom/2003.html
[15] National Electrical Manufacturers Association. *Digital Imaging and Communication in Medicine (DICOM), supplement 23 : structured reporting storage SOP classes.* Rosslyn, Va : NEMA, 2000.Available at : http://medical.nema.org

Address for correspondence :

Valerie Bertaud : valerie.bertaud@univ-rennes1.fr

Connecting Medical Informatics and Bio-Informatics
R. Engelbrecht et al. (Eds.)
IOS Press, 2005

Advanced Information Retrieval Using XML Standards

Ralf Schweiger[a], Simon Hölzer[a], Joachim Dudeck[a]

[a]*Institute for Medical Informatics, Justus-Liebig-University Giessen, Germany*

Abstract

The bulk of clinical data is available in an electronic form. About 80% of the electronic data, however, is narrative text and therefore limited with respect to machine interpretation. As a result, the discussion has shifted from "electronic versus paper based data" towards "structured versus unstructured electronic data". The XML technology of today paves a way towards more structured clinical data and several XML based standards such as the Clinical Document Architecture (CDA) emerge. The implementation of XML based applications is yet a challenge. This paper will focus on XML retrieval issues and describe the difficulties and prospects of such an approach. The result of our work is a search technique called "topic matching" that exploits structured data in order to provide a search quality that is superior to established text matching methods. With this solution we are able to utilize large numbers of heterogeneously structured documents with only a minimum of effort.

Keywords:
XML, Topic Maps, RSS, CDA, Semantic Web

1. Introduction

More and more healthcare data become available in an electronic form. The data range from weakly structured text to highly structured messages and databases. The eXtensible Markup Language (XML) seems to become the standard format for electronic data interchange. The Clinical Document Architecture (CDA), for example, provides an exchange model for clinical documents such as discharge summaries and pathology reports [1]. CDA documents are XML documents. The document-oriented view of XML corresponds well with the organization of healthcare data. In addition, XML is easy to process due to the growing number of free XML tools. The exploitation of electronic data, on the other hand, is still limited. Despite existing communication standards and commercial application systems clinical data are often not accessible and searchable at the clinical workstation. Most healthcare data is narrative text and requires structural preparation. Moreover, the relationships between the resources are often implicit and vary from site to site. We therefore developed a pragmatic and flexible approach, which is based on standards such as XML and Topic Maps. The approach aims to combine the simplicity of a web search with the accuracy of customized applications.

2. Methods and materials

Representing relationships between data using XML

In our use case model a healthcare professional simply enters search terms into a web browser and a search engine selects the "appropriate" information resources. A resource in this context is anything that has a Uniform Resource Identifier (URI), e.g. a document, an image or even a service. Existing text matching methods relate search terms to resources and have limitations to identify relationships between the terms. Search results are often inaccurate. Figure 1 illustrates the limitation of simple text matching. The pathology report contains two findings "Basaliom" and "Keratose" that refer to different sample excisions with the locations "Stirn" (forehead) and "Nase" (nose) respectively. Numbers 1, 2 are used to express the relationships between findings and locations. Existing search engines simply relate terms to document addresses, e.g. [basaliom]=>[report.txt], [keratose]=>[report.txt], [stirn]=>[report.txt] and [nase]=>[report.txt] where "report.txt" is the relative URI of the pathology report. If the clinical user now enters the query "Keratose Stirn" she or he probably wants to find those reports in which the given terms are related with each other. The document in Figure 1 is therefore less relevant to the query because the fnding "Keratose" relates to the wrong location "Nase". The search engine, on the other hand, relates the given terms to "report.txt" and returns the document as a relevant search result. Search engines have still severe limitations to automatically detect relationships between the terms within plain text documents. More sophisticated search engines consider the distance of the words in the text (proximity) as a relationship indicator. The proximity measure works well in many cases. In the pathology example, however, it fails.

Gießen, den 14. April 1999

Prof. Dr. med. A. Schulz
Institut für Pathologie
am Klinikum der Justus-Liebig-Universität

Institut für Pathologie
Langhansstraße 10
35385 Gießen

Sekretariat: +49-641-9941101
Prof. Dr. Glanz   Befundauskunft: +49-641-9941103
                                               Fax: +49-641-9941109
HNO-Klinik   Dr. Dreyer
Zentrum HNO und Augenheilkunde
Feulgenstr. 10

Patient: Thomas Müller, 10.04.1970

Einsendung vom 12. April 1999
Kennung 9907946
1 PE Stirn li.
2 PE Nasenflügel re.

Es handelt sich um ein multizentrisch wachsendes oberflächl. Basaliom (1)
sowie eine aktinische Keratose mit bis zu leichten Epitheldysplasien (2).

Figure 1: Is this pathology report relevant to the query „Keratose Stirn"?

The eXtensible Markup Language (XML) offers many possibilities to represent relationships between the data [2] in a way that a machine can understand. The markup <location id="2">Nase</location> and <finding ref="2">Keratose</finding>, for example, relates the finding "Keratose" to the right location "Nase". A search engine would now be able to detect the relationships between the findings and locations and return more accurate search results. Other XML standards such as the Resource Description Framework (RDF) allow to express even more sophisticated relationships between the data. XML structured documents consequently enable new search techniques that are superior to existing text matching methods.

The organizational cost of inserting XML markup into plain text documents has been described in [3]. Producing structure always requires some initial effort. The document oriented view of XML, however, suggests to structure the data in a stepwise, i.e. more flexible manner. The resulting structures are maintainable with web browsers (XML forms) and reusable in different applications. In this paper we will focus on retrieval issues. The subsequent section outlines a search method called "topic matching" that exploits XML structures to compute higher search quality and calls attention to the difficulties with such an approach.

3. Exploiting XML represented relationships using Topic Maps

Many XML standards have established since 1998 and search engines increasingly have to deal with structured data. At this point another limitation of existing search engines reveals. Search engines parse the given text into single words and directly relate the words to the address of the document in which they occur (indexing). More advanced search engines can also manage a list of synonymous terms. More complex relationships, however, can not be represented. The relationship between the finding "Keratose" and the location "Nase", for example, is not of type "synonym". Another example is the more precise location "Stirn links" (forehead left) which should be represented as one concept and related as a whole to the finding "Basaliom". We consequently need a data model for the representation of arbitrary relationships between terms and other resources. The International Organization for Standardization (ISO) provides a standardized notation, called Topic Maps (ISO13250), for interchangeably defining topics, and the relationships between topics [4]. **Fehler! Verweisquelle konnte nicht gefunden werden.** shows the fundamental elements of the Topic Maps model. Topics are perceived as abstract, meaningful and reusable concepts (subjects) described by a number of "meaningless" words (reification). Topics may be related to one another (associations) and to documents or other information resources such as databases (occurrences). Advanced Topic Maps elements such as "classifications" and "scopes" allow to express even more.

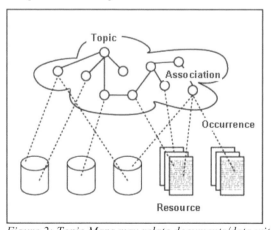

Figure 2: Topic Maps may relate documents/data with each other

specific relationships between the data items. The Topic Maps standard provides a simple, yet flexible data model to represent semantic networks that meaningfully link the data with each other.

The representation of data relationships is only part of the solution. We also need methods that exploit the given knowledge in an efficient way. Due to our experience semantic networks grow very fast and may comprise millions of single relationships. The challenge with such an approach is therefore the efficient searching and refreshing of very large semantic networks. Efficiency is a result of many details that will not be presented here. Figure 3, however, illustrates the basic idea of our search method that is referred to as "topic matching". The search method has been subdivided into two steps. The "association step" finds a set of topics that relate the search terms meaningfully with each other. The "occurrence step" relates the identified topics to resources such as documents and images. The search method consequently finds meaningful topics rather than meaningless words. Topic matching consequently captures more meaning than simple text matching and excludes irrelevant relationships very quickly.

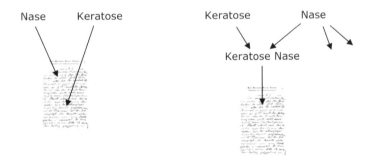

Figure 3: Text matching compared to „topic matching".

4. Results

Figure 4 shows a web browser interface of our search engine applied to drug information sources at our university hospital. The name of the search engine derives from XML and URI: LuMriX. The development of new search services is as simple as listing the addresses (URIs) of the documents that Lumrix is to search. Lumrix automatically identifies the topics within the documents and links them meaningfully with each other. Hyperlinks between the documents are considered as well. In addition, Lumrix controls modifications of the document space and informs the users if new documents emerge or existing documents have changed. The documents may be differently structured. The university hospital's pharmacy, for example, creates XML, HTML and PDF documents. Heterogeneous data are characteristic for a clinical environment. Clinical users simply enter search words into the text field and submit the query to the search engine using the "Suchen" button or pressing the return key. Lumrix tries to match the words with topics ("topic matching") and returns links to appropriate information sources which will be rendered on demand. With such an approach we are able to quickly search, link and utilize arbitrary document collections. The access rate to the drug documents, for example, has grown in our hospital from less than 50 accesses per month up to almost 200 accesses per day because the information of interest is only a search term or click away. It turned out that XML structures improve the search quality. In the meantime, the hospital's pharmacy maintains approximately 300 XML documents using web browsers and XML forms. The markup allows us to extract, for example, drug substances from the hospital's drug formulary and to search a given substance in the German drug formulary, which contains complementary information such as drug indications and drug interactions. Another use case illustrates the benefit of XML: If a physician enters a clinical diagnosis she or he probably searches for drug indications rather than drug contraindications. If the indications and contraindications of the drugs have been marked in the text Lumrix can specifically search the given diagnosis in the right context.

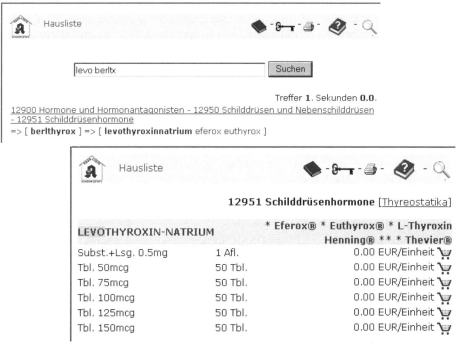

Figure 4: Application of our search engine LUMRIX to drug information sources.

Lumrix has been applied to many data such as medical code systems (ICD, SNOMED etc.), the university library and RSS (Really Simple Syndication) news on the web. The main difficulty in the development of search engines is the simultaneous optimization of different search criteria (fuzzy search, search recall, search precision, search performance etc.) that tend to run in the opposite direction. A very precise search, for example, often requires many recalls in order to find the information of interest. It turned out that XML may improve the situation. The key challenge in our approach, however, is the management of very large semantic networks. Lumrix is able to manage several millions of documents and data relationships using a single desktop computer. The average search time is always below a second. Furthermore, the search load may be distributed on many computers as the number of documents grows. The freshness of the semantic network is another challenge if the topics are highly interwoven. If an author modifies his/her document Lumrix must identify the document's topics and carefully analyze the relationships to other topics before it can update the network. Our work consequently meets the Semantic Web Initiative, which also addresses the management of very large semantic networks. Applications of Lumrix to SNOMED-CT, ICD-10, drug formularies, the German Law Code, the University

Library and RSS-structured news on the Web are accessible at http://www.lumrix.de/campus/suchdienst.html.

5. Discussion

There are other approaches to information retrieval that use XML. XML databases, for example, can be used to store and retrieve XML documents without the need to map hierarchical XML schemas onto relational database schemas. XML query languages may be used to select information from a set of XML resources [5]. XML databases and XML query languages provide a retrieval infrastructure for semi-structured XML data. Nonetheless, there are major differences to our approach. XML databases provide no inference method that directly relates search terms to resources. In addition, developers and users need to learn XML schemas. The key features of our approach are the ease of development and use. Our inference engine relies on the Topic Maps standard, which allows representing arbitrary relationships between resources. The relationships between the data are no longer fixed in the application logic. As a result, we can start with little requirements and establish new relationships between the data as they become available. New data relationships enable new ways of reasoning; i.e. the intelligence of the search engine grows continuously. Such relationships are often referred to as semantics. Another difference between XML databases and our approach is the level of decentralization. Databases tend to centralize data. Search engines, on the other hand, separate the index from the data; i.e. the data are usually located somewhere else and authored by different individuals. Pragmatism, flexibility, and decentralization are important features in little organized and distributed healthcare systems.

Another challenge is the insertion of XML markup into textual documents. The bulk of clinical information still resides in simple text files (unstructured data). Comparatively little data is stored and organized in clinical databases (structured data). It is not a challenge to create XML documents, e.g. CDA (Clinical Document Architecture) documents, from a clinical database for the purpose of interchange (preservation of structure). The structuring of so far unstructured text documents, on the other hand, entails a change of the established workflow (production of new structures) and changing a workflow is always a challenge. In our drug application the pharmacists enter the data into simple web forms which are translated into XML documents using the XML forms standard [6]. The document oriented approach seems to be more flexible than a database approach because it allows us to manage distributed and heterogeneously structured data that are difficult to map within a single database and to incrementally insert structure where needed.

6. References

[1] Clinical Document Architecture Framework Release 1.0, ANSI/HL7 CDA R1.0-2000, Health Level Seven, Inc. http://www.hl7.org, accessed 2003-02-23.

[2] Dudeck J, Schweiger R. Representation of Relationships between Data in Healthcare Documents. Stud Health Technol Inform. 2003;96:272-279.

[3] Schweiger R, Brumhard M, Hölzer S, Dudeck J. Implementing health care systems using XML standards. Int J Med Inform 2005;74:267-277.

[4] Pepper S, Moore G: XML Topic Maps (XTM) 1.0. http://www.topicmaps.org/xtm/1.0/, accessed 2003-02-23.

[5] Boag S, Chamberlin D, Fernandez MF, Florescu D, Robie J, Siméon J: XQuery 1.0: An XML Query Language, W3C Working Draft 15 November 2002.

[6] Dubinko, Micah, XForms Essentials O'Reilly, Sebastopol CA, 2003.

Connecting Medical Informatics and Bio-Informatics
R. Engelbrecht et al. (Eds.)
IOS Press, 2005
683

Refinement of an Automatic Method for Indexing Medical Literature – a Preliminary Study

Michel Joubert, Anne-Laure Peretti, Joanny Gouvernet, Marius Fieschi

LERTIM[1], Faculté de Médecine, Université de la Méditerranée, Marseille, France

Abstract

Objectives: to rank according to their significance MeSH terms automatically extracted from Internet sites in the framework of a French project, VUMeF, a contribution to the NLM' UMLS project. Material and methods: scores are affected to key-words of a given document on the basis of the Semantic Network of the UMLS and frequencies of co-occurring major terms in the Medline literature. If N is the number of major terms of a document, and n is the number of major terms retrieved in the N first terms ranked in descending order according to their scores, the measure of the achievement of the method is n/N. Results: a set of 1444 randomized documents have been extracted from Medline. For each document we computed the retrieved major terms among the first N terms with two methods: a statistical method using only frequencies given by co-occurrences, and our method that uses furthermore the UMLS semantic network. In 34% of cases corresponding to documents indexed by about 16 key-words, about 3 major terms among them, our method produces a better precision (7%) than the statistical method. Discussion: the rough calculation of the proportion of retrieved major terms should be enhanced by the use of a probability law allowing to enlarge the list of terms to select taking into account both the number of major terms and the total number of key-words used to index each document.

Keywords:
Medical Informatics; Documentation; Unified Medical Language System; Medical Subject Headings; Internet.

1. Introduction

The UMLS (Unified Medical Language System) of the U.S. National Library of Medicine is a huge project aiming at integrating the main nomenclatures of the biomedical domain inside a Metathesaurus which registers each biomedical concept as an only entity [1]. The project VUMeF[2] (*Vocabulaire Unifié Médical Fançais*) [2] aiming at extending the French involvement in the UMLS Metathesaurus with an improved French translation of an already present nomenclature (MeSH [3]), the introduction of the French translation of an

---

[1] Laboratoire d'Enseignement et de Recherche sur le Traitement de l'Information Médicale. Faculté de Médecine, Université de la Méditerranée, Marseille, France. http://cybertim.timone.univ-mrs.fr/lertim/.
[2] Project sponsored by the French « Ministère de la Jeunesse, de l'Education Nationale et de la Recherche – Direction des Technologies, RNTS », in 2004-2005.

already present nomenclature (SNOMED [4]), and the introduction of a French nomenclature: CCAM (*Classification Commune des Actes Médicaux*) [5].

In the framework of the project VUMeF, a task is dedicated to the automatic indexing of Internet sites providing high-quality information in the health domain. Health information is said of high-quality when it adheres to commonly accepted principles and today enacted by organizations such as HON (Health On the Net) [6], MedCIRCLE [7] or the Internet Health Coalition [8], for instance. Indexing of documents published on the Internet became quickly a necessity facing the amount of available information. The Dublin Core Metadata Initiative [9] initiated by librarians was a trailblazer in this domain, followed by the Medical Core Metadata [10] applied to biomedical documentation. Even if restricted to high-quality one, it is no more possible to humanely index health information published on the Internet.

The project VUMeF addresses this problem and, among other topics, intends to realize an automatic indexing of health high-quality Internet sites. In this framework a module has been realized that extracts MeSH terms from French-speaking Internet sites. This article presents, in addition to this functionality, the design and implementation of a ranking method of extracted terms according to their significance in a document. This method is based on UMLS knowledge sources and on results of previous research works [11, 12]. It consists in building a conceptual graph linking the extracted terms by the means of semantic relationships, evaluating the role of the terms in this graph and computing a score for each of them, and then organizing the terms according to their computed scores.

2. Material and Methods

The UMLS knowledge sources are made of, among others, a Metathesaurus which registers biomedical concepts in an only way and a semantic network composed by types of concepts, to which the concepts of the Metathesaurus are attached, linked by the means of binary semantic relationships. This provides with a base for applications intended to exploit biomedical concepts [13].

Another knowledge source from the UMLS registers in a table frequencies of co-occurrences of MeSH terms (notified as major by the indexers) in the Medline literature. More precisely, since the human indexers qualify terms by the means of *subheadings*, this knowledge source registers frequencies for pairs of <term/subheading>. In previous research works, we built a knowledge base that establishes relations between relationships of the UMLS semantic network and subheadings used by the indexers. For instance, the relationship *Diagnoses* applies to the two types of concepts *Diagnostic Procedure* and *Disease or Syndrome*, that is translated by the list of subheadings for this last one: *Pathology, Diagnosis, Radiography, Radionuclide imaging, Ultrasonography, Immunology, Microbiology, Virology*.

The method proposed here is intended to compute a score for each extracted term, that allows to rank them in decreasing order, the first ones are the more significant with regard to a document they participate to index. Two MeSH terms being given, then two concepts of the Metathesaurus, the following operations are processed:

- Identifying the types of concepts they are attached to in the semantic network,
- Identifying the semantic relationships that apply on these types,
- Translating the relationships in subheadings for each concept,
- Selecting for each pair of <term/subheading> the related lines in the co-occurrences table.

A first and implicit hypothesis made here is that if a relationship is not represented in the scientific literature (translated by subheadings associated to terms), then it does not apply to. A second hypothesis is that the more a concept is related with other identified ones, the more is it is important for a document description.

This provides us with a heuristics able to compute a score for each concept. The score affected to a concept is the sum of the frequencies of all the lines selected in the co-occurrences table for this concept.. This is illustrated by the schema of Figure 1. Two concepts C_1 and C_2 being given and linked to the concept C_3 by the way of semantic relationships the total of frequencies of which are f_1 and f_2 respectively, the score affected to the term T_1 issued from C_1 is f_1, the score affected to T_2 is f_2, and the score affected to T_3 is f_1+f_2. The principle here is that more a term is semantically linked to other ones in a same document, more it seems significant. In our example, if $f_1>f_2$, the ordered list of terms in significant decreasing order is: T_3, T_1, T_2.

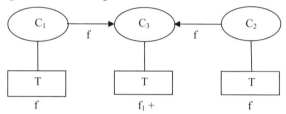

Figure 1. Principle of score calculation of terms.

With the intent to illustrate the interest of the method, let us consider an article indexed in Medline. Thus we have terms that describe it and major terms given by indexers. The major terms are starred. For instance, the article: « *Alternates to EBCT for coronary calcium* », has the list of MeSH key-words: *Tomography , X-Ray Computed* ; Calcinosis* ; Coronary Arteriosclerosis* ; User-Computer Interface ; Imaging, Three-Dimensional ; Calcium ; Endoscopy ; Human.* The conceptual graph built on the base of the UMLS semantic network is presented in Figure 2.

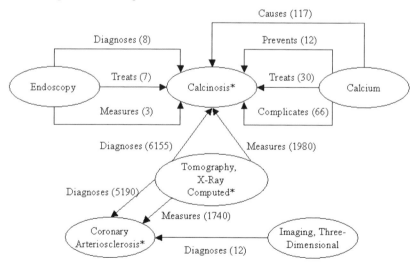

Figure 2. Scores computed and affected to terms concerning an example.

In the end, the algorithm produces the following list:

Tomography, X-Ray Computed*	15.065
Calcinosis*	8.378
Coronary Arteriosclerosis*	6.942
Calcium	225
Endoscopy	18
Imaging, Three-Dimensional	12
Human	0
User-Computer Interface	0

Let remark that the three first terms, initially considered as major terms and ranked in the three first positions by the algorithm, are in a central position in the graph of Figure 2, because they are targets of a lot of semantic relationships and that high frequencies are affected to these ones, and can be considered as main concepts in the document description.

Let also remark that *Human* and *User-Computer Interface* that are not referenced in our own knowledge source are not classified.

3. Results

The aim of our algorithm is to retrieve the most important MeSH terms of a document and to confront this result with the list of major terms proposed by human indexers. With the intent to validate our method we proceeded with documents indexed with MeSH terms by highly qualified human professionals who are the Medline indexers. We proceeded on 1444 randomized articles extracted from Medline irrespectively from origins and disciplines. The diagram of Figure 3 shows the distribution of major terms regarding the total number of key- words for each article.

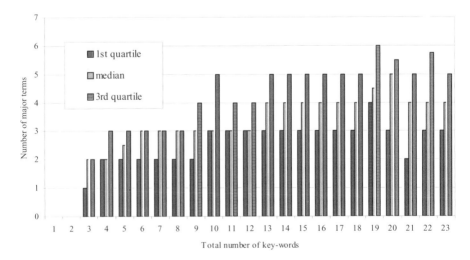

Figure 3. Number of major terms in documents vs total number of key-words.

We experimented on this corpus two methods for identifying major terms:

- a method only based on frequencies of co-occurrences as stored in a UMLS knowledge source,
- our heuristics-based method which furthermore takes into account the knowledge allowed by the UMLS semantic network.

In each case we represented the proportion of retrieved major terms among the total number of major terms. This means that if a document had N major terms, and if n of them have been ranked in the list of the N first terms, the proportion is n/N. Results are presented in the table of Figure 4. Each line represents a class of documents regarding the ration of major terms to the total of terms for each document (less than 10%, between 10 and 20%, etc., more than 50%).

Class (%)	Size	Average of the total number of terms	Average of major terms	Proportion of major terms retrieved with a basic method	Proportion of major terms retrieved with the semantic method
0-10	63	17,43	1,29	0,30	0,56
10-20	235	16,27	2,45	0,44	0,51
20-30	463	14,07	3,45	0,56	0,53
30-40	328	12,20	4,13	0,64	0,55
40-50	143	10,38	4,43	0,74	0,60
>50	212	7,51	4,27	0,86	0,70

Figure 4. Results of indexing 1444 documents issued from Medline with a method based on co-occurrences (basic method) and our method (semantic method).

The table of Figure 4 shows that our method produces a proportion of retrieved major terms greater than 10% as opposed to a method based on statistics only in the case of classes 0-10 and 10-20, corresponding to an important number of terms (more than 16) and a small number of major terms (about 2). If we try to extend these results to the class 20-30, they stay interesting but are not significant (3% of precision more). The boundary stands after the first half-part of the class 20-30 corresponding to a size of 34% of the total population, with an average of total number of terms of 16, an average of majors terms about 3, and a gain in proportion of retrieved major terms of 7%.

4. Discussion

We must have in mind that the scores resulting from our heuristic method are not absolute ones. The proposed method has the only objective to rank retrieved terms in separate documents. In the above example, but somewhat complex document indexation, this method proposes three concepts as major indexing terms. Its aim is not to decide that the first is most important for document description than the following ones. Its aim is to propose three (major) indexing terms among the three first identified ones, just as human indexers did.

The use of the semantic network of the UMLS is a positive contribution that must be refined. A more precise evaluation of the presented method with a different calculation of the proportions of retrieved major terms is on the way. It should be based on a probability law given a number N' (N'≥N) of terms to select in which major terms should be present. This "window" N' will take into account both the number of major terms and the total number of key-words used to index a document, that the rough method we presented here does not.

After this evaluation, we are thinking of testing it with a corpus of Internet sites registered by the portal CISMeF [14] and comparing the obtained results with those produced by the human indexers. In case of disagreement between them, the aim is to make the indexers react and to measure in what this kind of computer-aided indexation could be useful.

5. Acknowledgements

The authors thank the French « Ministère de la Jeunesse, de l'Education Nationale et de la Recherche – Direction des Technologies », which sponsored the project VUMeF, and the whole consortium of this project. They thank the U.S. National Library of Medicine which provided them with the UMLS knowledge sources (this work has been achieved with the 2004 release of the UMLS package).

6. References

[1]   Humphreys BL, Lindberg DAB. Building the Unified Medical Language System. *Proc. 13rd SCAMC.* IEEE Computer Society Press; 1989: 475-80.

[2]   Darmoni SJ, Jarrousse E, Zweigenbaum P, Le Beux P, Namer F, Baud R, Joubert M, Vallée H, Côté RA, Buemi A, Bourigault D, Recourcé G, Jeanneau S, Rodrigues JM. VUMeF: extending the French involvement in the UMLS metathesaurus. *Proc. AMIA Symp.* 2003: 824.

[3]   National Library of Medicine. *Medical Subject Headings.* http://www.nlm.nih.gov/mesh/

[4]   SNOMED International. http://www.snomed.org/

[5]   Classification Commune des Actes Médicaux. http://www.ccam.sante.fr/

[6]   Health on the net Foundation. *HON Code of Conduct.* http://www.hon.ch/HONcode/

[7]   MedCIRCLE. http://www.medcircle.org/

[8]   Internet Health Coalition. http://www.ihealthcoalition.org/

[9]   Dublin Core Metadata Initiative. http://dublincore.org/

[10] Malet G, Munoz F, Appleyard R, Hersh WR. A model for enhancing Internet medical document retrieval with "medical core metadata". *Am Med Inform Assoc.* 1999, 6: 183-208.

[11] Aymard S, Falco L, Dufour JC, Joubert M, Fieschi M. Modeling and implementing a health information provider on the Internet. *Proc. MIE2003.* IOS Press; 2003: 89-94.

[12] Gaudinat A, Joubert M, Aymard S, Falco L, Boyer C, Fieschi M. WRAPIN: new health search engine generation using UMLS Knowledge Sources for MeSH Term Extraction from Health Documentation. *Proc. Medinfo 2004.* IOS Press; 2004: 356-60.

[13] McCray AT, Nelson SJ. The Representation of Meaning in the UMLS. *Meth Inform Med.* 34; 1995: 193-201.

[14] Catalogue et Index des Sites Médicaux Francophones. http://www.chu-rouen.fr/cismef/

Address for correspondence

Michel Joubert
LERTIM
Faculté de Médecine
27, bld Jean Moulin
13385 Marseille Cedex 5
France
e-mail: mjoubert@ap-hm.fr
http://cybertim.timone.univ-mrs.fr/lertim/

Connecting Medical Informatics and Bio-Informatics
R. Engelbrecht et al. (Eds.)
IOS Press, 2005

689

Making Two-Level Standards Work in Legacy Communication Frameworks

Istvan Vassanyi, Jozsef Barcza, Tamas Tobak

University of Veszprém, Department of Information Systems
Veszprém, Hungary

Abstract

The research presented deals with the problem of how information technology can support the interconnection of medical information systems in practice. We apply a two-part structural standard that consists of a fixed Information Reference (IR) Model, and an Archetype Reference (AR) Model that uses the structures of the IR model. A very important problem with the real-world application of such a two-level model is that the high level (abstract) entities, structures and their connections must be somehow translated into lower level equivalents that legacy database information systems can actually use to program their standardised interface. Our choice for the lower level medium is XML, such that the standard appears as an XSD schema that can be used, in the usual way, to validate a message document. To test the viability of the above paradigm, we developed an archetype-XSD translator tool in the form of Protégé/OWL plugins and tested it on an industrial interface for exchanging medical episodes (MedQuery), using an implementation of openEHR. We found that the most important features: Containment, Cardinality, Named references to other instances, and References to external terminologies, could all be mapped to standard XSD constructs. We also developed a validator plugin to check external references. We plan to put the system at work in a heterogeneous medical messaging system (a descendant of the Budapest based MediNet system) in the near future.

Keywords:
Medical Records, Structural Mapping, Archetypes, XML

1. Introduction

The interconnection of medical information systems for automated information exchange is an ultimate goal to improve cost-efficiency and quality of service in the health care domain.

The difficulty is, however, that due to historic, economic and cultural reasons, the information systems in most European medical institutions, especially in Eastern Europe, were developed as a local initiative within the institution and without much effort for standardization [1]. This resulted in systems with totally different information models, even in the same area of specialization, sometimes even within the same institution. Recently, new structural standards by CEN, HL7 (v3 RIM), openEHR, etc. have appeared [2-4], and they are being applied in pilot research and industrial projects to implement new information systems e.g. [5, 6].

However, the question of *today* is how to interconnect heterogeneous legacy systems, based on huge relational databases. Existing system interconnection schemes can be classified into two broad categories:

1. Point-to-point programmed connection between two specific systems, with or without the application of a messaging standard (e.g. HL7). The standard, if used, does not specify the actual content, i.e. the DOCUMENT part of the message. This is the most commonly used scheme in practice, and also the most popular solution with legacy system vendors. This way a new ad-hoc interface must be specified and implemented for any two communicating parties.

2. A messaging standard is used in combination with a field level message content standard [7]. This solution means that programming a single interface for each communicating party is sufficient. However, the content standard usually has a fixed, flat–file structure and the correct interpretation of the fields depends on the programmers of the interfaces. The content standard cannot express sophisticated information structures (like that of all the data making up a cardiac episode) and does not support object references among sub-structures.

To improve the shortcomings of present-day solutions, structural standards should be used for the message content [8]. All major emerging healthcare standards have extensions to build such models. Among them, openEHR, the applicable standards of the CEN, and also the recently developed Hungarian national pre-standard adopts a two-level approach by splitting the structural model in two parts (Fig 1):

*   a fixed Information Reference (IR) Model, which contains a hierarchy of information structures like arrays, folders, etc., and

*   an Archetype Reference Model that builds upon the structures of the IR model, and that is edited and updated by a committee of medical experts. An example of an AR model is the structure and content of an inpatient episode at a hospital department.

The applicability of two-level standards was proven in several studies [9, 10]. Since the IR Model is fixed, software can be developed independent of changes in Archetype Models [2]. Due to the phenomena, as well as their relations, of medical science being very complex, Archetype Models must be defined at a high level of abstraction, preferably in the form of an ontology. In such an ontology, the classes normally form the IR model, and the instances of these classes form the archetypes. The focus of the research presented in this paper was on the practical application of archetype ontologies to build communication frameworks.

2. Methods

In our system model, messages from all communicating parties are sent via a data centre. The centre stores the archetype definitions, provides public access to them for all parties and for the development team of medical experts. Each message passing the centre references an archetype registered in the archetype store. The centre checks conformity with the referenced model and also checks the validity of the terminology references (for the role of terminologies, see Section 3.4).

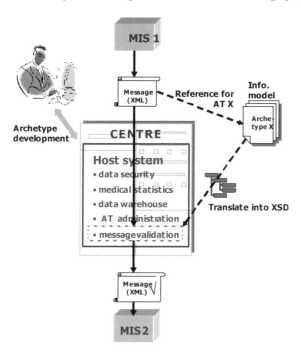

Fig 1: Model of the communication system (AT: Archetype, MIS: Medical information system)

Additional functions of the centre may include data security, medical data warehousing and data mining. These functions, especially data mining, contribute to the cost-effectiveness of the overall health system. An overview of the system is shown in Fig. 1. An example for such a centralized medical communication system, although without support for archetypes, is the experimental MEDINET system in Budapest that connects GPs to hospitals and service providers.

3. Results

The basic problem with the real-world application of an archetype is that the high level (abstract) entities and their connections must be somehow translated into a lower level equivalent that legacy systems can use to program their standardised interface for the archetype. Our choice for the lower level technology is XML. This means that the archetype appears as an XML schema that can be readily used to validate the message document. XML appears at a medium level between the archetype ontology and the relational database structures. Table 1 shows an overview of these three abstraction levels.

Table 1: Levels of structural modelling

Abstraction level	Model type	Model ownership
High	Archetype ontology	Medical standard
Medium	XML schema	IT standard
Low	Relational structures	Proprietary

XML also has a wide support across various database technologies, e.g. the MS SQL Server uses XSD Mapping Schema and XML Views for the XML-relational mapping. Although XML is at a significantly lower level of abstraction than the archetype ontology, the interface programmer of the medical information system must still augment the relational data with domain-specific knowledge to produce a valid message. This is illustrated in Fig 2.

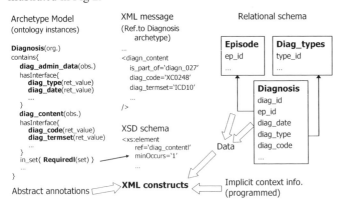

Fig 2: Example of mapping among different structural levels

In the figure, the "implicit contextual information" added by the interface programmer is the correct classification of the relational data. For example, the structural standard may prescribe separate folders for administrative and medical data items that are stored mixed in the same table.

Our basic goal was to examine how the crucial features of the ontology can be mapped to natural XML constructs. We identified four minimal features that the XML schema must be able to express: Containment, Cardinality, References to other instances within the message, and References to external terminologies.

3.1. Containment

Data structures in an archetype are normally nested into each other. For example, an observation called Primary diagnosis may be contained in an organizer called Anamnesis which in turn may be contained in a folder called Medical data. Containment appears in the archetype ontology as a special reference, called "Contains/Is_contained_by" between two instances within an archetype. This relation quite naturally maps into nested <element> XML structures. The nested structure makes the message easy to understand even for the human reader.

3.2. Cardinality

Cardinality means the allowable range of the number of references, contained items etc at any level. An ontology normally allows more freedom in specifying cardinality than XML which supports it only via the minOccurs/maxOccurs properties. However, our experiences show that very special cardinalities are not really necessary, nor used, in real-life archetypes. So, for this feature the basic XML construct will suffer.

3.3. References to other instances

An actual XML message references an archetype which defines its allowed structure. For example, we may prescribe that an organizer called "Diagnoses" must exist that must contain zero or more Diagnosis observations. The archetype model may also specify that there may/must be certain references among the objects making up the archetype. For example, a diagnosis may have a possibly multi-valued reference called "Contradicting diagnoses", pointing to other diagnoses. When using this feature, there will be more than one diagnosis instances in the same Diagnoses organizer in the actual XML message. To implement the reference as a property of the diagnosis element, we cannot use the key/keyref XML construct as this would not allow the reference to Diagnoses placed in other places of the document tree. So we had to resort to the old ID/IDref construct that requires a message-global identifier to be created for each element that can be referenced. The other, worse, solution would be placing all elements in the root of the tree, and thereby losing the visible containment structure. However, creating global identifiers from the object (archetype) name and database table identifier should not be a great pain for the interface programmers.

3.4. References to external terminologies

Term sets, code-dictionaries, hierarchical terminologies form a major part of all data contained in medical information systems. Some of these terminologies are used only locally, like the codes of the wards, some are also proprietary. The archetype must allow the message to contain all sorts of external references. XML by itself cannot guarantee the correctness and existence of an external terminology reference, which appears in the message as a simple text string. We propose that the Data Centre should validate external references instead. For this, the archetype must specify the type and URI of the referenced terminology. For proprietary or hidden terminologies, the validation may use a validator module (plugin) provided by the owner. This was the approach we took in our test implementation.

4. Discussion

To test the viability of the above principles, we implemented an archetype-XSD translator tool (called Schema Maker) and a separate Validator tool as Protégé plugins in a test system. The Information Reference Model we used was the openEHR class hierarchy in the implementation of Isabel Roman Martinez [11]. For the test archetype, we chose the relatively simple MedQuery industrial messaging standard, which we manually implemented with the openEHR information reference model. This standard is used in some medical information systems in Hungary to transfer all sorts of information on medical episodes in hospitals. The standard contained examples for all four modeling issues discussed above. The tools correctly produce the XML schema for the tested cases.

Why not simply use XML as the only means of defining structural standards? That way we would lose the power of the two-level approach that effectively constrains the possible archetype structures with the building blocks of the information reference model. However, it must be emphasized that our solution for the transform of the ontology into XML schema, although straightforward, is not the only one possible solution. In order for the programs to work, we needed to create and adhere to certain conventions like the configuration and naming of references in the archetype definition, or whether we prescribe the ID tags for all elements in the message that can be referenced, or only for those that are actually referenced, etc. In fact these conventions form a meta-standard on the interpretation of the ontology that would come otherwise in an ad hoc manner from the interface programmers.

5. Conclusions and future work

The paper analyzed the problem of how information technology can support the standardised transfer of structural information among health information systems. Adopting the principles of the archetype-based, two-level medical standards, we identified the correct interpretation of high level Archetype Model constructs as the most crucial aspect of practical industrial implementation.

In the demo system presented in the paper, we translate the archetype model ontology into a suitable middle level description (XML schema) that is already a useful and unambiguous standard for a programmer of legacy healthcare information systems, and that can easily be used for the validation of messages. We found that the most important features: Containment, Cardinality, References to other instances within the message, and References to external terminologies, could all be safely mapped to XSD constructs.

We plan use the concept and the tools in a heterogeneous medical messaging system (a descendant of the Budapest based MediNet system) soon.

6. Acknowledgements

The work presented was supported by the Hungarian Scientific Research Fund, grant no. F037416 and IKTA 142/2003.

7. References

[1]   Frieder Klein. What is the present status of electronic patient's record in Germany – a user's personal experience. *Proc. European Federation for Medical Informatics, Special Topic Conference*, Munich, Germany 13-16 June 2004, pp. 87-88.

[2]   The openEHR EHR Reference Model, http://www.openehr.org

[3]   CEN/TC 251, http://www.centc251.org

[4]   HL7 V3 Reference Information Model (Health Level Seven, Inc), http://www.hl7.org

[5]   Bernd Blobel. Advanced EHR architectures – promises or reality, Proc. *Eur. Federation for Medical Informatics, Special Topic Conference*. 13-16 June 2004, Munich, Germany, pp. 73-78.

[6]   Petr Hanzlicek, Josef Splidlen, Miroslav Nagy. Universal electronic health record MUDR, in: Duplaga M, Zielinski K, Ingram D, eds. *Transformation of Healthcare with Information Technologies*, IOS Press, 2004. pp. 190-201.

[7]   Stergiani Spyrou, Alexander Berlerb, Panagiotis Bamidis. Information System Interoperability in a Regional Health Care System Infrastructure: a pilot study using Health Care Information Standards. *Proc. XVIIIth International Congress of the European Federation for Medical Informatics (MIE'2003)*, Saint-Malo, France, 4-7 May 2003, pp. 364-369.

[8]   Frank Oemig, Bernd Bloebel. Making Messaging Standards Work: From Definition to Interoperability at Runtime. *Proc. MIE'2003*, pp. 679-683.

[9]   C.A.Brandt, K.Sun, P.Charpentier, P.M.Nadkarni. "Integration of Web-based and PC-based clinical research databases." *Methods Inf Med* 2004; 43: 287-95.

[10]   Knut Bernstein, Morten Bruun-Rasmussen, Soren Vingtoft, Stig Kjar Andersen, Christian Nohr. Modelling and implementing Electronic Health Records in Denmark. *Proc. MIE'2003*, pp. 245-250.

[11]   Isabel Roman Martinez. An implementation of the openEHR Information Reference Model. at http://trajano.us.es/%7Eisabel/EHR/

Address for correspondence

Istvan Vassanyi, University of Veszprem, Dept. Information Systems, Veszprem, Egyetem u. 10, H-8200, Hungary. Email: vassanyi@irt.vein.hu

Connecting Medical Informatics and Bio-Informatics
R. Engelbrecht et al. (Eds.)
IOS Press, 2005

Issues in the Classification of Disease Instances with Ontologies

Anita Burgun[a], Olivier Bodenreider[b], Christian Jacquelinet[c]

[a]*EA 3888, Laboratoire d'Informatique Médicale, Faculté de Médecine, IFR 140, Université de Rennes I, France*
[b]*U.S. National Library of Medicine, Bethesda, MD, USA*
[c]*Etablissement français des Greffes, Paris, France*

Abstract

Ontologies define classes of entities and their interrelations. They are used to organize data according to a theory of the domain. Towards that end, ontologies provide class definitions (i.e., the necessary and sufficient conditions for defining class membership). In medical ontologies, it is often difficult to establish such definitions for diseases. We use three examples (anemia, leukemia and schizophrenia) to illustrate the limitations of ontologies as classification resources. We show that eligibility criteria are often more useful than the Aristotelian definitions traditionally used in ontologies. Examples of eligibility criteria for diseases include complex predicates such as ' x is an instance of the class C when at least n criteria among m are verified' and 'symptoms must last at least one month if not treated, but less than one month, if effectively treated'. References to normality and abnormality are often found in disease definitions, but the operational definition of these references (i.e., the statistical and contextual information necessary to define them) is rarely provided. We conclude that knowledge bases that include probabilistic and statistical knowledge as well as rule-based criteria are more useful than Aristotelian definitions for representing the predicates defined by necessary and sufficient conditions. Rich knowledge bases are needed to clarify the relations between individuals and classes in various studies and applications. However, as ontologies represent relations among classes, they can play a supporting role in disease classification services built primarily on knowledge bases.

Keywords:
Ontologies; Medical domain; Knowledge bases; Knowledge representation; Classification; OpenGALEN; SNOMED CT; Diagnosis; Patient records.

1. Introduction

Biomedical ontology aims to study the kinds of entities (i.e., substances, qualities and processes) in reality which are of biomedical significance and the relations among them. One role played by ontologies is to organize data (instances) according to classificatory principles reflecting a theory of the domain. In the clinical domain, disease instances, i.e., the particular forms of diseases (as described in the records of patients suffering from these diseases) are expected to be associated with the relevant disease categories represented in biomedical ontologies [1]. One role of the classifiers (e.g., Racer, FaCT) developed for ontologies represented in Description Logics (DL)-

based systems is precisely the automatic classification of instances. From an operational viewpoint, an ontology can be seen as a set of concepts or types that are organized in such a way that knowledge can be processed automatically by computers. To achieve that goal, the underlying structure must be "well-formed" and based on formal criteria, and the semantics must be explicit and consistent. Definitions in ontologies often embrace the Aristotelian model of genus and differentiae. In practice, definitions rely on a set of primitive terms which are not defined but rather given as such, and a set of interconcept relationships whose nature must be explicitly stated. Clarity was already mentioned by Gruber [2]: "Definitions should be effective [...]. Where possible, a complete definition (a predicate defined by necessary and sufficient conditions) is preferred over a partial definition (defined by only necessary or sufficient conditions)".

Besides terminological issues and clinical convention in naming diseases (some phrases do not literally mean what they say) [3,4], getting an effective definition can be difficult. Applied to diseases, the classificatory principles and properties represented in ontologies may not be sufficient to classify instances. In this paper, we discuss two major limitations of current biomedical ontologies, preventing them from effectively classifying disease instances. First, some properties are too general to be useful in an operational setting (e.g., "presence of abnormal cells", where "abnormal cells" refers to an abstraction or interpretation rather than a piece of information present in medical records). Second, the definition of medical conditions is not always sharp. In practice, diagnostic criteria often include probabilistic components rather than the binary (presence/absence) elements recorded in most ontologies. For these reasons, we argue that biomedical ontologies should not be expected to provide operational definitions of diseases. Rather, they can be used as supporting resources for disease classification services developed primarily on systems including probabilistic and statistical knowledge as well as rule-based criteria. We use three examples (anemia, leukemia and schizophrenia) to illustrate the limitations of ontologies as instance classification resources.

2. Anemia

Anemia is defined as "a reduction below normal in the concentration of erythrocytes or hemoglobin in the blood [...]; it occurs when the equilibrium is disturbed between blood loss (through bleeding or destruction) and blood production" (Webster 30th ed.). This definition is not operational as it contains a reference to normal concentrations. The same source provides reference intervals for the interpretation of laboratory tests (p. 2182), including references for erythrocyte and hemoglobin concentration, with distinctions for several population groups, shown in Table 1. The definition, complemented by reference intervals, makes it clear that properties such as age and gender are required for the interpretation of blood concentrations of erythrocytes and hemoglobin. Interpreting "or" as a true alternative, a low concentration of either entity is sufficient to diagnose anemia.

Biomedical ontologies such as OpenGALEN[1] and SNOMED CT[2] differ from the dictionary definition in that they only refer to the concentration of either hemoglobin (OpenGALEN, see Figure 1) or erythrocytes (SNOMED CT, see Figure 2). However, all definitions have in common to refer to abnormally low concentrations.

---

[1] http://www.opengalen.org/
[2] http://www.snomed.org/

• Haemoglobin Concentration
• Low Concentration
• Low Biochemical Measurement   } parent classes
• Haematological Disorder
• Pathological Concentration

(Haemoglobin Concentration
  which < *has Quantity* (
    Level which < *has Magnitude* low Level >
) >)

Figure 1 – Representation of Anaemia in OpenGALEN

* *Is a*
    Red blood cell disorder
* *Finding site*
    Hematopoietic system structure
* *Finding site*
    Erythrocyte
* *Has definitional manifestation*
    Erythropenia

Figure 2 – Representation of Anemia in SNOMED CT

Table 1 – Reference intervals for the interpretation of blood concentrations of erythrocytes and hemoglobin (conventional units)

Population group	Erythrocytes (million/mm^3)	Hemoglobin (g/dl)
Males	4.6-6.2	13.0-18.0
Females	4.2-5.4	12.0-16.0
Children *	4.5-5.1	11.2-16.5
Newborns	-	16.5-19.5

* (varies with age)

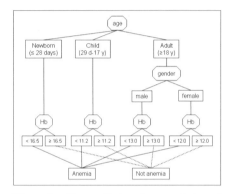

Figure 3 – Diagnostic tree for anemia based on age, gender and hemoglobin (Hb) concentration values

Not more than the textual definitions of dictionaries, the formal definitions of biomedical ontologies provide an operational definition of anemia, required for identifying anemic patients. A rule-based definition of anemia can be proposed instead, which would first consider *age* and then *gender* (for adults) before comparing *hemoglobin* (or erythrocytes) *concentration* values to the lowest bound of the reference interval for the corresponding population group. A diagnostic tree based on such rules (restricted to hemoglobin) is shown in Figure 3.

3. Leukemia

Leukemia is defined as 'a progressive, malignant disease of the blood-forming organs, characterized by distorted proliferation and development of leukocytes and their precursors in the blood and bone marrow' (Dorland, 28th ed). As for anemia, the textual definition uses references to abnormality but does not indicate precisely what kind of information is necessary to establish the diagnosis of leukemia. Examples of eligibility criteria for *acute leukemia* include the presence of at least 30% blasts (immature hematopoietic cells) in the bone marrow[3].

In both OpenGALEN (Figure 4) and SNOMED CT (Figure 5), leukemia is represented as a neoplastic disease with location to the hematological/lymphatic system. Children of *leukemia* in SNOMED CT include kinds of leukemia by cell type (e.g., *Myeloid leukemia*), by the degree of cell differentiation (e.g., *Acute leukemia*) and by the existence of an active disease (e.g., *Leukemia in remission*). Like the textual definitions above, these formal definitions fail to provide sufficient informations for classifying instances of leukemias based on patient data. Moreover, none of the classificatory criteria are represented explicitly, which makes it difficult – if at all possible – for users to automatically process knowledge.

Additionally, the example of *leukemia* raises two interesting issues. First, biomedical knowledge is evolving rapidly, often leading to changes in the theory of the domain. For example, knowledge of gene mutations related to leukemia may change the classification of leukemia (e.g. MLL rearrangements are correlated with poor prognosis in childhood acute myeloid leukemia[4]). Second, the categorization of *leukemia in remission* as a kind of *leukemia* in SNOMED CT is problematic. Remission means that the disease seems under control, but *leukemia in remission* has few of the characteristics of the active disease of which it should therefore not be considered a subtype. For example, the percentage of blasts in the bone marrow required to assess remission is generally less than 5% (as opposed to more than 30% in the acute form of the disease). Moreover, if *remission* is a valid classificatory principle, it is also surprising that a *remission* subclass is defined for only a few diseases (including some cancers) in SNOMED CT.

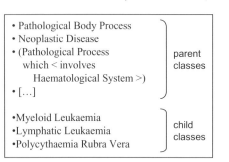

Figure 4 – Representation of Leukemia in OpenGALEN

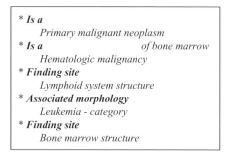

Figure 5 – Representation of Leukemia in SNOMED CT

4. Schizophrenia

The Diagnostic and Statistical Manual of Mental Disorders - 4th Edition (DSM-IV) is the main diagnostic reference thesaurus in psychiatry. For decades, psychiatrists have introduced in this classification diagnostic criteria for the most common mental disorders. Such criteria are needed to enable the consistent diagnosis of mental diseases in various contexts, including patient records, clinical trials and public health studies. Here is the definition provided for *schizophrenia* in DSM-IV: "a group of psychotic disorders characterized by disturbances in thought, perception, affect, behavior, and communication that last longer than 6 months". The following clinical

---

[3] http://www.cancer.org/docroot/cri/content/cri_2_4_3x_how_is_adult_acute_leukemia_diagnosed_57.asp?sitearea=&level=
[4] http://www.ncbi.nlm.nih.gov/entrez/query.fcgi?CMD=search&DB=omim

criteria are added to this general definition in order to create an operational definition: "For a material part of at least one month (or less, if effectively treated) the patient has had two or more of: (i) Delusions; (ii) Hallucinations; (iii) Speech that shows incoherence, derailment or other disorganization; (iv) Severely disorganized or catatonic behavior." The example of *schizophrenia* illustrates the following three issues:

- The eligibility criteria for schizophrenia in DSM-IV correspond to complex predicates: (i) at least n criteria among m must be verified; (ii) criteria may differ according to some condition: symptoms must last at least one month if not treated, but less than one month, if treated; (iii) exclusion criteria are needed for differential diagnosis (schizophrenia is not directly caused by a general medical condition or the use of substances). Such complex predicates are more likely to be present in knowledge bases designed to assist in diagnosis than in ontologies. In fact, the definitions of *schizophrenia* in OpenGALEN and SNOMED CT only specify that it is a kind of *Psychotic disorder*. Possible qualifiers (e.g., *acute*) are also listed in SNOMED CT.
- As it is often the case for diseases, references to normality are used in DSM-IV definitions. For example, when referring to "bizarre delusions", a typical example is provided ("being abducted in a space ship from the sun") rather than a formal definition. The use of typical examples in lieu of formal definition is not specific to psychiatric disease. For example, typical instances of skin lesion provide effective operational definitions in dermatology. Such alternatives to Aristotelian definition are usually not found in ontologies.
- The onset of schizophrenia may include a schizophrenic prodrome, i.e., a temporal part of a disease in which the manifestations are milder, preceding the main phase of the disease. In medical ontologies, schizophrenic prodrome is expected to be represented as a temporal part of schizophrenia, not as its subclass as it is the case in SNOMED CT.

5. Discussion

5.1. Knowledge bases vs. ontologies

Biomedical ontologies represent classes of diseases based on broad classificatory principles such as etiology and location. The classification is refined using ad hoc principles such as organism for infectious diseases or pharmacologic action for drug poisoning. While useful for organizing biomedical knowledge and supporting inference (i.e., reasoning about classes), ontologies do not generally contain the detailed information required for classifying disease instances and reasoning about them. In contrast, the methods used in knowledge bases designed for solving problems (e.g., rule-based systems, probabilistic systems) are more suitable for storing and processing the diagnostic information required for the classification of disease instances. For example, rules for the definition of anemia are illustrated by the decision tree presented in Figure 3. On the other hand, knowledge bases are created to support specific tasks, such as diagnosis. The relation *manifestation of* between a finding and a disease differs from the "necessary and sufficient conditions" in operational definitions. For example, the presence of *fever* and *necrotizing tonsillitis* would suggest the diagnosis of leukemia but are unlikely to be mentioned in its definition. Furthermore, ontologies of diseases in decision-support systems are hierarchies designed for specific application rather than formal reference ontologies that can serve any purpose. Finally, part of the knowledge needed to classify diseases is not represented in standard clinical decision-support systems, but rather in textbooks of medicine or in clinical genomics resources such as OMIM.

5.2. Applications to data integration

Eligibility criteria complement Aristotelian definitions as they clarify the meaning of the relation "is an instance of" and, in particular, make it distinct from the "isa" relation. Such criteria are required for the consistent classification of disease instances in clinical information systems. As a consequence, they also contribute to data integration by enabling disease instances recorded in heterogeneous systems to be reliably linked to disease ontologies. In practice, eligibility criteria may be linked to clinical databases, enabling the corresponding predicates to be instantiated with the clinical information stored in patient records (e.g., *hemoglobin concentration*, *age* and *gender* to classify instances of *anemia*). Moreover, as illustrated by the notions of remission (existence of a class *disease in remission*) and prodrome (existence of a class *disease prodrome*), further efforts are needed to clarify how the temporal dimension can be used as an organizing principle in ontologies and connected with information about the course of diseases in patients. A better representation of the temporal dimension of diseases would also contribute to data integration, for example by helping to distinguish between active diseases and diseases in remission.

5.3. Toward instance classification services

Classifying disease instances, i.e., linking patient records to disease classes, is a complex process requiring several types of resources. This finding is consistent with the characterization of resources proposed in [5], especially the distinction between terminology models (ontologies) and inference models (knowledge bases). While knowledge bases contain the predicates necessary to establish a diagnosis from phenotypic and genotypic criteria, these criteria may not be directly applicable to the data found in patient records. For example, equivalent criteria may be expressed in several different ways and ontologies can help bridge the semantic gap between knowledge bases and patient data. Along the same lines, there is a need for data expressed in one unit system to be compared to references expressed in another unit system (e.g., between traditional and international unit systems). Rather than the product of one resource, classifying disease instances can be thought of as a service based on both ontologies and knowledge bases. This view is analogous to that, promoted by GALEN, of terminology services based on ontologies [6].

6. References

[1]   Cimino JJ. From data to knowledge through concept-oriented terminologies: experience with the Medical Entities Dictionary. *J Am Med Inform Assoc.* 2000 May-Jun;7(3):288-97.

[2]   Gruber, T.R Toward Principles for the Design of Ontologies Used for Knowledge Sharing, *Int. Journal of Human-Computer Studies*, 1995, Vol. 43, pp.907-928.

[3]   Cimino JJ. Desiderata for controlled medical vocabularies in the twenty-first century. *Methods Inf Med.* 1998 Nov;37(4-5):394-403.

[4]   Rector AL. Clinical terminology: why is it so hard? *Methods Inf Med.* 1999 Dec;38(4-5):239-52.

[5]   Rector AL. The interface between information, terminology, and inference models. Medinfo. 2001;10(Pt 1):246-50.

[6]   Rector AL, Solomon WD, Nowlan WA, Rush TW, Zanstra PE, Claassen WM. A Terminology Server for medical language and medical information systems. *Methods Inf Med.* 1995 Mar;34(1-2):147-57..

Address for correspondence

Anita Burgun, EA 3888, DIM, CHRU Pontchaillou, 2, rue H Le Guilloux F-35033 Rennes Cedex, anita.burgun-parenthoine@univ-rennes1.fr

Connecting Medical Informatics and Bio-Informatics
R. Engelbrecht et al. (Eds.)
IOS Press, 2005

Terminological System Maintenance: A Procedures Framework and an Exploration of Current Practice

Ferishta Raiez [a], **Danielle Arts** [ab], **Ronald Cornet** [a]

[a] *Department of Medical Informatics,* [b]*Department of Intensive Care,*
Academic Medical Center, Universiteit van Amsterdam, the Netherlands

Abstract

The use of electronically stored data requires that the data is recorded in a structured and standardized manner. This has led to the development of terminological systems. The content of these medical terminological systems is subject to continuing changes as a consequence of the developments in the field of medicine.

By means of a literature study criteria were obtained for the maintenance of terminological systems. The criteria are used to develop a framework for the management of the maintenance process. The current practice of terminology maintenance was explored in a survey of twenty-seven organizations that currently maintain a terminological system. The results of the survey reveal the diversity and suboptimality of the current maintenance processes. The framework for the management of the maintenance process can be used to eliminate deficiencies in this process. This framework for terminology maintenance is an important step towards standardization of the maintenance of medical terminological systems.

Keywords:
Terminological systems, maintenance, process design

1. Introduction

For the use of electronically stored data it is important to have a structured and standardized way of data storage [1]. This has led to the development of numerous terminological systems. The dynamic character of medical knowledge makes the maintenance of medical terminological systems necessary [2]. However, with the regular changes in the content of terminological systems, incorrect representation of the knowledge might occur in the terminological system. In addition, frequent changes in the content of terminological systems can lead to difficulties in the processing and tracking of coded data [3]. Therefore it is necessary that the maintenance of terminological systems is performed in a structured way. Within this study we have summarized the criteria for the management of maintenance process of a terminological system in order to keep its knowledge consistent and up to date. Based on these criteria we have developed a framework which can serve as a guideline to design the maintenance process of (new) terminological systems. Organizations that are already maintaining a terminological system can use this framework to evaluate their maintenance process and, if necessary, to improve it.

To examine the current practice of maintenance in terminological systems, we held a survey among various organizations that currently maintain a terminological system. The results of the survey made it possible to compare current practice of maintenance process of terminological systems with the criteria within the framework.

2. Materials and methods

By means of a literature study we made an inventory of the most important aspects of the maintenance process and the criteria for good maintenance. Based on these criteria we have developed a framework.

To examine how maintenance takes place in real practice and to compare this current practice with the criteria found in the literature, we held an on-line questionnaire among administrators of some terminological systems. To compose the questionnaire we used the results of our literature study and the 'Terminology Questionnaire' which was held by the National Committee on Vital and Health Statistics (NCVHS) in February 2003.1 Our complete questionnaire was sent to the administrators of terminological systems included in the 'Unified Medical Language System Metathesaurus' that did not participate in the NCVHS survey (n = 46). Questions within our questionnaire that were not covered by the NCVHS survey were also sent to the participants of NCVHS survey (n = 37). The topics covered by the questionnaire were the structure, the content and the maintenance process of the terminological system.

3. Results

Based on the results of the literature study, we divided the maintenance process of a terminological system into four components; 1) 'process management', 2) 'change model' 3) 'execution' and 4) 'support'. Furthermore we summarized the criteria for maintenance mentioned in the literature and classified these criteria according to the four components of the maintenance process. Table 1 gives a summary of these criteria for each of the four components [2] [3] [2-16]. Finally, based on the results of the literature study and the criteria mentioned above, we have developed the framework for the maintenance process. A summarized version of the framework is displayed in figure 1. This framework summarizes the components of the maintenance process, the relations among them and the requirements to satisfy the related criteria. Within the framework the criteria are referred to by means of bracketed numbers. For instance the component 'execution' is based on a change model and is carried out according to some way of process management. The component 'execution' summarizes the sub processes of the maintenance process and describes how to carry out these sub processes. For instance the sub-process 'documentation' tells us what characteristics should be documented about changes made in the system and how to arrange this documentation. An extensive version of the framework with detailed descriptions of the components and sub-process is available from the authors.

1The National Committee on Vital and Health (http://www.ncvhs.hhs.gov)
2, GCL Maintenance Guide (http://www.wordmap.com/downloads/whitepapers/gcl_maintenance_guide.pdf)
3 Design/selection criteria for software used to handle controlled vocabularies (http://www.govtalk.gov.uk/documents/2004-01%20GCL%20softwareRequirements.pdf)

Table 1: Criteria for the maintenance of terminological systems and the extent to which the current practice of 27 organizations meets these requirements. N/A: Not available

	Criteria	#
Process Management	1. Assign a maintenance team, responsible for organization of the maintenance.	26
	2. The maintenance team must be easily accessible.	N/A
	3. The response time of the maintenance team on proposals and questions must be short.	N/A
	4. Different relevant disciplines should be involved within the maintenance team.	10
	5. Only qualified people should be able to make changes in the terminology content	N/A
Change model	6. The codes that are assigned to concepts must be non-significant.	7
	7. The codes that are assigned to concepts must be unique and should not be reused.	12
	8. Within the terminological system there must be no limitations for the number of concepts, hierarchic levels and terms that can be added.	N/A
	9. There must be a 'change model' which defines all changes that can occur in the content of a terminological system.	N/A
	10. Concepts that are no longer in use should not be removed from the terminological system. Instead, these concepts must remain in the terminological system and should be marked obsolete.	12
Execution	11. Proposals for changes in the terminology content must be standardized	16
	12. For each proposal, the consequences must be determined and thereupon anticipated.	N/A
	13. Proposals must be processed within a predetermined time period.	N/A
	14. Proposals for changes in the terminology content must be validated.	N/A
	15. Proposals for changes must be documented.	N/A
	16. Changes made in the terminology content must be validated.	24
	17. Changes made in the terminology content must be documented.	21
	18. Documentation must be structured and standardized.	18
	19. New versions of the terminological system must be provided with a unique identification number, including the publication date.	12
	20. Depending on the type of terminological system, on average twice a year a new version of the system must be launched.	18
Support	21. The administrators must use a supporting system for their maintenance process.	23
	a. The application must be secured with Login name and password.	*14*
	b. The application must support collecting the proposals for changes.	*17*
	c. The application must contain a module to enable the consensus process.	*18*
	d. The application must support the input of changes into the terminological system.	*19*
	e. The application must support the automatic validation controls.	*9*
	f. The application must generate reports for documentation.	*14*
	g. The application must support managing of different versions of the terminological system.	*7*
	h. The application must support editing of new versions for distribution.	*7*

Twenty-seven [4] of the eighty-three approached organizations filled in the questionnaire, which amounts to a response of 33 percent. Table 1 provides also a summary of the numbers of organizations that, according to the results of the questionnaire, satisfied the mentioned criteria. Because of the fact that the literature study and the survey were hold simultaneously, not al the criteria are covered by the questionnaire. If we compare the results of the questionnaire with the framework it appears that in daily practice none of the criteria is met by all organizations.

With respect to the 'process management', it appears that most of the participating institutions have organized their maintenance process properly.

---

[4] UMDNS, NTvG databank , MeSH, ICNP, DeCS, AOD Thesaurus , DICE, Medcin, NeuroNames, HHCC, DICOM Terminology, MED, SNOMED CT, Foundational Model of Anatomy, Omaha System , NANDA, Thesaurus of Psychological Index Terms , Diseases Database , PDQ Terminology, ABC codes V2004, FinMeSH, NCI Thesaurus , LOINC , NDF rt, RxNorm , Nursing Outcomes Classification, UMLS®

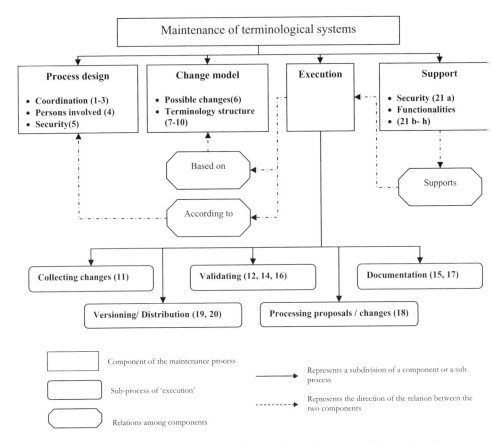

Figure 1: Framework for the maintenance of terminological systems. The numbers between the brackets refer to the related criteria from table 1.

With regard to the 'change model' we found that in many terminological systems (55%) the terms and concepts are completely removed from the content if they are no longer in use, which is undesirable according to the criteria. Furthermore, in twenty terminological systems (74%) significant codes are assigned, which means that the codes are not meaningless, as is required according to the criteria. Regarding this component ('change model') of the maintenance process most of the participating organizations could make improvements in their maintenance process. Also the component 'execution' has shown some shortcomings in real practice. For instance in contrast to the extensive dataset that is recommended for documentation of the changes and proposals in the literature, most organizations only document the date, the type and the executors ID. With respect to the component 'support' twenty-three organizations (85%) stated to use a supporting system for the maintenance process. If we compare the functionalities of these systems with the criteria mentioned in the literature, some improvements can be recommended.

In general the maintenance process in real practice is well organized. However, if we take a closer look at the maintenance process of the participating organizations separately, it appears that there are large differences between the different terminological systems. Some organizations satisfy most of the criteria, while others fail almost all criteria. Figure 2 gives an overview of the participating organizations and the number of criteria that are satisfied by their maintenance process.

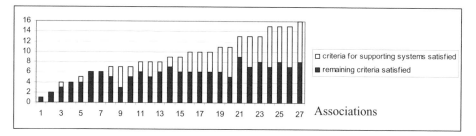

Figure 2: Number of criteria satisfied in the maintenance process of the 27 participating associations.

4. Discussion and Conclusions

Although the need for standardization of the maintenance process of medical terminological systems is recognized in literature, no large steps have been taken in this direction. Within this study we have tried to do so by developing a framework for the management of the maintenance process of medical terminological systems. This framework is based on criteria for the maintenance process that are mentioned in literature. Many publications considering the technical aspects of the maintenance process of medical terminological systems were available. For instance Cimino and Oliver have made an important contribution to this topic [2, 3, 4, 14]. However the design of the maintenance process has not yet been explored very well. The information found on this aspect of the maintenance process that was considered suitable and relevant for our study came mainly from publications outside the field of Medical Informatics.

Even though the number of 27 organizations that filled in our questionnaire appears to be relatively small, the participation of different kinds of terminological systems and of some of the well known large terminological systems makes the results representative.

The results of the survey reveal the diversity and incompleteness of the maintenance processes and thereby emphasizes the importance of the development of this framework. Terminological systems differ and the administrators do not always have the needs or possibilities to arrange the maintenance process optimally, for example because of budgetary constraints. For an advanced terminological system with a large number of users it is advisable to design the maintenance process optimally. However, for a local terminological system that is used by a limited number of users some of the criteria might be superfluous or too expensive. The framework presented here can be applied to every terminological system in conformity with the needs and the potentials of its administrators. The administrators can decide which criteria should be fulfilled. In the future the framework could be specified for the different types of terminological systems taking into account the structure and the size of the terminological systems. This could simplify the use of the framework for the administrators of terminological systems. This optimalization of the framework might be achieved by applying it to different terminological systems.

It can not be claimed that the framework guarantees the best management of the maintenance process. However, based on the contemporary literature, the framework provides the most complete management of the maintenance process of terminological systems. The framework, as it is, is an important step towards the standardization of the process of maintenance of medical terminological systems.

5. Acknowledgements

We thank the Authors of the NCVHS questionnaire for sharing the results of their study with us. We express our gratitude to the respondents of our questionnaire.

6. References

[1] Rose JS, Fisch BJ, Hogan WR, Levy B, Marshal P, Thomas DR, and Kirkley D. Common medical terminology comes of age, Part One: Standard language improves healthcare quality. *J Healthc Inf Manag*, 2001. 15(3): pp. 307-18.

[2] Oliver DE. *Change Management and Synchronization of Local and Shared Versions of a Controlled Medical Vocabulary. California: Department of Computer Science Stanford, 2000.*

[3] Cimino JJ and Clayton PD. Coping with changing controlled vocabularies. *Proc Annu Symp Comput Appl Med Care*, 1994: pp. 135-9.

[4] Cimino JJ. Desiderata for controlled medical vocabularies in the twenty-first century. *Methods Inf Med*, 1998. 37(4-5): pp. 394-403.

[5] Chute CG, Cohn SP, and Campbell JR . A framework for comprehensive health terminology systems in the United States: development guidelines, criteria for selection, and public policy implications. ANSI Healthcare Informatics Standards Board Vocabulary Working Group and the Computer-Based Patient Records Institute Working Group on Codes and Structures. *J Am Med Inform Assoc*, 1998. 5(6): pp. 503-10.

[6] Aryel RM, Cai J, Chueh HC and Barnett GO, Maintaining the integrity of a Web-based medical vocabulary glossary. *Proc AMIA Annu Fall Symp*, 1997: pp. 600-4.

[7] Pfleeger SL. *Software Engineering Theory and Practice. 2nd ed. Prentice Hal, 2001.*

[8] Zanstra PE, Haring v/d EJ and Cornet R. Introduction of a Clinical Terminology in the Netherlands. 2003, Nationaal ICT Instituut in de Zorg.

[9] IEC (International Electrotechnical Commission), Basic Aspects regarding Maintenance & Validation *Procedures of the IEC* 61360 reference Collection. 2000.

[10] Schmitz KD. Basic Requirements for Terminology Management within ISO Technical Committees. Language Resource Management. 2002

[11] Hartel FW, Fragoso G, Ong KL and Dionne R . Enhancing quality of retrieval through concept edit history. *Proc AMIA Symp*, 2003: pp. 279-83.

[12] Brown EG, Wood L and Wood S . The medical dictionary for regulatory activities (MedDRA). *Drug Saf*, 1999. 20(2): pp. 109-17.

[13] Schopen M. Consistency Checks for the maintenance of ICD-10. 200: WHO.

[14] Cimino JJ . Terminology tools: state of the art and practical lessons. *Methods Inf Med*, 2001. 40(4): pp. 298-306.

[15] Prins A, Arts D, Cornet R and de Keizer NF . Internet-based terminological Knowledge Maintenance,. *Medinfo*. 2004;2004(CD):1820

[16] Ganzman J . Criteria for the evaluation of thesaurus software by Jochen Ganzmann. *International Classification*, 1990. 17(1990) No. 3/4: pp. 148-157.

Address for correspondence

Dept. of Medical Informatics, J1b-121
Academic Medical Center, Universiteit van Amsterdam
P.O. Box 22700
1100 DE Amsterdam, the Netherlands
E- mail: f.raiez@amc.uva.nl

Connecting Medical Informatics and Bio-Informatics
R. Engelbrecht et al. (Eds.)
IOS Press, 2005

GALEN Based Formal Representation of ICD10

Gergely Héja[a], György Surján[b], Gergely Lukácsy[c], Péter Pallinger[a], Miklós Gergely[a]

[a] Budapest University of Technology and Economics, Department of Measurement and Information Systems
[b] National Institute for Strategic Health Research
[c] Budapest University of Technology and Economics, Department of Computer Science and Information Theory

Abstract

The authors present a formal representation of ICD10 based on GALEN CRM. The goal of the work is to create a coding support tool for coding clinical diagnoses to ICD10. The formal representation of the first two chapters of ICD10 has been almost completed. The paper presents the main aspects of the modelling, and the experienced problems. The constructed ontology has been converted to OWL, and a test system has been implemented in Prolog to verify the feasibility of the approach. The system successfully identified diseases in medical records from gastrointestinal oncology. The classifier module is still under development.

Keywords:
Ontology, ICD10, GALEN

1. Introduction

Indexing of medical diagnoses is a difficult and error-prone task. Providing assistance to manual coding is an important research area in medical informatics since many decades [1], still unsolved. Computer-assisted coding system can be basically classified into two groups.

Statistical systems do not "know" anything about the coding systems and the natural language, they classify the diagnoses based on statistical features of the training samples [2, 3]. Such systems are language-independent and easy to implement, since only well-controlled training samples are required. The usage of thesauri could significantly enhance the performance of such systems [4]. The drawback of this approach is that it can only cope with problems more or less masked by the training sample.

Knowledge-intensive systems represent formally both the coding system and the clinical text to be coded. The creation of the knowledge base is a resource intensive task, but the knowledge-based formal representation of medical narratives can support the reuse of information in various ways (clinical decision support, communication between different EPR systems, etc.) When the knowledge base describes both the clinical concepts and those of the coding system, the system can infer the possible codes even in those cases when the clinical expression uses different terms or even different concepts than the code category.

This paper presents a knowledge-intensive method for assisting ICD10 [5] coding. Both manual and computer-assisted coding processes may use clinical diagnoses as input information. This is a rational constraint (although it has some drawbacks [6]), because processing of the whole patient record would require a very complex model. In cases where the diagnosis is not specific enough, the user should consult the patient record.

2. Material and methods

2.1. ICD10

ICD10 is the most frequently used classification of diseases in Europe. It has been published in 1992 by WHO in 3 volumes. Our work is based on the first volume, which contains the ICD codes together with their natural language labels, definitions, (local) coding rules, etc. The second volume defines global coding rules and the third volume is a mere index to the first volume.

ICD10 is a hierarchical coding system, organised in 5 levels. The 21 chapters group together diseases according to major categories (location – e.g. cardiovascular diseases – and pathology – e.g. neoplasms). A separate chapter contains the international classification of oncology based on SNOMED [7]. Chapters contain sections grouping together similar diseases (like J10-J18 "Influenza and pneumonia"). Sections contain groups, which collect very similar diseases (like J10 "Influenza due to identified influenza virus"). Groups contain items, which define narrow groups of diseases (like J10.0 "Influenza with pneumonia, influenza virus identified"). In some cases items are subdivided on the fifth character (like H4411 "Endogenous uveitis"). 5th character subdivision is left for national purposes, however WHO itself defined some categories.

Each category has a name and may have (local) coding rules, definitions, and comments. Groups and items may have synonyms and dagger-asterisk cross-reference. Since our goal is to formally represent the meaning of the given category, these pieces of information is not directly represented in the ontology, but they have to be taken into account during modelling, since they may affect the meaning of the category.

Since the aim of ICD10 is to classify all possible diseases, there are a lot of "other" (e.g. J10.8 "Influenza with other manifestations, influenza virus identified") and "not otherwise specified" (e.g. J12.9 "Viral pneumonia, unspecified") categories. The later does not cause any problems, however the formal representation of "other" is a more difficult task. The problem is that it is not certain that an "other" category is defined by the exclusion of its siblings from its explicit parent category, therefore a detailed review of the coding system is required. The cause of this phenomenon is that the localisation of disease groups with similar (clinical) meanings may be in completely different parts of the hierarchy.

2.2. GALEN

The GALEN Core Reference Model (CRM) is designed to be a reusable application-independent and language-independent model of medical concepts to support EHRs, clinical user interfaces, decision support systems, classification and coding systems, etc [8]. The key feature of the GALEN approach is that it provides a model – a set of building blocks and constraints – from which concepts can be composed (in contrast to traditional classification systems). The classification of composite concepts is automatic and based on formal logical criteria. The structure of the GALEN has four logical layers: high-level ontology, CRM, subspecialty extensions and model of surgical procedures. For the representation of ICD10 only concepts from the first three layers were needed.

GRAIL is a description logic-like language [9] with special features to handle part-whole relations and other transitive relations needed to represent medical knowledge. These features are called role propagation and role composition in the description logic world, and the existing DL reasoning systems began to support them only recently [10]. It is related also to Conceptual Graphs, and to typed feature structures. Even so GRAIL is typically referred to in the literature as a description logic language. The main differences between GRAIL and a typical DL language are multi-level sanctioning and the lack of concept constructors without quantification.

Sanctioning is similar to canonical graphs in conceptual graph theory [11]. This notion means that an attribute (a role in DL) can only be used after it is allowed (in contrary to DLs where any relation can be used if it is not prohibited). Grammatical sanction is a statement that "an abstraction is useful for querying but not sufficiently constrained for generation". Sensible sanction means that the constraint can be used for generating complex concepts, but first it has to be permitted on grammatical level.

The lack of concept constructors without quantification is partially solved by elements in the ontology. Sets are represented by the concept **Collection** and there is a workaround for limited negation (introduced to represent conditions *with* or *without* other conditions, but it is implemented in the ontology, not in the grammar).

The role propagation in GRAIL can be asserted by the construct called *refinedAlong* (or *specialisedBy*), with the semantics:

r ° s ≡ ∀ x, y, z: r(x, y) AND s (y, z) → r(x, z)

where *r* and *s* are the relations, and *x*, *y* and *z* are classes. If this axiom is asserted between *hasLocation* and *partOf*, the reasoner can infer e.g. that a heart valve disease is a heart disease. This is a very important peculiarity of medical knowledge representation.

2.3. GALEN based formal representation of ICD10

The goal is to represent formally the meaning of each ICD category, using the concepts and attributes of GALEN CRM. Only the formal definition of the category (labelled by the ICD code) is represented. Since the other information (e.g. coding rules) give only additional information to the user, therefore they are separated from the formal representation. The hierarchical relations of ICD10 are also not represented in the ontology, since they may not always overlap with the hierarchy inferred from the formal definition.

According our view ICD categories can be defined by a multi-axial conceptual system:

- anatomy: location of the disease (if applicable). In case of the ICD anatomical entities are tissues, organ parts, organs, organ systems and regions.
- morphology: type of pathological alteration (e.g. inflammations and neoplasms)
- etiology: cause of the disease (if applicable, mostly organisms, chemical, physical and socio-environmental entities)

This classification is similar to SNOMED, which is the pathologist's view of medicine.

In case of certain categories additional axes are required, such as mode of diagnosis (e.g. A15 "Respiratory tuberculosis, bacteriologically and histologically confirmed"). By the way, this additional constraint has nothing to do with what is tuberculosis, thus it could be seen as a violation to original aim of ICD: to classify diseases.

Organisms can be further specified by e.g. type of transmission (A83 "Mosquito-borne viral encephalitis"). The disease may have complications (A98.5 "Hemorrhagic fever with renal syndrome") or be itself a complication of another disease (B01.0 "Varicella meningitis").

Thus categories are defined by formal relations among potentially complex entities:

MorphologicalEntity which
  hasLocation **AnatomicalEntity**
  isConsequenceOf **EtiologicalEntityOrDisease**
  isIdentifiedBy **DiagnosticProcedure**
  hasComplication **Disease**
  modifierAttribute **ModifierConcept**

In some cases GALEN contains a composite entity of anatomy and morphology (e.g. meningitis). A relation may be omitted if there is no constraint on the particular relation. The entities may be complex classes not present in the underlying core ontology (e.g. "**ArboVirus** which *isActedOnBy* (**Transmitting** which *hasSpecificPersonPerforming* **Mosquito**)"). The required modalities of the diseases (such as chronicity, laterality, disease state, acquisition mode, etc.) could be defined by using GALEN modifier concepts.

E.g. A81.1 "Subacute sclerosing panencephalitis", which is an autoimmune disease caused by measles infection is represented as:

> **Encephaliti***s* which *isConsequenceOf*
> (**AutoimmuneProcess** which *isConsequenceOf* (**InfectionProcess** which *isSpecificConsequenceOf* **MeaslesVirus**))

2.4. Transforming the ontology to OWL

The aforementioned "other" categories can be defined by the exclusion of its (logical) siblings from the parent concept. The parent concept is not always a defined ICD10 category (e.g. in case of A02 "Other salmonella infections", since there is no "Salmonella infections" in ICD10). This construction of exclusion cannot be represented in GRAIL.

This reason and the problems with reasoning support for GALEN led us to convert the ontology to the quasi-standard OWL [12]. We found that OWL is appropriate for the task, except for the definition of role propagation. Nevertheless we have chosen OWL, because we expect that role propagation would be added to it shortly.

Since there are cases when the reasoning on part-whole relation is important for ICD10 coding (e.g. S62.1 "Fracture of other carpal bone(s)" – clinical diagnosis "Fractura ossis lunati") the role propagation axioms have to be added to the ontology. It is advisable to store them in the OWL file, in the ontology header. Therefore the resulting OWL file is valid, available OWL reasoners can load it, and can reason about it (except role propagation based reasoning). If an own OWL interface is implemented above the reasoner (which supports role propagation), the system can also take the role propagation axioms into account.

The following GRAIL constructs have been transformed to OWL:

- The newSub / addSub / addSuper operators are used to define asserted subsumption. Their parallel in OWL is rdfs:subclassOf.

- The operators which / whichG formally define a category. We made no distinction between them in OWL. The "**A** which *hasX* **B**" concept is represented in OWL by the intersection of **A** with the (to **B**) restricted ObjectProperty *hasX*.

- The necessarily / topicNecessarily / valueNecessarily operators express the necessity of the criterion. ValueNecessarily is the inverse of topicNecessarily and necessarily asserts both criteria. A topicNecessarily *hasX* **B** is converted to a class (**A**) which is a subclass of an unnamed class with property restriction owl:someValuesFrom on the ObjectProperty *hasX*.

- Since sanctioning is only a tool supporting concise modelling it has not been converted to OWL yet. It is possible to convert sensible level sanctioning to owl:allValuesFrom.

The definition of "other" categories is achieved by the owl:disjoint construct.

2.5 Automatic coding tool

The NLP module of the system is a simple statistical component augmented with a thesaurus, since it has only to identify the expressions denoting diseases in texts. To allow easy implementation, the domain of the medical records has been constrained to gastrointestinal oncology. The whole text is searched for disease names, not only the "diagnoses" field. The sentences are analysed almost separately, no anaphora resolution is performed, only terms of a disease name located in adjacent sentences are contracted. The module contains a dictionary that translates Hungarian and Latin names of anatomical and morphological terms of the domain into English (which is the typical language of labels in GALEN). The relevant anatomical and morphological entities are stored in two lists.

First the text is broken down to sentences (boundary identified by the sequence "period-space-capital letter"), then the words are translated by the dictionary. Morphological analysis is not performed, only the statistical similarity of the word compared to the words in the thesaurus is computed. The candidates are ranked, and only the most relevant ones are considered. The found anatomical and morphological entities are combined into a disease, which is described in GRAIL. The diseases are displayed, together with the originating sentences and relevant words.

The medical records were manually analysed, the relevant diseases have been extracted, and manually coded to ICD10, thus allowing us to check the abilities of the NLP module. The module identifies 84% of the relevant diseases, however it also founds a lot of unnecessary diseases and locations, thus the precision is low: 45%.

The coding module – which classifies the found disease concepts into ICD10 categories – is still under development. The idea is that the found concepts are classified by the SILK DL reasoner [13] into ICD10 categories. If the two concepts are not totally identical, a similarity measure can be estimated. In most cases the found disease concept is a subclass of one or more ICD10 categories. However, frequently this subsumption relation can only be found out using role propagation. The used DL reasoner cannot cope with role propagation; therefore first of all it has to be augmented with this feature.

3. Results and discussion

The formal definition of the first two chapters of ICD10 (infectious diseases and neoplasms) has been almost completed. During the building of the ontology only the hierarchical relations have been taken into account as sibling concepts. After the completion of the formal representation of the whole ICD10 a review step is required to find the other related categories and the consistency errors.

During the work, some problems with GALEN CRM, as core ontology has been found. First, there were some required anatomical ("retroperitoneal lymphnode") and a lot of etiological ("enteropathogenic Escherichia Coli") concepts missing from GALEN. These concepts were added to the core ontology. Second, there were some concepts that could not be defined using GALEN CRM:

- The meaning of C10.4 "(malignant neoplasm of) branchial cleft" is a malignant neoplasm located on branchiogen cyst, which is a developmental residuum (thus a pathological structure). The definition of such concepts in GALEN would require the defoinition of (human) development, with concepts for temporary phenomena.
- The representation of C06.2 "(malignant neoplasm of) retromolar area" requires the definition of "retromolar region", which needs attributes describing 3D relations.

Based on these problems, we have decided that the project will be continued using FMA as core anatomy ontology [14]. FMA is a detailed ontology of human anatomy and development. The work up to now would not be lost: most of the references to anatomical concepts can be converted automatically. The conversion of FMA to OWL DL is underway. For computational effectiveness the enumerative approach of FMA is transformed to a composite approach (such as that of GALEN). The modeling of physiology, pathology, etc. is also required.

Some problems (in ontological sense) with ICD10 have also been found:

- C09 "Malignant neoplasm of tonsil", and C09.0 "Tonsillar fossa", which is not a part of the tonsil, but a structure formed by tonsillectomy. This example shows that the hierarchical relations in ICD not necessarily coincide with formal subsumption.
- In case of C86-C90 "Malignant neoplasms of ill-defined, secondary and unspecified sites" the formal definition of "ill defined site" is not realisable.

4. Conclusion

The formal representation of ICD10, together with the required NLP and inference tools could significantly enhance the quality of coding. The first step to this aim has been fulfilled: the development of a model of ICD10 based on GALEN. The formal definition of two chapters of ICD10 has been almost completed, with observations indicating that GALEN may not be the appropriate core ontology. A test system has been created to automatically classify oncological clinical diagnoses. The statistical NLP method has good recall, however the precision is quite low. The classifier module is still under development. The results indicate that the goal is realisable, although the used inference engine has to be supplemented by role propagation, and a more efficient NLP module should be used.

5. Acknowledgements

This work has been partially founded by the Hungarian Ministry of Education, contract No. IKTA 00126/2002 and by the Hungarian Ministry of Health. The kind help of dr. Gábor Csongor Kovács is highly appreciated.

6. References

[1] F. Wingert An indexing system for SNOMED, Meth Infom Med 1986; 25:22-30
[2] C. G. Chute, Y. Yang An overwiew of Statistical Methods for the Classification and Retrieval of Patient Events Methods of Information in Medicine (1995); 34:104-110
[3] G.Surján, G. Héja Maintenance of self-consistency of coding tables by statistical analysis of word co-occurrences Stud Health Technol Inform. 1999; 68:887-90.
[4] G. Héja, G. Surján: Analysing coding tables with thesaurus augmented statistical methods in CD ROM of MIE2003, XVIIIth International Congress of the European Federation for Medical Informatics, St. Malo, France, 4-7 May 2003.
[5] International Statistical Classification of Diseases and Health Related Problems, Who, Geneva, 1992
[6] G. Surján: Questions on validity of International Classification of Diseases-coded diagnoses, International Journal of Medical Informatics 54 (1999) 77-95
[7] Coté R.A. Rothwell D.J. et al. (eds.) SNOMED International, College of American Pathologists, Northfield Il. USA 1993
[8] Information materials about Galen can be found at http://www.opengalen.org/open/crm/index.html
[9] F. Bader et al. (editors): The Description Logic Handbook (Theory, Implementation and Applications), Cambridge University Press, 2003
[10] I. Horrocks, U. Sattler: Decidability of SHIQ with complex role inclusion axioms. Artificial Intelligence, 160(1-2):79-104, December 2004.
[11] J. F. Sowa Conceptual Structures: Knowledge Representation in Mind and Machine, John Wiley & Sons, New York, 1985
[12] Information materials about OWL can be found at http://www.w3.org/2004/owl
[13] T. Benkő, G. Lukácsy, A. Fokt, P. Szeredi, I. Kilián, P. Krauth: Information Integration through Reasoning on Meta-data, Proceedings of AI Moves to IA, Workshop on Artificial Intelligence, Information Access, and Mobile Computing", IJCAI'03, Acapulco, Mexico
[14] Information material about FMA can be found at http://sigpubs.biostr.washington.edu/view/projects/Foundational_Model_of_Anatomy.html

Address for correspondence

Budapest University of Technology and Economics, Dept. of Measurement and Information Systems, 2. Magyar tudósok körútja, Budapest, Hungary, H-1117, e-mail: heja@mit.bme.hu

Connecting Medical Informatics and Bio-Informatics
R. Engelbrecht et al. (Eds.)
IOS Press, 2005

713

Signe: A Geographic Information System on the Web for End-Stage Renal Disease

Jean-Baptiste Richard[a], Laurent Toubiana[b], Loïc Le Mignot[a], Mohamed Ben Said[a],
Claude Mugnier[a], Christine Le Bihan–Benjamin[a], Jean Philippe Jaïs[a], Paul Landais[a]

[a]Service de Biostatistique et d'Informatique Médicale, Hôpital Necker, Université Paris 5, France
[b]Inserm – U707, Faculté de Médecine St-Antoine, Paris, France

Abstract

A Web-based Geographic Information System (Web-GIS), the Signe (Système d'Information Géographique pour la Néphrologie), was designed for the Renal Epidemiology and Information Network (REIN) dedicated to End-Stage Renal Disease (ESRD). This Web-GIS was coupled to a data warehouse and embedded in an n-tier architecture designed as the Multi-Source Information System (MSIS). It allows to access views of ESRD concerning the epidemiology of the demand and the supply of care. It also provides maps matching the offer of care to the demand. It is presented with insights on the design and underlying technologies. It is dedicated to professionals and to public health care decision-makers in the domain of ESRD.

Keywords
Web-GIS; Multi-Source Information System; Data warehouse; End-Stage Renal Disease; Decision-making

1. Introduction

The qualitative and quantitative epidemiological changes of the last decade have shown that the incidence and the prevalence of End-Stage Renal Disease (ESRD) have increased. However, no coordinated information was available [1]. In order to increase medical, epidemiological and organisational knowledge of ESRD at a national level, a Multi-Source Information System (MSIS) has been set up as part of the Renal Epidemiology and Information Network (REIN) [2]. This program involves several organizations : Paris 5 University and Grenoble J. Fourier University, Société de Néphrologie, Société francophone de dialyse, Etablissement français des Greffes (EfG), INSERM, Institut de Veille Sanitaire, Caisse Nationale d'Asssurance Maladie, Direction de l'Hospitalisation et de l'Organisation des Soins, and representatives of patients' associations. Integrated to the MSIS application, SIGNe is a tool dedicated to dynamically visualize and analyse the ESRD data sets. Based upon new technologies such as Geographic Information Systems (GIS), Web-GIS, On-Line Analytical Processing (OLAP), SIGNe program aimed at analysing ESRD epidemiology, assessing resource allocation and improving public health decision-making.

2. Material and Methods

Data collection

The Multi-Source Information System (MSIS-REIN) is dedicated to collect all ESRD minimal patient records with their annual follow-up, the content of which were defined by a national consensus.the main variables of these records concern both epidemiological informations and description of the supply of care: age at first initiation of replacement therapy, type of initial nephropathy, type of dialysis, comorbidities, handicaps, remoteness from dialysis unit, characteristics of the units of care and territorial distribution of the nephrologists. The MSIS initially tested in two adminitrative regions in 2002, is currently running in six regions : Limousin, Languedoc-Roussillon, Champagne-Ardenne, Provence Alpes Côte d'Azur, Ile de France, Centre. The control of exhaustiveness and quality of the data is performed regionally by clinical research assistants. At present the data set gathers more than 9000 records.

MSIS architecture

The architecture of MSIS-REIN is based on an n-tier architecture (figure 1). A universal client (1st tier) connects to a dynamic Web server (2nd tier) that is in relation with several databases (3rd tier). The information system tier may access three types of databases: the identification database, the production database and a data warehouse. Collected data supply the production database. After exhaustiveness and quality control is performed, consolidated data are integrated to the data warehouse. A secure connection and the use of an identification server warrant confidentiality and security of patient informations according to the French law.

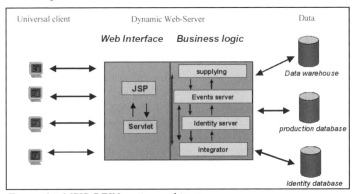

Figure 1 – MSIS-REIN n-tier architecture

Data Warehouse

A data warehouse [3] can be defined as a collection of data, which are subject-oriented, integrated, time variant, non-volatile and historicized. It allows reorganizing data imported from the production database in order to support analytical and decision processes. Data warehouse is often linked to data mining and On-Line Analytical Processing (OLAP) used in a decisional information system. This organization of ESRD data sets is helpful to create persistent views concerning different axes : temporal, age of patient, incidence, prevalence or other indexes.

SIGNe objectives and integration

Objectives

It is very useful and customary to divide the geography of health into two interrelated areas:

- the geography of disease, which covers the exploration, description and modelling of the spatio-temporal incidence and prevalence of disease, the detection and analysis of disease clusters and patterns;
- the geography of healthcare systems, which deals with the planning, management and delivery of suitable health services, after determining healthcare needs of the target community and service catchments zones.

The importance of Geographic Information System (GIS) for medical research and epidemiology has long been recognized [4,5,6,7]. Health geography plays an important role in public health surveillance, and can also help identifying interregional inequities in health service delivery, and in the efficiency of allocating and monitoring healthcare ressources. Thus geographical visualizations may be helpful for both studying spatial epidemiology and helping to assess the best distribution of healthcare units based on current needs.

SIGNe aims at answering distinct important questions: what is the temporal evolution of ESRD epidemiology? What is the spatial distribution of ESRD incidence and prevalence? What are the main chararcteristics of the ESRD population? What are the characteristics of the dialysis units? Are there any inequities in health care needs or accessibility to care?

In order to achieve these objectives, we developed a web-based interface aimed at ESRD professionals and decision-makers at a regional and national level. This interface includes tools that allow creating dynamically both maps and charts representing current data sets regarding epidemiological and care management aspects.

Web-GIS and OLAP

A GIS is a system composed of hardware and software used for storage, retrieval, mapping and analysis of spatially referenced (georeferenced) information. A GIS makes possible overlaying and integrating multi-source data. It helps discovering and visualizing new data patterns and relationships that otherwise would have remained invisible, by creating the link between spatial data and their related descriptive information. A Web-based GIS (Web-GIS) allow to reproduce on a Web-interface main functions of GIS: spatial analysis, navigation (zoom, pan), dynamic creation of map, layer overlaying, interactive querying. A Web-GIS is a new mean to dynamically share and represent spatial information, with a large access. A lot of Web-GIS have recently emerged (MapServer, ArcIMS, MapXtrem, Alov Map, GeoServer), using different displaying technologies : vector (SWF, SVG...), raster (PNG, JPEG...), server side or client side mapping. Regarding the interactivity, the database connection abilities and the costs of development, we chose to develop our interface with Flash MX™, Php™ and MySQL™.

Besides, we used tools to create dynamic charts in connection to the data warehouse. Different open-source programs allow to realize this on-line analytical processing (OLAP): JPGraph, PhP/SWF Chart, or owtchart. We used Php/SWF Chart, that create main chart types in a vector format (SWF) compatible with our Web-GIS system.

Integration to the MSIS

SIGNe interface was integrated as a new tool to the MSIS and to the data warehouse. The global architecture of the application is presented on figure 2. The MSIS supplies the data warehouse with consolidated data. Once the connection to the SIGNe established, the user send requests to the data warehouse that extracts current data.

SIGNe is being tested with three region data sets: Limousin, Languedoc-Roussillon and Champagne-Ardenne. Patients and dialysis units are georeferenced using their place of residence or their location, respectively.

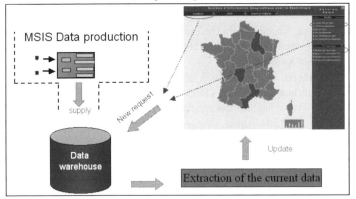

Figure 2 – SIGNe integration to MSIS

User interface

SIGNe offers representing on a single interface cartographical and statistical representations. The screen structure and the different functionalities are presented on figure 3. The user defines the theme (incidence, prevalence, survival....), the year and the region of interest (one region data set or the whole data set). A list of maps and charts is then updated, and eventually displayed on the representation area.

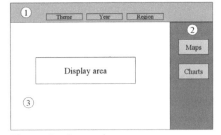

Figure 3 – *Screen layout structure*

3. Results

Epidemiological results

Examples of epidemiological results are presented on figure 4. The thematic map is a data visualization where the attributes of geographic features (here the incidence rates by region) are displayed on a map. It allows assessing the geographical distribution of new ESRD cases considering several French departments. Other thematic maps can be obtained for different themes (prevalence, mortality...), and also at a smaller scale. For instance, the user is able to map the disease distribution by district or even smaller administrative boundaries.

The bar chart aimed at defining more precisely the ESRD population. It represents the distribution of incidence cases by age group. Other similar representations can be created regarding the type of treatment, the co-morbidities or the handicaps

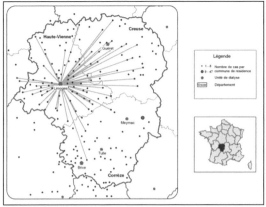

Figure 4 – Epidemiological representations.

Health care attractiveness

Figure 5 shows an example of both supply and demand of care representation. Patient's affiliations according to their district of residence (points) are linked to the location of their dialysis unit. It shows that Limoges hospital attracts patients beyond the limits of the Haute-Vienne department despite the presence of other dialysis units in the adjoining departments.

Such a map of several different types of data, provides medical professionals and administrators with information about the matching between the supply and demand of care for dialysis.

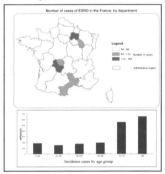

Figure 5 – Attractiveness of the Limoges Hospital dialysis unit.

4. Discussion

This study shows how Web-GIS and statistical tools can be useful to better respond to information needs concerning the demand and supply of care of ESRD. SIGNe offers an intuitive way of accessing and mining large health care informations. Besides the need of epidemiological knowledge regarding the demand of care, SIGNe helps describing the relationships between the location of care and the place of residence of ESRD patients. It may assist in better health care planning, aiming at more efficient and effective utilization of resources. The use of web-based interfaces including interactive mapping is growing in health geography. Such interfaces are usually developed in order to help public health surveillance and a better knowledge of disease geographical distribution, such as the application of the world health organization [8]. In the field of renal disease, the United

States Renal Data System has also developed an interactive atlas to share information about ESRD, the Renal Data Extraction and Referencing (RenDER) [9]. It is an online data querying application accessible through the USRDS website. Based upon user's query specification, it returns a table of data or an interactive map. SIGNe proposes a user-friendlier tool, including not only the demand of care but also the offer of care, at the interface of epidemiology and public health. The cost effectiveness of SIGNe has not been evaluated yet in this implementation and loading phase. It will be initiated considering macroscopic markers followed longitudinally: for instance, shortening patients' travel-time to their dialysis unit, or improvement of clinical performance measures (e.g. erythropoietin level according to European standards).

5. Conclusion

SIGNe is a GIS embedded in the Multi-Source Information System of the French Renal Information and Epidemiological Network. It was dedicated to representing the demand and the supply of care and their match at a regional level. Complementary tools are presently in preparation aiming at describing more precisely accessibility to health care units. For instance, works on model to determine the minimum travel time and distance to health care units are currently developed [10]. We'll adapt this approach and develop scenarios for renewed resource allocations. In effect, geographical access models have enormous potential for fruitful debate on how to achieve social equity of care access. These scenarios will be a useful information resource that can be used in health service delivery planning and assessment.

6. Acknowledgments

We thank the members of the participating regions to the MSIS. This research was funded by a grant from STIC-Santé-Inserm 2002, n°A02126ds, and by Paris 5 University. This work was also supported by grants provided by the Caisse Nationale d'Assurance Maladie des Travailleurs Salariés, the Institut de Veille Sanitaire and the Agence de la Biomédecine. Xavier Ferreira and Jean-Philippe Necker are acknowledged for their skilful help.

7. Reference

[1]   Landais P. L'insuffisance rénale terminale en France : offre de soins et prévention. *Presse Med*.2002; 31:176-85.

[2]   Landais P, Simonet A, Guillon D, Jacquelinet C, Ben Saïd M, Mugnier C, Simonet M. SIMS@REIN : Un Système d'Information Multi-Sources pour l'Insuffisance Rénale Terminale. *CR Biol* 2002;325:515-528.

[3]   J ones K. An Introduction to Data Warehousing: What Are the Implications for the Network? *Int. J. Network Mgmt* 1998; 8:42-56.

[4]   Croner CM. Public Health GIS and the Internet. *Annu Rev Public Health*. 2003; 24:57-82.

[5]   Cromley EK. GIS and Disease. *Annu Rev Publ Health* 2003; 24:7-24

[6]   Richards T.B. et al. Geographic information systems and public health: mapping the future. *Public Health Rep* 1999; 114: 359-60.

[7]   Bedard Y, Gosselin P, Rivest S, Proulx MJ et al. Integrating GIS components with knolewdge discovery technology for environmental health decision support. *Int J Med Inform* 2003; 70:79-94.

[8]   http://www.who.int/csr/mapping/en/

[9]   http://www.usrds.org/odr/xrender_home.asp

[10]   Brabyn L, Skelly C. Modeling population access to New Zealand public hospitals. *Int. J. of Health Geographics* 2002; 1:1-3.

Address for correspondance

Dr Paul Landais, Service de Biostatistique et d'Informatique Médicale, Hôpital Necker-Enfants Malades 149, rue de Sèvres, 75743 Paris cedex 15, e-mail : landais@necker.fr

Connecting Medical Informatics and Bio-Informatics
R. Engelbrecht et al. (Eds.)
IOS Press, 2005

Which Graphical Approaches should be Used to Represent Medical Knowledge?

Jean-Baptiste Lamy[a], Catherine Duclos[a], Vincent Rialle[b], Alain Venot[a]

[a] LIM&BIO (Laboratoire d'Informatique Médicale et de BIO-informatique), University of Paris 13, Bobigny, France
[b] TIMC, University of Grenoble 1, La Tronche, France

Abstract

Medical knowledge is growing both in quantity and complexity. Although sources of medical knowledge have been digitalized, the way the knowledge they contain is presented to users has not changed and is still highly text-based. However, it has been shown that this information could be presented more efficiently using graphical approaches, such as graphical languages and information visualization. We present here a survey of existing methods and applications, and discuss the potential value of these methods for medical practice. These graphical approaches have great potential for improving medical knowledge consultation, provided they are well-designed, well-evaluated and standardized for re-use.

Keywords:
Data Display; Nonverbal Communication; Visual Perception

1. Introduction

Medical knowledge is growing both in quantity and complexity, and it is becoming increasingly difficult to find the right information. Most medical knowledge sources have been digitalized, but the way knowledge is presented to the user has not changed, and still relies principally on text-based approaches. According to the well-known proverb, 'a picture is worth a thousand words', L. S. Elting et al. [1] showed that a picture can worth a thousand of medical words. Healthcare professionals need information in three different situations, each of which could benefit from graphical approaches:

- During a consultation: as the patient is present, the professional is stressed and lacks time but the information concerned is often simple. This situation is ideal for graphical approaches, which can reduce the volume of knowledge displayed and provide more rapid access to that knowledge.

- After a consultation, to investigate a specific point in greater detail: the professional is less stressed, and the knowledge involved may be complex. A graphical approach would probably not be accurate enough to represent the complex medical knowledge, but could make it easier to find the right reference text rapidly.

- In continuing education: a graphical approach could make the knowledge more accessible and attractive.

A literature review showed that two complementary approaches can be used: graphical languages and information visualization. We present here the various techniques, with their pros and cons. We also survey existing medical applications and discuss their potential value for use in medical practice.

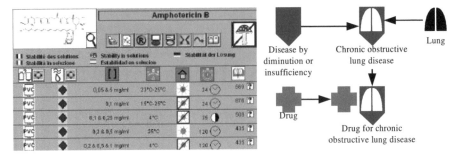

Figure 1: On the left, the stability of amphotericin B expressed in the graphical language of Stabilis 2 (reproduced with the agreement of the authors). On the right, example of pictogram construction in VCM.

2. Graphical languages

Graphical languages are found everywhere today, from traffic signs to computer software icons and modeling (unified modeling language, UML). As simple as they seem, these languages are governed by the complex rules of *semiotics*, the science of signs and sign systems. Graphical languages have several advantages over textual languages:

- They tend to be universal. They can be understood without learning by analogy: words have arbitrary meanings, but we can guess the meaning of pictures of concrete things. They are also independent of native languages, although it is difficult to achieve complete independence from cutural background.

- They are more concise and more attractive to the eye than text, and can be read faster. Under certain circumstances that allow pre-attentive perception, it is possible to search items in a picture very rapidly (< 200 ms), regardless of the number of items [2].

However, graphical languages have some drawbacks: they are less precise than native textual languages, and they often have greater technical requirements such as color printing or animated display. Graphical languages are therefore most appropriate for simple information that must be understood rapidly or universally. Graphical languages often optimize one of these two aspects. For example, chemical product labeling focuses on universal understanding, as everyone must be able to understand the labels, whereas traffic signs focus on the rapid transmission of information, as trained drivers must be able to assimilate the information conveyed by traffic signs as rapidly as possible. Graphical languages for use in medicine also falls into these two categories:

2.1 Graphical languages for patients

These languages involve simple information, convyed in a fashion that can be understood by everyone, using iconic pictures and few, if any grammatical structures. An example is provided by the United States Pharmacopeial Convention (USP) pictograms for drug patient leaflets [3]. These pictograms deal with dose planning, adverse effects, administration route, safe practices for administration, drug storage, interactions with food, contraindications, etc. The pictograms are in black and white and are followed by a sentence in English.

2.2 Graphical languages for health professionals

These languages aim at easing the access to complex medical information. They are specialized and may therefore require a learning period and a medical background, and thus they may use more abstract symbols. When they can't represent complex information, these graphical languages can be used in addition to text in order to take the advantages of both graphical and textual languages. Graphical languages are of particular value when the patient is present, as the professional may be short of time.

Stabilis 2 [4] is a knowledge base on the stability and compatibility of injectable drugs. For each drug, it provides information concerning drug's therapeutic classification, storage, stability in various solutions, incompatibilities, etc. (figure 1, left). It uses a graphical language of about 150 pictograms but has no real grammatical structures. These pictograms make Stabilis native language-independent, whereas most knowledge sources (medical literature, specialized reference books) are available only in English.

VCM (*Visualisation des Connaissances sur le Medicament*, Drug Knowledge Visualization) is a graphical language that we are developing at the LIM&BIO for representing drug knowledge, such as the Summary of Product's Characteristics (SPC) and the therapeutical parts of clinical guidelines (CG). The intended users are health professionals, such as physicians and pharmacists. VCM relies on solid cognitive and semiotic bases. It includes a set of pictograms (currently about a hundred) for anatomical sites, etiologies, pharmacological targets, and adjectives (such as 'forbidden', 'recommended' or 'risk of'), together with simple grammar to combine these pictograms and build 'composed pictograms' such as disease or drug pictograms, and then sentences concerning contraindications, adverse reactions, and so on (figure 1, right).

VCM has been designed to extend textual language but not to replace it, as it cannot achieve a similar level of precision. For example, specific concepts such as the diseases 'asthma' and 'chronic obstructive bronchitis' cannot be represented directly by the language. We use only more generic concepts, such as 'chronic obstructive lung disease', determined with the inheritance relations of medical classifications such as the International Classification of Diseases (ICD10). When more details are required, physicians should refer to the text version.

3. Information visualization

Information visualization (IV) aims to represent a given piece of information graphically, to make that information more accessible and, in some cases, to allow 'visual data-mining'. IV focuses on abstract information with no spatial or geometric properties, and thus no obvious graphical form. Many items of medical data and knowledge are neither spatial nor geometric and fall into the field of IV: for example drug knowledge, patient characteristics and antecedents, clinical results, whereas anatomy and anatomical examinations (e.g. X rays) do not. L. Chittaro [5] reviewed the use of IV in medicine, and K. Andrews [6] has produced an almost exhaustive list of IV systems.

IV relies on *interactivity* to involve users. *Fisheye* is used to generate this interactivity; it separates information into the *focus* (information interesting for the user) and the *context* (information less interesting for the user). The user interacts with the system to specify the focus and the context. The focus is then displayed in more detail than the context. There are two types of Fisheye: filtering and deforming Fisheyes. In the *filtering* Fisheye, the context is hidden, like in zoom-based technics. In the *deforming* Fisheye, a larger area of the screen surface is devoted to the focus than to the context. An example of deforming Fisheye is a 3D perspective in a virtual reality tool, in which the nearby objects are the focus and appear larger.

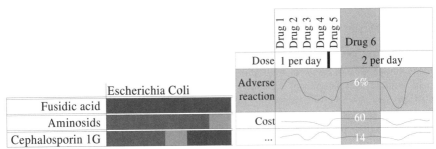

Figure 2: On the left, table displaying antibiotic spectra [8]. On the right, example of a table lens for drug comparison (the selected row and column in gray are the focus).

IV technics are traditionally classified according to the structure of the visualized information, as spatial/geometric properties in IV are often based on the structure of the information.

3.1 Texts

Several methods have been proposed for texts, including greeking and Fisheye, but these methods either deform the text or make it unreadable. As a consequence, none of them appears to be suitable for medical texts; we therefore suggest that graphical languages are the most appropriate way to represent texts.

3.2 N-dimensional data

2D and 3D graphics have been widely used to display medical data for overview or monitoring purposes. An example is provided by interactive parallel bar charts (IBPC), a system designed by L. Chittaro *et al.* [7] for visualization of the clinical data acquired by hemodialyzer devices. However, this system is less useful for the representation of medical knowledge.

3.3 Object-attribute matrices

In medicine, object-attribute matrices may be applied to patients (*e.g.* patients involved in a clinical trial), drugs, diseases and so on. Several visualization methods exist, and these methods highlight the differences or similarities between objects.

Tables can display object-attribute matrices with about 660 cells on screen. A *table lens* can multiply this number by 30. In a table lens, the user can choose how rows and columns are displayed: as numerical values or graphics. This method is highly suitable for highlighting the differences between objects. M. Spenke *et al.* [9] have successfully used the table lens method to display medical data, such as blood parameters, and C. Wroe *et al.* [10] have used such methods to display a drug ontology for authoring purposes. However, table lenses are also likely to be useful for clinical purposes, such as drug comparison. For example, C. Duclos [8] used tables to display antibiotic spectra. Each spectrum is represented by an horizontal bar, the length of which indicates the prevalence and the color of which indicates the susceptibility or resistance (figure 2).

Glyphs are an ideal method for finding similar objects. Each object is represented by a glyph, a small picture arbitrarily modified according to the object's attributes. Similar objects therefore have similar glyphs. L.S. Elting *et al.* [1] have evaluated the use of glyphs for monitoring purposes.

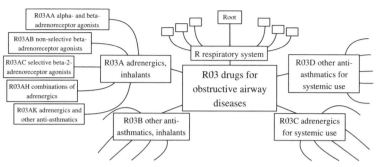

Figure 3: Part of the ATC classification displayed on an hyperbolic tree.

Gene Ontology

| Unknown | Enzyme | Transporter |

Figure 4: Genes (marked by 'X') classified according to ontology, inspired from [12].

3.4 Trees and networks : medical classifications

Medicine is full of hierarchical structures, such as medical classifications and ontologies. I. Herman *et al.* [11] reviewed tree visualization methods , but few IV methods deal with networks. Most focus on simplified forms of the network and try to turn them into trees. Two methods seem to be particularly interesting:

Hyperbolic trees are highly suitable for navigation, for medical classifications in particular. A hyperbolic tree is a radial tree in a hyperbolic plane. The hyperbolic geometry generates a deforming Fisheye, so more details are visible near the center than at the periphery. The user can navigate through the tree by deplacing the center (figure 3).

Tree-maps provides an overview of a tree, making it possible to discover recurrent patterns; B. Ketan [12] applied this method to the gene ontology. Tree-maps use all the available space; this space is divided horizontally or vertically into several rectangles, one for each node at the first level of the tree. The rectangle for each node is then divided into subrectanges corresponding to the daughter nodes, and so on (figure 4).

3.5 Similarity indices

This method is applied to a set of objects (often texts). A similarity index is then defined for each pair of objects within the set. Objects with high similarity indices are located close together on the screen, forming clusters. This makes it very easy to identify similar objects. In medicine, similarity indices could represent medical documents in a searching tool, or drugs in prescribing software. This would help physicians to find similar drugs when unable to prescribe their first-choice drug due to contraindications, for example. This method could also be used to find clusters of similar patients.

4. Discussion and conclusion

Many methods have been proposed for the graphical representation of knowledge. These methods have already been applied to medical knowledge, but most applications have been evaluated sufficiently and follow an 'intuitive approach' rather than a rational approach.

Graphical language design should take into account semiotics and the abilities of human visual perception. The standardization of medical graphical languages, as has been done for traffic signs, would help to create new languages by re-using some pictograms or some grammatical structures, and would reduce the time required to learn the new language.

It is difficult to choose the right IV method, and the structure-based classification presented above is of little help in practice. For example, drugs can be treated as texts (SPC), a tree (ATC classification), an object-attribute matrix (drug-drug property matrix) or similarity indices (extracted from SPC). It is therefore possible to use any of the methods described above. Methods should therefore not be selected on the basis of the structure of the information to be displayed. Instead, they should be chosen such that the method is appropriate for the intended use. Ideally, several methods should be combined and applied to the same knowledge, allowing the physician to choose the most appropriate method for a particular situation. For example, hyperbolic tree could be used to navigate to beta-blocking anti-hypertensive drugs; a table lens could then be used to compare these drugs, and finally a graphical langage could be used to obtain an overview of the SPC of the most interesting drugs.

In conclusion, there is a clear need for rigorous methodology based on semiotics and information vizualisation. We are currently far from the achievements in other domains, such as information retrieval, but this study has provided convincing evidence that graphical approaches are of value for the presentation of medical knowledge.

5. References

[1]   Elting LS, Bodey GP. Is a picture worth a thousand medical words ? A randomized trial of reporting formats for medical research data. *Methods of information in medicine* 1991;30:145–150.

[2]   Bertin J. *Semiology of graphics*. University of Wisconsin Press; 1983.

[3]   University of North Carolina at Chapel Hill Duke University. *Optimizing patient comprehension through medicine information leaflets*. United States Pharmacopeia; 1998. Http://www.uspdqi.org/pubs/other/PatientLeafletStudy.pdf

[4]   Vigneron J, Gindre I, Daouphars M, Monfort P, Georget S, Chenot E, *et al*. Stabilis 2: an international CD-ROM database on stability and compatibility of injectable drugs. *Journal of the European Association of Hospital Pharmacists (EJHP)* 2004;(2):59–60.

[5]   Chittaro L. Information visualization and its application to medicine. *Artificial Intelligence in Medicine* 2001;22(2):81–88.

[6]   Andrews K. *Information visualisation: tutorial notes*; 2002. Available from: http://www2.iicm.edu/ivis/ivis.pdf

[7]   Chittaro L, Combi C, Trapasso G. Data Mining on Temporal Data: a Visual Approach and its Clinical Application to Hemodialysis. *Journal of Visual Languages and Computing* 2003;14(6):591–620.

[8]   Duclos C, Cartolano GL, Ghez M, Venot A. Structured representation of the pharmacodynamics section of the Summary of Product Characteristics for antibiotics: application for automated extraction and visualization of their antimicrobial activity spectra. *Journal of the American Medical Informatics Association* 2004;11(4):285–293.

[9]   Spenke M. Visualization and interactive analysis of blood parameters with InfoZoom. *Artificial Intelligence in Medicine* 2001;22(2):159–172.

[10] Wroe C, Solomon W, Rector A, Rogers J. DOPAMINE: A Tool for Visualizing Clinical Properties of Generic Drugs. In: *Proceedings of the Fifth Workshop on Intelligent Data Analysis in Medicine and Pharmacology (IDAMAP)*; 2000.

[11] Herman I, Melançon G, Marshall MS. Graph Visualization and Navigation in Information Visualization: A Survey. *IEEE Transactions on Visualization and Computer Graphics* 2000;6(1):24–43.

[12] Ketan B. *Using Treemaps to Visualize Gene Ontologies*. Human Computer Interaction Lab and Institute for Systems Research. University of Maryland, College Park, MD USA; 2001. Http://www.cs.umd.edu/hcil/treemap/GeneOntologyTreemap.pdf.

Address for correspondence

Lamy Jean-Baptiste (jibalamy@free.fr), Laboratoire LIM&BIO, UFR de Santé, Médecine et Biologie Humaine (SMBH) – Léonard de Vinci, 74, rue Marcel Cachin, 93017 Bobigny Cedex France

Connecting Medical Informatics and Bio-Informatics
R. Engelbrecht et al. (Eds.)
IOS Press, 2005

mVisualizer: Easily Accessible Data Exploration for Clinicians

Nils Erichson, Olof Torgersson

Department of Computer Science and Engineering, Chalmers University of Technology, Göteborg, Sweden

Abstract:

> *In medical research and clinical work, having direct access to a large knowledge base of information about patients is very useful. Software for information visualisation can help the user browse, analyse and learn from such knowledge, thus providing new insights and accelerating research. However, when introducing new software to clinicians, who may have limited computer knowledge, adoption can be hindered by the complexity of the applications and the time investments necessary to learn them. By involving clinicians directly in the design process, we have developed mVisualizer, an application that provides a hands-on workspace to visualise and explore patient data. mVisualizer was designed for accessibility and simplicity, and to encourage users to explore the data in order to make discoveries and pose new questions relevant for knowledge gathering and research. The user-centered approach helped ensure that mVisualizer is understandable and easy to learn for clinicians. The application is in use by clinicians today, and its use has led to new discoveries and theories that will be the subject of future medical research. This leads to the conclusion that information visualisation software for exploring patient data can help clinicians and researchers by making the data more accessible, which stimulates research and learning.*

Keywords:
Access to Information; Data Display; Dental Informatics; Information Retrieval; Medical Informatics; Oral Medicine; Software Design; User-Computer Interface

1. Introduction

Since 1995, clinicians at the Clinic of Oral Medicine and Department of Endodontology/Oral Diagnosis at the Sahlgrenska Academy in Gothenburg have been using computer software to collect formal data about patients during examinations as part of the MedView project [1]. The data for each examination uses a protocol where values for observations are selected from a standardised set of values based on a formal model [2].

The purpose of collecting this data is to use it for learning and clinical research. Once data has been collected, clinicians need a way to access it. Traditional access methods such as browsing medical records, querying databases or generating reports, have the disadvantage of requiring a clearly defined question from the outset. If it is later discovered that additional information is needed, or that the question needs to be modified, the process must be restarted. This results in a high turn-around time when asking questions.

These problems can be solved by introducing interactive software for analytical viewing of the patient data, i.e. the activity of visually exploring the entire database to find patterns and relations that may warrant further investigation. To this end information visualisation is used, which can be defined as visualising and navigating abstract data and structures [3, 4].

Such software gives clinicians direct access to the patient information, which reduces the delay between asking a question and getting an answer. Another advantage is that questions can be formulated iteratively and on-the-fly during data exploration.

For these reasons, an application for exploring the collected patient data was developed. This paper details the design process, and the results of clinicians using the application in their daily work.

2. Design considerations

From analysing the problem, three major design goals were established to maximize the usefulness of the application to clinicians and researchers.

2.1. Goal 1: Simplicity

When introducing new software, adoption can be hindered by the time investment required to learn how to use the software. Clinicians are busy people and generally have limited computer knowledge. Because of this, they can be impatient and reluctant to invest the time necessary to learn new applications, especially complicated ones that demand a lot of the user. Previous attempts to create applications for visualisation of MedView data [5] have been made, but these have focused on creating new types of visualisation and have not been widely adopted by the clinicians due to being too complex or abstract. This reluctance to adopt complex applications highlights the need to keep new software for clinicians simple and easy to learn.

2.2. Goal 2: Accessibility

If a clinician gets a hunch or an idea which prompts a question, for example during a coffee break, it should be easy to walk over to a computer and follow up on the question immediately. If accessing the patient data is regarded as complex or time-consuming, the idea might be shelved until later, and in the worst case forgotten. In other words, having software that provides a simple and time-efficient way to access the patient data can stimulate research, as questions and ideas can be acted on immediately when they appear.

2.3. Goal 3: Exploration

The purpose of examining the collected data is not only to find the answers to questions, but also to discover new questions that may not have been asked before. Clinicians state that "The key to medical research is *asking the right question*". Thus the application should not only help in answering questions, but also help refine them and discover new ones. This can be achieved by encouraging the user to explore the patient data, creating visualisations to follow a train of thought and hopefully make new discoveries about the patient information. In other words, what is needed is not an application that provides answers, but a workspace that helps the user explore the data interactively. The users should feel that they are using the application as a supporting tool for exploring the data, not a device that automatically provides answers to given questions. To encourage such exploration, the interface should encourage the users to interact with the data and explore it, to feel empowered and realize that they are the ones doing the actual work.

3. Method

When developing the application, a user-centered design method [6] was used, based on short (1-2 weeks) iterations of developing ideas, prototyping them and later implementing them. This method was chosen as a response to the difficulties involved in getting the clinicians to adopt new software. By meeting regularly with the users to discuss their needs and evaluate the latest progress, development could be kept on track with respect to the established goals, and ideas and concepts that proved too complex or simply not useful could quickly be discarded or taken back to the drawing board.

4. Solution: mVisualizer

The result of the development is mVisualizer, an application which provides a visual workspace for exploring patient data (Figure 1). mVisualizer uses multiple views and an interaction method based on graphical selections and drag-and-drop operations. This type of interaction was inspired by Visage [7] by the SAGE Visualization group[1].

When mVisualizer is started, the user loads patient data into one or more initial *Data Groups*. This data can then be dragged to one or more *Views* for exploration (Figure 2). Several types of Views exist: Bar charts, Scatter plots, Frequency reports and Tables, and also some MedView-specific views such as the Photo View, which allows browsing of images taken during examinations, and the Summary View, which contains a computer-generated summary of the examination, similar to what a medical record may contain.

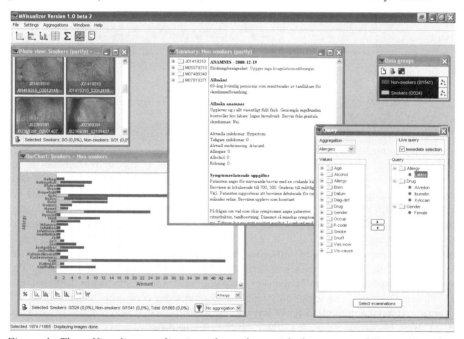

Figure 1: The mVisualizer application, shown here with three types of Views (Bar chart, Photos and Patient Summary), the Query Tool and the Data Group window.

[1] http://www-2.cs.cmu.edu/~sage/

By using multiple views in parallel, relationships that are not apparent from a single visualisation may be discovered [8]. Views are linked by visual cues such as *brushing* (elements selected in one view are marked in others) and colouring, which helps the user to keep track of which examinations correspond to each other in different Views.

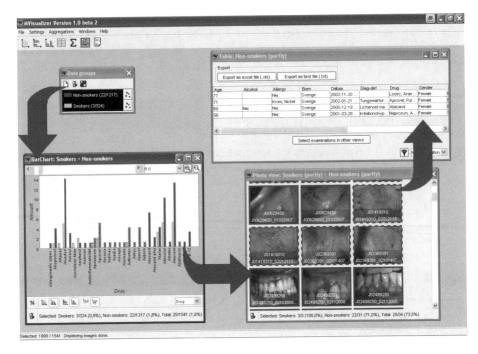

Figure 2: Example of how sets of examinations can be "drilled down" by selections and subsequent drag-and-drop operations between Views.

The basic way of working with mVisualizer is using Views of the patient data to select subsets of examinations that share some kind of relationship or common properties. Such subsets can then be dragged to other Views for new insights, or tagged as members of one or more Data Groups. Since elements in a View are rendered colour-coded by the Data Group they belong to, this is an effective way to compare how different sets of data are distributed in a View. If a detailed look at an examination is desired, the user can double-click on an examination at any moment to view the Summary of the examination and its associated images.

mVisualizer provides several different ways to ask questions or isolate sets of examinations. In addition to using selection and drag-and-drop operations to find interesting sets of data (Figure 2), the user can make formal queries by using the Query tool (see Figure 1), or use text search to single out examinations containing specific data. The advantage of having multiple ways of working is twofold: First, different kinds of questions (in the mind of the user) may lend themselves better to different ways of interacting with the data. Second, different users may choose to approach a question in different ways.

A problem when working with large and detailed sets of clinical data is that the value domain can become hard to survey, and/or may have a level of detail that is not relevant from the researchers' point of view. Some topics generate hundreds of possible values.

From the aspect of analysis, it would be extremely difficult to analyse the database if individual values could not be assembled into larger groups. For this purpose, *Aggregations* can be created to cluster input data into categories. One example where this is useful is to put individual drugs into larger categories such as "diuretics", "NSAIDs" or "steroids". The clustering can then be used as an analytical tool to detect patients with established criteria.

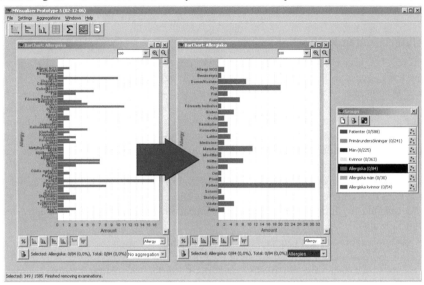

Figure 3: A bar chart View of allergies before and after aggregation. Note how the value domain and the amount of examinations per value have changed.

Aggregations can therefore also be applied in order to sample patients with similar professions, similar diagnoses, or in any situation where a clustering of parameters is regarded essential for the analysis.

In mVisualizer, Aggregations can be applied to any View at any time to unify the value domain (Figure 3). When the views thus become less scattered, common denominators or relationships that were not noticeable before may stand out. Aggregations are created by clinicians themselves, and can be re-used and shared with other users.

When discoveries have been made in mVisualizer and further, more formal research, is desired, data can be exported (to Excel or text format), which enables the user to continue working with the data in other applications such as spreadsheets or statistical tools.

5. Evaluation and practical use

The research use of mVisualizer at the Clinic for Oral Medicine proved itself early on, as correlations between estrogen levels and changes in the mucous membranes of patients diagnosed with Oral Lichen Planus were found using an early version of mVisualizer before development was finished. This indicated that the user-centered approach was working, and that we were on the right track.

When the development process was finished, mVisualizer was deployed at the Clinic for use by the clinicians. Giving a short demonstration of about 15 minutes is usually enough to get users started, and enthusiastic users tend to help other clinicians to learn the application. As of today, it is being used daily and its group of users is growing.

Recently, mVisualizer was used to examine a group of patients that shared a "burning sensation" in the mouth, which was caused by a kind of lesion. When surveying these patients in mVisualizer, originally looking at factors such as medication, smoking and allergies, it was discovered that the patients all shared certain characteristics: accumulations of calculus and decreased levels of saliva. This combination can cause increased amounts of bacterial plaque in the mouth. The conclusion drawn was that such conditions might be the cause of the lesions. The examination data that was used was exported for sharing with other clinics, and will be the subject of research in the near future.

6. Conclusions and future work

Through careful user-centered design, we have developed an application that gives clinicians easy access to the patient data for research and daily work at the clinic. Users state that *"mVisualizer provides us with new possibilities of getting insight into the patient data that we did not have before"*. The accessibility of the data enables them to quickly check out hypotheses, and the focus on exploration encourages finding new insights and relations between different aspects of the patient data. The application is now in daily use at the clinic, and has yielded several practical results in the form of new questions and discoveries about the patient data.

This leads to the conclusion that interactive information visualisation software that helps explore patient data can be very helpful to clinicians and researchers. When the patient data is made accessible to clinicians, learning from the patient information is made easier and research is stimulated.

Future development of mVisualizer will focus on providing additional types of visualisation and new perspectives. One such area is that clinicians want to be able to view overall trends in a larger time perspective, such as the effect of treatments over a longer time.

7. Acknowledgements

The work presented in this paper was supported by the Swedish Agency for Innovation Systems (VINNOVA).

8. References

[1] Jontell M, Mattsson U and Torgersson O. MedView: An instrument for clinical research and education in oral medicine. *Oral Surg. Oral Med. Oral Pathol. Oral Radiol. Endod.,* 99:55-63, 2005.

[2] Falkman G. and Torgersson O. Knowledge Acquisition and Modeling in Clinical Information Systems: A Case Study. In: Gómez-Pérez A and Benjamins VR, eds. *Knowledge Engineering and Knowledge Management: Ontologies and the Semantic Web. Proc. 13th Int. Conference, EKAW 2002, Siguenza, Spain, October 1-4, 2002.* vol. 2473 of LNAI. Springer-Verlag, 2002; pp. 96-101.

[3] Herman I, Marshall MS and Melançon G. Graph Visualisation and Navigation in Information Visualisation: A Survey. *IEEE T. Vis. Comput. Gr. 2000:* 6, 24-43.

[4] Gershon N, Eick S and Card S. Information Visualization. *Interactions.* 1998:2(5), 9-15.

[5] Falkman, G. Information visualization in clinical odontology. *Artificial Intelligence in Medicine.* 2001: 2(22), 133-158.

[6] Vredenburg K, Isensee S and Righi C. *User-Centered Design: An Integrated Approach.* Prentice Hall, 2001.

[7] Roth S, Lucas P, Senn J, Gomberg C, Burks M, Stroffolino P, Kolojejchick J and Dunmire C. Visage: A user interface environment for exploring information. In *Proceedings of Information Visualization.* San Francisco: IEEE, 1996; pp. 3-12.

[8] Baldonado MQW, Woodruff A and Kuchinsky A. Guidelines for using multiple views in information visualization. In: *Advanced Visual Interfaces.* 2000; pp. 110-119.

Address for Correspondence

Nils Erichson, Department of Computer Science and Engineering, Chalmers University of Technology, SE-412 96 Gothenburg, Sweden. E-mail: erichson@cs.chalmers.se

Connecting Medical Informatics and Bio-Informatics
R. Engelbrecht et al. (Eds.)
IOS Press, 2005

A Knowledge Management Framework to Morph Clinical Cases with Clinical Practice Guidelines

Fehmida Hussain[a], Syed Sibte Raza Abidi[b]

[a]Institute of Business Administration, Karachi Pakistan
[b]Dalhousie University, Halifax, Nova Scotia, Canada

Abstract

In this paper we present a knowledge management framework that allows the automatic linking/mapping of contextually and functionally similar medical knowledge that may originate from different sources and be represented in diverse modalities. Our tacit-explicit knowledge morphing framework supports the extraction of tacit knowledge from past cases stored in a case-base and maps it to corresponding explicit knowledge stored in clinical practice guidelines. The novelty of our approach is inherent in the fact that it allows practitioners to simultaneously refer to explicit knowledge—i.e. clinical practice guidelines—and experiential knowledge—i.e. past clinical cases. Here we present the system design and intended functionality of our knowledge morphing framework.

Keywords:
Knowledge Management, Clinical Practice Guidelines, Clinical Cases, Tacit Knowledge

1. Introduction

Medical knowledge can be differentiated along the lines of *explicit* and *tacit knowledge* [1, 2], where each knowledge modality provides a specific kind of input in addressing a clinical problem. The emergence of knowledge management as a discipline has highlighted the importance of capturing and operationalizing knowledge to support decision support, learning/training and improving operational workflows and outcomes [3, 4]. This has precipitated the development of methodologies, tools, and frameworks to capture the different knowledge modalities, given their inherent existential and operational constraints, and an attempt to automate the captured knowledge through knowledge management systems. We note with interest that the current knowledge management systems are largely designed to deal with a single knowledge modality, for instance some variation of explicit knowledge represented as either documents, guidelines/workflows, symbolic rules and so on; or a type of tacit knowledge represented either as cases, scenarios or peer discussions [5,6]. Given the diversity of knowledge modalities that encompass any given topic/problem it is reasonable to demand access and use of all available knowledge, irrespective of their representation modality, to derive a knowledge-mediated solution.

Typically, medical practitioners tend to make use of a single knowledge modality—either explicit or tacit—when solving a problem, as most decision support systems do not support the synthesis of heterogeneous knowledge sources. The prevailing situation leads to a knowledge gap in clinical decision support systems. In our work we attempt to address this knowledge gap by developing a knowledge management framework that allows the automatic synthesis of contextually and functionally similar knowledge elements albeit in different modalities. The objective is to provide practitioners 'holistic' medical knowledge that has its origin in both tacit and explicit modalities of knowledge. For instance, whilst referring to past clinical cases that withhold the tacit knowledge, clinicians should be able to relate them to explicit knowledge resources such as clinical practice guidelines/medical literature or vice versa.

In this paper, we firstly introduce the novel concept of *knowledge morphing* to characterize the mapping of contextually similar knowledge modalities. To demonstrate the working of the proposed knowledge morphing framework, we present a system that (a) captures clinical case-based tacit knowledge in terms of structured case representation with respect to a case-based reasoning system; (b) computerizes Clinical Practice Guidelines (CPG) in the XML-based Guideline Element Model (GEM); and (c) automatically links user-specified aspects of a clinical case with related and relevant clinical evidence within a CPG.

2. The Case for Knowledge Morphing

Knowledge morphing is defined as "the intelligent and autonomous fusion/integration of contextually, conceptually and functionally related knowledge objects that may exist in different representation modalities and formalisms, in order to establish a comprehensive, multi-faceted and networked view of all knowledge pertaining to a domain-specific problem" [7].

In medicine, the need for leveraging all possible resources of medical knowledge is paramount, as there is the need and realization to give clinical care that is grounded in best evidence. From a pragmatic decision-support point of view, what medical practitioners require is "comprehensive, contextually-relevant knowledge that is both congruent with the evolution of the patient and at an appropriate level of abstraction" [7]. We contend that knowledge gaps in clinical decision making can be addressed by linking heterogeneous knowledge modalities through a knowledge morphing framework. In the past, knowledge morphing has been successfully achieved by linking CPG with related clinical evidence published in medical articles at PUBMED [8]. Further literature search also reveals work directly or indirectly related to the concept proposed here [9-14].

3. Our Research Methodology

In this section we present the detailed design of the morphing system proposed in this research work. The explicit modality of knowledge used in this context is clinical practice guidelines and the tacit modality of knowledge which is morphed with the explicit side is past clinical cases. Our goal is to be able to link these two different modalities of clinical knowledge by leveraging upon the contextual similarities of both modalities. Clinical practice guidelines are computerized (referred to as C-CPG) and the clinical cases are rendered computable using some case base reasoning representation (referred to as CBR-CC). The knowledge contained in CPG is strictly explicit and in accordance with the belief that it advocates the practice of evidence based medicine [15]. On the other hand, clinical case are tacit in nature because it captures clinical episodes which depicts the expertise of the expert. Our research methodology identifies a sequence of steps that involve both the transformation of the knowledge resources into formats that render them computable, and the forging of morphing linkages between the C-CPG and CBR-CC as illustrated in figure

1. Linkages between the two modalities lead to the following situations:

C-CPG to CBR-CC: In this case, the user wants to find corresponding experiential and tacit knowledge for some aspect of a CPG in question. The user, therefore, highlights the C-CPG content in question for which corresponding tacit knowledge, in terms of clinical cases, within CBR-CC is sought. Based on the normalized medical terms identified within the selected C-CPG content we generate a term-based search query for selecting the relevant CBR-CCs. CBR-mediated case similarity assessment methods that cater for both numeric and text based features are used to establish the similarity between the search query and the problem-description component of the CBR-CC.

CBR-CC to C-CPG: In this case, the user wants to find the clinical evidence for some clinical action noted in the CBR-CC. In this case, a set of case-defining feature-value pairs are selected by the user to form the basis for establishing the linkage with specific elements of C-CPG. The case-defining features are transformed to a search query using a standing information retrieval based vector support model. The search query is applied to the C-CPG with pre-set similarity measurement criterion, and sections of the CPG that relate to the search query are retrieved.

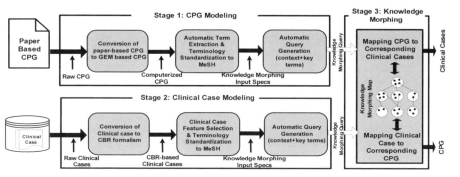

Figure 1: Schematic of our Knowledge Morphing methodology

We explain below some of the steps of our methodology in detail:

3.1 Operationalization of Explicit Knowledge

The explicit modality of knowledge used here are clinical practice guidelines. Clinical Practice Guidelines (CPG) are systematically prepared statement to help the physician with best decision making with regards to a certain medical condition. As mentioned earlier, the knowledge contained in CPG is explicit in nature and synonymously referred to as evidence-based guidelines. There are various guideline representation models which include the Arden Syntax, the Asbru model, the EON model, the GLIF model, the PROforma model, the GUIDE model, the GASTON mode, the Guideline element model (GEM) model etc [16]. GEM was developed at the Yale Center for Medical Informatics and was designed to provide structure for marking up any CPG in XML. In our work we use the Guideline element model (GEM). We convert the textual CPG using the Guideline Element model (GEM). The guideline selected for use here is the evidence-based guideline for weaning and discontinuation of ventilatory support (www.rcjournal.com/online_resources/cpgs/ebgwdscpg.asp). This guideline broadly covers recommendations for the management of mechanically ventilated patients, assessing the possibility of weaning the patients, managing patients who have failed spontaneous breathing trials, role of tracheotomy and the role of long term care facilities for such patients. Keeping these in mind, our domain expert (who is a fellow in pulmonary and critical care medicine) has provided us with clinical cases covering the above mentioned scenarios.

3.2 Operationalization of Tacit Knowledge

The tacit modality of knowledge used in this context is clinical cases which contain the innate knowledge of medical experts. Though the majority of healthcare knowledge is found in published journal articles, structured reviews, and practice guidelines; it is strongly believed that the tacit knowledge of the expert also contributes significantly towards optimal decision making [17-18].

The operationalization strategy used here is simple but effective which uses the clinical cases as the tacit modality of knowledge. Cases are marked up using XML tags to represent case structure illustrated in figure 2, as verified by the domain expert. This has also been proposed and successfully implemented in literature [19]. The objective here is to convert a text-based case into a format such that it could be mapped with the knowledge components in the CPG.

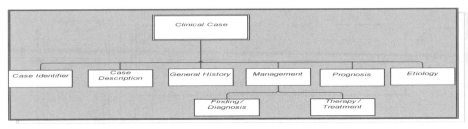

Figure 2: Data Type Definition of a generic Clinical Case

3.3   Morphing of explicit and tacit knowledge

Morphing of explicit and tacit knowledge modalities will involve (a) understanding and establishing a conceptual mapping of the DTD of a clinical case and GEM tags of the CPG; (b) developing an input module for interfacing with the user; (c) search query generation and execution; finally (d) displaying resultant output.

The idea of drawing a conceptual mapping of CPG elements to corresponding clinical case elements (performed by a domain expert) is to relate corresponding elements of these two different knowledge modalities, both refereeing to the same problem domain, in order to facilitate knowledge morphing. Once that is done then we will be required to build an interface with the user whereby the user can select text from the CPG or the case for which supplementary information is being sought. For text selected, we need to normalize the terms to standardized biomedical vocabulary and determine semantic types for each term. The Meta Map Transfer tool- MMTx is used to normalize terms before generating query, that is find synonyms of the MeSH(Medical Subject Headings) terms and find semantic types of the selected terms. The MMTx program takes as input sentence and separates it into phrases, identifies the medical concepts and assigns proper semantic categories to them according to knowledge embedded in UMLS. The output of MMTx would give us the MeSH terms together with UMLS semantic types. All these tools are downloadable from the UMLS Knowledge Servers found at NLMs website which are made available for research purposes only. [www.mmtx.nlm.gov/].

Once the candidate terms are identified, search query needs to be generated. The search query generation strategy is adapted from the original work by Abidi et al with respect to the BiRD system [20]. The BirD search strategy is as follows: (a) categorize queries based on a set of a priori defined query types [21]; (b) the search query is a combination of query type and candidate MeSH terms. Search query should only comprise of MeSH terms thus leading to the generation of optimum search queries [22]. The Search query generation is summarized as follows: (a) Parsing the string through MMTx for determining semantic types - query categorization; (b) Parsing of string through MMTx for identifying synonyms or alternate terms - query expansion; (c) Filtering out words which are not MeSH terms, i.e. the terms which do not have a definition in the MeSH vocabulary identifying them as extras and stripping them off. Also, terms which have semantic types other than the ones identified in the process of conceptual mapping of CPG and cases are also omitted. – term filtering; (c) For terms which already have semantic types identified, compose query to look up that string in the associated XML tags (according to semantic type category). Thus the candidate terms are used to generate queries generated using XQuery Language - query composer. Finally the result from the execution of the query is displayed for the user to review.

4. Conclusions and Future Work

Here we have presented a novel approach for linking of semantically, contextually and functionally similar knowledge element, albeit in different knowledge representation modalities, to realize a holistic knowledge resource for a particular medical problem. This paper presents an interesting working of the knowledge morphing concept in order to supplement explicit forms of knowledge with tacit knowledge and vice versa. This can further be extended to morph other modalities of knowledge or even more than two modalities at the same time. The work is still underway and therefore complete implementation details and evaluation which will be carried out with the help of the domain expert has not been covered in this paper.

5. Acknowledgements

We wish to thank Syed Ali Raza for his support in pursuing this research. We would also like to extend our appreciation to Dr. Rubina Kerawala who is the domain expert for our project.

6. References

[1] Wyatt JC. Management of explicit and tacit knowledge. *Journal of the Royal Society of Medicine*, Vol. 94, 2001

[2] Yu-N C, Abidi SSR. The role of information technology in the explication and crystallization of tacit healthcare knowledge. *Health Informatics J* 2001; 7(3/4): 158-167.

[3] Pavia L, The era of knowledge in Health-care", Healthcare strategic Management, Vol. 19, pp 12-13, 20001

[4] Alavi M, Leidner D. Knowledge Management System: issues, challenges and benefits. Communications of the Association for Information Systems, Vol 1 No 7, pp 1-37,1999-

[5] Jones B, Abidi SSR, Ying W. Using Computerized Clinical Practice Guidelines to Generate Tailored Patient Education Materials. 38th Hawaii IEEE International Conference on System Sciences (HICSS-38), Hawaii, 2005

[6] Abidi SSR, Finley GA, Milios E, Shepherd M, Zitner D. Knowledge Management in Pediatric Pain: Mapping On-line Expert Discussions to Medical Literature. 11th World Congress on Medical Informatics (MEDINFO'2004), San Francisco, 7-11 Sept. 2004

[7]   S.S.R. Abidi, "Medical Knowledge Morphing: Towards Case-Specific Integration of Heterogeneous Medical Knowledge Resources", 18th IEEE International Symposium on Computer-Based Medical Systems, Dublin, June 23-24 2005

[8]   S.S.R. Abidi, M. Kershaw M, E. Milios, "Augmenting GEM-Encoded Clinical Practice Guidelines with Relevant Best-Evidence Autonomously Retrieved from MEDLINE", *Health Informatics Journal*, Vol. 11(1), pp. 57–72, 2005

[9]   Lusignan-de D, Pritchard K, Chan T, A Knolwedge Management model for Clinical Practice., Journal of Postgraduate Medicine, 2002, vol 48, issue , pg 297-303

[10]   Cheah Yu-N, Rashid FA, Abidi SSR, An approach to enrich online medical problem-based learning with tacit healthcare knowledge. 18th international congress of the European Federation for Medical Informatics Medical Informatics in Europe(MIE 2003), St Malo(France), 4-7 May 2003

[11]   Abidi SSR. A case for supplementing evidence base medicine with inductive clinical knowledge: towards a technology-enriched integrated clinical evidence system.14th IEEE symposium on computer based medical systems (CBMS'2001), 26-27 July, Bethesda (USA).

[12]   Jones B, Abidi SSR, Ying Winston. An approach to generating patient education materials from a GEM-based clinical practice guidelines. 38th Hawaii IEEE International Conference on System Sciences (HICSS-38), Hawaii, January 3-6 2005

[13]   Moody DL. Using knowledge management and the internet to support evidence based practice: A medical case study. Proc of 10th Australasian conference on information systems, 1999.

[14]   Goldstein MK, Hofman BB, Coleman RW, Musen MA, Tu SW, Advani A, Shankar R, O'Connor M. Implementing clinical practice guidelines while taking account of changing evidence:ATHENA DSS, an easily modifiable decision-support system for managing hypertension in primary care. Proc AMIA Symp 2000; 300-4

[15]   Field MJ, Lohr KN (Eds). Guidelines for clinical practice: from development to use. Institute of Medicine, Washington, D.C. National Academy Press, 1992.

[16]   Peleg M, Tu S, Comparing computer interpretable guideline models: A case-study approach. *J Am Med Inform Assoc.* 2003; 10: 52-68

[17]   Davenport TH, Prusak L. Working Knowledge: How organizations manage what they know, Harward Press:Cambridge. 1997

[18]   Suchman L. Manage work Visible, Communications of the ACM, 38(9), 1995

[19]   Coyle L, Hayes C, Cunningham P .Representing Cases for CBR in XML. Proceedings of 7th UKCBR Workshop, Peterhouse, Cambridge, UK, 2002

[20]   20 S.S.R. ABIDI, M. Kershaw, E. Milios. BiRD: A Strategy to Autonomously Supplement Clinical Practice Guidelines with Related Clinical Studies. 38th IEEE Hawaii International Conference on System Sciences (HICSS-38), Hawaii, January 3-6 2005.

[21]   Haynes B, A Wilczynski, , McKibbon A, Walker C, Sinclair J. Developing optimal search strategies for detecting clinically sound studies in MEDLINE. Journal of American Medical Informatics Association, pp. 447-458, 1994

[22]   Cimino J, Mendonca E. Automated Knowledge extraction from MEDLINE citations. Proceedings of AMIA Symposim, pp. 575-9, 2000

Address for correspondence

Center for Computer Studies, Institute of Business Administration, M. A. Jinnah Road, Karachi, Pakistan.
Email: fhussain@iba.edu.pk

Connecting Medical Informatics and Bio-Informatics
R. Engelbrecht et al. (Eds.)
IOS Press, 2005

The Significance of SNODENT

Louis J Goldberg[a], Werner Ceusters[b], John Eisner[c], Barry Smith[d]

[a]Department of Oral Diagnostic Sciences, School of Dental Medicine, University at Buffalo
[b]European Center for Ontological Research Saarland University, Germany
[c]Department of Pediatric and Community Dentistry, School of Dental Medicine, University at Buffalo
[d]Department of Philosophy, University at Buffalo and Institute for Formal Ontology, Saarland University, Germany

Abstracts

SNODENT is a dental diagnostic vocabulary incompletely integrated in SNOMED-CT. Nevertheless, SNODENT could become the de facto standard for dental diagnostic coding. SNODENT's manageable size, the fact that it is administratively self-contained, and relates to a well-understood domain provides valuable opportunities to formulate and test, in controlled experiments, a series of hypothesis concerning diagnostic systems. Of particular interest are questions related to establishing appropriate quality assurance methods for its optimal level of detail in content, its ontological structure, its construction and maintenance. This paper builds on previous–software-based methodologies designed to assess the quality of SNOMED-CT. When applied to SNODENT several deficiencies were uncovered. 9.52% of SNODENT terms point to concepts in SNOMED-CT that have some problem. 18.53% of SNODENT terms point to SNOMED-CT concepts do not have, in SNOMED, the term used by SNODENT. Other findings include the absence of a clear specification of the exact relationship between a term and a termcode in SNODENT and the improper assignment of the same termcode to terms with significantly different meanings. An analysis of the way in which SNODENT is structurally integrated into SNOMED resulted in the generation of 1081 new termcodes reflecting entities not present in the SNOMED tables but required by SNOMED's own description logic based classification principles. Our results show that SNODENT requires considerable enhancements in content, quality of coding, quality of ontological structure and the manner in which it is integrated and aligned with SNOMED. We believe that methods for the analysis of the quality of diagnostic coding systems must be developed and employed if such systems are to be used effectively in both clinical practice and clinical research.

Keywords:
Diagnostic coding systems; SNODENT; SNOMED; Quality Assurance; Ontology

1. Background

As a means of providing free access to a reputable clinical coding system, the US Department of Health and Human Services purchased rights to SNOMED Clinical Terms (hereafter: SNOMED-CT) from the College of American Pathologists in the summer of 2003. The first release of SNOMED-CT included 375,000+ concepts, 957,000+ descriptions or synonyms and 1,370,000+ relationships. Embedded in this January 2004 release was a 6,000+ term dental diagnostic vocabulary, known within the dental community as SNODENT. It was designed as a diagnostic companion to the Current Dental Terminology (CDT) treatment codes of the American Dental Association. Of these 6000+ terms approximately 1600 were contributed by the American Dental Association while the remainder were dental terms already contained within SNOMED.

This is an example in which in which two separate groups (CAP and the ADA) designed two distinct diagnostic coding systems for one specific domain (dentistry). As far as we know there was no significant communication between the groups and no attempts to evaluate the quality of either diagnostic coding system.

It should, therefore, be no surprise that SNODENT is imperfectly integrated into the SNOMED-CT environment. Nonetheless, in the absence of established alternatives, SNODENT could well become the *de facto* standard for dental diagnostic coding. Its imminent release thus provides a unique dual research opportunity of potentially high significance. SNODENT's manageable size, the fact that it is administratively self-contained, and relates to a well-understood domain suggest that it might well provide valuable opportunities to formulate and test, in controlled experiments, a series of hypotheses concerning clinical coding systems.

Medical coding systems need to have a maximal degree of permanence in order to facilitate the cost-efficient training of coders and to avoid over-frequent updates. Yet at the same time they need to have the flexibility to take account of changes in medical knowledge while dealing with the nuances of actual cases encountered at the point of care.

While almost all medical coding systems have been designed and subsequently maintained with *content* as primary focus, it has more recently been shown that, even in addition to the use of DL-style formal definitions, adherence to good coding principles [1-3] can bring significant advantages. It is generally recognized further that errors in medical coding can have important consequences for the quality of health care. Moreover the increasing alignment of terminologies and ontologies from different parts of biomedicine, and the increasing use of coding systems in the annotation of gene product and other data, means that the correction of code-based errors has an increasingly high cost, since errors in one coding system propagate through all the many other data resources into which information expressed using the relevant codes has been absorbed or annotated.

Clearly, these factors point in competing directions [4], and they make it clear that a methodology for quality assurance of clinical coding systems cannot focus narrowly on the elimination of errors in the formulation of content and on the creation of structural architectures which enjoy a high degree of elegance but bring no further benefits in efficiency or reliability of coding. Rather, as [5] points out, theoretically inspired moves towards fine-tuned representations of reality should be accompanied by empirical demonstrations of usefulness. In our view, the assessment and enhancement of SNODENT should focus on repeated statistical measures comparing the effectiveness in a real-world coding environments of the original (baseline) SNODENT codes with a series of controlled enhancements. No comprehensive methodologies for the quality assurance of medical coding systems have thus far been proposed, and we believe that such an analysis can break new ground not merely in testing methodologies for improving code sets in controlled experiments but also in measuring the costs and benefits brought about by such improvements. The enhancements we are working on relate to three levels: encompassing (i) broadening dental content, (ii) adding Description Logic architecture, and (iii) improving structural/ontological organization. We concentrate here on level (iii) – the alignment of SNODENT within SNOMED.

2. Methods and Results

We have been working for two years on testing a variety of software-based methodologies for the management and quality assurance of medical terminologies. The methodology described in [6] which was first to applied to the January 2003 and July 2003 versions of SNOMED-CT, was also used to analyze SNODENT using SNOMED as the gold standard. The basic idea is that it is possible to search for errors in a terminology by comparing different ways in which information can be extracted from its terms, concepts, descriptions, and definitions. To that end, the inter-concept relationships that are expressed in a terminology are first organised in a graph. This graph is then expanded in two ways. First, it is overlaid by a graph that represents the lexical relationships between all the terms in the system. Second, concepts that are formally *described*, but not *defined* (and hence are declared to be *primitive* in the original version of the terminology) are given a defined version, which then subsumes the undefined version. After reclassification, more concepts might be found to be subsumed by the defined version. Error discovery is then reduced to a process that seeks unexplainable differences in the semantic distances between concepts computed over the lexical graph as compared to the original concept graph, and a search for idiosyncratic patterns in the expanded concept graph.

2.1. Problems in the Calibration of SNODENT and SNOMED

Our initial findings related to calibration include:

618 (9.52%) of SNODENT **terms**, involving 208 (5.38%) termcodes, point to **concepts** in SNOMED-CT that have a "watch out" status, distributed as follows: *retired* 86, *duplicate* 15, *ambiguous* 517. 1203 (18.53%) SNODENT terms point to SNOMED-CT concepts that are labelled as *active*, but that do not have (in SNOMED) the term used by SNODENT. This means that if SNOMED-CT would be taken as the gold standard to compare term usage within SNODENT, 18.53% of the SNODENT terms must be considered to be inappropriate. If SNODENT would be taken as gold standard, SNOMED-CT would lack 18.53% of the accepted terms in SNODENT.

368 (5.67%) SNODENT **terms** are not found in SNOMED, although the corresponding **concept** does exist in both systems (and with the same code). The extra terms can be divided into a number of categories, such as: adjectival form, use of a determiner, use of "NOS", eponyms, and spelling variants.

While SNODENT enforces just a single meaning for terms that are in and of themselves polysemous, SNOMED allows terms to be used in a variety of meanings. 437 (6.73%) SNODENT terms are used in SNOMED with different meanings, the majority reflecting a (systematic) oddity of SNOMED rather than of SNODENT. Some examples are given in Table 1.

Table 1: Examples of single terms in SNODENT used with plural meanings in SNOMED

SNODENT term	SNODENT enomen	SNOMED concept name
Bruise	M-14200	Bruise (finding)
Bruise	M-14200	Contusion – lesion (morphologic abnormality)
Alveolar arch of mandible	T-11182	Structure of alveolar arch of mandible (body structure)
Alveolar arch of mandible	T-11182	Entire alveolar arch of mandible (body structure)
Bloody discharge	M-36860	Bloody discharge (morphologic abnormality)
Bloody discharge	M-36860	Bloody discharge (substance)
Chemotherapy	P2-67010	Chemotherapy (procedure)
Chemotherapy	P2-67010	Drug therapy (procedure)
Chemotherapy	P2-67010	Antineoplastic chemotherapy regimen (regime/therapy)
Chemotherapy	P2-67010	Administration of antineoplastic agent (procedure)

It is clear from the above that, at the time of our initial analyses (May 2004), all of the SNODENT terms have not yet been incorporated into SNOMED-CT.

2.2 Terms and Conceptcodes in SNODENT

For the work described here we used the SNODENT version received from the American Dental Association in March 2004, and the July 2003 version of SNOMED-CT.

The SNODENT file contained 6491 unique records, relating to 6491 unique terms (called enomens in SNODENT) and 3863 unique concept codes (called termcodes in SNODENT). A first problem concerns the absence of a clear specification of the exact relationship between a term and a termcode in SNODENT. Most examples suggest a relation of synonymy, as in:

- D5-10000   Dental disease, NOS
- D5-10000   Disease of teeth, NOS
- D5-10000   Tooth disorder, NOS
- F-51540   Expectoration of bloody sputum
- F-51540   Expectoration of hemorrhagic sputum

Other examples, however, suggest that terms receive the same termcode also where detailed differences are irrelevant for the purposes to which SNODENT is to be put. Thus all of the following refer to the same SNODENT termcode:

- F-A3692   Adverse taste perception
- F-A3692   Chorda tympani disorder
- F-A3692   Dysgeusia
- F-A3692   Neurologic unpleasant taste
- F-A3692   Parageusia
- F-A3692   Perversion of sense of taste
- F-A3692   Primary taste disorder

A *chorda tympani disorder* does not need to involve *a taste disorder. Dysgeusia* and *parageusia* are related, but different disorders, while a *primary taste disorder* subsumes *absence of taste* which is not the case with *neurologic unpleasant taste*.

Another example of the same phenomenon is:

- T-53120   Dorsal surface of anterior two-thirds of tongue
- T-53120   Dorsal surface of tongue
- T-53120   Dorsum of anterior tongue

There are cases in which the exact meaning of a term cannot be captured without inspecting the other terms in its immediate neighborhood. As an example: *facial nerve function* could refer to the function of any nerve in the face or to the function of that nerve which is called *the facial nerve*:

- F-A3610   Facial nerve function, NOS
- F-A3610   Seventh cranial nerve function, NOS

2. 3. Analysis of Structural and Ontological Problems in SNODENT

There are also problems in SNODENT caused by the failure to follow ontological principles of good coding. [5]. Thus there are closely related, though ontologically completely different, entities which receive the same termcode. *Cheilodynia* is *pain in the lips*, hence a pain; while *painful lips* are lips. Yet these entities receive the same termcode in SNODENT:

- D5-22070   Cheilodynia
- D5-22070   Painful lips

Another example of the same phenomenon is:

- D5-10578   Sensitive dentin
- D5-10578   Tooth sensitivity

Of course there is nothing wrong with assigning the same code to different entities if the differences at issue are irrelevant for a specific objective. And certainly pain in the lips and lips that are painful are closely associated (the entire sensation is cortical under either heading). Our studies have shown, however, that when a terminology is structured in accordance with what ontologists have called the principle of **disjointness**, so that ontologically distinct top-level categories do not overlap in the classes they subsume, then this brings significant benefits in avoiding error propagation, and also supports alignment with external data and information sources. [7]

2.4. Analysis of SNODENT relative to SNOMED-CT

In order to arrive at a well-founded understanding of the way in which SNODENT is integrated structurally within the wider SNOMED framework, it is necessary to employ a methodology which begins by tracing paths from all SNODENT concepts to SNOMED-CT's *topconcept*, following only the relationships available in SNOMED. The resulting sub-graph represents some 2% of the total SNOMED graph structure.

By applying the algorithm described above to this sub-graph we were able to identify via a comparison of the original subsumption hierarchy with the generated one cases of both under- and overspecification of entities. We subjected each of these cases to detailed analysis in order to isolate the precise types of problems with which they are associated.

In all some **1081** new termcodes were generated by this method, reflecting entities not present in the SNOMED-CT tables but required by SNOMED's own classification principles. To give an example, consider the hierarchy generated for the SNODENT-concept *Moon's molar teeth*. We found this concept to subsumed by the generated concept which subsumes in its turn the concepts *congenital anomaly of molar tooth* and a third generated concept with the defined meaning: *congenital developmental tooth disorder of size and form*. Inspection of the generated concepts in context reveals that the concept *taurodontism* is underspecified, since it does not contain any other information than that carried by its parent concept. This contravenes a structural principle underlying DL-based terminologies (and also a central structural principle of good terminology building practice).

This example points to a number of tasks to be carried out in the enhancement of SNODENT, including:

- assessing which generated concepts should be included in an enhanced version of the SNODENT codes and which should be excluded
- assigning a fully specified name to the included concepts
- subjecting the differentiating criteria which led to the excluded concepts to a critical analysis and revising them accordingly
- verifying for the included concepts that they subsume all concepts that they should subsume. (Thus an experienced dentist might expect disorders other than *taurodontism* and *tuberculum paramolare* to be subsumed by the corresponding generated concept.) This may lead to the observation that the disclosed disorders need to be added to the system, or that they are currently underspecified or classified in the wrong place.

To give an impression of the size of the task, we note that the **1081** generated concepts themselves subsume between 1 and 37 concepts. Many of the generated concepts that subsume only one concept have a meaning identical to that of the existing SNOMED-CT concept. This feature is typical of concepts high in the subsumption hierarchy. This method allows us to look for other significant patterns as well, such as generated concepts that are subsumed by non-generated concepts that also subsume other non-generated concepts. So we discovered that *tooth finding* erroneously does not have the criteria for *tooth structure* and *jaw region*, which is clearly an underspecification in SNOMED. That is SNOMED currently treats *tooth finding* as if it were associated with the locations: *digestive structure* and *oral cavity structure* but *not* with the locations: *tooth structure* and *jaw region structure*.

3. Conclusion

Dentistry is one of the health care professions and has a number subspecialties within it. It has its own educational institutions (dental schools), governing bodies (e.g., the American Dental Association in the US), and specialty boards (e.g., Periodontics, Orthodontics). Dentists in private practice and in health care institutions use billing systems that are specifically designed for dental procedures, however, diagnostic codes are not in use in dentistry.

SNODENT is a set of diagnostic codes that was specifically designed to serve the field of dentistry. It is hoped that SNODENT will become an effective tool in enhancing the clinical practice of dentistry. It is also hoped that SNODENT will become a resource for both basic and clinical research into issues that involve oral health and the interaction of orofacial systems with other systems in the body.

SNODENT has now, appropriately, been included in SNOMED-CT. If SNODENT is to become widely used in dentistry, and fulfill the hopes regarding the benefits it can bring to the dental profession, its patients and to the research community, a great many problems will have to be overcome. Our results show that SNODENT requires considerable enhancements in content, quality of coding, quality of ontological structure and the manner in which it is integrated and aligned with SNOMED. We believe that methods for the analysis of the quality of diagnostic coding systems must be developed and employed if such systems are to reach their full potential.

4. References

[1] Smith B, Köhler J, Kumar A. On the application of formal principles to life science data: A case study in the Gene Ontology, Proc DILS 2004 (Data Integration in the Life Sciences), (Lecture Notes in Bioinformatics 2994), Berlin: Springer, 2004, 79–94.

[2] Smith B, Rosse C. The role of foundational relations in the alignment of biomedical ontologies, Proc Medinfo, 2004.

[3] Guarino N. Some ontological principles for designing upper level lexical resources. In: Rubio A, Gallardo N, Castro R, Tejada A, editors. Proceedings of First International Conference on Language Resources and Evaluation. ELRA European Language Resources Association, Granada, Spain; 1998. 527-534.

[4] Cimino JJ. Desiderata for controlled medical vocabularies in the twenty-first century. Methods of Information in Medicine; 1998;37(4-5):394-403

[5] Spackman KA, Reynoso G. Examining SNOMED from the perspective of formal ontological principles. KR-MED 2004.

[6] Ceusters W, Smith B, Kumar A, Dhaen C. Ontology-based error detection in SNOMED-CT. Proc Medinfo 2004 (in press).

[7] Ceusters W, Buekens F, De Moor G, Waagmeester A. The distinction between linguistic and conceptual semantics in medical terminology and its implications for NLP-based knowledge acquisition. Met Inform Med 1998; 37(4/5): 327-33.

Address for correspondence:

Louis J. Goldberg, Department of Oral Diagnostic Sciences, School of Dentistry, University at Buffalo , Buffalo, New York, 14216, USA, goldberg@buffalo.edu

Connecting Medical Informatics and Bio-Informatics
R. Engelbrecht et al. (Eds.)
IOS Press, 2005

Representing Clinical Knowledge in Oral Medicine Using Ontologies[1]

Marie Gustafsson, Göran Falkman

School of Humanities and Informatics, University of Skövde, Skövde, Sweden

Abstract:

How can information technology be used to model and handle clinical knowledge in everyday work so that clinicians can more systematically learn from collected clinical data? Ontology is a crucial element in answering this question. Based on nearly ten years of clinical experience, fundamental requirements of an ontology for oral medicine are presented. The use of the proposed W3C standards RDF and OWL for the design and implementation of an ontology for oral medicine is then described and discussed. The reported work contributes to knowledge representation in oral medicine by presenting the pioneering work towards an ontology for oral medicine using RDF/OWL, thereby testing the latter on a new domain.

Keywords:
Oral Medicine; Dental Informatics; Information Dissemination; Evidence-Based Medicine; Internet; Knowledge Representation; Ontology; RDF; OWL

1. Introduction

The MedView computer system [1] is an implementation of evidence-based oral medicine based on the view that health care should be built on finding, validating and using the latest research results as a basis of clinical decisions. In order to provide support for subsequent analysis and validation, key issues in evidence-based medicine are the collection of the 'right' clinical data and the possibility of sharing the information generated thereby.

It has been argued that medical informatics is the bridge between the domain of medicine and practitioner psychology [2]. Ontologies [3] are a crucial element in building this bridge, in that ontologies try to capture the best existing medical knowledge, through the systematic and explicit representation of medical definitions, concepts and processes, and by providing methodologies and tools for constructing computer support systems that help clinicians to perform clinical tasks more effectively and efficiently. Over the past decade, there has been much research in using ontologies in different medical disciplines.

Recently, both the Resource Description Framework (RDF) [4] and the Web Ontology Language (OWL) [5] have become World Wide Web Consortium (W3C) recommendations for representing information, exchanging knowledge and for publishing and sharing ontologies. There has been much activity in developing applications and programming frameworks for creating and managing ontologies using RDF/OWL, although, so far, limited research connected to the medical domain has been reported. Despite these current developments, there is to our knowledge no previously reported work on ontology for oral medicine, and especially no work in which RDF/OWL have been used.

---

[1] The work presented in this paper was supported by the Swedish Agency for Innovation Systems (VINNOVA)

We therefore propose the use of ontologies in dealing with problems faced by a system for evidence-based oral medicine such as MedView. Further, we argue that adapting to standards such as RDF and OWL will increase possibilities of knowledge sharing, as well as giving the possibility of using external tools. The reported work contributes to knowledge representation in oral medicine by presenting the preliminary work towards an ontology for oral medicine using RDF/OWL, thereby testing the latter on a new domain.

1.1. MedView

MedView is the product of nearly ten years of cooperation between the Chalmers University of Technology, the Clinic of Oral Medicine at the Sahlgrenska Academy in Göteborg and the University of Skövde. The overall goal is to develop models, methods and tools to support clinicians in their daily work and research. A central question is how information technology can be used to model and handle clinical knowledge in everyday work so that clinicians can more systematically learn from collected clinical data.

The knowledge base built in the MedView project currently contains data from over 8000 clinical examinations, covering more than 2000 different cases. The main knowledge base is located at the Clinic of Oral Medicine at the Sahlgrenska Academy. Clinics within the Swedish Oral Medicine Network (SOMNET) and various non-Swedish clinics have local knowledge bases, which are regularly added to a central knowledge base, so that the entire amount of data collected can be accessed through one common knowledge base.

1.2. Overview

The article identifies some important problems concerning the representation of knowledge in oral medicine. Given these problems, we describe how a preliminary ontology for oral medicine can be designed and implemented,, and investigate whether an approach using RDF and OWL might be fruitful in developing this ontology.

2. Knowledge Representation in Oral Medicine

Based on the experience gained during the first decade of the use of MedView and on recent interviews with domain experts and developers, the following requirements of an ontology for oral medicine have been identified:

- We must be able to utilise external sources of knowledge, e.g., general medical vocabularies and taxonomies of diseases and medications. Faster sharing of information is a prerequisite for effective evidence-based medicine [6].
- The relation between the conceptual models of fundamental clinical concepts, e.g., examination templates, lists of approved values for terms and groups of related terms, and their corresponding concrete entities must be formally examined.
- Relations and interactions between different entities of the ontology must be captured, e.g., that a certain answer to a specific question in an examination template triggers another question. By limiting the amount of questions to be answered, a potential barrier to clinicians entering the relevant information is diminished.
- A strong typing of elements is needed. We must be able to enforce that a given term only has values that are, e.g., numeric or a certain enumerated domain. The problem is amplified by the general problem in medicine of agreeing on canonical terms [7].
- We must be able to capture different kinds of meta-data, e.g., who is the creator of a specific examination template and what the purpose (scientific or clinical) is of the introduction of a specific examination template [8, 9].

- We need to differentiate between different 'views' of the underlying data, e.g., a patient, time or quantitative oriented view. The provision of different 'views' and the manipulation of these views are an intrinsic part of ontology management [10].
- The localisation of data has to be addressed rigorously. How can different language-based versions of the defined concepts, definitions and terms be provided? This is important since the transparent transition between language borders is a presumption of evidence-based medicine and knowledge sharing at a global level.
- An increasingly larger portion of medical data has its origin in images. The enormous amount of information obtainable from images is, however, difficult to grasp for the unaided human mind [7]. Thus, information contained in images, e.g., photos taken during the examination of patients, must be captured and represented.

3. Towards an Ontology for Oral Medicine

We will in the following introduce RDF and OWL and describe the design and the status of the implementation of the SOMWeb (Swedish Oral Medicine Web) ontology.

3.1. OWL and RDF

Essentially, RDF is a data-model, with subject-attribute-object triples, called statements, as its basic building blocks. Statements are graphs, where subjects and objects are nodes linked by attributes as the arcs. The abstract data model of RDF is most commonly described using XML (eXtensible Markup Language). Core concepts of RDF are resources and properties. Resources are the things we want to talk about, e.g., diagnoses, medications and allergies. Properties, a special kind of resources, describe relations between resources.

OWL is designed to be the standardised and broadly accepted language for describing ontologies, allowing users to write explicit, formal conceptualisations of domain models. OWL builds on RDF and uses RDF's XML-based syntax. Some language elements of OWL are classes, properties and property restrictions. We can state that classes are equivalent, what a property's domain, range and inverse property are, and make restrictions on what values a certain property can take, among other things.

For constructing ontologies, an ontology editor can be used. Of the graphical editors, Protégé [11] is one of the more widely used. Among the plugins available for Protégé are tools for reasoning and visualisation, as well as an OWL-plugin [12]. Further, there are several query languages for RDF, which can be used for finding instances fulfilling criteria of interest, as well as programming frameworks to interact with RDF and OWL content.

3.2. Designing the Ontology

The different 'views' supported by the ontology should be chosen based on how well they support real-life clinical tasks [13]. Our MedView experience has shown that the concept of a 'clinical examination' is the natural starting point for an ontology for oral medicine. In this respect, our methodology for building the SOMWeb ontology can best be described as a 'middle-out' approach [8], based on real-life scenarios, e.g., an examination situation.

3.3. Implementing the Ontology

3.3.1. Examinations, Terms, Values and Classes

In the SOMWeb ontology, OWL classes are used to represent clinical terms, e.g., *Allergy*, and parts of examination templates, e.g., *GeneralAnamnesis*. Term values, e.g., *Peanuts*, are represented as RDF instances of these OWL classes (see upper part of Figure 1 below). A concrete examination record, created by the user filling in a form based on an examination template, is represented as an RDF document, part of which can be seen in the lower part of Figure 1 below.

OWL object properties, e.g., *hasAllergy*, are associated with terms, where the range gives the term the property it is related to, e.g., *Allergy*, and the domain gives the part of the examination it is connected with, e.g., *GeneralAnamnesis* (see Figure 2 below).

```
<rdf:Description rdf:ID="Peanuts">
    <rdf:type>"somwebOntology#Allergy"</rdf:type>
    <rdfs:label xml:lang="en">Peanuts</rdfs:label>
    <rdfs:label xml:lang="sv">Jordnötter</rdfs:label>
    <dc:creator>"somwebPeople#Jontell"</dc:creator>
</rdf:Description>

<somweb:GeneralAnamnesis rdf:ID="GeneralAnamnesis_32_041115">
    <somweb:hasAllergy rdf:resource="somwebOntology#Apricot"/>
    <somweb:takesDrug rdf:resource="somwebOntology#Losec"/>
    <somweb:goodHealth
rdf:datatype="http://www.w3.org/2001/XMLSchema#boolean">
        true</somweb:goodHealth>
</somweb:GeneralAnamnesis>
```

Figure1 – RDF/XML for part of the values for the term Allergy *and for part of the* GeneralAnamnesis *section of the examination record* 32_041115

```
<owl:ObjectProperty rdf:ID="hasAllergy">
    <rdfs:comment xml:lang="en">What allergies do you have?</rdfs:comment>
    <rdfs:comment xml:lang="sv">Är du allergisk mot något?</rdfs:comment>
    <rdfs:range rdf:resource="somwebOntology#Allergy"/>
    <rdfs:domain rdf:resource="somwebOntology#GeneralAnamnesis"/>
</owl:ObjectProperty>
```

Figure 2 – OWL example for the object property hasAllergy

Classifying related terms is an important way for users to categorise different aspects of the data, e.g., different types of allergies. This can be accomplished using RDF/OWL at different levels. One way is to rigorously define subclasses, e.g., by defining *FoodAllergy* as a subclass of *Allergy*. We can also create descriptions of categories, e.g., for smoking habits, where an OWL restriction can be created for what it means to be a heavy smoker.

3.3.2. Using External Sources

An important contribution of using ontologies, and one of OWL's central features, is the ability to reuse existing ontologies. Currently, we are looking into importing ontologies for countries, units, medications and diagnoses. The Dublin Core, which is an ontology defining a standard for information resource description, will also be used.

3.3.3. Typing of Elements

Several methods in RDF and OWL can be used in aiding the typing of terms and values. Apart from object properties, which relate objects to other objects, OWL also supports data type properties, which relate objects to data type values. A good candidate for a data type property is *hasGoodHealth*, taking a value of true or false. For OWL data type properties, XML Schema data types can be used, so *hasGoodHealth* would have range XMLSchema#boolean, as defined by W3C (see lower part of Figure 1).

On the issue of units, OWL and RDF provide good support. We have applied the Semantic Web Best Practices and Deployment Working Group's working draft for defining *n*-ary relations[2]. For example, smoking habits could be represented as follows:

---

[2] http://www.w3.org/TR/swbp-n-aryRelations/

```
<SmokingRelation rdf:ID="Relation_1">
    <smokingValue rdf:datatype="http://www.w3.org/2001/XMLSchema#int">
    4</smokingValue>
    <hasTobaccoType rdf:resource="#Cigarette_Filter"/>
    <hasTimeUnit rdf:resource="timeOnt#Day"/>
</SmokingRelation>
```

This gives a separation of quantities and units, using fictive external time ontology. There are several initiatives for ontologies for units, which the SOMWeb ontology could use.

3.3.4. Meta-Data

For managing the multitude of terms, values and templates, using metadata is necessary. The SOMWeb ontology captures who created a term, value or template, and their reason for doing so. The Dublin Core includes elements such as creator, subject and description. In Figure 1, the creator element is used to describe who entered the value described.

3.3.5. Localisation of Data

We are especially interested in support for different languages. In the case of a value, e.g., *Peanuts*, and questions associated with the properties, e.g., *hasAllergy*, different labels can be specified for different languages using xml:lang (see Figure 1 and 2). Applications will use this to choose either the Swedish or the English labels and questions.

4. Discussion

Although ontologies may ease both knowledge sharing and the process of ontology construction, it is not a trivial process. Pinto and Martins [14] give an overview of methodologies for ontology construction and different processes of ontology reuse. Our approach is based on the observation that one success factor for bringing knowledge-based systems into daily clinical use is the careful planning of the introduction of the system in the clinical setting, in cooperation with end-users [15]. Right from the start, MedView was set up as a close collaboration between domain experts and computer scientists, in order to ensure that the developed systems were directly integrated into the clinical 'workflow' [17, 15, 9, 16]. Another key success factor is that the resulting system uses 'real' clinical data [13], a factor that is definitely met in MedView. Along the lines with previous research, we have started our work on constructing an ontology for oral medicine by focusing on a specific perspective of knowledge in oral medicine [9, 10], namely the concept of an 'examination'.

Three requirements listed in Section 2 have not been thoroughly explored: In catering for perspectives other than 'examination', e.g., 'patient' and 'time', the possibility to focus on different parts of the graph structure of RDF and OWL could be used. Inverse properties could also be defined to aid in moving in both directions on the graph. For example, the *hasAllergy* property may need an inverse property *allergyOf*. For representing relations and interactions between different parts of the model, OWL rule languages, e.g., [18], could be used. When it comes to representing information in photos, there are several initiatives for annotating photos using RDF/OWL. Using one of these, information ranging from simple descriptors referring to the diagnosis and quality of the photo, to marking regions of interest could be added. Another aspect we wish to explore is user modelling, needed to support users of different familiarity with computers, different roles and working in different departments. This can be a way to cope with the problem of getting the end-user to feel comfortable with the application, meaning a greater chance of data being entered [19].

5. Conclusions and Future Work

We have identified requirements faced in representing knowledge in oral medicine. Key issues here are the adherence to proposed standards, the utilisation of external data sources, and the amplitude of conceptual entities that have to be formally represented. We have described how these requirements can be fulfilled by constructing an ontology implemented in RDF and OWL. We have also begun identifying ontologies of interest for reuse.

During the initial implementation of this ontology, it has become apparent that RDF and OWL are applicable in fulfilling the requirements identified in Section 2. This work will be continued with further modelling of examinations and related concepts. Ontologies to be imported will be identified and hopefully successfully incorporated. As a case study, an existing MedView application will be adapted to using RDF and OWL, though the use of RDF and OWL will not be apparent to the end user. The new application will be tested as part of a more general evaluation of the RDF/OWL approach. Although reasoning is not our focus at present, advances on reasoning about instances may be relevant in the future.

As RDF and OWL are becoming widely used, we propose that these be used in the implementation of the SOMWeb ontology. By applying international standards, sharing knowledge and connecting ontologies should be achieved more easily. Further, the array of existing development tools will aid us in this implementation, and ensure that other ontology creators will have an equivalent ease of development.

6. References

[1] Jontell M, Mattsson U, and Torgersson O. MedView: An instrument for clinical research and education in oral medicine. *Oral Surg. Oral Med. Oral Pathol. Oral Radiol. Endod.* 2005: 99, 55–63.
[2] Hajdukiewicz JR, VicenteKJ, Doyle DJ, Milgram P, and Burns CM. Modeling a medical environment: An ontology for integrated medical informatics design. *Int. J. Med. Inform.* 2001: 62(1), 79–99.
[3] Gruber TR. A translation approach to portable ontologies. *Knowl. Acquis.* 1993: 5(2), 199–220.
[4] Manola F and Miller E, eds. *RDF Primer: W3C Recommendation 10 February 2004*. Created 2004. Retrieved December 28, 2004. Available at: http://www.w3.org/TR/2004/REC-rdf-primer-20040210/.
[5] Smith M, Welty C, and McGuinness D. *OWL Web Ontology Language Guide*. Created 2004. Retrieved December 28, 2004. Available at: http://www.w3.org/TR/2004/REC-owl-guide-20040210/.
[6] Mendonça EA, Cimino JJ, Johnson SB, and Seol YH. Accessing heterogeneous sources of evidence to answer clinical questions. *J. Biomed. Inform.* 2001: 34(2), 85–98.
[7] Cios KJ and Moore GW. Uniqueness of medical data mining. *Artif. Intell. Med.* 2002: 26(1–2), 1–24.
[8] Fernández-López M and Gómez-Pérez A. Overview and analysis of methodologies for building ontologies. *Knowl. Engin. Rev.* 2002: 17(2), 129–156.
[9] Edgington T, Beomjin C, Henson K, Raghu TS, and Vinze A. Adopting ontology to facilitate knowledge sharing. *Commun. ACM* 2004: 47(11), 85–90.
[10] Noy NF and Musen MA. Specifying ontology views by traversal. In: McIlraith SA et al., eds. *Proc. ISWC'04*. Springer, 2004; pp 713–725.
[11] Noy NF, Sintek M, Decker S, Crubezy M, Fergerson RW, and Musen MA. Creating semantic web contents with Protégé-2000. *IEEE Intell. Syst.* 2001: 2(16), 60–71.
[12] Knublauch H, Fergerson RW, Noy NF, and Musen MA. The Protégé OWL plugin: An open development environment for semantic web applications. In: McIlraith SA et al., eds. *Proc. ISWC'04*. Springer, 2004; pp 229–243.
[13] Zeng Q and Cimino JJ. A knowledge-based, concept-oriented view generation system for clinical data. *J. Biomed. Inform.* 2001: 34(2), 112–128.
[14] Pinto HS and Martins JP. Ontologies: How can they be built? *Knowl. Inform. Syst.* 2004: 6(4), 441–464.
[15] Wetter T. Lessons learnt from bringing knowledge-based systems into routine use. *Artif. Intell. Med.* 2002: 24(3), 195–203.
[16] Mendonça EA. Clinical decision support systems: Perspectives in dentistry. *J. Dent. Edu.* 2004: 68, 589–597.
[17] Sutherland SE. The building blocks of evidence-based dentistry. *J. Can. Dent. Assoc.* 2000: 66, 241–244.
[18] Horrocks I and Patel-Schneider PF. A proposal for an OWL rules language. In: *Proc. 13th International Conference on World Wide Web*. ACM Press, 2004; pp 723–731.
[19] Razmerita L, Angehrn AA, and Maedche A. Ontology-based user modeling for knowledge management systems. In: Brusilovsky P, Corbett AT, and de Rosis F, eds. *User Modeling*. Springer, 2003; pp 213–217.

Address for Correspondence

Marie Gustafsson, School of Humanities and Informatics, University of Skövde, PO Box 408
SE-541 28 Skövde, Sweden. Email: marie.gustafsson@his.se

Connecting Medical Informatics and Bio-Informatics
R. Engelbrecht et al. (Eds.)
IOS Press, 2005

The Epistemological-Ontological Divide in Clinical Radiology

Dirk Marwede[a,b], Matthew Fielding[a]

[a]Institute of Formal Ontology and Medical Information Science, Saarland University, Saarbrücken, Germany
[b]Department of Diagnostic Radiology, Leipzig University Hospital, Leipzig, Germany

Abstract

Medical ontologies like GALEN, the FMA or SNOMED represent a kind of "100% certain" medical knowledge which is not inherent to all medical sub-domains. Clinical radiology uses computerized imaging techniques to make the human body visible and interprets the imaging findings in a clinical context delivering a textual report. For clinical radiology few standardized vocabularies are available. We examined the definitions given in the glossary of terms for thoracic radiology published by the Fleischner Society. We further classified these terms with regard to their definitions in terms of (a) describing visible structures on the image itself, (b) referring to ontological entities of the body (anatomical or pathological), and (c) terms imposing knowledge on structures visible on the image, epistemologically representing ontological entities of the body. Each ontological/epistemological definition was rated on a scale of vague/weak-sound/strong and put in context with the evaluation comments for the use of the terms given in the glossary itself. The result of this distinction shows that clinical radiology uses many terms referring to ontological entities valid for representation in a medical ontology. However, many epistemological terms exist in the terminology which impose epistemological knowledge on ontological entities. The analysis of the evaluation comments reveals that terms classified as sound (ontologically) and strong (epistemologically) are evaluated higher than terms bearing vague or weak definitions. On the basis of this, we argue that the distinction between ontological and epistemological definitions is necessary in order to construct epistemologically-sensitive application ontologies for medical sub-domains, like clinical radiology, where knowledge is fragmented in terms of description, inferred from a description, concluded on the basis of imaging, or other additional information with varying degrees of certainty.

Keywords:
Controlled vocabularies, medical ontology, clinical radiology, conceptual modelling

1. Introduction

With the development of medical ontologies such as GALEN [1], SNOMED-CT [2] and the Foundational Model of Anatomy (FMA) [3], medical knowledge from different medical sub-domains has been captured representing entities and relations between those entities. Knowledge modelling in a particular domain is based on the exploration of terms used in that particular domain and the definition of entities (universals) in a hierarchical structure. In the domain of clinical radiology this process is confronted by a difficulty: the large reliance on specifically epistemic and epistemically-qualified terms. When dealing with an image of the body, as in chest x-ray or computertomography (CT) for instance, we would like to claim that radiologists use the image on the film in order to describe clear and distinct entities within the body directly. However, more often radiologists are required to describe the complexes of shadows, densities and contrast enhancements subsequently providing what amounts to the appearance of a body structure in a clinical context and what those appearances represent in reality (anatomically as well as pathologically). Even if interpretation of those appearances represents highly specialized medical domain knowledge terms used in radiologic reports are of both kinds, ontological and epistemological. The purpose of this paper is two fold. We here return to the Fleischner Society's "Glossary of Terms for Thoracic Radiology" [4] in order to:

- draw out the implicit ontological and epistemological commitments of these terms and thereby making them explicit to the informatics community in order to aid the development of "epistemic-sensitive" ontologies;
- investigate any possible relationships between these ontological and epistemological commitments (previously unstated) and the explicit evaluations of the terms proposed in the glossary itself.

We aim to demonstrate how these commitments, once they have been made explicit, may increase the ability of these terms to satisfy the strict restraints in the development of application-ontologies and to further propagate the use of this glossary among radiologists.

1.1   The Epistemological/Ontological Divide

Ontology has famously been defined as the "science of what is." This philosophical understanding of ontology will only underlie our discussion here insofar as it will serve to make the epistemic/ontological divide clearer. Primarily, we will concern ourselves with that notion of ontology employed by the various sorts of biomedical ontologies of the medical informatics community such as GALEN, SNOMED or the FMA. Application ontologies, of the biomedical sort such as these, are commonly designed around the principle that there are pure and certain objectifiable classes (also called 'universals' – organized according to the substumption/parent-child/IS-A relationships) with any number of more specific relations that may be mapped between these classes, horizontally (i.e. *is-participant-of*) and vertically (i.e. *is-part-of*). The idea being that any given particular instantiation of these classes will invariably conform to these class mappings [5]

Epistemology, on the other hand, deals with questions of knowledge, certainty, and ways we have of accessing those entities in the world [6]. In other words, questions of epitemology encompass the various methods by which doctors and clinicians come to know about those anatomical and pathological entities that are the focus of their discipline. Epistemological questions are very rarely dealt with in the literature aimed at an informatics audience, and understandably so. When designing an ontology it is rarely profitable to introduce such questions as: "how do we know that's a tumor?", for however a particular physician, dealing with a particular patient, comes to know a particular tumor, bears little on the so-called 'universal' structures of tumors. That all tumors arise from a particular type of cellular tissue, may be benign or malignant, may spread by metastasis, etc, is true ontologically, regardless of whether there really exists a tumor in an particular instance. However, such ontological commitments are difficult to achieve in radiology.

1.2   Imaging the Human Body

Clinical radiology uses different techniques like conventional x-ray, computertomography (CT), magnetic resonance imaging (MRI) or ultrasound to deliver images of the human body. Deciding on which imaging technique to use is crucial to getting the proper results, on the basis of which a radiologist may make or exclude a particular diagnosis. The results of an examination in clinical radiology are stated in a report, which yields a description of the imaging findings and a conclusion. For the interpretation of imaging findings the individual perception, knowledge and experience about the appearance of anatomical or pathological structures with regard to the technique applied and the clinical information at hand is crucial. Radiology departments nowadays represent highly computerized environments where digital images are compiled, processed by software and stored in huge picture archiving repositories. Image interpretation is usually done on computer workstation where the findings are reported, in recent years utilizing speech and language recognition software.

1.3 Terms Used in Radiology and Concept Modelling

Despite the increasing use of computers in radiology, the content of radiology reports which serves as the basis for the communication of results of imaging examinations to colleagues, has not been affected by these technologies [7]. For the description of imaging findings and their interpretation no general standardized terminology is available. Some efforts have been undertaken to compose standardized vocabularies for specialized reporting tasks like the BIRADS classification for mammography reporting [8] or the glossary of terms for thoracic imaging proposed by the Fleischner Society. Some studies have extracted terms from radiographic reports to develop a concept model of the content of those reports [9, 10]. However, the integration of those terms in an application-ontology dealing with imaging domain knowledge has not been done.

2. Materials and Methods

Definitions stated in the "Glossary of Terms for Thoracic Radiology" published by the Fleischner Society were examined. The glossary of thoracic imaging contains definitions for 176 terms used in thoracic radiology. One term can have more than one definition. Each definition is classified by category, most frequent used categories are: *Radiology, Radiology physics, Pathophysiology, Physiology, Pathology and Anatomy*. If a term has the same definition in different categories, a composite category is used, e.g. *Anatomy/Radiology*. Few terms have definitions for which no category is specified. For most definitions an *evaluation* comment is given. The *evaluation* indicates whether the term is recommended or not, useful or not and whether the term represents an *inferred* or *diagnostic* conclusion.

2.1 Analysis

For this paper we focus on term definitions in the category of *Radiology*, for which we further specified the terms as purely *ontological* or *epistemological*. In a second step the *ontological* definitions were classified on an ordinal scale as *vague, intermediate,* or *sound*. *Epistemological* definitions were similarly classified as *weak, intermediate,* or *strong*, respectively. The evaluative comments were further classified as *positive, negative,* or *not stated explicitly* and the results were compared with regard to the ontological/epistemological distinction described above.

2.2 Ontological/Epistmological Classification

On the *ontological level of the body* we see terms, radiological as well as general anatomical, such as: "**parenchyma**. The lung exclusive of visible pulmonary vessels and airways," as well as common radiological instruments and tools such as: "**contrast medium.** An agent administered to render the lumen of a hollow structure, vessels, or viscus more or less opaque than its surrounding for the purpose of radiographic imaging." For the most part, terms of this categorization were of the *sound* distinction and highly evaluated.

Those terms which properly isolate themselves to the *ontological level of the image* are termed "features of radiological anatomy," elements which may serve to orient the radiologist but may not necessarily represent any *bona fide* entity within the body itself. Here we see such terms as: "**posterior tracheal stripe.** A vertically oriented, linear opacity ranging from the thoracic inlet to the bifurcation of the trachea and visible only in lateral radiographs of the chest. It is situated between the air shadows of the trachea and the right lung and is formed by the posterior tracheal wall and contiguous mediastinal interstitial tissue." Terms at this level are generally categorized as *sound*.

The second category we call *epistemological* which represents those cases where an inference has been made from specific features of the image to specific entities within the body. Here we categorize term definitions such as: "**coin lesion.** A sharply defined, circular opacity within the lung, suggestive of a coin and usually representing a spherical or nodular lesion." The term is further qualified however, "The term *coin* may be descriptive of the shadow, but certainly not of the lesion producing it," and hence the evaluation, "A radiologic descriptor, the use of which is to be condemned. This term is categorized as *weak* epistemological. However, an example for a *strong* epistemological definition is: "**pneumopericardium.** The presence of gas within the pericardium; visible only where the gas shadow is seen in profile: laterally in the frontal view, anteriorly or posteriorly in the laterial projection." Terms of this category are generally evaluated on the degree to which they are appropriately based on radiographic evidence. Those conclusions not appropriately based on radiographic findings alone are generally rated as *weak* (or *intermediate* if the term is cautioned against and its use restricted).

3. Results

166 definitions in the category of *Radiology* were classified. Table 1 shows the number of terms classified as *ontological* or *epistemological* with regard to the strength/soundness of the definition. Overall 109 terms were classified as *ontological* and 58 terms as *epistemological*. From terms classified ontological most terms were rated *sound* ontological (94). Few ontological terms were rated *intermediate* (12) and only three terms were rated *vague* (3). In contrast, terms classified epistemological showed moderate difference on the rating scale: 24 terms were rated *strong*, 23 *intermediate* and 11 *weak*.

Table 1 Number of ontological and epistemological radiologic definitions.

Soundness/Strength	Ontological	Epistemological
Sound/strong	94	24
Intermediate	12	23
Vague/weak	3	11
Sum	109	58

Evaluation comments given in the glossary by the authors are displayed in Table 2 with respect to the ontological/epistemological classification.

Table 2 Evaluation comments on ontological and epistemological definitions

Evaluation comment	Ontological (%)			Epistemological (%)		
	vague	intermediate	sound	weak	intermediate	strong
positive	0	8 (7)	73 (67)	0	7 (12)	20 (34)
Not stated explicitly	0	3 (3)	15 (14)	3 (5)	14 (24)	3 (5)
negative	3 (3)	1 (1)	6 (6)	8 (14)	2 (3)	1 (2)

Table 2 shows that most of the terms classified as ontologically *sound* or epistemologically *strong* had a *positive* evaluation comment. In contrast, none of the *vague* or *weak* ontological or epistemological classified terms was rated *positive* by the authors. However, ontological terms classified as *intermediate* were more positive evaluated as epistemological terms which frequently did no have an evaluation comment in the glossary.

4. Conclusions and Discussion

The glossary for thoracic radiology published by the Fleischner society is a valuable resource for terms used in thoracic radiology and a recommendation of their use in radiologic reports. Even if the distinction between ontological and epistemological terms is not given explicitly in the glossary, the definitions and the evaluation comments stated give a detailed view on the origin, the usefulness, and the value of each term in radiology.

Ontological considerations in medical information science leads towards a greater perspicuity in our definitions of body entities via a sound understanding of their place within a class hierarchy as well as the relationships that exist between these entities and others. This applies equally to radiology as to other medical domains like biology, anatomy or genomics. Clear ontological definitions of terms used in radiology would facilitate the exchange of information between radiologists and those reading their reports. Our study revealed that many terms used in radiology have a sound ontological definition independently of the entity they refer to, an entity on the image (e.g. posterior tracheal stripe) or the body itself (e.g. parenchyma). Additionally, most terms with sound ontological definitions were rated positive by the authors and their use is recommended. They represent valid entities for the construction of an imaging ontology or for incorporating into an existing ontology dealing with entities of the body (e.g. the FMA).

Terms with epistemological definitions are less frequent in the glossary but strong epistemological definitions were mostly rated positive, even if there were a remarkable high number of epistemological definitions which were intermediate ranked. While the epistemological status of many terms cannot be changed, it must be cleared up which epistemological terms are inferred, which terms are diagnostic conclusions and which are descriptors. This would not improve the precision of the terms itself but restrict their use to the appropriate context.

Terminology used in clinical radiology consists of both epistemological evidence and ontological entities. In particular, terms which deliver epistemological evidence about ontological entities seem to represent a large portion of terms used in radiology reporting. However, future medical ontologies with the aim of representing knowledge about certain medical sub-domains, like clinical radiology, have to find ways to integrate terms containing epistemological evidence about ontological entities with varied levels of certainty.

5. Acknowledgements

The present paper was written under the auspices of the Wolfgang Paul Program of the Alexander von Humboldt Foundation, the Network of Excellence in Semantic Interoperability and Data Mining in Biomedicine of the European Union, and the project Forms of Life sponsored by the Volkswagen Foundation.

6. References

[1]   Rector AL,Nowlan WA. The GALEN project. *Comput Methods Programs Biomed* 1994;45(1-2):75-8.

[2]   American College of Pathologists. *Snomed Clinical Terms Technical Reference Guide*; 2003.

[3]   Rosse C ,Mejino JL Jr. A reference ontology for biomedical informatics: the Foundational Model of Anatomy. *J Biomed Inform* 2003;36(6):478-500.

[4]   Tuddenham WJ. Glossary of terms for thoracic radiology: recommendations of the Nomenclature Committee of the Fleischner Society. *AJR Am J Roentgenol* 1984;143(3):509-17.

[5]   Smith B. The Logic of Biological Classification abd the Foundations of Biomedical Ontology. In: *Invited Papers from the 10th International Conference in Logic Methodology and the Philsoph of Science*; 2003; Oviedo, Spain; 2003. p. forthcoming.

[6]   Bodenreider O, Smith B, Burgun A. The Ontology-Epistemology Divide: A Case Study in Medical Terminology. In: Vieu Laure, editor. *International Conference on Formal Ontology and Information Systems*; 2004; Torino, Italy; 2004.

[7]   Langlotz CP. Automatic structuring of radiology reports: harbinger of a second information revolution in radiology. *Radiology* 2002;224(1):5-7.

[8]   Liberman L, Menell JH. Breast imaging reporting and data system (BI-RADS). *Radiol Clin North Am* 2002;40(3):409-30, v.

[9]   Bell DS, Pattison-Gordon E, Greenes RA. Experiments in concept modeling for radiographic image reports. *J Am Med Inform Assoc* 1994;1(3):249-62.

[10] Friedman C,Cimino JJ, Johnson SB. A schema for representing medical language applied to clinical radiology. *J Am Med Inform Assoc* 1994;1(3):233-48.

7. Correspondence:

Dirk Marwede, IFOMIS, Saarland University, Postfach 151150
66041 Saarbruecken, Germany.
Email: dmarwed@gwdg.de

Connecting Medical Informatics and Bio-Informatics
R. Engelbrecht et al. (Eds.)
IOS Press, 2005

Representation of Medical Informatics in the Wikipedia and its Perspectives

Udo Altmann

Institute of Medical Informatics
University of Gießen, Heinrich-Buff-Ring 44, D-35392 Gießen

Abstract

A wiki is a technique for collaborative development of documents on the web. The Wikipedia is a comprehensive free online encyclopaedia based on this technique which has gained increasing popularity and quality. This paper's work explored the representation of Medical Informatics in the Wikipedia by a search of specific and less specific terms used in Medical Informatics and shows the potential uses of wikis and the Wikipedia for the specialty. Test entries into the Wikipedia showed that the practical use of the so-called WikiMedia software is convenient. Yet Medical Informatics is not represented sufficiently since a number of important topics is missing. The Medical Informatics communities should consider a more systematic use of these techniques for disseminating knowledge about the specialty for the public as well as for internal and educational purposes.

Keywords:
Wiki,;Wikipedia; Encyclopaedia; Medical Informatics

1. Introduction

"A wiki is a website (or other hypertext document collection) that allows a user to add content, like on an Internet forum, but also allows that content to be edited by anybody " (Definition for "wiki" in the Wikipedia [1]). The name "wiki" is based on an Hawaiian word for "quick". Web pages can be put into an edit mode which means that an HTML form (text area) is displayed where text is entered in a specific syntax. The syntax can easily be learned and is much more compact than HTML syntax (although some wiki engines also allow input of HTML). Thereby collaborative documents can be edited quickly with one author complementing and improving the other author's work.

Based on these ideas wikis are used for projects where documents have to be edited collaboratively, preferably for presentation on the Web or for the compilation of help pages. The first wiki initiated by Ward Cunningham was about sharing and developing ideas about programming in 1995. Meanwhile, a large variety of wikis exist, e.g., for different aspects of lifestyle, scientific issues, program languages, user documentation for programs, and, for encyclopaedic projects. The largest of the encyclopaedic projects is the "Wikipedia" that exists in many languages. Among these the English language project is the largest (437086 entries, start in January 2001, status on January 1st, 2005) and the German language project is the second largest one (183012 entries, start in May 2001). The project's mission is to provide free encyclopaedic information with a license for using the text that has similarities to free software license models.

Since anybody can contribute to articles there is much concern about quality issues (including so-called "vandalism" of contents). A test carried out by a German computer magazine in October 2004 showed, that overall quality is good comparing the contents of the German Wikipedia to commercial products [2].

Other authors promote or use wikis for knowledge management in work groups [3] or as part of an interactive, web-based programming environment that enables biologists to analyze biological systems by combining knowledge and data through direct end-user programming [4].

This contribution shall explore the potential of Wiki techniques with respect to public and specialist knowledge about Medical Informatics.

2. Methods

To investigate the coverage of Medical Informatics topics by the English language Wikipedia, a number of terms (57) were selected mainly from the table of contents of the "Handbook of Medical Informatics" [5]. They comprised of terms closely related to Medical Informatics as well as of general informatics topics. For each search term, a full text search was performed to get a most specific (with respect to Medical Informatics) result. The full list of search terms can be seen in the results table.

The Wikipedia website (http://www.wikipedia.org) was visited systematically on two days (October 17th, 2004 and January 2nd, 2005). On these days the terms were searched and their existence or non-existence was recorded.

In case of existence the date of entry, the date of last change and the number of changes were recorded on occasion of the January visit according to the Wikipedia's built-in "history" function. Since changes of contents are often followed by a number of small immediate corrections, one author was only counted once per day. This count shall give a rough measurement of activity on this term.

In few cases the author added new entries on October 17th (Medical Subject Headings, Hospital Information System, Nursing Informatics, Medical Classification, Cancer Registry). The intention was not only to give new input to the encyclopaedia but to observe what happens to new articles.

Articles entered or modified by the author were put on a so-called "watchlist" that allows a quick overview of articles that were recently modified. Thus authors can quickly react if something undesired (for example vandalism) happens to these articles.

The selection of terms claims not be representative for Medical Informatics. Therefore results of the investigation are interpreted textually and the few counts and calculations have only limited value.

3. Results

Table 1 shows the result of the search. The column "Search Term" contains the initial term that was searched. The next column shows one ore more terms that were found during the search. For these terms, the date when they were entered and when they were changed for the last time is listed as well as the number of changes during this time. The last column contains the intensity of changes as calculation of: number of changes / (last change – date entered + 1).

Table 1 – Search Terms and Results

Search term	Found term	Entered	Last change	Days	Length	Changes	Intensity
Medical Informatics	Medical Informatics	28.10.2003	28.12.2004	428	4763	34	0,08
Nursing Informatics	Nursing Informatics	17.10.2004	04.11.2004	19	3508	8	0,42
Hospital Information System	VA Kernel (but not VistA)	22.02.2003	22.02.2003	1	828	0	0,00
	Hospital Information System	17.10.2004	17.10.2004	1	622	1	1,00
	Laboratory information system	16.12.2004	01.01.2005	17	5288	10	0,59
Clinical Information System	Not found						
Patient Record	Medical record	27.10.2004	31.12.2004	66	8094	11	0,17
	Medical privacy	28.11.2003	28.11.2003	1	1588	2	2,00
	HIPAA	01.12.2003	17.11.2004	353	2057	16	0,05
Electronic medical record	Electronic medical record	25.08.2004	25.12.2004	123	2566	11	0,09
Electronic Patient Record	see Electronic medical record						
Computer-based Medical Record	Not found						
Electronic Health Record	Not found						
Health Level Seven	HL7	01.12.2003	23.11.2004	359	2524	7	0,02
Primary Care	Primary Care	17.03.2004	01.08.2004	138	1493	2	0,01
Shared Care	Not found						
Information	Information	25.02.2002	15.04.2004	781	9434	92	0,12
Communication	Communication	07.11.2001	01.01.2005	1152	5311	120	0,10
Completeness	Completeness	10.06.2002	16.12.2004	921	4561	23	0,02
Accuracy	Accuracy and precision	26.02.2002	28.12.2004	1037	3395	11	0,01
Precision	Precision	25.02.2002	31.08.2004	919	1430	13	0,01
Coding	Coding	25.02.2002	17.10.2004	966	1839	11	0,01
Free Text	Not found						
Data Entry	see Data processing						
User Interface	User Interface	21.03.2002	08.12.2004	994	5134	16	0,02
Information Processing	Information Processing	10.09.2003	08.12.2004	456	2159	14	0,03
Data Processing	Data Processing	26.02.2002	02.12.2004	1011	1827	14	0,01
Data Presentation	Presentation (disambiguation)	25.04.2004	17.10.2004	176	1076	7	0,04
	Small multiple	16.03.2004	16.03.2004	1	594	0	0,00
	Markup (computing)	20.10.2003	21.11.2004	399	1231	11	0,03
Data Model	Data Model	09.09.2002	12.12.2004	826	2643	12	0,01
Data Structure	Data Structure	27.10.2002	24.11.2004	1125	3714	80	0,07
Classification	Classification	23.05.2003	27.12.2004	585	1651	23	0,04
Nomenclature	Nomenclature	07.12.2003	29.12.2004	389	1139	14	0,04
Thesaurus	Thesaurus	06.12.2001	31.12.2004	1122	2521	24	0,02
Taxonomy	Taxonomy	10.08.2001	18.12.2004	1227	3299	43	0,04
Nosology	Nosology	11.08.2002	01.11.2004	814	745	11	0,01
ICD	International Statistical Classification of Diseases and Related Health Problems	30.12.2001	06.11.2004	1043	3603	21	0,02
SNOMED	Medical Informatics						
ICD-O	Not found						
ICPM	Not found						
MeSH	Medical Subject Headings	17.10.2004	17.10.2004	1	892	2	2,00
DRG	Diagnosis-related group	13.03.2003	03.10.2004	571	3196	15	0,03
UMLS	SPECIALIST lexicon	15.05.2004	09.11.2004	179	5389	4	0,02
	Medical Classification	17.10.2004	06.11.2004	21	1794	3	0,14
Biosignal	Signal Processing	25.02.2002	25.12.2004	1035	922	14	0,01
Medical Imaging	Medical Imaging	27.05.2003	31.12.2004	585	4819	30	0,05
Ultrasound	Medical ultrasonography	02.11.2002	01.12.2004	761	6132	24	0,03
Computer Tomography	Computed axial tomography	01.05.2002	25.11.2004	940	4872	44	0,05
MRI	Magnetic resonance imaging	03.08.2001	20.12.2004	1236	10629	79	0,06
Medical Image Processing	Medical Imaging						
Decision Support	Decision support system	14.02.2004	19.12.2004	310	11223	18	0,06
Bayes' Rule	Bayes' theorem	18.04.2002	10.11.2004	938	13708	79	0,08
Arden Syntax	Not found						
Neural Network	Neural Network	02.10.2001	31.12.2004	1187	19649	128	0,11
Guideline	Guideline (medical)	18.12.2004	18.12.2004	1	2998	1	0,00
Data Protection	Not found						
Data Security	Privacy	02.01.2002	28.12.2004	1092	2919	31	0,03
	Data Security	11.11.2004	15.12.2004	35	688	2	0,06
	Medical privacy	28.11.2003	28.11.2003	1	1588	2	2,00
Confidentiality	Confidentiality	31.10.2003	28.12.2004	425	1982	15	0,04
Health Telematics	Telematics	29.07.2004	19.12.2004	144	1474	8	0,06
Registry	Registry	30.09.2003	31.12.2004	459	2376	24	0,05
Cancer Registry	Cancer Registry	17.10.2004	19.11.2004	34	1663	1	0,03
Hospital Cancer Registry	Not found						
Population-based Cancer Registry	Not found						

Coverage / Missing Terms

The more general "informatics" topics were covered well, but important rather specific "Medical Informatics" terms could not be found on the first visit:

- Nursing Informatics
- Hospital Information System, Clinical Information System
- ICD-O, ICPM
- Biosignal
- Arden Syntax, Guideline
- Health Telematics
- Cancer Registry

Some of the terms that were missing on the first visit were added by the author. "Medical guideline" was entered between the first and second visit by other authors as well as the terms "Laboratory information system" and "Data Security".

Variation of terminology

Some topics could not be found by the original term but by variations. The largest variation exists for "Electronic Medical Record".

Intensity of work on terms

Usually activity on terms is high during the first time after the term was entered. After excluding terms with a short period (20 days) between entry and last change, the arithmetic mean value for intensity is 0.047 (with a range from 0.01 – 0.17) which means that the terms of this set were changed approximately once per twenty days on average. Terms with high activity were

- Medical record, Medical Classification ("medical terms")
- Information, Neural Network, Communication ("informatics" terms)

From the terms that were entered by the author only "Nursing Informatics" was changed frequently.

Quality of entries

This paper has no focus on the quality of specific articles. Where possible improvements were obvious and the author felt competent they were introduced usually without negative response by other contributing authors. In some cases (Data model, Classification) the intention was to introduce a more common language use into rather expert/technical definitions. The Wikipedia software offers a possibility to discuss articles with other authors (Talk pages) that helped to explain this intention to the previous authors and to develop formulations that could be accepted by all active authors.

During the period of observance no vandalism could be observed to the articles on the author's watchlist.

4. Discussion

In October 2005, the German computer magazine c't published a comparison between two commercial encyclopaedias (Microsoft Encarta Pro and Brockhaus) and the Wikipedia (all

German versions). Terms with different degrees of difficulty from different areas of science, society and culture were searched and compared by length and quality. The overall quality of the Wikipedia was better than the one of the commercial products although there were also articles of poor quality and there exist shortcomings with respect to specific multimedia functions (e.g. interactive maps). One of the most evident disadvantages that also could frequently be observed by the author was a slow response time of the servers due to capacity overload. According to information from the project, this is mainly caused by limited hardware resources. To sum up the magazine's evaluation shows that the ideas "wiki" and "Wikipedia" work well, and that it is worthwhile thinking about their significance for Medical Informatics.

Representation of Medical Informatics in the Wikipedia

The results of this paper's work show that Medical Informatics topics are not very well represented in the Wikipedia currently. This can mean that

- there is low awareness of / few knowledge about the Wikipedia project in the Medical Informatics "community"
- there exist no resources to contribute to the project
- the project is not estimated as a possibility to transfer knowledge about Medical Informatics to the public

One can indeed question whether and to what extent Medical Informatics should be represented in such a project. What are the options to obtain knowledge about Medical Information on the internet? Web portals of organizations like the International Medical Informatics Association (IMIA, http://www.imia.org) and European Federation for Medical Informatics (EFMI, http://www.efmi.org) are often designed to support organisational issues and don't explain what this specialty contributes to society and science. Using search engines internet users can obtain extensive information but with the disadvantage that search engines cannot measure quality and the user himself has to decide what information is best for him within an often large search result. Although it doesn't guarantee quality per se an encyclopaedia offers a more systematic access to knowledge. Yet as the mentioned experiences with "Data model" and "Classification" show, there is a risk of using a technical language that cannot be understood by the readers. Actually we have to deal with at least two major groups of readers.

The first group are people with no or few knowledge about Medical Informatics who might come across terms e.g. in newspapers or consider studying the profession. Articles for this public should be easily understandable. Since they won't provide very detailed information the frequency of changes will be low.

The second group are people with at least basic knowledge about Medical Informatics who want to learn more about another area. They will expect more detailed and up to date information than the first group. The advantage of wikis is that everybody can contribute to them and that information can easily be actualised in contrast to books.

How To Build Up A Wiki For Medical Informatics

The own experiences affirm that the Wikipedia's project software (MediaWiki, open source) works well and allows convenient editing of articles. The culture of collaboration leads to usually continually improving articles. Since obviously the area of Medical Informatics has not been worked on systematically in the Wikipedia, it is more or less left to chance whether an article is further developed or not (e.g. "Nursing Informatics" versus "Cancer Registry").

Writing articles for the Wikipedia can be very labour-intensive. A starting point to a more systematic approach to put Medical Informatics contents into a wiki like the Wikipedia could be its use in education and training. Students often have to do homeworks or presentations on specific topics. The same techniques they learn by these works – learning through active acquiring and presentation of knowledge, use of neutral point of view language, correct composition of papers, developing exact and understandable formulations – can also be trained by building up articles (at least for parts of their work, e.g. introductions and glossaries). The review that is necessary to improve quality of articles can be done by the teachers who would have to revise and assess the work anyway or by a group of students collaboratively. Using the built-in revision history, the contributions of the author or the state of a document can easily be tracked.

Although such wikis could be hosted on local servers, the best integration would be implementing them as part of the Wikipedia project. In this case, providing some funding should be considered to support the expansion of the currently limited resources.

As soon as authors from different institutions contribute to one article, one can anticipate that conflicts will arise from different opinions regarding a topic, e.g. the correct definition of a term. The WikiMedia software offers a medium to discuss these opinions through the already mentioned talk pages. A discussion on a topic remains linked to it and helps following readers or authors of the topic to interpret the contents and to understand the crux of the matter.

5. Conclusion

Wiki techniques offer new perspectives for collaborative work including the dissemination of knowledge. The Wikipedia project has gained an impressive volume with an overall good quality. Yet this potential is currently not used sufficiently by Medical Informatics for its representation neither to the general public nor to specialists. A means to improve this situation efficiently could be to use wikis or the Wikipedia for education and get articles as by-product of student works.

6. References

[1] http://en.wikipedia.org/wiki/Wiki on January 2nd, 2005

[2] Kurzidim M. Wissenswettstreit – Die kostenlose Wikipedia tritt gegen Marktführer Encarta und Brockhaus an. c't Magazin für Computertechnik, Heise-Verlag, Hannover, Heft 21, pp 132-139

[3] Kosuch HT; Porth AJ. Wissensmanagement in der Medizin mit "Wikis". Kooperative Versorgung - Vernetzte Forschung - Ubiquitäre Information. 49. Jahrestagung der Deutschen Gesellschaft für Medizinische Informatik, Biometrie und Epidemiologie (gmds), 19. Jahrestagung der Schweizerischen Gesellschaft für Medizinische Informatik (SGMI) und Jahrestagung 2004 des Arbeitskreises Medizinische Informatik (ÖAKMI) der Österreichischen Computer Gesellschaft (OCG) und der Österreichischen Gesellschaft für Biomedizinische Technik (ÖGBMT). Innsbruck, 26.-30.09.2004. Düsseldorf, Köln: German Medical Science; 2004. Doc 04gmds371 (http://www.egms.de:80/en/meetings/gmds2004/04gmds371.shtml)

[4] Massar JP, Travers M, Elhai J, Shrager J. BioLingua: a programmable knowledge environment for biologists. Bioinformatics. 2004 Aug 12; [Epub ahead of print]

[5] van Bemmel JH, Musen MA (eds). Handbook of Medical Informatics. Springer, Houten/Diegem 1997

Address for correspondence

Dr. med. Udo Altmann, Institute of Medical Informatics, University of Gießen, Heinrich-Buff-Ring 44 D-35392 Gießen, Tel. ++49 641 99-41380, Fax. ++49 641 99-41359, e-Mail: Udo.Altmann@informatik.med.uni-giessen.de

Connecting Medical Informatics and Bio-Informatics
R. Engelbrecht et al. (Eds.)
IOS Press, 2005

761

Does HL7 Go towards an Architecture Standard?

Frank Oemig[a], Bernd Blobel[b]

[a] *Ringholm GmbH, Essen, Germany*
[b] *Fraunhofer Institute Integrated Circuits, Erlangen, Germany*

Abstract

Starting as a rather simple message standard to be used within hospitals, the scope of HL7 has been extended to covering all domains and institutions in health. The most important development of the HL7 standard set was its development towards a model-based message specification methodology and the further movement towards a unified development process: HL7 Version 3. The focus was design for interoperability, which is also the driving aspect of architectural standards such as OMG's CORBA or the CEN EN 13606 Electronic Health Record Communication. The paper gives an overview about the HL7 standard set, comparing it with the principles of advanced information systems architecture.

Keywords:
Health telematics; HL7, Model driven architecture; Electronic health record architecture

1. Introduction

The health systems of all industrial countries are faced with the challenge of improving quality and efficiency of health delivery. The way for meeting these requirements is the introduction of shared care, which is bound to extended communication and cooperation between all healthcare establishments and their information systems. Such communication and collaboration can be provided at different levels of interoperability as shown in the next section. If communication focuses on message exchange, collaboration depends on the applications' behaviour and functions. Therefore, the application architecture defines the level of interoperability and usability of applications. An architecture describes the system to be designed, its objectives, its elements, their inter-relationships and functionalities.

Documenting observations regarding data and procedures provides the basic part of health related information. Applications recording, storing and processing such information are Electronic Health Records (EHRs). That information can be used for many different purposes by many different departments and their applications. Following, the EHR is called the core application in healthcare settings.

The paper investigates HL7 from the aspect of advanced interoperability.

2. The HL7 Communication Standard

Following, the HL7 communication standard will be shortly discussed. For more information see [1-4].

2.1   General Principles

The advent of an increasing number of computer systems in combination with complex applications from different vendors raised the challenge to connect those systems which can be done at different levels of interoperability: At the lowest level, mechanical plugs including the voltage and the signals used have been harmonised. We are talking of technical interoperability. At the next level, the data exchanged have been standardised providing data level interoperability. Nevertheless, different terminologies might be used. Therefore, at the next level, terminology must be agreed on. For realising a common understanding, the semantic of terms must be harmonised providing semantic interoperability. At the highest level, concepts and context of information exchanged are harmonised including the service realised based on that information. We call this highest level service oriented interoperability. Furthermore, the design process of systems meeting that level of interoperability must be comprehensively defined and standardised.

HL7, an ANSI accredited standards development organisation with close liaison to ISO TC 215, specifies communication contents and exchange formats on the application layer. In the communication model of ISO for interconnection of open systems (Open System Interconnection, OSI), this layer is the seventh, which led to the name HL7. It is important that the communication solution is independent from the software used as well as the underlying hardware and the chosen network. Thus, the user has the freedom to realize a solution best suited to his needs.

The HL7 communication standard was developed especially for the health care environment and enables communication between meanwhile almost all institutions and fields of health care. With HL7, all important communication tasks of a hospital can be handled and the efficiency of the communication process is decidedly improved.

2.2   HL7 Version 3

HL7 Version 3 means much more than being a new version in the course of development of the standard. HL7 Version 3 follows a new paradigm. And this paradigm change was not a short step but a long term and contradictory process. This has been demonstrated not only by the frequent change of direction and the obviously endless series of versions of its basic elements. What is the new HL7 Version 3 paradigm's characteristic?

2.2.1   HL7 Version 3 Basics

The HL7 Version 3 communication standard is based on a new and comprehensive development methodology, which has been called the Version 3 Message Development Framework1 (MDF) covering the whole life cycle of the standard specification from development through adaptation and maintenance up to the implementation, use and testing of messages. For that purpose, first techniques of modern software engineering have been deployed within a standard development process such as object-oriented analysis and object-oriented design as well as formal modelling. Following, the development process of HL7 Version 3, its development methodology, available tools to specify HL7 Version 3 messages as well as further perspectives will be considered.

If HL7 Version 2.x strictly follows the message paradigm including ad hoc development and extensions, HL7 Version 3 implies the following different principles:

- Stepwise movement from message to architecture paradigm driving towards the HL7 Development Framework (HDF) and

---

1 Because HL7 is now moving from a communication standard based on the communication paradigm towards a comprehensive set of interoperability standards including architectural concepts, decision procedures, visual integration, implementation specifications, etc., this framework is currently extended to the HL7 Development Framework (HDF).

- Introduction of model-based specification of messages on the basis of a Reference Information Model (RIM).

2.2.2   HL7 RIM

The development of HL7 Version 3 has been performed in different phases characterised by important changes. In the first phase, the RIM has been a presentation of all the elements specified in the standard by using a partially object-oriented methodology. Items belonging together due to their properties, their use, etc. have been grouped into object classes and modelled as attributes of those classes. Additionally and step by step, Use Case Models and Sequence Diagrams have been introduced. Following the message paradigm (also called integration type "Interfacing"), only attributes have been specified but no operations. Because all instances specified in the standard have been defined as RIM object classes, the HL7 modelling approach was a one model approach. Problems bound to that approach became obvious in extensions performed, frequently leading to a re-arrangement of attributes or even classes. Thus, the model was hardly maintainable and extendable. As a consequence, in the second phase the RIM has been changed towards a stepwise abstraction of the RIM reducing it to only a few generic core classes and a movement towards a service paradigm by introducing the Unified Service Action Model (USAM).

The resulting RIM describes six core classes for objects of the health domain as well as the associations between those classes and their specialisations:

Entities, i.e. the physical information objects or better the actors of the domain (e.g. organisation, living subject, materials, location);

Roles, played by those entities and therefore assigning them the competence to perform specific actions (e.g. patient, provider, employee, specimen, practitioner);

Participations of role playing entities in specific acts (e.g. performer, author, subject, destination, witness);

Acts (e.g. observation, procedure, supply, medication);

Role Relationships to manage interactions between entities in their corresponding roles;

Act Relationships chaining different acts.

The core classes contain some basic attributes such as Type_CD (Class_CD), Concept_Descriptor, Time, Mood (determiner), Status, ID. It is obvious that the core classes for Roles and Participations are specialisations of the corresponding entities, whereby Roles represent competence-related specialisations and Participations represent action-related specialisations.

2.2.3   Definition of Domain-Specific Messages

First, the scenario considered for a specific communication or co-operation must be highlighted. This is performed by the graphical representation of scenarios using UML Use Case Diagrams. Additionally, the scenario may be described verbally, which is called the HL7 Storyboard. For describing the outcome of actions related to role-specific specialisations, state diagrams or state transition diagrams are used. After reaching clarifications on the general issues of messages, we may proceed to specify specific messages. Starting point is always the HL7 RIM.

2.2.4   Domain-Specific Models

For generating a message, the information (attributes) about the objects (classes) involved must be established, connected in a proper way, and instantiated. The link between RIM classes and the selection or completion of attributes of the corresponding classes depends on legal, organisational, functional, and technological conditions in the related communicating application domains, i.e., of their policies, their concepts, rules, and the knowledge.

For developing domain-specific messages therefore, the classes needed according to the information requirements must be selected and their attributes have to be updated, i.e., non-required attributes must be cancelled and missing attributes must be added: For defining a doctor's order message related to a specific patient, the relation between an entity person playing the role of a physician (instantiated as „Dr. Smith") participating as „order/requester" of an act „Laboratory result" (instantiated as "Blood Test") and an entity person playing the role of a patient (instantiated as „Mr. Miller") with the participation observant must be designed. For that reason, we have to clone the classes from the RIM and update the attributes properly (DMIM).

2.2.5   Reusable Message Fragments - the CMETs

This short introduction clearly shows the complexity of the method. Furthermore, such messages across domains are hardly to standardise. In that context, certain classes, their specialisations and associations are described as domain-specific information model. If those models of characteristic objects und their relations can be standardised, a set of Common Message Element Types (CMETs) can be established which are re-used in different domains.

CMETs are multi-domain information models based on RIM core classes and appropriate associations. Thus, HL7 is moving from one-model approach to a multi-model approach. The advantage of such a procedure is obvious:

Domain-specific requirements and conditions can be consistently described by the RIM using object-oriented and UML-based methods. The resulting architectural components are part of the standard. They can easily be updated or replaced (by local definitions) without any implications on the usability of the other components. Thereby, an open, scalable, maintainable, component-oriented specification can be provided.

The standard's development can happen step by step extendable to any level of complexity. CMETs represent concepts and knowledge, so enabling interoperability at the level of concepts and knowledge.

Use cases (scenarios) or their verbal variant – the story board are the starting point for message development in HL7 version 3. The harmonisation between globally active developers and implementers at the one hand and the continuous extension regarding the involved domains (chapters) at the other hand is realised via a unique reference model of health care – the HL7 Reference Information Model (RIM). Besides that generic RIM as well as its domain-specific specialisation as the Domain Message Information Model (DMIM), the Refined Message Information Model (RMIM) can be derived. Dynamic and procedural aspects are described using sequence diagrams, state diagrams, activity diagrams, etc.

2.2.6   Hierarchical Message Description (HMD)

Starting from models described, the resulting message related to a defined trigger event must be specified. For that purpose, the relation between the different vocabularies, „graphical description of components", „verbal description of components", and presentation using "XML exchange format" must be provided. One opportunity for doing that has been given by the XML Standard Set with its XML Metadata Interchange (XMI) specification as described, e.g., in [5]. Another way is the use of specific tools as practised in HL7. Please mention that not only a UML-like graphical modelling is used by the HL7 community, but also special tools such as Rose Tree© and Microsoft's Visio© (stencils) for message design via Refined Message Information Models (RMIMs) (e.g. for correct, RIM-adequate modelling of the domain models or CMETs). RMIMs are results of the walk through the graph (RIM) with its clones and refinements related to classes and attributes. The transformation of a Rational Rose© UML information model as well as the transformation of Visio© Templates by a graphical walk through into a Hierarchical Message Description (HMD) is provided using Woody Beeler's Rose Tree© tools.

The information managed concerns classes, subclasses (Specialisations), their attributes and data types, associations as well as the latter's cardinalities (multiplicities), which lead to nested message structures and their required or optional components. The HMD of the related message structure is finally transferred into an equivalent XML schema definition using a self-developed schema generator.

2.2.7   Specialisation vs. Standardisation

HL7's version 3 strategy of model-based message definition reduces optionality by modelling and defining every message according to its specific requirements and conditions. Thus, all specified components are required and are being served, resulting in a set of similar but specific messages. Therefore, the interoperability striven for may be taken into question. The way out of this dilemma should be provided by the following principles:

• Reference to a globally acknowledged Reference Information Model
• Specification of an accepted and binding vocabulary for all reference components as well as all domain concepts (knowledge concepts) (definition in the framework of RIM, all DMIMs, RMIMs etc.)
• Development of Application Roles for characterising the participation in message interchange
• Definition of requirements profiles, which lead to Conformance Statements.

2.2.8   Application Roles

Requirements and conditions of interoperating applications related to their data and functionality have to be clearly defined in order to assure communication between them. This includes besides mandatory data also the specification of messages and trigger events needed. That specification of functional and data-related requirements and conditions of applications is also called Application Roles.

2.2.9   Conformance Statements

For providing interoperability in a very complex and divergent world, interesting solutions have been developed. Mostly known is DICOM (Digital Imaging and Communication in Medicine, [7]), which is the globally established image communication standard. Contrary to HL7, DICOM realises interoperability not only at the level of message exchange independent of the level of semantic interpretation, but also at the level of service-oriented interoperability. That linking of communicated data and functions has been defined as Service Object Pairs (SOP) for different modalities within a client-server environment. By that way, an optimal coding (interpretation of the message at the originator side is the same as that at the receiver side) has been guaranteed. The needed equivalence of SOPs, client and server properties, protocols, presentation instructions, etc, is defined by the Conformance Statements. Two communicating applications have to meet the corresponding mutual Conformance Statements.

HL7 Version 3 is using an analogue way of defining Conformance Statements. References to a global RIM and a binding vocabulary, messages between two interoperable applications have to follow the corresponding Application Roles as sender and receiver including the assigned responsibilities.

In that context, the current specification of Clinical Templates as well as the work on CDA Level 2 are especially important.

2.2.10   Contents and Specifications of the HL7 Standard

For assuring interoperability between applications based on the HL7 Version 3 Standard, all messages must be based on the HL7 RIM, on agreed data types as well as on a binding vocabulary. At the domain-specific level, CMETs, RMIMs, the temporal and procedural conditions expressed by Interaction Diagrams or State Diagrams as well as Application Roles, from which trigger events and interactions result, must be standardised.

Because of their different character, standard components are managed in different ways. The HL7 Version 3 methodology, the HL7 RIM as well as the HL7 vocabulary are reference materials of HL7 Version 3 and not ballot issue. Information about HL7 data types, Implementable Technology Specifications (ITS) as well as the chapters containing domain-related specifications are normative part of the HL7 Version 3 Standard. They need the affirmation of HL7 members.

The Version 3 Publication is an automated process provided on the basis of the artefacts from HL7 Technical Committees (TCs) and Special Interest Groups (SIGs) collected in HL7 databases (repositories). For assuring the consistency of the standard, all specifications are verified with existing specification stored in such a repository. After successful verification, the new specification can be added to the repository.

3. Conclusions

HL7 Version 3 evolved towards a standard set developed according to the clearly defined process, the HDF. All components and functions of architectural standards have been meanwhile established such as reference models and terminologies (RIM, vocabulary), domain-specific references (DMIM), building blocks (CMETs), implementation rules (application roles, ITS) as well as conformance statements for providing practical semantic interoperability. All architectural views needed are meanwhile defined in HL7 Version 3 starting from scenarios up to maintenance and education, including the tools for automatically or at least semi-automatically to define the pieces and aggregate them to running systems [4].

4. References

[1]   Health Level Seven, Inc.: http://www.hl7.org
[2]   Heitmann KU, Blobel B, Dudeck J: *HL7 Communication standard in medicine. Short introduction and information.* Köln: Verlag Alexander Mönch, 1999. (completely revised and extended edition)
[3]   Hinchley A: *Understanding Version 3 – A primer on the HL7 Version 3 Communication Standard.* Köln: Verlag Alexander Mönch, 2003
[4]   Blobel B: *Analysis, Design and Implementation of Secure and Interoperable Distributed Health Information Systems.* Series Studies in Health Technology and Informatics, Amsterdam: Vol. 89. IOS Press, 2002
[5]   Jeckle M: Entwurf von XML Sprachen, *Java Spectrum* 6/2000, 56-60
[6]   Blobel B: Application of the Component Paradigm for Analysis and Design of Advanced Health System Architectures. *International Journal of Medical Informatics* 60 (3) (2000) 281-301
[7]   DICOM: "Digital Imaging and Communication in Medicine", 2003, http://www.rsna.org

Address for correspondence

Frank Oemig, Ringholm GmbH Integration Consulting, Amselstr.12, D-45472 Mülheim, Germany
E-mail: Frank.Oemig@ringholm.de, URL: http://www.ringholm.de

Connecting Medical Informatics and Bio-Informatics
R. Engelbrecht et al. (Eds.)
IOS Press, 2005

Integrating the Modelling of EN 1828 and Galen CCAM Ontologies with Protégé: towards a Knowledge Acquisition Tool for Surgical Procedures

J M Rodrigues[a], B Trombert Paviot[a], C Martin[a], P Vercherin[a]

[a] Dpt de Santé Publique et d'Information Médicale, Université de Saint Etienne, France

Abstract

The presentation assess the usability of the ontology platform protégé integrated with the terminology reasoning tool RACER to represent different terminology systems as the CEN European standard EN 1828 which is a categorical structure and the extensive French coding system CCAM supported by a GALEN representation. We present the 2 systems and some results showing the easiness to test the consistence of the ontology or of instances of terminology systems.

This type of software tool which is accessible as open source could support a convergent "reference terminology representation" approach. Based on a formal representation development and allowing diversity in linguistic expressiveness of end users this approach can associate shared knowledge acquisition in the public domain and competing systems, software developers and researchers.

Keywords:
Ontology; Formal representation; Software; Standards; Coding system; Healthcare; Surgical procedures;

1. Introduction

The semantic interoperability is becoming the top challenge to the implementation of the electronic healthcare record. There are a lot of divergent initiatives addressing the different aspects of interoperability: information models (HL7 Reference Information Model RIM, CEN Continuity of care, et.), architectures (HL7 Common Document Architecture CDA, CEN EHRcom, et.), context (Templates or Archetypes, et.) and the forest of "pragmatic" or "reference" clinical terminologies for different national languages.

Since 15 years advanced information technologies have enable more complex approaches using artificial intelligence tools. There are named terminologies servers architecture where data ware house are connected to knowledge bases used to browse and extract increasing volume data bases shared by increasing numbers of users for an increasing number of goals [1]. These knowledge bases are representing multiple concepts hierarchies and semantic links subsuming the logical meaning of their networking. These knowledge representations are named ontology [2] which is a term coming from metaphysics but are in fact formal logic using mathematical expressions. These representations need specific software tools and natural language processing of knowledge embedded in the ambiguous lexicons from different national languages [3].

Amongst the pragmatic output of this approach can be quoted several achievements: 2 full terminology standards have been produced in Europe (CEN/TC251) [4] and internationally (ISO/TC215) [5] and 5 more are in the final approval process .On the other hand a EU and France funded consortium has finalised the formal representation of a new coding system for surgical procedures named CCAM [6]. This formal representation is available as open source at [7]. Other consortiums in UK have produced representations for drugs [8] and in the US for Snomed CT [9].

To ease manual developments and implementations of such representation the University of Manchester and Stanford University have developed an ontology editor named Protégé [10] associated with a terminology reasoning tool named RACER [11].

We propose here the representation of the European standard EN 1828 [4] and Galen CCAM [6] with the Protégé editor. We show their communality and differences and their specific roles to discuss how these tools can help to integrate and extend the third generation terminologies of surgical procedures.

2. Material

2.1 EN 1828 Categorial structure for classifications and coding systems for surgical procedures

The standardisation in health informatics started in 1990, in Europe with CEN (Comité Européen de Normalisation) and internationally in 1998 with ISO (International Standard Organisation). The process supporting the electronic health record of the patients (EHR) was encompassing messages, architecture, security, and a definition of the minimum requirements a terminology (controlled vocabularies, nomenclatures, coding systems and classifications) must comply with to support interoperability between different informatics systems.

MOSE [12] presents a categorial structure (or reference terminology model) as "a minimal set of domain constraints for representing concepts systems in a precise domain to achieve a precise goal". It is a semantic representation.

Four information types are needed:
   a) The list of semantic categories,
   b) The goal of the categorial structure,
   c) The list of relevant associated semantic links,
   d) The minimum combinatorial rules allowing the generation and validation of well formed concepts systems.

This must allow comparison, reuse of so costly to produce information and to prevent the development of data "cemeteries".

This methodology has been applied by CEN for the coding systems and classifications of surgical procedures [4] and by ISO for nursing diagnostics and procedures [5]. The standardisation processes are on going for clinical laboratories, medical devices, medicinal products and continuity of care.

2.2 Galen CCAM

A very short definition of ontology for terminology as proposed in [2] « explicit representation of a concept system » can be widely accepted. There is less agreement with a more specific definition.

First the level must be distinguished between meta-ontology not far from the metaphysics studying the different entities of the universe, top-ontology, central or reference ontology, specific knowledge and... until the very diverse and ambiguous linguistic expressions for sub domains and for different goals [13].

The main issue is that the representation must be rigorous using software and languages able to express constraining mathematical statements and consistent reasoning across the different domains which often overlap in medical informatics.

The new French coding system for surgical procedures CCAM has been developed using a dual methodology: the traditional domain expert consensus and the formal representation GALEN [12].

The GALEN formal representation [7] is made of around 52000 entities, with 800 included links.

To represent the 7478 CCAM surgical procedures in the GRAIL (Galen Representation and Integration Language) formal language, 2400 concepts descriptors and 59 semantic links were used. Amongst these 2400 descriptors, 1297 are from the semantic category Anatomy, 271 from Pathology, 231 from Device, 186 from Deed. Amongst the 59 semantic links 27 are for the 4 previous categories and 7 only for Pathology.

3. Method

We applied Protégé integrated to the terminology reasoning tool RACER on one hand to the European standard EN 1828 [4] and on the other hand to the GALEN ontology representing the French CCAM [6]. This representation is a subset of the whole GALEN representation [7].

The goals are:

- To test the flexibility and easiness of using Protégé,
- To validate the conformity of a classification or coding system to the standard EN 1828,
- To compare the standard EN 1828 and the GALEN CCAM representation for knowledge and consistence.

4. Results

4.1 EN 1828

Tab 1 and Tab 2 show the hierarchies of the semantic categories and their associated semantic links.

Tab 1 EN1828 Semantic categories   *Tab 2 EN 1828 Semantic links*

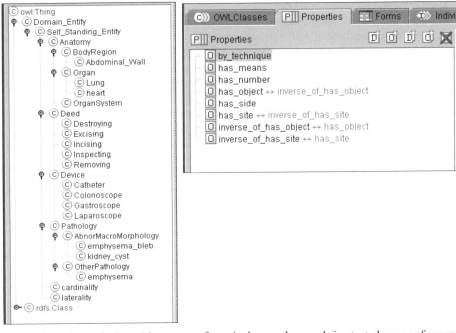

Tab 3 show that only 3 to 6 instances of surgical procedures rubrics tested are conformant with the standard . The 3 red circled one are considered non consistent by RACER and this output conformity test is aligned with the rule.

Tab 3 EN 1828 Conformity test

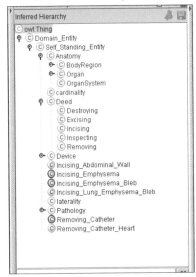

4.2 Galen CCAM

The Diagram 1 (EN 1828) and 2 (Galen CCAM) show that the second representation has more semantic categories namely in anatomy than the first one and is considered to be consistent with the EN1828 by RACER. The first one has the same 3 non consistent red circled instances.

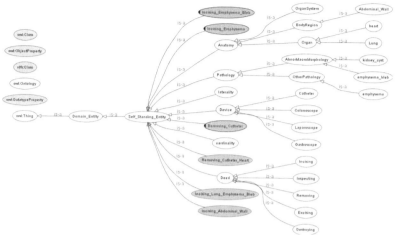

Diagram 1 EN1828

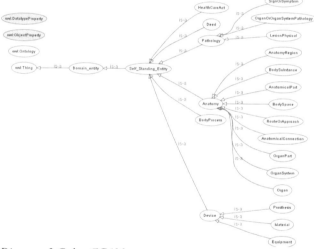

Diagram 2 Galen CCAM

5. Conclusion

5.1 The Protégé platform is assessed as being flexible for a reduced formal representation of the European standard EN 1828 and for more complex ones like the Galen CCAM. The easiness of use is real with the support of information available at the open source Stanford web site [15].

5.2 The Protégé RACER platform allows to test the conformity of classifications and coding systems to the standard EN 1828.

5.3 It is possible to compare the different representations and to test their cross consistence.

Protégé can be considered as a support tool for convergence of 3rd generation terminology systems and for quality insurance.

5.4   The availability of tools and knowledge as open sources like Galen and Protégé is a good argument in favour of the setting of an open international network developing a terminology formal representation approach to support extensive medical knowledge acquisition.

Such an organisation could benefit to national and international coding centres, developers and researchers on the base of their participation to the knowledge acquisition.

6. Acknowledgements

We wish to thank Alan Rector and Jeremy Rogers from the University of Manchester which trained us in Protégé after having developed the Galen formal representation for the French CCAM, the Stanford team for their kindness and the open quality of their website. Special thanks to our partners in the GALEN program and namely the University of Nijmeguen and the University of Geneva.

7. References

[1]   Rector AL, Johnson PD, Tu S, Wroe C, Rogers J. Interface of inference models with concept and medical record models. In: Quaglini S, Barahona P, Andreassen S, editors. Artificial Intelligence in Medicine Europe (AIME); 2001; Cascais, Portugal: Springer Verlag; 2001. p. 314-323.

[2]   Gruber T. A translation approach to potable ontology specifications. Knowledge Acquisition 1993; 5(2):199-220.

[3]   Smith B, Ceusters W. Towards industrial strength philosophy :how analytical ontology can help medical informatics. Interdisciplinary Science Reviews 2003; 28:106-11.

[4]   CEN AFNOR EN NF 1828:2002. Health informatics – Categorial Structure for classifications and coding systems of surgical procedures .

[5]   EN ISO 18104 2003. Integration of a Reference Terminology Model for Nursing.

[6]   Trombert-Paviot B, Rodrigues J-M, Rogers J, Baud R, van der Haring E, Rassinoux A-M, Abrial V, Clavel L, Idir H. GALEN: a third-generation terminology tool to support a multipurpose national coding system for surgical procedures. International Journal of Medical Informatics 2000; 58–9: 71–85.

[7]   http://www.opengalen.org/

[8]   Solomon W, Wroe C, Rogers JE, Rector A. A reference terminology for drugs. Journal of the American Medical Informatics Association 1999((Fall Symposium Special Issue)):152-155.

[9]   Dolin RH, Huff SM, Rocha RA, Spackman KA, Campbell KE. Evaluation of a « lexically assign logically refine »strategy for semi-automated integration of overlapping terminologies.J Am Med Informatics Assoc 1998 ;5 :203-213

[10]   Noy NF , Fergerson RW , Musen MA   . The knowledge model of Protege-2000: Combining interoperability and flexibility. 2th International Conference on Knowledge Engineering and Knowledge Management (EKAW'2000), Juan-les-Pins, France. 2000.

[11]   Haarslev V, Möller R. Description of the RACER system and its applications. Proceedings of the International Workshop on Description Logics 2001;1.-3 ,132-41.Stanford USA.

[12]   CEN/TC251/prEN 12264:2004 Health informatics - Categorial structures of concepts systems .

[13]   Rector AL, Zanstra PE, Solomon WD, Rogers JE, Baud R, Ceusters W, et al. Reconciling Users' Needs and FormalRequirements: Issues in developing a Re-Usable Ontology   for Medicine. IEEE Transactions on Information Technology in BioMedicine 1999;2(4):229-242.

[14]   Trombert-Paviot B, Rodrigues J-M, Rogers J, Baud R, Martin C . Les standards en terminologie de santé peuvent ils faciliter le développent et l'harmonisation des système de codage ? Un exemple franco-européen . Proceedings des Journées Francophones d'Informatique Médicale 2002 Québec Canada .

[15]   http://www.stanford.edu

Address for correspondence

JM Rodrigues, CHU de St Etienne SSPIM, Hôpital St Jean Bonnefonds, 42 650 St Jean Bonnefonds, France. rodrigues@univ-st-etienne.fr

Connecting Medical Informatics and Bio-Informatics
R. Engelbrecht et al. (Eds.)
IOS Press, 2005

773

Semantic Clarification of the Representation of Procedures and Diseases in SNOMED® CT

Stefan Schulz[a], Udo Hahn[b], Jeremy Rogers[c]

[a] *Department of Medical Informatics, Freiburg University, Germany*
[b] *Language And Information Engineering Lab, Jena University, Germany*
[c] *School of Computer Science, Manchester University, United Kingdom*

Abstract

SNOMED® CT is emerging as a reference terminology for the entire health care process. It claims to be founded on logic-based modeling principles. In this work we analyze a special encoding scheme for SNOMED disease and procedure entities, the so-called relationship groups which had been devised in order to avoid ambiguities in entity definitions. We show that these artifacts may represent hidden mereological relations. We also report discrepancies encountered between the defined semantics of many SNOMED® CT entity terms and their intuitive meaning, and inconsistencies detected between the definition of some complex composed entities and the definition of their top-level parents. As a result we formulate recommendations for improvements of SNOMED® CT.

Keywords:
SNOMED, Knowledge Representation, Logic

1. Introduction

SNOMED® Clinical Terms (SNOMED® CT) is a huge clinical terminology constructed by merging, expanding, and restructuring the previous SNOMED version RT and the Clinical Terms Version 3 (former Read Codes). SNOMED® CT contains around 364,000 concepts, 984,000 terms and 1.45 million defined relationships between concepts[1]. In the coming years it will be deployed for routine usage in several countries (U.S., U.K., Denmark), and it is intensively being analyzed by medical terminologists and decision makers in many other countries.

SNOMED® CT is a concept-oriented controlled vocabulary which has been designed according to previously suggested criteria for computer-based medical terminologies [1]. SNOMED® CT is described as a clinical reference terminology, i.e. "a set of concepts and relationships that provides a common reference point for comparison and aggregation of data about the entire health care process" [2]. SNOMED® CT concepts belong to multiple is-a hierarchies and are related with one another by various semantic relationships such as *"is-a"*, *"has-associated topography"*, *"has-action"*, *"has-associated morphology"*. Interestingly, SNOMED® CT explicitly encodes *"part-of"* relationships only between

---

[1] http://www.snomed.org

anatomic entities [3]. There is no relation with which to describe partonomy between diseases or procedure entities.

2. Relationship groups[2] in SNOMED®

SNOMED® NT and CT follow a formal semantics based on KRSS, an early description logic [4], and have used a terminological classifier for terminology development [5,6]. In the UMLS distribution, however, the relational format of the MRREL table requires SNOMED® CT content to be compressed into the common OAV (object – attribute – value triplets) format. For a logic-based model such a representation is ambiguous because it (i) obscures which attribute-value pairs are sufficient for the entity3 definitions, (ii) lacks role quantifications, and (iii) does not indicate whether sets of related attribute-value pairs should be interpreted as disjunction, conjunction or optional. Table 1 gives an example:

Table 1. Example of OAV (object –attribute-value) format of SNOMED® CT entities such as distributed via the UMLS Metathesaurus

SNOMED® Concept 1	SNOMED® Relationship	SNOMED® Concept 2
Renal glomerular disease	*has_finding_site*	*Kidney*
Renal glomerular disease	*has_onset*	*Gradual onset*
Renal glomerular disease	*has_onset*	*Sudden onset*

Since 2004, the UMLS Rich Release Format (RRF) has encoded further information in the MRSAT table, including which entities are defined or primitive, which OAV triplets are optional (qualifiers) and which are restrictions, and which relationship group each belongs to.

The purpose of relationship groups such as introduced by SNOMED® is best explained by an example: *Removal of foreign body from the stomach by incision* involves *Stomach structure* and *Digestive structure* as values of the attribute *has_procedure_site*, and both *Incision* and *Removal* as values of the attribute *has_method*. However, such a simplistic representation is ambiguous: it could also be interpreted as *Removal of the stomach and incision of a foreign body*. Relationship groups declare associations between sets of OAV triplets (see Table 2). Although each group has an integer value, this does not imply any temporal or other ordering between groups.

The *SNOMED® CT Technical Implementation and Technical Reference* makes the following statement about relationship groups:

"Relationships, for a concept that are logically associated with each other.
The Relationship group field in the Relationships Table is used to group these
rows together for a concept".

As relationship groups occur in about 17,000 disease entities and 13,000 procedure entities, according to [5], this phenomenon constitutes a major issue in SNOMED® CT. In [5], Spackman *et al.* propose a description logics representation for relationship groups, in which they are expressed by an anonymous relation, named *rg*. From an ontological point of view, the proposed solution is, however, rather obscure. In the following we therefore explore the possible semantics of SNOMED® CT relationship groups. We show that some basic assumptions of SNOMED® CT are ontologically problematic, and we propose a

---

[2] also called „role groups" [5]
[3] Many ontological assumptions of SNOMED CT are still unclear. E.g., different things like „Foot", „Absent Foot", „Football (qualifier value)", „Europe", „Love",„mmol", „Yin excess", „Kiel Classification", are „concepts" in SNOMED® CT. Hence we use – for the sake of neutrality – the term „entity" for what SNOMED names „concept".

solution for clarification which will be mostly compatible with the current SNOMED® CT architecture.

Table 2. Entries in the SNOMED® CT core relationships table for the entity "64550003: Removal of foreign body from the stomach by incision", using three relationship groups

SNOMED® Concept 1	SNOMED® Relationship	SNOMED® Concept 2	RG
Removal of Foreign Body from the Stomach by Incision	*Access*	*Open Approach*	*0*
	Is A	*Removal of foreign body from digestive system*	*0*
	Is A	*Removal of foreign body from stomach*	*0*
	Is A	*Incision of stomach*	*0*
	Method	*Removal - action*	*1*
	Direct Morphology	*Foreign body*	*1*
	Procedure site-Indirect	*Digestive structure*	*1*
	Method	*Incision - action*	*2*
	Procedure site	*Stomach Structure*	*2*

3. Ontological Analysis of Relationship Groups

We refer to the same parsimonious variant of description logics as used by [5]. Entity names are characterized by initial capital letters. They can be joined by the AND operator. As an example, the expression *AcuteDigestiveSystemDisorder AND AcuteInflammatoryDisease* denotes inflammatory diseases of the digestive system, i.e. the intersection of entities subsumed by AcuteDigestiveSystemDisorder with all those subsumed by the entity AcuteInflammatoryDisease (or the set of all entities subsumed by both). Relation symbols begin with lower case, e.g. *hasAssociatedMorphology*. Roles are formed by a quantifier (here only the existential quantifier, $\exists$, is used), a relation symbol, followed by a dot and an entity symbol. For example,

$\exists hasAssociatedMorphology.Inflammation$ denotes the entity whose instantiation is the set of all individuals related to an instance of *Inflammation* by the relation *hasAssociatedMorphology*. We can therefore rewrite the role group 1 and 2 entries in Table 2:

$$RemovalOfForeignBodyFromTheStomachByIncision \text{ IMPLIES}$$
$$\exists rg.(\exists hasProcedureSite.StomachStructure \text{ AND}$$
$$\exists hasMethod.IncisionAction) \qquad \text{ AND}$$
$$\exists rg.(\exists hasProcedureSite.DigestiveStructure \text{ AND}$$
$$\exists hasDirectMorphology.ForeignBody \text{ AND}$$
$$\exists hasMethod.RemovalAction)$$
(1)

Let us now look at the parent entities, *RemovalOfForeignBodyFromDigestiveSystem* and *IncisionOfStomach* [4]. The first is an *is-a* descendent of *RemovalProcedure*, and the latter an *is-a* descendent of *IncisionProcedure*. Consequently, all instances of the entity *RemovalOfForeignBodyFromTheStomachByIncision* are instances of both *IncisionProcedure* and *RemovalProcedure* and as a result must therefore inherit the properties of both *Incision* and *Removal*. This is hardly imaginable: In this case, objects

---

[4] As contained in the SNOMED® CT sources from the UMLS, or visualized by the SNOMED® CT Browser at http://snomed.vetmed.vt.edu/sct/menu.cfm

would be equally incised and removed. In a strict upper level ontology *Incision* and *Removal* are expected to be mutually exclusive. In reality, the surgeon first performs the incision and then the removal: *Incision* and *Removal* are two separate sub-procedures and so are properly not **parents** but **parts**[5] of the entity *RemovalOfForeignBodyFromTheStomachByIncision*.

Fig. 1 gives a graphic outline of this procedure which begins with the incision of the wall of the stomach, followed by the removal action and the closure of the wound (the latter is not mentioned in the procedure definition). These time-dependent sub-procedures stand to the main procedure in a *part-of* relationship. This is concordant with the commonly accepted mereological (*part-whole*) view of actions and processes, which are, according to [8] characterized by time-dependent parts. Having this in mind it seems straightforward to re-interpret the relationship group attribute *rg* in (1) as the mereological primitive *has-part*:

$$
\begin{aligned}
&RemovalOfForeignBodyFromTheStomachByIncision\ IMPLIES\\
&\quad \exists\, has\text{-}part.(\exists\ hasProcedureSite.StomachStructure\ AND\\
&\quad\quad \exists\, hasMethod.IncisionAction) \qquad\qquad AND\\
&\quad \exists\, has\text{-}part.(\exists\ hasProcedureSite.\ DigestiveStructure\ AND\\
&\quad\quad \exists\, hasDirectMorphology.ForeignBody\ AND\\
&\quad\quad \exists\, hasMethod.RemovalAction) \qquad\qquad (2)
\end{aligned}
$$

Similarly, for the parent entities we obtain:

$$
\begin{aligned}
&IncisionOfStomach\ IMPLIES\\
&\quad \exists\, has\text{-}part.(\exists\ hasProcedureSite.StomachStructure\ AND\\
&\quad\quad \exists\, hasMethod.IncisionAction) \qquad\qquad (3)
\end{aligned}
$$

$$
\begin{aligned}
&RemovalOfForeignBodyFromDigestiveSystem\ IMPLIES\\
&\quad \exists\, has\text{-}part.(\exists\ hasProcedureSite.\ DigestiveStructure\ AND\\
&\quad\quad \exists\, hasDirectMorphology.ForeignBody\ AND\\
&\quad\quad \exists\, hasMethod.RemovalAction) \qquad\qquad (4)
\end{aligned}
$$

Looking up the SNOMED® CT hierarchy, we obtain exactly these definitions after replacing *rg* by *has-part*. At a first glance this seems strange, since the main rationale for relationship groups, *viz.* the avoidance of ambiguities, makes no sense, here. Entity names such as *Incision of Stomach*, suggest definitions without the *has-part* role:

$$
\begin{aligned}
&IncisingAStomach\ IMPLIES\ \exists\ hasProcedureSite.StomachStructure\ AND\\
&\quad \exists\, hasMethod.IncisionAction \qquad\qquad (5)
\end{aligned}
$$

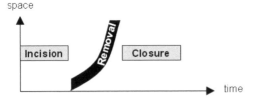

Fig. 1. Graphical Representation of the Process Removal of Foreign Body from the Stomach by Incision"

---

[5] Entity *A* has *B* as part is equivalent to the DL expression *A IMPLIES ∃has-part.B*,

The semantic difference is the following: Whereas *IncisingAStomach* denotes the atomic procedure of performing an incision onto a stomach, SNOMED's *IncisionOfStomach* subsumes any complex procedure during which an incision of stomach is being performed. Analogously, *RemovalOfForeignBodyFromDigestiveSystem* subsumes any complex procedure during which a foreign body is extracted from the digestive system.

Looking still higher up the SNOMED® CT hierarchy, *IncisionOfStomach* is a child entity of *IncisionProcedure, which is* itself related to an *Incision action* by the relation *has_method*:

$$IncisionProcedure\ IMPLIES\ \exists\ rg.(\exists\ hasMethod.IncisionAction)$$
$$(6)$$

As indicated above, the semantics of *rg* may be improved to derive:

$$IncisionProcedure\ IMPLIES\ \exists\ has\text{-}part.(\exists\ hasMethod.IncisionAction)$$
$$(7)$$

An *IncisionProcedure* is, therefore, any procedure which has a part characterized by the enactment of an *Incision*. Only this broader definition justifies *IncisionProcedure* being the ancestor of nearly one thousand entities: so many distinct flavours of incision do not exist, but more than one thousand surgical procedures have an incision as part of their description. We have taken our example from the "procedure" branch of SNOMED® CT. We could have used, as well, numerous examples from the "disease / disorders" branch, e.g. *Acute Perforated Appendicitis*, which is subsumed by both *Inflammation* and *Perforation* (in the above sense).

However, there may be situations in SNOMED where the translation of *rg* as *has-part* would not be correct. For example, within the current SNOMED content, it is possible to construct the post-coordinated composition of an *urgent swab of the left eye*, by adding the urgent and left qualifiers as appropriate. The flattened (not role grouped) representation that would result would be:

Entity 1	Relationship	Entity2
	isA	*Specimen from Conjunctiva*
	specimenSourceTopography	*Conjunctival Structure*
Urgent Swab of the Left Eye	*specimenProcedure*	*Taking of Swab*
	priority	*Urgent*
	laterality	*Left*

Here it would then be impossible to tell whether the attribute *Left* should be applied to the swab or the eye. So, we might want to formalize:

UrgentSwabOfLeftEye IMPLIES
Specimen from Conjunctiva AND
$\exists rg.(\exists specimenSourceTopography.ConjunctivalStructure\ AND$
$\quad \exists Laterality.Left)\ AND$
$\exists rg.(\exists specimenProcedure.TakingOffSwab\ AND\ \exists.Priority.Urgent)$
(8)

4. Conclusion

Our analysis of relationship groups in SNOMED® CT revealed weaknesses which motivated us to make some recommendations which would improve SNOMED® CT in clarity and which would remove inconsistencies from the terminology. These suggestions would encompass only minor modifications of the SNOMED® CT architecture:

- Rename the relationship group attribute *rg* by *has-part* or *has-subprocess* where it appears between a complex process and its subprocesses (i.e. especially in the disease and procedure chapters of SNOMED® CT).

- Make a clearer distinction between atomic entities (such as *IncisionAction*) and those entities which have atomic entities as parts (such as *IncisionProcess*). The present entity names are misleading.

Finally, one has to take into account, there are scenarios in which the use of relationship groups seem adequate, without, however, corresponding to a mereological relation. A more detailed ontological inquiry of these cases is still due.

5. Acknowledgments

This work was supported by the *EU Network of Excellence Semantic Interoperability and Data Mining in Biomedicine* (NoE 507505), cf. http://www.semanticmining.org. We also thank Ulrike Sattler (Manchester, UK) and Kent Spackman (Portland, OR, U.S.), for their helpful discussions.

6. References

[1]   Cimino JJ. Desiderata for controlled medical vocabularies in the twenty-first century. *Methods of Information in Medicine*, 1998: 37(4/5):394-403.

[2]   Spackman KA, Campbell K, and Cote RA. SNOMED RT: A reference terminology for health care. In Daniel R. Masys, editor, *AMIA'97 - Proceedings of the 1997 AMIA Annual Fall Symposium*, pp. 640-644. Philadelphia, PA: Hanley & Belfus, 1997.

[3]   Spackman KA and Reynoso G. Examining SNOMED from the perspective of formal ontological principles: Some preliminary analysis and observations. In Hahn U, Schulz S, and Cornet S, editors, *KR-MED 2004 - Proceedings of the 1st International Workshop on Formal Biomedical Knowledge Representation, Collocated with the 9th International Conference on the Principles of Knowledge Representation and Reasoning (KR 2004)*, pp. 81-87. Whistler, B.C., Canada, June 1, 2004. Bethesda, MD: American Medical Informatics Association (AMIA), 2004. Published via http://CEUR-WS.org/Vol-102/.

[4]   Baader F, Calvanese D, McGuinness D, Nardi D, Patel-Schneider P. *The Description Logic Handbook. Theory, Implementation and Applications.* Cambridge, U.K. Cambridge University Press.

[5]   Spackman KA, Dionne R, Mays E, and Weis J. Role grouping as an extension to the description logic of ONTYLOG, motivated by entity modeling in SNOMED. In Kohane IS, editor, *AMIA 2002 - Proceedings of the Annual Symposium of the American Medical Informatics Association,* pp. 712-716. Philadelphia, PA: Hanley & Belfus, 2002.

[6]   Spackman KA and Campbell KE. Compositional entity representation using SNOMED: Towards further convergence of clinical terminologies. In Chute CG, editor, *AMIA'98 - Proceedings of the 1998 AMIA Annual Fall Symposium*, pp. 740-744. Philadelphia, PA: Hanley & Belfus, 1998.

[7]   Schulz S and Hahn U. Medical knowledge reengineering: Converting major portions of the UMLS into a terminological knowledge base. *International Journal of Medical Informatics* 2001: 64(2/3):207-221.

[8]   Simons P. *Parts: A Study in Ontology.* Oxford: Clarendon Press, 1987.

Address for correspondence

PD Dr. med. Stefan Schulz, Abteilung Medizinische Informatik, Universtätsklinikum Freiburg Stefan-Meier-Str. 26, D-79106 Freiburg (Germany), stschulz@uni-freiburg.de, http://www.imbi.uni-freiburg.de/medinf/~schulz.htm

Connecting Medical Informatics and Bio-Informatics
R. Engelbrecht et al. (Eds.)
IOS Press, 2005
779

Method of GLIF Model Construction and Implementation

D Buchtela[a,b], J Peleska[a,c], A Vesely[a,b], J Zvarova[a,b]

[a]*EuroMISE Center, Prague, Czech Republic*
[b]*Dept. of Medical Informatics, Institute of Computer Science AS CR, Prague, CR*
[c]*2nd Dept. of Medicine, General University Hospital, Prague, CR*

Abstract

Knowledge acquired in medicine is possible to represent by medical guidelines. The most important and nowadays mostly used for formalisation of guidelines is the GLIF (Guideline Interchange Format) model. Final model can be coded in XML (eXtensible Markup Language). Some situations can be modelled only very hard or no ways in a practice use. This paper describes a method of GLIF model construction and implementation in XML. The method specializes in risks of whole process and tries to find a solution to problematical model situations. The GLIF model universality is kept for any medical guidelines.

Keywords:
Medical guidelines, GLIF model, XML implementation

1. Introduction

Knowledge acquired in medicine is possible to represent by medical guidelines, which make decision process in concrete cause easy and in a harmony with guidelines. For computer implementation and processing, it is necessary to have guidelines explicitly structured. The most important and nowadays mostly used is the GLIF (*Guideline Interchange Format*) model. The GLIF model is result of collaboration among Columbia University, Harvard University, McGill University and Stanford University. The main goal of GLIF was to enable sharing of guidelines among institutions and across computer applications.

2. Design and methods

GLIF model

GLIF specifies an object-oriented model for guidelines representation and syntax for guidelines utilization in software systems as well as for their transport. GLIF guidelines are mostly given as a flowchart representing a temporarily ordered sequence of steps. The nodes of the graph are guideline steps and edges represent continuation from one step to the other one. Guideline steps are an *action step, decision step, branch and synchronization steps* and a *patient state step* [1], [2].

- **Action steps** specify clinical actions that are to be performed. It can be an application of some therapy, carrying out some examination or measurement etc. Action step also may name sub-guidelines, which provide a detail for the action.
- **Decision steps** are used for conditional branching. There are two kinds of decision steps: **Case step** is used, when branching is determined by evaluation of defined logical criteria based on data items. **Choice step** is used when the decision cannot be precisely specified in guidelines themselves and decision should be made by the user.
- **Branch** and **synchronization steps** enable concurrence in the model. Guideline steps that follow branch step can be performed concurrently. Branches with root in branch step eventually converge in a synchronization step. In this step all branches are synchronized after evaluation of synchronizing condition.
- Patient **state step** characterizes a patient's clinical state.

Criteria of conditions

The decision step specifies several criteria of condition for each decision option:

- The **strict-in** criterion is used to specify a decision condition that could be computed automatically (for example if systolic blood pressure is 130 or greater). If a strict-in is true then the control flows to the guideline step that is specified by that decision option's destination

- The **strict-out** criterion is analogous to an absolute contraindication (for example if a patient is gouty he could not be cured by thiazides diuretics). If a strict-out is true then the decision option's destination is forbidden.

- The **rule-in** criteria rank a choice as the best among several options. For example, when there are competing diagnoses for a disease, a pathognomonic condition would be a rule-in for the disease. This criterion is analogous to conditions favouring the use (indications).

- A **rule-out** takes precedence over rule-in when ranking options. If an option contains both a rule-in criterion and a rule-out criterion, and both are evaluated as true, then that option should be the last choice. This criterion is analogous to contra-indications.

The *strict-out* criterion is evaluated at first. If *strict-out* criterion is evaluated as true the rest of criteria is not evaluated. This option is forbidden. In opposite case the *strict-in* criterion is evaluated. If *strict-in* criterion is false too, the *rule-in* and *rule-out* criteria are evaluated. The ranking of *rule-ins* and *rule-outs* is left to the user who may use his or her clinical judgment or may develop their own ranking schemes.

GLIF implementation in XML

GLIF model is graphical so it is necessary to code it in XML form. Syntax for guideline describing language is a part of guideline model specification. In a language form encoded guidelines consist of a sequence of guideline steps. Some attributes of a guideline step contain next guideline steps. It enables sequential representation of a graph structure in the guideline language [3].

```
<GLIF>
<Step>              = start of step
        <name>      = name of step – identification (ID)
        <type>      = type of step:        action
                                           case
                                           state
                                           subgraph
        <note>      = short description of step
        <text>      = text in a graphical symbol of step
        <tag>       = shadow actions
                <T>
                        <ttype>     get     = input parameter get
                                    put     = output parameter set
                                    open    = open of subgraph or HTML file
                                    run     = service application run
                        <tparam>            = list of parameters
                </T>
                <T>
                ...     next shadow actions
                </T>
        <x>         = x-coordinate of graphical symbol
        <y>         = y-coordinate of graphical symbol
        <w>         = width of graphical symbol
        <h>         = height of graphical symbol
        <focus>     = highlighting of step:    0 = no
                                               1 = yes
        <status>    = status of step:          1 = start step of a graph
                                               2 = end step of a graph
                                               0 = the rest of steps
        <next>      = next step(s)
                <F>         = one of option attributes
                        <nname>     = identification of option
                        <nstep>     = name of destination (target step)
                        <ncaption>  = caption of option
                        <nnote>     = description of option
                        <nline>     = coordinates of line to target step
                        <priority>  = priority of option
                        <nstrictin> = strict-in criteria
                        <nstrictout>= strict-out criterion
                        <nrulein>   = rule-in criterion
                        <nruleout>  = rule-out criterion
                </F>
                <F>
                ...     = other options
                </F>
        </next>
</Step>              = end of step
<Step>
...                  = next steps
</Step>
</GLIF>
```

Figure 1: XML syntax of GLIF model

3. Results and discussion

A GLIF model construction and implementation of text guidelines is not easy. The whole process can be divided to a several stages (see fig.2).

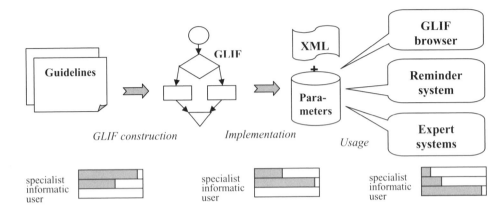

Figure 2: Process of GLIF model construction, implementation and usage

GLIF model construction stage

In a stage of GLIF model construction from text guidelines, it is important to find a logical and process structure of guidelines, all fundamental parameters and their interrelationships. Some data mining method for free text can be used for this construction. However, it's required allow to multiword connections in a automatic search. The search process becomes more complicated and error prone. Cooperation of information and medical specialist (the author of text guidelines is preferred) is more effective.

The result of this cooperation is graphic GLIF model that corresponds to text guidelines. The construction stage is the most important and difficult of all stages.

GLIF model implementation stage

In a stage of GLIF model implementation, the graphic model of guidelines is coded into XML. Besides a list of basic and derived parameters is created. Basic parameters represent directly measurable values. Derived parameters are obtained in arithmetical, logical or logically-arithmetical operation above basic parameters. Informatics and expert's cooperation plays an important role in creation of basic and derived parameters list too.

The result is data model that serves as interface between GLIF model and real input data stored in HER (*Electronic Health Record*). It is important to pay attention to definition of all criteria of condition (*strict-in, strict-out, rule-in, rule-out*) for each decision option. In this criteria evaluation, it often happens that input parameters values are not known. Therefore the criteria are evaluated in three-value (or multi-value) logic.

Well-designed model has to fulfil several conditions for each decision step:

- At most one *strict-in* criterion can be evaluated as true for all possible values of input parameters.
- At least one *strict-out* criterion must be evaluated as false for all possible values of input parameters.

- *Strict-in* or *rule-in* criteria must be evaluated as true at least in one option.
- At least *strict-in* and *strict-out* criteria evaluation should be definite (true or false). If some *strict-in* or *strict-out* criterion is evaluated as unknown, the user will have to insert missing data.

A quantity of essential data is dependent on order of single option evaluations. Therefore it is necessary to set an order of evaluation i.e. to set priority of decision options. The priority is chosen by specialist (see Fig.3).

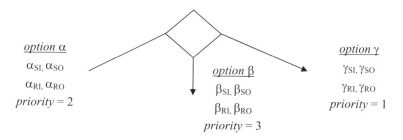

Figure 3: Set of option priority

In modelling of parallel GLIF model branches it is necessary to specify which branch is fixed and which one is optional. That is why the synchronisation conditions are set for each synchronisation step (see Fig.4).

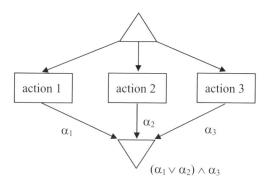

Figure 4: Set of synchronisation condition

GLIF model usage stage

GLIF model coded in XML can be used in several types of applications (see [3],[4]):

- **GLIF browser** - Formalized medical guidelines offer to users a more accessible form of knowledge presentation than a classical text. Moreover, it can show explanatory information with different levels of details. It can be used for education of students and as a decision support system in medical practice.
- **Reminder system** - System checks if input data values are in accordance with medical knowledge. Usually the system verifies if the input value is inside defined

interval. If a stated diagnosis or a chosen treatment is not in agreement with common medical guidelines, the system warns the user and suggests diagnosis that is more probable or more appropriate action.

- **Expert system** – GLIF model or a set of GLIF models create knowledge base of the expert system.

In the EuroMISE Center was developed a general GLIF browser for a few Czech and European medical guidelines as Formalized 2003 European Guidelines on Cardiovascular Disease Prevention in Clinical Practice, 2003 ESH – ESC guidelines for the management of arterial hypertension and others (see http://www.euromise.cz/new/guidelines.php).

4. Conclusion

The GLIF model is designed as a general tool that can present any formalized medical guidelines in a user-friendly manner. In modelling of text guidelines it is necessary to observe some principles. A method of GLIF model construction and implementation in XML contained in this paper describes important aspects and rules for each stage whole process. The result of observance of these rules is well-designed GLIF model, which is usable in several practical applications.

5. Acknowledgement

Research was partially supported by the project AV0Z10300504 of the Academy of Sciences CR.

6. References

[1] Ohno-Machado L., Gennari J. H., Murphy S.,N., Jain N.,L., Tu S., W., Oliver D., et al.: *The GuideLine Interchange Format: A model for representing guidelines*, Journal of the American Medical Informatics Association 1998, 5(4), pp. 357-372.

[2] Ash N., Bernstam E., Greenes R.A., Lacson R., Mork P.,Shortliffe E.H.: *Guideline Interchange Format 3.5 Technical Specification* , online - 12.12.2002, In: http://smi-web.stanford.edu/projects/intermed-web/guidelines/

[3] Buchtela D., Peleska J., Vesely A., Zvarova J.: *Presentation of Medical Guidelines on a Computer*, Transformation of Healthcare with Information Technologies, Ed.: Zielinski K., Duplaga M., Ingram D., IOS Press, Amsterdam, 2004, pp.166-171, ISBN 1-58603-438-3.

[4] Vesely A., Anger Z., Buchtela D., Peleska J., Zvarova J.: *Medical Guidelines Presentation and Comparing with Electronic Health Record*, International Joint Meeting EuroMISE 2004 Proceeding, Ed.: Zvarova J., Hanzlicek P., Peleska J., Preckova P., Svatek V., Valenta Z., Praha, 2004, pp.53, ISBN 80-903431-0-4.

Contact:

Ing. David Buchtela
EuroMISE Center - Cardio
Institute of Computer Science
Pod Vodarenskou vezi 2, Praha 8
Czech Republic
e-mail: buchtela@euromise.cz
url: http://www.euromise.cz

Section 10

Natural Language, Text Mining and Information Retrieval

Connecting Medical Informatics and Bio-Informatics
R. Engelbrecht et al. (Eds.)
IOS Press, 2005

Grepator: Accents & Case Mix for Thesaurus

Vincent Mary, Pierre Le Beux

Laboratoire d'Informatique Médicale, University of Rennes, France

Abstract

There is a real need among researchers and students for pedagogical resources. In France, information retrieval techniques have been developed, for example in the Doc'CISMeF web site. As Pubmed, documents are indexed with (French) MeSH terms, one of the problems discovered, in quality studies, is the inadequacies between the user requests and the MeSH controlled vocabulary. Moreover, French (but also Greek or Spanish), pose specific problems for indexing, due to the diacritic characters.
In this article, we present the Grepator project. The main goal is to transform any thesaurus (or any entry) in case mix and accentuated characters, for a specific domain. Furthermore, Grepator has to complete MeSH terms according to their usual form in natural language and finally, to correct user spelling mistakes. Grepator is based on a statistical approach. A large French medical corpus has been constituted from pedagogical resources indexed in CISMeF. Using regular expressions, Grepator searches the more usual ways to spell the word.. Seventy five percent of MeSH terms are found in the corpus, using this method, with less than one mistake for a hundred words. This first evaluation of the tools is analyzed and we discuss further steps that might be developed.

Keywords:
Natural language processing, Controlled Vocabulary, Language, Algorithms, MeSH

1. Introduction

The growth and development of information and communication technologies has led to a huge mass of information available on internet. Some information retrieval systems such as PubMed [1] use controlled vocabulary, like MeSH [2], but information retrieval (IR) in medicine is still a difficulty for students or professionals. MeSH poses three problems in IR systems.

The two first of them result from a lack of well-established conventions for typing characters, like the Unicode standard [3] now used by SNOMED [4] and UMLS (since 2004AB).

On the one hand, that means that up until recently, MeSH, like other thesaurus (e.g.: the French ADM [5] Aide au Diagnostic Médical)) were done in upper case. Concepts can be recognised wrongly in the indexing process : "IL" and "AIT" are ambiguous in French : "IL" could be interpreted as "Interleukin" and "he"; "AIT" matches both the "Accident ischémique transitoire" and the "have" verb.

On the other hand, the MeSH does not use diacritic characters: "cote", "côte" and "coté" have three different meanings in French for example. This situation is tolerable for a human reader, but indexing engines have to recognise the correct one during the indexing process.

Automatic accent insertion is the problem of reinserting accents (diacritics), if needed, into a term.

The third problem is that MeSH terms are not represented as found in medical documents (i.e., in the usual form). Analysing web server logs of one of the most popular French websites in this domain, CISMeF, Grabar [6] and Soualmia [7] remind us that students' requests are not even MeSH terms : 40 % of those requests send back nothing (inadequacies between MeSH and users terms). There is a real pedagogical need to reduce this silence.

With regard to the case mix and automatic accent insertion problems, previous studies, based on lexical analyses [8], learning tools [9] or the stochastic language model [10], do not try to register complex terms such as *legal abortion,* but break them into their lexemes *legal* and *abortion*. Our objective is, in this first step, to explore a new approach by keeping the whole term in the case mix and accentuation process. We want to keep the link between words that can exist in the medical domain. In what follows, we introduce an original automatic accent insertion method (specific to one domain), bind to a case mix restoring method. We have developed a program, called Grepator, which uses regular expressions from a very large corpus to search for one concept using the right way to spell it.

Furthermore, we want to develop Grepator as a complete tool which can facilitate research on the web in the medical domain by translating a MeSH term into its usual form, and at the same time, correcting user requests (typing errors or spelling mistakes). Previous studies, based on bigrams [11] or phonetization (*soundex*)[12][13], try in some cases to detect mistakes or to correct them. Grepator aims to do both at the same time, using Levenshtein algorithms [14][15]. Levenshtein algorithms are also used to accord queries to the nearest MeSH term. This tool should be easily integrated into any search engine.

2. Materials and methods

2.1 Creating the corpus

Our French medical corpus was constituted with PDF documents from two sources: pedagogical resources linked within the CISMeF and within the pedagogical network web site of Rennes University. We only kept the PDF files because we supposed that pdf's authors would pay more attention to spelling than for other formats like HTML. Thus, as our method is statistically based, it is more important to have a few but correct documents, than a very large collection of documents with mistakes. A Perl script parses both databases, downloads the 1700 PDF files and converts them using the Unix pdftotext tools. The whole corpus (150 Mb) contains 22,861,962 words, as counted by the standard wc UNIX program.

2.2 MeSH and ADM

Although Grepator accepts any thesaurus in any language as input, we used two French terminological systems : the MeSH French version, included in the 2044AA MULS version, and another knowledge base : the ADM. This knowledge base contains information on more than 10,000 diseases from all pathological fields, using more than 100,000 signs or symptoms.

3. Methods

Grepator takes a term as input (any entry or a ADM or MeSH term), and parses the corpus to look for the most popular way to spell it. For each entry, Grepator follows the following steps.

3.1 Hypotheses generation

3.1.1. Regular expressions : case mix and 'diacritization'

Each term is translated into a regular expression to generate hypotheses. This generates a list of possible alternatives for a term. For example, *SYSTEME ABO* is translated into :

syst[eèéêë]m[eèéêë] [aâäà]b[oôö]

3.1.2. Regular expressions : completing the terms

To maximize the chance of detecting a MeSH term in a user's query, it is important to accord the MeSH terms to their usual forms. For example, the query *ANGINE DE POITRINE* (*angor* whose Concept Unique Identifier is C0002962 in UMLS) has to be matched to the *ANGINE POITRINE* MeSH concept. Some information retrieval engines could detect the two concepts *ANGINE* (~*tonsilitis* CUI C0040425) and *POITRINE* (*breast* CUI C0006141) incorrectly, while the association has a different meaning. The regular expression is completed so that articles like *le, la, les, du, des, à, par, pour* as well as *d'* and *l'* can be found between terms :

syst[eèéêë]m[eèéêë][leasduàpro]{1,7}['][aâäà]b[oôö]

3.2 Candidate selection

3.2.1. Mapping the corpus

We mapped the entire corpus with the unix Grep command.

Grep -Piow "syst[eèéêë]m[eèéêë[leasduàpro]{1,7}['][aâäà]b[oôö]"

To improve results, we searched twice :

1. First, with an exact cover, i.e. with the whole term, so that we do not lose the links between words in a term such as *HeLa cells*. In French, *HeLa* can refer to the *to hail* verb. By keeping the whole term, Grepator aims to limit noise.

2. If a term is not found within the first method, we break the term into his components, using spaces as delimiters. Grepator then launches the search again, in a complete cover.

Finally, the most popular way to spell a term is inserted into the database.

3.2.2. Unknown terms

A term is unknown when it is not found by Grepator in our corpus. In this case, Grepator perl scripts using the Google search engine to ask and download documents relative to the unknown terms. Grepator downloads the 10 first PDF documents, transforms them into text, adds them to the corpus and reuses the regular expression. Finally, the document's links are stored in a MySQL database, so that Grepator does not download them again.

3.3 Implementation

3.3.1. Mapping queries to MeSH

A prototype of Grepator was integrated into a simple web page. User queries can be mapped to MeSH or ADM terms: for each MeSH or ADM term, Grepator keeps the frequently used forms from medical documents in the database. For example, the MeSH term *INTERRUPTION GROSSESSE* can be spelt in different ways in the corpus (*interruption de grosse, interruption de la grosse, interruption de sa grosse...*). Conversely, for a user query, Grepator will find the corresponding MeSH term.

3.3.2. Detect incorrect query

The levenshtein distance (LD) is defined as the minimal number of characters to replace, insert or delete in order to transform a term into another one. For example, the LD between *rhynofarynx* and *rhinopharynx* is 3. If no MeSH term can be mapped to a user query, Grepator uses Levenshtein algorithms to find the nearest MeSH term. We aim to correct spelling mistakes (*rhinofaringite / rhinopharyngite* LD = 3) and inflection problems (*fémur / fémurs* : LD = 1).

4. Results

For each terminology we extract two sets: 1600 of the accentuated part, and 1600 others which have been mixed case. Terms are manually checked, as no gold standard is available. Table 1 summarizes the validation results obtained on the two terminologies. The recall is the part of MeSH (or ADM) that has been found in the corpus. The two other lines shown the mistake frequency for each catagory. An example of the candidate selection process is illustrated in Table 2.

Table 1 - Results

	MeSH	**ADM**
Recall / Silence	73.1 % / 26.9 %	68.6 % / 31.4 %
Accentuation process	1/200	1/140
Case mix process	1/100	1/88

Table 2 - Terms found for INTERRUPTION GROSSESSE

Frequency	*Term's form*
123	interruption de grossesse
26	interruption de la grossesse
8	interruptions de grossesse
4	INTERRUPTIONS DE GROSSESSE
2	Interruption de sa grossesse

5. Discussion

With regards to the silence, the thesaurus is more often found in the corpus thanks to the term completion. For example the *INTERRUPTION GROSSESSE* term is not directly found, but we found *interruption de grosse* (123 times), *interruption de la grosse* (26 times)... Silence is still important, but consequently it concern terms that are not often used. The CISMeF team only use 5500 MeSH terms during the indexing process. It could be interesting to reduce silence by increasing corpus size with DOC or RTF files.

The exact cover step, during the mapping process is important. For example, *FRACTURE DE COTE* (*rib fracture* CUI C0035522) is properly spelt : *fracture de côte* (found 5 times). We do not evaluate the real contribution but several mistakes made in complete cover could be avoided. We could evaluate this contribution by comparing our results to other accentuated MeSH versions (CISMeF, INSERM, STIM from AP-HP...). However, Grepator is the only one that manages case mix at the same time. The whole process takes one week.

Levenshtein algorithms have been easily integrated into our user interface, and we are planning to integrate our results into the French medical university web site. By analysing the search engine logs, we could assess their contribution.

6. Conclusion

By adding complementary processes to previous studies, our method proposes an original way, allowed by even faster computers. For a first evaluation, the results are very promising. Other applications are planned by detecting mistakes in terminology information, using the UMLF [16]. Grepator will be released under the GPL license, to allow researchers to test and improve it.

7. References

[1]   AR. Aronson, O Bodenreider, FH. Chang, SM. Humphrey, J Mork, SJ. Nelson, TC. Rindflesch et JW. Wilbur. The nlm indexing initiative. Journal of the American Medical Informatics Association, 7(suppl) :17 21, 2000.

[2]   National Library Of Medicine. Medical subject headings. National Library Of Medicine, 1986.

[3]   Mark Needleman. The unicode standard. Serials Review, 2 :51 54, Aout 2000.

[4]   J. Kilbourne et T Williams. Unicode, UTF-8, ASCII, and SNOMED CT(R). page 892, 2003.

[5]   P. Lenoir, JR. Michel, C. Frangeul et G. Chales. Realisation, développement et maintenance de la base de donnees ADM. Medecine informatique, 6 :51 6, 1981.

[6]   Nathalie Grabar, Pierre Zweigenbaum, Lina Soualmia et Stefan J. Darmoni. Les utilisateurs de Doc CISMeF peuvent ils trouver ce qu ils cherchent ? Une étude de l'adéquation du vocabulaire des requêtes des utilisateurs au MeSH. In : IXemes Journees Francophones d'Informatique Medicale (JFIM), pages 158 - 69, May 2002.

[7]   L.F. Soualmia and S.J. Darmoni. Projection de requêtes pour une recherche d'information intelligente sur le web. RCJA, (in press), Juillet 2003.

[8]   T Spriet et M ElBèze. Re accentuation automatique de textes. Besançon, France, 1997.

[9]   Pierre Zweigenbaum et Nathalie Grabar. Restoring accents in unknown biomedical words : application to the French MeSH thesaurus. Int J Med Inf, 67(1-3) :113 26, Dec 2002.

[10]   M. Simard. Re accentuation automatique de textes francais. In : Centre d'innovation en technologies de l'information, Laval, Canada. 1996.

[11]   B. Thomson McInnes, S.V. Pakhomov, T. Perdersen et C.G. Chute. Incorporating bigram statistics to spelling correction tools. 11th World Congress on Medical Informatics (Medinfo 2004), (in press), septembre 2004.

[12]   J Keene, L. Swift, S. Bailey et G. Janacek. Shared patients : multiple health and social care contact. Health Soc Care Community, 9(4) :205 - 14, Juillet 2001.

[13]   RV. Sideli et C. Friedman. Validating patient names in an integrated clinical information system. In : Proc Annu Symp Comput Appl Med Care, pages 588 - 92, 1991.

[14]   V.I. Levenshtein, Binary codes capable of correcting deletions, insertions and reversals, Cyber. Contr. Theory 10 (8) (1966) 707-710.

[15]   B. Lambert. Predicting look-alike and sound-alike medication errors. Am J Health Syst Pharm, 54(10):1161-71, May 97.

[16] Pierre Zweigenbaum, Robert Baud, Anita Burgun, Fiammetta Namer, Eric Jarrousse, Nathalie Grabar, Patrick Ruch, Franck Le- Duff, Benoit Thirion et Stefan Darmoni. Towards a united medical lexicon for french. In : The New Navigators : from Professionals to Patients. Proceedings of MIE 2003, volume 95 *in* : Studies in Health Technology and Informatics, pages 415 420. IOS Press, mai 2003.

8. Address for correspondence

Vincent MARY
Laboratoire d'informatique médicale, Faculté de Médecine
2 rue PR. Léon Bernard, 35000 Rennes, France
vincent.mary@univ-rennes1.fr

Connecting Medical Informatics and Bio-Informatics
R. Engelbrecht et al. (Eds.)
IOS Press, 2005

793

Predicting Lexical Relations between Biomedical Terms: towards a Multilingual Morphosemantics-based System

Fiammetta Namer[a], Robert Baud[b]

[a] *UMR ATILF CNRS & University of Nancy2, Nancy, France*

[b] *Hôpitaux Universitaires de Genève, Geneva, Switzerland*

Abstract

This paper addresses the issue of how semantic information can be automatically assigned to compound terms, i.e. both a definition and a set of semantic relations. This issue is particularly crucial when elaborating multilingual databases and when developing cross-language information retrieval systems. The paper shows how morpho-semantics can contribute in the constitution of multilingual lexical networks in biomedical corpora. It presents a system capable of labelling terms with morphologically related words, i.e. providing them with a definition, and grouping them according to synonymy, hyponymy and proximity relations. The approach requires the interaction of three techniques: (1) a language-specific morphosemantic parser, (2) a multilingual table defining basic relations between word roots, and (3) a set of language-independant rules to draw up the list of related terms. This approach has been fully implemented for French, on an about 29,000 terms biomedical lexicon, resulting to more than 3,000 lexical families.

Keywords:
Natural Language Processing; Semantics; Language; Multilingualism; Neoclassical Compounds; Morphosemantics for French; Semantic Relations; Biomedical lexical database.

1. Introduction

The approach and the results presented here[1] intend to contribute in developing a multilingual structuration of biomedical lexicons by the use of a morpho-semantics based approach, i.e. which provides morphologically complex words with a definition as well as with lexical relations. Our objective with such semantically tagged terms is to enrich thesauri and ontologies, to enable cross-language question-answering and to multilingually extend information retrieval requests to neighbour concepts, that is at least synonyms, hyponyms, and morphologically related terms. The fundamental principle is that semantic information is acquired on morphologically complex words through the joint action of lexical data, a morphosemantic parser and lexical relation computation rules. This leads to the calculation of several types of lexical relations: first, each complex word is defined with

---

[1] Methods and results reported here are supported by projects UMLF (coordination: P. Zweigenbaum, grant from French Ministry for Research and Education, 2002-2004) [1], and VumeF (coordination: S. Darmoni, grant from French Ministry for Research, National Network of Health Technologies, 2003-2005) [2].

respect to its base (i.e. its morphologically related word); second, pairs of complex word may be bound by synonymy, hyponymy or proximity links. The developed system relies on **three** hypotheses. **First**, complex words form more than 60% of the new terms found in technico-scientific domains, and especially in the biomedical field ([3]). It is therefore impossible for dictionaries to collect all neologisms. On the other hand, linguistic-driven constraint-based morphosemantic systems are suitable techniques to define words meaning with respect to the meaning of their parts: for instance, whereas Dorland's medical dictionary proposes the following definition for the adjective *anticephalalgic*[2]: "inhibiting headache", a morphosemantic parser, such as DériF for French (see §3) is able to provide it with the following definition: "which is against head pain". **Second** observation is that whatever the involved European language[3], complex words in biomedical field make use of latin and greek roots, which are called here combining forms (CF) following [4]. CFs inherit their part-of-speech tag from the modern language words they substitute for (stomach,N → gastr,N). Additionally, CF realizations are simple graphic variants from a language to another. Moreover, very similar word formation rules are at play in all these languages to build words belonging to specialized terminologies. Both CFs and complex word structures are therefore likely to be identified by neutral representations, which abstract away differences between languages: VASCUL--ITE[4] = *vascul--ite*$_{FR}$ = *Vascul--itis*$_{GE}$ = *vascol--ite*$_{IT}$ = *vascul--itis*$_{ES/EN}$. **Third** assumption deals with biomedical classifications: just like words they substitute for, abstract CFs can be ranked according to sound hierarchies (SNOMED, MesH…), in such a way that they can be labelled by descriptors such as *anatomy* (GASTR), *physiology* (TAXI) or *symptoms* (ALGI). Consequently, CFs may be combined by links: synonymy = (e.g. OPT=OPHTALM, vision), hyponymy < (e.g. BLAST, embryonal cell < CYT, cell), meronymy ← (e.g. CORO, pupil ← OCUL, eye) and proximity ~ (e.g. RHIN, nose ~ OTO, ear). How are these three background hypotheses exploited in order to reach our goal: elaborating a multilingual approach in order to supply biomedical terms with semantic information and to prove the feasibility of the method by implementing it for French.

2. Materials and Methods

2.1 Language specific resources: As we shall see, the quality of the results mainly depends on lexicon size. Therefore large-scale monolingual lexica are required in order to optimize lexical content and coverage. On the other hand, only one resource among the three of which our methodology relies on is fully language-specific, namely the **word formation parser**. Linguistic-driven constrained-based morphological analysis, i.e., the process of decomposing a complex word into its constituent parts, is a language dependent task. It has proved useful to avoid the need for costly, repetitive maintenance of specialized dictionaries to account for new terms ([5],[6],[7]); morover it can additionally enrich the decomposition of each word with semantic knowledge, as described in ([8],[9]). For biomedecine, units that compose complex words often are CFs: in suffixation *epatico*$_{IT,ES}$ (hepatic), prefixation *Hypothermie*$_{GE}$ (hypothermia), as well as in compounding *thermo--taxy*$_{EN}$, *stomac--odynie*$_{FR}$ (stomach--odynia). Unlike affixation, which builds a complex word by applying a suffix (-*ico*$_{IT,ES}$) or a prefix (*hypo*-$_{GE,FR,EN}$) to a base word or CF, compounding constructs a new word by associating two words or CFs. In so-called neoclassical compounds, which the paper focuses on, the rightmost component, which is called *head* (noted **X**), governs the left hand component, called *modifier* (noted **Y**).

---

[2] Though we said the system currently runs for French, examples are given in English whenever necessary, for sake of readability.
[3] This claim is illustrated here with exemples in German (GE), English (EN), French (FR), Italian (IT) and Spanish(ES)
[4] Throughout the paper, abstract CFs are written in small capitals, CF to CF boundaries are represented by '--'

2.2 Multilingual CF Table: The second and third hypotheses of §1 lead to the design of a 900 rows table sampled in Table1. Part-of-speech tag (3), SNOMED head chapters (4) and basic lexical relations (5) refer to CF abstract representations whereas instantiation (2) deals with CFs (1) respective realizations[5] and translations in each language (see [10]).

Table 1 - Multilingual Combining Forms Table

CF (1)		Instanciation (2)					POS (3)	Semantic Type (4)	Lexical relation (5)
		English	German	French	Italian	Spanish			=STOMAC,
GASTR	realization	gastr	Gastr	gastr	gastr	gastr	N	*ANATOMY*	←ABDOMIN,
	translation	stomach	Magen	estomac	stomaco	estomago			~ENTER , ~HEPAT, ~PANCREAT
ALGI	realization	algia/algy	algie	algie	algia	algia	N	*SYMPTOM*	=ODYN, ~ITE,
	translation	pain	Schmerz	douleur	dolore	dolor			~OSE
ITE	realization	itis	ite	ite	ite	itis	N	*SYMPTOM*	~ALGI,
	translation	inflammation	Inflammation	inflammation	infiammazione	inflamación			~ODYN
PHLEB	realization	phleb	Phleb	phléb	fleb	fleb	N	*ANATOMY*	=VEN,
	translation	vein	Vene	veine	vena	vena			<ANGI, <VASCUL
ANGI	realization	angio	Angio	angio	angio	angio	N	*ANATOMY*	=VASCUL,
	translation	blood vessel	Blutader	vaisseau sanguin	vaso sanguigno	vaso sanguíneo			~VAS
ECTOMI	realization	ectomy	ektomie	ectomie	ectomia	ectomía	N	*MEDICAL ACT*	~TOMI,
	translation	ablation	Ablation	ablation	ablazione	ablación			~STOMI

2.3 Language independent Lexical Relation Computation Rules: The third technique required to perform cross-language semantic tagging on compounds is a set of rules capable of propagating basic lexical relations attached to CFs, and encoded in the CF Table, onto words which are composed with these CFs. There are currently four rules that only deal with compound words, as indicated in Table 2. Extensions are on progress to account for affixed words as well. To explain briefly how the rules work, let us paraphrase the second one. Assume two compound words A and B. Their respective head component, X_A and X_B are synonyms (ALGI equals ODYNI). So, if Y_A refers to a part of Y_B (ENTER ← ABDOMIN) then A is a hyponym of B (*enteralgia* is a special type of *abdominodynia*). Otherwise, if Y_A and Y_B hold any other basic relation (ABDOMIN equals LAPAR, ALBUMIN is a subtype of PROTEIN, XER is an approximation of SCLER) then A and B share the same relation as Y_A and Y_B, whatever the language.

Table 2 - Language independent Lexical Relation Computation Rules

Rule	Example		
	Y	X	$[Y_A X_A]$ R $[Y_B X_B]$
A = $[Y_A X]$ and B=$[Y_B X]$			
	PROCTO ← COLO	RRAGIE	EN: proctorrhagia < colorrhagia
If Y_A ← Y_B then A < B	LEUCO ← HÉMATO	GRAMME	GE: Leukogramm < Hämatogramm
else	ABDOMIN=LAPAR	SCOPIE	FR: abdominoscopie = laparoscopie
if Y_A R Y_B and R is { =, <, ~}	ALBUMIN<PROTEIN	EMIE	IT: albuminemia < proteinemia
then A R B	XER ~SCLER	OPHTALMIE	ES: xerophtalmia ~sclerophtalmia

---

[5] According to the language in consideration, CFs may have ambiguous written forms: so in Franch 'aur' means either *gold* (*aurithérapie$_N$*: "gold therapy" or *ear* (*auriforme$_A$*: "ear shaped"). Abstract CF desambiguisation is ensured by the other field values in the CF Table

A = [Y_AX_A] and B=[Y_BX_B] and		X_A = X_B		
X_A = X_B	ENTER←ABDOMIN	ALGIE = ODYNIE	**EN:** enteralgia < abdominodynia	
If Y_A ← Y_B then A < B	MORT = THANAT	FERE = GENE	**IT:** mortifero = tanatogeno	
else if Y_A R Y_B and R is { =, <, ~}	API < ENTOMO	VORE = PHAGE	**FR:** apivore < entomophage	
then A R B	CANCER ~CARCIN	FORME = OÏDE	**GE:** cancriformis ~Karzinoïd	
A = [YX_A] and B=[YX_B]	BACTÉR	OÏDE = FORME	**FR:** bactérioïde = bactériforme	
if X_A R X_B and R is {=, <, ~}	OTO	RRAGIE < RRHEE	**GE:** Otorrhagie < Otorrhö	
then A R B	ARTHR	ALGIE ~ITE	**ES:** artralgia ~artritis	
A = [Y_AX_A] and B=[Y_BX_B] and		Y_A = Y_B		
Y_A = Y_B	ORTHO = RECTI	DONTE = DENT	**FR:** orthodonte = rectident	
if X_A R X_B and R is {=, <, ~}	MÉTR = HYSTÉR	RRAGIE < RRHEE	**FR:** métrorragie < hystérorrée	
then A R B	LIP = ADIP	MATOSE ~OME	**EN:** lipomatosis ~adipoma	

The interaction between morpho-semantic **parser, CF table** and **lexical** relation computation **rules** results in a processing chain which leads to the tagging of compounds by means of the =, < and ~ lexical relations. (1) The **parser** analyses an input word and provides it with a definition with respect of the word components; it also feeds **lexical rules** with CFs the input word is composed with. (2) **Lexical rules** try to match these CFs against the **CF Table** content, in order to identify the abstract roots basically related to them. (3) According to these collected basic relations, **lexical rules** predict all the "possible words" the input may be lexically linked to. (4) The last task is then to filter out unattested words from this candidates list. This is what has been fully realized for French, as described in the next section.

3. Results

Results for French have been obtained on a 29,000 nouns, verbs and adjectives specialized input lexicon. The language specific morpho-semantic parser for French (§2.1) is DériF ("Dérivation en Français") ([11]), which makes use of the CF Table content (§2.2) to provide each input lemma with a linguistic-based ([12]) recursive and hierarchical analysis, whose result is threefold: it includes the parsing trace, under square brackets, the ordered list of results, from the input to an undecomposable unit, and the definition of the input, expressing in natural language the semantic relation between the input and its morphological base (Table 3 (1)). Lexical relation computation rules (§2.3) are then applied to (Y,X) CF pairs, which correspond to DériF analysis of each compound word input A, in order to collect all possible (Y',X') links, by matching Y and X against the appropriate entries in the CF Table. Each computed relation is displayed together with the corresponding candidate (Y',X') pairs (Table 3 (2)). To identify which of the candidate (Y',X') relations are actual words, the system first instanciates (Y',X') into the French pair (Y'_FR, X'_FR) according to CF Table. Then it examines each of the parsing results from the input lexicon. For each compound word B, (Y'_FR,X'_FR) is compared to B components. In case of Y'_FR/Y_B and X'_FR/X_B identity, B is added to the semantic family of A, with the appropriate relation (Table 3 (3)).

Table 3 - Analysis and lexical family for hystérrorragie (hysterrorrhagia)

(1)	hystérorragie=>[[hystéro N*] [rragie N*] N] , (hystérorragie/N, rragie/N*), "uterus bleeding"
(2)	Constituents = /hystéro/rragie/ Type = symptom
R_POSS:Y',X'	**Poss. Rels :** (=:HYSTER/RRHAGI), (<:HYSTER/RRHE), (=:METR/RRAGI),(=:UTER/RRAGI), (~:COLP/RRAGI,) (~:FALLOP/RRAGI)
(3)	hystérorragie/N (symptom) , " bleeding of the uterus "
R_ACT:Y_B,X_B	**Actual Relations : synonym of** métrorragie/N; **subtype of** hystérorrhée/N, métrorrhée/N; **see also** colporragie/N

From a quantitative point of view, the following can be said about results obtained so far for French. First, DériF implement various WF processes, that comprise about 30 suffixation, prefixation and compounding rules. It analyses 17,240 lemmas as complex words, out of the 29,000 lemmas, and each of them is provided with a definition relating it to its base, or to its components. Finally, the processing chain defines more than 3,000 lexical families among compound nouns and adjectives that are included in the 29,000 input lexicon.

4. Discussion

[6] and [7] approaches already makes use of word decomposition and CF (they call 'subwords') in order to enhance IR recall. But the originality of our (linguistic-based) approach lays in the computation of cross-linguistic lexical relations, in addition to the computed definition each decomposed word is provided with. Of course, in counterpart, its strongest drawback ([13]) is that it requires lists of exception to be accounted for: a human validation is therefore necessary, first to check the appropriateness of morphological decompositions, second to validate computed definitions, and finally to verify the basic relations in the CF Table[6]. On one hand, this task is delicate, because basic lexical relations between CFs must be compatible with all medical terms they can occur in; LABI (lip) < BUCC (mouth) is e.g. too much a powerful assumption, since LABI can be used in ginecology: *inguino-labial*$_{EN}$: the wrong relation between CFs would be propagated through rules, and *inguino-labial* would record somewhere that it has to do with the mouth. On the other hand, this task has to be performed once and for all, whatever the language.

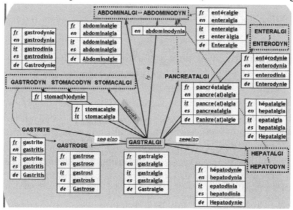

Fig.1 - Abstract cross-language family of GASTRALGI

Extending the approach to other languages requires only the availability of **language-dependent morphosemantic parsers**, that can be reduced e.g. to simple stemmers in a first approach, as their primary task is to recognize Y and X components for compound words[7]. As soon as it is available for EN, GE, IT and ES, together with monolingual lexical resources necessary to feed the system, the processing chain, already operative for French, will produce a set of lexical families as illustred in Fig.1: each label (GASTRALGI) identifies a group of words that hold one of the =,<, ~ relations with other multilingual group of words, when attested in the monolingual lexicon.

5. Conclusion

---

[6] Among them, proximity relations have to be dealt with carefully in the CF Table, in order to reduce discutable projections, e.g. *gastr* ~ *hépat* implying *gastritis* ~ *hepatitis*.
[7] The fact that German makes less use of CFs than the other European languages (e.g. *Schädigung* is employed instead of *pathie*, in *Chorioschädigung* (*choriopathy*)) may imply in the end a less important amount of lexical links with this language.

The approach enables to group morphologically compound words belonging to the medical sublanguage into semantic families, according to a basic multilingual classification (the CF table) set up on the basis of international terminologies of the biomedical domain. A few language-independent lexical relation computation rules is required to project the basic CF relations onto the words containing these CFs. Results obtained so far for French are use to enrich terminology descriptions, and to enhance term matching systems by creating new links, e.g. between *traitement contre la **fièvre*** (fever treatment) and *traitement antipyrétique* (antipyretic treatment). Another possible application is to use hyponymy links in order to solve discourse anaphora (*"... **gastralgy**. Treating this **pain** ... "*). Families and lexical relations could furthermore enrich already existing French information retrieval systems. Once available, some of the possible applications for the obtained multiple translations (see Fig. 1) are straightforwards: cross-linguistic question-answering or information retrieval, multilingual terminological enhancing etc.; moreover, relations between abstract labels are likely to play other roles. Let us take *stomachodynie*$_{FR}$ which seems the sole instance of STOMACODYNI, according to Fig.1. However, synonymy relations between STOMACODYNI STOMACALGI, GASTRODYNI and GASTRALGI indirectly provide it synonymy links with terms of other languages, e.g. *gastralgia*$_{ES}$, *stomacalgia*$_{IT}$, *Gastrodynie*$_{GE}$ and *gastrodynia*$_{EN}$: lexical relation between abstract terms may be used as plurilingual translators.

6. Acknowledgments

Thanks to UMLF project members for insights and guidance: S. Darmoni and P. Zweigenbaum.

7. References

[1]   Zweigenbaum P, Baud R, Burgun A, et al. Towards a unified medical lexicon for French. In: Baud R, Fieschi M, Le Beux P, P. R, eds. *Stud Health Technol Inform*; 2003. p. 415-20.
[2]   Darmoni SJ, Jarrousse E, Zweigenbaum P, et al. VumeF: Extending the French part of the UMLS. In: Musen M, ed. *Proc AMIA Symp 2003*, Washington, DC: AMIA; 2003. p. 824 (poster).
[3]   Lovis C, Baud R, Rassinoux A-M, Michel PA, Scherrer JR. Medical dictionaries for patient encoding systems: a methodology. *Artif Intell Med* 1998;14:201-14.
[4]   Iacobini C. Distinguishing derivational prefixes from initial combining forms. In: Booij G, Ralli A, Scalise S, eds. *Proc 1st Mediterranean Morphology Meeting*. Mytilene (Greece); 1999. p. 132-40.
[5]   Lovis C, Michel PA, Baud R, Scherrer J-R. Word segmentation processing: a way to exponentially extend medical dictionaries. In: Greenes RA, Peterson HE, Protti DJ, eds. *8th World Congress on Medical Informatics*; 1995. p. 28-32.
[6]   Schulz S, Romacker M, Franz P et al. Towards a multilingual morpheme thesaurus for medical free-text retrieval. In: *Proceedings of MIE'99*; Ljubljana, Slovenia: IOS Press; 1999. p. 891-4.
[7]   Hahn U, Honeck M, Piotrowski M, Schulz S. Subword segmentation: Leveling out morphological variations for medical document retrieval. *J Am Med Inform Assoc* 2001;8(suppl):229-33.
[8]   Daille B, Fabre C, Sébillot P. Applications of computational morphology. In: Boucher P, ed. *Many Morphologies*. Somerville, MA: Cascadilla Press; 2002. p. 210-34.
[9]   Namer F, Zweigenbaum P. Acquiring meaning for French Medical Terminology: contribution of Morphosemantics. In: *MEDINFO*; San Francisco, CA; 2004. p. 535-9.
[10] Namer F. Acquiring Lexical Classes in Biomedical Lexicons: a Morphosemantics-based Multilingual Approach. In: *Word Structure and Lexical Systems;* Pavia, Italy; 2004. (poster).
[11] Namer F. Automatiser l'analyse morpho-sémantique non affixale: le système DériF. In: Hathout N, Roché M, eds. *Cahiers de Grammaire*. Toulouse: 2003. p. 31-48.
[12] Corbin D. *Morphologie dérivationnelle et structuration du lexique*. Lille: Presses Universitaires de Lille; 1987.
[13] Baud R, Rassinoux A-M, Ruch P, Lovis C, Scherrer J-R. The power and limits of a rule-based morpho-semantic parser. *J American Med Inform Assoc* 1999;6(suppl):22-6.

Address for correspondence

Fiammetta Namer, UMR 7118 "ATILF" & Université Nancy2 - CLSH – 23 Boulevard Albert 1er, BP3397 – 54015 Nancy Cedex. email: *Fiammetta.Namer@univ-nancy2.fr*; URL:http://www.univ-nancy2.fr/pers/namer

Connecting Medical Informatics and Bio-Informatics
R. Engelbrecht et al. (Eds.)
IOS Press, 2005

Simplified Representation of Concepts and Relations on Screen

Hans Rudolf Straub[a], Norbert Frei[b], Hugo Mosimann[a], Csaba Perger[a], Annette Ulrich[a]

[a]Semfinder AG, Kreuzlingen, Schweiz
[b]University of Applied Sciences St. Gallen (FHS), St. Gallen, Schweiz

Abstract

The fully automated generation of diagnostic codes requires a knowledge-based system which is capable of interpreting noun phrases. The sense content of the words must be analysed and represented for this purpose. The codes are then generated based on this representation.
In comparison with other knowledge-based systems, a system of this kind places the emphasis on the data structures and not on the calculus; coding itself is a simple matter compared to the much more difficult task of incorporating the complex information contained in the words used in natural language in a systematic data model. Initial attempts were based on the assumption that each word was linked to one conceptual meaning, whereas such a naive viewpoint certainly no longer applies today. The notation of concepts and their relations is the task at hand.
Existing notation methods include predicate logic, conceptual graphs (CGs) as proposed by J. F. Sowa [2], GRAIL as used by the GALEN Project [1] and methods developed as part of the WWW consortium, e.g. RDF's (Resource Description Frameworks). For the purpose of coding, we developed a notation system using "concept particles" back in 1989 [3]. In 1996, the resulting experience led us to represent "concept molecules" (CM), with which both complex data structures and multi-branched rules can be denoted in a simple manner [4]. In this paper we shall explain the principles behind this notation and compare it with another modern concept representation system, conceptual graphs.

Keywords:
Natural Language Processing, Expert Systems, Classification, International Classification of Diseases

1. The dual demands made on concept notation

For concept notation in our text interpreter, we drew up the following requirements:

1. The notation system must be able to reproduce all the necessary structures.
2. The number of formal elements should be kept as low as possible.
3. The notation system must be unambiguous (one representation for one meaning).
4. Concept representation must be expandable (no "closed world").
5. It must be easy and intuitive to read on the screen.
6. It should be as compact as possible, i.e. show as much content per screen as possible.

These requirements are the result of the dual demands imposed on concept notation, i.e. that it should be easy to read, both for the machine and for humans. For machines, the notation system must be mathematically clear. Humans also impose the additional demand that the rules should be quick and easy to read; this is even more important with larger and more complex rule bases for expert systems. A system which is mathematically perfect, but which does not satisfy conditions 4 to 6, will inevitably fail, as it can no longer be maintained once it exceeds a certain size. This is why the last three points are so important.

The semantic interpreter which we have developed for coding purposes uses a notation system which fulfils the specified conditions. This was possible thanks to the introduction of *concept molecules* which use the two-dimensional nature of the screen to depict complex concept structures.

2. The role of relations: atomic concepts and concept molecules (CM)

Concepts are the meanings which we combine with words. However, it is not just the concepts themselves which play a role: how the concepts are linked together is the crucial element in formulating knowledge. The relations – i.e. the links between the concepts – contain the actual knowledge and must be capable of being represented explicitly in each concept representation.

In our representation, we see concepts as indivisible units, i.e. as atoms. Everything that is said about a concept is said in the form of relations to other concepts. If the knowledge is extended, the concept does not change, merely the bundle of relations connected with the concept.

When concepts are linked together, they form clusters. These clusters are represented on the screen in a strictly regulated fashion. Just as atoms in chemistry have binding sites via which they can bind with other atoms, our atomic concepts also have precisely defined binding sites via which they can form bindings with other precisely defined atoms. We call the resulting concept clusters concept molecules (CM).

3. Atomic concepts: both type and value

In order to deal systematically with concepts, they are classified. This leads to two kinds of expressions, namely types (classes) and values. These two kinds of expressions are clearly differentiated in databases, where the type corresponds to the column in the database and the value corresponds to the value of a specific field in the column. In a "diagnosis" column, "angina pectoris", "bronchogenic carcinoma" and "lung TB" are possible values. In Sowa's conceptual graphs (CG) [2] a concept may, for example, consist of a type-value pair. The colon in the left-hand rectangle on Figure 1 denotes the relation of type to value.

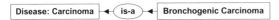

Figure 1 - Class and instance, as shown by conceptual graphs

In the CM representation, the information is shown as follows:

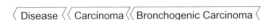

Figure 2 - The information from Figure 1 shown as a chain of 3 atomic concepts

The concept "carcinoma" is both the type and the value in Figure 2, i.e. the type for its subordinate concept ("bronchogenic carcinoma") and the value for its superordinate concept ("disease"). In this context, we talk about the bifaciality of the atomic concept.

Each concept can – depending on its constellation – be a type (class) or a value, or both at the same time.

In Section 1 we impose the requirement that the semantic net (overall concept representation) should represent an "open world" and must therefore be expandable at any point. The bifaciality of atomic concepts fits in well with this, in that the concept chains can be opened at any point and intermediate concepts can be inserted.

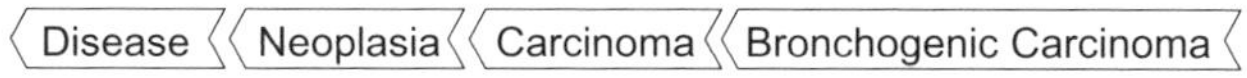

⟨ Disease ⟨⟨ Neoplasia ⟨⟨ Carcinoma ⟨⟨ Bronchogenic Carcinoma ⟨

Figure 3 - The CM from Figure 2 - extended by adding an intermediate concept

Figures 2 and 3 show quite clearly how the number of formal elements is reduced with CM: we can manage with one formal element, whilst Figure 1 requires four, including a rectangle, oval, arrow and colon.

4. Implicit representation of relators

The fact that we are able to manage with one formal element in Figure 3 is thanks to a kind of "trick". The information conveyed by the oval or colon in the conceptual graph (Figure 1) is represented *implicitly* in the CM: whenever two concepts are side by side on the same line, it means that there is an "is-a" relation between them. The left-hand concept is the superordinate concept in this case and the right-hand concept is the subordinate concept. This hierarchical ("is-a") relationship can be extended over any number of stages. The resulting representation is easy to read and saves space. We aim to show below that implicit representation of relators is also possible for additional relators.

5. The two basic relations: hierarchy and attribution

In CM's the links can be traced back to two basic relations:

1. The hierarchical relation (= "is-a") is represented horizontally.
2. The attributive relation (= "has-a") is represented vertically.

Both relationships are asymmetrical, i.e. the two linked concepts cannot be exchanged for one another. The relation includes a direction which cannot be reversed. This direction is defined on the screen by the left-right axis:

Table 1 - the two basic relations are asymmetrical

	Left	Right
Hierarchy	superordinate concept	subordinate concept
Attribution	attributed concept	attribute

With the aid of attributes, branched CM's can be drawn:

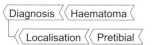

Figure 4 - A branched CM with a "has-a" relation

In Figure 4, the concept "diagnosis" has one attribute, i.e. "localisation". It is linked to the attribute via an attributive relation which is shown by the little hook beneath "diagnosis".

A conventional concept representation might show the situation as follows:

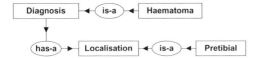

Figure 5 - The content of Figure 4 in conventional notation

Fig. 5 does not merely contain more elements than Fig. 4, but also does not have a standardised spatial configuration. Several possible spatial arrangements of the concepts are possible.

6. Benefits of the strict spatial configuration within the CM

The standardised spatial configuration in CM's has more to recommend it to knowledge base engineers than the convenience of customary practice. The strict systematic nature of CM's improves readability and processing quality:

1. Each line only contains concepts from one hierarchy.
2. As soon as the line is changed, the semantic dimension (i.e. semantic type) is also changed.
3. The number of lines thus also always displays the number of semantic dimensions (types).
4. The most general concept of the corresponding semantic dimension is always at the left of each line.
5. The root of the overall CM, i.e. the concept to which all the other concepts in the molecule are subordinate, be they hierarchical or attributive, is always at the top left-hand side.
6. Since a molecule, including all its branches, always has a tree structure (see Figure 9), it can be simply and systematically processed by a computer program.

The last point shows how a representation which facilitates readability for humans can also improve readability for machines.

7. Converting the named relators into unnamed relators

The two basic relators for CM's, the hierarchical relator and the attributive relator, can be recognised by their position. Other relators are converted into a combination of attributive and hierarchical relations:

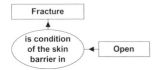

Figure 6: Conceptual graph with a named relator

The named relator is converted into a combination of 1 concept and 2 basic relators:

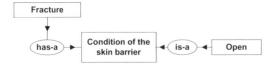

Figure 7 - Information from Figure 7 using solely the two basic relators

This information is then written as follows using a CM:

Figure 8 - Information from Figure 7, represented in a CM

Figure 8 is shorter and easier to read than Figure 6 or Figure 7. The concept "condition of the skin barrier" is omitted however. This is admissible because, in CM's, the binding sites - even if they are not named - are clearly defined in the semantic net. In our current knowledge base, the concept "fracture" has ten different attributive binding sites, for example. The two concepts "open" and "closed" are linked exclusively to one of these binding sites, whilst the two concepts "intraarticular" and "extraarticular" are linked to another. Although the binding sites are unnamed, the knowledge engineer can immediately see the content-related meaning of the binding site from the linked concepts (see Figure 9). This has the following benefits:

1. The engineer does not need to worry about relator names - often lengthy and arbitrary.
2. Representation with CM's (Figure 8) takes up less space on the screen.
3. It is thus quicker and easier to read.
4. More information can be taken in at a glance.
5. Despite this, the information is always clear.
6. The conclusions which the computer draws from the CM's are always unambiguous and relate only to a specific binding site.

An additional benefit is associated with fundamental semantic considerations. The two basic relators – the hierarchical and the attributive - do in fact correspond to the two fundamental relationships which two values within the semantic framework can have (see Section 3.3 in [4]). In addition, concepts in CM's and OOP object types display surprising affinities (see Section 8 in [4]). Furthermore, practical research shows that CM's without named relators work, provide accurate results and make it possible to compile and maintain large and complex knowledge bases.

8. Multi-branched CM's

Figure 10 shows the interaction between hierarchical and attributive relations in a concrete diagnosis. The example contains 9 lines and thus has 9 hierarchies (or dimensions or axes).

The diagram could have been obtained from the following noun phrase: "Suspected simple, extraarticular and not dislocated left distal radial fracture". The phrase can also be formulated in quite a different manner. In addition to the clarity of its form, the representation shown in Figure 10 also has the following benefits over the noun phrase:

1. The implicit meanings are reconstructed ("forearm", "bone"). Implicit meanings can be crucial for coding or querying in a data warehouse.
2. The links are much clearer. Thus, "distal" belongs to the "bone<radius" group and not to the fracture group. The inference machine for coding purposes is based on this clear, multi-dimensional **and** multifocal [5] structuring of the underlying data structure and could not function without it.
3. This structuring is a considerable help to the knowledge engineer in reviewing the knowledge base.

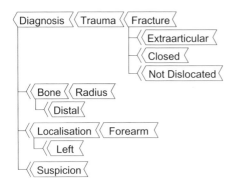

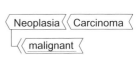

Figure 9 - An average branched CM   *Figure 10 – A simple rule*

9. Representation of processing rules

Figure 9 shows concepts in a specific configuration and represents an information status at a given moment in time. Such a status is amended by a processing rule. The rule causes a specific previous status (an "if") to be converted to a subsequent status (a "then"). Rules are written as CM's with operators which are allocated to the individual atoms in the CM's. In Figure 10 the "then-add" operator (underlined in green on the screen) causes the concept "malignant" to be added to the two other atoms.

10. Results

On the basis of the CM's described above we have created a rule editor, an inference machine and an extensive knowledge base for coding freely formulated diagnosis texts. This system (Semfinder®) permits fully automated coding (one-step coding) and was in everyday use in over 100 hospitals in Germany by the end of 2004.

11. References

[1] Rector A et al. A Terminolgy Server for Medical Language and Medical Information Systems. *Methods of Information in Medicine 34*, 1995: 147-157.

[2] Sowa JF: *Knowledge Representation: Logical, Philosophical and Computational Foundations*. Pacific Grove: Brooks/Cole, 2000.

[3] Straub, HR. Wissensbasierte Interpretation, Kontrolle und Auswertung elektronischer Patientendossiers. In: *Kongressband der IX. Jahrestagung der SGMI. Schweizerische Gesellschaft für Medizininformatik*, Nottwil, SGMI, 1994, pp. 81-87.

[4] Straub HR: *Das interpretierende System - Wortverständnis und Begriffsrepräsentation in Mensch und Maschine, mit einem Beispiel zur Diagnose-Codierung*. Wolfertswil: Z/I/M-Verlag, 2001

[5] Straub HR. Four Different Types of Classification Models. In: Grütter R, ed. *Knowledge Media in Health Care: Opportunities and Challenges*. Herskey / London: Idea Group Publishing, 2002, pp. 58 – 82.

12. Address for correspondence

Hans Rudolf Straub, Semfinder AG, Hauptstrasse 23, CH-8280 Kreuzlingen, Schweiz
straub@semfinder.com
http://www.semfinder.com/methode

Connecting Medical Informatics and Bio-Informatics
R. Engelbrecht et al. (Eds.)
IOS Press, 2005

Indexing UMLS Semantic Types for Medical Question-Answering

Thierry Delbecque[a], Pierre Jacquemart[a], Pierre Zweigenbaum[a,b,c]

[a] INSERM, U729, Paris, France
[b] Assistance Publique – Hôpitaux de Paris, STIM/DSI, Paris, France
[c] INALCO, CRIM, Paris, France

Abstract

Open-domain Question-Answering (QA) systems heavily rely on named entities, a set of general-purpose semantic types which generally cover names of persons, organizations and locations, dates and amounts, etc. If we are to build medical QA systems, a set of medically relevant named entities must be used. In this paper, we explore the use of the UMLS (Unified Medical Language System) Semantic Network semantic types for this purpose. We present an experiment where the French part of the UMLS Metathesaurus, together with the associated semantic types, is used as a resource for a medically-specific named entity tagger. We also explore the detection of Semantic Network relations for answering specific types of medical questions. We present results and evaluations on a corpus of French-language medical documents that was used in the EQueR Question-Answering evaluation forum. We show, using statistical studies, that strategies for using these new tags in a QA context are to take in account the individual origin of documents.

Keywords:
Natural Language Processing; Information Retrieval; Language; France; UMLS; Funding, Non-US Government

1. Introduction

An increasing volume of good-quality textual knowledge bases is available in the medical domain, mostly through the development of the Web. Whereas the largest part of these documents is in English, an increasing proportion uses other languages. For instance, high-quality medical documents in French are available through the CISMeF catalog of French medical web sites [1]. The interest of Medical Question-Answering (henceforth QA) systems, which aim to bring precise, short answers to medical questions [2], has been highlighted recently [3]. These systems should benefit from these large document collections.

QA systems generally rely on an indexing of *named entities* [4] (names of persons and locations, dates and amounts, etc.), which are the focus of most questions in open-domain QA. In medical QA, we consider that named entities (henceforth NE) should be adapted to the domain [3]. An appropriate set of classes of entities is therefore necessary: we propose to use the UMLS semantic types for this purpose.

In this paper, we describe an experiment in indexing a French-language medical text collection, obtained from health-oriented Web sites, with UMLS (Unified Medical

Language System) concepts and semantic types. We evaluate the quality of these indexes both intrinsically (appropriateness of UMLS tags *wrt* the corresponding text) and in a goal-oriented task (relevance to help answer a specific question). We show that strategies for using these new tags in a QA context are to take in account the individual origin of documents.

2. Material and Methods

2.1 Material

Our corpus is the text collection prepared for the EQueR 2004 evaluation of French QA systems [5] (http://www.technolangue.net/article61.html). It consists of the documents indexed by the CISMeF catalog for nine sites (see table 1), extended with the documents to which they point (through HTML links) on the same sites. In the UMLS, we used the French terms and their associated concepts from the Metathesaurus 2002AA, together with their semantic types in the Semantic Network.

Table 1: Web sites from which the corpus was collected

[CANCER]	www.fnclcc.fr & www.fnclcc.com : French national federation of anti-cancer centers
[DOCFRA]	www.ladocfrancaise.gouv.fr & www.ladocumentationfrancaise.fr : French official documentation institute
[AFSSAPS]	afssaps.sante.fr : French agency for health safety of health products (former Drug Agency)
[ANAES]	www.anaes.fr : National agency for accreditation and evaluation in health
[ORPHA]	www.orpha.net : Information on rare diseases
[SENAT]	www.senat.fr : official site of the French Senate
[CHUROUEN]	www.chu-rouen.fr : Rouen School of Medicine
[UROUEN]	www.univ-rouen.fr : Rouen University, medical branch
[CANADA]	www.hc-sc.gc.ca : bilingual site of Health Canada, federal department of information on health

2.2 Tagging UMLS Semantic Types in French Texts

The first step of our method consists in locating occurrences of UMLS semantic types inside the corpus. For the English language, there exist UMLS linguistic companion tools such as the Specialist Lexicon [6], which can be used for instance in UMLS-oriented indexing tasks [7]. In contrast, the French language cannot benefit today from such tools (this situation should improve, nevertheless, thanks to the recent UMLF initiative [8]). Therefore, we resort to a mixture of general-purpose tools and specifically-developed methods.

We first tag the corpus with part-of-speech (POS) information (noun, verb, etc.) with Tree-Tagger   (http://www.ims.uni-stuttgart.de/projekte/corplex/TreeTagger/DecisionTreeTagger.html). We then use POS patterns to locate noun phrases [9]. Then, for each located noun phrase, we look for all the French strings in the UMLS Metathesaurus that contain at least one common word with the phrase. This builds a lattice of terms, from which only the maximal elements are retained: those that share the maximum number of words with a Metathesaurus term. The phrase is then tagged with the concepts and the semantic types associated with these maximal elements. This method allows for example to locate the UMLS concept for *oedème papillaire* (CUI = C0030353, *Papillary edema*) inside the phrase "oedème bilatéral papillaire" (bilateral papillary edema), though the latter is not an UMLS string.

After noun-phrase processing, our system tries to extract *clauses* from the corpus, a *clause* being a segment of text that is roughly structured as **[Subject part][Verb part][Complement part]**. Relying on punctuation-based segmentation was not possible due to a lot of noise in the corpus. Therefore the system uses, here again, part-of-speech patterns. Clauses aim to define regions within which we want to detect the cooccurrence of previously located semantic types. If such a cooccurrence occurs, and the two semantic types are linked by a possible semantic relation in the UMLS Semantic Network, the clause is tagged with this possible semantic relation. This completes the tagging step.

2.3 Quantitative Evaluations of the Tagging Process

French language is poorly represented in the UMLS (this situation should also evolve, thanks to the VuMEF initiative [10]). This may cause the above tagging procedure to remain silent in some cases (missing tags). In the same time, a lot of general terms are associated with UMLS concepts, which may cause false tagging. We have evaluated these two aspects of the tagging process by evaluating, on the one hand, for missing tags, the proportion of:

- **false negatives**: phrases that were not tagged, but should have been, given their medical meaning meaning (*e.g.*, "curage ganglionnaire" – *lymph node dissection*);
- **true negatives**: phrases that were rightly not tagged ("cadre stratégique national" for instance);
- **indecision**: ambiguous cases, for which we preferred not to decide ("enfermement familial",or"entourage ultraviolent" for instance).

and on the other hand, for false tagging, the proportion of:

- **correct**: phrases that were tagged according to their meanings;
- **incomplete**: phrases for which not all aspects of the meaning were tagged; *e.g.*, tagging "atteinte gastrointestinale" with T047 (*disease or syndrome*) is incomplete since "atteinte" is tagged, but not "gastrointestinal";
- **incorrect**: phrases for which the meaning of the semantic type is clearly different from the intended meaning of the phrase.

2.4 Selection of a Semantic Relation as a Named Entity, and Performance Analysis

Our experiment aimed at evaluating the performance of UMLS semantic relations as named entities in a QA context. As 53 semantic relations was a too big number for an exhaustive study in a preliminary work, we decided to focus our efforts on a specifically selected relation. The goodness of fit of the corpus tagging with the semantic relation was the main criterion of our selection.

In order to assess this goodness of fit, we assume that the meaning of a clause is closely related to the meaning of its verbal part. Exploratory Data Analysis techniques are natural tools to reveal relationships between the verbs and the projected semantic relations. We tried correspondence analysis and clustering techniques [11, 12], and we finally kept the latter as a selection tool.

In a QA context, the above-chosen semantic relation is used as a criterion to select clauses as answers to medical questions, here related to suitable treatments given some symptoms. The last step of our study therefore consisted in evaluating the precision of answers obtained through this semantic relation.

3. Results

3.1 Quantitative Measures of the Tagging

Table 2a gives the overall density of tags in the corpus. It shows that about 37 % of the noun phrases have been attached to at least one semantic type. The proportion of *missing tags* was evaluated by manually inspecting a random sample of untagged noun phrases. In the same way, the *false tagging* proportion was evaluated by examining a random sample of tagged noun phrases. In each case, the size of the sample was 300 phrases. The results can be read in tables 2, and can roughly been summarized by saying that about half of the phrases were correctly tagged.

Table 2: Evaluation of the tagging

Item	Number
Noun phrases occurrences	4101404
Distinct noun phrases	393966
... tagged	147007
... not tagged	246959

(a) Density of tags in the corpus

Item	Rate
True negatives	45 %
False negatives	25 %
Indecision	30 %

(b) Missing tags

Item	Rate
Correct	52 %
Incomplete	32 %
Incorrect	16 %

(c) Tags correctness

3.2 Semantic Relations and Clause Verbs

An Ascending Hierarchical Classification of the semantic relations, according to the verbs of the clauses in which these relations are suspected to occur (due to the cooccurrence of semantic types) allowed us to investigate the match between the meaning of the relations and the meaning of the clauses. The overall aspect of the obtained dendrogram showed us the most relevant clusters of relations. For each of these groups, we looked for the verbs that contributed the most to the eccentricity of the group. We have postulated that the match was good when the meanings of these verbs were clearly related to the meanings of the relations inside the group.

This analysis led us to focus on the cluster made up by relations *treats* and *prevent*. Table 3 shows the most contributive verbs for that group. French readers can convince themselves of the fit between the medical usage of these verbs and the meaning of the two relations. Finally, we kept only the *treats* relation to pursue our study.

Table 3: Most contributive verbs for {treats, prevents}

Verb	Eccentricity fraction	Cumulated eccent. Frac.	Verb	Eccentricity fraction	Cumulated eccent. Frac.
Envisager (to envisage)	0.0599	0.0599	Modifier (to modify)	0.0275	0.2325
Traiter (to treat)	0.0465	0.1064	Rédiger (to write)	0.0264	0.2589
Justifier (to justify)	0.0360	0.1424	Proposer (to propose)	0.0241	0.2830
Discuter (to discuss)	0.0331	0.1755	Recommander (to recommend)	0.0209	0.3039
Donner (to give)	0.0295	0.2020			

3.3 The treats Relation as a Named Entity

On a random sample, we estimated the precision of the tags obtained thank to the *treats* relation, when it is used alone to extract answers to questions such as "what is the treatment for ..." (which is one of the question types that usually arise during a consultation [2]). We consider that an extraction is successful when the extracted clause contains both the treatment and the symptom or the pathology, and that it fails when the extracted clause is not related to the question, or only contains a truncated answer (for example because of anaphoric references).

A separate sample was drawn from each source making up the corpus. The source by source results are shown in table 4.

Table 4: Precision of treats *in extracting treatment-sign associations, ordered by increasing success rate*

Source	Noun phrases number	treats-tagged noun phrases number	Sampling	Successful (%)	(%)
SENAT	199372	1265 (0.6 %)	200	10	2.1
CANADA	90986	2743 (3.0 %)	200	16	2.6
CHUROUEN	10232	230 (2.2 %)	200	19	2.8
UROUEN	14799	621 (4.2 %)	200	20	2.8
AFSSAPS	5187	202 (3.9 %)	202	20	0.0
ANAES	125659	4174 (3.3 %)	200	22	2.9
ORPHA	1460	25 (1.7 %)	25	27	0.0
CANCER	47356	2325 (4.9 %)	200	32	3.3

We can see that tagging with the *treats* relation behaves quite differently depending on the original source to which it is applied. Extreme cases are **[SENAT]** (low tagging rate, and low success rate) and **[CANCER]** (higher tagging rate, and good precision).

The natures of the original sources are quite different from each other: **[SENAT]** is rather legislation-oriented, **[CANADA]** is medically oriented, and aimed to the general public. At the opposite end, **[CANCER]** is a very focused site, intended for specialists. Table 4 shows that the performance of *treats* increases as the intended skills of the users grow higher. Correspondence Analysis, computed on the tagged corpus, has given us more insight of this phenomena, by revealing the structure of the tagged corpus [9].

It is interesting to notice that the differences we have measured among the distinct sources do not come from differences in the density of tagging, but really from differences in the level of specialization of the language used in the documents of each specific source.

4. Discussion and Conclusion

We have presented an experiment in tagging a French corpus with UMLS concepts and, to some extent, with semantic relations, in the context of a Question-Answering system. The amount of incorrect tags (noise) or of missing tags (silence) was evaluated, but a more useful evaluation is linked to an actual task, here QA: the precision of answers generated for *treats*-type questions. A conclusion of this study is that when using the *treats* relation, one is to take into account the individual origin of the documents in which the search is done. Search strategies including this fact now have to be worked out.

Given the status of French in the version of the UMLS that we used, UMLS concept-tagging is very close to MeSH-tagging. The techniques used in the current English- or French-MeSH taggers (see, *e.g.*, [7, 13]) would therefore also be useful in the present task. Besides, the inclusion of an increasing number of French terms and synonyms in the UMLS should enhance the content coverage of French texts; UMLS version 2004AC contains 57,571 French strings, which can be further extended with terms from ICD-10 and from the French translation of SNOMED International [10].

Further work indeed still needs to be done to improve the tagging process, by using more elaborate linguistic tools. This should allow us (i) to use syntactic structures that could be more complex than the approximate clause structure we have used here; (ii) to be able to assert more precisely the presence of a semantic relation in the text, not only by using cooccurrences between semantic types, but also by using dependency analysis of the text; and (iii) to try to take into account anaphora, when this is tractable.

Besides, all statistical aspects of the tagged corpus have not been investigated yet; the dendrogram of the Ascending Hierarchical Classification shows other potentially interesting candidates to study, such as for example the *causes* and *diagnoses* relations. Entities based on these relations may be used to find answers to questions relative to diagnosis.

5. References

[1]   Darmoni SJ, Leroy JP, Thirion B, et al. CISMeF: a structured health resource guide. Methods Inf Med 2000;39(1):30–5.

[2]   Alper BS, Stevermer JJ, White DS, and Ewigman BG. Answering family physicians' clinical questions using electronic medical databases. J Fam Pract 2001;50(11):960–5. Available at http://www.jfponline.com/content/2001/11/jfp110109600.asp.

[3]   Zweigenbaum P. Question answering in biomedicine. In: de Rijke M and Webber B, eds, Proceedings Workshop on Natural Language Processing for Question Answering, EACL 2003, Budapest. ACL, 2003:1–4.

[4]   Harabagiu S and Moldovan D. Tutorial on open-domain textual question answering. In: Proceedings of the 19th COLING, Taipei, Taiwan. 24 August– 1 September 2002.

[5]   Grau B. EQueR: Évaluation de systèmes de Questions Réponses. Project definition, LIMSI-CNRS, Orsay, France, 2002. Part of the EVALDA evaluation initiative, ELDA, Paris, France.

[6]   McCray AT and Nelson SJ. The semantics of the UMLS knowledge sources. Methods Inf Med 1995;34(1/2).

[7]   Aronson AR. Effective mapping of biomedical text to the UMLS Metathesaurus: The MetaMap program. J Am Med Inform Assoc 2001;8(suppl).

[8]   Zweigenbaum P, Baud R, Burgun A, et al. A unified medical lexicon for French. International Journal of Medical Informatics 2004. To appear.

[9]   Delbecque T. Structuration de corpus médicaux par l'UMLS. Utilisabilité comme source d'entités nommées pour les systèmes de questions-réponses. Rapport de DEA, Informatique Médicale, Université Paris 5, 2004.

[10] Darmoni SJ, Jarrousse E, Zweigenbaum P, et al. Extending the French part of the UMLS. In: Musen M, ed, Proceedings AMIA Annual Fall Symposium 2003, Washington, DC. AMIA, November 2003:824–. (poster).

[11] Benzécri JP. Correspondances, (vol2). Dunod, 1979.

[12] Benzécri JP. La taxinomie, (vol1). Dunod, 1984.

[13] Ruch P, Baud R, and Geissbühler A. Learning-free text categorization. In: Dojat M, ed, 9th Conference on Artificial Intelligence in Medicine Europe, Cyprus. 2003:199–204.

Address for correspondence

Pierre Zweigenbaum, Mission de recherche en Sciences et Technologies de l'Information Médicale, STIM/DSI, Hôpital Broussais, 96, rue Didot, 75674 Paris Cedex 14, France
E-mail: pz@biomath.jussieu.fr Url: http://www.biomath.jussieu.fr/~pz/

Breaking the Language Barrier: Machine Assisted Diagnosis Using the Medical Speech Translator

Marianne Starlander[a], Pierrette Bouillon[a], Manny Rayner[a,b], Nikos Chatzichrisafis[a],

Beth Ann Hockey[b], Hitoshi Isahara[c], Kyoko Kanzaki[c], Yukie Nakao[c],

Marianne Santaholma[a]

[a]University of Geneva, TIM/ISSCO, Geneva, Switzerland
[b]UCSC/NASA Ames Research Center,
Moffett Field,California, USA
[c]NICT, Kyoto, Japan

Abstract

In this paper, we describe and evaluate an Open Source medical speech translation system (MedSLT) intended for safety-critical applications. The aim of this system is to eliminate the language barriers in emergency situation. It translates spoken questions from English into French, Japanese and Finnish in three medical sub-domains (headache, chest pain and abdominal pain), using a vocabulary of about 250-400 words per sub-domain. The architecture is a compromise between fixed-phrase translation on one hand and complex linguistically-based systems on the other. Recognition is guided by a Context Free Grammar Language Model compiled from a general unification grammar, automatically specialised for the domain. We present an evaluation of this initial prototype that shows the advantages of this grammar-based approach for this particular translation task in term of both reliability and use.

Keywords
Medical informatics; Diagnosis, computer assisted; Natural language processing; speech translation.

1. Introduction

Language is crucial to medical diagnosis. During the initial evaluation of a patient in an emergency department, obtaining an accurate history of the chief complaint is of equal importance to the physical examination. However, this physician-patient communication is often made substantially difficult because of language barriers: in many parts of the world there are large recent immigrant populations that require medical care but are unable to communicate fluently in the local language.

One solution to this problem would be to use human translators. Unfortunately, trained interpreters are only too rarely available in emergency cases, as it is quite expensive to provide every hospital with medical interpretation resources (see [1] for a description of the situation in the USA). Most of the time doctors have to rely on improvised translators such as relatives, acquaintances or hospital employees with no medical training that happen to speak the language in question. This situation can be dramatic for the patient. In particular, the study by Glenn Flores, Professor of Paediatrics at the Boston University Schools of Medicine, shows that errors of interpretation are often responsible for errors in diagnosis [2]. It is therefore crucial to find a reliable and cost-effective alternative to the more expensive solution of providing a pool of trained emergency interpreters for each hospital. Our system is designed to address this problem using *spoken machine translation*.

Designing a spoken translation system to obtain a detailed medical history would be well beyond state of the art if we had to build a general system capable of translating anything the doctor or patient might wish to say. The reason that the use of spoken translation technology is feasible is because what is actually needed in the emergency setting is more limited. Since medical histories traditionally are obtained through two-way physician-patient conversations that are mostly physician initiative, there is a pre-established limiting structure that we can follow in designing the translation system. Our starting point is that this limited structure allows a physician to successfully use one way translation to elicit and restrict the range of patient responses while still obtaining the necessary information.

Another helpful constraint is that examinations can be divided into smaller sub-domains based on symptom types, for example headaches, chest pains, abdominal pains, and so on. This gives the possibility of further constraining the range of utterances that needs to be recognized at any point in the dialogue. For example, standard examination questions about chest pain include intensity, location, duration, quality of pain, and factors that increase or decrease the pain. The answers to these questions can be successfully communicated by a limited number of one or two word responses (e.g. yes/no, left/right, numbers) or even gestures (e.g. nodding or shaking the head, pointing to an area of the body). The above observations suggest that this is a domain in which the constraints of the task are sufficient for a limited domain, one way spoken translation system to be a useful tool.

The aim of this paper is to describe an Open Source toolkit (MedSLT, [3]) supporting quick development of this kind of speech translation systems for limited emergency diagnosis sub-domains. Although most spoken translation systems use statistical speech recognition [4], we show that a grammar-based approach is more suitable for this kind of task. This approach produces greater speech recognition accuracy, which is more important in the medical setting than robustness.

2. The MedSLT system

MedSLT [3] is an Open Source project which is developing a generic platform for building medical speech translation systems; early versions are described in [5], [6]. The basic philosophy behind the MedSLT system architecture is to attempt an intelligent compromise between fixed-phrase translation on one hand (e.g. (Phraselator [7]) and linguistically motivated grammar-based processing on the other (e.g. Verbmobil [8]) and Spoken Language Translator [9].

At run-time, the system behaves essentially like a phrasal translator which allows some variation in the input language. This is close in spirit to the approach used in most normal phrase-books, which typically allow "slots" in at least some phrases ("How do I get to---?"). However, in order to minimize the overhead associated with defining and maintaining large sets of phrasal patterns, these patterns are derived from a single large linguistically motivated unification grammar, using the Open Source Regulus platform [6], [10], which implements an example-based specialisation method driven by small corpora of examples.

The linguistically motivated compile-time architecture makes the system easy to extend and modify. In particular, it makes it easy to port the grammar between different medical sub-domains, which seem to be quite convergent. For example, the first version of the system covered only the headache sub-domain; when we ported the English grammar to the new chest pain sub-domain, over 80% of the training sentences could be analysed correctly as soon as we had added the relevant new vocabulary.

The translation module is implemented in SICStus Prolog, and is interlingua-based. Translation consists of four stages illustrated in Figure 1: (1) mapping from the source representation to interlingua; (2) ellipsis processing; (3) mapping from interlingua to the target representation and (4) generation, using a suitably compiled Regulus grammar for the target language. In accordance with the generally minimalist design philosophy of the project, semantic representations have been kept as simple as possible, namely a flat list of attribute-value pairs.

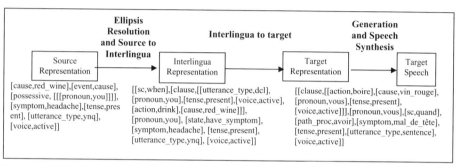

Figure 1: Translation flow in MedSLT for the source sentence: "Does red wine cause your headaches"
Target: "Avez-vous vos maux de tête quand vous buvez du vin rouge"

The run time system provides a GUI based interface, which allows the user to select the input and output languages and the sub-domain. The user initiates speech recognition through a push-to-talk interface.

Both the string of words produced by the speech recognizer (what the system heard) and a back-translation from the interlingua (what the system understood), are displayed on the screen, after which the user can choose either to proceed with the translation or to abort in the case of apparently unsuccessful speech understanding. Output speech is produced using either pre-recorded waveforms or the Nuance VocalizerTM TTS engine, depending on the output language. It is important to realise that the recognised words and the back-translation can be quite different, particularly when translating incomplete utterances. For example, if the previous utterance was "Do the headaches typically last more than an hour?", the follow-on question "More than two hours?" would be back-translated as "Do the headaches usually last more than two hours?".

If the system is unable to produce any translation, the system invokes a simple context-sensitive help module. This uses the result of traditional recognition using a statistical language model (SLM) to display a list of in-coverage example sentences. Examples are selected from a predefined list, using a heuristic which prioritises sentences maximizing the number of words and phrases shared with those extracted from the SLM recognition result.

The current prototype covers the three subdomains of headaches, chest pains, and abdominal pains, and can translate from English into French, Japanese and Finnish. The Finnish version is still under development, and is not as mature as the other two. Initial versions supporting translation from Japanese, French and Spanish and to Spanish are also available. Some examples of English-French translations are given in Table 1.

Table 1: Examples of collected data and translation by MedSLT

Source language	Target language
'Do sudden head movements make the pain worse?'	'La douleur empire-t-elle quand vous bougez soudainement la tête ?'
'Is your headache relieved by sleep?'	'Vos maux de tête s'améliorent-ils quand vous dormez ?'

3. Evaluation

In the long-term, the real question we would like to answer when evaluating the prototype is whether this system is practically useful for doctors. As a first step, we compare the performance of the grammar-based architecture on the medical examination task with that of a second version of the system. This version was built using a statistical language model (SLM) created with the help of the Nuance SayAnything tool [11], and trained on the same data as the GLM version. In the following sections, we present a comparison of these two versions of the MedSLT system. It is striking to see that the two systems give nearly the same results on the training data, but that when judged on a real task the GLM version clearly outperforms the SLM. We used the headache version of the Open Source MedSLT system [3] to perform our experiments. Both versions of the recogniser were trained from the same corpus of 575 standard examination questions put together by Dr. Vol Van Dalsem III[1].

We collected data from 12 native speakers of English. Each subject was first given a short acclimatization session, where they used a prepared list of ten in-coverage sentences to learn how to use the microphone and the push-to-talk interface. They were then encouraged to play the part of a doctor, and conduct an examination interview, through the system, on a team member who simulated a patient suffering from a specific type of headache. The subject's task was to identify the type correctly out of a list of eight possibilities. Half of the subjects used the grammar-based version of the system, and half used the SLM based version. We collected a total of 870 recorded utterances.

The recorded data was first transcribed, and then processed through offline versions of both the grammar-based (GLM) and statistical SLM processing paths in the system. This was done as follows. We first set the system to translate from English into English (via the interlingua), and then had an English-speaking judge evaluate each back-translation. Utterances for which the back-translation was judged acceptable were regarded as correctly recognised, and were then translated further into the target languages French and Japanese.

Translations to French and Japanese were judged for acceptability by native speaker judges for each language: there were six judges for French, and three for Japanese. Judges were asked to categorise translations as "good", "ok" or "bad". For each target language, and each processing method (GLM or SLM), we consolidated the results using a majority voting scheme. If two-thirds of the judges (i.e. four for French, or two for Japanese) agreed that the translation was clearly "good" or "bad", we counted the translation as belonging to the appropriate category. Otherwise, we counted it as "ok". The results of this judging are shown below.

---

[1] El Camino Hospital, Mountain View, California.

Table 2: Recognition and Translation quality

		GLM	SLM		GLM	SLM	
French	Bad recognition	54.6%	59.8%	**Japanese**	54.6%	59.8%	Bad recognition
	Good translation	34.4%	30.8%		36.4%	32.8%	Good translation
	Ok translation	8.7%	7.7%		3.6%	3.3%	Ok translation
	Bad translation	0.3%	0.2%		0.5%	0.5%	Bad translation
	No translation	2.0%	1.5%		4.9%	3.7%	No translation

4. Discussion

We will now attempt to draw some general conclusions about the relative performance of GLM and SLM processing in these experiments. As shown in Table 2, the GLM produces fewer recognition errors (54.6%) than the SLM (59.8%). Although these figures are quite high for both systems, these results should be interpreted in the light of further results (cf. [12]) clearly showing the difference in performance between the two recognisers on in-coverage data. The GLM (5.7%) clearly out-performs the SLM (12.7%) on in-coverage sentences measured in terms of WER. This pattern is inverted for the out of coverage sentences, where the SLM outscores the GLM by 47.8% to 57.5%.

This confirms our intuition that the SLM version is more robust than the GLM but that the GLM is more precise. If a sentence is in the coverage of the GLM, global constraints usually insure that the sentence is well recognised and translated. The extra robustness offered by the SLM does indeed result in a lower word error rate on the out-of-coverage data, but what counts in this type of medical speech translation task, where partial translations are worse than useless, is to achieve a correct output on in-coverage data.

The ratio of in-coverage to out-of-coverage in the dataset is however mainly a function of how familiar the subjects are with the system's coverage. An experienced user will produce mostly in-coverage data; a novice user will produce mostly out-of-coverage data.

Table 3: Learning effect: improvement of recognition quality.

		GLM	SLM			GLM	SLM
Help	All data	54.0%	61.1%	Help	All data	55.3%	58.4%
system	First quarter	58.6%	65.8%	system	First quarter	63.1%	64.1%
OFF	Last quarter	52.1%	58.1%	ON	Last quarter	45.9%	56.0%
	Improvement	6.5%	7.7%		Improvement	17.2%	8.1%

A critical point is thus the capacity of the subjects to improve their performance with increased familiarity. This improvement is especially noticeable for the subjects using the GLM system: as people become more expert, they gravitate towards the intended coverage, and robustness becomes less important. We can get some idea of what's happening here by contrasting performance for the two architectures averaged over the first and last quarters of each session. Table 3 presents the recognition scores for the GLM and SLM comparing the start of a session to the end of the session. A lot of the improvement seems to be due to the help system. Subjects with access to the help system improved much more between the first quarter session and the last. The difference in improvement only occurs if the GLM system is being used, not surprisingly since the help system is steering users towards the grammar's coverage.

5. Conclusion

We have described an approach to automatic limited medical speech translation, and compared two different architectures. We conclude that a grammar-based architecture is more effective for the task, particularly when combined with the inclusion of an intelligent help component. With the grammar-based architecture and the help component, Table 3 shows a dramatic improvement in subjects' performance even over short sessions averaging 60 utterances in length. These results, and other informal studies we have conducted, suggest that a new user would be able to achieve a useful level of performance after only a few hours of practice with the system. Within the next few months, we hope to be able to gain more data on the system's utility as we begin to test it in a simulated emergency room setting.

6. Acknowledments

The MedSLT project is funded by the Fonds National de la Recherche Suisse (FNRS) and the Japanese National Institute of Information and Communications Technology. Finally we would like to thank Vol Van Dalsem for his expert advice.

7. References

[1]   Loviglio, J. Interpreters Lower Risks in Hospitals, Article by Associated Press writer published on various internet news sites on 21 November 2004

[2]   Flores G, Laws B, Mayo S, Zuckerman B, Abreu M, Medina L, and Hardt EJ. Errors in medical interpretation and their potential clinical consequences in pediatric encounters. *Pediatrics* 2003:111 pp: 6-14.

[3]   MedSLT, http://sourceforge.net/projects/medslt/. As of 12 January 2005.

[4]   Akiba Y, Federico M, Kando N, Nakaiwa H, Paul M and Tsujii J. Overview of the IWSLT04 Evaluation Campaign. In: *Proceedings of the International Workshop on Spoken Language Translation IWSLT04*, Kyoto, Japan, pp. 1-12.

[5]   Rayner M, Bouillon P. A flexible Speech to Speech Phrasebook Translator. In: *Proceedings of the 40th Annual Meeting of the Association for Computational Linguistics Workshop on Speech-to-Speech Translation: Algorithms and Systems*, Philadelphia, PA, 2002, pp. 69-76.

[6]   Rayner M, Hockey BA and Dowding J. An Open Source Environment for Compiling Typed Unification Grammars into Speech Recognisers. In: *Proceedings of the 10th European Association for Computational Linguistics (demo track)*, Budapest, Hungary, 2003, pp. 223-226.

[7]   Phraselator, http://www.phraselator.com. As of 12 January 2005.

[8]   Wahlster W. *Verbmobil: Foundations of Speech-to-Speech Translation*, Springer, 2000.

[9]   Rayner M, Carter D, Bouillon P, Digalakis V and Wirén M, eds. *The Spoken Language Translator*, Cambridge University Press, 2000.

[10]   Regulus, http://sourceforge.net/projects/regulus/. As of 12 January 2005.

[11]   Nuance, http://www.nuance.com. As of 12 January 2005.

[12]   Bouillon P, Rayner M, Chatzichrisafis N, Hockey BA, Santaholma M, Starlander M, Nakao Y, Kanzaki K, Isahara H. A Generic Multi-Lingual Open Source Platform for Limited-Domain Medical Speech Translation. In: Proceedings of the 10th International Conference of the European Association for Machine Translation, Budapest, Hungary, 2005.

Address for correspondence

Marianne Starlander, University of Geneva, ETI/TIM/ISSCO, 40, bd. du Pont d'Arve, 1211 Genève 4, Tel. ++41.22.379.86.78 Email. Marianne.starlander@eti.unige.ch http://www.issco.unige.ch/projects/medslt/

Connecting Medical Informatics and Bio-Informatics
R. Engelbrecht et al. (Eds.)
IOS Press, 2005

Automatic Annotation of Medical Records

Ján Antolík

Institute of Computer Science AS CR, Department of the Medical Informatics, Prague, Czech Republic

Abstract

One of the research projects running at the medical informatics department of the Institute of Computer Science AS CR explores the problem of medical information representation and development of electronic health record (EHR). With respect to this effort an interesting problem arises: how to transfer knowledge from a medical record written in a free text form into a structured electronic format represented by the EHR. Currently, this task was solved by writing extraction rules (regular expressions) for every element of information that is to be extracted from the medical record. However, such approach is very time consuming and requires supervision of a skilled programmer whenever the target area of medicine is changed. In this article we explore the possibility to mechanize this process by automatically generating the extraction rules from a pre-annotated corpus of medical records. Since we are currently in the phase of data acquisition and preliminary tests we will not present any final results, rather we will sketch the technologies we intend to use and describe the tools that were developed so far as a part of this project.

Keywords:
Natural Language Processing; Medical Records; Artificial Intelligence

1. Introduction

Development of Electronic Health Record (EHR) is one of the key projects running within the scope of research at the Medical Informatics department of Institute of Computer Science AS CR. In EHR, knowledge contained in a medical record is stored in a structured form suitable for computer processing. This is an important prerequisite for any further development of applications that are capable to process medical information in a more intelligent manner. However, the development of EHR reveals a new problem: how to extract relevant information from medical record written by a physician in a free text form. A straightforward solution would be to write a separate extraction rule for every single element of information that we are concerned with. However, such solution has some obvious disadvantages. First of all writing of these rules might be very time consuming, especially if we consider the fact, that the number of entries we need to collect can reach hundreds only within the scope of single medical area such as cardiology. Another problem that is sometimes overlooked is the fact that the process of creation of the extraction rules requires a close cooperation of the programmer and specialists within the target medical area. Such cooperation, however, might often turn out problematic and slow down the development even further. The final observation is that whenever the list of collected data elements is changed we have to repeat the whole process again.

As a consequence of the previous facts, we would like to automate the process of generation of the extraction rules and thus eliminate the involvement of programmer from the process. Naturally, specialists from the target area are still required, because we will always need some source of information from which the extraction rules can be deduced. In this article we will discuss our effort to build such automated system. Finally, let us note that our project focuses on the Czech language, which is a natural consequence of the fact that it is the language in which we are capable to collect the pre-annotated medical records from the cooperating physicians. However, since many problems we came across so far are beyond the language barriers, we believe that the knowledge collected in this project will be applicable also to systems working with different languages.

2. Information extraction

Information extraction (IE) is a field of computer science that studies automatic extraction of information from textual sources usually written in natural language. As the description of this discipline indicates it is of great interest for us since it may offer techniques that can help us solve the problem identified in the previous section. In fact several algorithms for automatic generation of extraction rules have been developed in this field such as RAPIER [1], SRV [2], WHISK [3], $(LP)^2$ [4] etc. In such systems the background knowledge comes in the form of pre-annotated corpus of texts. An annotation includes data about the start and end of subtext in the document and the type of information that is stored in this subtext (e.g. pulse rate). Such corpus is then fed to the system, which after several iterations over the corpus offers the learned extraction rules as the output, where each of these extraction rules corresponds to a single type of information that is to be extracted.

For our project we have decided to use the AMILCARE [5] system developed by Fabio Ciravegna at Department of Computer Science, University of Sheffield. AMILCARE is based on the $(LP)^2$ algorithm, which is a supervised algorithm that falls into a class of Wrapper Induction Systems using LazyNLP [6]. In the rest of this section we will briefly discuss the facts that supported our decision to use this particular system.

Probably the most important argument for integrating the AMILCARE system into our project is the performance of $(LP)^2$ algorithm compared to his other counterparts [5]. Another reason is that the AMILCARE system provides us with several means allowing us to supply it with some additional knowledge. For example gazetteers can be inserted into the system (for example a list of pharmaceutics or a list of possible diagnosis) or the input text can be extended with various tags that may help in the learning process. Another advantage is that the NLP pre-processing phase is separated from the main system and thus allows us to use custom tools, which is especially important with respect to the fact that we will work with texts written in Czech language. Finally AMILCARE contains also a Java API, which enables us to easily integrate the extraction rules produced by the system into our own application. Generally, to our best knowledge, AMILCARE is currently the most mature system for automatic extraction rule generation, ready to be deployed in real world problems.

3. Information extraction in medical records

Generally straightforward application of IE systems to biomedical data is problematic. The main reason comes from the fact that the performance of most IE systems depends on the performance of Natural Language Processing (NLP) tools that do the pre-processing of the input text and supply the IE system with additional information. Since these NLP tools are usually developed and tested over corpuses of more common types of texts such as newspaper articles, they do not achieve full performance when applied to biomedical data [8]. This fallback in performance naturally propagates further in the given IE system. Although there already are promising results in retraining some NLP tools over biomedical corpuses it is unlikely that such applications will soon be available for less widespread languages such as Czech, because the costs of collecting appropriate annotated training data are high.

Unfortunately, even further problems arise when we focus our attention to the medical health records. The most important difference between them and the majority of other analysed biomedical documents is that medical records are not written for the purpose of publication. Consequently the overall quality of the captured text is significantly lower. One of the most important negative effects is that medical health records are usually poorly structured. Further they contain a large number of typing errors that are very hard to detect by the IE tools. The use of character '*O*' instead of '*0*' or '*l*' instead of '*1*' is just another example of inconsistencies commonly contained in medical records. The virtual non-existence of division of the text into proper sentences prevents the application of more advanced NLP techniques such as part of speech tagging, which normally supply the IE system with valuable information. One of the most important goals of our projects is to find techniques that will overcome these problems specific to the medical health records.

Let us also note that system based solely on extraction rules restricts the type of information possibly retrieved from the medical record to such that is explicitly contained in the text as a string of characters. Therefore this approach helps us solve the problem only partially and the project discussed in this paper has to be viewed as the initial stage, preceding a system capable of extracting all required information from any medical record. However we believe that extraction rules will be capable to fill majority of the most common slots occurring in medical records and provide us with a good basis for the following stages of development, for example by identifying parts of text that are probably relevant with respect to the given more complicated type of information that we need to extract.

4. The state of the project

Within the scope of the discussed project, there were already few particular steps conducted. First of all, our collaborating physicians have built a list of medical concepts that are frequently explicitly expressed in medical health records in the area of cardiology. Next, before we can proceed to the learning phase, we need to collect the training set – the corpus of pre-annotated medical records that will be presented to the AMILCARE system. To date we have collected a corpus containing approximately 300 health records, enriched with more than 100 different types of medical annotations. For this purpose we have looked for a suitable existing tool, especially with respect to a simple user interface. Unfortunately, we were not successful. Therefore, we have decided to build our own annotation application, which we call simply *Anotátor*. The purpose of this application is to enable physicians insert annotations into the medical health records. The input of the application is a set of text documents (in our case the medical health records). The output is the original set of documents and a corresponding set of files containing the annotation information.

The main focus while developing this application was to make the annotation process as simple and as fast as possible. This is reflected by the very simple, yet efficient architecture of the application. It consists of a single main window that is divided into two main areas. On the left user can see the window containing the list of all information elements we intend to extract. Each such item may have several particular annotations attached. In the right part of the main window resides the view of the currently annotated document. All annotations are colourfully highlighted in the text. User can simply add annotations by selecting the given text with mouse and selecting the target annotation in the left view. In order to speed up the annotation process it is possible to load multiple texts into the system and then quickly scroll between them. Reader can see a screenshot of the *Anotátor* application on Figure 1.

The process of preparation of the training corpus for the AMILCARE system continues. Every medical record has to be enriched with NLP information in order to provide additional tokens that can be exploited in the formation of the extraction rules, thus possibly increasing the performance of the final system. For this purpose we use the Free Morfology [8] toolkit developed by Jan Hajič at the Institute of Formal and Applied Linguistics, School of Computer Science, Faculty of Mathematics and Physics of the Charles University. This tool is capable of extracting various linguistic information from a textual source. Currently, we use primarily the lemmatization engine and also word class identifiers. Further we add some simple flags such as *capitalized* word etc. The final step of the preprocessing phase is the integration of the NLP information, the annotations and the original texts into a single large file that serves as the input to the AMILCARE system. All the above described steps are mechanized by means of several interleaving PERL scripts. This way we have built a tool that recieves the list of all original texts and annotations data as the input and outputs a single large file that serves as the input to the AMILCARE system.

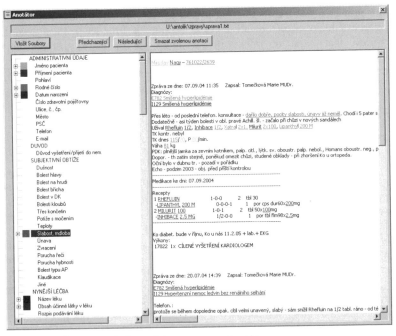

Figure1 - The main window of the program Anotátor

5. Preliminary results

Currently we have run the learning process for the first time with the basic settings and pre-processing as described in the previous section. We have not done deeper analysis of the results yet. Therefore, let us present only few initial observations. The first important fact is that out of the more than 100 different types of medical data that were selected for extraction only 41 had occurrence higher than 10 in the approximately 300 medical records included in the testing corpus. This means that we can build a system that may substantially reduce the amount of work physician have to conduct by looking only at relatively small subset of the collected data elements. On the other hand, in our experiments we face the problem of insufficient data for the more than 60 other data elements. In the rest of this section let us discuss only the more frequently occurring types of extracted information. This group subdivides into two subgroups – those cases where the performance of recall and precision reaches reasonable values and those which appear to be problematic (F-measure below 10). It is interesting that there are very few cases between these two groups – those with the F-measure in the range [10-50]. Another encouraging fact is that those cases which have reasonable values of F-measure thus are potentially useable already after this first preliminary training reach very high values of precession (but not necessarily also recall). This is a favourable condition, because it is usually acceptable for users when only partial help is provided, but it is frustrating to correct additional mistakes produced by the software. Finally let us present a table containing the list of more frequently occurring annotations with various performance statistics: Table 1.

Table 1 – A shortened table of annotations with their performance statistics system.

TAG	Possible	Actual	Correct	Wrong	Partial	Missing	Precision	Recall	F-mes
First name	146	119	113	1	5	28	94	80	86
Surname	142	89	83	5	1	58	93	58	72
Birth number	102	27	25	0	2	75	92	25	39
Birth date	42	31	28	2	1	13	90	68	77
Insurance company nummber	62	65	57	6	2	3	87	95	91
Address : street	82	14	12	1	1	69	85	14	25
Address: city	87	29	23	1	5	59	79	28	41
Address: postal code	38	37	30	4	3	5	81	85	83
Education	10	0	0	0	0	10	0	0	0
Physical activity	13	0	0	0	0	13	0	0	0
Alergies to drugs	18	0	0	0	0	18	0	0	0
Smoking	41	17	16	0	1	24	94	40	56
Smoking quantity	14	0	0	0	0	14	0	0	0
Subjective bothers	17	0	0	0	0	17	0	0	0
Weight	94	87	76	9	2	16	87	82	84
Height	65	60	54	4	2	9	90	85	87
Pulse	82	39	33	6	0	49	84	40	54
Right arm systolic presure	94	71	62	3	6	26	87	70	77
Right arm diastolic presure	88	68	63	4	1	24	92	72	81
Left arm systolic presure	36	10	10	0	0	26	100	27	43
Right arm diastolic presure	36	10	6	1	3	27	60	18	27
Cholesterol total	44	2	1	0	1	42	50	2	4
Cholesterol hdl	49	48	32	7	9	8	66	80	72
Cholest ldl	37	31	25	5	1	11	80	69	74
Hypertension	43	22	16	2	4	23	72	41	52
Hypertension treatment	10	0	0	0	0	10	0	0	0
Diagnosis	32	26	26	0	0	6	100	81	89
Treatment : drug	23	2	1	0	1	21	50	4	8
Treatment : drug dosage	13	0	0	0	0	13	0	0	0
Father	25	27	24	3	0	1	88	96	92
Mother	23	23	22	1	0	1	95	95	95
Sibling	12	13	12	1	0	0	92	100	96

6. Conclusions

In this paper we have discussed the problem of transforming a medical health record into structured form. We are developing a system that should assist the physician in this activity by applying extraction rules to the free text medical records. As the means for building such system we use techniques and tools from the field of IE and NLP. We have also discussed several specific problems that arise when these systems are applied to the free text medical records. One of the main aims of this project is to analyse and possibly overcome these obstacles and successfully apply the IE tools. Although we are currently only in the initial phase of the experiments we have reported the preliminary results with few basic insights. We believe that a deeper analysis of these results will allow as modifying the various tools and parameters involved in the training process such that the performance will rise. Apart from finishing the experiments and building the full system, in the future we would like to explore the possibility of enabling the training of the system also during its deployment, thus allowing it to adapt to a particular user.

7. Acknowledgments

The work was supported by the grant number 1ET200300413 of the Academy of Sciences of the Czech Republic.

8. References

[1]   Freitag D.: Multistrategy learning for information extraction. In: *Proceedings 15th International Conf. on Machine Learning*, 1998, pp. 161—169.

[2]   Califf M., Mooney.: Relational learning of patternmatch rules for information extraction, *Working Papers of the ACL-97 Workshop in Natural Language Learning, pp. 9—15.*

[3]   Soderland S.: *Learning Information Extraction Rules for Semi-structured and Free Text*, Machine Learning. 1999.

[4]   Ciravegna F.: (LP)², an Adaptive Algorithm for Information Extraction from Web-related Texts. In: *Proceedings of the IJCAI-2001 Workshop on Adaptive Text Extraction and Mining, held in conjunction with the 17th International Conference on Artificial Intelligence (IJCAI-01)*, Seattle, August, 2001.

[5]   Ciravegna F.: Adaptive Information Extraction from Text by Rule Induction and Generalization. In: *Proceedings of 17th International Join Conference on Artificial Intelligence (IJCAI 2001)*, Seattle, August 2001.

[6]   AMILCARE Homepage: http://nlp.shef.ac.uk/amilcare/lp2.html

[7]   Campbell DA., Johnson SB.: Comparing syntactic complexity in medical and non-medical corpora. In: Suzanne Bakken, (Ed.), *AMIA 2001 – Proceedings of the Annual Symposium of the American Medical Informatics Association. A Medical Informatics Odyssey: Visions of the Future and Lessons from the Past*, pages 90–94.Washington, D.C., November 3-7, 1. Philadelphia, PA: Hanley & Belfus, 2001.

[8]   Hajic J.: *Disambiguation of Rich Inflection - Computational Morphology of Czech.* Charles University Press - Karolinum, in press

Address for correspondence

Ján Antolík,
Institute of Computer Science AS CR
Pod Vodarenskou vezi 2, 182 07 Prague 8, Czech Republic
antolik@euromise.cz
http://www.euromise.org

Connecting Medical Informatics and Bio-Informatics
R. Engelbrecht et al. (Eds.)
IOS Press, 2005

Evaluation of Medical Problem Extraction from Electronic Clinical Documents Using MetaMap Transfer (MMTx)

Stéphane Meystre, Peter J Haug

Department of Medical Informatics, University of Utah School of Medicine, Salt Lake City, Utah, U.S.

Abstract

To improve the use and quality of the electronic Problem List, which is at the heart of the problem-oriented medical record in development in our institution (Intermountain Health Care, Utah, U.S.), we developed an Automated Problem List system using Natural Language Processing (NLP) technologies. A key part of this system is a module that automatically extracts potential medical problems from free-text clinical documents. The NLP module uses MMTx, developed at the U.S. National Library of Medicine. Negation detection was added to this application by adapting a negation detection algorithm called NegEx. To evaluate the adequacy of the performance of the NLP module for our Automated Problem List system, we evaluated it with 160 electronic clinical documents of different types. Two different data sets for MMTx were used: the default full UMLS data set and a customised subset adapted to detect the set of 80 medical problems we are interested in. With the default data set, we measured a recall of 0.74 (95% CI 0.68-0.8) and a precision of 0.76 (0.69-0.82). The customised subset had a significantly better recall of 0.9 (0.85-0.94), and a non-significantly different precision of 0.69 (0.63-0.75).

Keywords:
Program Evaluation; Natural Language Processing; Medical Records, Problem-Oriented.

1. Introduction

The Medical Problem List is an important piece of the medical record as well as a central component of the problem-oriented medical record in development in our institution. To serve the functions it is designed for, the Problem List has to be as accurate and timely as possible. The Problem List application that is used currently is typically incomplete or inaccurate, and is often unused. To address this deficiency, we extended this tool with components designed to make the Problem List easy and efficient to maintain. We developed an application using Natural Language Processing (NLP) to harvest potential Problem List entries from the multiple free-text electronic documents available in our EMR (Electronic Medical Record). These proposed problems drive an application designed for management of the Problem List, and are proposed to the physicians for addition to the official Problem List. Physicians then accept the problems proposed by changing their state to *active*, *inactive*, or *resolved*, or reject them by changing their state to *error*. The global aim of our project is to automate the process of creating and maintaining a Problem List for hospitalised patients and thereby to help guarantee the timeliness, accuracy and completeness of this information.

The problem-oriented, Computer-based Patient Record (CPR) and the Problem List have seen renewed interest as an organisational tool in the recent years [1,2]. Advantages to the

Problem List are that it can be the central place for clinicians to obtain a concise view of all patients problems, that it facilitates associating clinical information in the record to a specific problem, and that it can encourage an orderly process of clinical problem solving and clinical judgement. The Problem List in a problem–oriented patient record also provides a context in which continuity of care is supported, preventing both redundant and repeated actions [1].

Since problems of interest are frequently referenced in clinical documents collected electronically, we chose to supplement the practice of manually entering problems by developing an application built with Natural Language Processing tools. Several systems designed to automatically map clinical text concepts to standardised vocabularies have been reported, like MetaMap [3] and IndexFinder [4]. MetaMap was developed by the U.S. National Library of Medicine (NLM), and is used to index text or to map information in the analysed text to UMLS concepts. The mapped concepts are ranked, but no negation detection is performed. Five steps are needed, beginning with noun phrases identification using the SPECIALIST minimal commitment parser[1], followed by variants generation, candidate phrases retrieval, and computing of a score for each candidate by comparing it with the input phrase, and ending with the mapping and ranking using the computed score. MetaMap has been shown to identify most concepts present in MEDLINE titles [5]. It has been used for Information Extraction in biomedical text [5,6] and has been shown capable of extracting the most critical findings in 91% of the documents in a prior study [7]. Independent negation detection is required when using MetaMap. The application does not discriminate between present and absent concepts. In the medical domain this is important due to the fact that findings and diseases are often described as absent. A few negation detection algorithms have been developed, like NegEx, a computationally simple algorithm using regular expressions [8], or the more complex general-purpose Negfinder [9]. These algorithms have been evaluated and have shown good results. NegEx has been shown to have a sensitivity of 94.5% and a specificity of 77.8% [8].

2. Materials and Methods

As mentioned earlier, the Automated Problem List (APL) system extracts potential medical problems from free-text medical documents, and uses NLP to achieve this task. The APL system is made of two main components: a background application and the Problem List management application. The background application does all the text processing and analysis and stores extracted problems in the central clinical database, called CDR (Clinical Data Repository). These problems can then be accessed by the Problem List management application integrated in our Clinical Information System. We are currently evaluating a prototype in which the background application looks for 80 different problems, principally diagnoses, that were selected based on their frequency of use in our field of evaluation (cardiovascular and general medicine). Document processing starts with detection of sections and sentences, and is followed by a text restructuring step, to prepare it for the NLP module. This module uses MMTx, the Java™ version of MetaMap. Some processing to reduce ambiguity is also required, to avoid confusion with common acronyms (e.g. "Mr." detected as mitral regurgitation). Since we are currently interested in 80 different problems, and not in the entire UMLS Metathesaurus content (UMLS version 2004AA contains over 1 million concepts[2]), we created a subset of the Metathesaurus adapted to our system. The selection process resulted in a reduction to about 0.25% of the original data set (from more than a million to about 2,500 concepts). This reduction made the NLP module

---

[1] http://ii.nlm.nih.gov/MTI/phrasex.shtml
[2] http://www.nlm.nih.gov/pubs/factsheets/umlsmeta.html

more than 3 times faster, and also improved accuracy. The process of selecting relevant concepts first consisted in the use of MetamorphoSys[3], an application provided with the UMLS that allows filtering the Metathesaurus based on source vocabularies, semantic types and other filters. To subset it further, we loaded the data into a MySQL[4] database for subsequent processing. A mapping table was manually built to link the 80 selected concepts with all related subconcepts (e.g. *Right Bundle Branch Block* was mapped to *Incomplete Right Bundle Branch Block, Complete Right Bundle Branch Block,* and *Other or unspecified Right Bundle Branch Block*). This table was built manually and was used to select relevant concepts in the UMLS subset. The final step was the creation of the MMTx data files. A tool called MMTx Data File Builder[5] is provided with MMTx and allows the creation of these files from UMLS Metathesaurus subsets or from custom built data sets.

As mentioned above, MMTx lacks negation detection: concepts are mapped the same way whether they are described as present or as absent. We therefore had to add this feature. To this end, the NLP module actually works in two steps: a first step uses MMTx to extract each potential medical problem, and a second step infers the state of each of those problems. During the first step, phrases recognised by MMTx are replaced by a tag containing the corresponding UMLS identifier (CUI). This transformed version of the sentence is then passed to a negation detection algorithm that infers the state of the mapped concept. In this second phase, we adapted the NegEx algorithm described above, and implemented it in Java. We used the improved version of NegEx, called NegEx 2[6].

Study design:

To determine the success of our approach, we conducted a descriptive laboratory resource's function study. Two standard measures were used to evaluate the accuracy of this Natural Language Processing system: precision, the proportion of problems found that were correct (equivalent to positive predictive value here), and recall, the proportion of problems present in the documents that were actually found (equivalent to sensitivity here). Another typical value combining precision (P) and recall (R) – the F-measure (equal to $(\beta^2+1)PR / (\beta^2P)+R)$ – was also calculated.

A medical problem was considered present if mentioned in the text as probable or certain in the present or the past (e.g. "the patient has asthma"; "past history positive for asthma"; "pulmonary oedema is probable"), and considered absent if negated in the text or not mentioned at all (e.g. "this test excluded diabetes…"; "he denies any asthma").

We randomly selected 160 clinical documents from a study population of adult inpatients seen in a cardiovascular unit of the LDS Hospital during the year 2002. Subjects were restricted to those who had stayed for at least 48 hours. These clinical documents were of various types, like radiology reports, procedure reports, history and physical exam reports, pathology reports, discharge summaries, progress notes, etc. They were processed by our background application, using the MMTxAPI and MMTx version 2.3.C. The system processed each document twice: once with the default data set, and once with our customised subset. The extracted problems and a transformed XML version of the document were then stored in a local database. This transformed version of the document uses an information model described in another publication [10]. It is used by the web-based review application mentioned below. A reference standard for problems present in these documents was created using an electronic chart review by physicians. Two independent physicians reviewed each electronic document using a web-based review

---

[3] http://www.nlm.nih.gov/research/umls/meta6.html
[4] http://www.mysql.com
[5] http://mmtx.nlm.nih.gov
[6] http://web.cbmi.pitt.edu/chapman/NegEx.html

application. When the two reviewers disagreed, a third physician determined the presence or absence of the disputed problem. To reduce the potential disagreement between reviewers, they were trained and tested on selected sample cases before the formal review, and were provided a set of standardised instructions. We also used a medical record review technique called *structured implicit review* that focuses the reviewers' attention on specific issues (our list of selected problems) on which judgement is to be based [11]. This technique is associated with higher inter-rater reliability than *implicit review*, where reviewers use only their knowledge or beliefs to make judgements. This focus was achieved in the review application by displaying the document to review beside a list of the 80 problems to look for. Reviewers checked the problems present in the document and submitted these as an initial review. To improve the quality of the review, these first results were compared in real-time with the results of the NLP module. Reviewers were then asked whether they wanted to keep a problem that wasn't found by NLP, or add a problem that was found only by NLP. During this second phase, the document was displayed with the sentences containing the problem text highlighted in red for faster reading. After responding to the suggestions from the application, the reviewers submitted their final list of the problems present. The two reviews of each document were compared and, if disagreement was found, a third reviewer used the same web-based application to select the disputed problems he considered present in the document.

3. Results

Eight physicians participated in the review process to create the reference standard. Five were board-certified physicians, and three were residents with two or more years of training. With the web-based application described above, reviewers spent an average of 93 to 189 seconds per document. Reviewers' overall agreement was almost perfect, with a Cohen's kappa of 0.9 and a Finn's R of 0.985. This latter value is more representative of the agreement, our agreement table being strongly skewed, with far more true negatives than true positives.

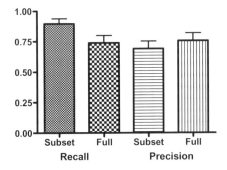

Figure 1: Graphical display of recall and precision
(Subset is customised subset; Full is full data set)

Recall and precision were measured with means and 0.95 confidence intervals. The F-measure was calculated with a value of 1 (same weight for recall and precision), and a value of 2, to give more importance to the recall, the most important feature for our system. Indeed, our aim is to detect as many medical problems present as possible.

Statistical evaluation of these results showed that the recall was significantly higher (two-tailed p < 0.0001) for the customised subset than the full data set. Precision was not significantly different (two-tailed p = 0.0797) (Figure 1 and Table 1). When only considering certain types of clinical documents analysed with the customised data subset, no significant difference was found, except a significantly higher precision with discharge summaries when compared to history and physical exam reports. The test used for this analysis was Mann-Whitney U-statistic, to compensate for lack of normality.

Table 1: NLP module evaluation results

Measurements	Full default data set	Customised data subset	Radiology reports	H&P reports	Discharge summaries
Recall	0.740 *	0.896 *	0.802	0.918	0.878
	(0.680-0.8)	(0.854-0.949)	(0.667-0.937)	(0.854-0.982)	(0.786-0.971)
Precision	0.756	0.691	0.624	0.648 □	0.821 □
	(0.694-0.819)	(0.63-0.752)	(0.477-0.771)	(0.524-0.772)	(0.714-0.928)
F-Measure (β = 1)	0.748	0.78	0.701	0.76	0.849
F-Measure (β = 2)	0.743	0.846	0.759	0.847	0.866

* Extremely significant difference (p < 0.0001); □ Significant difference (p = 0.0368)

4. Discussion

To reduce biases and improve the generalisability of this evaluation, we tried respecting criteria for effective evaluation of NLP systems [12]. Most criteria were respected. However, the developer of the system also participated in the evaluation. To minimise this problem, documents were randomly selected after the system was frozen for evaluation, and reviewers did their task fully independently.

The results of this evaluation show good recall and satisfying precision, both at a level that fulfils our requirements for the NLP module of our Automated Problem List system in a clinical setting. A sufficient recall is required to significantly improve the quality of the Problem List, and a sufficient precision is desirable to avoid overloading the Problem List with false positives. Our application was developed to maximise recall, to the expense of a lower precision. We suppose that about 30% of false positives will be acceptable by users of the problem list. Our results compare favourably with another evaluation of MMTx, where a recall of 53% was reported. However, this latter result has to be considered cautiously because of small sample size and other reasons [13]. Also, our system only extracted a limited set of concepts, and all children of those concepts were matched to the parent ones, therefore improving the recall. Other NLP systems extracting UMLS concepts from free-text have been reported, like MetaMap with exact-match recall of 52.8% and exact-match precision of 27.7% [5]; this study evaluated detection of all biomedical concepts in title phrases. MedLEE has been recently evaluated when extracting UMLS concepts from medical text documents, achieving 83% recall and 89% precision [14].

The excellent agreement among reviewers allows a reference standard of good quality, therefore giving accurate results for the set of randomly selected test documents. A limitation is the fact that the developer of the system also designed and led its evaluation, therefore reducing the generalisability of this study. The limited set of 80 targeted medical problems also limits the generalisability of the study. The sample size was sufficient to show significantly different recall between the two data sets used with MMTx, but a larger sample could have reduced confidence intervals and possibly allowed detection of differences in precision.

5. Conclusion

We developed tools to automate the Problem List using NLP to extract potential medical problems from free-text documents in a patient's EMR. This system's goal is to improve the Problem List's quality by increasing its completeness, accuracy and timeliness. We have evaluated the NLP module developed with MMTx and shown reasonable performance for clinical use in our system. The effect of our system on the quality of actual Problem Lists will be evaluated. We anticipate that, by automatically proposing appropriate additions to the list of problems, we will see an increased proportion of correct problems, a reduced proportion of incorrect problems, and a reduced time between problem identification and addition to the Problem List. This will help to guarantee the quality of this central component for our problem-oriented Electronic Medical Record. Further analysis of the NLP module is planned including a comparison to other Natural Language Processing tools present in our laboratory.

6. Acknowledgements

This work is supported by a Deseret Foundation Grant (Salt Lake City, Utah, U.S.).

7. References

[1]   Bayegan E, Tu S. The helpful patient record system: problem oriented and knowledge based. *Proc AMIA Symp* 2002:36-40.

[2]   Elkin PL, Mohr DN, Tuttle MS, Cole WG, Atkin GE, Keck K, et al. Standardized problem list generation, utilizing the Mayo canonical vocabulary embedded within the Unified Medical Language System. *Proc AMIA Annu Fall Symp* 1997:500-4.

[3]   Aronson AR. Effective mapping of biomedical text to the UMLS Metathesaurus: the MetaMap program. *Proc AMIA Symp* 2001:17-21.

[4]   Zou Q, Chu WW, Morioka C, Leazer GH, Kangarloo H. IndexFinder: A Method of Extracting Key Concepts from Clinical Texts for Indexing. *Proc AMIA Symp* 2003:763-7.

[5]   Pratt W, Yetisgen-Yildiz M. A Study of Biomedical Concept Identification: MetaMap vs. People. *Proc AMIA Symp* 2003:529-33.

[6]   Weeber M, Klein H, Aronson AR, Mork JG, de Jong-van den Berg LT, Vos R. Text-based discovery in biomedicine: the architecture of the DAD-system. *Proc AMIA Symp* 2000:903-7.

[7]   Shadow G, McDonald C. Extracting structured information from free text pathology reports. In: *Proc AMIA Symp* 2003. p. 584-588.

[8]   Chapman WW, Bridewell W, Hanbury P, Cooper GF, Buchanan BG. A simple algorithm for identifying negated findings and diseases in discharge summaries. *J Biomed Inform* 2001;34(5):301-10.

[9]   Mutalik PG, Deshpande A, Nadkarni PM. Use of general-purpose negation detection to augment concept indexing of medical documents: a quantitative study using the UMLS. *J Am Med Inform Assoc* 2001;8(6):598-609.

[10] Meystre S, Haug PJ. Medical problem and document model for natural language understanding. *Proc AMIA Symp* 2003:455-9.

[11] Ashton CM, Kuykendall DH, Johnson ML, Wray NP. An empirical assessment of the validity of explicit and implicit process-of-care criteria for quality assessment. Med Care 1999;37(8):798-808.

[12] Friedman C, Hripcsak G. Evaluating natural language processors in the clinical domain. *Methods Inf Med* 1998;37(4-5):334-44.

[13] Divita G, Tse T, Roth L. Failure Analysis of MetaMap Transfer (MMTx). *Medinfo*2004;2004:763-7.

[14] Friedman C, Shagina L, Lussier Y, Hripcsak G. Automated Encoding of Clinical Documents Based on Natural Language Processing. *J Am Med Inform Assoc* 2004.

Address for correspondence:

Stéphane Meystre
Department of Medical Informatics
University of Utah School of Medicine, Room AB194
Salt Lake City, UT 84132-2913, USA
s.meystre@utah.edu or smeystre@bluewin.ch

Connecting Medical Informatics and Bio-Informatics
R. Engelbrecht et al. (Eds.)
IOS Press, 2005

Automatic Lexicon Acquisition for a Medical Cross-Language Information Retrieval System

Kornél Markó[a,b], Stefan Schulz[a], Udo Hahn[b]

[a]Medical Informatics Department, Freiburg University Hospital, Germany
[b]Jena University Language & Information Engineering Lab, Germany

Abstract

We present a method for the automated acquisition of a multilingual medical lexicon (for Spanish and Swedish) to be used within the framework of a medical cross-language text retrieval system. We incorporate seed lexicons and parallel corpora derived from the UMLS Metathesaurus. The seed lexicons for Spanish and Swedish are automatically generated from (previously manually constructed) Portuguese, German and English sources. Lexical and semantic hypotheses are then validated making iterative use of co-occurrence patterns of hypothesized translation synonyms in the parallel corpora.

Keywords:
Medical Informatics; Information Storage and Retrieval; Multilingualism; Vocabulary, Controlled

1. Introduction

The access to medical documents (from medical narratives, research articles, web-based health portals, etc.) is typically characterized by a mix of natural languages. While English is the primary (though not only) language of scientific communication for medicine, medical specialists and general practitioners use their native language(s) for medical reports of any sort. For non-English native speakers, even those familiar with English medical terminology, this diversity tends to create a problem to properly express their information needs. Therefore, automatically performed intra- and interlingual lexical mappings or transformations of equivalent expressions become crucial for adequate medical information supply.

We respond to these challenges in terms of the MORPHOSAURUS system.[1] It is centered around a new type of lexicon, in which the entries are subwords, i.e., semantically minimal, morpheme-style units [1]. Language-specific subwords are linked by intralingual as well as interlingual synonymy and grouped into concept-like equivalence classes at the layer of a language-independent interlingua. Our claim that this approach is useful for the purpose of cross-lingual text retrieval and document classification has already been experimentally supported [2].

---

[1] Acronym for MORpheme TheSAURUS, see http://www.morphosaurus.net

The quality of cross-lingual indexing and retrieval crucially depends on the underlying lexicons and the thesaurus in which equivalence classes are organized. As their manual construction and maintenance is costly and error-prone, we here propose an approach to automatically acquire Spanish and Swedish lexicons, starting from already available Portuguese, English, and German lexicons. We then evaluate our approach on a Spanish-Swedish parallel medical corpus.

2. Multilingual Lexicon Acquisition

Our work starts from the assumption that neither fully inflected nor automatically stemmed words constitute the appropriate granularity level for lexicalized content description. In the medical sublanguage, we observe a high frequency of domain-specific suffixes (e.g., '*-itis*', '*-ectomia*') and complex word forms such as in '*pseudo◊hypo◊para◊thyroid◊ism*'.[2] Morpheme-style subwords are lexical entities capable of dealing with these phenomena in a particularly adequate manner. They are assembled in a multilingual lexicon and thesaurus, which contain lexemes, their attributes, synonym classes and semantic relations between them, according to the following considerations:

- Subwords are registered in 7-bit ASCII (with few exceptions for Swedish), together with their attributes such as language and subword type (stem, prefix, suffix, invariant). Each lexicon entry is assigned a unique identifier representing one synonymy class, the MORPHOSAURUS identifier (MID).

- Synonymy classes which contain intralingual synonyms and interlingual translations of subwords are fused. Equivalence is judged within the context of medicine only.

- Semantic links between synonymy classes are added. We subscribe to a shallow approach in which semantic relations are restricted to a single paradigmatic relation *has-meaning*, which relates one ambiguous class to its specific readings,[3] and a syntagmatic relation *expands-to*, which consists of predefined segmentations in case of utterly short subwords.[4]

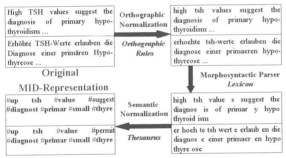

Figure 1- Morpho-semantic normalization pipeline

Figure 1 depicts how source documents (topleft) are converted into an interlingual representation. First, each input word is orthographically normalized according to language-specific rules for the transcription of diacritics (topright). Next, words are segmented into sequences of subwords (bottom-right). The segmentation results are checked for morphological plausibility using a finite-state automaton in order to reject invalid segmentations (e.g., segmentations without stems

---

[2] '◊'denotes the concatenation operator.
[3] For instance, {*head*} → {*zephal,kopf,caput,cephal,cabec,cefal*} OR {*leader,boss,lider,chefe*}
[4] For instance, {*myalg*} → {*muscle,muskel,muscul*}◊{*schmerz,pain,dor*}

or beginning with a suffix). Finally, each meaning-bearing subword is replaced by a language-independent semantic identifier, the MORPHOSAURUS identifier (MID) (bottom-left). In Figure 1, bold-faced MIDs co-occur in both document fragments.

The manual construction of a trilingual lexicon and the thesaurus has consumed three and a half person years. The combined subword lexicon contains 59,288 entries, with 22,041 for English, 22,385 for German and 14,862 for Portuguese. In an effort to further expand the language coverage of our system by Spanish and Swedish, we wanted to reuse the already available resources for Portuguese, English, and German in order to speed up and to ease the lexicon acquisition process.

For the initialization of the Spanish and Swedish subword lexicons we proceed as follows: From the PORtuguese (alternatively, ENGlish and GERman) lexicon, identical and similarly spelled SPAnish (SWEedish) subword candidates are generated. For example, the Portuguese word stem *'estomag'* [*'stomach'*] is identical with its Spanish cognate, while *'mulher'* [*'woman'*] (Portuguese) is similar to *'mujer'* (Spanish). Similar subword candidates are generated by applying a set of string substitution rules, some of which are listed in Table 1. In total, we formulated 44 rules for the Portuguese-Spanish pair, 19 rules for German-Swedish and 6 for English-Swedish. Some of these substitution patterns cannot be applied to starting or ending sequences of characters in the source subword. This constraint is captured by a wildcard ('+' in Table 1).

Table 1- Some String Substitution Rules

Rule	POR	SPA	Rule	GER	SWE	Rule	ENG	SWE
ss→s	fra*css*	fra*cas*	ei→e	B*ein*	b*en*	c→k	*c*ramp	*k*ramp
lh→j	mu*lh*er	mu*j*er	+aa→a	S*aal*	s*al*	ph→f	*ph*os*ph*or	*f*os*f*or
+ca→za	cabe*ca*	cabe*za*	+u→ö	br*u*st	br*ö*st	ce→s	*ce*land	*s*land

Based on these rules and the already available (Portuguese, English, German) subword lexicons, for each subword, all possible Spanish and Swedish variant strings were generated. All resulting subword variants were subsequently compared with target language (Spanish and Swedish) text corpora we acquired from the Web. Wherever a (subword-) variant matched a word in the target corpus, the matching string was listed as a potential Spanish (Swedish) cognate of the Portuguese (alternatively, English and German) subword it originated from. Whenever several substitution alternatives for a source subword had to be considered, that particular alternative was chosen, which had the most similar lexical distribution in the corpora considered. All other candidates were discarded. As a result, we obtained a list of putative Spanish (Swedish) subwords, each linked by the associated MID to their grounding source cognate in the Portuguese (alternatively, English and German) lexicon.

Table 2- Selected Cognates (Union in Brackets)

Language Pair	Source Lexicon	Variants	Selected Cognates	Linked MIDs
Portuguese-Spanish	14,004	123,235	8,644	6,036
German-Swedish	21,705	145,423	4,249 (6,086)	3,308 (4,157)
English-Swedish	21,501	68,803	4,140 (6,086)	3,208 (4,157)

Starting from 14,004 Portuguese, 21,705 German and 21,501 English stems (affixes were excluded), a total of 123,235 Spanish subword variants were created using the string substitution rules. For Swedish, 145,423 variants were derived from German and 68,803 from English. Matching these variants against the Spanish and Swedish corpora and allowing for a maximum of one candidate per source subword, we identified 8,644 tentative Spanish and (combining English and German evidence) 6,086 tentative Swedish cognates (cf. Table 2). Spanish candidates are linked to a total of 6,036 MIDs from their Portuguese correlates (hence, 2,608 synonym relationships have also been hypothesized), whilst Swedish candidates are associated with 4,157 MIDs from their German and English correlates.

We then wanted to identify *false friends*, i.e., similar words in different languages with different meanings. In our experiments, we found, e.g., the Spanish subword candidate *'crianz'* for the Portuguese *'crianc'* [*'child'*] (the normalized stem of *'criança'*). The correct translation of Portuguese *'crianc'* to Spanish, however, would have been *'nin'* (the stem of *'niño'*), whilst the Spanish *'crianz'* refers to *'criac'* [*'breed'*] (stem of *'criação'* in Portuguese). For eliminating such false friends, we relied on parallel corpora made available by the *Unified Medical Language System* (UMLS) *Metathesaurus*. Unfortunately, word-to-word translation occurs only in very few cases. Much more common are more or less complex noun phrases with a similarly complex semantic structure. Examples for typical English-Spanish alignments are *"Cell Growth"* aligned with *"Crecimiento Celular"*, or *"Heart transplant, with or without recipient cardiectomy"* aligned with *"Trasplante cardiaco, con o sin cardiectomia en el receptor"*.

We use English as the pivot language for our experiments, since it has the broadest lexical coverage in the UMLS. The size of the corpora derived from the linkages of the English UMLS to other languages amounts to 60,526 alignments for English-Spanish (only *preferred entries* in the UMLS MRCONSO table) and 10,953 alignments for English-Swedish. The parallel corpora of the aligned UMLS expressions were morpho-semantically processed as described in Figure 1. Whenever a MID occurred on both sides after this simultaneous bilingual processing, the appropriate Spanish (Swedish) subword entry that led to this particular MID is taken to be a valid entry. This approach is a reasonable way, since it is highly unlikely that a false friend occurs within the same translation context. All translation hypotheses that never matched in this validation procedure were rejected from the candidate lexicons. As a result, 3,230 of the original Spanish (37%) and 1,565 of the Swedish hypotheses are kept (26%) (cf. also Table 2 & 3).

These supported cognates now serve as the seed lexicons (in the following, *L(0)*) for acquiring additional lexicon entries, which are *not* cognates to elements of any of the source lexicons. To illustrate this process, assume the Swedish subword *'blod'* was identified as being a cognate to the English subword *'blood'* (and, therefore, is included in *L(0)*). Then, the yet unknown Swedish word *'Blodtryck'*, which has the English translation *'blood pressure'* in the UMLS Metathesaurus gets (invalidly) segmented into [ST:*blod*|UK:*t*|SF:*r*|UK:*yck*], with ST being a marker for a stem, SF for a suffix and UK for an unknown sequence. At the same time, the morpho-semantic normalization of *'blood pressure'* leads to the sequence of MIDs [#*blood* #*tense*], whilst the normalization of *'Blodtryck'* leads to [#*blood*], since *'tryck'* is not yet part of the Swedish lexicon.

Comparing these two representations, exactly one MID resulting from English cannot be found in the Swedish normalization result. In this case, the invalid segment is then reconstructed (leading to *'tryck'*) by eliminating those substrings that led to a matching MID (*'blod'*) in the aligned unit (*'Blodtryck'*). The supernumerary MID resulting from the English normalization is then assigned to the reconstructed substring. After processing all UMLS alignments, this new entry is then incorporated in the Swedish lexicon as a stem, resulting in the lexicon *L(1)*.

Next, all UMLS alignments are recursively processed once again. The newly derived lexicon entry may now serve for extracting, e.g., the Swedish word *'luft'* with its identifier #*aero* from the UMLS entry *'Air Pressure'* (indexed to [#*aero* #*tense*]) linked to *'Lufttryck'* (Swedish), and so on. When no new entries can be generated in one run of processing the whole UMLS-derived alignments, the recursive algorithm stops. Table 3 depicts the growth steps of the target lexicons for the entire bootstrapping process. After 14 runs, learning comes to an end with 7,154 lexemes generated for Spanish, while after 8 runs 4,148 lexicon entries for Swedish are acquired.

For multilingual lexicon acquisition, we referred to English-Spanish and English-Swedish corpora compiled out of the UMLS Metathesaurus. To estimate the quality of the interlingual connections between the newly derived lexicons, we now compare the results after running MORPHOSAURUS on these collections. We are aware that these results probably include overfitting phenomena. Therefore, we additionally extracted a Spanish-Swedish parallel corpus from the UMLS. This corpus has 8,993 alignments ranging, again, from word-to-word translations (e.g., *'Pierna'* to *'Ben'* [*'leg'*]) to complex noun phrases, which sometimes correspond to a single word in the other language, e.g., the Spanish phrase *'Enfermedad virica transmitida por artropodos, no especificada'* maps to the Swedish *'Arbovirusinfektioner'* [*'Arbovirus Infections'*] in the UMLS.

Table 3- Lexicon Growth Steps for Spanish (left) and Swedish (right)

Lexicon	Spanish	Lexicon	Spanish	Lexicon	Swedish	Lexicon	Swedish
L(0)	3,230	L(6)	7,110	L(0)	1,565	L(6)	4,142
L(1)	6,817	L(7)	7,111	L(1)	2,324	L(7)	4,147
L(2)	7,001	L(8)	7,114	L(2)	3,685	L(8)	4,148
L(3)	7,094	L(9)	7,126	L(3)	4,013	-	-
L(4)	7,108	...	...	L(4)	4,119	-	-
L(5)	7,109	L(14)	7,154	L(5)	4,136	-	-

However, we rely on these resources for evaluation only. Rather than simply measuring the coverage, we wanted to estimate the quality of the generated lexicons, i.e., the validity of the interlingual synonymy relations we stipulate. For this goal, we indexed the English-Spanish and English-Swedish corpora employing the MORPHOSAURUS routines, for each lexicon level $L(0)$-$L(14)$. Furthermore, the Spanish-Swedish corpus – previously unseen by the learning algorithm – was processed accordingly. For each alignment unit of the parallel corpus, we then compared the resulting MIDs. In order to determine the fit of the two representations, we used a measure of indexing *consistency* proposed by Hooper (1965) [3]: $C_{AU(i)} = (100*A)/(A+N+M)$. The indexing consistency of one alignment unit $AU(i)$ of the parallel corpus, $C_{AU(i)}$, is dependent on A, the number of MIDs that co-occur on both sides of that unit in the parallel corpus and the number of MIDs that occur only on one side, N or M . To express the overall consistency, the arithmetic mean of all alignment units ($C_{AU(i)}$) of the corpus is calculated.

3. Results

Table 4 depicts the over-all consistency values (columns 2, 5 and 8) starting from lexicon $L(0)$ (only validated cognates) to lexicon $L(5)$ for the Spanish and Swedish lexical acquisition (improvements after that step are only marginal, cf. Table 3). When processing the English-Spanish corpus, consistency is already about 40%, only considering cognates. Adding those entries acquired from recursively bootstrapping the same corpus, consistency climbs to a maximum of 52%. As a reference item, the processing of an English-German corpus, which is also derived from UMLS, yields 57% consistency – keeping in mind that English and German lexicons were generated manually and provide a real good coverage [2]. For English-Swedish, consistency ranges from 27% (only cognates) to 56% (after five cycles). The processing of Spanish-Swedish is particularly interesting, since the underlying corpus was not involved at all in the lexical acquisition. With consistency starting from 21% for cognates, 46% is reached after five cycles of generating the non-English lexicons by processing parallel corpora aligned to English only.

Coverage was measured by counting those cases in which at least one MID occurs on both sides of the alignment units considered. For Spanish cognates only ($L(0)$ in Table 4), alignments to English can be observed for 88% of the corpus. This value increases to 96% after five runs of bootstrapping the Spanish lexicon. For English-Swedish, coverage reaches 86% and for Spanish-Swedish 84%. Again, as a reference, the processing of the English-German corpus yields 97% coverage. The number of cases in which both sides are indexed *identically*, range from 6% to 12% for English-Spanish, from 12% to 43% for English-Swedish and from 9% to 27% for Spanish-Swedish. The reference data for these values is 30% for English-German.

Table 4- Indexing Consistency (C), Coverage (Cov.) of Lexicons and Number of Identical Indexes (Ident.) at each Stage of Lexicon Generation.

Lexicon	English-Spanish: n=60,526			English-Swedish: n=10,953			Spanish-Swedish: n=8,993		
	C	Cov.(%)	Ident.(%)	C	Cov.(%)	Ident.(%)	C	Cov(%)	Ident.(%)
L(0)	39.6	87.6	6.1	27.4	60.0	11.7	21.4	53.8	8.9
L(1)	47.5	95.5	9.7	29.8	63.3	18.4	29.8	77.1	18.4
L(2)	51.0	95.6	11.8	50.7	81.8	39.9	40.6	80.1	23.9
L(3)	51.3	95.6	12.1	55.4	84.8	41.4	44.6	83.2	25.8
L(4)	52.0	95.6	12.3	56.0	85.4	42.2	45.6	83.7	26.7
L(5)	52.0	95.7	12.4	56.3	85.6	42.6	45.9	83.8	26.9

4. Discussion and Conclusion

We have shown that a significant amount of Portuguese, English and German subwords from the medical domain can be mapped to Spanish and Swedish cognates by simple string transformations. With these seeds, we further enlarge the Spanish and Swedish cognate lexicons by subwords which are *not* cognates. For the latter task, we used the UMLS Metathesaurus, and extracted those non-cognates in a bootstrapping way. Most alternative automatic approaches to multilingual lexical acquisition either employ heavy linguistic parsing machinery [4] or use statistical methods, such as context vector comparison [5] which require a seed lexicon of *trusted* translations. We derived such a seed lexicon via a generative method to cognate mapping. Déjean et al. [6] incorporate hierarchical information from MeSH for combining different evidence for lexical acquisition.

5. References

[1] Honeck M, Hahn U, Klar R, Schulz, S: Text retrieval based on medical subwords. In *Health Data in the Information Society. Proceedings of MIE 2002*. Budapest, Hungary, August 2002; 241-245.

[2] Markó K, Hahn U, Schulz S, Daumke P, Nohama P: Interlingual indexing across different languages. In *Conference Proceedings of the 7th RIAO Conference*. Avignon, France, April 26-28, 2004; 82-99.

[3] Hooper RS: *Indexer Consistency Tests: Origin, Measurement, Results, and Utilization*. Bethesda, MD: IBM Corporation, 1965.

[4] Hersh WR, Campbell EH, Evans DA, Brownlow ND: Empirical, automated vocabulary discovery using large text corpora and advanced language processing tools. In *Proceedings of the 1996 AMIA Annual Fall Symposium*. Washington DC 1996; 159-163.

[5] Widdows D, Dorow B., Chan C-K: Using parallel corpora to enrich multilingual lexical resources. In *Proceedings of the 3rd International Conference on Language Resources and Evaluation - LREC 2002*. Las Palmas de Gran Canaria, 2002; 240-245.

[6] Déjean H, Gaussier E, Sadat, F: An approach based on multilingual thesauri and model combination for bilingual lexicon extraction. In *Proceedings of the 18th International Conference on Computational Linguistics- COLING 2002*.2002; 218-224.

Address for correspondence

Kornél Markó, marko@coling.uni-freiburg.de, Medical Informatics Department, Freiburg University Hospital, Stefan-Meier-Str. 26, 79104 Freiburg, Germany

Connecting Medical Informatics and Bio-Informatics
R. Engelbrecht et al. (Eds.)
IOS Press, 2005

Extracting Key Sentences with Latent Argumentative Structuring

Patrick Ruch [a], Robert Baud [a], Christine Chichester [c],
Antoine Geissbühler[a], Frédérique Lisacek [c], Johann Marty[ad],
Dietrich Rebholz-Schuhmann[e], Imad Tbahriti [abe], Anne-Lise Veuthey [b]

[a]SIM, University Hospitals of Geneva, Geneva, CH
[b]Swiss-Prot, Swiss Institute of Bioinformatics, Geneva, CH;
[d]Health-on-the-Net Foundation, Geneva, CH; [e] European Bioinformatics Institute ,Hinxton, UK

Abstract

PROBLEM: Key word assignment has been largely used in MEDLINE to provide an indicative "gist" of the content of articles. Abstracts are also used for this purpose. However with usually more than 300 words, abstracts can still be regarded as long documents; therefore we design a system to select a unique key sentence. This key sentence must be indicative of the article's content and we assume that abstract's conclusions are good candidates. We design and assess the performance of an automatic key sentence selector, which classifies sentences into 4 argumentative moves: PURPOSE, METHODS, RESULTS and CONCLUSION. METHODS: We rely on Bayesian classifiers trained on automatically acquired data. Features representation, selection and weighting are reported and classification effectiveness is evaluated on the four classes using confusion matrices. We also explore the use of simple heuristics to take the position of sentences into account. Recall, precision and F-scores are computed for the CONCLUSION class. For the CONCLUSION class, the F-score reaches 84%. Automatic argumentative classification is feasible on MEDLINE abstracts and should help user navigation in such repositories.

Keywords:
Machine Learning; Abstracting and Indexing; Information Storage and Retrieval; Natural Language Processing; Digital Libraries.

1. Introduction

Systems for text mining are becoming increasingly important in biomedicine because of the exponential growth of knowledge. The mass of scientific literature needs to be filtered and categorized to provide for the most efficient use of the data. The problem of accessing this increasing volume of data demands the development of systems that can extract pertinent information from unstructured texts, hence the importance of key words extraction, as well as key sentence extraction. While the former task has been largely addressed in text categorization studies [1], the current status of the latter is the matter of this report. Defining what is a key sentence is a complex task because more than key words, key sentences are dependent on the domain and dependent on the point of view of the reader; however like for key words, which can comprehensively be provided through a controlled vocabulary, we believe it is possible to propose criteria to define key sentences. Applying key words mapping methods to extract the informative content is a well-known technique to navigate digital documents [2][3], but sentences provide additional materials and therefore suggest original strategies. As stated in professional guidelines (ANSI/NISO Z39. 14-1979), articles in experimental sciences tend to respect strict argumentative patterns with at least 4 sections: purpose-methods-results-conclusion. These 4 moves –leaving aside minor variation of labels- are reported to be very stable across different scientific genres (chemistry, anthropology, computer sciences, linguistics...) [4], and are confirmed in biomedical abstracts and articles [5][6][29]. Following recent developments in information retrieval [7][27], which show that conclusion sentences are the most content-bearing to perform related articles search and index pruning tasks in MEDLINE, we assume that conclusion sentences would be good candidates for such key sentences in scientific texts.

2. Background and Methods

Selecting argumentative contents is formally a classification task: for each piece of text the system will have to decide whether it is a relevant conclusion or not. Sentences are natural candidate segments for such classification [8], because they are more self-containing than phrases; however anaphoric phenomena may demand larger segments [9].

2.1 Summarization has a related task

Modern summarization systems use annotated corpora in order to acquire appropriate knowledge; based on textual features summarization tools are able to conduct general summarization tasks. Thus, Kupiec and al. [10] report that in abstracts produced by professionals, 80% of sentences are also found in the source document. In such systems, the complex abstracting task is recast into a more modest sentences' selection problem. To do so, experts identify a set of relevant sentences into large corpora; these sentences are then used to train the learning system. Complementary to machine learning approaches, Teufel and al. in [23], who design a task very similar to our one, combine a set of manually crafted triggered expression, such as *finally, we have shown that, we conclude that...* to classify sentences into 7 argumentative classes.

2.2 Basic classifiers, features selection and weighting

Choosing a priori an appropriate classifier for a given task is a fairly difficult task; therefore, empirical comparisons are often necessary. Among state-of-the-art classifiers for text categorization, such as k-NN [11], SVM [12][28], neural networks [13], and rule-induction systems [14], Bayesian classifiers [15] show a linear complexity, while most top performing algorithms have quadratic complexity; therefore they are often more adapted for rapid application developments and exploratory studies [16] [24]. The basic features in text categorization are usually word-based. Possible variants are stems, which often implies stop-words removal, and/or sequences of stems, such as bi- or trigrams of stems. Examples of stemming algorithms are provided in Table 1. Our preliminary studies confirmed that elaborated string normalization and stop word removal strategies such as Porter and Lovins did not outperformed simpler approaches, such as plural normalization, which process morphological variations of plural forms (-s, -ies). This strategy appears sufficient to help the classifiers to generalize without removing interesting features, such as verb tense (as suggested in [4]), which is usually removed by stemming (cf. Table 1).

Table 1: String Normalization Methods

	Type of Normalization			
Token	Lovins	Porter	Plural Stemming	Lemmatization
genetic	genet	genet	genetic	genetic
genetically	genet	genetically	genetically	genetically
genetics	genet	genet	genetic	genetics
gene	gene	gene	gene	gene
genes	gene	gene	gene	gene
homogeneous	gene	homogen	homogeneous	homogeneous
plaid	plai	plai	plaid	play
play	plai	plai	play	play

The last step concerns feature weighting. Indeed naive Bayes classifiers combines the log-likelihood of each features in order to select the most probable category, however the real frequency observed in training corpora can follow different refinement and smoothing processes, known as feature weighting [11]. We tested 3 weighting methods tf-idf (term frequency-inverse document frequency), chi-2, df-thresholding (only features appearing frequenty in each class are selected). Our conclusion is that chi-2 and df-thresholding perform similarly, while tf-idf weighting should be avoided. Indeed, tf-idf weighting is appropriate for weighting content-bearing features, while argumentative content is supported by functional words. Three types of features are linearly combined to get a final probability ranking per class: stems; stem bigrams and stem trigrams. As in [15], length normalization of sentences as been applied in order to master biases introduced by too long or too short sentences.

2.3 Training and Test Data

In text classification tasks, two types of strategies are competing: expert-driven and data-driven approaches. While the former, which rely on a domain expert, are often time and labour-intensive, the latter are directly dependent on the availability of large training sets. Fortunately, training data for our task can be acquired in a cheap manner. Most abstracts in MEDLINE are unstructured (i.e. provided without explicit argumentative markers, such as METHODS, PURPOSES…), but fortunately, a significant fraction of these abstracts contain explicit argumentative markers. Using PubMed and its Boolean query interface, we collected a set of 12000 MEDLINE citations containing strings such as "PURPOSE:", "METHODS:", "RESULTS", "CONCLUSION:". This fully automatic data collection process introduces some argumentative noise, since some of the explicit markers gather additional argumentative content. Thus, explicit markers such as "BACKGROUND AND PURPOSES:" were also collected as pure "PURPOSES:" markers by this simple method. The collection was then split into two sets:

- set A (10800 abstracts) was used for training and validation purposed,

- set B (1200) was used for the final assessment.

In addition to sets A and B, we also collected a smaller set (C) of marker-free abstracts (100 items). Then, two human annotators were asked to manually annotate this set, using the four selected argumentative classes. In contrast with the automatically acquired sets, here we do not assume that argumentative segments and sentences are overlapping items. As shown in figure 2, some sentences in set C receive more than one label, because they may express two different argumentative moves in the same sentence. In such cases, we do not attempt to identify segment boundaries (like explored in [18] and [19]) and instead ask the system to provide any of the relevant classes. The interannotator agreement on the C set for argumentative segments is 0.81, when measured by kappa statistics, which indicates that agreement is good.

> *INTRODUCTION:* Chromophobe renal cell carcinoma (CCRC) comprises 5% of neoplasms of renal tubular epithelium. CCRC may have a slightly better prognosis than clear cell carcinoma, but outcome data are limited. *PURPOSE:* In this study, we analyzed 250 renal cell carcinomas to a) determine frequency of CCRC at our Hospital and b) analyze clinical and pathologic features of CCRCs. *METHODS:* A total of 250 renal carcinomas were analyzed between March 1990 and March 1999. Tumors were classified according to well-established histologic criteria to determine stage of disease; the system proposed by Robson was used. *RESULTS:* Of 250 renal cell carcinomas analyzed, 36 were classified as chromophobe renal cell carcinoma, representing 14% of the group studied. The tumors had an average diameter of 14 cm. Robson staging was possible in all cases, and 10 patients were stage 1) 11 stage II; 10 stage III, and five stage IV. The average follow-up period was 4 years and 18 (53%) patients were alive without disease. *CONCLUSION:* The highly favorable pathologic stage (RI-RII, 58%) and the fact that the majority of patients were alive and disease-free suggested a more favorable prognosis for this type of renal cell carcinoma.

Figure 1: Example of explicitly structured abstracts in MEDLINE. We observe that the 4-class model is sometimes split into different classes in training data, cf. the INTRODUCTION marker.

<CONCLUSION> Skin surface proteolytic activity in the living animal was detected </CONCLUSION> <METHODS> by a sensitive, non-invasive methodol. developed in our laboratory</METHODS>. <METHODS>A non-leaky well was constructed on the shaved back of an anesthetized guinea pig. The well contained the reaction mixture including the substrate   125I-S-carboxymethylated <GPN> insulin B-chain</GPN> (<GPN>ICMI</GPN>)</METHODS>. <RESULTS>The proteolytic activity was shown to be time-dependent. The activity was strongly inhibited by <ASP_GPN>pepstatin A</ASP_GPN>, indicating the involvement of aspartic proteinase(s) such as <ASP_GPN>cathepsin D</ASP_GPN> and/or <ASP_GPN>E</ASP_GPN>. Pretreatment of the skin with propylene glycol blocked the proteolytic activity</RESULTS>. <CONCLUSION>The present study demonstrates the presence of proteolytic activity located on skin surface<CONCLUSION> <METHODS>using a unique, non-invasive method for in situ proteinase detn. in the living animal</METHODS>.

Figure 2: Example of structured abstracts. Four argumentative classes are annotated with XML tags; Gene and Protein Names (GPN and ASP_GPN), are also annotated.

As mentioned above, our goal is to extract conclusion sentences, but because the information is available in our training data, this binary task has been modified into a 4-class problem: {PURPOSE, METHODS, RESULTS, CONCLUSION}. We expect that working with more classes will help the system to discriminate between classes that have been reported to be lexically similar [4][21], such as PURPOSE and CONCLUSION. In the data sets used for the evaluation (B and C), explicit argumentative markers have been removed.

2.4 Combining positions of segments

Optionally, we also investigated the sentence position's impact on the classification effectiveness through assigning a relative position to each sentence. Thus, if there were ten sentences in an abstract: the first sentence has a relative position of 0.1, while the sentence in position 5 receives a relative position of 0.5, and the last sentence has a relative position of 1. The following distributional heuristics are encoded in a distributional model: 1) if a sentence has a relative score strictly inferior to 0.4 and is classified as CONCLUSION, then its class becomes PURPOSE; 2) if a sentence has a relative score strictly superior to 0.6 and is classified as PURPOSE, then its class is rewritten as CONCLUSION.

CONCLUSION|00160116| The highly favorable pathologic stage (RI-RII, 58%) and the fact that the majority of patients were alive and disease-free suggested a more favorable prognosis for this type of renal cell carcinoma.

METHODS|00160119| Tumors were classified according to well-established histologic criteria to determine stage of disease; the system proposed by Robson was used.

METHODS|00162303| Of 250 renal cell carcinomas analyzed, 36 were classified as chromophobe renal cell carcinoma, representing 14% of the group studied.

PURPOSE|00156456| In this study, we analyzed 250 renal cell carcinomas to a) determine frequency of CCRC at our Hospital and b) analyze clinical and pathologic features of CCRCs.

PURPOSE|00167817|Chromophobe renal cell carcinoma (CCRC) comprises 5% of neoplasms of renal tubular epithelium. CCRC may have a slightly better prognosis than clear cell carcinoma, but outcome data are limited.

RESULTS|00155338| Robson staging was possible in all cases, and 10 patienhts were stage 1) 11 stage II; 10 stage III, and five stage IV.

Figure 3: example of classification for the abstract in figure 1: the attributed class comes first, then the score obtained by the class, and finally the text segment is provided.

3. Results and Conclusion

In this section, we report on evaluation of the classification task on sets B and C, using the naive Bayes classifier with and without using positional information. Results in table 2 give the confusion matrices between what was expected (columns) and the class proposed by the classifier (row): the diagonal (top left to bottom right) indicates the rate of well classified segments for each of the classes. On the input text, sentence splitting is performed via a set of manually crafted regular expressions. An example of the output is given in Figure 3. Confusion matrices help to identify cross-class confusion: thus, in benchmark B it is observed that RESULTS are often misclassified into CONCLUSION (15.56%); while METHODS are sometimes misclassified into PURPOSES (4.64%). It is also observed that combining our classifier with the positional heuristics does not result in a significant improvement for this benchmark. The opposite occurs for benchmark C, where classification on CONCLUSION and PURPOSES classes is improved when heuristics are used: from 80.65% to 93.55% for PURPOSES and from 79.55 to 95.45 for CONCLUSION. Unfortunately, we see that for the RESULTS class, effectiveness is highly affected. More generally, this class seems less appropriately separated by the classifier.

Table 2: Classification with and without position on structured and unstructured data.

	Structured benchmark (B) without position				Structured benchmark (B) with position			
	PURP	METH	RESU	CONC	PURP	METH	RESU	CONC
PURP	93.24%	0.76%	1.00%	5.00%	96.24%	0.58%	1.00%	2.18%
METH	4.64%	93.67%	0.00%	1.69%	6.33%	93.67%	0.00%	0.00%
RESU	4.30%	8.94%	71.19%	15.56%	2.65%	8.94%	71.19%	17.22%
CONC	1.72%	0.00%	0.72%	97.56%	1.11%	0.00%	0.72%	98.17%
	Unstructured benchmark (C) without position				Unstructured benchmark (C) with position			
PURP	80.65%	0%	3.23%	16%	93.55%	0%	3.23%	3%
METH	10%	70%	10%	10%	30%	70%	0%	0%
RESU	18.58%	5.31%	63.89%	12.21%	12.43%	5.31%	79.25%	24.25%
CONC	18.18%	0%	2.27%	79.55%	2.27%	0%	2.27%	95.45%

Finally, with an F-score (i.e the harmonic mean, with recall and precision having the same importance; cf [22]) above 85%, recall and precision measures are competitive with the trigger-based approach proposed by Teufel and al [23] (F-score ~ 68%), and the SVM learner used in McKnight and Srinivasan [25] (F-score ~ 80%). While recall show excellent effectiveness, precision could still be improved: conclusion segments are well classified, but some non-conclusion sentences are classified as conclusion (false positives). This is problematic for RESULTS segments, which is found ill-defined by the classifier, but looking at the corpus, the distinction between RESULTS and CONCLUSION appears questionable, so that merging these two classes could be both beneficial and legitimate. Naive Bayes classifiers provide an adapted framework to perform argumentative classification, outperforming expert-driven approaches. The improvement brought by adding positional heuristics is useful for unstructured abstracts, which are fortunately the most frequent type of abstracts in MEDLINE, and further developments based on generalization of distributional features using a Markov model, that have proved effective for classifying textual data based on positional features [26].

4. Acknowledgments

The study has been supported by the EU-IST program (SemanticMining Grant 507505 - Swiss OFES Grant 03.0399). We would like to thank C. Boyer, T. de la Charrière, and A. Gaudinat for the user feedback of the final system (WRAPIN portal: www.wrapin.org).

5. References

[1]   F Sebastiani, Machine learning in automated text categorization. ACM Computing Surveys 34(1): 1-47, 2002.
[2]   A Aronson, O Bodenreider, H Chang, S Humphrey, J Mork, S Nelson, T Rindflesch, W Wilbur, The NLM Indexing Initiative. Proc AMIA Symp. 2000;:17-21.
[3]   P Ruch, R Baud, and A Geissbühler. Learning-free Text Categorization, AIME 2003, LNCS 2780.
[4]   C Orasan, Patterns in scientific abstracts, in Proceedings of Corpus Linguistics 2001 Conference, Lancaster University, Lancaster, UK, pp. 433 - 443, 2001.
[5]   J Swales, Genre Analysis: English in academic and research settings, Cambridge University Press, 1990.
[6]   F Salanger-Meyer, Discoursal movements in medical English abstracts and their linguistic exponents: a genre analysis study, INTERFACE: Journal of Applied Linguistics 4(2), 1990, pp. 107 - 124
[7]   Tbahriti, C Chichester, F Lisacek and P Ruch. Using Argumentation to Retrieve Articles with Similar Citations: an Inquiry into Improving Related Articles Search in the MEDLINE Digital Library. *Int J Med Inf*, 2005 (to appear)
[8]   Ruch, C Chichester, G Cohen, G Coray, F Ehrler, H Ghorbel, H Müller, V Pallotta. Report on the TREC 2003 Experiment: Genomic Track, *TREC* 2003.
[9]   U Hahn, M Romacker, S Schulz, Why discourse structures in medical reports matter for J Kupiec, J Pedersen and F Chen: A Trainable Document Summarizer, SIGIR 1995, p. 55-60.
[10] Y Yang, An evaluation of statistical approaches to text categorization. Journal of Information Retrieval 1 (1999) p. 67-88.
[11] S Dumais, J Platt, D Sahami: Inductive learning algorithms and representations for text categorization. In: CIKM, ACM (1998) p. 148-155.
[12] K Ming Adam Chai, Hai Leong Chieu, Hwee Tou Ng, Bayesian online classifiers for text classification and filtering, SIGIR 2002, p. 89-96.
[13] D Beeferman, A Berger, and J Lafferty, Statistical models for text segmentation. Machine Learning, (34):177-210, 1999. Special Issue on Natural Language Learning (C. Cardie and R. Mooney, eds).
[14] D Lewis and M Ringuette, M.: A comparison of two learning algorithms for text categorization. In: SDAIR. 1994, p. 81-93
[15] P Domingos and M Pazzani, On the Optimality of the Simple Bayesian Classifier under Zero-One Loss, Machine Learning, 29 (2-3), 1997, p. 103-130.
[16] Y Yang, J Pedersen, A Comparative Study on Feature Selection in Text Categorization, Proceedings of ICML, 14th International Conference on Machine Learning, 1997, p. 114-121.
[17] K Nigam, J Lafferty and A McCallum. Using maximum entropy for text classification. In IJCAI Workshop on Machine Learning for Information Filtering, pages 61-67, 1999.
[18] M Hearst, Multi-Paragraph Segmentation of Expository Text. Proceedings of the 32nd Meeting of the Association for Computational Linguistics, 1994, p. 79-94.
[19] J Reynar and A Ratnaparkhi. A maximum entropy approach to identifying sentence boundaries. In Proceedings of the Fifth Conference on Applied Natural Language Processing, pages 16-19, 1997. ACL
[20] S Teufel and M Moens, Argumentative classification of extracted sentences as a first step towards flexible abstracting. Mani, M. Maybury (eds), Advances in automatic text summarization, MIT, 1999.
[21] C van Rijsbergen, Information Retrieval. Buttersworth, 1979.
[22] S Teufel and M Moens, Sentence Extraction and rhetorical classification for flexible abstracts, AAAI Spring Symposium on Intelligent Text summarization, 1998, p. 89-97.
[23] P Ruch, L Perret and J Savoy. Feature Combination for Extraction of Gene Functions. ECIR 2005. Springer LNCS, 112-126.
[24] L McKnight and P Srinivasan. Categorization of Sentence Types in Medical Abstracts. *AMIA* 2003.
[25] P Ruch, R Baud, P Bouillon, and G Robert. Minimal Commitment and Full Lexical Disambiguation: Balancing Rules and Hidden Markov Models. CoNLL-2000, pages 111-115.
[26] P Ruch, R Baud, and A Geissbühler. Latent Argumentative Pruning for Compact MEDLINE Indexing, AIME 2005, Springer LNCS (to appear)
[27] G Cohen, P Ruch, M Hilario: Model Selection for Support Vector Classifiers via Direct Simplex Search. FLAIRS 2005: 431-435.
[28] Y Mizuta and N Collier: Zone Identification in Biology Articles as a Basis for Information Extraction, In Porceedings of JNLPBA (NLPBA/BioNLP), 28-29 August, Geneva, Switzerland.

Address for correspondence

Patrick Ruch, University Hospitals of Geneva, 24 Micheli du Crest, CH-1211 Geneva, Switzerland,
Tel: +41 22 372 61 64, patrick.ruch@sim.hcuge.ch

Section 11

Online Health Information & Patient Empowerment

Connecting Medical Informatics and Bio-Informatics
R. Engelbrecht et al. (Eds.)
IOS Press, 2005

Physicians' Use of Clinical Information Systems in the Discharge Process: An Observational Study

Inger Dybdahl Sørby[a,b], Øystein Nytrø[a,b], Amund Tveit[a,b], Eivind Vedvik [a,c]

[a]Norwegian Centre for Electronic Patient Records, Trondheim, Norway
[b]Department of Computer and Information Science, Norwegian University of Science and Technology, Trondheim, Norway
[c]Faculty of Medicine, Norwegian University of Science and Technology, Trondheim, Norway

Abstract

This study has been performed in order to categorize and measure usage of different information sources and types in a well defined stage of clinical work. The underlying motivation is to improve computer-supported presentation and retrieval of relevant information and to be able to evaluate the functionality of a future improved interface to the electronic patient record (EPR). By observing and analyzing 52 discharge processes, we have seen that the EPR is primarily used for background information and verification. There is a large potential for improved EPR systems that support the clinicians in the plan/future part of the discharge.

Keywords:
Observational Study; Clinical Information Systems; Electronic Patient Records; The Discharge Process

1. Introduction

The study presented in this paper was conducted in order to investigate to what extent clinical information systems – in particular the EPR system – support clinicians in critical and information intensive tasks such as the discharge process. The discharge process includes writing a preliminary summary, having a discharge conversation with the patient, and writing or dictating a final summary. The discharge summary serves as a basis for further treatment and follow-up of the patient when transferred from the hospital specialist to primary care. By studying how and where relevant information is represented in current clinical information systems and the cost of retrieving the information, we can get an impression of how the EPR supports (or does not support) the physicians in the discharge process. This is a step towards a more complete survey of information usage in specific situations, which is necessary for future situation-aware and helpful user interfaces to clinical information systems.

2. Background

EPR systems have been used in Norwegian hospitals for several years, but paper-based information systems are still essential in most patient-centred work [1]. The most apparent reasons are that today's EPR systems do not support the health-care workers' real needs as the systems are not always available, they are not integrated with other clinical systems, they do not support the clinical procedures performed by the different health care workers, and they are not context sensitive or adaptable to individual needs [2, 3]. The quality and content of discharge summaries have been discussed in several studies [8,9,10,11]. However, few systematic evaluations have been performed to investigate why EPR systems are not more extensively used in the discharge process. In order to be able to develop EPR interfaces that really support physicians in the discharge of patients, it is necessary to investigate how current information systems are used.

The main research questions we wanted to answer by conducting this study were as follows:

1. To what extent does the EPR system support the physicians in the discharge process?
2. Is the physicians' work related to the discharge of patients characterized by regularity?
3. What areas of this process can be improved by appropriate computer support?

Our main hypothesis was that the EPR system does not in particular support the physicians' information needs in the discharge process, and thus is not preferable to other information systems. We also presumed that the discharge process to a certain extent is characterized by regularity. Our third hypothesis was that certain areas of the discharge process can be improved by appropriate computer support.

3. Study design and methods

The study was conducted at Department of Cardiology at a large Norwegian university hospital (922 beds) during the period March – June 2004. Two medical students performed non- participatory observations of physicians during the discharge process, including preparations, discharge conversations with the patients, and dictating discharge summaries. The students spent totally 100 hours in one ward, observing the discharge of 52 patients. Every physician working in one particular ward (15 beds) during the study period participated in the study. The participants included two chief physicians with many years experience in the ward, three medium experienced residents, three young residents who had just began working in the ward, and one house physician. The patients followed in this study were mainly suffering from angina pectoris or heart failure, and the investigation of their heart diseases typically led to hospital stays of 3-5 days.

In the initial phase of the study, the two observers worked together in order to co-ordinate their observation notes and to agree on a "standard" for the remaining observations. The observers used a note-taking form partly based on a form described in a textbook on task analysis for interface design [4], pp. 270-271. The form was divided into three main parts. The first part included nine columns, one for each known/expected information source. The sources were *Patient record (paper-based), Electronic patient record (EPR), the patient chart, ICD-10 code overview, X-rays reports or pictures (including other picture results like CT and MR), Patient Administrative System (PAS, not integrated with the EPR), Physicians' Desk Reference (PDR), Colleagues, and Patient.* Personal notes were an important additional information source for some physicians. During the observations, the appropriate table cells were marked 'X' with an exception for the ICD-10 codes and the PDR which existed both on paper ('P') and electronic ('E') medium. In addition, the columns marked "Supplementary

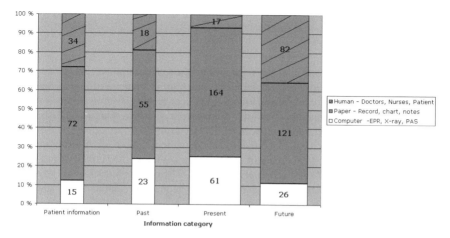

Figure 1 – Usage of human, paper-based, and electronic information sources. Numbers are distinct information elements (totally 688). Column width indicates the total number of information elements in each information category.

information" could be used if several sources were used to find, control, verify, or check consistency of some information. *However, in order to focus on patient-specific information, and eliminate regular use of static reference tools, we have omitted PDR and ICD-10 usage from the further analysis.*

The second main part of the form was used to describe the information that was retrieved from the selected information source. The last main part included a field for the observers' personal comments or questions, as it is important to separate their own thoughts and interpretations from the "objective" observations noted in the "Information" column [4]. The forms were filled in chronologically, from top to bottom. In addition to the notes taken by the observers, a few of the discharge processes were videotaped for further analysis.

The contents of the 52 observation forms were coded into matrices (one matrix per observation) containing information sources versus information categories. The information categories were taken from a discharge summary template suggested by the Norwegian Centre for Medical Informatics (KITH) [5]. During analysis of the results, the information categories were first divided into four disjunctive groups of different temporal significance:

Future: Information that pertains to plans and future care. This group contains categories assessment, follow-up, medications, info to next of kin, and medical certificate.

Present: Information about current state and hospital treatment. This group contains the categories: Diagnosis and procedure, progress and treatment, findings and examination results.

Past: Historic/permanent patient information. This group contains the categories: Allergies, previous illnesses, and reason for referral.

Patient information: Information not related to the patient's current hospital stay: Biographical data and family/social history.

During the 52 discharge processes, a total of 735 information elements were identified, 688 of these were patient specific and belonged to one of the four information categories mentioned above. Figure 1 shows the relative distribution of the information elements retrieved from the different sources.

4. Findings

In the following sections we comment on some of our findings, ordered according to information category and source.

4.1 Information categories

Patient information is very static, and has surprisingly low reliance upon electronic sources (12%), main sources are the paper record and chart. The high percentage of human sources can be interpreted as a validation of information (and patient identity).

Past: Historic patient information is mainly from paper sources, which is costly and difficult to find in old, and often large, records.

Present: The paper chart is obviously the most convenient source of information, in addition to actually remembering the patient and the course of actions. Human sources are surprisingly little used, even if they are easily available. There is considerable variation in work style; we have seen an effect of physicians writing personal notes, later used in addition to chart and other tools.

Future: Much of this information is about plans and medication (involving colleagues and the patient), and the necessary assessment and decisions are often made during the discharge process. We have also seen that development of medication plans and prescriptions involve search in *many* separate sources that frequently are inconsistent and incomplete [7].

4.2 Information sources

The EPR was used as information source in 27 of the 52 observed discharge situations, while the patient chart was used in 51 of 52 situations. The number of sources used in the discharge processes varied from 1 to 9 (average: 3.77 sources). Figure 2 shows mean first use of the various information source types in the observed discharge processes. The figure shows that paper based information systems are most often selected as primary sources in the discharge process. The electronic sources were often used as secondary sources if the physicians could not find the expected information in the papers. The confidence interval (CI) is quite large for these information sources, and to what extent the electronic information sources were used varied a lot, depending on the individual physicians. The younger physicians showed a tendency to use the EPR as primary information source more often than the more experienced and older physicians. The human information sources where mainly used as third choice, often in order to verify data collected from other information sources.

5. Discussion

The study presented in this paper was performed in order to investigate how physicians, exemplified by cardiologists, use various information sources in the discharge process. All the patients in the study had been treated for similar heart diseases like angina pectoris or heart failure, but there were large variations in their previous medical history and thus the volume of the patient records and for instance the amounts of medications of each patient. Consequently, these factors had implications for how complicated the physicians' work regarding the discharge process was. This is clearly shown in the individual observational notes, as they vary from only 2 information elements to 25. Another aspect when analyzing the results is that due to limited time of the students performing the observations, not every observation included the entire discharge process. Most of the observations, however, included the physician's preparation for the discharge conversation, including writing a preliminary discharge summary. Most observations also included the discharge conversations, but due to time pressure of the physicians, the final discharge summaries were not always written immediately after the discharge conversations, and hence some observations do not include the writing/dictating of these summaries. However, this also

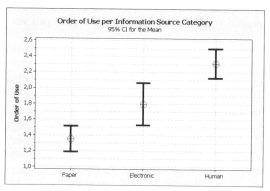

Figure 2 – Order of use per information source

means that some discharge summaries are written separately, some time after the patient left the hospital and possibly by a different physician than the one that performed the actual discharge of the patient. A few of these situations were also observed and are included in the analysis.

The nine physicians that participated in the study varied in age, gender, and experience, both as clinicians and at the specific ward. Every physician had his or her own established working pattern, and this varied a lot from individual to individual. Even though the number of physicians participating in the study is limited, the sample is fairly representative as they included every physician working in the specific ward during the study period. In similar studies, prospective participants have been excluded if they had less than for instance one month of experience in the ward being studied [6]. In our study, however, no such exclusion criteria were used, as we regard physicians with little experience of particular interest since they are even more dependent on appropriate information systems than the more experienced physicians.

The quality of observational studies depends to a large extent on the observers; their knowledge of the domain, and their ability to transform the observations into data/written information that can be analyzed. The subjects being observed might also be affected by the presence of the observers, however, by using medical students as observers this problem was hopefully minimized, as the physicians are used to being followed by students and house physicians. The note-taking form that was developed prior to and iterated during the study helped the students structuring their observations, and at the same time it allowed for comments and questions that could be discussed later. The form was changed two times during the study, based on the students' experiences and feedback. The changes of the form only led to easier note-taking for the students, and had no effect on the content or the quality of the resulting observation forms. The observation forms were coded into tables of information categories versus information sources. In order to ensure consistency, one of the students performed the coding of all the observation forms.

Despite the weaknesses mentioned above about the methods used in the study, the analysis of more than 50 different discharge processes gives a good impression of how the various information sources are used in the discharge process at the department of cardiology. Even though this is a very limited study based on only one hospital ward, this department is one of the most complex departments of the hospital, characterized by high activity and large variations in the patients' illness patterns, and thus hopefully it is fairly representative for several hospital departments.

The analysis of the results has so far not been used for more qualitative descriptions of the discharge process. However, the preliminary analysis shows that there is an obvious need for an improved interface to the EPR system that makes it easier for the physicians to retrieve and produce relevant information when preparing and performing the discharge of patients.

6. Conclusion

Our research hypotheses were to a large extent confirmed. The analysis of the observations shows that today's EPR system is not preferable to paper based information systems, as the current EPR system was not designed to support the discharge process in particular. The analysis also shows that the discharge process to a certain degree is predictable but with large individual variations due to different working patterns of the various physicians, and also due to large variations in the patients' illness histories. We have seen examples of discharge processes where the physician has known the patient well and most information has been retrieved from the physician's memory, while other situations have required the physician to search for information in up to nine different information sources. A new and improved EPR system should be preferred by every physician in every discharge situation; hence it has to be simple and easy to use but also flexible and adaptable in order to support the different working styles of the individual users.

7. Acknowledgments

We would like to thank the staff at the Department of Cardiology at the University Hospital of Trondheim for their cooperation during the observational studies. This research was financed by the strategic research area Medical Technology (http://www.ntnu.no/medtek) at NTNU and the NTNU Innovation Fund for Business and Industry (http://www.ntnu.no/idefondet/).

8. References

[1]   Lærum H, Ellingsen G, Faxvaag A. Doctors' use of electronic medical records systems in hospitals: cross sectional survey. *BMJ 2001;323(7325):1344-1348.*

[2]   Dahl Y, Sørby ID, Nytrø Ø. Context In Care - Requirements For Mobile Context-Aware Patient Charts. In: *MedInfo 2004; 2004; San Francisco, California, USA;* 2004.

[3]   Sørby ID, Melby L, Nytrø Ø. Characterising Cooperation in The Ward: A Framework for Producing Requirements to Mobile Electronic Healthcare Records. In: *Second International Conference on the Management of Healthcare and Medical Technology: The Hospital of the Future; 2002; Chicago, Illinois, USA;* 2002.

[4]   Hackos J, Redish JC. *User and task analysis for interface design.* New York: John Wiley & Sons, Inc.; 1998.

[5]   Ree, AO. Medical information in discharge summaries - 'the good discharge summary'. *Guideline (in Norwegian) 2002-12-31, KITH 32/02, KITH,* December 2002.

[6]   Brown PJ, Borowitz SM, Novicoff W. Information exchange in the NICU: what sources of patient data do physicians prefer to use? *International Journal of Medical Informatics 2004; 73 (4): 349-355.*

[7]   Rognstad, S and Straand, J. Do general practitioners know what medication community nurses give their shared patients? (In Norwegian). *Tidsskrift for den Norske Lægeforening, 124(6):810–812,* March 2004.

[8]   Archbold, RA, Laji, K, Suliman, A, Ranjadayalan, K, Hemingway, H, and Timmis, AD. Evaluation of a computer-generated discharge summary for patients with acute coronary syndromes. *Br J Gen Pract., 48(429):1163–1164,* April 1998.

[9]   Solomon, JK, Maxwell, RB, and Hopkins, AP. Content of a discharge summary for a medical ward: views of general practioners and hospital doctors. *J R Coll Physicians Lond., 29(4):307–310,* August 1995.

[10] van Walraven, C. and Rokosh, E. What is necessary for high-quality discharge summaries. *Am J Med Qual., 14(4):160–169,* July 1999.

[11] Wilson, S, Ruscoe, W, Chapman, M, and Miller, R. General Practitioner-hospital communications: a review of discharge summaries. *Journal of Quality in Clinical Practice, 21(4):104–108,* December 2001.

Address for correspondence

Inger Dybdahl Sørby, IDI, NTNU, NO-7491 Trondheim, E-mail: inger.sorby@idi.ntnu.no

Connecting Medical Informatics and Bio-Informatics
R. Engelbrecht et al. (Eds.)
IOS Press, 2005

Cost-effective Ambulatory Monitoring

Pantelis Angelidis, Markela Psymarnou

Vidavo Ltd., Thessaloniki, Greece

Abstract

The Mobinet service concept emerged, as points of care move closer to the patient and the citizen/patient undertakes a more active role in healthcare monitoring and prevention. Today's advances in monitoring devices and telecommunication networks have made possible a viable solution regarding the provision of continuous health monitoring services, seamlessly from the patients' point of view. The Mobinet concept has been tested under various clinical, technical and business pilots throughout Europe and is currently set for commercial launch in Greece.

Keywords:
Telemonitoring; Patient empowerment

1. Introduction

As healthcare infrastructure matures, the sector is able to support a wide range of advanced applications. The healthcare actors reform their healthcare provision models in order to remain competitive in a demanding landscape and in order to reach rising customer expectations for improved services, while maintaining economic efficiency.

Disease management and treatment plans consisted the core of the healthcare processes, prior to the evolution of new practices due to IT developments in the framework of the information era. The development of novel back-office applications or telemedicine solutions and other services addressing demanding patient needs triggered patient centric processes, mainly focusing on prevention rather than treatment. Additionally, it has been shown that better patient education and self-management on heart failure and other chronic diseases may increase the mean time to re-admission and decrease the number of days in hospital and the annual health care cost per patient [1].

Further to the new approaches in the provision of healthcare services in the frame of ehealth, wireless developments create new opportunities, for the healthcare professionals, individuals and organizations, patients and health authorities. Mobile health advances generate new capabilities in patient self-care. Cost effective solutions minimize effort in monetary and human input terms, whereas creating new communication modes, facilitating both the healthcare professionals and the patients.

The Mobinet service concept aims to explore the dynamics of interactive continuous chronic patient and citizen monitoring. The pilot application particularly focused on the telemonitoring impact on the patients' quality of life, the patients' active involvement in their own care and accordingly, the impact on the overall quality of healthcare provision, as well as the benefits for the healthcare providers (time management, patient management, savings, etc). Utilizing the ICT and medical industry advances, Mobinet will exploit a modular telemedicine platform, in order to achieve remote vital signs' diagnosis. The Mobinet concept was piloted in Greece and developed a sound business case regarding the provision of innovative telemedicine services to citizens with chronic conditions, as well as those who want to monitor their health more closely for "wellness" purposes, since Mobinet is directed at the "chronically ill" as well as the "worried well" citizens.

2. Mobinet Ambulatory Monitoring

2.1 Mobinet concept

The Mobinet service concept emerged, as points of care move closer to the patient and the citizen/patient undertakes a more active role in healthcare monitoring and prevention. The need to provide cost-effective healthcare services for continuous telemonitoring of vital signs to remote or on the move patients has been early identified, to bridge the gap in healthcare provision. This gap is created by the inability of healthcare providers to offer continuous monitoring, seamlessly to chronic patients.

2.2 Mobinet service description

Mobinet allows the physician to design the personalized care protocol of each patient, to monitor the application of the protocol and the measurements already taken by the patient. Two major subsystems, the patient's module and the server, compose the overall Mobinet service concept.

The patient's module consists of one or more monitoring devices. The patient or a nurse/carer, following the care protocol created by the physician, takes the measurements. The data are then sent to the server (multiple routes were tested including PSTN, GPRS and TCP/IP), where it is examined by the physician. A number of pilots were set to test the concept from a clinical and a business point of view. Two of them were partially supported by the EC under the IST and eTEN programmes of DG INFSO between 2000 and 2004 [2] [3].

During the clinical tests the service was provided to patients with chronic cardiac and pulmonary diseases, such as arrhythmias, Coronary Heart Disease (CHD), asthma and Chronic Obstructive Pulmonary Disease (COPD). The patients were equipped with the appropriate monitoring devices and recorded their vital signs (ECG and/or lung function parameters as FVC) on a pre-defined basis. The physician at the medical center reviewed and processed the measurements, providing then feedback to the patient.

In a full-scale commercial operation, physicians and patients will have access to the service from PC, PDA's or mobile phones connected to the Internet.

2.3 Customer typology and benefits

The two main user groups of the telemonitoring services are the healthcare professionals and the citizens/patients. Each user group is divided into several sub-groups. More specifically, the Mobinet service concept targets:

- *Healthcare professionals:* including cardiologists, pulmonary specialists, GPs, and/or family doctors. Depending on the vital data to be measured by the patient and monitored remotely, this group of users can be easily expanded to address further specialties (i.e. *endocrinology*). The healthcare professionals, either individuals in private practice or entities can expand via the Mobinet concept their customer base, address remote geographical markets, and manage more effectively resources.

- *Citizens / Chronically ill patients*: including patients with heart or pulmonary diseases as well as citizens wishing to maintain an optimal physical condition. Mobinet empowers citizens/patients to actively monitor their health status and enjoy autonomy and an elevated quality of life.

Besides the main user categories identified, other actors include diagnostic centers, private insurance companies, private clinics / hospitals, free-lance doctors, pharmaceutical companies, private clinics for the elderly or athletes that may utilize ambulatory monitoring services in order to expand their service portfolio, while reducing costs.

3. Results

3.1 Service evaluation

The service was tested in various settings (i.e. diagnostics centers, hospitals, residential homes, doctors' offices in private practice, and individual patients) throughout Europe, by a total of ninety-four users, enabling continuous health monitoring and patient-physician interaction. Healthcare professionals and chronic patients comprised the core of the group that validated the service.

The health status of the patients was closely monitored, when they were at home, work, vacation, etc. The majority of the patients responded positively to the service and highly valued the enhanced feeling of safety they experienced via Mobinet. The latter was even more intense in the case for the female population participating in the service concept evaluation. Additionally, all patients (both with cardiac and pulmonary diseases) reported that the Mobinet process of ambulatory monitoring is particularly easy for the inexperienced users.

Patients located in remote areas in particular and utilizing the service, such as monks at the Holy Mountain Athos, appraised the time and money savings deriving from the remote monitoring, instead of visiting the closest urban center, in order to contact specialized healthcare professionals.

The healthcare professionals acknowledged the Mobinet contribution in facilitating their everyday tasks. A larger base of patients is handled in a straightforward manner. The cardiologists viewed the service as a valuable tool for monitoring heart diseases and depicting a change in the patient's condition. In the case of arrhythmias in particular, Mobinet contributes to the evaluation of the patients' description of symptoms that cannot be diagnosed for example at the doctor's office, but only at the time they occur.

The pulmonologists pointed out that in the case of asthma patients, Mobinet has diagnostic value, which is to be furthered explored and tested. Via Mobinet, the basic measurement reflecting the narrowing of the airways, is monitored and provides input for differentiating between obstructive and restrictive patterns, for asthma diagnosis (via the vital signs' variability), for assessing the severity of the condition and monitoring the patient's response to a pre-specified treatment plan, for monitoring the severity of COPD and also assessing the suitability of patients for oxygen therapy. As the major problem with asthma and COPD patients is that may be asymptomatic, when they visit their doctor and have exacerbations when they are at home, via Mobinet the doctor ensures that the complete image of the patient condition is considered.

Following the healthcare professionals feedback on the use of the service, the following application areas were identified for the Mobinet concept deployment: a) diagnosis, b) monitoring, c) treatment, and d) follow-up.

It should be noted at this point, that only the healthcare professionals familiar to new technologies were initially positive towards the Mobinet service implementation. Techno phobia can comprise a remarkable constraining factor to the Mobinet concept success. Healthcare professionals unaware of the information society capabilities and their impact on the practice of medicine view the Mobinet concept as a potentially competing service that will compel them to reduce their patient base. On the other hand, the only way to appeal to the majority of the patients is to reach them via their attendant physician.

3.2 Financial Feasibility

The successful completion of the clinical trials and the service attributes highly valued by the users, contributed to the preliminary business considerations and the development of a complete implementation plan for commercial operation in Greece. The business plan was technically based on the Cardguard PMP® solution, the only currently world-wide commercially available solution matching the Mobinet concept requirements. Based on the business planning elements, the service has a significant potential in the local Greek market, but also, on a pan-European basis as well. It is crucial to address with novel healthcare services the cardiology and pulmonary fields of medicine, as they comprise diseases that affect a great amount of the population on local and European levels. CHD and COPD for example, constitute in cases not only life-threatening health conditions, but additionally entail a series of associated socio-economic costs (e.g. negative impact on the patient's overall quality of life, hospitalisation expenses, insurance expenses, etc) [4].

The business plan focuses on the peculiarities of the local health market, explores the potential of telemonitoring services and draws the business, financial and marketing strategies for the successful penetration to the Greek market.

Based on the Mobinet business planning considerations, telemonitoring services can prove to be cost-effective either in the public or the private healthcare provision domain. On the one-hand public healthcare providers are able to reach remote isolated areas and possibly reduce hospitalisation expenditures in the long run. On the other hand, individual citizens may benefit from the service. Undertaking the cost of telemonitoring can save them the time and money previously allocated to visits at private medical establishments for the conduction of routine diagnostic tests. Additionally, when the service is provided by a private healthcare provider, it is considered as an added-value service to its existing portfolio of services, meaning that it can attract a wider customer base.

Although the market is still immature, the financial benefits generated for all parties involved create the potential for appealing to the general public. Nevertheless, there is still uncertainty about the impact telemonitoring will have when used in routine practice. The wider economic implications have not been comprehensively quantified and valued. In addition, long-term sustainable telemedicine programs must be consistent with business objectives and strategic plans, which is not always evident in the area of current applications [5].

4. Discussion

The Mobinet concept generates significant social benefits, including improvement in the provision of healthcare services and elevation of the patient quality of life. Mobinet enables healthcare professionals to allocate their time in an efficient and effective manner, as they are able to manage more patients, since telemonitoring allows the simultaneous monitoring of the health status of multiple patients. Patient management and also, data management for each patient is improved, facilitating medication management and the completion of administrative tasks for the healthcare professionals.

Mobinet is a novel service concept within the Greek market and it is expected that part of the costs previously allocated to home visits and/or visits to the hospital will be allocated to Mobinet. Therefore, it is anticipated that the full market deployment of Mobinet will positively impact hospitalization duration and according expenses and that it will improve patient's morale since s/he will have an active role in monitoring his/her health condition.

The service feasibility in Greece has been validated and the outcome so far creates expectations for the full market deployment. The Mobinet concept in Greece directly targets citizens that reimburse the primary healthcare services they receive, via out-of-pocket payments. Whereas virtually all Greek citizens have coverage for healthcare services through statutory insurance or the National Healthcare System, there is a large private sector consisting of consultations with physicians in private practice, visits to private diagnostic centers, as well as private hospitals for in-patient care. This is due to dissatisfaction with publicly provided services. Nevertheless, public insurance funds, sooner or later, are expected to notice the advantages of (the Mobinet concept and other) telematic services and, overcoming their reluctance towards innovative technological systems, employ them. This allows a perspective of a much wider user base in the future.

5. Conclusion

Services like the Mobinet concept enable patient-doctor continuous interaction, regardless of location and any other geographical limitation. Following the trend for healthcare service provision away of the traditional nursing areas (i.e. at the patient's homecare setting, work environment, or event at vacation, etc), ambulatory telemonitoring services have a direct impact on the patient's overall quality of life.

The enhanced monitoring capabilities of the Mobinet service concept are expected to have a positive impact on the time saving and the cost efficiency of the healthcare professionals, as the service enables the simultaneous monitoring of the health status of multiple patients. Patient management and also, data management for each patient will be improved, facilitating medication management and the completion of administrative tasks for the healthcare professionals. Additionally, Mobinet is anticipated to positively impact hospitalisation duration and costs, and also, to minimize transportation costs allocated by patients / citizens in remote areas to doctor visits for routine examination.

The Mobinet service when deployed is expected to promote the wellness concept at the chronically ill and worried well market segments.

6. Acknowledgements

The authors would like to thank the medical center IASIS and Dr. Chrysoula Kourtidou-Papadeli in particular for her contribution in the conduction and evaluation of the Mobinet service clinical trials. In addition, the authors would like to thank the representatives of the Business Development and Global Marketing Department of Cardguard, and in particular Mr. Reuven Freudinger, for their support and contribution towards the Mobinet business case.

7. References

[1]   Cline CMJ, Israelsson BYA, Willenheimer RB, Broms K, Erhardt LR. Cost effective management programme for heart failure reduces hospitalisation. *Heart*, 1998;80:442-6

[2]   CHS project, "Distance Information Technologies for Home Care," contract number IST-1999-13352

[3]   e-Vital project, "Cost-Effective Health Services for Interactive Continuous Monitoring of Vital Signs Parameters," contract number C27979

[4]   *European White Book on Lung Disease*, to be published by the European Respiratory Society and the European Lung Foundation

[5]   Andriana Prentza, Pantelis Angelidis, Lefteris Leondaridis and Dimitris Koutsouris, Cost-Effective Health Services for Interactive Continuous Monitoring of Vital Signs Parameters – the e-Vital Concept, *International Congress on Medical and Care Compunetics*, The Hague, The Netherlands, June 2-4, 2004

8. Address for correspondence

Pantelis Angelidis
9th km Thessaloniki – Thermi road
57001 Thessaloniki, Greece
Tel/Fax: (30-2310) 486951
e-mail: pantelis@vidavo.gr
www.vidavo.gr

Connecting Medical Informatics and Bio-Informatics
R. Engelbrecht et al. (Eds.)
IOS Press, 2005

Health Information Systems Evaluation: A Focus on Clinical Decision Supports System

Maryati Mohd. Yusof, Ray J Paul, Lampros Stergioulas

School of Information Systems, Computing and Mathematics, Brunel University, United Kingdom

Abstract

In a review of selected literature on Health Information Systems (HIS) evaluation, a specific focus on Clinical Decision Support Systems (CDSS) is taken because of their relative popularity. This paper discusses the issues and problems of CDSS evaluation such as methods, adoption and barriers. The limited use and evaluation of CDSS are still debated. Clinical evaluations of CDSS performed in the actual clinical settings may provide better understanding of their adoption, particularly in the diagnostic function. New HIS evaluation frameworks that incorporate technological, human and organisational issues may be useful to complement existing ones.

Keywords:
Information Systems, Evaluation, Clinical Decision Support Systems

1. Introduction

Health Information Systems (HIS) evaluation seeks to answer the *why, who, when, what* and *how* questions that relate to technological, human and organisational issues surrounding it. In addition to this complexity, HIS evaluation is also unclear and confusing [1]. Hence, this paper seeks to discuss the issues and problems of HIS evaluation that are highlighted in the selected health informatics literature. A specific focus on clinical decision support systems (CDSS) evaluation is taken because of their relative popularity [17,19]. CDSS have been controversial – they are still not widely used despite their potential usefulness [2,3]. Yet, a large number of CDSS have continued to develop.

HIS range from simple systems, such as transaction processing systems, to complex systems such as clinical decision support systems. Different types of HIS are defined in various terms in health informatics literature; the same term is –sometimes- used for different types of systems, which can create confusion. A classification of different types of health information systems is therefore proposed to distinguish between them.

This paper is organised into four sections. The following section provides a brief description of HIS and their classification. Section three presents the features of HIS evaluation and a discussion of early evaluation studies using CDSS as an example. Finally, the conclusion and suggestions for further research are given in section four.

2. Health Information Systems

HIS are used extensively in the healthcare organisations to support various task such as conventional data processing tasks that include patient billing, accounting, inventory control, statistics calculation, and patient history maintenance (See Table 1). They are also used for scheduling, automating nurse stations, monitoring intensive care patients, and providing preliminary diagnoses [4].

Table 1: Classification of Health Information Systems

Information Systems	Descriptions	Characteristics	References
Patient Centred Information Systems	They are the electronic version of patients' information. Different terms are used to refer to these systems including Electronic Patient Record (EPR), Electronic Medical Record (EMR) and Computer based Patient Record (CPR)	• Manage comprehensive patient care information such as medical records, appointment scheduling, theatre management and ward reporting • Have entry and retrieval functions for medical records and clinical procedures	[4]
Administrative Information Systems	Record the main business processes and routine transactions of organisations such as patient admission, discharge and transfer, bill processing, reporting and other management purposes.	• May constitute accounting subsystems, financial subsystems, inventory subsystems, equipment subsystems and general management subsystems tailored to the clinical environment	[4,5]
Clinical Information Systems (CIS)	Represent separate systems in specialized service of clinical departments.	• Perform specific tasks including collection of specific data for patient care, research, management, planning and maintenance of national data repositories • Specific tasks operate in departments such as internal medicine, cardiology, neurology, obstetrics, surgery and psychiatry • CIS are used for administrative support, patient data collection, decision support, picture archiving, image analysis, monitoring, reporting, assessment and research	[4,6]
Radiology Information Systems	Support the acquisition and analysis of radiological images as well as administrative functions of radiology department. Example: Picture Archiving and Communication Systems (PACS)	• May be stand alone or integrated in hospital information systems	[6]
Laboratory Information Systems	Perform data validation, administration, electronic transmission and computer storage.	• In high demand when a large number of tests generate large data. Samples are analysed fully automatically, and the results are computer generated. • Support clinician to analyse trends to assess treatment effects	[6]
Pharmacy Information Systems	Maintain medication information	• Include functions such as keeping patients' medication records, checking prescriptions, and providing drug prescriptions and administration to physicians and nurses	[6]
Telemedicine	Telemedicine provides and supports healthcare services and education across distances via electronic communications and IT	• Facilitates exchange between primary care physicians and specialists as well as patients from disperse locations • "Allows physicians to practise medicine at a distance"	[3,4,7]
Clinical Decision Support Systems	Designed specifically to aid clinical decision making	• Common functions: alerting, reminding, critiquing, interpreting, predicting, diagnosing, assisting and suggesting.	[8,9]
Hospital Information Systems	Consist of integrated hospital information processing systems. Examples: Computerized Physician Order Entry (CPOE), Patient Care Information Systems, nursing (bedside) documentation systems	• Support healthcare activities at the operational, tactical and strategic levels. • Encompass patient management, administration, facilities management and medical applications. • Contain database systems, data communication facilities and terminal or workstations	[4,6,10]

Patient Centred Information Systems are the core system in healthcare organisations; they are usually linked to other HIS to provide patients' information and their medical history. Clinical Information Systems are designed uniquely according to each clinical department. A number of systems are identified as clinical support information systems including Radiology Information Systems, Laboratory Information Systems and Pharmacy Information Systems [6]. Hospital Information Systems refer to general systems that comprise several hospital information processing systems.

3. Health Information Systems Evaluation

Health Information Systems evaluation is defined as "the act of measuring or exploring attributes of a HIS (in planning, development, implementation, or operation), the result of which informs a decision to be made concerning that system in a specific context" [11]. Evaluation serves different purposes. Given the unpredictable characteristics of Information Systems (IS) in general and the purpose of improving clinical performance and patient outcomes in particular, evaluation is performed to understand system performance [6]. Essentially, the evaluation of health informatics applications has the potential to improve the quality of care, its costs and certify HIS as safe and effective [12,6].

As mentioned above, evaluation seeks to answer the *why* (objective of evaluation), *who* (which stakeholders' perspective is going to be evaluated), *when* (which phase in the system development life cycle), *what* (aspects or focus of evaluation) and *how* (methods of evaluation) questions.

The *Who*. Evaluation involves many stakeholders who have different views on the systems. The usefulness of the evaluation results varies among different individuals. Common types of stakeholders of HIS include developer, user, patient and purchaser [13]. The potential of HIS to improve patient care and the performance of clinicians is often thwarted by the users' reluctance to accept and adopt it [14]. Therefore, the usefulness of HIS depends largely on users (customers), because they are the experts in their work, not the developers (designers) [15].

The *When*. In general, apart from the feasibility study, evaluation can be carried out during four main system development phases – pre-implementation (development), during implementation, post-implementation or routine operation [16]. From the health informatics domain, four evaluation phases are defined: preliminary, validity, functionality and impact [17]. Each phase addresses specific evaluation aspects. Based on these phases, evaluation can be distinguished into two types of studies, formative and summative. The aim of formative evaluation is to improve the system under development or during implementation; thus, problems can be identified as they emerge and the system can be improved as it is being developed. On the other hand, the aim of summative evaluation is to assess a system in operation and overall system effectiveness to provide information for determining system continuation [18].

The *What*. Many aspects of HIS can be evaluated. Evaluation involves human, technology, organisations and interaction between them [19,20]. Hence, evaluation can hold technical, professional, organisational, economic, ethical and legal domains [21]. The four evaluation phases are also individually associated with these aspects of evaluation: feasibility, technical verification, usability and impact [17].

The *How*. Evaluators ask various questions and use a variety of methods to address them. Evaluation approach is mainly classified into two types, which are objectivist and subjectivist. The limitation of the objectivist approach suggests the subjectivist approach is a better alternative [22]. It is viewed as being holistic, thorough, rigorous, economical, and time efficient as opposed to the objectivist approach, which is viewed as being both financially and time consuming and labour intensive. In addition, "difficulties in conducting objectivist studies make it difficult to conduct such studies in the first place". Evaluation can also be performed using quantitative and qualitative methods or a combination of both methods.

3.1 Early Studies on Evaluation

Early studies on HIS evaluation are listed in Table 2. HIS evaluation faces a number of barriers and problems that pose challenges to its evaluators [1,13,20,23]. It is argued that while HIS is being increasingly developed, the number of published evaluations is limited [10]. In addition, an existing strong foundation for good evaluation theory and practice is yet to be disseminated in an understandable form [11]. However, it seems that such problems regarding evaluation methods in health informatics can be improved [23]. Therefore, new methods and extensions of the existing methods for health informatics may be useful to complement the existing ones [22].

Table 2: Early Studies on HIS Evaluation

References	Theme	Findings/Conclusions
[11,23]	Problems and challenges of HIS evaluation	Research in Health Informatics evaluation is still in its infancy and what constitutes 'good' HIS is still unclear. It seems desirable to have a broadly accepted, detailed evaluation framework that could guide researchers to undertake evaluation studies.
[22]	Comparison between objectivist and subjectivist approach	Subjectivist approach has advantages over the limitations of objectivist approach.
[24]	Critiques for randomized controlled clinical trials (RCT) and experimental approaches	The limitations of RCT/experimental approaches to evaluation call for alternative approaches that address contextual issues such as social interactionist.
[9]	Review the effects of CDSS on physician performance and patient outcome based on the assessment of RCT	There was a rapid increase in published CDSS studies with improved quality. The benefits of CDSS in enhancing clinical performances can be seen in drug dosing, preventive care and other aspects of health care but not convincingly in diagnosis. The studies on CDSS effects on patient outcomes are limited.
[2]	Review CDSS literature concerning evaluation	Although CDSS is acknowledged for its potential to improve care, evidence is unclear in its diagnostic function. There is a general consensus on limited use of CDSS despite its proven or potential benefits. Most studies use experimental or RCT approach but very few studies involve field tests and almost none take place in actual clinical settings. Most studies focus on physicians and exclude other clinicians. Studies in understanding issues surrounding development, implementation and use of CDSS are lacking.
[1]	The importance of human factors in HIS evaluation	Human factors are central to HIS evaluation.
[18,25,26]	Review papers on human, organisational and social issues in HIS evaluation	Human, organisational and social issues are important to address during overall system development. Newer evaluation trends are focusing more on these non-technical issues.

A large number of CDSS have been developed; yet their use are still limited, although they have been adopted by a number of institutions, mostly from academic hospitals [2,3,6]. While most studies noted the low adoption rate of CDSS, one study argued that numerous CDSS are used in clinical work, most of which are small systems but which contribute to care [27]. It is interesting to note the similarities in barriers in the use of Decision Support Systems (DSS) in both management and healthcare domain. It can be inferred that in general, the reluctance to use DSS is mainly because decision makers feel challenged by their role and authority in making decisions [28]. On the other hand, CDSS are yet to be successful in application because they are not practical, and do not match with the settings where they are implemented and the manner in which tasks are performed by physicians [2,10,27,29]. The success of a specific system in a specific setting can only be shown from a rigorous evaluation [10]. However, apart from their limited use, CDSS are also acknowledged for their limited clinical evaluation [2,3,6].

Two reviews on CDSS indicate that evidences regarding improved diagnostic function for CDSS are still unconvincing [2,9]. A relevant question to ask is whether physicians really need CDSS to diagnose their patients. Nevertheless, the benefits of CDSS in other medical areas including patient safety, quality of care and efficiency in health care delivery have been reported [3,27]. CDSS have also known to aid reducing two types of errors, in particular, medication and diagnostic errors [27]. A further review of CDSS evaluation literature was carried out in early 2000 [2]. It appears that CDSS evaluation studies are not linked to other informatics applications. As a result, the understanding of the effectiveness of CDSS is impeded by insufficient information from other informatics evaluations, and this results in less informed decisions about CDSS and other health informatics applications. Further, this review shows that studies have focused on these aspects of CDSS: system accuracy, user performance, system functionality, and patient care.

A number of evaluation studies including those on impact, fit, comparison, usability, design and organisational, ethical and adoption influence have been performed [1,18,25,26]. These studies show the importance of human and organisational issues such as organisational and human factors, cognitive factors, readiness, diffusion of innovation, workflow, change management, clinical context and methods of development and dissemination in influencing system success. Hence, evaluation should not only address the "how well a system works, but also how well it works with particular users in a particular setting"[26]. More works on these areas have been called for as most existing evaluation studies tend to focus on the technical issues or clinical processes [2,24,25,26,27,29].

4. Conclusion

This paper has taken a closer look at combined technical and non-technical issues of HIS evaluation to provide a better understanding of the complexity and issues surrounding this area. This review has identified a number of research needs in HIS evaluation. HIS evaluation methods have room for improvement; new HIS evaluation frameworks that incorporate technological, human and organisational factors may be useful to complement existing ones. The combination of techniques and methods in HIS evaluation may be combined with those of other disciplines to explore and expand the other aspects of their usefulness. Meanwhile, the limited use and evaluation of CDSS are still being debated. Thus, clinical evaluations of CDSS performed in the actual clinical settings may provide better understanding of their adoption and the identification of features that make them more effective, particularly in the diagnostic function.

5. References

[1] Gremy F, Fessler JM, Bonnin M. Information systems evaluation and subjectivity. *Int J Med Inform* 1999; 56(1-3):13-23.

[2] Kaplan B. Evaluating informatics applications—clinical decision support systems literature review. *Int J Med Inform* 2001a; 64(1):15-37.

[3] Gawande AA, Bates DW. The Use of Information Technology in Improving Medical Performance – Physician-Support Tools. *MedGenMed* 2000;2(1 Pt 2).

[4] Smith J. *Health Management Information Systems: A Handbook for Decision Makers*. Buckingham: Open, University Press; 2000.

[5]   Glandon GL, Buck TL. Cost-benefit analysis of medical information systems: a critique. In: Anderson JG, Aydin CE, Jay SJ, editors. *Evaluating Health Care Information Systems: Methods and Applications.* Newbury Park: Sage Publications; 1994. p. 164-89.

[6]   Van Bemmel JH, Musen MA editors. *Handbook of Medical Informatics.* Heidelberg: Springer–Verlag. 1997.

[7]   Parrino T. Information Technology and Primary Care at the VA: Making Good Things Better, Health Service Research & Development 2003. [cited 2004 21 July]. Available from: URL: http://www.hsrd.research.va.gov/publications/internal/forum10_03.pdf

[8]   Randolph AG, Haynes RB, Wyatt JC, Cook DJ, Guyatt GH. Users' Guides to the Medical Literature: XVIII. How to Use an Article Evaluating the Clinical Impact of a Computer-Based Clinical Decision Support System. *JAMA* 1999;282(1): 67-74.

[9]   Hunt D, Haynes RB, Hanna S, Smith K. Effects of computer-based clinical decision support systems on physician performance and patient outcomes. *JAMA* 1998;280(15):1339-46.

[10] Van Der Meidjen MJ, Tange HJ, Troost J, Hasman A. Determinants of Success of Inpatient Clinical Information Systems: A Literature Review. *JAMA* 2003;10(3): 235-43.

[11] Ammenwerth E, Brender J, Nykanen P, Prokosch HU, Rigby M, Talmon J, HIS-EVAL Workshop Participants. Visions and strategies to improve evaluation of health information systems: Reflectionsand lessons based on the HIS-EVAL workshop in Innsbruck. *Int J Med Inform* 2004;73(6):479-91.

[12] Kuhn KA, Giuse, DA. From Hospital Information Systems to Health Information Systems – Problems, Challenges, Perspective. *Yearbook of Medical Informatics 2001*: 63-76.

[13] Friedman CP, Wyatt JC. *Evaluation Methods in Medical Informatics.* New York: Springer-Verlag; 1997.

[14] Williamson M. (2004). How do I evaluate user acceptance of an electronic decision support system, Australian Health Information Council 2004 [cited 2004 23 December]. Available from http://www.ahic.org.au/evaluation/user.htm

[15] Beyer HR, Holtzblatt K. Apprenticing with the Customer. *Commun ACM* 1995;38(5): 45-52.

[16] Willcocks L. Managing technology evaluation - techniques and processes. In: Galliers RD, Baker BSH, editors. *Strategic Information Management: Challenges and strategies in managing information systems.* Oxford: Butterworth Heinemann; 1994. p. 365-81.

[17] Brender J. *Methodology for Assessment of Medical IT-Based Systems.* Amsterdam: IOS Press; 1997.

[18] Kaplan B. Addressing Organizational Issues into the Evaluation of Medical Systems. *JAMA* 1997;4(2): 94-101.

[19] Ammenwerth E, De Keizer N. An inventory of evaluation studies of information technology in health care: trends in evaluation research 1982-2002. *Medinfo 2004*;2004 Sep 7-11; San Francisco, CA,USA. IOS Press; 2004. p.1289-94.

[20] Wyatt JC, Wyatt SM. When and how to evaluate health information systems? *Int J Med Inform* 2003; 69(2-3):251-59.

[21] Stoop AP, Berg M. Integrating Quantitative and Qualitative Methods in Patient Care Information Systems Evaluation: Guidance for the Organizational Decision Maker. *Int J Med Inform* 2004:42(4): 458-62.

[22] Moehr JR. Evaluation: salvation or nemesis of medical informatics? *Comput Biol Med* 2002: 32(3): 113-25.

[23] Ammenwerth E, Graber S, Hermann G, Burkle T, Konig J. Evaluation of health information systems – problems and challenges. *Int J Med Infom* 2003 Sep;71(2-3):125-35. Review.

[24] Kaplan B. Evaluating informatics applications—some alternative approaches: theory, social interactionism, and call for methodological pluralism. *Int J Med Inform* 2001b; 64(1): 39-56.

[25] Kaplan B, Shaw NT. Future directions in evaluation research: people, organisational, and social issues. *Methods Inf Med* 2004;43(3):215-31.

[26] Kaplan B, Shaw NT. People, organizational, and social issues: Evaluation as an exemplar. *Yearbook of Medical Informatics 2002* (Review Paper): 91-102.

[27] Coiera E. *Guide to Health Informatics.* 2nd ed. London: Hodder Arnold; 2003.

[28] Jiang JJ, Muhanna WA, Klenin G. User resistance and strategies for promoting acceptance across system types. *Information & Management* 2000;37(1):25-36.

[29] Brender J, Nøhr C, McNair P. Research needs and priorities in health informatics. *Int J Med Inform* 2000;58-59:257-89.

Acknowledgements:
Alison Cheetam, Herbert W. Daly.

Address for correspondence:
Maryati.Yusof@brunel.ac.uk; maryati226@yahoo.com

Connecting Medical Informatics and Bio-Informatics
R. Engelbrecht et al. (Eds.)
IOS Press, 2005

User Acceptance of and Satisfaction with a Personal Electronic Health Record

A Ertmer, F Ückert

Department of Medical Informatics and Biomathematics, University Hospital Münster, Germany

Abstract

Objective: With akteonline.de a patient owned Electronic Health Record (EHR) has been implemented that combines both data from clinical information systems and data entered by the patient. In addition the EHR supports information exchange/communication controlled by the user. The EHR thus offers the potential to place the patient into a more empowered position. This impact on patient empowerment and the implementation of additional features is to be investigated. Additionally, the user satisfaction is to be evaluated regarding patients' acceptance and utilization of the system. Method: Users were divided into three groups, two of which received different training on the functionalities of akteonline.de. A quantitative study employing an online-questionnaire and considering all registered users was conducted. Results: Users evaluated the internet based system to be feasible and the navigation to be suitable, yet additional training for users regarding particular features seems to be required and also for hospital staff in general. The proposed add-ons were approved of. The study also showed positive effects on patient empowerment.

Keywords:
Patient empowerment; Evaluation; Electronic health record; Personal electronic record; EHR

1. Introduction

The concept of patient empowerment has numerous roots of which enabling and supporting the patient's position as an active member in a team with health care professionals for shared care is only one. Nevertheless it is, next to financial, legal and informational aspects, one of the main reasons for patients to change their health behaviour and use new technological methods, which are made available to them by medical and bio-medical informatics. As one example for those new technologies the Electronic Health Record (EHR) *akteonline.de* was already presented and awarded several times, but until today has not proven its value by a formal user evaluation.

A renowned model for this purpose is the technology acceptance model (TAM) by Davis [1], correlating perceived usefulness, perceived ease of use, attitude towards using, and actual system use. In general, user acceptance is seen to reflect whether a system adequately applies to the characteristics of the users and the characteristics of the task which is to be performed. Thus, user acceptance can be seen as an adequate indicator whether an information system really supports users and therefore can be taken as an overall indicator for a system's success [2].

2. Materials and Methods

The underlying EHR *akteonline.de* is a collection of medical data of one patient, accessible via the internet. The in- and output of data uses web technology or data interchange from the hospital information system (HIS). Internal structures enable the patient to handle a complex access management system with different authorization levels for different persons. As one special access method the patient can create transaction numbers (TAN) with specific access rights and give them away for one-time access.

Study Aims

Goals of the conducted study can be divided into the following sections:
a) Evaluation of: 1. User acceptance (retro- and prospectively); 2. Perceived ease of use; 3. Training of users, training video vs. training brochure
b) Implications on patient empowerment

Study Method

The conducted study was mainly a retrospective, quantitative study, but also contained items regarding future implementation of additional functionalities. In order to study differences between training materials and non-training n=64 users were assigned to one of three groups. EX1 (n=29) received a CD-Rom which contained a self-extracting 30 min video file, addressing all applications in *akteonline.de* and guiding the user through every single functionality, step-by-step. Likewise users in EX2 (n=24) were sent a brochure comprehending the identical information, yet to illustrate the functionalities the brochure contained extensive screen-shots. K3 (n=11) was conceived to be the control group and therefore obtained no training materials. Users in EX1 and EX2 were assigned randomly, however K3 consisted of users who, according to log files had not used the system frequently. It was hypothesized they would not be as interested in taking part in the study as other users. Because of the relatively small sample size K3 was constructed smaller than EX1 and EX2. EX1 was created slightly larger than EX2 as it was expected that hardware problems might occur concerning the video file and therefore users of EX1 might have to be shifted to EX2. A self-administered online-questionnaire was constructed utilizing PHPSurveyor, regarding guidelines by ADM, ASI, D.G.O.F. and BVM [3], applying Dillmann's Tailored Design Method [4] and pre-tested successfully. Users received an invitation via email, including a link for personal one-time access to the questionnaire in order to control participation. The online-questionnaire contained identical items for EX1 and EX2, for K3 items regarding training materials were excluded. The online-questionnaire included branching according to the user's previous answer to an item, so the maximum number of items displayed to EX1 and EX2 was n= 54, the modified version for K3 contained n=47 items. All items were divided into six groups: A: General profile of system use, B: Assessment of system functions, C: Utilization of internet/ Computer knowledge, D: Doctor-Patient relationship, E: Training materials and F: Demographic data. Apart from statements that were to be rated on a four-point, respectively three-point scale and demographic data, the questionnaire also contained free-text questions to provide qualitative data.

Course of study

Initially the time period to be covered by the study was planned 01.07.2004-23.07.2004. As the database contained only n=31 data sets to that date, the trial was extended another 14 days, including a follow-up by telephone. In the end n=50 data sets were included in the analysis using SPSS 11.0.

3. Results

An overall return of 78% was put into effect, ranging from, as expected, relatively low in K3 (38%), 83% in EX1 to 92% in EX2. Ever since the start of this implementation of *akteonline.de* in September 2003 users logged in on average every two months.

Evaluation of user acceptance

Retrospective Evaluation

The items showed a very high internal consistency: Reliability analysis for items assessing system functions resulted in Cronbach's Alpha=0,8282 and standardized item alpha=0,8301. In total users demonstrated a very high level of satisfaction with the system's features:

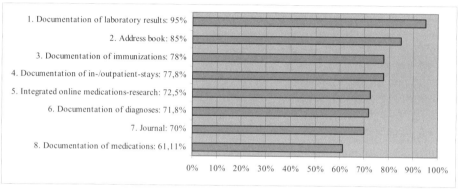

1. Documentation of laboratory results: 95%
2. Address book: 85%
3. Documentation of immunizations: 78%
4. Documentation of in-/outpatient-stays: 77,8%
5. Integrated online medications-research: 72,5%
6. Documentation of diagnoses: 71,8%
7. Journal: 70%
8. Documentation of medications: 61,11%

Figure 1-Positive assessment of system features (in %)

Statements regarding the items were to be rated on a uniformly distributed scale. "Unable to provide an answer" was coded as a missing value. The following values indicate accumulated percentages. Users evaluated the EHR's world-wide access via the internet to be very useful. The unique functionality of controlled one-time access via transaction numbers (TAN) for healthcare providers etc. was found to be highly approved, although only seven users indicated they had made use of that feature in the past.

Table 1 - Evaluation of utility

Item	"very useful"	"rather useful"	"less useful"	"not useful at all"	Missing values
World-wide access	53,2%	31,9%	14,9%	0%	3
Controlled one-time access via TAN for healthcare providers	40,4%	29,8%	21,3%	8,5%	3

Prospective evaluation

Regarding the extension of the presently implemented system it can be stated, that the proposed features should be welcomed by the users.

Table 2 - Prospective evaluation

Item	"very useful"	"rather useful"	"less useful"	"not useful at all"	Missing values
Reminder-service via email	81,6%	12,2%	6,2%	0%	1
Personalized wellness-information	35,6%	24,4%	35,6	4,4%	5
Personalized health-information	61,7%	34%	4,3%	0%	3

Currently akteonline.de is available for patients of the University Hospital of Münster free of charge. Willingness to pay for this service was assumed to be an indicator for user acceptance as it was presumed that only content users would accept a relatively small fee. Users were offered categories ranging from 0 EUR, and max. 30, 40 or 50 EUR per year. 42 users provided an answer, the vast majority of accumulated 71,4% stated they would not be willing to pay, 23,8% offered 30 EUR and each 2,4% stated they would be willing to pay 40, respectively 50 EUR. It should be taken into consideration, that accumulated 70,8% of the users shop online "occasionally" to "rarely", only 12,5% "often", and 16,7% indicated "never".

Perceived ease of use

The following values indicate accumulated percentages. Users indicate they are able to navigate their way through the system and rate the online-help provided sufficient.

Table 3 - Perceived ease of use

Item	agree completely	rather agree	rather disagree	disagree completely	Missing values
System-navigation is complicated	6,3%	16,7%	39,5%	37,5%	2
Help feature is sufficient	26,1%	69,6%	4,3%	0%	4
Well-oriented in system	35,7%	54,8%	7,1%	2,4%	8

However, free-text comments provided an interesting insight, namely that users do need and ask for personal assistance.

Evaluation of training

Rating of distributed training materials
Reliability analysis for items regarding training materials resulted in Cronbach's Alpha=0,8379 and standardized item alpha=0,8474. Due to the small sample size no statistically significant results could be obtained by comparison of mean values. Yet a trend could be established: the training video was rated slightly better than the training brochure regarding the lucidity of presentation, intelligibility, information content, information amount and design. Also the communication of system features appears to result in better understanding via a training video. With Eta=0,456 a comparison of mean values resulted in a better rating of the training video regarding user's interest.

Training effects

Due to the small sample size no statistically significant results could be obtained by comparison of mean values. However a trend was observed for the training brochure to be slightly more effective regarding orientation and navigation. Comparison of users' safety concerns resulted in less safety concerns due to the presentation of the system's safety concept via training video with Eta=0,436 and a difference Δ=0,5 scale points concerning video vs. brochure.

Table 4 - Safety concerns

group	Mean value	N	Standard deviation
EX1 (video)	3,45	22	,671
EX2 (brochure)	2,95	19	,705
K3 (control group)	4,00	3	,000
total	3,27	44	,727

Implications on patient empowerment

Investigated possible implications of a patient-administered, internet-based EHR on the patient-doctor relationship and resulting implications on patient empowerment indicate that users appreciate the possibility to take a more active role in their health management.

Table 5 - Patient as "health manager"

Item	agree completely	rather agree	rather disagree	disagree completely	Missing values
akteonline.de improves my understanding of therapy/diagnosis	22%	34,1%	34,1%	9,8%	9
Expect *akteonline.de* to be helpful when switching health provider	69,6%	26,1%	2,15%	2,15%	4

This is also indicated in the behaviour of users regarding informed health choices they base on internet research. Users do keep a critical distance to online information and therefore also rely on other sources. In a multiple-answer item of n=138 answers 33% stated they sought information of each "experts" and "books", another 18,1% stated "friends", "TV" 13,8%, "magazines" 12,2% and "other" 8%.

Table 6 - Role of internet in information acquisition

Item	agree completely	rather agree	rather disagree	disagree completely	Missing values
Internet is an important source for medical information	35,4%	18,8%	37,5%	8,3%	2
I trust information found on the internet	14,9%	63,8%	21,3%	0%	3

It should be noted that users' affinity to the internet is above the German average [6]: 41,7% indicate they use the internet at home on a daily basis, 31,3% 3-4 times/week, an additional 16,7% state 3-4 times/month and the remaining 10,3% less than that.

4. Discussion and Conclusion

Standardized questionnaires can be seen as a reliable and valid method to measure certain psychological attributes such as user satisfaction and thus provide quantitative results [2], the utilized online-questionnaire proved to be reliable. It should be noted that the results might contain a certain bias: prior to participating in the study, users had to register online for access to their own *akteonline.de*. Therefore it can be supposed, that users hold a certain degree of basic internet/computer knowledge and are familiar with navigation of web-sites and accounts. Also the follow-up by telephone resembled more of an interview-situation and a lot of users took advantage of the opportunity of personal contact and complained about firstly the lack of a contact person and secondly about the missing training of hospital staff concerning *akteonline.de*.

Users indicate a high acceptance of *akteonline.de*, especially the possibility to view and store laboratory results is highly approved. However in free-text entries users also state they'd appreciate the inclusion of more clinical data in their EHR. In addition users specified they would approve of the proposed additional functionalities whose implementation should therefore be considered.

The evaluation results indicate the user interface being operated intuitively and that the system appears to be relatively easy to use. Nevertheless users did note in free-text entries they'd welcome more information on how to use all features. In combination with the information derived from the follow-up this leads to the conclusion that both utilizing parties, namely registered users (patients) and hospital staff, need to be provided with information and training: A combination of training video, potentially via live-stream over the internet, and training brochure seems to be a favorable way.

Regarding the EHR as a tool for patient empowerment *akteonline.de* proves to be a step forward. The system is to be considered the benchmark concerning autonomy of the patient as the manager of his health, no other system provides the patient with equal functionality [6,7]. Furthermore world-wide access to health data and the possibility to share that information with other healthcare providers is highly appraised by users, although they're not yet willing to pay for that benefit. This result is consistent with findings of a general decrease of internet user's willingness to pay for online-services [8]. Further research is needed to evaluate if the implementation of the proposed supplementary functionalities in addition to training facilities will change that attitude.

Maintaining an EHR to educate on therapy and diagnosis with users being in full possession of their own health data is appreciated by users and considered helpful. This awareness could shift the patient-role towards the patient being an active contributor in medical decision making [9]. Since both data provided by the clinical information system and data entered by the patient are integrated in *akteonline.de* the patient is equipped with the opportunity to form an integral part of the healthcare-team. In addition to resulting benefits such as better compliance, the possibility to create a longitudinal patient record that incorporates all health data of a patient over the span of a life-time can be expected to optimize healthcare in general [10] and furthermore enhance clinical decision making [11]. Consequently an EHR appears to be on the right track to encourage further development of patient empowerment and improve healthcare at large.

5. References:

[1] Davis F. User acceptance of information technology: System characteristics, user perceptions and behavioral impacts. In: *Int J Man-Machine Studies* 1993; 38:475-487.

[2] Ammenwerth E, Kaiser, F, Wilhelm, I, Höfer, S. Evaluation of user acceptance of information systems in health care. The value of questionnaires. In: Baud, R, Fieschi, M, Le Beux, P, Ruch, P, eds. *The New Navigators: from Professionals to Patients. Proceedings of Medical Informatics Europe (MIE 2003)*, 4 – 7 May 2003, St. Malo, France. *Stud Health Technol Informat.* Volume 95. Amsterdam, Berlin, Oxford: IOS Press: 643-648.

[3] ADM, ASI, BVM, D.G.O.F. Richtlinie für Online-Befragungen. 2000. Online available: http://www.adm-ev.de/pdf/R08_D.pdf (cited 18.08.04 18:00 MEZ).

[4] Dillman, DA. Mail and Internet Surveys- the Tailored Design Method, New York: John Wiley&Sons, 1999.

[5] Van Eimeren B, Gerhard H, Frees B. ARD/ZDF-Online-Studie 2003. Internetverbreitung in Deutschland: Unerwartet hoher Zuwachs. In: *Mediaperspektiven* 8/2003: 338-358.

[6] Ückert F, Görz M, Ataian M, Tessmann S, Prokosch HU. The new Navigation in EHRs: Enabling Teamwork of Professionals and Patients. In: Baud, R, Fieschi, M, Le Beux, P, Ruch, P, eds. *The New Navigators: from Professionals to Patients. Proceedings of Medical Informatics Europe (MIE 2003)*, 4 – 7 May 2003, St. Malo, France. *Stud Health Technol Inform.* Volume 95. Amsterdam, Berlin, Oxford: IOS Press: 334-339.

[7] Sittig, DF. Personal health records on the internet: a snapshot of the pioneers at the end of the 20th century. In: *Int J Med Inform.* 2002 Apr; 65(1):1-6.

[8] Van Eimeren B, Gerhard H, Frees B. ARD/ZDF-Online-Studie 2004. Internetverbreitung in Deutschland: Potenzial vorerst ausgeschöpft? In: *Mediaperspektiven* 8/2004: 350-370. Online available: http://www.daserste.de/service/ardonl04.pdf (cited 20.11.04 17:10 MEZ).

[9] Winkelmann, WJ, Leonard, KJ. Overcoming Structural Constraints to Patient Utilization of Medical Records: A Critical Review and Proposal for an Evaluation Framework. In: *J of Am Med Inf Assoc.* 2004; 11: 151-161.

[10] van der Haak M, Mludek V, Wolff AC, Bulzebruck H, Oetzel D, Zierhut D, Drings P, Wannenmacher M, Haux R. Networking in Shared Care- First Steps towards a Shared Electronic Patient Record for Cancer Patients. In: *Methods Inf Med* 2002; 41: 419-425.

[11] Kimura, M. What can we currently expect from patient records? Synopsis. In: Haux R, Kulikowski C, eds. *Yearbook of Medical Informatics*, Stuttgart: Schattauer Verlagsgesellschaft GmbH 2002: 329-331.

Address

University Hospital Muenster, Department for Medical Informatics and Biomathematics, Andrea Ertmer, Domagkstrasse 9, D-48129 Münster, Germany, ertmer@imfl.de

Connecting Medical Informatics and Bio-Informatics
R. Engelbrecht et al. (Eds.)
IOS Press, 2005

Experimenting with Case-Based Reasoning to Present Educative Health Information on the Internet: The Example of SeniorGezond

Nicole P M Ezendam[a], Laurence L Alpay[a], Ton A J M Rövekamp[b], Pieter J Toussaint[a]

[a] *Clinical Informatics, Leiden University Medical Center, The Netherlands*
[b] *Technology in Health Care, TNO Quality of life, The Netherlands*

Abstract

Background: Information about health prevention can contribute to the awareness and the knowledge of consumers and patients about their own health. Messages originating from other users (cases) can be perceived as more credible and hence more persuasive. With this in mind, we have developed an informative website called SeniorGezond, which includes a case-based tailoring component, in the domain area of fall incidences. **Objectives:** *To investigate whether the use of cases is suitable for presenting and tailoring educative health information; and to gain insights in the user's opinion about the use of cases to provide tailored preventive information.* **Methods:** *We conducted a qualitative study using questionnaires, focus group discussions, interviews, and observations. Participants were elderly, family caregivers and healthcare professionals.* **Results:** *Users were able to find relevant cases for their problems, but had a mixed reaction on the usefulness and appreciation of the cases.* **Conclusions:** *There is a need for a delicate balance between a recognizable story with all the important health information and good readable and concise information. A good text structure is required to support this. While cases do have potential in health education, further research is needed in order to identify the necessary requirements which will make the cases successful.*

Keywords:
Case-based reasoning; Internet; Public health informatics; Health education; Elderly; Accidental falls

1. Introduction

Falls are a major health problem among the elderly. Approximately 30% of the community-dwelling persons aged 65 and older fall at least once per year. The consequences of falling are dramatic both in personal health loss as well as in economic costs [1]. This stresses the importance of preventing the elderly from falling.

More and more the Internet is used for disseminating information about preventive health activities. The use of the technology to improve patient's knowledge and to involve them in their own health promotion can lead to better health outcomes [2].

Rimal and Adkins [3] have hypothesized that messages originating from other users would be perceived as more credible and hence more persuasive when similar to their own situations. Case-based reasoning is an approach to problem solving and learning. It utilizes the specific knowledge of previous experienced, concrete problem situations [4]. Finding a similar case, which is reused in this new problem situation, solves the problem of a user.

There are many different health promotion websites using an information tailoring approach [5]. However, as far as we know, none of these websites uses cases to present health information. However, Kreuter et al. proposed the idea of using narrative stories to tailor information [6]. Case-based reasoning might be considered as a way of presenting tailored information.

We have been interested in exploring the use of cases within a health information system. For our purpose, this meant compiling a database with cases on falling problems. Because falling incidents are often 'caused' by multiple health problems together, cases reflect multiple health and environment problems in different combinations.

This article reports on a study with two objectives: (1) To investigate whether the use of cases is suitable for presenting and tailoring educative health information; (2) To gain insights in the user's opinion about the use of cases to provide tailored preventive information.

2. Methods

2.1. The instrument: The website SeniorGezond

The website SeniorGezond (SeniorHealth) contains information about falling and possible interventions. Target audience of the website are the elderly who are at risk from falling, family caregivers and healthcare professionals. We developed a prototype [7], which incorporates twenty cases, covering a limited part of the actual domain knowledge. We adapted an existing case-based reasoning system and prepared case titles on the basis of gender, age, main (health) problem, and solution. Our assumption was that the user could identify him/herself with one or more cases and learn from them.

Users could enter their query in natural language. We assumed that the use of natural language would provide good results, since no specific knowledge of query formulation is required [8]. After formulating their problem users received in order of relevance a list of cases matching their problem. A case contained a description of a similar problem that the user experiences, possible solutions, and options to search for further information such as facts about relevant topics and more information about actions a person can take.

2.2. Study design

We conducted a usability test, using questionnaires, focus group meetings, interviews, and observations. In total 28 people participated in the evaluation of the prototype. This included 18 elderly, aged 55 years or older (one however did not comply), 5 family caregivers and 5 healthcare professionals. The elderly were experienced with using the computer; a majority (n=13) was also familiar with the Internet. The elderly and two of five family caregivers tested the website in a laboratory situation, while three family caregivers and all the healthcare professionals (nurse, physician, and policy makers) used the website either at home or at work. The elderly and the family caregivers tested the website by carrying out four scenarios. Each scenario contained a problem regarding falling.

2.3. Data collection

Each participant filled in a questionnaire of 57 questions, about the interface, the content, and usability. The options were mainly multiple choice. Participants could also add comments and explanations if needed. The elderly and two family caregivers were observed while using the system. Observation was carried out using an "observation form" wherein points of attention could be recorded. Focus group sessions and interviews were used to gather additional information.

3. Results

3.1. Usefulness of cases

We were interested in finding out whether a suitable case could be found for a given scenario the participant had to work with. Eleven out of 16 seniors (69%) found a suitable case for their scenario. In the focus group discussions and the interviews the following question was discussed: "What do you think about the search facility to find relevant cases?". This question on the use of cases provoked a mixed reaction. Interestingly all healthcare professionals, some family caregivers and some seniors thought cases would be useful *for others but not for themselves*. Results are summarized in table 1.

Table 1 - The table summarizes the reactions of the participants on the use and relevance of the cases.

	Questionnaires	Focus groups / interviews	Observations
Seniors	11 out of 16 positive (2 not responded)	Do not need cases Patronizing, unnecessary, a total failure and not realistic Like the recognition	Some experienced difficulties searching for a suitable case
Family caregivers	4 out of 5 positive	Useful and reassuring Cases contain useful tips	-
Healthcare professionals	1 out of 5 positive (4 not responded)	Important facility Good for elderly	-

3.2. Structure of cases

Fourteen out of 16 seniors (88%) found the cases well structured (question A in table 2) and 12 out of 16 seniors (75%) found the information well readable (question B in table 2). In the focus group discussions and the interviews the following question was discussed: "What do you think about the website's lay out?". Participants were critical about the structure. They wanted to have smaller pages or more structure within one page using for instance bold accents. Important aspects were that the case titles did not reflect the whole content of the cases and that the cases were too specific. Stories contained too many details and were too long-winded. There is a great discrepancy between the user's overall opinion given in the questionnaire and the comments made during the focus groups and the interviews. It is likely that during the focus groups negative critics were given, with less attention being given to positive comments. Table 2 shows the results about the content structure.

Table 2 - The table summarizes the reactions of the participants on the content structure.

	Questionnaires		Focus groups / interviews	Observations
	Question A (structure)	**Question B (readable)**		
Seniors	14 out of 16 positive (2 not responded)	12 out of 16 positive (2 not responded)	Title does not reflect the case content Cases need to be more general Cases need to be less specific, so more users can recognize themselves Cases are too long-winded The text need to be more to the point (some did not agree) Text is too long, more telegram style is needed Comforting such descriptive stories	Critics on the amount of text
Family caregivers	3 out of 5 positive	4 out of 5 positive	Stories are too long More accentuation of keywords within the text	Due to the amount of text user sometimes does not see everything on one page
Healthcare professionals	3 out of 5 positive (2 not responded)	4 out of 5 positive (1 not responded)	No good match between the questions asked and the answer in the case	-

3.3. Finding the cases

Users were asked about their preferred ways of searching (multiple answers could be given). Three out of 18 seniors (17%) preferred searching by entering a sentence in natural language, while, whereas 13 out of 18 (72%) preferred to search by keyword (not in table). Indeed, some participants reported their difficulty in formulating their request in natural language and it often took them a long time to enter a query (as also observed in the sessions). As a result, some participants tended to use keywords instead of queries in natural language. Users also had trouble interpreting case titles and therefore had difficulties determining the most relevant case in the list. Table 3 shows more detailed information about user's search preferences.

Table 3 - The table summarizes the reactions of the participants on case search.

	Questionnaires	Focus groups / interviews	Observations
Seniors	3 out of 17 positive (1 not responded)	Difficult to formulate a question It might be good for people who fall Not clear you could choose from the case list Formulating query took a lot of time	It was very clear that some users found it difficult to enter questions in natural language. They were instead entering keywords During the sessions, participants commented on how much it would cost if they had to do this at home, because it took them such a long time
Family caregivers	1 out of 5 positive	Nice to formulate a question like this Difficult to formulate and think what words to enter Takes a lot of time Useful for others Often only a small part of the case applicable to oneself	-
Healthcare professionals	2 out of 5 positive	Good for family members and seniors themselves Nice to formulate a question	-

4. Discussion

In order to propose relevant cases to the user, the website first needs to be able to accurately identify the user's problems. In our context, the participants had problems entering whole queries in natural language, and spent a lot of time trying to do so. It is thus not surprising that they did not favour searching via natural language input and rather opted for a keyword search. However, we found no literature regarding users having problems using natural language on the Internet.

Cases often turned out to be too specific for the users. Too many details in the problem description made cases less recognizable for the user, and not all the information matched the user's profile. As a result, users had some trouble identifying themselves with the persons portrayed in the cases. It is indeed acknowledged that user's identification with information is important. For example, the fall prevention project at Queen Mary's School of Medicine and Dentistry [9] used images of rooms to illustrate risk for falling. However, the user's concentration weakened if a room looked significantly different from their own room. This study indicates that if users have trouble in identifying themselves with the cases this might influence the case's persuasiveness for behavioural change.

Some comments were made about too much text being presented in single pages. Less information within one page might be more suitable and helps the users identify better with the case. In addition, when there is less information within the case the information can be better reflected in the case title. However, it needs to be stressed that cases have a descriptive nature and larger text pages are often inevitable. Altering this, might counter balance the essence of case stories.

We found that collecting realistic cases for SeniorGezond was not easy. Often cases were too medical for a website about fall prevention targeted at lay people. In addition, it appeared difficult to cover the whole problem domain of fall incidents in cases.

5. Conclusions

The participants in our study (especially the elderly users) often did not prefer using natural language to formulate their problems and find relevant cases. The target audience must thus be carefully considered when designing search facilities within a website. There needs to be a delicate balance between a recognizable story with all the important health information and good readable and concise information. A good text structure is required to support this. Furthermore, the content must not be too specific in order to help the user identify with the case and to compose case titles that fit the content. While cases do have potential in health education, further research is needed in order to identify the necessary requirements which will make cases more successful.

6. Acknowledgements

The SeniorGezond project is funded by OGZ and Zorg en Zekerheid. The authors thank all the participants of the evaluation and all project members: K.L. Chan, W.C. Graafmans (TNO Quality of Life), A.M. Kamper and J.H.M. Zwetsloot-Schonk (Leiden University Medical Center).

7. References

[1] Tromp AM, Pluijm SM, Smit JH, Deeg DJ, Bouter LM, Lips P. Fall-risk screening test: a prospective study on predictors for falls in community-dwelling elderly. J Clin Epidemiol 2001; 54(8):837-844.

[2] Lewis D. Computer-based approaches to patient education: A review of the literature. J Am Med Inform Assoc 1999; 6(4):272-282.

[3] Rimal RN, Adkins AD. Using computers to narrowcast health messages: the role of audience segmentation, targeting and tailoring in health promotion. In: Thompson TL, Dorsey AM, Miller KI, Parrott R, editors. Handbook of health communication. Lawrence Erlbaum; 2003. 497-513.

[4] Aamodt A, Plaza E. Case-based reasoning: foundational issues, methodological variations, and system approaches. Artificial intelligence communications 1994; 7(1):39-59.

[5] Casebeer LL, Strasser SM, Spettell CM, Wall TC, Weissman N, Ray MN et al. Designing tailored Web-based instruction to improve practicing physicians' preventive practices. J Med Internet Res 2003; 5(3):e20.

[6] Kreuter MW, Holt CL. How do people process health information? Applications in an age of individualized communication. Curr Dir Psychol Sci 2001; 10(6):206-209.

[7] Alpay LL, Toussaint PJ, Ezendam NPM, Rovekamp T, Graafmans W, Westendorp R. Easing internet access of health information for the elderly users: design considerations and usability. Health Informatics Journal 2004; 10(3):185-194.

[8] Sutcliffe A, Ennis M. Towards a cognitive theory of information retrieval. Interact Comput 1998; 10(3):321-351.

[9] Wilmes, B, Radhamanohar, M, Vogel, M, Bennett, G, and Underwood, M. Involving users in the development of consumer health information on falls: outcomes and experiences. URL : http://www.smd.qmul.ac.uk/hcop/research/falls.htm [accessed 2004 Aug 23

8. Address for correspondence

Nicole Ezendam, MSc
Clinical Informatics, Leiden University Medical Center
PO Box 9600, 2300 RC, Leiden, The Netherlands
E-mail: n.p.m.ezendam@lumc.nl

Connecting Medical Informatics and Bio-Informatics
R. Engelbrecht et al. (Eds.)
IOS Press, 2005

Log Analysis of a Turkish Web Portal; Febrile Neutropenia

Kemal Hakan Gülkesen[a], Hamdi Akan[b], Murat Akova[c], Tamer Çalıkoğlu[d]

[a]Akdeniz University, Antalya, Turkey, [b]Ankara University, Ankara, Turkey
[c]Hacettepe University, Ankara, Turkey, [d]Oncology Hospital, Ankara, Turkey

Abstract

In the last years, a lot of health portals have emerged which give service to health professionals. Neither number nor usage patterns of these portals have been well known. In this study, we analysed the usage patterns of a Turkish health portal. The main theme of the portal is febrile neutropenia.
In a six months period, 714 users had visited the web site. 595 (83 %) of these users had three or more visits. During this period, 428 new web pages had entered the system. The most frequently visited pages were education materials and guidelines, whereas the least frequently visited pages were reviews and news. One hundred and ninety nine (27.8 %) of the users had one or more visit every week. After the web page was published, the mean of total number of the visits in first week was 40.1. The mean number fell to 1.0 in the fifth week.
The users preferred to read concentrated resources as education materials and guidelines. Possibly they could not find sufficient time to read detailed texts in daily routine. Another result of our analysis is that, a web page gets "old" when it is one month old. The editors inform the users about the new pages by the e-mail postings. So, preparation of good content may not be sufficient alone, and the presence of the pages must be announced to possible readers.

Keywords
Internet; Information Systems; Attitude of Health Personnel; Neutropenia

1. Introduction

The internet users reach large numbers in last years. At the beginning, internet applications were simulating the traditional paper based resources. The most widely known applications were e-mail and web. However, the use of internet evolves by the time. Nearly every type of computer applications is integrated into web interfaces; various applications such as discussion lists, instant messaging emerged and the internet has created its own style of use. One of the services that have growing popularity is web portal. A web portal is a web site or service that offers a broad array of resources and services, such as e-mail, forums, search engines, and on-line shopping malls. Web portals may be general or on specific subjects such as commerce, health, or designed for groups of people such as women, youth, students, singles, and people of a city.

The number of internet users also grows. There are several studies about profiles and usage patterns of the health professionals [1, 2]. In the last years, a lot of health portals emerged which give service to lay people or health professionals. The use of the portals was also reported in medical literature [3]. The portals may be designed for assisting the patients [4-6], or reaching organized resources for professionals [7-9].

The presence of a lot of web portals for the physicians is known. These portals may be general or on specific medical subjects. Neither number nor usage patterns of these portals have been well known. In our opinion, a substantial number of health professionals use some portals, and behaviours of the users must be well known to have better designed web portals. When we better understand the profile of the users and the factors that affect their visit to pages, more ergonomic and more popular sites may be designed.

In this study, we examined the usage patterns of a Turkish health portal (http://www.febrilnotropeni.net/). The main theme of the portal is febrile neutropenia. We tried to define the user profile, and analyse their behaviour pattern.

2. Methods

The web portal is sponsored by five pharmaceutical companies and regulated by Turkish Febrile Neutropenia Working Group. The health professionals usually learn about the portal from their colleagues and the portal is announced in some scientific meetings. The health professionals can use the portal by subscription without a fee. They have to give some personal information on a web interface during the subscription. They can log in using their password anytime after subscription. The content of the portal is mainly composed of announcements, news, Turkish translation of abstracts, articles and reviews, original reviews, guidelines, and education materials. Weekly e-mails from portal editor inform all the subscribers about new content of the portal.

Data about the visits of the subscribers is recorded and kept in a database which is maintained by a IT company (Pleksus IT, Ankara, Turkey), and the personal data of the users is not shared with the sponsor companies or any third parties.

Statistical analysis is performed by SPSS 10.0 software. Mann-Whitney U test or Kruskal-Wallis test were applied. Bonferroni correction was used when required. Data is usually shown as median and statistical significance is set to 0.05.

3. Results

In a six months period, 714 users had visited the web site. Five hundred and ninety-five (83 %) of these users who are considered as active users had three ore more visits. The total number of visits was 18285. The mean number of visits were 3048 and 102 by a monthly and daily basis respectively. When the recurrent visits were excluded from the total, 13915 visits had been made by the users in six months with monthly 2319 and daily 77 averages. During this period, 428 new web pages or applications had entered the system. In table 1, the most frequently visited five web pages are shown.

The frequency of visits according to category is shown in table 2. The most frequently visited pages are education materials and guidelines, the least frequently visited pages are reviews and news. Table 3 demonstrates visit frequency according to subjects.

In the analysis of visit frequency of the users, it is seen that some users (16.7 %) did not efficiently use the system. Their monthly frequency of visits was below 0.5. On the other hand, 199 (27.8 %) of the users had one or more visit every week.

Table 1-The most frequently visited five links. Mean visit: The mean number of visits by each user.

	Title	Category	Subject	n	Mean visit
1	3rd Postgraduate Febrile Neutropenia Course	About scientific meetings	Febrile neutropenia	308	3.0
2	Diagnosis and therapy guidelines in febrile neutropenic patients Part one	Guidelines	Febrile neutropenia	178	1.9
3	Crimean-Congo Hemorrhagic Fever in Turkey	News	Viral infections	144	1.6
4	Guidelines for writing and reviewing scientific articles	Guidelines	Research/ article writing	137	1.2
5	The second highest number of contributions to 14th ECCMID Congress is from Turkey	About scientific meetings	Infections	125	1.2

*Table 2-The frequency of visits according to web page category. *less frequently visited than guidelines. **less frequently visited than education materials, guidelines, articles, and contests. (p<0.05, Mann Whitney U test and Bonferroni correction)*

Category	n	Median	Minimum	Maximum
Education material	14	37,5	8	101
Guideline	25	34,0	5	178
Article	169	28,0	3	112
Contest	12	25,0	10	64
Meeting announcement	14	16,0	3	308
Review*	127	11,0	3	101
News**	66	6,0	3	144
Other	1	65	65	65
Total	428	22	3	308

Table 3-The frequency of visits according to subject. Data belonging to the subjects that have less than 10 web pages are not shown.

	n	median	minimum	maximum
General medicine	50	45,0	3	101
Systemic infections	12	40,0	3	107
Transplantation	18	39,0	4	101
Respiratory infections.	19	39,0	4	82
Fungal infections	15	26,0	4	82
Contests, questionnaires	14	25,0	10	65
Haematology/oncology	26	24,5	3	71
antibacterial agents	35	23,0	3	90
Resistance	53	21,0	3	93
Febrile neutropenia	31	21,0	3	308
Sepsis	17	9,0	3	89
Hepatitis	24	8,0	3	107
Antifungal agents	12	4,0	3	72
Total	428	22,0	3	308

Table 4 shows the number of visits according to gender. The web site is slightly more frequently visited by male users, but the difference is not statistically significant.

The frequency of monthly visit number according to academic titles were 3.7, 2.9, 2.8, 2.5, 2.2, 1.8 for assistant professors, professors, associate professors, research assistants, specialists, and others respectively. There is a significant difference between assistant professors and "others" (p<0.05, Mann Whitney U test and Bonferroni correction. The users whose monthly visit frequency is under 0.5 were not included).

Table 4-Number of visits according to gender (The users whose monthly visit frequency is under 0.5 is not included, p=0,147, Mann-Whitney U test).

Gender	n (%)	mean	median
Female	274 (46)	3,7	2,2
Male	309 (52)	4,0	2,8
Unknown	12 (2)	-	-
Total	595 (100)	3.9	2.5

Table 5 demonstrates visit frequency according to speciality of the users. Infectious disease specialists are the most frequent users of the portal.

Table 5-Monthly frequency of the visits according to speciality (The users whose monthly visit frequency is under 0.5 were not included, *higher than "other medical speciality", pharmaceutical company workers, non-physician health professionals, ** higher than "other medical speciality". p<0.05, Mann Whitney U test and Bonferroni correction)

Speciality of the user	n (%)	Median
Infectious disease*	196 (33)	3.8
Haematology	54 (9)	2.9
Paediatric Haematology	32 (5)	2.8
Paediatrics	17 (3)	2.3
Clinical microbiology**	112 (19)	2.3
Internal medicine	42 (7)	2.3
Pharmaceutical company workers	49 (8)	1.8
Paediatric Oncology	14 (2)	1.8
Other medical speciality	41 (7)	1.5
Non-physician health professionals	19 (3)	1.5
Oncology	12 (2)	1.3
General practitioners	7 (1)	1.0
Total	595 (100)	2.5

The information related to time of visits after the page entered to the portal is showed in figures 1 and 2. The mean number of first visits in the first week was 26.4. The mean numbers of first visits were 5.4, 1.3, and 0.9 in 2nd, 3rd, and 4th weeks respectively. The mean number fell to 0.7 in the fifth week and it was below this figure in subsequent weeks. The mean of total number of the visits in first week was 40.1. The numbers of total visits were 9.0, 2.4, and 1.7 in 2nd, 3rd, and 4th weeks respectively. The mean number fell to 1.0 in the fifth week and it was below this figure in subsequent weeks.

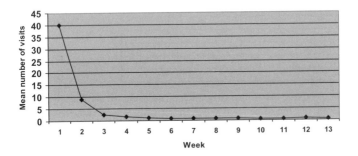

Figure 1-Mean visit number according to the week of the first visit after the web page entered to the system (evaluation of 131 pages that have 13 weeks of visit logs and at least 10 visits).

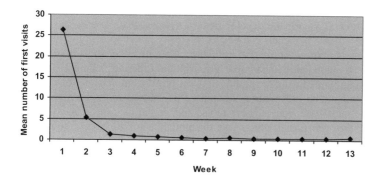

Figure 2-Mean visit number according to the week of all visits after the web page is entered to the system (evaluation of 148 pages that have 13 weeks of visit logs and at least 20 visits).

4. Discussion

Internet provides some new tools for education and communication of health professionals. Web portals are suitable "gates" providing updated information, news, announcements and education material for the health professionals. Portals have also advantage of using nearly all possibilities of information technology to help keep interest of users and compose virtual communities. To examine and understand usage patterns and personal characteristics of the users would certainly help the design of better health portals.

In this study, we examined a Turkish health portal on a specific subject, febrile neutropenia. Most of the users were specialist physicians, and 595 of 714 users were using the system three times or more in a six month period. Approximately one fourth of the users visited the portal every week or more frequently. The system has recorded mean 102 visits everyday. The mentioned figures show a relatively frequent use of the system.

The users had most frequently visited web pages containing education materials and guidelines. This finding suggests that the users prefer to read concentrated resources. Possibly they cannot find sufficient time to read detailed texts in daily routine. When the pages were classified according to subjects, the more general subjects have taken more hits. This may be explained by the heterogeneous expertise of the users, thus the more general subjects may take attention of more users.

An important proportion (46 %) of the users was females, and we could not detect a statistical difference of visit frequency between two sexes. Assistant professors had higher visit frequency than associate professors and professors but the difference was not statistically different. We do not have the ages of the users, but assistant professors are generally younger than the others. In a previous study, physicians younger than 50 years old who had full- or part-time academic affiliation reported using computers more frequently for medical applications [10]. The most frequent first three groups by title were academic staff. Visit numbers of research assistants, specialists and other users were lower than these academic people, but the only statistical difference was between assistant professors and "others".

Another result of our analysis is that, a web page gets "old" when it is one month old. The mean number of visits was 40 in the first week of publishing, and it fell under 1.0 after the fifth week. These figures may be explained by the e-mail postings of the editors, who inform the users about the new pages. So, preparation of good content may not be sufficient alone, and the presence of the pages must be announced to possible readers.

Current technologies now allow for the development of systems that cover a physician's entire professional experience. Physicians can be electronically linked to many or all of the information and communication systems that influence their practice, including patient medical record systems, knowledge databases, prescription ordering, clinical decision support tools, and continuing medical education [11]. User profile and behaviour should be better known for designing such information systems. This study examines a web portal that mainly contains clinical decision support tools, and continuing medical education material. In summary, the web portal which was examined seems to have a significant traffic. We observed that the "health portal user" tends to be relatively young, no sex difference is observed. They frequently use concentrated sources such as clinical guidelines and education materials. The users seem to be activated by announcement of new material by e-mail, and reading rate of the pages substantially decreases after one month.

6. Acknowledgements

The authors wish to thank Dr. Buket Cinemre for revising the English of this article. This research is supported by Akdeniz University Research Foundation.

7. References

[1] Lorenzo S, Mira JJ. Are Spanish physicians ready to take advantage of the Internet? *World Hosp Health Serv*. 2004;40(3):31-5, 41-3.

[2] Koller M, Grutter R, Peltenburg M, Fischer JE, Steurer J. Use of the Internet by medical doctors in Switzerland. *Swiss Med Wkly*. 2001; 131: 251-4.

[3] Pankaskie M, Sullivan J. Health care Web portals. *J Am Pharm Assoc* (Wash). 2000; 40: 117-8.

[4] Do N, Marinkovich A, Koisch J, Wheeler G. Electronic access to care system: improving patient's access to clinical information through an Interactive Voice Response (IVR) system and Web portal. *AMIA Annu Symp Proc*. 2003; 830.

[5] Farrell SP, Mahone IH, Guilbaud P. Web technology for persons with serious mental illness. *Arch Psychiatr Nurs*. 2004; 18: 121-5.

[6] Wald JS, Bates DW, Middleton B. A Patient-controlled Journal for an Electronic Medical Record: Issues and Challenges. *Medinfo*. 2004; 2004: 1166-72.

[7] Aymard S, Falco L, Dufour JC, Joubert M, Fieschi M. Modeling and implementing a health information provider on the Internet. *Stud Health Technol Inform*. 2003; 95: 89-94..

[8] Crass T, Antes I, etal The Helmholtz Network for Bioinformatics: an integrative web portal for bioinformatics resources. *Bioinformatics*. 2004; 20: 268-70.

[9] Cognetti G, Cecere L. E-oncology and health portals: instructions and standards for the evaluation, production organisation and use. *J Exp Clin Cancer Res*. 2003; 22: 677-86.

[10] Lacher D, Nelson E, Bylsma W, Spena R. Computer use and needs of internists: a survey of members of the American College of Physicians-American Society of Internal Medicine. *Proc AMIA Symp*. 2000; 453-6.

[11] Selsky DB, Eisenberg FP, Spena RP, Hersh W, Price SL, Buitendijk HJ. Knowledge integration: insight through the E-portal. J Healthc Inf Manag. 2001; 15: 13-24.

Address for Correspondence

Dr. K. Hakan Gulkesen, Akdeniz Universitesi Tip Fakultesi , Biyoistatistik AD, Antalya, Turkey.
hgulkesen@akdeniz.edu.tr

Connecting Medical Informatics and Bio-Informatics
R. Engelbrecht et al. (Eds.)
IOS Press, 2005

Collaborative Approaches to e-Health: Valuable for Users and Non-users

Charles Safran,[a] Grace Pompilio-Weitzner,[b] Kathryn D Emery[c], Lou Hampers[c]

[a]Harvard Medical School, Boston MA
[b]Emerson Hospital, Concord, MA
[c]University of Colorado School of Medicine, Denver, CO

Abstract

Objective: To describe parental use of an Internet-based educational and emotional support system, in a regional NICU program. Methods: Baby CareLink was installed in NICUs in 4 Denver area hospitals in 2003. Parents were offered access from hospital terminals and from any other Internet access point. Data on use of the program was collected by the computer system. Discharge status was verified by Colorado's Department of Public Assistance. Results: Of the 388 families admitted to Denver area NICUs with Baby CareLink during the study period, 135 (34.8%) were identified as Medicaid families (needing public assistance). After exclusions, data for 81 Medicaid and 154 non-Medicaid families were available for analysis. Medicaid families who accessed 3 or more Baby CareLink web pages per day took their infants home 17.5 days sooner than families who used Baby CareLink less often (p=0.03). Among the non-Medicaid families, more frequent users of Baby CareLink took their infants home 14.3 days sooner (p=0.04). Conclusions: Internet portals will be used by both Medicaid and non-Medicaid parents with children in NICUs to meet educational needs. More frequent use of Baby CareLink was associated with significantly shorter length of stay. Self-help tools for parents may free nursing resource for families with greater needs.

Keywords
Internet Portals; eHealth; Home Care; Collaborative Healthware; Care Management; NICU; Neonatal care; Infants; Parents; Education

1. Introduction

New parents with children in the neonatal intensive care unit (NICU) are frequently surprised by the outcome of their pregnancies and emotionally and educationally ill-equipped to be full participants in their child's care (1-3). Brazy and colleagues showed that most parents in this situation spent more than 20 hours of the first week in information seeking behavior (4). Moreover, even after 4 weeks of hospitalization a third of parents with children in the NICU still spend 20 hours or more seeking information about their child's condition and future care. "Information seekers" is now a term applied to Internet searchers, and researchers have estimated that about 50% of all Internet searches are health related. While physicians have expressed concern about the quality of information on the "web" (5), consumers of healthcare are increasingly turning to the Internet for information and answers (6-9).

Trends and surveys clearly show an increasing demand by healthcare consumers for educational and emotional support on the Internet (10,11). However, little is known about how such support systems work in the context of complex care and how these systems actually affect care delivery and costs (12). Even less is known about how such systems are used by medically indigent healthcare consumers (13,14).

Baby CareLink, an educational and emotional support system for parents with children in the NICU, has been previously described (15,16). This system was shown in a randomized controlled trial to improve parent satisfaction with care and tended to shorten length of stay (LOS) for very small infants with prolonged hospital stays (15). This paper reports an observational study of this Internet application in 4 Denver area hospitals as part of a state initiative to improve neonatal care management. We hypothesized that use of this application by information-seeking parents would be associated with decreased NICU LOS's.

2. Methods

Baby CareLink was an Internet-based application to support the educational and emotional needs of families with premature infants requiring prolonged hospitalization in the NICU. Using the Baby CareLink system, parents could receive daily updates from the NICU, track information about their baby's health, see recent pictures of their baby, communicate with NICU staff, access a personalized knowledge base for newborn care, and provide feedback regarding the care process. Using Baby CareLink, NICU nurses could communicate with families, personalize discharge planning and baby care education, and access a medical reference library. Following discharge, Baby CareLink was used to support care coordination, follow-up monitoring and ongoing communication with parents, with the goal of reducing emergency department visits and re-hospitalization. Baby CareLink was available in English and Spanish, uses simple language, and leveraged multimedia to accommodate parents with little or no Internet experience and low reading and health literacy. The company providing Baby CareLink no longer exists and hence Baby CareLink is no longer in operations.

Baby CareLink was installed in 4 Denver area hospitals starting in January 2003. The NICU staff in each hospital was trained in the use of Baby CareLink. Parents signed consent to be registered in the Baby CareLink system. Each parent had their own computer ID and password. Data were analyzed from all parent sessions that could be linked to a single infant. In the case of twins or triplets, the infant with the lowest medical record number (e.g., probably the first born) was chosen for analysis. If multiple computer keys were linked to an infant (as would be the case when a parent forgot his/her ID and password or when both a mother and father had separate IDs and password) the activities of the two keys were summed. Medicaid status was verified by chart review. Access to each secure web-page is logged in an audit trail recording time of day and the computer key of the end-user. Since Baby CareLink can dynamically generate over 80,000 different web-pages, for the purpose of analysis we classified the type of page by the intended use for the page. These uses were 1) for a parent to see a picture of their baby, 2) to communicate and collaborate with the NICU staff, 3) or to get clinical information about their child's condition. Examples of communication and collaboration would be messages concerning one of the sixty discharge educational modules that the clinical staff could prescribe for the parents. Examples of clinical information would be a parent access to the NICUpedia to lookup information about retinopathy of prematurity.

The intensity of Baby CareLink use was analyzed with regard to LOS using a simple linear regression model. Variables considered in the model were gestational age, weight at birth, Medicaid or non-Medicaid status, and the total number of web pages viewed by parents. LOS comparisons were made using Student's t-test for unequal variance.

3. Results

In the four study hospitals a total of 133 singletons and 2 sets of twins were admitted and identified as Medicaid infants. Eight infants died, 19 were transferred to other hospitals, and 27 infants were registered but their parents never used Baby CareLink, leaving 81 records for analysis. Similarly, 234 singletons, 17 sets of twins, and 2 sets of triplets were identified as non-Medicaid infants. Of these, 12 infants died, 26 were transferred, and 51 infants were registered but their parents never used Baby CareLink, leaving 154 non-Medicaid infants records for analysis. The average length of stay for Medicaid infants was 46.5 days versus 39.4 days for non-Medicaid infants, but this difference was not significant. Length of stay between hospitals was not significantly different.

Table 1 shows the average weight, gestational age, and LOS for infants as well as their parents' usage of Baby CareLink in terms of the average number of logins, Baby CareLink web pages viewed, and the average number of pages viewed per day of NICU stay. In comparing Medicaid to non-Medicaid, only the number of parent logins (29.44 vs. 44.48 p=0.04) represents a significant difference.

Table 1 Descriptive Statistics of Infants and Parental use of Baby CareLink.

Medicaid (n=81)	Weight	GA	LOS	Logins	Pages	Pages/day
Mean	2016.16	33.45	46.53	29.44	165.36	5.28
Standard Error	102.89	0.50	4.70	5.13	22.35	0.74
Median	2000.00	34.29	29.00	14.00	85.00	2.95
Range	4413.00	16.71	171.00	213.00	953.00	38.17
Minimum	350.00	24.00	4.00	1.00	5.00	0.08
Maximum	4763.00	40.71	175.00	214.00	958.00	38.25
Non-Medicaid (n=154)						
Mean	2090.94	33.79	39.38	44.48†	198.21	6.27
Standard Error	78.21	0.38	2.53	5.51	24.40	0.67
Median	1901.00	33.79	32.50	17.50	78.00	2.85
Range	4420.00	19.00	130.00	510.00	1916.00	61.22
Minimum	350.00	23.00	3.00	1.00	2.00	0.03
Maximum	4770.00	42.00	133.00	511.00	1918.00	61.25

†p=0.04

In order to analyze the impact of Baby CareLink on the cost of care, we chose to analyze LOS as a surrogate for resource consumption. Since all hospitals in our study offered Baby CareLink to their patients, we did not have a concurrent control for comparison. Regression analysis shows that the intensity of Baby CareLink use (pages viewed per NICU day) was significantly correlated with decreased LOS for both Medicaid and non-Medicaid families.

Table 2 shows a decrease in length of stay for infants <1500 grams and infants ≥1500 grams when comparing parents who viewed fewer than three Baby CareLink pages per day of their infants hospitalization to those parents who viewed three or more Baby CareLink pages per day.

Baby CareLink has thousands of pages that a parent can access. These dynamically generated web pages can be categorized into three categories: 1) Seeing your baby (parents viewing digital pictures of their infant), 2) Communication and Collaboration Tools such as the message center, and 3) Access to Knowledge and Information such as the discharge learning modules. When a parent logs onto Baby CareLink, the program records the Internet Protocol (IP) address of the user. Based upon the IP address we determine if the parent is using Baby CareLink from within the hospital's network or from outside the hospital's network (i.e., home or at work.)

Table 2 Length of Stay by Baby CareLink Use and Birthweight

All Colorado (n=235)	< 3 page/d	≥3 page/d	Reduction in	
<1500	81.3 (n=40)	64.0 (n=31)	17.3	p=0.03
≥1500	33.4 (n=80)	22.9 (n=80)	10.5	p=0.002
	49.4 (n=120)	34 (n=115)	15.4	p=0.001
Medicaid (n=81) <1500	94.6 (n=13)	78.2 (n=10)	16.4	
≥1500	36.9 (n=28)	24.2 (n=30)	12.7	p=0.04
	55.2 (n=41)	37.7 (n=40)	17.5	p=0.03
Non-Medicaid (n=154) <1500	74.8 (n=27)	57.2 (n=21)	17.6	p=0.03
≥1500	31.6 (n=52)	22.2 (n=54)	9.4	p=0.01
	46.3 (n=79)	32.0 (n=75)	14.3	p=0.04

31% of their time looking at pictures of their infants, but Medicaid parents tend to access knowledge and information resources more often (18% vs. 11%) where non-Medicaid parents use the communication and collaboration tools of Baby CareLink (58% vs. 51%) more often.

Table 3 Pages viewed by parents

Out of Hospital	See Your Baby	Communication and Collaboration Tools	Access to Knowledge and Information	
Medicaid (n=68)	2334 (27%)	5180 (59%)	1289 (15%)	8803
Non Medicaid (n=146)	7723 (30%)	15153 (60%)	2580 (10%)	25456
Total	10057	20333	3869	34259
In Hospital				
Medicaid (n=52)	1724 (41%)	1472 (35%)	1027 (24%)	4223
Non Medicaid (n=79)	1377 (32%)	2181 (51%)	760 (18%)	4318
Total	3101	3653	1787	8541
Total Usage				
Medicaid (n=81)	4058 (31%)	6652 (51%)	2316 (18%)	13026
Non-Medicaid (n=154)	9100 (31%)	17334 (58%)	3340 (11%)	29774
Total	**13158**	**23986**	**5656**	**42800**

4. Discussion

Having a baby in the NICU is one of the most stressful events in the life of any parent. NICU parents experience many different emotions including denial, guilt, anger, and, ultimately, acceptance of their baby's situation (17). In addressing family-centered needs of NICU parents (18,19), Baby CareLink provides information for parents who have a need for greater understanding of their baby's condition (present and future) and a need for access to resources beyond those available in the NICU (state and community resources). Our data demonstrate information-seeking behavior by NICU parents, both in the Medicaid and non-Medicaid population.

In this study, parents who viewed more than 3 pages of Baby CareLink per day during their baby's NICU hospitalization, took their babies home an average of 15.4 days sooner than parents who used Baby CareLink less frequently. In the Medicaid population, this length of stay reduction was even greater, 17.5 days. This correlation between Baby CareLink use and reduction in LOS is both highly statistically and economically significant.

Parents who use Baby CareLink may be more motivated in general, and more likely to actively participate in their baby's care. However, the magnitude of the LOS differences observed suggest that use of Baby CareLink was a major factor in this outcome. Parents with frequent Baby CareLink use (as defined by viewing three or more pages of Baby CareLink per hospital day) used Baby CareLink to look at a recently updated picture of their infant, communicate with their care team in the NICU, and view information specifically selected by the NICU team to augment their understanding of their infant's condition and post discharge needs. About half of all families (Medicaid and non-Medicaid) used Baby CareLink in this fashion.

Medicaid families tend to look at information related to their baby's care more often than non-Medicaid families. This finding suggests that medically indigent families may be using this application to meet their educational needs to an even greater extent than families with more resources.

Of the 42,000 pages of Baby CareLink information delivered to the 235 Colorado families in the pilot study, 13% were focused on health education and discharge learning. Although fewer than the number of "See Your Baby" pages displayed, frequency of use is not the same as potential impact on health behaviors. Baby CareLink employs technology designed to support just-in-time learning. Baby CareLink is designed to deliver written and/or multimedia (video or voice over) information that can support a parent's need-to-know and result in improved quality of care at lower cost. Baby CareLink fosters parent participation and collaboration in care, presenting information at a time when parents may be most receptive. Thus, displaying or reading a single intensely personalized paragraph of information at the right time could have a much greater effect on health related outcomes than the volumes of less specific web pages. Never-the-less, infant pictures are popular and one of the reasons families visit and revisit the website.

These tertiary care centers in Denver draw from a vast geographic area. Although their data were excluded from the study analysis, parents from Kansas, Wyoming, and Montana utilized Baby CareLink. Premature babies remain hospitalized for so long that the parents may not be able to remain in the area for the entire length of their baby's NICU stay. Distance impacts these parents' ability to visit the NICU, see their baby's progress, and get frequent face-to-face updates from the NICU team. This is true not only for out-of-state parents, but for many parents who live outside of the Denver-metro area. In this regard, "See Your Baby" has an unparalleled benefit to parents who can see their infant's progress without being physically present in the NICU.

Likewise, for Spanish-speaking parents, Baby CareLink offers an opportunity to have access to educational information that is written in their native language. As presented in the case studies above, Spanish-speaking parents can access information through Baby CareLink that is explained in their language of comfort, in a private and unhurried environment.

Our study is limited by the observational design and the lack of detailed information about the parents' background such as educational level, prior experience with a computer, and other important socio-economic factors. Data from families who did not use Baby CareLink or who were excluded were not analyzed. The two NICU's contributing the majority of infant families accept complex infants with congenital heart disease in transfer and hence may have longer lengths of stay than community-based NICU's.

Concerns about Internet access among the Medicaid population were addressed through a laptop lending program which gave NICUs the ability to lend laptop computers to families who did not have access to the Internet at home, but were motivated to use the Baby CareLink system. This study showed that 84% of Medicaid families who chose to use Baby CareLink found access outside the hospital. While Medicaid families may log on to Baby CareLink less often, the magnitude of the effect on LOS is greater.

We have shown that an educational support tool provided by a NICU to their parents is heavily used by about half of the families and that these participatory parents take their children home much sooner than less participatory parents. Maybe those families who can use tools like Baby CareLink would have had shorter stays in the NICU anyway. Even so, a reliable method to identify such families would allow scarce nursing time to be focused on those families at greater risk for prolonged stays.

Perhaps our most striking result is the parents are parents. A stereotype of the Medicaid parent as one who would not embrace the digital advantage of Internet resources when appropriately designed is not supported by our observations. The circumstance of being poor and perhaps not having prior experience with the Internet does not negate the measured benefit of a tool like Baby CareLink. In fact, the lack of traditional access to medical support seems to predict a wider benefit.

5. Acknowledgments

Supported by a grant from Johnson and Johnson and the Colorado Department of Public Assistance.

6. References

[1]   Perlman NB, Freedman JL, Abramovitch R, Whyte H, Kirpalani H, Perlman M. Informational needs of parents of sick neonates. *Pediatrics*. 1991; 88(3): 512-518.
[2]   McKim EM. The information and support needs of mothers of premature infants. *Journal of Pediatric Nursing*. 1993; 8(4): 233-244.
[3]   Singer LT, Salvator AMS, Guo S, Collin M, Lilien L, Baley J. Maternal psychological distress and parenting stress after the birth of a very low-birth-weight infant. *The Journal of the American Medical Association*. 1999; 281(9): 799-805.
[4]   Brazy JE, Anderson BMH, Becker PT, Becker M. How parents of premature infants gather information and obtain support. *Neonatal Network*. 2001; 20(2): 41-48.
[5]   Dhillon AS, Albersheim SG, Alsaad S, Pargass NS, Zupancic JAF. Internet use and perceptions of information reliability by parents in a neonatal intensive care unit. *Journal of Perinatology*. 2003; 23: 420-424.
[6]   Eng, T., & Gustafson, D. (Eds). (1999). *Wired for health and well being: The emergence of interactive health communication*. Washington DC: US Department of Health and Human Services.
[7]   Eng, T.R., Maxfield, A., Patrick, K., Deering, M.J., Ratzan, S., & Gustafson, D. (1998). Access to health information and support: a public highway or a private road? *JAMA*, 280, 1371-1375.
[8]   Ferguson, T. (1995). Consumer Health Informatics. *HealthCare Forum*, 28-33.
[9]   Ferguson, T. (2000). Online patient-helpers and physicians working together: A new patient collaboration for high quality health care. *BMJ*, 321(7269), 1129-32.
[10]   Donna M. D'Alessandro and Nienke P. Dosa. Empowering Children and Families With Information TechnologyArch Pediatr Adolesc Med, Oct 2001; 155: 1131 - 1136.
[11]   Lamp JM, Howard PA. Guiding parents' use of the Internet for newborn education. *The American Journal of Maternal/Child Nursing*. 1999; 24(1): 33-36.
[12]   Qavi T, Corley L, Kay S. Nursing staff requirements for telemedicine in the neonatal intensive care unit. *Journal of End User Computing*. 2001; 13(3): 5-13.
[13]   Gustafson, D.H., McTavish, F., Boberg, E., et al. (1999). Empowering patients using computer based health support systems. *Quality Health Care*, 8(1), 49-56.
[14]   Safran, C. The collaborative edge: Patient empowerment for vulnerable populations. *International Journal of Medical Informatics*, 2003 (69):185-190.
[15]   Gray JE, Safran C, Davis RB, Pompilio-Weitzner G, Stewart JE, Zaccagnini L, Pursley DW. Baby CareLink: Using the Internet and telemedicine to improve care for high-risk infants. *Pediatrics*. 2000; 106(6): 1318-1324.
[16]   Goldsmith DM, Safran C. Collaborative Healthware. Chapter in: Nelson R, Ball MJ. *Consumer Informatics: Applications and Strategies in Cyber Health Care*. New York: Springer-Verlag, 2004; pp 9-19.
[17]   Kenner C. Caring for the NICU parent. *The Journal of Perinatal and Neonatal Nursing*. 1990; 4(3): 78-87.
[18]   Cisneros Moore KA, Coker K, DuBuisson AB, Swett B, Edwards WH. Implementing potentially better practices for improving family-centered care in neonatal intensive care units: Successes and challenges. *Pediatrics*. April 2003; 111(4): e450-e460.
[19]   Harrison H. The principles for family-centered neonatal care. *Pediatrics*. 1993; 92(5): 643-650.

Address for correspondence

Charles Safran, MD Harvard Medical School, 56 Park Lane, Newton, MA 02459 charles@safran.org

Connecting Medical Informatics and Bio-Informatics
R. Engelbrecht et al. (Eds.)
IOS Press, 2005

Health Information on the Internet: Evaluating Greek Health Portals and Depicting Users' Attitudes in West Macedonia, Greece

Panagiotis Bamidis, Fotis Kerassidis, Kostas Pappas

Lab of Medical Informatics, Medical School, University of Thessaloniki, Thessaloniki, Greece

Abstract

The increasing use of communication networks help individuals, organizations and governments to access this information as an every day practice to support their decision-making procedures. Information seekers use the web to get hold of information that exists on the Internet. A lot of times this information has to do health. The existence of health portals has made life easier for the people that need this information. However, the quality of portal interfaces as well as the portal content has many times been in doubt. Many surveys have obtained results that are negative as far as health portal quality is concerned. The purpose of this paper is to evaluate a representative selection of Greek health portals from the actual users' point of view. The evaluation takes place at a small town of North-West Greece called Ptolemais. Questionnaires and interviews as well as interface evaluation techniques are used. The outcome seems positive for the Greek health portals. The study is extended to get some estimate of simple and professional users' attitudes upon seeking health related information on the internet in Greek. The conclusions of this study regarding information preferences of health information seekers are compared to international surveys.

Keywords:
Web site Evaluation, health portal, information seeker attitude, internet, on line information assessment

1. Introduction

Information is a term that can take many meanings depending on the case it is used. It can contain "news, intelligence, facts and ideas that are acquired and passed on as knowledge" [1]. Universally accepted standards for storing, retrieving, formatting and displaying information are used in the internet environment to offer new possibilities in information transactions. The existence of the Web has made Internet browsing an every day action for many people around the world. Information seekers make use of search machines or portals to access information. Any form of data, text, audio, and/or video that describe how to stay well or prevent oneself from a disease, how to take care of a disease, or make any decisions that relate to health and health care, and in the same time contains information of health products and health services is defined as Health Information [2].

A health portal, as an interactive service or entry point site to the Web, offers information resources related to health subjects like hospital and doctor information, nutrition, health guide, daily care, health tests, latest published research work, health articles on nearly every subject, health electronic libraries and athletics. Services offered include search engines, links to health portals around the world, e-mail, chatting, news about the pharmaceutical industry and a part with medical information for the people that practice medicine. According to Ahmann, an increasing number of health care consumers are using the Internet for health-related research. Out of one half of the adult population in the United States that use the Internet, three fourths have searched for health information online, the main reason being to find answers to their health questions [3]. In Greece, and according to the World Fact Book [4], 13.13% of the overall population were internet users in 2003.

Two of the major problems in the field of health information on the Internet are the difficulty in searching for information through the various web site or portal interfaces, as well as, the intricacy to decide for the validity of the retrieved information [5,6]. As a great variation in both quality and accessibility is usually realised in various contexts [7], there is a need for specific studies worldwide to exploit the richness of the local socio-economic variability affecting the users' behaviours. Thus, the purpose of this exploratory study is twofold: firstly, to examine a representative set of Greek health portals and provide their evaluation. Secondly, to evaluate the portal Resources and obtain a picture of the user preferences by examining health information-seeking practices among health professionals and non-professionals in a small town in West Macedonia, Greece, called Ptolemais.

2. Context

The study was performed in the Greek country side, in Ptolemais, a small town in the region of West Macedonia in the north of Greece. The Ptolemais tableland is a heavily industrialized area. Big open brown coal mines cover a very large percentage of the agricultural area that existed forty years ago. In two generations people have turned from agricultural workers into industrial workers. Heavy winters and high mountains make life and transportation quite difficult for at least three-four months per year. Continuous advancement of the communications infrastructure accounts, at the moment, for a moderate Internet speed. Cultural life does not provide many alternatives and the largest percentage of the teenagers leave the area after school for good. The Internet is, therefore, very much accepted by the local people, at least the younger ones, because it is a very good means of communicating with the rest of the world. The whole study was therefore adapted to the "environment" of the Ptolemais inhabitants.

3. Background

Web site quality evaluation has been proved to be not trivial task, as many methodologies and methods with a wide variation have appeared to date [8]. The National Cancer Institute proposed ten questions that are thought to cover all-important issues in evaluation [9]. In [10], a table of twenty-four Web sites and five journal articles was provided that contained explicit criteria for assessing health related Web sites. Of the 165 criteria in total, 80% were grouped under 12 categories and 20% were grouped as miscellaneous. The most common criterion group is that of "content" of the site, which includes concepts related to the quality, reliability and accuracy of the site resources. The group criteria that follow have to do with design and aesthetics of the site, disclosure of authors, sponsors, currency of information, authority of source and ease of use. In another effort, an agreement of a subset of Internet rating systems was sought [11], with the conclusion that some web sites characteristics such as number of daily visits, resources updating frequency and number of other web sites linked to them, could be processed to produce quality indicators about the sites in concern. In addition, Web evaluation tools may be used to assist site evaluations. Finally, classical techniques of interface design and evaluation, like *Heuristic Evaluation*, and *Cognitive Walkthrough*, may be adopted to be used in various contexts.

4. Materials and Methods

4.1 Stages and scope of the study

Three stages were involved in this study. The available Greek health portals had to be found and searched thoroughly. A representative number of portals were selected using certain criteria. The cognitive walkthrough and the heuristic evaluation techniques were chosen to be used for the interface evaluation of these portals. In the next stage, this exploratory study goes a little further aiming to evaluate the portal Resources; it is conducted using a set of questions answered by a number of people from Ptolemais, and provides a picture of the user preferences. Finally in the last stage, semi-structured interviews were conducted in Greek over a small number of individuals practicing medical or pharmaceutical professions. Interviews lasted for about twenty minutes each, and envisaged to elicit incidents of both purposive seeking and accidental encountering of health information, but also to outline the professionals' opinion on health portals.

4.2 Portal selection

The available Greek health portals were found mainly using the Greek search engine Robby. The main reason for choosing it was that it works in the Greek and English languages. Each portal was thoroughly examined for the type of information offered, the services offered, the general presentation and, when available, the number of user visits. Having in mind the definition of a health portal given in the introduction, three portals were chosen for further evaluation. These were: http://care.flash.gr (P1), http://health.in.gr (P2) and http://www.iatronet.gr (P3). These three portals (or vortals) constitute about 30% of the total number of eleven portals found at the time the study took place (2003). P2 is owned by large press organisations in Greece. As a result, health news is updated very often (intraday). Visit statistics prove that this portal is a very popular, if not the most popular health portal in Greece. Similarly, P1 belongs to another mass media organization. Health news is also updated within the same day here too. On the other hand, P3 offers basically standard information about certain health matters, and is only updated when something new has come up in the scientific world.

4.3 Portal Interface Evaluation

Interface evaluation was performed by Cognitive Walkthrough and Heuristic evaluation. Both tests were performed for the same task, which was the search of the same subject "Stomach Ulcer". Cognitive walkthrough is a method of evaluation that establishes how easy is for the user to learn the system under assessment. The method was applied by one of the authors, who pretended to be a naive user in the task and portals set. Heuristic evaluation, makes use of a set of 10 heuristics to structure the critique of a system. The evolution of Web technology resulted in a few more heuristics, the classic ten, plus a few more concerning Web site evaluation [12]. This method was applied by the authors, acting as a group of experts.

4.4 Portal Resource Evaluation

Portal resources were evaluated with two groups of criteria. First, is the *Credibility* group, which contains *Source* of information, *Currency* of the document, *Relevance* to what is claimed to be offered and *Review* process. Second, is the *Content* group, which refers to *Accuracy* of content, *Disclaimer* of purpose *(authority) limitations*, and *Completeness* of presentation. Both of these groups were compiled into a set of questions, as simple as possible, and as short in required response time as possibly achievable. On the top of the questionnaire an explanation of what the questionnaire was about and the three chosen sites for evaluation were given. The only personal questions asked were those of age and gender. The rest of the questions had to be answered by ticking on the side of one of the provided answers. Questionnaires were handed out all on the same day and collected back after one week. Response rate was 65%, the number of returned questionnaires was 108 in total, 8 of which were unusable. Although 60% of the sample were younger than 20 years old, the sample was acceptable considering that this is also the main part of the population mostly using the internet in this area, thereby usually undertaking the task of seeking for family health related queries. Finally, all professional interviewees (ten (10) doctors and four (4) pharmacists) were in the age range of 35 – 50 years old. As the majority of them were male (10 M – 4 F), a gender analysis of the results was not attempted.

5. Results

The main results of the interface evaluation are shown in Tables 1 and 2. Qualitative analysis of the first four questions of questionnaires showed that, 88% have visited a health portal at least once (27 M – 17 F). From these, 57% (34 M - 16F) visit a health portal once a week, 16% (10 M – 4 F) once per month, and 27% (10 M - 14 F) just a few times per year.

Table 1 Health Portal Interface Evaluations using Cognitive Walkthrough

Questions asked	Results
Will the user be trying to produce whatever effect the action has?	The user has nothing to produce in all portals. The search ability of the sites is already a complete action and nothing else (for example indexing) needs to be done
Will users be able to notice that the correct action is available?	In P1 and P2 the user notices immediately on the top of the screen the available space to enter the theme words. In P3, the user sees a button with the label SEARCH.
Once correct action is found, will they know that it is the right one for the effect they are trying to produce?	For P1 and P2 things are very simple. A search label and the empty space (box) next to it for writing the theme words. The user is sure about the action. For P3, user becomes certain, because after pressing the button SEARCH, a new page (search page) opens and requires entry of theme words
After the action is taken, will the users understand the feedback they get?	After the action, all portals provide a new page with a list of articles containing the theme words mentioned. Therefore the users understand very well the feedback they get.

The **Credibility** criteria were satisfied by nearly 90% of the sample. Females seemed to be more satisfied by a very small percentage. **Content** criteria were satisfied by a percentage of 96% (space limitations do not allow for a detailed presentation of these). One question of the questionnaire produced an indication of users' preferences on health subject topics. Their relative distribution is illustrated in Figure 1. The last question gave an indication for the induced change of behaviour. Only 8% have changed habits after seeking information from the Internet.

Finally, the majority of medical professional interviewees (60% of doctors) indicated Internet use, awareness of the Web health portals, and at least one visit to all available Greek health portals. They make use of the Greek, but also international, health sites mostly to find bibliography or generally references about subjects of their professional interests. All of them stated that they have come across patients, who make use of Web health resources. Their constant advice to all those were that, they can educate themselves in whatever way they like, but, they should never attempt to practice medicine themselves. Last, interviewed pharmacists indicated Internet use and awareness of health portals, but no professional use (i.e. information for pharmaceutics). All of them, however, would be ready to make professional use (logistics, information, etc) if it were required by their central pharmaceutical suppliers.

Table 2 Health Portal Interface Evaluations using Heuristics Evaluation

Criteria checked	Results
Match between system and real world	True, because the language used in all portals is simple without any special jargon terms
Consistency & standards	In P3 the user finds the British flag indicating that text in English will appear as soon as the flag is pressed. For P1 and P2 many different little pictures are used to indicate the encyclopaedia, the counters and many other selections
Aesthetic & Minimalist design	True, as all portals have interfaces with simple design and only present relevant information. P3 has the simplest interface and P2 has the most information rich interface
Avoid Gratuitous use of features	Moving banners in all sites used for advertisements do not violate this
Keep download and response times low	The transfer from one page to the next in all portals takes place very quickly and printing of an article is a very fast. As soon as the little printer picture is pressed the printer starts to print.
Information chunking	Information on the screens is grouped satisfying the heuristic
Important information belongs above the fold	True, as the most important action (search), is kept high in the screen. For P1 and P2, search is on the horizontal menu
Scan able pages	In all portals text on the screen can be read nearly at a glance

6. Discussion and Conclusions

The successful cognitive walkthrough, as well as, the satisfaction of the most important heuristics, indicate that portal interfaces are properly designed. Furthermore, the satisfaction of the two groups of criteria indicates that people generally consider that Internet Health Resources are accurate. In a RAND study on the quality of health information on the Internet funded by the Californian HealthCare Foundation [13], it was argued that although seek results are usually incomplete, when information is provided, it is generally accurate. As years go by, Internet user numbers rapidly increase, thereby proportionally increasing health portal users. The high volume of research work in quality portal evaluation seems to have produced positive results. Another result that this study produced, was that younger people use the Internet for health information more than the older ones. The most popular subjects to them are "body" related, that is sex health, fitness and gymnastics. This is also confirmed in reports worldwide. Finally, obvious limitations stem from the size of the samples, age, gender and education related misdistributions.

However, the study is part of a survey which is undertaken by the authors in the region of South East Europe, and is envisaged to produce more accurate and quantitative results. As information literacy proves to be an ambiguous concept [6], and the need for medicine to fit patients' social and language contexts [5] grows, the importance of studies like the one in this paper is obvious.

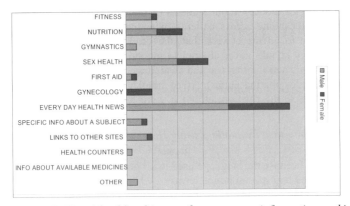

Figure 1: Users' health subject preferences upon information seeking

7. References

[1] Cambell, J., "Grammatical Man: Information, Entropy, Language and Life", Simon & Schuster, New York, 1982.

[2] Health Informatics Europe, "eHealth Code of Ethics." www.hi-europe.info/files/2000/ehealth_code.htm

[3] Ahmann, E. (2000), "Supporting Families' Savvy Use of Internet for Health Research", Ped.Nurs., Vol.26:419-424.

[4] The World Fact Book 2003 (2004), www.bartleby.com/151/country.html [Feb 2004]

[5] Birru M., Steinman R.A, "Online Health Information and low-literacy African Americans", J.Med.Int.Res 6(3):e26.

[6] Saranto K., Hovenga E.J.S., "Information literacy – what is it about? Literature review of the concept and the context", Int. J. Medical Informatics, 2004; 73:503-513.

[7] Greenberg L., D'Andrea G., Lorence D., "Setting the public agenda for online health search: a white paper and action agenda", J Med Internet Res 2004; 6(2):e18.

[8] Eysenbach, G., "A framework for evaluating e-health: systematic review of studies assessing the quality of health information and services for patients on the Internet", J Med Internet Res 2000, 3(suppl2):e9.

[9] National Cancer Institute (1999), "10 things to know about evaluating medical resources on the web" cancertrials.nci.nih.gov/beyond/evaluating .html, [Oct 2002]

[10] Kim P., Eng R.T., Deering J.M., Maxfield A. (1999), "Published criteria for evaluating health related web sites: review", www.bmj.com/cgi/content/full/318/7184/647, [Feb 2003]

[11] Hernandez-Borges, A.A., et al, "Can Examination of WWW Usage Statistics and other Indirect Quality Indicators Help to Distinguish the Relative Quality Of Medical websites?" J Med Inter Res 1999; 1:e1.

[12] Pearrow, M., "Web Site Usability Handbook", Charles River Media Inc., 2000.

[13] RAND report, "Evaluation of English and Spanish Information on the Internet", www.chcf.org, [Mar 2003]

Address for correspondence

Panagiotis D. Bamidis, Lecturer, Lab of Medical Informatics, The Medical School, Aristotle University of Thessaloniki, Tel: +30 2310 999310, Fax: +30 2310 999263, e-mail: bamidis@med.auth.gr.

Connecting Medical Informatics and Bio-Informatics
R. Engelbrecht et al. (Eds.)
IOS Press, 2005

A Decade Devoted to Improving Online Health Information Quality

Celia Boyer[a], Antoine Geissbuhler[a, b]

[a]*Health On the Net Foundation, Switzerland,* [b]*Geneva University Hospital, Switzerland*

Abstract

Created in 1995 in response to consumer enthusiasm for the World Wide Web, Health On the Net Foundation[1] has developed solutions to address the problem of potentially dangerous online health and medical information. Then as now, no international legal framework regulated online content, and consumers needed to be given the means to check the reliability and the relevance of health information [[1]]. HON was first to introduce a code of conduct for online health and medical publishers, the HONcode [[2],[3],[4]], which was readily adopted by webmasters aware of the need for credibility in the new, competitive online space. HON went on to develop Web applications to enhance access to reliable information, making use of innovative NLP-based and semantic search technologies.

This paper describes the implementation of a quality standard for online information (HONcode) based on the information production process; its evolution through nearly 10 years of effectiveness, its challenges and results. Today, over 4,700 HON-accredited websites, respecting minimum standards for disclosure and responsibility in online medical publishing, constitute the largest voluntary accreditation network on the Web.

Keywords:
Trustworthiness; Quality; Medical Internet, Medical information, Credibility

1. Background

Health On the Net Foundation was created in 1995 by Prof. Jean-Raoul Scherrer, former director of the Geneva University Hospital; Donald Lindberg, Director of the U.S. National Library of Medecine, Michel Carpentier, former director of the European Commission DGXIII and Guy-Olivier Second, former Director-General of the Geneva Ministry of Health. They foresaw that consumers, newly empowered to research their own medical conditions, could easily fall prey to misleading advice [[1], [5]]. New information technologies have given online publishers the means to replicate and re-use digital content, and the public can now access previously hard to find material. With no international legal framework to regulate online content, consumers urgently needed to be given the means to assess the reliability and the relevance of health information, and be provided with enhanced access to information of the highest quality.

Persistent medical controversies meant that multiple information sources needed to be considered, weighed and analysed.

Health On the Net Foundation was created to fill this role. Its stated mission is to "guide the growing online community of healthcare consumers and information providers to sound, reliable medical information and expertise". Over a ten-year period, HON has developed strategies to improve information quality addressed to content creators, and

---

[1] Health On the Net Foundation: http://www.healthonnet.org/

technologies to enhance access to reliable information intended for the general public. HON has devised analytical tools that infer reliability from the information production process itself. The HONcode, discussed in the following section, is a strategic, human, pedagogic and consumer-oriented effort aimed at two target audiences: web publishers and the general public. HON's MedHunt search engine, HONselect directory and WRAPIN next-generation search tool complement the human-based ethical approach with technological means [[6],[7],[8],[9]].

2. Objectives and solutions set up by Health On the Net Foundation

Establishing trust is crucial in any relationship between a patient and a provider of health services. This applies not only to doctors and other caregivers, but also to information providers. This approach to the promotion of best practices in eHealth would only be possible if web masters could be motivated to voluntarily adopt an initiative aimed in improving the quality of health/medical information on the web.

Requesting transparency on the operational level of providing online health information infers awareness of responsibility from the information provider. To achieve this, HON first needed to reach a consensus among information providers, medical experts and consumers, to define criteria for trustworthy health information websites.

The HONcode was the first code of conduct developed in 1996 for online medical and health information providers, with a voluntary accreditation programme setting out eight criteria that any well-intentioned webmaster could follow [Text Box 1].

Text Box 1. The HONcode is now translated in 29 languages. The HONcode obliges Websites to respect and disclose the following information:

Authority
Is medical advice given by a medical professional?

Complementarity
Information should support, not replace, the doctor-patient relationship

Privacy
What use is made of personal data collected through the Web site

Attribution
Refer accurately to source information

Justifiability
Site must back up claims about benefits & performance

Transparency
Accessible presentation, identities of editor & webmaster, email contact

Financial disclosure
Identify sources of funding

Sponsorship
Clearly distinguish advertising from editorial content

The accreditation process was designed not only to protect the public, but to educate the webmaster and improve online information quality by requiring the addition of meta information, including complete citations and revision dates, and through the labelling of advertising or commercially-oriented content. User confidence would be enhanced by the disclosure of potential conflicts of interest, as the web publisher was required to declare the funding sources of the web site.

HONcode
The HONcode Code of Conduct consists of elementary rules that any conscientious webmaster can easily adopt [Text Box 1]. It is a voluntary accreditation system based on an

"active seal" concept. Site administrators must take the initiative to apply for HONcode accreditation. HON found that some 90% of sites did not fully or correctly apply the Code of Conduct and many sites did not follow instructions in their display of the HONcode seal. To promote accountability and combat fraudulent use of the HONcode logo, a unique certificate was assigned to each accredited site, appearing when a user clicked on the accreditation seal.

Review Process

Each request for accreditation is examined by a member of the HONcode review team. HON makes a thorough visit of the site and verifies that all eight of the HONcode ethical principles are respected according to the HONcode accreditation guidelines [[10]]. The site is accredited by HON when the site not only complies with the HONcode principles but also demonstrates how each principle is implemented. As the result of the HONcode accreditation the site which is found to respect the eight HONcode principles is given a unique, active seal' to place on their pages. The presence of the distinctive blue and red HONcode seal on subscribing sites helps users identify sources of reliable information. The term 'active seal' refers to the link which webmasters are required to maintain from the HONcode seal to a certificate attesting to their accreditation status, residing on the HON site. Tampering with the seal is prohibited by the HONcode agreement. Visitors are encouraged to 'Click to verify' the HONcode status, which can be revoked at any time.

The HONcode accreditation process is strengthened by regular monitoring. An accredited site receives a check-up visit periodically, beginning one year after initial accreditation, or following a complaint or technical malfunction detected by our monitoring services. The HONcode has undergone one revision since its introduction in 1996 [[11]], and an elaborate system has been built to support the reviewing process, dubbed HONuser. This system provides a workflow for administrators and manages the many interactions among teams of scattered reviewers and webmasters.

Regionalisation

To more effectively extend HONcode accreditation to websites targeting regional, and in particular, non-English language audiences, HON is extending its reviewing activities in European countries, North America and Africa. In addition to linguistic support, this initiative aims to preserve cultural diversity. HON has already formed a reviewing team based in Valencia, Spain [12], and new teams are being set up in Mali and Romania, to carry out reviewing and to promote online health information quality to content creators and the public. Despite the global reach of the Internet and the fact that international websites are often produced in English, HON's regional initiatives are a necessary response to the growth of Internet use in the target regions, allowing HON to remain sensitive to questions of health and culture and more easily conform to differences in legal requirements. The question of financial support is not yet resolved we believe that the new regional activities should be supported by local and regional authorities.

Search engine and other technologies

Internet users commonly use a single preferred general-purpose search engine to locate Web pages on any subject [13]. Beginning in 1996, HON opted for a restricted-domain approach to search only medical resources [14]. The generic robot, MARVIN, (Multi-Agent Retrieval Vagabond on Information Network), combines crawler and extraction technologies. MARVIN uses a multilingual glossary (Dutch, English, French, German, Italian, Polish, Spanish, and Portuguese) to reinforce the 33,000 Medical Subject Headings (MeSH) as it indexes and automatically extracts MeSH terms, feeding HON's databases [[6]]. MARVIN searches from the complete database of over 4,700 HONcode accredited sites, offering a specialized search engine for trustworthy Web sites named HONcodeHunt.

The next-generation search tool, WRAPIN (Worldwide Reliable Advice to Patients and Individuals), is a set of technologies developed within the framework of a two-year EU project (IST–2001-33260) [[8], [9]].. WRAPIN was developed to identify relevant documents and make assertions as to their trustworthiness. The system, powered by Natural Language Processing, is able to identify the main scientific concepts contained in a text, and performs 'background checks' on a document to ascertain the origins and relations of the ideas it contains. A reference database of trustworthy sources includes MEDLINE (U.S. National Library of Medicine), Clinical Trials (US National Health Institute), FDA Drug Information (U.S. Food Drug Administration), UROFrance (French Association of Urology) and OESO (World Organ. for Specialised Studies on Diseases of the Esophagus) and HON's databases. The result is a semi-automatic editorial policy engine which aims to enhance access to the knowledge contained within a collection of scientific documents.

3. Results

When initially applying for HONcode accreditation, not all Websites are compliant with all eight HONcode principles. Currently, 78% of web sites applying for HONcode accreditation respect Principle 1, which requires that the author or editor of the information be named (Principle 1: Authority). In the study of Hernández Borges [[15]], which evaluated a sample of 159 paediatrics web sites, this number was 65%.

Some 76% of web sites with health information clearly stated the goal of the site and its target audiences (Principle 2 Complementarity). The sources of medical information are clearly established in 81% of the sites. Often, the date provided in the web site is not the date of last modification, but is set to automatically display the current date. A credible date of last modification is only stated in 70% of sites (Principle 4: Attribution). Very few web sites (less than 6%) made claims on a specific treatment (Principle 5: Justifiability).

Over the years, HON has noted a significant change in the provision of a confidentiality policy. 65% of the web sites have a confidentiality policy (Principle 3: Confidentiality), as opposed to 24% in the previous study. Some 99% of sites provided a means of contacting their webmasters (Principle 6: Transparency of Authorship). Finally, 52% of webmasters clearly stated their sources of financial support (Principle 7: Transparency of sponsorship). Only 41% declared that they host advertising on their site (Principle 8: Honesty in Advertising and Editorial Policy).

This showed a mean rate of compliance with the HON principles of 73.6%. 7.5% of applicants were rejected due to inappropriate content or to an impossibility to respect the HONcode. At the initial application, despite the voluntary nature of the accreditation process, only 23% of sites were fully compliant with the HONcode However, following communications between the webmaster and the HONcode staff, 99% of sites that decided to continue the accreditation process were brought into compliance with the eight HONcode principles.

Outstanding web sites such as Medline, PubMed Central, aids.org, American Cancer Society, , National Institute of Mental Health, The American Council for Headache Education, Guillain Barré Syndrome Support Group, Healthfinder, InteliHealth, MayoClinic, Meningitis Research Foundation, Multiple Sclerosis Foundation, WebMd, Stop-tabac and others are all HONcode subscribers.

According to the 'Web Impact Factor' of Alta Vista, over 800,000 quality web pages link to the HON web site in 72 countries. HONcode accredited Web sites are categorized under more than 33,000 subject headings, covering both most common and rare diseases. The language coverage of HONcode web sites is 55% for English, 15% for French, 12% for Spanish, 7% for Italian.

In an outreach to the public, HON released a multifunctional browser toolbar (a plugin named the HON Toolbar) [[16]] which, when activated, automatically displays a site's HONcode status. This toolbar was implemented in order to assist Web surfers to access trustworthy Web sites. The HONcode tool bar is used by more than 20,000 persons each day.

4. Discussion and Conclusion

Comforting the HONcode initiative, in 2001 the European Commission has released Quality Criteria for Health related Websites recommending to members states to respect elementary rules [[17]]. This recommendation has been developed in collaboration with HON. Inspired by HON, other recent nationals initiatives to promote health website accreditation have been initiated in US and in Germany respectively in 2001 and 2003[[18], [19]]. These initiatives choose a different economic model than the one adopted by HON. URAC accreditation is based on a yearly fee proportionally to the organisation (around USD 13'000 per year – difficult to find the exact cost on [18]), while the AFGIS, intended to the German language web sites, is based on a membership fee (around EURO 150 per year) trying to build a community. As a neutral, standards-setting body, HON retains the confidence of all concerned parties. HON is free of commercial influence and perceived by the public and the industry as free of influence. The HONcode accreditation is free.

The introduction of the HONcode in 1996 was a milestone for online health information, as evidenced by numerous references to the HONcode in the Health Informatics literature. The HONcode has often been shown to be a major indicator of accuracy in content in scientific studies [[21], [22], [23], [24], [24]]. The need for online information quality standards arose concurrently with the popularity of the World Wide Web. Ten years on, substantive discussion of Internet Governance is just beginning. The approach pioneered by HON has received wide support from government, industry, and citizens/patients groups; HON was the winner of the Best Content in e-Health category of the World Summit Awards, attributed in December 2003, for a comprehensive overview of best practices in e-content and creativity, within the framework of the World Summit on the Information Society (WSIS). In May 2004, HON was named winner of the eEurope Award for eHealth, in the category "eHealth Information tools and services for citizens." at the EU High-Level Conference on eHealth held in Cork, Ireland [[25]].

5. Acknowledgments

Health On the Net Foundation is a Non-Governmental Organization under the aegis of the Direction générale de la santé Département de l'Action Sociale et de Santé (DASS - République et canton de Genève, Switzerland). The WRAPIN (Worldwide online Reliable Advice to Patients and Individuals) project, IST-2001-33260, is supported by the EC and the "Office Fédéral de l'Education et la Science" (OFES, Switzerland). The authors wish to thank all HONcode members, collaborators and friends for their contributions to the development and achievements of HON. HON servers are powered by Sun Microsystems.

6. References

[1] Impicciatore P, Pandolfini C, Casella N, Bonati M. Reliability of health information for the public on the world wide web: systematic survey of advice on managing fever in children at home. *BMJ* 1997; 314: 1875-1879

[2] HONcode principles. In Health On the Net Foundation. Retrieved Jan 21 2004, from http://www.hon.ch/HONcode/

[3] Selby M., Boyer C., Jenefski D.A., Appel R.D. Health On the Net Foundation Code of Conduct for Medical and Health Websites. *MEDNET96 - European Congress on the Internet in Medicine*, Brighton, U.K., Oct. 14 to 17, 1996.

[4] Boyer C., Selby M., Appel R.D. The Health On the Net code of conduct for medical and health web sites. *MEDINFO 98, Seoul, 9th World Congress on Medical Informatics*, vol 2, 1163-1166, August 98.

[5] Chiara Pandolfini and Maurizio Bonati, Follow up of quality of public oriented health information on the world wide web: systematic re-evaluation *BMJ* 2002 324: 582-583

[6] Baujard O., Baujard V., Aurel S., Boyer C., Appel R.D. A multi-agent softbot to retrieve medical information on Internet. *MEDINFO 98*, Seoul, 9th World Congress on Medical Informatics, vol 1, 150-154, August 98.

[7] C Boyer, V Baujard, JR Scherrer, HONselect: Multilingual Assistant Search Engine Operated by a Concept-based Interface System to Decentralized Heterogeneous Sources. *Medinfo, 2001*

[8] Gaudinat A, Joubert M, Aymard S, Falco L, Boyer C, Fieschi M. WRAPIN: New Generation Health Search Engine Using UMLS Knowledge Sources for MeSH Term Extraction from Health Documentation. *Medinfo. 2004*; 2004:356-60.

[9] WRAPIN- Worldwide online Reliable Advice to Patients and Individuals European Project : IST-2001-33260. Retrieved Jan 21 2004, from http://www.wrapin.org

[10] Accreditation Guidelines for the HON Code of Conduct (HONcode). Accessed Jan. 21 2005, from: http://www.hon.ch/HONcode/Guidelines/guidelines.html

[11] HONcode first version in 1996,. Retrieved Jan. 21 2005 from http://www.hon.ch/HONcode/ConductVs1_5.html

[12] García S, Montesinos E, Baujard V, Boyer C. Health on The Net Foundation, Geneva Switzerland. *MedNet 2003* 3-7 December 2003. A descriptive analysis of strategies in Spain for internet biomedical content evaluation

[13] *Pew Internet and American Life*: Report on Internet Health Resources, July 2003, http://www.pewinternet.org/pdfs/PIP_Health_Report_July_2003.pdf (accessed 17 feb 2005)

[14] Supporting families' savvy use of the Internet for health research. Ahmann E. *Pediatr Nurs.* 2000 Jul-Aug; 26(4): 419-23.

[15] Hernández Borges AA, Macías Cervi P, Torres Álvarez de Arcaya ML, Gaspar Guardado MA, Ruíz Rabaza A, Jiménez Sosa A. Rate of compliance with the HON code of conduct versus number of inbound links as quality markers of pediatric web sites. *Proceedings of the 6th world congress on the internet in medicine, Udine, Italy, Nov 29-2 Dec 2001*. http://mednet2001.drmm.uniud.it/proceedings/paper.php?id=75 (accessed 2005 Jan 21).

[16] HONcode tool bar: Health Information you can trust (Jan 2004). In Health On the Net Foundation. Accessed Jan 21 2004, from http://www.hon.ch/HONcode/Plugin/Plugins.html

[17] European Union recommendation: Quality Criteria for Health related Websites http://www.hon.ch/HONcode/HON_CCE_intro.htm

[18] URAC: http://www.urac.org/

[19] AFGIS: http://www.afgis.de/

[20] Petra Wilson, How to find the good and avoid the bad or ugly: a short guide to tools for rating quality of health information on the internet, *BMJ*, Mar 2002; 324: 598 - 602.

[21] Diabetes websites accredited by the Health On the Net Foundation Code of Conduct: readable or not? Kusec S, Brborovic O, Schillinger D. *Stud, Health Technol Inform*. 2003; 95: 655-60.

[22] "Trust-building Measures: A Review of Consumer HEALTH PORTALS Health Web sites are employ a medley of trust-building approaches. But does a definitive formula exist for winning consumer trust?" by Wenhong Luo and Mohammad Najdawi, *COMMUNICATIONS OF THE ACM* January 2004/Vol. 47, No. 1 109 - 113

[23] Search Engine Retrieval Effectiveness For Medical Information Queries, IST 637 Research Project - Group Elmo by Linda Galloway, Nicole Chase-Iverson, Glen Wiley, Gerrit Vander Sluis (March 2003 - http://web.syr.edu/~gevander/ "In order to determine authoritativeness of the medical information returned by each search engine, adherence to the HON (Health on the Net) Code was used as a measure."

[24] Fallis D, and Fricke M., Indicators of accuracy of consumer health information on the Internet: a study of indicators relating to information for managing fever in children in the home. *JAMIA*, 2002 Jan-Feb;9(1):73-9.

[25] 2004 eEurope Award for eHealth http://www.hon.ch/Global/eHealth2004/winner.html

Address for correspondence

Health On the Net Foundation, 24 rue Micheli-du-crest, 1211 Geneva 14, Email:
Celia.Boyer@healthonnet.org

Connecting Medical Informatics and Bio-Informatics
R. Engelbrecht et al. (Eds.)
IOS Press, 2005

Construction of an Instrument for Measuring Medical Student Satisfaction with Virtual Campus

Ziad EL Balaa[a], **Henri-Jean Philippe**[a], **Christelle Volteau**[b], **Pierre Le Beux**[c] , **Jean-Michel Nguyen**[b]

[a]*Faculty of Medicine, Nantes, France*
[b]*PIMESP – Nantes Hospital, Nantes, France*
[c]*University of Rennes1, Rennes, France*

Abstract

In France, the virtual campus became a pedagogical tool used in the medical education in year 2000. Therefore, it is appropriate to measure the student satisfaction, user of virtual campus. The objective of this research was to develop a student satisfaction instrument adapted to the medical field. Based on the literature, we obtained 36-item questionnaire, using 5-point Likert-type scale. 80 students in the Faculty of Medicine at the Nantes University participated to this survey. In this study, two analyses were conducted, the first included all the items and the second excluded items for which a high rate of non response were found. The results show that the instrument contains three dimensions: 'self evaluation – tutorial', 'appropriateness of content' and 'user-friendliness'. Nevertheless, this exploratory study need to be validated with a greater sample of students.

Keywords:
Student satisfaction; Instrument development; Measurement; Electronic learning; Virtual campus; Medical Informatics

1. Introduction

The evolution of medical knowledge imposes techniques of diffusion which have a great reactivity. The virtual campuses represent a pedagogical approach allowing a fast update and less expensive than the traditional support (e.g., book, CD-Rom, etc.).

The virtual campus was set up in France in 2000 [1]. Its integration within the higher education is increasingly important especially in the medical field. Little assessment were carried out in a particular with regard to medical student satisfaction.

To our knowledge, there is not validated instrument for measuring the satisfaction with virtual medical campus in France, whereas in other fields such as engineering these instruments was developed [2-8] .

The goal of our study is to develop, in France, a student satisfaction instrument.

The first part of this study consists in analysing the common points with the other existing instruments. Our strategy is to extract common information from the other instruments which can be applicable in medicine. No specific hypothesis is suggested in our survey.

2. Review of related Literature

During the last years, several instruments have been developed to measure user satisfaction, although the student can be regarded as Information System (IS) user in a particular e-learning system.

Wang [9] developed a new instrument, from the User Information Satisfaction (UIS) and End User Computing Satisfaction (EUCS), to measure the E-Leaning Satisfaction (ELS). This instrument contains 17 items using 7-point Likert-type scale. These items representing 4 factors were interpreted as learner interface, learning community, content and personalisation. Wang proved that the 2 factors, learning community and personalisation, are specific factors to the ELS and are excluded from UIS and EUCS. The sample of this study is formed of the employees having used an e-learning system.

The satisfaction survey of Stokes [10] contains 16 items selected from the review of literature. 3 factors are described; temperament, satisfaction and demographic characteristics. The students were the target population for this research. These students represent the Colleges of Commerce and Business Administration, Education, Arts and Sciences.

Hong [11] used an instrument of a previous study to measure student satisfaction. The items were grouped under 3 factors (computer experience, learning style, and perceptions of the Web-based course) with 5-point Likert scale. The subjects in this study consisted of students in Master of Science.

The instrument of D'Ambra and Rice [12] was based on the literature, focus groups and pilot surveys. They administrated three surveys to develop and validate a questionnaire containing 50 items. Items ranges were 1 (strongly disagree) to 5 (strongly agree). 9 factors was retained as following; training, interests, information, shopping cost, difficult information, fun, social influence, identity control and use control. Students were sample of this study.

Chen, Lin and Kinshuk [13] used the critical incident technique (CIT) to collect data about the user satisfaction. They developed a new instrument adopted from the previous studies applied in various fields: marketing, public transport services [14,15] and education. The instrument consisted of three parts. The first part represented overall cumulative satisfaction (OCS) and attribute-specific cumulative satisfaction (ASCS). For each item, a 7-point Likert scale ranging from "strongly unsatisfied" to "strongly satisfied" was given. The second part consisted of a description of the frequency of negative critical incidents (FNCI). For each item, a 5-point Likert scale ranging from "never" to "always" was attributed. The third part contained demographic items. The items were divided into 4 factors; administration, functionality, instruction and interaction. The subjects of this study were students taking Master's online.

3. Research Methodology

Sample survey

Our target population was the 5th year students in the Faculty of Medicine at the Nantes University who used the virtual campus.

The teaching in the 5th year of medicine is divided into 4 subjects (Gynaecology obstetrics, Pediatry, Cancerology and Dermatology), each subject contains several courses and propose a virtual campus. The students participate into a training in the morning at the hospital and the afternoon follow courses at the Faculty. They use the virtual campus as an option, completing their traditional courses (face-to-face).

Construction of satisfaction instrument

A review of the literature made possible to identify the e-learning satisfaction instrument and the used items. The construction of our instrument consists to collect all the items of all the recent instruments in the e-learning system [9, 10, 12, 13, 16,17] and to test them by using Principal Component Factor Analysis (PCA).

The redundant items between the instruments were deleted, we retained 36 items, table 1 presents the list of the questions. All items are represented by a 5-point Likert-type scale ranging from 1 (strongly unsatisfied) to 5 (strongly satisfied).

Data collection

During the class, the 80 students received the survey package containing the questionnaire and a cover letter explaining the objective of the study and its importance about their satisfaction with virtual campus. The participation in this study was voluntary. The questionnaire is anonymous and confidentially guaranteed. Answers are given individually, the whole questionnaire needs 7-9 minutes to be filled in. An online questionnaire was suggested for all the other French-speaking universities.

Statistical analysis

Principal Component Factor Analysis was done using varimax rotation on the correlation matrix, Cronbach's alpha coefficient were calculated for each dimension. Two analyses were conducted. The first included all the items and the second excluded items for which a high rate of non response were found. All analyses were done using SPAD and SPLUS.

4. Results

The first analysis was conducted with 36 items, missing data were not considered. For these 36 items, 55 students gave exhaustive responses. More than half of them used the campus less than 2 hours, indicating their inexperience.

Three factors were identified explaining 59.2% of the variance. The first 'self evaluation – tutorial' (14 items) accounting for 41.1% of the variance, the second 'Content', 11.4% (6 items) and the third 'user-friendliness' (6 items) 6.7% of the variance.

In the second analysis, 6 items (Q10, Q11, Q12, Q13, Q14, Q15) were excluded. These were about information of the relation between students and professor. Two factors were identified, explaining 47.9% of the variance. The first dimension concerned the 'self evaluation, tutorial and content' (6 items and 38.5% of the variance explained) and the second 'user-friendliness' (7 items and 9.43% of the variance explained).

Cronbach's alpha coefficients were respectively 96% and 94% for the two analyses.

Mean scores were respectively 69.1+/-13 and 71.3+/-12.8 for the two scales.

5. Discussion

The students in great majority used the campus less than 2 hours. For these students, the first reason is the lack of time. Indeed, a timetable shared between the morning devoted to the training course at the hospital and the afternoon devoted to courses, gives little availability to the students to use the virtual campus. The second major obstacle is the lack of comfort and their inexperience towards computer or Internet. Third, the virtual campus is optional. Those 3 reasons explain the results we developed above.

Conceived to assess a virtual campus, the questionnaire contained initially 36 items based on the whole satisfaction instrument, in the literature, with e-learning system. This lead to the inadequation of a few questions that were not related to our virtual campus (items about the follow-up and the evaluation of student and relationship with theirs tutor). 17 subjects were thus excluded.

We eliminated from the first analysis the items concerning interaction and communication between the professor and the students. This dimension is not developed in the French medical virtual campus, explaining the number of non responses, whereas in the others education fields, the interaction student-teacher and students-students via the virtual campus were more developed and related to the student satisfaction [18].

Two dimensions emerged from the second analysis. The first dimension explores the possibilities of self evaluation of the virtual campus. This information seems essential to us. Indeed, the students' objective is to pass their examination. The virtual campuses are thus particularly appreciated if they allow a good preparation to the examinations. Beyond the contents, the student search, firstly, a high level position in the examination. Although the quality of contents is expected to be very high [17,19,20], the virtual campus is not to be mistaken with a knowledge encyclopaedia. The second dimension seems to focus on the ease of use, the design aspect, and the interface. The interface is a key element in the virtual campus and is closely related to the students' satisfaction. Johnson, Zhang, Tang, and Turely [21] confirm this point of view and prove that the interface maximizes the benefits courseware user satisfaction and that it is important to the e-learning system.

This study allowed us to develop a student satisfaction instrument with medical virtual campus, but limits may have affected the results. First, the small sample size (80 students participated to this study). Second, our instrument is based on existing scale developed in other domains. Thus, a specific dimension of medical courses cannot be explored. This could be done using open questionnaires.

6. Conclusion and future research

The results suggest that such an instrument must be limited to ensure that the content is appropriate to the student's needs, to ask questions about the possibility of self evaluation and about the ease of use of the virtual campus. The other domains are too specific and must be evaluated by specific scale like students' interaction with their tutors or student follow-up by tutors.

Starting from the overall of items used in the literature, we identified a tool exploring 3 dimensions of the student satisfaction. It related to the possibilities of self evaluation and tutorial, the appropriateness of the content and the facility of use of the virtual campus. Further studies are needed to confirm our results and to explore other dimension of medical student satisfaction.

7. Acknowledgments

The authors would like to thank the TICEM team at the Faculty of medicine – Nantes for his contribution to the data collection and the French Virtual Medical University (UMVF) for his cooperation.

Table 1 – List of items

Q1 - The virtual campus is easy to use
Q2 - The virtual campus is user-friendly
Q3 - The operation of the virtual campus is stable
Q4 - The virtual campus is accurate
Q5 - The output information is clear
Q6 - The virtual campus makes it easy for me to find the content I need
Q7 - The output is presented in a useful format
Q8 - The course planning and design are clear
Q9 - The virtual campus makes it easy for me to discuss questions with my teachers
Q10 - The virtual campus makes it easy for me to discuss questions with other students
Q11 - The interaction for office-hour
Q12 - The virtual campus makes it easy the interaction among students
Q13 - I am satisfied with the degree of contact I have with my teacher through the virtual campus
Q14 - The virtual campus provides content that exactly fits my needs
Q15 - The virtual campus provides content that easy to understand
Q16 - The virtual campus provides useful content
Q17 - The virtual campus provides sufficient content
Q18- The virtual campus provides up-to-date content
Q19 - The virtual campus responds to my requests fast enough
Q20 - The virtual campus enables me to control my learning progress
Q21 - The virtual campus records my learning progress and performance
Q22 - The virtual campus provides the personalized learning support
Q23 - The virtual campus enables me to learn the content I need
Q24 - The virtual campus enables me to choose what I want to learn
Q25 - I am able to access a computer with an Internet connection to do my work
Q26 - The resources I need are readily available through the virtual campus
Q27 - My technology knowledge level is sufficient for learning in the virtual campus
Q28 - I am feeling somewhat isolated when I learn in the virtual campus
Q29 - I would prefer to take more courses through the virtual campus
Q30 - The virtual campus has allowed me more flexibility in my daily activities
Q31 - I would prefer the face-to-face courses to the virtual campus
Q32 - The virtual campus enables me to take a more active role in the learning process
Q33 - The virtual campus is providing me with skills that I can use in other courses
Q34 - The virtual campus is preparing me for technology use in my profession
Q35 - The testing methods provided by the virtual campus are easy to understand
Q36 - The virtual campus provides testing results promptly

8. References

[1] Philippe HJ, El Balaa Z, Ploteau S, Philippe M. Modélisation d'un campus numérique pour les études en médecine à partir de l'expérience française en gynécologie-obstétrique. *Pédagogie Médicale* 2003; 4: 235-41.

[2] Chin JP, Diehl VA, Norman KL. Development of an instrument measuring user satisfaction of the human-computer interface. *Proceedings of the CHI'88 Conference: Human Factors in Computing Systems;* 1988 May 15-19; Washington DC, USA. New York: ACM press; 1988; pp. 213-8.

[3] Chin WW, Lee MKO. On The Formation of End-User Computing Satisfaction: A Proposed Model And Measurement Instrument. *Proceedings of the 21st International Conference On Information Systems;* 2000 Dec 10-13; Brisbane, Australia; 2000.

[4] Delucchi M, editor. *Student satisfaction with higher education during the 1970s- a decade of social change.* New York: The Edwin Mellen Press, 2003.

[5] Lazar J, Norico A. End-user Satisfaction in Training Novice Users to surf the Web. *Proceedings of the WebNet2001.*

World Conference on the WWW and Internet; 2001 Oct 23-27; Orlando, USA; 2001.

[6] Ong CS, Lai JY. Developing an instrument for measuring user satisfaction with knowledge management systems. *Proceeding of the 37th International Conference on System Sciences*; 2004 Jan 05-08; Big Island, Hawaii; 2004.

[7] Torkzadeh G, Cios KJ, Pflughoeft KA. Inductive machine learning for instrument development. *Information and Management* 1996; 31: 47-55.

[8] Xiao L, Dasgupta S. Measurement of user satisfaction with Web-Based information systems: An empirical study. In: Zhang P, editor. *Proceeding of the 8th Americas Conference on Information Systems*; 2002 Aug 9-11; Dallas, USA. New York; 2002; pp. 1149-55.

[9] Wang YS. Assessment of learner satisfaction with asynchronous electronic learning systems. *Information and Management* 2003; 41: 75-86.

[10] Stokes SP. Satisfaction of college students with the digital learning environment. Do learner's temperaments make a difference?. *Internet and Higher Education* 2001; 4: 31-44.

[11] Hong KS. Relationships between student's and instructional variables with satisfaction and learning from a Web-based course. *Internet and Higher Education* 2002; 5: 267-81.

[12] D'Ambra J, Rice RE. Emerging factors in user evaluation of the World Wide Web. *Information and Management* 2001; 38: 373-84.

[13] Chen NS, Lin KM, Kinshuk. Assessment of E-Learning Satisfaction from Critical Incidents Perspective. *Proceedings of the 6th Conference on Enterprise Information Systems*, 2004 Apr 14-17; Porto, Portugal. Porto: INSTICC press; 2004; pp. 27-34.

[14] Friman M, Edvardsson B, Gärling T. Frequency of negative critical incidents and satisfaction with public transport services I. *Journal of Retailing and Consumer Services* 2001; 8: 95-104.

[15] Friman M, Gärling T. Frequency of negative critical incidents and satisfaction with public transport services II. *Journal of Retailing and Consumer Services* 2001; 8: 105-14.

[16] McHaney R, Hightower R, Pearson J. A validation of the end-user satisfaction instrument in Taiwan. *Information and Management* 2002; 36: 503-11.

[17] McGorry SY. Measuring quality in online programs. *Internet and Higher Education* 2003; 6: 159-77.

[18] Irons LR, Jung DJ, Keel RO. Interactivity in Distance Learning: The Digital Divide and Student Satisfaction. Educational *Technology and Society* 2002; 5 (3) pp: 175-88.

[19] Cox J, Dale BG. Key quality factors in Web site design and use: an examination. *International Journal of Quality and Reliability Management* 2002; 19 (7) pp: 862-88.

20] Iwaarden JV, Wiele TV, Ball L, Millen R. Perceptions about the quality of web sites: a survey amongst students at Northeastern University and Erasmus University. *Information and Management* 2004; 41: 947-59.

[21] Johnson TR, Zhang J, Tang Z, Johnson C, Turley JP. Assessing informatics student's satisfaction with a web-based courseware system. *Int J Med Inform* 2004; 73:181-87.

9. Address for correspondence

Ziad EL BALAA
T.I.C.E.M – Faculty of Medicine
1, rue Gaston Veil
44035 Nantes cedex 01 – France
Tel : 00 33 2 40 41 29 92
Ziad.Elbalaa@univ-nantes.fr

Section 12

Organization Change, Information Needs

Connecting Medical Informatics and Bio-Informatics
R. Engelbrecht et al. (Eds.)
IOS Press, 2005

The Data-Gathering Broker – A User-Based Approach to Viable EPR Systems

Michael Rigby [a], David Budgen [b], Pearl Brereton [b], Keith Bennett [c], Michelle Russell [a], Mark Turner [b], Ioannis Kotsiopoulos [d], Paul Layzell [d], John Keane [d], Fujun Zhu [e]

[a] *Centre for Health Planning and Management, Keele University;*
[b] *School of Computing and Mathematics, Keele University;*
[c] *School of Engineering, University of Durham;*
[d] *School of Informatics, University of Manchester*
[e] *Department of Computer Science, University of Durham.*

Abstract

With the continued expansion of Electronic Patient Record systems ahead of comprehensive evidence, metrics, or future-proofing, European health informatics is embarking on a faith-driven adventure that also risks data swamping of end-users. An alternative approach is an information broker system, drawing from departmental data sources. A three-year study in health and social care has produced a first demonstrator which can search for specified information in heterogeneous distributed data stores, with source-specific permission can copy it, and then merge the search results in a real-time process.

Keywords:
Electronic patient records; Information broker; Departmental systems, Pervasive technology; Enterprise systems; Information swamping

1. Introduction

One of the biggest drives in health informatics in Europe is the development of Electronic Patient Records (Eprs). These have built upon a series of innovations in both primary and secondary care in many countries, not least the Netherlands, Finland and the United Kingdom, but have been encouraged forward by the seminal study of the US Institute of Medicine [1].

This unswerving drive forward seems obvious, and yet is unsupported. The obviousness comes from the powerful support to clinical diagnosis and healthcare delivery through the marshalling, analysis, searching, and representation of clinical data in a way which is totally impossible with paper-based records. Yet EPR systems are as much built on faith and instinct as balanced evidence. The Institute of Medicine Report [1] showed a high level vision, but was remarkably devoid of facts: there is no mention of record size, volume of transactions, or likely areas of further development. There are many instances of successful EPR developments, at practitioner level, institutional, and generic commercial level. Yet there are also cautionary tales of over-stretching [2], as well as a considerable literature on sub-optimal use. It is thus difficult to determine whether European health systems are embarking on a vision, a dream, or a nightmare.

2. Inexorable Growth of Vision

A further challenge is that as EPR systems develop, so there is a multi-dimensional inexorable growth extending the vision in many uncoordinated directions, principally:

Vertical integration – primary care and secondary care records are seen as of much greater benefit when they are linked into one single shared view of the patient.

Horizontal integration – records based on a single institution can lead to fragmentation of care, hence a move to regional records.

Temporal integration – previous medical history is often important in diagnosis, hence the interest in the concept of the electronic cradle-to-grave record.

Thus three dimensions of extension are leading towards vastly larger EPRs, yet it is claimed no system is yet complete [3]. However, even this is not the full story.

3. Expansion to Unsustainability?

These dimensions of integration are challenging in that they take record size, record storage, and transactions to previously unforeseen volumes. There are, though, further extensions, as current healthcare and diagnostic techniques themselves are growing inexorably, in very data-hungry ways, as is 'pervasive' technology potential. The following trends all cause further rapid expansion of EPR requirements:

Digitisation of Investigations – increasingly, x-rays, pathology results, ultrasound scans, and other diagnostic technologies are digitised in space-hungry formats.

Volume of Investigations – efficiencies from avoiding duplicate investigations are offset by the drive to undertake more investigations, particularly scans and traces.

Population Longevity – average life expectancy is increasing, and old age leads to increasing healthcare support and monitoring, increasing record size exponentially.

Genetic Analysis –genetic information increasingly is used as part of diagnosis and treatment, but detailed genetic code is large and therefore storage-hungry.

Designer Drugs – increasingly drugs will be tailored to the individual, and also "orphan" drugs will be utilised for patients with rare conditions. The prescribing part of records will grow rapidly to accommodate person-specific pharmaceuticals.

Domestic Environment Monitoring – as those with health conditions affecting their independent living are encouraged to live in their own homes, so "intelligent" housing monitoring systems will expand, and must be seen as part of the health record.

Continuous in vivo Monitoring – wearable monitoring devices and intelligent clothing are being developed both for diagnosis and to monitor daily living. The results must be part of health record, expanding far beyond current telemetry data.

Remote Service Delivery – increasingly telemedicine and other forms of remote healthcare delivery will be utilised, and must be included in the EPR.

The consequence of these cumulative drivers is rapid inflation of record size and the volume of transactions. Is this the uncontrolled evolution of a dinosaur which ultimately cannot be sustained? Experience from commerce is not encouraging, with large integrated enterprise systems proving vulnerability to instability and failure.

4. User Challenges

The physical growth of the EPR causes challenges for end users from the sheer complexity of the record, with increasing skill needed to navigate all the material – a typical incomplete

EPR system having 27 000 screen formats, 10 000 being used by ward nurses [4]. Data swamping is as much a potential risk as data shortage.

5. Is Doomsday upon Us?

This analysis is salutary, in that it makes the current instinctive drive forward to the integrated EPR vision look like a rush to an unsustainable solution. It is time to ask whether alternatives are possible. The motive of getting the relevant information to the right clinician at the right time is entirely laudable, and with the recent rapid developments in storage and communication powers the integrated record has seemed the natural solution, but expectations are now moving beyond the original vision.

At the same time, new means of searching for, retrieving, and handling data mean that much smaller record stores can be utilised as a virtual large facility if harnessed appropriately. For instance, though every airline runs its own reservations system, the consumer can now use services that present an integrated picture of all the possible routes between any two destinations for a specified date and time, then look for seat availability and prices for any option [5]. This is done not through data warehousing, but by accessing all the autonomous systems in real time and presenting to the end user in a standard display. The autonomy, and the different data formats, of the individual systems are not compromised, but the user receives an integrated picture.

6. The Broker or Data Gatherer

The new tool which achieves this vision is a broker - software which can register all potential data sources, find the relevant ones to meet a specific user query, and with approved permissions read the required data to create a real time picture. Of course, health is complex, with highly tuned requirements for confidentiality, and rich and varied sets of data items stored in many formats. However, a demonstrator broker has now been developed in the health and social care setting.

7. The IBHIS Project

This project was the Integration Broker for Heterogeneous Information Systems (IBHIS) project of the Universities of Keele, Durham, and UMIST* working as a consortium, funded by the UK Engineering and Physical Sciences Research Council (EPSRC) from 2002-2004. A web-based demonstrator linking data sets in real time now exists. Papers and presentations have been made to Medinfo 2004 [6] and UK Health Computing 2005 [7], to healthcare audiences, and international software and web service conferences [8,9].

The Information Broker solution rests on developing two key principles - that the end-user has situation-specific information requirements which need external data, and that local "departmental" record systems are generally robust. With paper records these two principles were in conflict, but the electronic information broker achieves the hitherto impossible. It acts as the user's agent, seeking defined information on demand about an identified patient, and presenting it in collated form without compromising the source systems' integrity. The work of the IBHIS team demonstrates this is possible in the health domain. If this were to be the architecture of the future, clinicians could have rich but relevant information at the point of decision-making, whilst the data could be held in

---

* From October 1st 2004, UMIST and the Victoria University of Manchester have merged to become The University of Manchester.

departmental and small systems, and new component record paradigms could be added without any overall change.

8. The Components of IBHIS

Because of the health domain demands the IBHIS broker has many components, listed below and shown in Figure 1:

- User authorisation (to access IBHIS)
- System authorisation (to gain access to a remote system, with its controls)
- Customised user screens (to meet different user needs).
- System and data inventories (to know who holds what, in what form).
- Ontology encyclopaedias (to record and translate data formats).
- Audit trails (to know who has used the system, with what results).

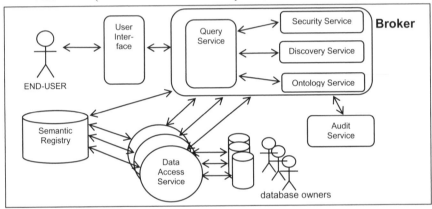

Figure 1: Conceptual Design of the IBHIS Enquiry Process [7]

9. The Vision of IBHIS in Action

Once the user has logged on, identified the patient by one of a number of identifiers, and stated the type of information required, the ability of the IBHIS system is to:

1. verify that the user's enquiry matched their permissions (permissions depend on identity, assigned roles, team membership, and the contexts of the access);
2. visit all the participating data repositories and identify all possible relevant matches for that identity;
3. visit (with permission) those systems to extract the data items requested;
4. using the ontology encyclopaedia, bring together the data items;
5. finally, check that the data aggregation would not create unauthorised disclosure of information by inference; and then
6. display the result, whilst the audit function would record not only the enquiry made, but the result as displayed

10. Purposeful Technical Components

The core components of the IBHIS broker are summarised in Figure 2:

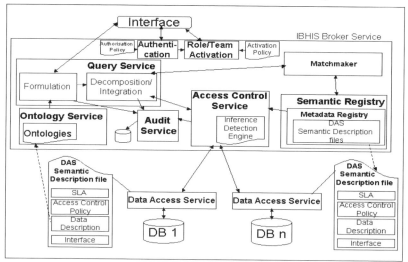

Figure 2: Conceptual Architecture of the IBHIS Broker [7]

The operational system comprises the following key components:

1. **Graphical User Interface (GUI)** – through a login screen authenticates the user, allows the user to navigate the domain ontology and guides him/her through query formulation, passes the query to the Query Service, and displays the results.

2. **Access Control Service (ACS)** - responsible for user authentication and authorisation, (special research having been done on service-based access control).

3. **Ontology Service (OS)** - consulted during the query decomposition and integration process.

4. **Query Service (QS)** - comprising two sub-modules:
   - *Query Decomposer* decomposes the Query into a set of local queries, in consultation with the matchmaker and the semantic registry which holds the semantic descriptions of the Export Schemas.
   - • *Query Integrator* - receives and integrates the individual results from the DASs.

5. **Audit Service (AS)** - comprised of two sub-modules, which keep track of every action of IBHIS that needs to be recreated or audited in the future.
   - • *User Audit* (per session): holds information such as: user log-in date, time, IP, logout, sequence of Queries, sequence of Results, etc.
   - • *System Audit* (per Registration): holds information about Data Source (e.g. registration date and time, intervals of availability, etc) and User Setup (e.g. time stamped creation, deletion, profile update, user registration/deletion etc)

6. **Data Access Service (DAS)** - the operational core, constructed using Web services. For each enquiry the QS decomposes the enquiry into a set of sub-queries, uses the Registry Service (see below) to look for DASs that provide the required data outputs; then uses the DAS description to bind with the data services.

The system is set by loading the **Registry Service** with details of available data sources, and the **Matchmaker Service** with the roles, users and access rules. The **Ontology Service** holds relevant ontologies harmonising results.

11. Current Status – Emerging Results

The IBHIS project team has now completed three years' work, at the end of which a laptop-based demonstrator is available for use anywhere with a telephone line, running live on distributed autonomous dummy data systems. Interest is being shown in a number of health and care domains, including child protection, an acute hospital (several ideas for collating local distributed information), and a primary care team.

12. Conclusion

The health information broker appears to offer a viable future alternative to the meta-enterprise very large EPR system. It would have the advantages of enabling users to feel in charge of their information support and the data systems. It could support European citizen mobility. Moreover, as new functions such as genetic records, pervasive technology and personalised drugs come into use, recording of these can be in dedicated systems yet fully accessible to end-users as and when necessary.

13. Acknowledgements

Solihull Primary Care NHS Trust, and particularly its field staff, provided initial input into the creation of the picture of user needs. The project was funded by the United Kingdom EPSRC Distributed Information Management (DIM) programme.

14. References

[1] Institute of Medicine (Dick R, Steen E eds.) The Computer Based Patient Record - An Essential Technology for Healthcare; National Academy Press, Washington DC, 1991.

[2] Hasselbring W, Peterson R, Smits M, Spanjers R. Strategic Information Management for a Dutch University Hospital, in Hasman A et al (eds.): Medical Infobahn for Europe: Proceedings of MIE2000 and GMDS2000, IOS Press, Amsterdam, 2000, 969-973.

[3] Wilson P, Leitner C, Mousalli A. Mapping the Potential of eHealth – Empowering the citizen through eHealth tools and services; European Institute of Public Administration, Maastricht, 2004.

[4] Goorman E, Berg M. Modelling Nursing Activities: electronic patient records and their discontents; Nursing Inquiry, 2000, 7(1), 3-9.

[5] www.travelocity.com

[6] Rigby M et al. The IBHIS Project: Reframing of EPR Systems Logic to Focus on the End User – A Vision and a Potential Broker Solution. In M Fieschi, E Coiera, Y-C J Li (eds.). Medinfo 2004 – Proceedings, IOS Press, Amsterdam, ISBN 1 58603 444 8 (CD ROM), 2004, 1831.

[7] Rigby et al. A Dynamic Data-Gatherer as an Emergent Alternative to Supra-Enterprise EPR Systems - paper accepted for HC 05, 2005 (in press).

[8] Kotsiopoulos I, et al. IBHIS: Integration Broker for Heterogeneous Information Sources, Proceedings of COMPSAC'03, IEEE Computer Society Press, 2003.

[9] Turner M, et al. Using Web Service Technologies to create an Information Broker: An Experience Report; Proceedings of 26th International Conference on Software Engineering, IEEE Computer Society Press, 552—561, 2004.

Address for Correspondence

Michael Rigby, Professor of Health Information Strategy, Centre for Health Planning and Management Darwin Building, Keele University, Keele, Staffordshire, ST5 5BG, United Kingdom, m.j.rigby@hpm.keele.ac.uk, tel. + 44 1782 583193; fax + 44 1782 711737

Connecting Medical Informatics and Bio-Informatics
R. Engelbrecht et al. (Eds.)
IOS Press, 2005

Towards Patient-Related Information Needs

Loes Braun[a], Floris Wiesman[b], Jaap van den Herik[a], Arie Hasman[b], Erik Korsten[c]

[a]Institute for Knowledge and Agent Technology, University Maastricht, The Netherlands
[b]AMC, University of Amsterdam, The Netherlands
[c]Catharina-ziekenhuis, Eindhoven, The Netherlands

Abstract

The quality of health care depends, among others, on the quality of a physician's domain knowledge. Since it is impossible to keep up with all new findings and developments, physicians usually have gaps in their domain knowledge. To handle exceptional cases, access to the full range of medical literature is required. The specific literature needed for appropriate treatment of the patient is described by a physician's information need. Physicians are often unaware of their information needs. To support them, this paper[1] aims at presenting a first step towards automatically formulating patient-related information needs. We start investigating how we can model a physician's information needs in general. Then we propose an approach to instantiate the model into a representation of a physician's information needs using the patient data as stored in a medical record. Our experiments show that this approach is feasible. Since the number of formulated patient-related information needs is rather high, we propose the use of filters. Future research will focus on the combination of personalization and filtering. It is expected that the resultant set of information needs will have a manageable size and contributes to the quality of health care.

Keywords:
Medical Records Systems, Computerized; Information Storage and Retrieval; Quality of Health Care

1. Introduction

We start with an example that precisely illustrates the need for knowledge of patient-related literature.

An 84-year-old woman was brought into the emergency department of a hospital, suffering from dyspnea and loss of consciousness. Five days earlier she had visited her general practitioner who diagnosed her with suspected respiratory tract infection and prescribed a drug called Clarithromycin. However, instead of improving, her condition worsened. In the hospital the diagnosis pneumonia was considered and she was treated accordingly, but without any effect. Upon her family's request, the patient was not admitted to the intensive care unit and she died one day after she was admitted to the hospital. Surprisingly, an autopsy revealed that the cause of death was not pneumonia, but a case of severe acute pancreatitis. The autopsy also revealed that the most plausible cause for the pancreatitis was the use of Clarithromycin, since pancreatitis is a (rare) side effect of the use of Clarithromycin [1].

Since the incidence of Clarithromycin-induced pancreatitis is quite low, it is

---

[1] This research is part of the MIA project (Medical Information Agent), which is funded by NWO (grant number 634.000.021).

understandable (but still undesirable) that the physician in the example above was not aware of this possible side effect. If the physician had performed a literature search in Medline on the side effects of Clarithromycin, he[2] probably would have found an article by Leibovitch, Levy, and Shoenfeld [2], in which another case of Clarithromycin-induced pancreatitis is discussed. If he had read this article, he probably would have ordered additional diagnostic tests to exclude pancreatitis (e.g., blood amylase) and he could have started the appropriate treatment immediately.

We define an *information need* as a formulation of missing information needed to perform a particular task. In our example the physician's information need was *What are the side effects of Clarithomycin?* However, the physician was not aware of his information need. Therefore, we call the information need *implicit*, as opposed to an *explicit* information need of which one *is* aware. Since the physician's information need was implicit, he had no incentive to search for information on the topic. Hence, our conclusion from the example is that information needs should be made explicit automatically in order to perform an appropriate literature search.

The example above clearly illustrates that (automatic) retrieval of relevant, patient-related literature is vital to the quality of care (cf. [3]). Various articles discuss information-retrieval (IR) systems that provide such literature (e.g., [4, 5, 6, 7]); our research roughly follows the contents of these articles. However, in our opinion the overall shortcoming of the systems mentioned in the articles is that the degree of necessary interaction with the systems is too high. This is especially true in the area of making information needs explicit. Therefore, our main research objectives are (1) to investigate to what extent a physician's implicit information needs can be made explicit automatically, and (2) to implement our approach together with some filters into a computer system supporting physicians in their daily work.

Section 2 describes how we determine a physician's information needs and how we model these needs. Section 3 presents our approach to formulate patient-related information needs (i.e., based on the patient and the physician's current activities with respect to the patient). In section 4 experiments and results are shown and briefly discussed. Section 5 provides our conclusions and directions for future research.

2. Modelling a Physician's Information Needs

Our approach to make a physician's information needs explicit is to anticipate them. As a starting point for this process, we need a set of a physician's potential information needs. However, such a set can never be complete, since it is impossible to capture all of a physician's information needs. Moreover, a physician generates new information needs over time, which should be added to the set. This is hard to facilitate.

One solution is to build a *model* of a physician's information needs. As long as the model represents information needs on a more abstract level it can be considered complete, meanwhile anticipating future information needs. Modelling a physician's information needs involves two steps described below: (1) identifying a physician's information needs (subsection 2.1) and (2) abstracting the identified information needs (subsection 2.2).

2.1 Identifying a Physician's Information Needs

To identify a physician's information needs, we used two methods, viz. (1) a literature survey and (2) interviews. Both identification methods are briefly described below. Table 1 summarizes the sources, the identification domains, and the number of information needs identified.

---

[2] For brevity we will use the pronoun 'he' ('his') where 'he or she' ('his or her') is meant.

Table 1 - Number of information needs identified by a literature survey and interviews.

Identification method	Source	Identification domain	# INs identified
Literature survey	[8]	Outpatient care, inpatient care, internal medicine	16
	[9]	General practice, cardiology, pulmonology, allergology	77
	[10]	Family care	10
	[11]	Primary care	16
	[12]	Various	32
	[13]	Various	10
	[14]	Surgical care	2
	[15]	Primary care	8
Interviews		Anaesthesiology	2
		Cardiology	1
		Neurology	0
		Pulmonology	3
		Surgery	3

In our literature survey, we searched for articles presenting information needs that are general, i.e., not specific for a particular group of physicians or for a particular geographical area. We found only eight such articles [8-15]. This set of articles covered a large number of medical domains from which the information needs were identified. In total we arrived at 171 information needs.

To obtain a set of information needs that is as diverse as possible, we succeeded in interviewing five physicians in five different medical specialisms: (1) anaesthesiology, (2) cardiology, (3) neurology, (4) pulmonology, and (5) surgery. The physicians were interrogated by means of an interview scheme composed in advance. This led to 9 additional information needs.[3]

2.2 Abstracting the Identified Information Needs

The identified information needs are highly context-dependent, which may render them useless in another (different) context. To reduce context-dependency, we abstracted the information needs, so as to make them context-independent. For the abstraction we used an approach similar to the one used by Ely, Osheroff, and Ebell [10]. We replaced each medical concept in the information needs by its semantic type, which is a high-level description of the medical concept (e.g., the concept 'Pneumonia' has the semantic type DISEASE OR SYNDROME). We obtained the semantic types of the concepts from the Semantic Network of the Unified Medical Language System (UMLS) that comprises 135 types [16].

The abstraction resulted in a general class of information needs, called *information-need templates*. Some information needs resulted in the same information-need template. For example, *Does Morphine cause rash?* and *Does Clarithromycin cause high blood pressure?* both resulted in the information-need template *Does [CHEMICAL] cause [SIGN OR SYMPTOM]?* To obtain a proper *set* of information-need templates, we removed all doubles. Currently, the set comprises 167 information-need templates.

3. Instantiating Templates into Patient-Related Information Needs

To represent a patient-related information need, an information-need template has to be instantiated with a patient's medical data. The data are acquired from the EPR (Electronic

---

3 Since we have to search English literature and several information needs were in Dutch, we translated the Dutch information needs into English.

Patient Record) of the specific patient. In our research we employed the *Intensive Care Information System*,[4] used at the Intensive Care Unit of the Catharina-ziekenhuis in Eindhoven.

Our approach of converting an information-need template into the representation of a patient-related information need comprises three steps, viz. (1) select EPR-queries that indicate the appropriate patient data[5] in the EPR, (2) execute the selected EPR-queries: the desired data are extracted from the EPR, and (3) instantiate the information-need template with the results of the executed queries.

In the first step, we start determining which semantic types occur in the information-need template. To convert the information-need template into an information need, each of these semantic types has to be instantiated with patient data. Consequently, an EPR-query has to be selected for each semantic type in the information-need template. The EPR-queries are selected from a list of EPR-queries, formulated in advance. Each EPR-query in this list specifies how to find the patient data associated with the corresponding semantic type. Assume we have the template *What are the side effects of [CHEMICAL]?* Based on (1) the semantic type CHEMICAL, (2) the information structure of our EPR, and (3) the patient number of the specific patient, the following EPR-query is selected (the names of the database tables are in Dutch) *SELECT Medicijn FROM Medicatie WHERE PatientNummer=1234567890*. To facilitate easy adaptation to other EPR-systems, all potential EPR-queries for a specific EPR-system are specified in a model, which is runtime consulted by the system and can be easily reformulated.

The second step is to execute the selected queries to extract the desired patient data from the EPR. The actual query-execution process is handled by the database itself. Each result that an EPR-query returns for a semantic type is called an *active concept* of that specific semantic type. Assume that our patient is taking three different medications. Then, our EPR-query has three results and consequently, the semantic type CHEMICAL has three active concepts, e.g., (1) *Clarithromycine,* (2) *Amoxi/Clavulaan,* and (3) *Furosemide-iv.* Since all terms from the EPR (and consequently also all active concepts) are in Dutch, we mapped them manually to UMLS concepts, which are then translated into English by means of the UMLS Metathesaurus.

The third step is to instantiate the information-need template with the data obtained from the EPR (active concepts of the semantic types). We call an information-need template *applicable* (i.e., it can be instantiated with patient data) if each semantic type within the information-need template has one or more active concepts. If the template is applicable, it is instantiated by systematically replacing each semantic type by one of its active concepts, until all possible combinations are used. The total number of resulting information needs is the product of the numbers of active concepts of all semantic types in the template. For the three active concepts of the semantic type CHEMICAL, our information-need template is instantiated three times, viz. (1) *What are the side effects of Clarithromycin?,* (2) *What are the side effects of Amoxicillin-Clavulanic Acid?,* and (3) *What are the side effects of Furosemide?* If a literature search were conducted, based on the above information needs, patient-related literature would be found. The approach described above was implemented in a computer system.

---

[4] Intensive Care Informatie Systeem, Version 2.8. INAD Computers & Software B.V. Eindhoven, Werkgroep ICIS Afd. Intensive Care, Dienst Informatie Voorziening, Catharina-ziekenhuis Eindhoven.

[5] All patient data used in the examples of section 3 are fictitious.

4. Experiments and Results

To establish the feasibility of our approach for instantiating information-need templates, we let our system formulate patient-related information needs based on the EPRs of 82 patients. Each EPR contained information about *all* hospital adm sions (in the hospital under consideration) of a patient. After each separate data entry, new information needs were formulated based on the added data (possibly in combination with already available data). We used our complete set of 167 information-need templates. For each patient, we calculated the average number of information needs formulated per data entry. Each patient was placed into one of four categories, based on the average number of information needs formulated, viz. (i) no information needs, (ii) a manageable number of information needs (1-100), (iii) a hardly manageable number of information needs (101-1000), and (iv) and

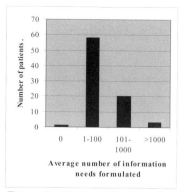

Figure 1 - Number of patients for which a specific number of information needs is formulated.

unmanageable number of information needs (>1000).

Figure 1 shows how many patients were placed in each category. As can be seen in figure 1, in 71% of the cases a manageable number of information needs is formulated. However, for 28% of the cases the number of information needs formulated is hardly manageable or even unmanageable. If a literature search were conducted for all these information needs, the set of retrieved literature would be unmanageably high for these cases. Since we do not want to overload physicians with literature, the number of information needs should be reduced by filtering. In the ideal situation, all patients would be in category 1-100 information needs.

To reduce the number of formulated information needs two filters can be used. The first one is the *stage of the medical process*. Not all information needs might apply to the current stage of the medical process. For example, when a physician has already selected chemotherapy as the appropriate treatment for a lung-cancer patient, he is assumed not to have information needs concerning the selection of a treatment, such as *What is the treatment for lung cancer for this patient?* Yet, he might have information needs concerning the execution of the selected treatment, such as *How high is the dose of chemotherapy for lung cancer for this patient?* The second filter is the *specialism of the physician*. Since a physician's information needs are probably connected to his specialism, we might ignore several information needs, because they are not linked to the physician's specialism. Ignoring the information needs is solely based on the patient data with which the corresponding information-need templates were instantiated. As information-need templates contain no patient data, templates cannot be ignored in advance. A series of future experiments may clarify to what extent the two filters are appropriate for a reduction of the number of information needs.

5. Conclusions

The cooperation with physicians, described in section 2, showed that we succeeded in identifying a physician's potential information needs and in modelling them into 167 information-need templates by using 135 semantic types.

In section 3 we designed an approach to convert information-need templates into patient-related information needs by taking patient data into account. From the experiments, we may conclude that our approach is adequate and can be generalized to other EPR-systems, as long as they use a suitable information structure. The number of automatically formulated, patient-related information needs per patient is still high (section 4), but may be reduced by taking the *stage of the medical process* and the *specialism of the physician* into account.

When using the automatically formulated information needs as a starting point for literature retrieval, patient-related literature can be provided to the physician automatically, thereby potentially contributing to an improvement in the quality of health care.

6. References

[1]   Schouwenberg BJJW and Deinum J. Acute pancreatitis after a course of Clarithromycin. *The Netherlands Journal of Medicine* 2003: 61(7) pp. 266–267.
[2]   Leibovitch L, Levy Y, and Shoenfeld, Y. Pancreatitis induced by Clarithromycin. *Ann Intern Med* 1996: 125(8) pp. 701.
[3]   Gamble S. Hospital libraries enhance patient care and save money. *Journal of the Alberta Association of Library Technicians* 1996: 23(2) pp. 10–12.
[4]   Miller RA, Jamnback L, Giuse NB, and Masarie FE. Extending the capabilities of diagnostic decision support programs through links to bibliographic searching: Addition of 'canned MeSH logic' to the Quick Medical Reference (QMR) program for use with Grateful Med. In Clayton P, ed. *Proc Annu Symp Comp App Med Care*. McGraw-Hill Inc., 1991; pp. 150–155.
[5]   Rada R, Barlow J, Bijstra D, Potharst J, de Vries Robbé P, and Zanstra P. OAR: Open architecture for reasoning applied to connection patient records to medical literature. In Noothoven van Goor J and Christensen JP, eds. *Advances in Medical Informatics*. Amsterdam: IOS Press, 1992; pp. 287–294.
[6]   Van Mulligen EM. UMLS-based access to CPR data. *Int J Med Inf* 1999: 53(2–3) pp. 125–131.
[7]   Cimino JJ, Johnson SB, Aguirre A, Roderer N, and Clayton PD. The Medline Button. *Proc Annu Symp Comput Appl Med Care* 1992; pp. 81-85.
[8]   Cucina RJ, Shah MK, Berrios DC, and Fagan LM. Empirical formulation of a generic query set for clinical information retrieval systems. In Patel V, Rogers R, and Haux R, eds. *Proc MedInfo2001*. Amsterdam: IOS Press, 2001; pp. 181–185.
[9]   De Vries Robbé PF, Beckers WPA, and Zanstra PE. *MEDES. Het prototype*. Groningen: Onderzoeksgroep Medische Informatie- en Besliskunde, Academisch Ziekenhuis Groningen, 1988. (In Dutch).
[10] Ely JW, Osheroff JA, and Ebell MH. Analysis of questions asked by family doctors regarding patient care. *BMJ* 1999: 319(7206) pp. 358–361.
[11] Gorman PN. Information needs of physicians. *J Am Soc Inf Sci* 1995: 46(10) pp. 729–736.
[12] Grundmeijer HGLM, Reenders K, and Rutten GEHM, eds. *Het Geneeskundig Proces. Van Klacht naar Therapie*. Maarssen: Elsevier Gezondheidszorg, 1999. (In Dutch).
[13] Jerome RN, Giuse NB, Gish KW, Sathe NA, and Dietrich MS. Information needs of clinical teams: analysis of questions received by the clinical informatics consult service. *Bull Med Lib Assoc* 2001: 89(2) pp. 177–185.
[14] Reddy MC, Pratt W, Dourish P, and Shabot MM. Asking questions: Information needs in a surgical intensive care unit. In Kohane IS, ed. *Proc AMIA '02*. Philadelphia: Hanley and Belfus Inc., 2002: pp. 647–651, 2002.
[15] Smith R. What clinical information do doctors need? *BMJ* 1996: 313(7064) pp. 1062–1068.
[16] U.S. National Library of Medicine. Unified Medical Language System, 2003. http://www.nlm.nih.gov/research/umls/.

Address for correspondence

Drs. L.M.M. Braun, Institute for Knowledge and Agent Technology, University Maastricht, P.O. Box 616, 6200 MD Maastricht, The Netherlands, L.Braun@cs.unimaas.nl.

Connecting Medical Informatics and Bio-Informatics
R. Engelbrecht et al. (Eds.)
IOS Press, 2005

Establishing a Regional Contact & Service Centre for Public Health Care: The Case in Central Macedonia, Greece

Dimitrios Vartzopoulos[a], Stergiani Spyrou[a], Eirini Minaoglou[a], Viktoria Karolidou[a],
Panagiotis D Bamidis[b]

[a] 2nd Regional Healthcare System Authority of Central Macedonia, Greece
[b] Lab of Medical Informatics, Medical School, Aristotle University of Thessaloniki, Thessaloniki, Greece

Abstract

Regional Healthcare System Authorities (RHSAs) run under the Ministry of Health and Welfare in Greece, aim is to improve the level of quality that health care organizations offer as well as to control the expenditure of health care services provided by the health care organizations. In this article we present the considerations taken during the establishment of the first Regional Contact & Service Center for Public Health in Greece in two of the RHSAs. In this respect, the current piece of work provides an up-to-date experience in establishing and setting the RCSC in its organizational context, an outline of its conceptual model and design, an outlook of the first quarterly results of its use, and a discussion of its potential impact.

Keywords:
Regional Contact Centre; Regional Service Centre; Health Information System, Regional Health Authority

1. Introduction

During the past couple of decades, public trust in western governments has continued to diminish due to various administrative, political, socio-cultural, and economic causes. The health care sector is unambiguously indicated as one of the primary dissatisfaction points in the public opinion. One of the contributing factors to the decline of public trust is associated with the gap between public expectation and perceived governmental performance. Information and Communication Technology (ICT) can be used to improve services and enhance some of the primary administrative values like efficiency, effectiveness, and responsiveness, so as to improve public trust in health care government by direct or indirect manners [1].

Moreover, information exchange and communication are intricate concepts in health care that have been given much attention over the last decade. In medical informatics, communication is seen as the exchange of messages, with an explicit or implicit intention, between actors, in a specific situation or a given certain task [2]. Furthermore, the capacity of countries, and organisations to develop and manage knowledge assets is a major determinant of effectiveness, competitiveness and economic growth. In this context, it has become common knowledge that the use of ICT may serve as an important influence and catalyst in facilitating the approach of the Greek Health Care System (GHCS) to EU health policies and the bridging of gaps in the development of an information based society with social cohesion [3]. To draw threads towards these direction lines, the 1st and 2nd Regional Healthcare System Authorities (RHSAs) of Central Macedonia, Greece, have established their Regional Contact & Service Centre (RCSC) for Public Health Care. The goal is to eliminate the need for citizens to visit the Centre by exploiting the ICT infrastructure of the Centre and obtaining persistent information from anywhere (e.g. home based) about procedures they should follow in the Health System.

The aim of this paper is, therefore, to share the up-to-date experience in establishing and setting the RCSC in its organizational context, to outline its conceptual model and design, to provide the first quarterly results of its use, and discuss the potential impact it may have for the RHSAs and the GHCS as a whole.

2. Background

Literature search shows that similar attempts in the health care arena can be found in most of the developed countries, where a number of Private Companies offer resembling services to the Health Organisations. The provided services are often offered through insurance companies, telephone centres or via Internet. In this way, citizens can obtain information, advice and guidance in relation to health procedures. They arrange and handle appointments in various health units or gain awareness about specific health professionals or special clinical treatment provided in hospitals [4].

One of the most common technologies used in Public Health Care Contact & Service Centres is the Voice Portal that permits citizens to obtain information and services via a telephone number that acts as an access portal [5]. In addition, there exist Health Care Systems that encompass regional integrated hospital-territory networks that allow the placement of family doctors and specialists on-line. Offered e-services include: 1) Referrals to specialists, 2) Prescriptions for medicines, 3) Consultation of lab and radiology reports, 4) Continued assistance for recovering patients and for patients with supplementary home-care assistance, 5) Regional indexing of clinical events [6].

3. The Greek Context

The 1st and 2nd RHSAs of Central Macedonia are two of the seventeen public RHSAs founded in Greece back in 2001. Each of them aims to improve the level of health care quality offered by their corresponding comprising organizations, as well as, to control the expenditure of health care services provided by the health care organizations. The two RHSAs cover a population of about 1,872,000 in Central Macedonia in total and manage twenty one (21) hospitals, thirty two (32) primary health units, a substantial number of rural health units and several welfare units, as well.

The concept of the Regional Contact & Service Centre is not new in Greece. The Greek government, after the success of the Citizen Service Centres (KEP in Greek) of the Ministry of Internal Affairs, decided to push the idea forward under the auspices of other Ministries and establish new Citizen Contact and Service Centres. Such examples are the Services Centre in the District Office in Athens, the Town-Planning office in Athens and others. All these are designed to operate in an internally oriented manner and have no reconciliation with other Offices [8].

However, the idea for the establishment of RCSC is new for the Greek Regional Public Health Care. In this case, the RCSC can be defined as "*an intra-organizational regional centre hosted at the Regional Health Care Authorities, that is supported by organizational arrangements in order to manage and integrate the flow of information for health services for all health care customers, with the ultimate aim of improving customer services and organizational efficiency in health-related issues. They are meant to integrate personal visits to the Centre and electronic communication by means of telephone or Internet".* The first pilot RCSC was established in the city of Thessaloniki by the two RHSAs of Central Macedonia, under the directions of the Greek Ministry of Health and Welfare.

The RCSC provides services posterior to those of the Citizen Service Centres (KEP), and complementary to those offered by smaller citizen service Offices founded in each hospital since 2001. The main aim of the latter is threefold: a) to inform citizens about their rights and obligations inside the Hospital; b) to inform them about relative legislation concerning the patient service during admission sessions; and c) to manage various complaints as reported by patients. These Offices, though, provide services regarding each hospital only and demand the physical visit of the health care customer to the Hospital. RCSC, on the contrary, may be thought of as a centralized, at regional level office, that can serve citizens/patients before their actual visits to health units. RCSCs, as official units, will be organised in all Health Regions of the Country, with the intention of limiting beaurocracy and avoiding unnecessary citizen and document shifting from one unit office to another. The services, offered by the RCSC, are given via collaboration of all Public Services and are briefly: 1) Formal - Administrative operations like ratification of copies etc, 2) Electronic Services providing information, concerning appointments or clinical services, via a web portal, and 3) additional Services associated with the retrieval of information via the telephone centre, the ability to mediate with other Public Services, the recording of citizens' complaints and their subsequent transmission to the suitable services or Ministries [7].

4. Materials and Methods

As it is the case in the development of every information system, during RCSC's project life cycle emphasis had to be placed in each of the three constituent pillars, namely, technology, humans, and organisational structures. The focal point of this new service is the citizen; technology is engaged to assist citizen-health care system interactions; the project is constrained by the RHSAs organisational structures and should be seen in the light of their actual engagement and support they can provide. With this in mind, the centre was divided in five sections according to the services provided, which are:

1. Information section (internet based; concerning services provided by regional hospitals and welfare institutes)
2. Section of Structural elements' system (procedures that the citizen has to follow in order to be served faster in health and welfare matters)
3. Complaints section (admission of citizen's opinion/complaints about the effectiveness of the provided health and welfare services)
4. Section for Suggestions for improvements
5. Volunteer network

To organize these sections, the two RHSAs had to constitute four work groups. Their work was first to create a process map by collecting information about the procedures followed in the various health units and welfare services (through the use of a structured questionnaire), and then to design applications that would support the electronic provision of information for all health services.. After a six-month period of analysis, the pilot operation of the Health Service Centre began a few months ago, while work groups still elaborate on research work regarding the effective design of the centre's information workflow.

The following list of actions was taken to assure achievement of the goals set: Implementation of an electronic protocol aiming to improve document management and request handling.

1. Implementation of a "Human Resources" Information System capable of informing citizens about vacancies in health units and welfare services, but also to handling requests for intra-regional exchanges of personnel.

2. Implementation of a software suite enabling the display of "Day of duty or emergencies/ Appointments at Outpatients' department", which will help patients in finding faster the hospitals on call, but also allow them to schedule appointments at the Outpatients' department.

3. Installation of an info Kiosk for the citizens from which they could gain information for almost all the previously mentioned points

4. Creation of a web portal that will represent the main locus of searching and retrieving citizen information.

A simplistic conceptual model of services request may be seen in Figure 1, while in figure 2, the ICT infrastructure for the RCSC is presented. Health units have access to the central administration system of RHSA via leased lines. The information system of the RCSC has all the infrastructure prerequisites for a secure access of citizen information by the health and welfare services (i.e. Application, Database, Mail, Web Server, and Firewall). Citizens can receive the health services by using the portal or the Info Kiosk without having to visit the Regional Contact & Service Centre for Public Health Care. Nevertheless, for those who are not keen on new technologies or are technology illiterate, there is still the option of visiting in person and being served by the agents.

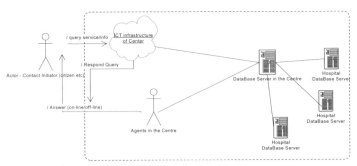

Figure 1: The conceptual model of the RCSC

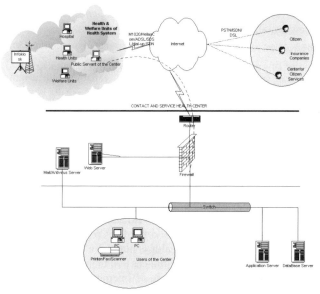

Figure 2: ICT infrastructure for the Centre

5. Results

After the first seven-month period of pilot operation of the RCSC, citizen requests may be split into four main categories as illustrated in Figure 3. The results are examined to improve the services provided by the Centre and to determine the basic set of requirements for the implementation of the Centres in other health regions of the country. Extended periods are of course required to make conclusions.

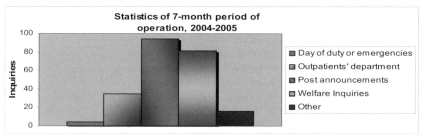

Figure 3: Three month pilot run of RCSC: relative distribution of main categories of requests

6. Discussion - Conclusions

It is vital to think about the impact of systems and technologies on the people that use them, as some of the worst mistakes made happen if this is neglected. In addition, if one wants to influence the way society is shaped, then factors affecting it need to be identified and studied. The RCSC has involved changes in the Public Administration but also in the society. Improvement in existing health infrastructures will be considered as procedures of the health services may be redesigned under the scope of decentralization of the services, resulting in the improvement of the State - Citizen relationship. In this new effort of the

RCSC establishment, there were reactions and reflections, due to the:

- lack of knowledge of new practices of change,
- lack of collaboration between institutions,
- limited education capacity of employees, affecting the way they respond to citizen needs,
- incorrect and invalid briefing of the RCSC by the Services of non-health related sectors.

However, the operation of the RCSCs for Citizens constitutes an innovative effort for the Greek Public Health Care Administration. The locomotive force for the successful completion of this attempt lies with the import of new information technologies that creates the conditions for the envisaged decentralization. Clearly, management and organizational factors, as well as effective technological mechanisms, affect the ability to maintain service quality. Much is dependent on the ICT infrastructure of a country of course, but the case for Greece looks promising [11]. Moreover, RCSC should be extensively evaluated given special evaluation frameworks [9]. However, there is also a need for regional studies and projects on information seekers behaviours, internet health content evaluation strategies, and analysis of the social supply of health information to citizens and their ability to use the information they receive [10]. To conclude, access and use of internet may be seen as a facilitator of social inclusion, democracy and liberalisation as a number of services become, through internet, more open to the wide public. ICT may be the catalyst for improving social relations as it enables easy social interaction among people without excluding those with special needs or living in deprived neighbourhoods. However, ICT policy makers should make sure that the digital divide is properly resolved in order to fully exploit the benefits [3].

7. References

[1] M. Jae Moon, "Can IT Help Government to Restore Public Trust? Declining Public Trust and Potential Prospects of IT in the Public Sector". In: Proceedings of the 36th Hawaii International Conference on System Sciences, IEEE, 2002.

[2] P.J. Toussaint, J. Verhoef, T.P.M. Vlieland, J.H.M. Zwetsloot-Schonk, "Improving the quality of communication in health care". In: R. Baud et al (eds), Proceedings of MIE 2003, pp. 857-862, IOS Press, 2003.

[3] P. Ketikidis, P. Bamidis, "The role of Research in Information Technology and Regional Policy Development: considerations and challenges in SEE". SEERC Bulletin, Vol 1(2): 10-12, June 2004, (www.seerc.info).

[4] NHS Direct, http://www.nhsdirect.nhs.uk/, visited on 05-01-2005

[5] Reina Suomi, Jarmo Tahkapaa, "Establishing a Contact Centre for Public Health Care", Proceedings of the 36th Hawaii International Conference on System Sciences, IEEE 2002.

[6] http://www.medicare.gov, http://www.uihealthcare.com, http://medineuvo.com, accessed 03-01-2005

[7] http://www.kep.gov.gr, accessed 03-01-2005

[8] L. Orfanidis, P.D. Bamidis and B. Eaglestone, 2004, "Data Quality Issues in Electronic Health Records: An adaptation framework for the Greek Health System", Health Informatics Journal, 10(1): 23–36.

[9] P. Turunen, "A framework for evaluation of medical information systems". In: R. Baud et al (eds), Proceedings of MIE 2003, pp. 611-616, IOS Press, 2003.

[10] M Ginman, "Social capital as a communicative paradigm", 2003, Health Informatics Journal, 9(1): 57-64.

Address for correspondence

Stergiani Spyrou, IT Manager of 2nd Regional Health Care Authority of Central Macedonia, Greece,. Tel: +302310368822, Fax:+302310368808, e-mail: spirou@med.auth.gr

Connecting Medical Informatics and Bio-Informatics
R. Engelbrecht et al. (Eds.)
IOS Press, 2005

923

Integration of the Cognitive Knowledge of Activity in a Service Oriented Architecture in the Home Care Context

N Bricon-Souf, E Dufresne, L Watbled

CERIM, Université de Lille, Faculté de Médecine

Abstract.

> The complex nature of a home care (HC) situation induces an important need for cooperation between the health care professionals. But even if this need is sometimes evocated in reports on HC issues, it is more difficult to get precise knowledge on this cooperative activity, and, consequently, propositions for computerized HC organization and management systems. We did some researches on this topic area. Previous phases of work let us highlight the actual need for cooperation, and obtain precise information on the HC activity processes and data. In this paper, we focused on the integration of this cognitive knowledge on the design of a HC cooperation architecture. Different levels of requirements for the cooperative system are mentioned: coordination, communication of information, delegation of activity, integration of services and personal access to the tasks to perform. A description of the usefulness and use of the cognitive knowledge is proposed, the architecture design, modular, distributed, and able to integrate external services is presented, and the results of a validation test of the implemented prototype, performed with actual HC professionals in an evaluation laboratory are presented.

Keywords:
Medical information technologies; Cooperation; Coordination ; Information; Communication; Homecare

1. Context

The need for the Home Care cooperation.

Most countries encounter an increase in the number of elderly people and the importance of HC services in the follow-up of chronic diseases or end-of-life situations [1,2], and at the same time, encounter major problems with health care costs and ratios of Health Care professionals. So, improving HC as an alternative to classical hospitalization appears as one of the main challenges for the 21st century. Good coordination of healthcare professionals is known as an essential element in quality health care. In HC settings, the improvement of the cooperation of workers becomes highly essential : first we observed that most of the requirements of the HC workers deals with the organization and management of the homecare system, second that HC induces a complex cooperation. A flexible and temporary therapeutic team works with rare common meetings, in asynchronous way, and includes new actors such as family, coordinator and equipment providers. In the context of homecare, researches are mainly focused on the ability to improve the follow-up of the patient or invent some distant care via less or more sophisticated tools such as video camera, captors, intelligent houses ; some control on the medication via intelligent pill boxes, and so on. [3,4,5,6]. Different reports relate the importance of homecare cooperation to improve the continuity of care between acute and home care and the improve the quality of home care[7,8]. But home care applications able to manage cooperation are still rare.

So we decided to perform a cognitive analysis of the homecare process and to use the results to model then implement and test a prototype : the Home Care Cooperation Platform. Previous papers detail our analyses[9,10], so they are presented very briefly. In the current paper we present the requirements for the architecture, we focus on how we used the description of information in such a system and how we modeled the activity management, so that distant applications could be launched and visualization of the processes could be used. Then we describe the first tests which were performed and discuss about the associated results.

Analysis of the Home Care processes.
We realized a cognitive analysis of the HC activities in order to define the main requirements for the development of a computerized tool for HC. We got different results : 1°) Description of the processes of HC : HC is built from two processes, i) the logistical process: decision for and organization of HC, supervised by coordinators, ii) the care process which manages the therapeutics activities. 2°) Description of each phases of both processes. 3°) Description of the information used and on the way it is used.

Some requirements for the home care architecture.
To improve the coordination of HC, one HC application (i) has to provide an easy access for all the HC participants given that it may be used by different workers, with different devices, at different places; (ii) has to help the participants to organize and launch the complex coordination activities (iii) must be capable of linkage to different and distributed applications, and may be called upon to interconnect different information systems (IS): hospital IS, GP's IS, laboratory IS, etc.; (iv) has to provide secure exchanges of data. We refined these requirements using our cognitive analyses to select some strong requirements for the HC system:

- *Coordination* - Proposing a coordination tool that could inform about the state of the HC processes: what are the performed tasks and what are the known information, could help the HC workers to control these processes. For the health care providers, it is highly important to maintain a common frame of reference about their patients. Care workers should also find some information or some help on what tasks are to perform and how to perform it. It is really important to propose such help in the social context of HC: due to a lack of experienced and very well organized HC organization, and due to the increase of HC needs, it could happen that unused people are devoted to the organization on the HC.

- *Delegation of activity* - Proposing some way to delegate the activity. It is well known that one individual could not know all the information about the patient or on what to do, and one important activity of the coordinators in HC situation is to ask some information to other people (GPs, hospital physicians, family) until they could gather enough data to organize the care in good conditions. Nowadays, most of such delegations or requests are made through phone calls, but phone calls are often disruptive and, as they are synchronous, the availability of both caller and requested people is needed. It is possible to use a computerized system to delegate some activities to other people. For example, it seems relatively easy to send a request to the GP so that she/he could give some complementary information on the medical history of the patient.

- *Communication of information.* Medical information comes from different Information Systems, different people, and it should be communicated in a secure manner and be easily integrated in the HC information systems.

- *Integration of services.* To perform the HC processes, a huge amount of different tasks should be performed. But it is not always necessary to know all the details about how to perform such tasks, the objective of the cooperation platform is not to deal with the specific abilities of each HC worker, but to aggregate the indispensable information required to manage efficiently the care. For example, the care coordinator doesn't mind how a medical bed provider inform about the availability of such a bed, but just want to know if it is possible to book such a bed. And it could exist as many ways of knowing about the availability of the bed, as the number of medical bed providers. The feasibility of the cooperation platform for HC is strongly linked to its ability to interoperate with external systems. The platform is in charge to explain which activity should be perform and which data are requested. Nowadays, a promising way to deal with these issues is to use Service-oriented Architecture (SOA) to *"address problems related to the integration of heterogeneous applications in a distributed environment"* [11]. Each activity could be performed by an external service, which may be complex, and should return the expected information. As most of the time, the activity deals with entering of new information in the system, the simplest services to propose are forms.

- *Personal access to the tasks to perform.* Each HC worker should be individually informed about the tasks he has to deal with.

Cognitive knowledge.
Three main types of knowledge descriptions have been extracted from the cognitive analyses: HC activities, HC information, and information linked to each activity (characteristics such as the address of the patient is very important for the decision of acceptance of the care during the request phase and it would be a priority to transfer it).

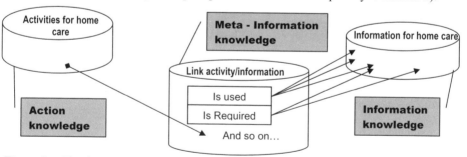

Figure 1. - The three types of knowledge on the homecare processes.

Such meta knowledge, issued from the activity analysis, is used to develop "user's activity oriented" system. In particular, the supervision interface could adapt the display of information, not only to the one who is connected, like in most of the current health care systems, but also to the current phase of the HC process. This point is important to help the user to focus on new or useful information, to build an efficient cognitive representation of the patient's state. Moreover, for each activity, one can find a description of the associated context needed to perform it, such as who could be asked to perform the tasks or what are the needed information. This point is important to build the exchanges between external services and the HC cooperation system.

1.1. .The system architecture

Such requirements have been implemented with a system architecture organized in different levels :

- *coordination level* which highlights the state of the processes, and the pertinent information,
- *routage level* to choose which activity to perform and to delegate information to right people,
- *activation level* to launch the services,
- *transport level* to safely communicate information,
- *access level* to reach to-do-lists.

Exchange For Activity (EFA) messages are defined and used to communicate between the different application, the different Information System and the HC System.

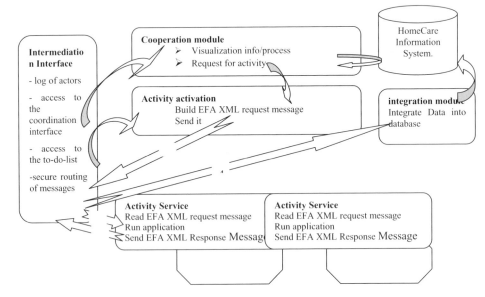

Figure 2. - The enactment loop in the Coquas architecture.

Different modules compose the system architecture:

- the *cooperation module*, it proposes a common and share representation of i) the HC process, ii) the evolution of the HC phases and iii) the related information. It describes recursively the different HC phases.
- The *activity activation module* is in charge of choosing who to request, it builds a request message devoted to launch an activity.
- The *intermediation interface* is done through a commercial system (Rithme^{TM}), and provides health care professionals' directory, patients' directory, security management, notification and data formatting. It connects the HC workers either to the coordination interface or to their personal to-do-lists.

- The *activity services*, it actually "runs" the HC tasks. Sometimes very complex, they are similar to services in SOA architectures, basic ones are automatically defined, using the description on the needed information associated to each description of activity, and propose some simple but dynamically generated forms.
- The *integration module* integrates the new data in the *homecare information system*.

2. Prototype.

A prototype has been implemented. It does not cover all the HC situations but tests the main functionalities. The coordination interface displays the HC processes and activities and the information, according to the actual activity. The whole cycle of communication is implemented : hospital extraction of data, integration in the homecare coordination system and the access through the coordination interface or through a to-do-list of the actions to perform. External applications can be launched from the coordination interface. Delegation of activities have been tested. Different technologies and languages are used to perform the complex system (JAVA, XML, ASP, MYSQL, Xforms, LDAP,…).

3. Validation Tests.

We have performed a validation of this prototype. This evaluation aimed to: 1°)Validate the interest of the functionalities implemented in the prototype: display of the whole process in one page, data entry via forms, the capability of asking someone else to complete missing information electronically, integration of the data sent by another individual in the right section, and display of information entered in one section in other sections if pertinent. 2°) Evaluate the feasibility of integrating this prototype in any center for HC.

This evaluation was performed in the Evaluation Laboratory of the faculty of Medicine in Lille, with three HC coordinators, two nurses and a physician, from different organizations. This laboratory allows us to accurately reproduce a work setting (an office in this case), to observe and guide the users (via video cameras, one-way mirrors, and microphones), and to record dialogs, facial expressions, gestures, etc. First the prototype was presented to the users, and they were told what was expected of them. The prototype was then tested through a scenario drawn from their usual activities. At the end of the test, the users were extensively debriefed on their experience and opinions of the prototype.

Video records have been analyzed. The users' comments were very positive: The system matches with the actual activity; they felt that it could avoid some waste of time, and could make coordination easier. Moreover, those positive comments came from people working in different structures which have completely different organizations (200 employees vs 4) and whose jobs are different (nurses vs. physician). The navigation through the interface seems to be intuitive. Required improvements concern some surface ergonomic aspects and could be easily modified in a future version.

4. Conclusion

HC is a complex cooperative situation. Multi-modal, distributed, multi-participant, asynchronous, the organization and the management of the care must nevertheless satisfy some criteria of quality, confidentiality, security, and so on. We did a cognitive analysis of HC users' activities to better understand how the actual homecare works and to be able to present some requirements to computerize the cooperation of the health professionals in such an activity. We got some interesting knowledge upon the HC, highlighted the need for cooperation, proposed some requirement for the system architecture, implemented a prototype and tested it with actual HC professionals. We hope that this research could help to define efficient HC applications in the future. During the test, the positive comments of the users encourage to continue with such architecture and to promote the integration of the cognitive knowledge in the future developments.

5. Acknowledgement

This work was realised with grants from the Région Nord-Pas-de-Calais within the Project TELECOS (CPER « TACT »), and from the Ministry of Research in the project COQUAS (RNTS 2000).

6. References

[1]   C. Arundel, S. Glouberman, L. Kun, Telehealth and the global health network in the 21st century. From home care to public health informatics in Computer Substudy 15 (2001) [Online: http://www.home carestudy.com/reports/full-text/substudy-15-final_report.pdf].

[2]   Mason, Lui, & Braun. The probability of using an aged care home over a lifetime (1999–00), Welfare Division Working Paper No. 36. AIHW Cat. no. AGE 21. AIHW, Canberra, 2001.

[3]   N. Maglaveras, V. Koutkias, I. Chouvard, D.G. Goulis, A. Avramides, D. Adamidis, G. Louridas, E.A. Balas, Home care delivery through the mobile telecommunications platform: the Citizen Health System (CHS) perspective, International Journal of Medical Informatics 68 (2002) 99 –111.

[4]   A. Mihailidis, B. Carmichael, J. Boger, G. Fernie, An Intelligent Environment to Support Aging-in-Place, Safety, and Independence of Older Adults with Dementia. In: proceedings of UbiHealth2003, The 2nd International Workshop on Ubiquitous Computing for Pervasive Healthcare Applications, Seattle, 2003, [Online: http://www.healthcare.pervasive.dk/ubicomp2003/papers/].

[5]   V. Rialle, N. Noury and T. Herve, An experimental health smart home and its distributed internet-based information and communication system: first steps of a research project, Medinfo 10 (2001) 1479–1483.

[6]   European Project Topcare: Implementation of a telematic Home care Platform in Cooperative Health Care Provider Networks [Online http://www.topcare.info/].

[7]   C. Woodward, J. Abelson, B. Hutchison, A My home is not my home anymore: Improving Continuity of Care in Home care, The Canadian Health Services Research Foundation web site [nline: www.chrsf.ca], Dec 2001.

[8]   Report of the workshop on home care Technologies for the 21st Century- Catholic University of America - granted by Food and Drug Administration, National Science Fundation. [Online http://www.eng.mu.edu /wintersj /HCTWorkshop /HCTW_report.htm].

[9]   N. Bricon-Souf, M-C Beuscart-Zéphir, L. Watbled, F. Anceaux, R. Beuscart, Information and Logistics for Homecare In proceesings of MIE 2002, Budapest , Hungary, 2002

[10] N. Bricon-Souf, E. Dufresne, MC. Beuscart-Zéphir, R. Beuscart, Communication of information in the homecare context, Stud. Health Technol. Inform. 8 (2003) 95-113.

[11] N Mukhi, R. Konuru, F. Curbera Cooperative Middleware Specialization for Service Oriented Architecture, in: Proceedings of WWW2004, 2004, pp. 206-215.

Address for correspondance :

Nathalie BRICON SOUF, nsouf@univ-lille2.fr, CERIM, Faculté de Médecine, 1 place de Verdun, F-59045 Lille Cedex - France

Connecting Medical Informatics and Bio-Informatics
R. Engelbrecht et al. (Eds.)
IOS Press, 2005

Cognitive Analysis of Physicians' Medication Ordering Activity

Sylvia Pelayo[a], Nicolas Leroy[a], Sandra Guerlinger[a], Patrice Degoulet[b], Jean-Jacques Meaux[c], Marie-Catherine Beuscart-Zéphir[a]

[a] *EVALAB, EA 2694, Faculty of Medicine, Lille, France*
[b] *Medical Informatics Department, Georges Pompidou University Hospital, Paris, France*
[c] *Medasys R&D, Gif sur Yvette, France*

Abstract

Computerized Physician Order Entry (CPOE) addresses critical functions in healthcare systems. As the name clearly indicates, these systems focus on order ***entry****. With regard to medication orders, such systems generally force physicians to enter exhaustively documented orders. But a cognitive analysis of the physician's medication ordering task shows that order* ***entry*** *is the last (and least) important step of the entire cognitive therapeutic decision making task. We performed a comparative analysis of these complex cognitive tasks in two working environments, computer-based and paper-based. The results showed that information gathering, selection and interpretation are critical cognitive functions to support the therapeutic decision making. Thus the most important requirement from the physician's perspective would be an efficient display of relevant information provided first in the form of a summarized view of the patient's current treatment, followed by in a more detailed focused display of those items pertinent to the current situation. The CPOE system examined obviously failed to provide the physicians this critical summarized view. Following these results, consistent with users' complaints, the Company decided to engage in a significant re-engineering process of their application.*

Keywords:
Medication ordering; Cognitive aspects; CPO; Usability engineering Human factors

1. Introduction

Medication ordering, dispensing and administration are key functions in healthcare, particularly in hospital settings. Survey studies of this process have identified concerns about patient safety and medical errors [1]. In this context, the automation of the medication process supported by CPOE systems has been widely considered "the right thing to do" [2] in order to standardize the entire workflow. The objectives of such systems are:

- to support the physician's decision making by integrating guidelines in the systems to prevent Adverse Drug Events and medication overuse;
- to get the physician to enter his orders himself and sign them instead of dictating them to the nurse;

- to constrain the physician to enter exhaustively documented and legible orders to (i) reduce medication errors due to ill documented orders and (ii) get orders precise enough to automatically inform the pharmacy for the dispensing task, allow the pharmacist to control the medication orders, and to automatically populate the nurses' Medication Administration Record (MAR).

With this kind of solution, the additional workload attached with the improvement of the quality of the process falls mostly on the physician, due to the requirement for exhaustively documented orders. In parallel, the design of CPOE systems has been focused strongly on this critical function of orders documentation, aiming at rigorously documented and exhaustive orders.

Indeed, most of the systematic survey studies have proven effective in reducing medication errors [3], assisting nursing tasks and improving patient safety [4]. But implementation of such systems remains difficult [5], physicians being particularly reluctant to use these applications to enter their orders. The discrepancy between the physicians' actual work processes and the model of work implemented in the systems has been cited to explain implementation failures [6, 7]. In this context, cognitive analysis of the physicians' medication ordering task could shed considerable light on the sources of physicians reluctance to use CPOE systems. From the physician's viewpoint, medication order **entry** is the last step (and probably subjectively the least important one) of a decision making process taking place in a dynamic environment [8]. When a physician takes responsibility for a patient, the healthcare process he has to manage takes place over a given period of time. During this period the patient's physiological status inevitably evolves, thus creating a dynamic environment in which the therapeutic decision making takes place.

At each encounter with the patient, the physician needs a rapid, summary display of relevant information in order to support and update his current representation of the patient's physiological status. As a consequence, information gathering, selection and interpretation are critical cognitive functions supporting the therapeutic decision making which ultimately results in a medication order. Thus, the most important requirement concerning the physician's cognitive activity for therapeutic decision making and medication ordering would be an efficient display of relevant information.

From this point of view, paper based systems seem to be more usable and efficient than CPOE systems. Our hypothesis is that this weakness of CPOE systems contributes to physicians' reluctance to use these systems. In this paper, we describe a comparative analysis of physicians' activity with paper based and computer based systems for therapeutic decision making, focusing on cognitive tasks such as information gathering and information interpretation. This cognitive analysis was combined with a usability evaluation of information display in the CPOE application. As a result of this study, we were able to make recommendations that led to partial re-engineering of the system's Human-Computer Interaction (HCI).

2. Materials and Methods

2.1.Activity analysis

We used standard methods from cognitive ergonomics:

- Semi-structured and structured interviews of physicians,
- Participant observations of physicians performing medication ordering tasks during their medical rounds, parts of these observations being audio-taped,

- Self-confrontation interviews: physicians were asked to comment on and mentally replay the processes involved in therapeutic decision making.

2.2. Usability assessment

- Usability Inspection: Three independent evaluators inspected the application's Graphic User Interface (GUI) according to a set of ergonomic criteria [9].
- Usability Tests: we performed on-site usability tests using portable labs equipped with a converter, a video recorder and a microphone connected to a laptop which was installed on the medical cart used by physicians during their rounds.

2.3. Context of the study

This study took place in 3 different French hospitals:

- The University Hospital of Lille, which is a 3000 bed hospital. Users' activity was analysed in the Nephrology and Neurosurgery departments, with paper-based systems.
- The Denain Public Hospital (413 beds). The activity analysis was carried out on three sites mainly: Respirology, Surgery and Convalescence, with paper-based systems.
- The Georges Pompidou University Hospital (HEGP) of 825 beds. The hospital has a complete Patient Care Information System (PCIS) including the MEDASYS DxCare® component. It combines the functions of a CPOE and a patient record, and it is interfaced with a pharmacy system. CPOE functions are available for laboratory, radiology and medication orders and for nurses' orders. At the time of the study the medication ordering functionalities of the DxC@re® software package was being used on two pilot sites, with a mobile at the bed of the patient. Activity analysis was carried out on these two sites, Nephrology and Immunology.

3. Results

3.1. Paper-based system

10 physicians were interviewed, 20 medical rounds were observed and 6 were audio-taped. In the hospital setting, medical decision making takes place mainly during the physician's rounds. For each patient, the physician gathers relevant information, focusing on last changes in the current treatment, orders or complementary exams pending, physiological and behavioural reactions of the patient. Most often, the nurse (or a house officer) accompanies the physician on his medical rounds. She summarizes the patient's case, sorts out the relevant paper files, and hands the physician the proper document if he asks for details. When on his own, the physician seeks himself relevant information in the paper record. Loose sheets allow him to lay out all the necessary information and make easier the information gathering.

 Then the physician turns to the actual medication management, and focuses on the patient's current treatment. To do so he almost always consults the MAR, but very rarely uses the order sheets itself. The MAR (cf. figure 1) is in effect the only document which provides a synthesized global view of the patient's current treatment. All the information the physician needs to get a complete picture of the current treatment is displayed on a single page. The treatments are summarized with a temporal axis which permits the physician to obtain, at a glance, a global, summarized view of the patients' current medication. At this stage, all he needs is the list of medications, with an indication of dosage. These observations were confirmed with self-confrontation interviews during which all the physicians spontaneously stressed the necessity of a global synthesised view of the current treatment.

From this representation he may then proceed to a greater level of detail for specific pertinent items. Thus therapeutic decisions invariably follow this two steps process: first a synthesized view of the current treatments, followed by a more detailed focussed examination of medication items pertinent to the current situation.

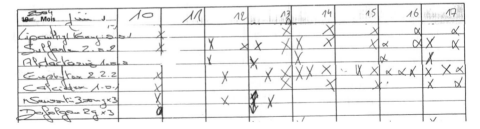

Figure 1 - Excerpt from a Medication Administration Record, Neurosurgery (site 1)

Typ	Avis	Libellés [med.chm.prf/en cours]	Début	Fin	Stat
MED		LIPANTHYL 100MG GELULE NSFP REMPLACEE PAR LIPANTHYL 67MG GELULE 1 GELULE/jour pendant 8 jours par voie ORALE 1 GELULE à 18h	26/01/2005 18:00	02/02/2005 18:00	EC
MED		SULFARLEM 12,5MG CPR ENR JAUNE ORANGE 4 COMPRIME/jour pendant 8 jours par voie ORALE 2 COMPRIME à 8h - 2 COMPRIME à 18h	26/01/2005 18:00	02/02/2005 18:00	EC
MED		ALDACTAZINE CPR ENR SECABLE BLANC 1 COMPRIME/jour pendant 8 jours par voie ORALE 1 COMPRIME à 8h	27/01/2005 08:00	03/02/2005 08:00	EC

Figure 2 - Display of the list of a patient's current treatments in the DxC@re® application under physician's profile

3.2. Computer-based system

4 physicians were interviewed, 7 medical rounds observed and 5 recorded. In the CPOE situation, the nurse usually does not accompany the physician during his rounds. With the computerised system, the physicians is forced to switch among several windows and screens to get all of the relevant information. The system provides him with alarms when new complementary exams or lab results are available, thus efficiently guiding him in his information gathering task. These functions are highly appreciated by all the physicians.

However, when the physician turns to medication management, he gets but one screen for the display of current treatments, which come out in the form of a list of overly detailed orders. Some usability problems emerge here. While the MAR is effectively reproduced, it is not readily available to the physicians. Access to the MAR requires three clicks and going through three different screens, and three more clicks and screens to get back to the list of orders and to order entry functions. Moreover, in the application, the information displayed in the MAR would not fill all the physician's needs in terms of information supporting the decision making.

Physicians are forced by default to use the list of medications ordered in the system (cf. figure 2), in which the display of information is flawed by (1) inclusion of considerable detail (such as the colour of the tablets) which obscures the global view and (2) considerable redundancy.

In addition to this critical loss of summarized global view, the specific program which we examined suffered from further usability problems. We present here two examples of such problems.

- The medications are listed chronologically by start date. The physicians in fact are interested primarily in the most recent intervention because they want to know whether they had had the desired effect. As the most recent orders appear at the bottom of the list, the doctors are forced to search through the list of meds with extensive scrolling.

- The length of time the patient had been taking the medication proved to be a critical piece of information in the physician's decision making process. This is absent in the computerised display, forcing the doctors to perform this calculation themselves.

4. Discussion

The cognitive analysis allowed us to identify the users' needs and demonstrated that the physicians' medication decision making process relies in two distinct steps for information gathering: (i) a global synthesized view of current treatments, followed by (ii) a detailed focus on specific pertinent items. In the paper-based situation the physician spontaneously refers to the MAR for information gathering instead of referring to the order sheets. The failure of the system to provide ready access to such a summarized view of the patient's current treatment contributes to resistance to the use of the system. This represents but a particular example of a weakness all to frequent in currently available systems, as noted by many authors [10].

On-site usability tests proved that medication order **entry** was efficient and fast enough with the DxCare® application. But physicians kept complaining about the "loss of overview" [10] of the patient's medical case and more particularly of his current treatment. Acknowledging this complaint, perfectly consistent with the cognitive analysis and usability assessment, the Company engaged in a re-engineering program of the application and its HCI.

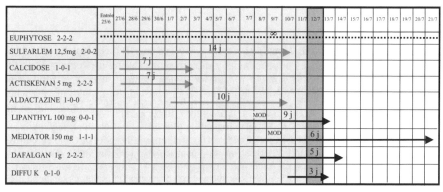

LEGENDE :
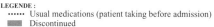 Usual medications (patient taking before admission)   MOD : Modified order
▨ Discontinued   N days : N days / medication administered
▮ Current medications

Figure 3- Suggested display providing global view

Relying on the cognitive analysis of the physicians medication ordering task, we provided the Company with a set of recommendations illustrated in a schematic mock-up (figure 3). This mock-up was designed so that the physician could view all the current treatments on one screen, and, at a glance, identify for each medication its dosage and actual/expected duration. Based on this analysis, a collaborative design process has now been undertaken, involving the Company designers and computer scientists, representatives of the users (particularly the physicians) from all the 38 hospital sites where the application is currently installed, and usability engineers. Indeed, the re-design process is far from terminated and a number of key functions such as the format of representation of the medication and its dose regimen, and the default order of display of medications must be precisely defined and agreed upon by all the participants in the re-design process. For example, all the physicians ask for a function allowing them to sort the current orders according to the patient's pathological process each medication cares for. To be reliable, such a sorting would require a more complex data model and an intelligent medication database. For the time being, in order to compensate for the faulty display of relevant information and to answer to the physicians' complaint, the Company has developed additional sorting functions by therapeutic class and route of administration. A direct access to the nurses' MAR from the physician's screens is also under development.

5. Conclusion

All these analyses make it possible to give usability recommendations and general orientations which will guide the later process of re-engineering. In complex work situations which are in the process of computerization, an activity analysis makes it possible to attain a level of comprehension and modeling of the work situation, and this is relevant: (i) to interpret the problems observed as well as users' requests, (ii) to guide and justify re-engineering decisions.

6. Acknowledgments

This research was supported by the French Ministry of Research (RNTS project). We thank the healthcare professionals (physicians, nurses and head nurses) of the Denain General Hospital, the University Hospital of Lille and the University Hospital Georges Pompidou for their close cooperation.

7. References

[1]   Kohn LT, Corrigan JM, Donaldson MS, *To Err is Human*, Washington, DC. National Academy Press, 1999.
[2]   Metzger J., Fortin J., *Computerized Physician Order Entry in Community Hospitals: lessons from the field*. CHCF & First Consulting Group, www.chcf.org, June 2003.
[3]   Bates DW., Evans RS., Murff H., Stetson PD., Pizziferri L., Hripcsak G., Detecting Adverse Events using information Technology, *J Am Med Inform Assoc*, 2003, 10 (2), pp. 115-128.
[4]   Ball MJ, Weaver C., and Abbott PA., Enabling technology to revitalize the role of nursing in a era of patient's safety, *Int J Med Inform*. 2003; 69, 29-38.
[5]   Ash J.S., Gorman P.N., Seshadri V., Hersh W.R., Computerized Physician Order Entry in U.S. Hospitals: Results of a 2002 Survey, J Am Med Inform Assoc. 2004; 11 (2): 95-99.
[6]   Gorman P.N., Lavelle M.B., Ash J.S., Order creation and communication in healthcare, *Meth Inf Med*. 2003; 42: 376-84.
[7]   Beuscart-Zéphir M.C., Pelayo S., Degoulet P., Anceaux F., Guerlinger S., Meaux J.J., *A usability study of CPOE medication administration functions : impact on physician-nurse cooperation. Proceeding Medinfo* 2004: 1018-22.
[8]   Hoc, J. M. & Amalberti, R. (1995). Diagnosis: some theoretical questions raised by applied research. *Current Psychology of Cognition, 14,* 73-101.
[9]   Bastien, C, Scapin, D.L. *Critères ergonomiques pour l'évaluation des Interfaces Utilisateurs*, Rapport Technique 156, INRIA, Rocquencourt, 1993.
[10] Ash J.S., Berg M., Coiera E., Some unintended consequences of information technology in healthcare: the nature of patient care information system-related errors, *J Am Med Inform Assoc*. 2004; 11: 104-112.

Address for correspondence

Sylvia Pelayo, EVALAB-CERIM, Faculté de Médecine, 1, Place de Verdun, 59045 Lille Cedex, France
spelayo@univ-lille2.fr

Connecting Medical Informatics and Bio-Informatics
R. Engelbrecht et al. (Eds.)
IOS Press, 2005

935

The MammoGrid Virtual Organisation - Federating Distributed Mammograms

Florida Estrella[a], **Richard McClatchey**[a], **Dmitry Rogulin**[a, b]

[a]*University of the West of England (UWE), Bristol, United Kingdom*

[b]*European Centre for Nuclear Research (CERN), Geneva, Switzerland*

Abstract

The MammoGrid project aims to deliver a prototype which enables the effective collaboration between radiologists using grid, service-orientation and database solutions. The grid technologies and service-based database management solution provide the platform for integrating diverse and distributed resources, creating what is called a 'virtual organisation'. The MammoGrid Virtual Organisation facilitates the sharing and coordinated access to mammography data, medical imaging software and computing resources of participating hospitals. Hospitals manage their local database of mammograms, but in addition, radiologists who are part of this organisation can share mammograms, reports, results and image analysis software. The MammoGrid Virtual Organisation is a federation of autonomous multi-centres sites which transcends national boundaries. This paper outlines the service-based approach in the creation and management of the federated distributed mammography database and discusses the role of virtual organisations in distributed image analysis.

Keywords:
Medical Informatics; Grid; Service-Orientation

1. Introduction

The medical community has been exploring collaborative approaches for managing mammographic image data and the Grid technology [1] is a promising approach in enabling distributed analysis across medical institutions without the necessity for the clinicians to co-locate. The EU-funded MammoGrid project [2] aims to use existing Grids technologies in developing a European wide database of mammograms to support effective co-working among healthcare professionals across the EU. The project has been active since late 2002 and involves hospitals in the UK and Italy, medical imaging experts and academics with experience of implementing grid-based database solutions.

One of the deliverables of this project is a software prototype using open-source Grid middleware and service-based database management system that is capable of managing federated mammogram databases distributed across Europe. The proposed solution is a medical information infrastructure delivered on a service-based, grid-aware framework, encompassing geographical regions of varying protocols, lifestyles and diagnostic procedures.

The prototype will allow, among other things

   a) mammogram data mining,

b) diverse and complex epidemiological studies,
c) statistical and computer aided detection (CAde) analyses, and
d) deployment of versions of the image standardization software Standard Mammogram Form (SMF).

The MammoGrid collaboration is composed of the following partners:

- Mirada Solutions and the University of Oxford – medical image analysis expertise, acquisition system and the SMF software
- University of the West of England and the European Centre for Particle Physics (CERN) – Grid and database service provision
- Udine Hospital – including a database of several thousand mammograms
- Addenbrookes Hospital – sourcing a database of around 2,000 mammogram cases
- Universities of Pisa and Sassari – delivering Computer Aided Detection (CAde) software.

2. The Grid Technologies

The grid is defined as *"flexible, secure, coordinated resource sharing among dynamic collections of individuals, institutions and resources"* [1]. Geographically separated but working together to solve a problem, groups of people can be organised in collaborations, referred to as virtual organisations (VO), and use the shared resources of the grid.

The Grid can provide a virtual platform for large-scale, resource-intensive and distributed applications. It offers a connectivity environment allowing management and coordination of diverse and dispersed resources. The Grid enables access to increased storage and computing capacity providing mechanisms for sharing and transferring large amounts of data as well as aggregating distributed resources for running computationally expensive procedures. Another important point is that the Grid utilizes a common infrastructure based on open standards thus providing a platform for interoperability and interfacing between different Grid-based applications from the particular domain.

Grid technology can potentially provide medical applications an architecture for easy and transparent access to distributed heterogeneous resources (like data storage, networks, computational resources) across different organizations and administrative domains. The Grid offers a configurable environment allowing grid structures to be reorganized dynamically without disturbing any overall active Grid processing.

In particular the Grid can address some of the following issues relevant to medical domains:

Data distribution: The Grid provides a connectivity environment for medical data distributed over different sites. It solves the location transparency issue by providing mechanisms which permit seamless access to and the management of distributed data. These mechanisms include services which deal with virtualization of distributed data regardless of their location.

Heterogeneity: The Grid addresses the issue of heterogeneity by developing common interfaces for access and integration of diverse data sources. Such generic interfaces for consistent access to existing, autonomously managed databases that are independent of underlying data models are defined by the Global Grid Forum Database Access and Integration Services (GGF-DAIS) [3] working group. These interfaces can be used to represent an abstract view of data sources which can permit homogeneous access to heterogeneous medical data sets.

Data processing and analysis: The Grid offers a platform for transparent resource management in medical analysis. This allows the virtualization and sharing of all resources (e.g. computing resources, data storage, etc.) connected to the grid. For handling computationally intensive procedures (e.g. CADe), the platform provides automatic resource allocation and scheduling and algorithm execution, depending on the availability, capacity and location of resources.

Security and confidentiality: Enabling secure data exchange between hospitals distributed across networks is one of the major concerns of medical applications. Grid addresses security issues by providing a common infrastructure for secure access and communication between grid-connected sites. This infrastructure includes authentication and authorization mechanisms, among other things, supporting security across organizational boundaries.

Standardization and compliance: Grid technologies are increasingly being based on a common set of open standards (such as XML, SOAP, WSDL, HTTP etc.) and this is promising for future medical image analysis standards.

The next section discusses the MammoGrid Virtual Organization.

3. The MammoGrid Virtual Organisation

The MammoGrid Virtual Organisation (MGVO) is composed of three mammography centres – Addenbrookes Hospital (UK), Udine Hospital (Italy) and Oxford University (UK). These centres are autonomous and independent of each other with respect to their local data management and ownership. The Addenbrookes and Udine hospitals have locally managed databases of mammograms, with several thousand cases between them. As part of the MGVO, registered clinicians have access to (suitably anonymised) mammograms, results, diagnosis and imaging software from other centres. Access is coordinated by the MGVO central node at CERN. See Figure 1.

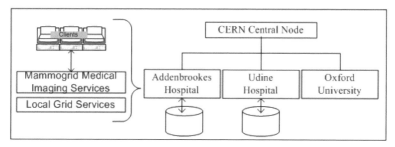

Figure 1 – MammoGrid Virtual Organisation

The adopted Grid implementation is the ALICE Environment (AliEn) [4] component of the EGEE-gLite middleware. gLite [5] is the middleware for grid computing of the EU-funded EGEE project [6]. The following AliEn services are used in the MammoGrid software:

a) Authentication for checking user credentials
b) Resource broker for resource management
c) Storage Element for file management
d) Computing Element for process management
e) File transfer for transferring files between nodes

A service-based approach to federate distributed mammography databases is employed [7]. A service-oriented approach permits the interconnection of communicating entities, called services, which provide some capabilities through exchange of messages. The services are 'orchestrated' in terms of service interactions – how services are discovered, how services are invoked, what can be invoked, the sequence of service invocations, and who can execute. The MammoGrid Services (MGS) are a set of services for managing mammography images and associated patient data on the grid.

The MGS are:
- a) Add for uploading files (DICOM [8] images and structured reports) to the grid system
- b) Retrieve for downloading files from the grid system
- c) Query for querying the federated database of mammograms
- d) AddAlgorithm for uploading executable code (e.g. SMF, CADe) to the grid system
- e) ExecuteAlgorithm for executing grid-resident executable code on grid-resident files on the grid system
- f) *Authenticate* for logging into the MGVO

Figure 2 illustrates the services that make up the MGVO. For simplicity, the Oxford University is not included.

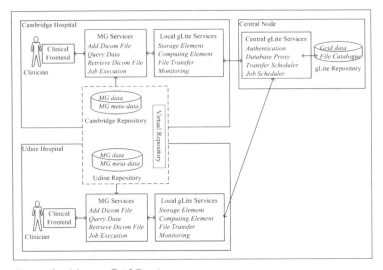

Figure 2 – MammoGrid Services

4. Query Handling

The MammoGrid project aims to provide a proof-of-concept demonstrator that allows clinicians to analyze mammograms resident on a Grid infrastructure. Clinicians define their mammogram analysis in terms of queries they wish to be resolved across the collection of data repositories. Queries can be categorized into simple queries (mainly against associated data stored in the database as simple attributes) and complex queries which require derived data to be interrogated or an algorithm to be executed on a (sub-)set of distributed images. The important aspect is that image and data distribution are transparent for radiologists so queries are formulated and executed as if these images were locally resident.

Queries are executed at the location where the relevant data resides, i.e. sub-queries are moved to the data, rather than large quantities of data being moved to the clinician, which can be prohibitively expensive given the quantities of data. Figure 3 illustrates how queries are handled in MammoGrid.

The *Query Analyzer* takes a formal query representation and decomposes into (a) a formal query for local processing, and (b) a formal query for remote processing. It then forwards these decomposed queries to the *Local Query Handler* and the appropriate *Remote Query Handler* for the resolution of the request. The *Local Query Handler* generates query language statements (e.g. SQL) in the query language of the associated Local DB (e.g. MySQL). The result set is converted to XML and routed to the Result Handler. The *Remote Query Handler* is a portal for propagating queries and results between sites. This handler forwards the formal query for remote processing to the Query Analyzer of the remote site. The remote query result set is converted to XML and routed to the Result Handler. See also [9].

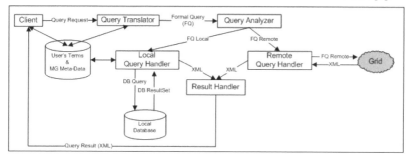

Figure 3 – Query Handling

5. Results

As of this writing the MGVO holds:

Site	Number of Patients	Number of Image Files	Number of SMF Files	Associated Database Size	File Storage Size
Cambridge	813	2798	2738	29 Mb	70 Gb
Udine	489	4663	2372	37 Mb	85 Gb

The average processing time for the core services are: (1) *Add* 8Mb DICOM file takes 7 seconds (2) *Retrieve* 8Mb DICOM file from a remote site takes 14 seconds (3) SMF workflow of *ExecuteAlgorithm* and *Add* takes 200 seconds. For querying:

Query	Cambridge	Udine	Num images	Num patients
By Id: Cambridge patient	2.654 sec	2.563 sec	8	1
By Id: Udine patient	2.844	3.225	16	1
All female	103	91	12571	1510
Age [50,60] and ImageLaterality=L	19.489	22.673	1764	357

Clinicians are still in the process of scanning and annotating cases contributing to several ongoing studies. These include (1) Cancers versus Control study: breast density study using SMF standard (2) Dose/Density study: exploring the relationship between mammographic density, age, breast size and radiation dose (3) CADe and validation of SMF in association with CADe. These studies aim to show how health professionals can work together without co-locating, and the MammoGrid approach provides a suitable environment for new forms of clinical collaboration.

6. Conclusions

The MammoGrid project has recently delivered its first proof-of-concept prototype enabling clinicians to store mammograms along with appropriately anonymised patient meta-data and to provide controlled access to mammograms both locally and remotely stored. A typical database comprising several thousand mammograms is being created for user tests of the query handler. The prototype comprises a high-quality clinician visualization workstation used for data acquisition and inspection, a DICOM-compliant interface to a set of medical services (annotation, security, image analysis, data storage and querying services) residing on a so-called 'Grid-box' and secure access to a network of other Grid-boxes connected through Grids middleware.

The MammoGrid Virtual Organisation is a distributed computing environment for harnessing the use of and access to massive amounts of mammography data across Europe. The MammoGrid approach uses grid technologies, service-orientation and database management techniques to federate distributed mammography databases allowing healthcare professional to collaborate without co-locating.

In the last couple of years, several Grid projects have been funded on health related issues at national and European levels (e.g. [10], [11]). These projects have a limited lifetime, from 3 to 5 years, and a crucial issue is to maximize their cross fertilization. Indeed, the HealthGrid [12] is a long term vision that needs to build on the contribution of all projects. The HealthGrid initiative, represented by the HealthGrid association, was initiated to bring the necessary long term continuity. Currently the HealthGrid Association is compiling an extensive White Paper on the requirements for Grids in biomedical healthcare [13].

Grid computing is a promising distributed computing paradigm that can facilitate the management of federated medical images. This technology spans locations, organizations, architectures and has the potential to provide computing power, collaboration and information access to everyone connected to the Grid. Grid-based applications like the MammoGrid project benefit from this solution being based on open-internet standards. These applications are potentially cross platform compatible, cross programming interoperable and widely accepted, deployed and adopted.

7. Acknowledgments

The authors thank their home institutes, the European Commission and acknowledge the support of the following MammoGrid Collaboration members: Prof R. Amendolia (formerly CERN), T. Solomonides, T. Hauer, D. Manset, W. Hassan (UWE), Dr R. Warren, I. Warsi (Addenbrookes Hospital), Dr C. Del Frate (Udine Hospital), Prof. M. Brady, C. Tromans (Oxford Univ.), M. Cordell, T. Reading (Mirada Solutions), Drs E. Fantacci (Pisa Univ.)& P. Oliva (Sassari Univ.), Dr A. Retico (Torino) and Dr P. Buncic and P. Saiz (CERN,AliEn).

8. References

[1]   Foster I and Kesselman C. The Grid: Blueprint for a New Computing Infrastructure. Morgan Kaufmann, 1998.
[2]   The Information Societies Technology Project: MammoGrid – A European Federated Mammogram Database Implemented on a Grid Insfrastructure. EU Contract IST 2001-37614. http://mammogrid.vitamib.com.
[3]   Global Grid Forum Data Access and Integration Services (GGF-DAIS) Working Group. http://www.cs.man.ac.uk/grid-db/
[4]   Buncic P, et. al. The AliEn System, Status and Perspectives. San Diego. Proceedings of the CHEP 2003.
[5]   gLite: Lightweight Middleware for Grid Computing. http://glite.web.cern.ch/glite
[6]   EGEE: Enabling Grids for E-Science in Europe. http://public.eu-egee.org
[7]   Amendolia R et al. Deployment of a Grid-based Medical Imaging Application Proceedings of the 3rd International HeathGrid 2005 Conference. To appear in the IOS Press. Oxford UK April 2005.
[8]   DICOM: Digital Imaging and Communications in Medicine. http://medical.nema.org
[9]   Estrella F, et.al. A Service-Based Approach for Managing Mammography Data. Accepted in the 11th World Congress on Medical Informatics (MedInfo'04). San Francisco, 2004.
[10] GEMSS: Grid-Enabled Medical Simulation Services. http://www.gemss.de
[11] Pereira AS, Maojo V, et. al. The Infogenmed Project. ICBME 2002. December 2002.
[12] Nørager S and Paindaveine Y. The HealthGrid Terms of Reference, EU Report Version 1.0, 20th September 2002.
[13] The HealthGrid White Paper, currently under preparation. Draft available from: http://www.heathgrid.org.

Address for correspondence:

Dr Florida Estrella, DSU-TT Group, CERN, Geneva 23, Switzerland 1211, Florida.Estrella@cern.ch

Connecting Medical Informatics and Bio-Informatics
R. Engelbrecht et al. (Eds.)
IOS Press, 2005

Ontological Definition of Population for Public Health Databases

György Surján

National Institute for Strategic Health Research

Abstract

This paper discusses available definitions of population and criticise them against some basic rules of ontology. None of the found definition satisfies the requirement of an ontology that supports building consistent public heath databases. Most definitions define population on territorial bases or as reproductive communities. The author argues that populations are systems (its members must be in connection to each other) and individuals forming the population must share a common resource. Proper usage of the definitions may help to build consistent ontology for public health indicators and consistent databases.

Keywords:

Population, Public health, Health Status Indicators, Ontology

1. Introduction

Public health data (often called health indicators) are used to measure, characterise and compare the health condition of various populations. Population is a fundamental category of public health. However it has many contradicting definitions. Looking at the various definitions of population found in the Web, we can be convinced that this category is unclear, and it is worthwhile to find some way to clarify it at least for our own specific purpose. This purpose is to build up consistent and comparable public health databases, which is an important, central task of several international and national organisations. In Hungary our institute is responsible to publish such a database on the Internet, and we are also responsible for reporting Hungarian data to various international organisations, like OECD (Organisation for Economic Co-operation and Development) and WHO (World Health Organisation).

Beyond the theoretical importance of having clear categories, a precise definition of population is absolutely necessary to have comparable public health indicators. Many of those indicators are ratios: a number of an observable phenomenon is divided by the number of relevant people. E.g. 'female death rate' in a population is the number of females who died in a period (a year) divided by number of female persons in the population. Different interpretations of population may result in different and incomparable values of the public health indicators. Perhaps the numeric differences arising from different definitions are sometimes not too high, but any unclear variations in the values decrease in the credibility of our data. To avoid this, it seems to be worthwhile to define precisely, what is meant by population. Our goal in this study was to look at various available definitions of population, analyse them according to some basic rules of ontology, and finally to propose a definition flexible enough to meet various needs and precise enough to be used in formal onotologies.

An exhaustive formal ontological representation of population can be a task of further studies. Such representation should be built on a formal top level ontology. Top level ontologies represent basic ontological classes independently form any domain specific applications. This is a research task of several groups [1][2]. We do not see at this moment whether their work will converge to a generally accepted top level ontology or which of them will be tailored so that it will be suitable for public health domain ontologies.

2. Material and method

A Google search was performed with the words: "population definition". From the first ten hits it was possible to derive 27 at least slightly different definitions. The MESH database also was searched for the term "population". Definitions of the word "population" and also of several related terms, like "Population characteristics" or "Population control", were also found. Their definitions were also retrieved. Some of the found definitions defined population as a basic concept of statistics. Since these definitions speak about a totally different thing, which has no direct relevance to public health, we excluded them from the study.

The collected definitions were then analysed manually. We tried to identified the "genus proximum" (i.e. the closest IsA category) used in each definition, and also the differentiating criteria. For instance if a definition says: *'the people who inhabit a territory or state'* then it states that 'population' <IsA> 'people', while the differentiating criterion is 'inhabiting a territory or state'

According to another definition population is *'a group of organisms of the same species inhabiting a particular geographical area at a particular time.'* In this case 'population' <IsA> 'group', while the differentiating criteria are:

*   being an organism

*   inhabiting a geographical area

*   inhabiting at a particular time

These IsA statements and differentia then were criticised against some rules found in the literature of formal ontology. Guarino and Welty [3] emphasise, that most of the problems are around the IsA relations.

3. Results

Critique on IsA statements

Just a few definitions state, that population is a set (set of persons, set of individuals). According to set theory, sets are defined by their elements. Two sets are identical if, and only if, they have exactly the same elements. If populations would be sets, than we had to state, that two populations are the same, if they consist of exactly the same persons. Contrary to that, a population remains the same while persons forming the population change continuously by birth, death and migration.

One third of the definitions state, that population is a group. This was the most frequent IsA statement. None of those definitions explains what should be meant by group. If group is a sort of set than it is not acceptable for the same reason. If not, then we have to know what a group is, and what identity criteria should be used.

We have found some other IsA statements, like population is an *aggregation, collection, entirety* etc. which are more or less synonymous to group, and show the same problem.

A large number of definitions says that population is a number (number of inhabitants, individuals, people). It is clear that the word population is often used instead of *size of the population*. This would be acceptable, if the term would be used consistently, but this is not the case. E.g. MESH database says that population is " the total number of individuals inhabiting a particular region or area" But it also states that 'Population Control: Includes mechanisms or programs which control the numbers of individuals in a population of humans or animals.' If we replace the term population in this statement with the definition of population we get the following strange statement:

> *Population Control: Includes mechanisms or programs which control the numbers of individuals in* {the total number of individuals inhabiting a particular region or area} *of humans or animals.*

One definition says that population is an act. This is again a word usage problem: the word population is used instead of act of populating.

We found also some tautological statements, like '*population is a people*' or even '*population is a population*'.

None of these IsA statements are fully acceptable. The best ones are those, that say that population is a group or collection, provided that not a sort of set is meant by these terms.

Critique on the differentiating criteria

The far most frequent differentiating criterion was that people or individuals forming a population must inhabit (reside, live in) a geographical area. Since all differentiating criteria should be necessary conditions, then it means, that persons living far from each other can not be a member of the same population. This seems to be convincing, but it is not true for all sensible interpretations of population, as we will show. Some definitions add that the individual must live in the given territory at the same time (or even at a particular moment in time).This again would mean that whenever an individual dies or another is born, the population becomes different.

The second frequent criterion was that individuals of a population must belong to the same species. Really a community of living beings belonging to different species not used to called population. This is an acceptable necessary but not sufficient condition. (However in public health we restrict our thinking to human populations, so this criterion says nothing.)

Fewer definitions view population as a reproductive community. According to these, members of the population are more likely to breed with another member than with a non member. Beyond the foolish interpretation of this condition, that in this case two males or two females never could belong to the same population, the problem is that not all populations are reproductive. One can think of e.g. a child-population or a population of elderly people.

We found two definitions very interesting. One states that individuals belonging to a population share a gene pool. The other says that persons belonging to a population must have at least one common property of interest. Although the former is very special, the latter is too general (not all people who have some common property form a population), these two definitions show us, how it is possible to bring all these different definitions under a common umbrella and improve ontological precision at the same time. This is shown in the following.

The proposed definition

If we leave open the question what a group is – but stress again that it is not a set – we could draw the following definition: *A population (in public health) is a group of persons sharing a common resource.* This definition covers the two major group of definitions presented above:

those which define population by territory (in this case the shared resource is the territory) or by interbreeding (the shared resource is a common gene pool). Beyond that it is possible to define populations in many other different ways (people having the same workplace, using the same water supply etc.) The proposed criterion defines who belongs to the group forming the population and who not. Now we have to say something about what is meant by group.

Let us say, that the shared resource is a territory. It can happen that one population using the territory dies out or moves away and later another comes in. The time difference is not sufficient to decide that these are different populations, since as we mentioned, it is not a necessary condition that all members of a population must live at the same time. If the mentioned change happens slowly and gradually, we could accept that this is just one population. What is the difference? (This problem is similar to the identity of artefacts, like machines: If I change one part of my computer in each year, after a certain time nothing original remains, but I still may say this is the same computer. If I do it in one step, it is a totally new computer.) In the former case people belonging to the different population never had any connection to or interaction with each other. (The same is the case with the computer: if I change the parts in one step, new parts will be never connected to the old ones.)

Along this way we can use Bertalanffy's definition of system. He says that system is a complex of interacting parts. [4] Smith criticise this definition as too general [5], but we do not see any reason why not use this for our recent purpose. (The question whether or not Bertalanffy's whole theory is too general is totally irrelevant here). So our final proposition is the following:

A population is a system formed by people sharing a common resource

Replacing the word *people* by the term *individual organisms* allows us to extend this public health definition to be used for non-human populations as well.

4. Discussion

This proposed definition seems to be flexible enough to meet various needs in public health. Of course it is more general than necessary. The proper selection of the resource is important. It is possible to find many resources which are totally irrelevant for public health. The corresponding populations can be foolish. For instance people who read the War and Peace form a population according to our definition (provided that they interact in some way), which is obviously of less importance in public health. Choosing appropriate resources to define actual populations that are relevant for public health is a task of public health experts. However they must be aware, what using or sharing a resource means. It is important to see the difference between 'populating a given area' and 'using a given area as a resource'. The first expression does not explain clearly the relation between the individuals and the given area. When we are speaking about using something as a resource, it is more imprecise and unclear, because an area can be used in many ways. (We can cultivate an area, or just stay there, or live there etc.) When we define a given population along our proposed general definition, we always have to tell, for what purpose the given resource is used. E.g. the population which uses the territory of Hungary for living there is different from the population which uses the same territory for staying there during summer holidays. Specifying the used resource clearly shows us, that "Hungarian population" is also an ambiguous term. The population who uses the territory of Hungary for living there and the population who uses the State of Hungary to obtain citizen's benefits are definitely different. Within the European Union such differences will become more significant in the future as we expect more and more people moving from their own country and living in another one while still remaining citizens of their own.

Another benefit of the proposed definition, that it makes clear that there are two different ways of definition of subpopulations. It is possible to define sub-population by partitioning the used resource, and by attributes of the individuals. Let us take the population which uses the territory of Hungary for living there. A subpopulation of this can be defined as the population which uses the Trans-Danubian part of Hungary. Defining subpopulations by the attributes of people leads to male and female, adult and child subpopulations etc. However these two kinds of subpopulations are different and perhaps it would be beneficial two name them differently. The discussion of this problem exceeds the limitation of this paper.

5. Conclusion

The proposed definition can solve some essential problems about the ontological representation of populations in public health databases. It makes clear that the population is not a set or sum of people having a certain property. Instead of that a population can gain and loose members without loosing its identity. This makes possible to speak about changing the health status of a given population over a period of time. The identity of population is not based on the identity of the people who form the population but on the resource which is shared by the people forming the population. The number of persons in a population represents the size of the population which may change over time. For that very reason it is not critical to count very precisely the number of individuals forming the population. (It is enough to know the expected statistical error of that value). The proposed definition is flexible enough to cover the two main traditional definitions of population, i.e. the territory based and the reproduction related definitions.

6. Acknowledgments

This work was partly supported by the EU 6FW IST507505 project. The author thanks to Arie Hasman for revising this paper carefully.

7. References

[1]   Grenon P, Smith B, Goldberg G, Biodunamic Ontology: Applying BFO in the Biomedical Domain. Stud Health Technol Inform. 2004;102:20-38

[2]   Stefano Borgo Paulo Leitão The Role of Foundational Ontologies in Manufacturing Domain Applications In R. Meersman, Z. Tari et al. (eds.) OTM Confederated International Conferences, ODBASE 2004, Ayia Napa, Cyprus, October 29, 2004, LNCS 3290, Proceedings Part 10, Springer Verlag, pp. 670-688

[3]   Guarino, N. and Welty, C. A Formal Ontology of Properties In R. Dieng, O. Corby (eds.), Knowledge Engineering and Knowledge Management: Methods, Models and Tools. 12th International Conference, EKAW2000. Springer Verlag, pp. 97-112

[4]   von Bertalanffy L General System Theory Allen Lane The Pinguin Press, London 1971

[5]   Smtih B Munn K Papakin I Bodily Systems and thge Spacial-Functional Structure of Human Body Stud Health Technol Inform. 2004;102:39-63

Address for correspondence

György Surján National Institute for Strategic Health Research. Budapest Hungary
e mail: surjan@eski.hu, http://www.eski.hu/surjan

Section 13

Public Health Informatics, Clinical Trials

Connecting Medical Informatics and Bio-Informatics
R. Engelbrecht et al. (Eds.)
IOS Press, 2005

Proposal for the Creation of a European Healthcare Identifier

Catherine Quantin[a], François-André Allaert[b],
Béatrice Gouyon[a], Olivier Cohen[c]

[a] *Department of Biostatistics and Medical Informatics. Dijon University Hospital, France*
[b] *W2 "data security" European Federation of Medical Informatics Dijon, France.*
[c] *Laboratory TIMC-IMAG UMR 5525, CNRS University of Joseph Fourier Medical School of Grenoble.*
France

Abstract:

In France, the European health card was created in June 2004 to increase the quality of healthcare granted to european citizen anywhere in europe and to facilitate the reimbursement of the healthcare costs. The patient identifier included in this card is essentially based on the healthcare insurance number of the patient and does not allow any linkage with his (her) previous health care data if he (she) is affiliated to another national healthcare insurance system when working for a long duration outside France. The purpose of this paper is to present the concept of a personal identifier based on familial components which has been validated by the French authority for personal data protection in the framework of a genetic study. Results issued from the Burgundy perinatal network demonstrate the interest and the faisability of adding a maternal component to the individual component of the new-born to allow Mother/new-born healthcare data linkage after anonymization. The advantage of adding a familial component to the healthcare insurance number is debated. This proposal will permit to link the data of a patient even when residing outside his country in Europe. It will also contribute to establish european public health statistics by matching healthcare data of the patients' records with other administrative data (mortality, social information ...) after anonymisation of these data in accordance with the European directive on data protection.

Keywords: Data linkage, Human identification, Confidentiality, Hash coding, European health card, Genetics, Perinatology

1. Introduction

Even if the harmonization of healthcare system will still take time, as soon as 1996 the European parliament recommended the development of a European health card in order to allow any European citizens to benefit of adequate care everywhere in Europe and above all when moving from one country to another one. Following the work conducted in the framework of the European project "Netcard" the European health card was created in June 2004. Thus, all French citizens will not use anymore the E111 form when travelling abroad inside Europe but will carry with them their European healthcard which is distributed by the French health insurance system. Today this is still a paper document but it should rapidly move towards a smart card [1]. The setting up of such a European health card intends to simplify the healthcare reimbursement for all European citizens which are travelling for leisure or work but also wants to contribute to a better quality of care by making easier an European access to medical data in the respect of its legal framework. The creation of this card gives also some new possibilities to gather the medical data needed to conduct epidemiological studies at the European level and to provide the global information required to manage public health at a European level. Such statistics would require to be able to match different categories of data issued from different origins, not only from the personal medical record we try to implement by the GPs in ambulatory care but also from hospital, cancer registers and governmental mortality data, according to some models which have been already used in the United Kingdom [2], in northern European countries and in the USA [3,4], or in Australia [5], This could also offer the possibility to conduct inter countries comparisons inside Europe. However, this data collection requires solving two main difficulties. First it must respect the European directive on data protection and must provide high guaranties concerning the quality of the linkage of the data of an individual. It implies that the chosen identifier must be sufficiently discriminating to avoid the risk of gathering the data of two set of information belonging to two different patients. The European health card already includes the social insurance number which has been given to the person in his own country. Unfortunately, this number is not an identifier sufficiently powerful to satisfy the objectives previously described: the patient may be also registered in the insurance system of another European country if he works there. Finally, even in the country where this social insurance number is the main identifier in the health domain, epidemiologists agree [6,7], on the fact that this identifier is not by itself sufficient to link healthcare data issued from the medical records with mortality statistics. The purpose of this paper is to describe the concept of family-based identifier. This will allow to show the interest of introducing this identifier in the European health card, apart from the social insurance number, in order to link all the data of a patient even when he moves and permit the production of public health statistics at the European level.

2. Proposal for a family-based identifier.

The French authority for data protection has validated this proposal for the linkage of genetic data.

Principle: The development of medical genetics has pointed out the importance of the familial dimension of the medical information and the need for introducing a familial component in the individual record of the patient. The interest of such familial component is supported by the identification of genetic factors influencing the outcome of some diseases or the therapeutic response to the drugs. In this framework we have set up an Internet application which gives the possibility to authorised geneticians and researchers to gather all the medical data concerning a patient with a genetic disease. By the use of anonymised family-based identifiers, data concerning the patient will be gathered along with the information issued from the medical records of the other members of his family. With the patient's agreement, this anonymised identifier is transmitted by a secured system to the data centre called HC-Forum platform [8] with all his medical data. Thus the patient will benefit from a medical record accessible from any medical centre. This record will be regularly updated with his own information and those of his family. In this data centre, for statistical purpose, this identifier will be anonymised a second time in order to avoid any kind of dictionary attacks [9]. The rules governing the information system are strictly in accordance with the European directive for data protection in order to guarantee the confidentiality of his data and of his relatives, and to grant the subject the right to obtain the rectification, of data. The French National Data Protection Authority (CNIL) validated this project in March 2004 (advice n° 04-006). A patent was filed to the French Patent Office in September 2004.

Composition of the family-based identifier: The choice of the criteria included in the individual part of the patients' identifier is based on a previous work we have conducted, with the French Department for the Modernization of Health Information Systems, which have demonstrated that the key information for patient identification are his first and last names and his date of birth [10,11,12]. The first name is the first one recorded in the register of birth and the last name is the family name which means for the women their maiden name and not their marital name for example. The familial components (last name, first name and date of birth of the mother and the father) were added to the individual component following the work conducted by our department on the linkage of the mother and her babies medical records in the Burgundy perinatal network [13] which has pointed out the necessity of introducing the maternal component in the individual identifier of the baby. However, we also need a paternal component to rebuild the genealogic tree.

Anonymisation of the family-based identifier: Hash algorithms are not reversible and cannot be deciphered and one of the most reliable [18,14] and freely available one is the Standard Hash Algorithm (SHA). The three key variables included in the individual part of the patient identifier (Last name, first name and date of birth) are separately hashed in order to maintain a higher security level. For the individual component, we have three variables: Hn: anonymous number corresponding to the last name of the subject; Hp: anonymous number corresponding to the first name of the subject; Hdn: anonymous number corresponding to the subject's date of birth. The family based identifier includes 9 variables. This anonymisation is made locally before any kind of data flows in such a way that only anonymised data are sent and made available on the HC forum data centre.

Familial linkage: By using the link existing between the identifiers of the subjects of a same family, the genealogic tree of the patient can be described. Thanks to this linkage, one can thus build the family tree from a "vertical" point of view, i.e. ascending/descending of an individual. This linkage also makes it possible to build the family tree from an "horizontal" point of view, i.e. within the same generation, for the following cases: - the phratry: by sorting the dates of birth of all the individuals having the same parents; - half-brothers and sisters: by sorting the dates of birth of all the individuals having the same father or the same mother;

3. Results obtained in the Burgundy perinatal network

The Burgundy perinatal network was initiated in 1992 to improve the quality of perinatal care in Burgundy, a French region with 1.800.000 inhabitants and 18.500 annual births and including 18 private and public hospitals. A multidisciplinary working group previously chose and precisely defined specific indicators20. These items could be mainly obtained from the discharge abstracts mandatory for each hospitalised patient in both public and private hospitals in France. These data are previously rendered anonymous before being sent from each hospital to the committee in charge of the assessment of the perinatal network's performance. The use of the ANONYMAT software has been authorised by the French Department for Information System Security (SCSSI) and the management of perinatal data in Burgundy was specifically authorised in 1998 by the CNIL. An optimal assessment of perinatal care obviously needs an effective linkage between maternal and neonatal data. Indeed, taking into account the mechanisms of neonatal diseases made essential the linkage between:1) abstracts of a mother and her corresponding neonate even if they were not cared for in the same hospital, 2) all discharge abstracts obtained from the same patient, who may have several discharge abstracts from different hospitals. We present here the results of the performance assessment of the file-linkage process of maternal and neonatal data used for the evaluation of the Burgundy perinatal network.

Population: All deliveries and newborn births, whenever alive or not, are considered in the perinatal network if the gestational age is at least of 20 weeks in pregnancy and/or if the birth weight is greater than 500g. For the purpose of this study, we took into account the population included since 1998, year of the beginning of the data collection, up to 2003. In

1998, only nine hospitals participated into the data collection, whereas since 2001 all the 18 hospitals involved in the regional perinatal care have provided items for 100 % of the 18.500 annual births.

Data Collection: Apart from discharge abstracts collected for all mothers and all neonates, five identification items (maiden names, first names and of dates of birth of mothers, first names and of dates of birth of neonates) have been added for both mothers and neonates to allow the linkage between their discharge abstracts. This identifier corresponds thus to the family-based identifier previously described, except for the identification of the father. The last name of the baby was not recorded as this name often changes during the first days after birth.

File linkage Once rendered anonymous, data were transmitted to the regional audit committee located in the University Hospital of Dijon (France) and were included in a regional database. A statistical model, taking into account the five identification variables, accomplished the linkage[15]. Three sets of possible decisions can be determined as follows: 1) the pair is matched, 2) no determination is made, 3) the pair is not matched. In case of no determination, a paediatrician validated the linkage by checking the data accuracy of the five identification variables as well as all medical information contained in the discharge abstracts of the neonate(s) and the mother.

Data validation: The exhaustiveness for the number of mothers and neonates registered in the regional database was assessed from hand-written notebooks which are used in each hospital for the registration of birth and/or admission of sick neonates in units caring for these infants. The quality of both medical items and linkage items were monitored as follows: 1) Exhaustiveness for the five linkage items was controlled for each discharge abstract; 2) Exhaustiveness for gestational age and birth weight was controlled for each neonatal discharge abstract; 3) For each patient, a paediatrician looked for inconsistency between medical data or between dates of exit and admission for successive hospitalisations. Computerized procedures have been developed to disclose those discrepancies. Correction of erroneous data was then performed on the nominative files in each hospital.

Reliability of the Linkage Procedure It was assumed that an erroneous link between a mother and a non-corresponding neonate was excluded in the case of a perfect agreement between two records on the five identification items. Indeed, it was highly unlikely that in the same maternity hospital, two women having the same maiden name, the same first name, the same date of birth would give birth the same day to babies with the same first name. Additionally, the risk for an homonym error was very low (10^{-48}) with the standard hash algorithm [11]. In a perinatal network, it is obvious that every neonate has a mother and vice versa. So, the fact that no link was found between a neonate and a mother will indicate either a linkage error or the lack of the mother record. The identification of linkage errors was performed using again the linkage method on the basis of only five items or even four. To verify these potential links, each hospital was asked to control the identification items of the records corresponding to the given anonymous numbers. The corrected data were rendered anonymous before being sent again from the hospitals to the regional database. Finally, the linkage is only performed if the five identification items are perfectly identical in the mother's and neonate's records.

Results: In 1998, 9 hospitals were involved in the collection of discharge abstracts. The percentage of mothers retrieved in the regional database after the validation procedure was 99.1 % of all eligible mothers; those percentages were of 98.7 % for neonates. In 2003, 18 hospitals were involved in the collection of discharge abstracts and the overall exhaustiveness for both mothers and neonates was 100 % after validation procedure. In 1998, the five items used for the linkage procedure were recorded in 80 % of discharge abstracts before validation and in 99 % after. In 2003, the exhaustiveness of these items were 93.7% before and 100% after validation. Before validation, the percentage of neonates linked to their corresponding mothers on the basis of the identification items were 71% in 1998, and 86,3% in 2003. After validation, 99.9% of neonates were linked to their mothers whatever the year concerned.

4. Discussion

4.1 Discussion of the result obtained in the burgundy perinatal network.

Optimal assessment of perinatal care needs a linkage procedure between successive files from the same patient and between files of the mothers and their corresponding neonate(s). This latter linkage was found to be mandatory in assessing the postnatal consequences of antenatal risk factors and maternal diseases. For instance, one maternity hospital showed in 1999 a significant increase both in the rates of Caesarean section and of neonatal hospitalisation for respiratory distress as compared with regional and national data rates. The linkage procedure disclosed that the excess in neonatal hospitalisation rate was related to an excess in caesarean section rate. This finding was a strong argument in reducing the Caesarean section rate in this hospital. The fact that at each mother corresponded a neonate and vice versa was particularly helpful in testing the linkage procedure. Indeed, coupling the direct linkage of anonymous data files to the validation procedure gave very satisfactory results, on a regional scale, with 99,9% of neonates linked with their mothers. Different types of errors were found during the validation procedure. The most frequent one corresponded to errors in spelling names leading to phonetic changes not subsequently corrected by the spelling process included in the ANONYMAT software. The inversion of the married name and the maiden name was also responsible for linkage failures. These results thus demonstrate the importance of a specific validation of the patient's identification, within each hospital databases, before the extraction of any information to the perinatal network committee, using appropriate methods for the reduction of the doubloon's rate [17, 18].

4.2 Proposal for using the family-based identifier to create a unique European identifier.

We propose to add in the European health card, apart from the national social insurance number of the patient in each country, a family-based identifier which could contribute to harmonise patients' identification at the European level. This solution would lead to the creation of a European health identifier which would allow to gather data patients anywhere in Europe, whatever their location, even if their social insurance number change according to their country of residence. This will be useful, at the individual level, to provide higher quality in health care due to a better follow-up of the patient and to facilitate the reimbursement of health care costs. At the community level, this will increase the reliability of public health statistics. The great advantage of this European health identifier based on the family component is to be founded on very basic information available for everybody, easily checkable and permanent during all the patient's life which is not the case for the social insurance number. To fulfil the rules of the European directive on data protection and of the medical deontology, the use of hash algorithms [22] with different keys would allow to create, from the information of the family-based identifier, different anonymised identifiers for a same patient which could be used in the different countries for different applications ie Medical personal record, healthcare network, epidemiological or clinical studies. The fact that all these anonymised identification numbers are issued from the same initial information will facilitate the linkage of the data of a same patient, coming from different health information systems, in a secure environment. If an error occurs on one of the identification criteria (Last name, first name or date of birth) of the patient or of the parents, the use of a probabilistic linkage algorithm [20] as described for the Burgundy perinatal network, could be used to recreate the link with the other parts of the medical information and to rebuild for example the medical record of a patient. This is not always possible today when there is an error in the social insurance number, particularly when this number is not significant, meaning that it is not made using characteristics of the patient (date of birth, gender …).

5. Conclusion

Our proposal for using the family-based identifier to create a unique European identifier will permit to link the data of a patient even when residing outside his country in Europe. It will also contribute to establish European public health statistics by matching healthcare data of the patients' records with other administrative data (mortality, social inform,) after anonymisation of these data in accordance with the European directive on data protection.

6. References

[1]   ENEL P. Relation internationale : vers une carte de santé européenne. Bulletin de l'ordre des médecins, décembre 2000.

[2]   MORGAN CL, KERR MP. Estimated cost of inpatient admissions and outpatient appointments for a population with epilepsy : a record linkage study. Epilepsia, 2004 ; 45 (7) : 849-854.

[3]   COOPER GS, VIRNIG B, KLABUNDE CN, SCHUSSLER N, FREEMAN J, WARREN JL. Use of SEER-Medicare data for measuring cancer surgery. Medical Care, 2002;40(8 Suppl):43-48.

[4]   VIRNIG BA, WARREN JL, COOPER GS, KLABUNDE CN, SCHUSSLER N, FREEMAN J. Studying radiation therapy using SEER-Medicare linked data. Medical Care, 2002; 40(8 Suppl):49-54.

[5]   BARTU A, FREEMAN NC, GAWTHORNE GS, CODDE JP, D'ARCY C, HOLMAN J. Mortality in a cohort of opiate and amphetamine users in Perth, Western Australia. Society for the Study of Addiction, 2004;99:53-60.

[6]   GRANNIS SJ, OVERHAGE JM, MC DONALD C. Real world performance of approximate string comparators for use in patient matching. MEDINFO 2004, Amsterdam.

[7]   GRANNIS SJ, OVERHAGE JM, MC DONALD C. Analysis of a probabilistic record linkage technique without human review. In: proceedings of American Medical Informatics Association Fall Symposium; 2003; Washington, DC.

[8]   COHEN O, MERMET MA, DEMONGEOT J. HC Forum® : a web site based on an international human cytogenetic database. Nucleic Acids Research 2001;29:305-307.

[9]   QUANTIN C, BINQUET C, BOURQUARD K, PATTISINA R, GOUYON-CORNET B, FERDYNUS C, GOUYON JB, ALLAERT FA. Which are the best identifiers for record linkage? Medical Informatics and the Internet Medicine, 2004;29 (3-4):221-227.

[10] QUANTIN C, BINQUET C, ALLAERT FA, CORNET B, PATTISINA R, LE TEUFF G, FERDYNUS C, GOUYON JB. Decision analysis for the assessment of a record linkage procedure: application to a perinatal network. Methods of Information in Medicine 2005 (in Press).

[11] QUANTIN C., BOUZELAT H., ALLAERT F.A., BENHAMICHE A.M., FAIVRE J., DUSSERRE L. How to ensure data security of an epidemiological follow-up : quality assessment of an anonymous record linkage procedure, International Journal of Medical Informatics. 1998; 49:117-122.

[12] CORNET B, GOUYON JB, BINQUET C, SAGOT P, FERDYNUS C, MÉTRAL P, QUANTIN C. Using discharge abstracts as a bool to assess a regional perinatal network. Revue Epidemiologie et Santé Publique 2001; 49:583-93.

[13] JARO M. Probabilistic linkage of large public health data files. Stat Med 1995;14:491-8.

[14] WINKLER W. String comparator metrics and enhanced decision rules in the Fellegi-Sunter model or record linkage. In: Proceedings of the section on Survey Research Methods: American Statistical Association; 2000. p. 354-9.

[15] FALKOE E, RASMUSSEN KB, MACLURE M, SCHROLL H. Statistical linkage of treatment to diagnosis for research and monitoring of practice patterns. Methods Informatic Medicine, 2004;43:282-6.

Address for correspondence

Professeur Catherine QUANTIN, Service de Biostatistique et Informatique Médicale, Centre Hospitalier Universitaire, BP 77908 21079 DIJON CEDEX, Tel: 33 3 80 29 36 29, Fax: 33 3 80 29 39 73
Email: catherine.quantin@chu-dijon.fr

Connecting Medical Informatics and Bio-Informatics
R. Engelbrecht et al. (Eds.)
IOS Press, 2005

Linking Primary Care Information Systems and Public Health Information Networks: Lessons from the Philippines

Herman Tolentino[a,c,] Alvin Marcelo[a,c], Portia Marcelo[a,b], Inocencio Maramba[a,c]

[a] *University of the Philippines Manila College of Medicine*
[b] *Department of Family and Community Medicine*
[c] *Medical Informatics Unit*

Abstract

Community-based primary care information systems are one of the building blocks for national health information systems. In the Philippines, after the devolution of health care to local governments, we observed "health information system islands" connected to national vertical programs being implemented in devolved health units. These structures lead to a huge amount of "information work" in the transformation of health information at the community level. This paper describes work done to develop and implement the open-source Community Based Health Information Tracking System (CHITS) Project, which was implemented to address this information management problem and its outcomes. Several lessons learned from the field as well as software development strategies are highlighted in building community level information systems that link to national level health information systems.

Keywords:
Public health informatics; Information management; Primary health care, Community networks

1. Introduction

The delivery of health care services in the Philippines was devolved to local government units in 1998 under the Health Sector Reform Agenda (HSRA) carried out by the Department of Health [1]. In the course of the devolution, there was not enough time to cede health information management functions to local government units (LGUs) for them to carry out data collection, integration and presentation in a seamless, distributed and coordinated manner. National vertical health programs remained in place, however, each with its own complement of logbooks, and reporting forms and protocols, and sometimes personnel. The Philippine vertical programs include among others, Child Care and Development, Maternal Care, the National TB Program, Family Planning, and the Expanded Program for Immunization. In busy community health centers, data entry of patient information over several logbooks can be inefficient and is characterized by redundant and inaccurate entries. As early as 1995, a case study of Philippine public health information systems by Jayasuria revealed proliferation of reports consuming 40% of the time of field personnel, high levels of duplication and delays due to manual processing [2], a situation that seems to have persisted for the last decade. Currently, there are no data quality control and validation procedures where paper forms are used and community health workers generally do not get feedback from reports that they submit. The collection of large amounts of health data without feedback to the collectors seems to be the practice not only in the Philippines but in other settings where national vertical programs of this type are used [3]. Vertical programs are generally useful particularly when there is a need to urgently address a public health problem like HIV-AIDS [4, 5] and smallpox [6] because they can achieve economies of scale and focus resources and manpower on a specific problem. In this particular situation, to make information management efficient and to ensure a good supply of quality information, we needed to integrate existing interfaces to vertical programs at the community level, as we work our way upwards for higher level integration of information systems to the level of the city health office. In addition to the information management situation above, an alarming trend is emerging in the Philippine health care scene. As early as 2003, thousands of physicians nationwide, including an undetermined number of government physicians, have been retraining as nurses to become part of the eligible health workforce migrating to developed countries [7, 8]. Intra- and inter-country migration of health workers potentially compromises the quality of health service delivery by creating uneven distributions of providers in relation to populations [9]. The scenario of having health centers without doctors required that the community-based information system should be usable by community-based or indigenous health workers.

It is in this context that in 2003 we conceptualized the project and submitted a proposal for funding to PANASIA-ICT [10] to implement the Community Health Information Tracking System, or CHITS (http://www.chits.info), a primary health care information system. The backdrop of this proposal is a bigger goal to build a national health information infrastructure within the next five years. The community-based information system can contribute to this bigger goal by improving health information management at the community level.

We deemed the following four objectives important for project success:

1. To design and develop a generic, reusable, open-source framework for community level health information systems for primary health care services
2. To determine the feasibility of integrating vertical programs at the community level.
3. To enable and empower community health center staff to use this community based health information system through the development of certificate training courses for community-based data managers.
4. To harness community resources for the sustainability of health information management activities

2. Methodology

Lorenzi enumerated four cornerstones of health informatics [11] and we deemed it important to embellish these to address the objectives above as follows:

Cornerstone 1: Producing structures to represent data and knowledge so that complex relationships may be visualized. To develop a generic, reusable, open-source framework for primary care level information systems (first objective) and integrate vertical programs at the community level (second objective), we needed to: (1) create an information system architecture based on conceptual data models revolving around national vertical programs and primary health care services at the community level; (2) build software functionality around data models directly related to health care services and vertical programs; and, (3) design this architecture such that it protects the health information system from extensive code and database revisions that may arise without software modularity.

Cornerstone 2: Developing methods for acquisition and presentation of data so that overload can be avoided. To carry out integration of data collection, integration and presentation activities of the different vertical programs at the user interface level and eliminate paper reporting (second objective), we needed to examine all health center forms and logbooks identified with the different vertical programs and subsequently map out intersecting and unique data elements for each program.

Cornerstone 3: Managing change among people, process and information technology so that the use of information is optimized. To empower community health center staff (third objective), we needed to: (1) determine work motivation factors; and (2) immerse ourselves in the milieu of health center activities for six weeks. To meet the fourth objective, aside from building rapport and a working relationship with the local government units, we needed to: (1) set up partnerships with external resources to create a "bandwagon effect"; and, (2) build external alliances around the project to create an ecosystem of similar applications that support project objectives.

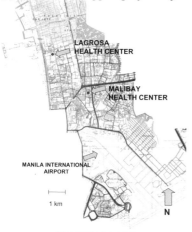

MAP OF PASAY CITY

Figure 1 - Map of Pasay City showing the location of the two health centers in the study

Cornerstone 4: Integrating information from diverse sources to provide more than the sum of the parts and integrating information into work processes so that it can be acted upon when it can have the largest effect. To address the first and second objective, we needed to (1) employ modular, object-oriented software development methods and adapted open-source software created by other developers for integration; (2) model the application from health center workflows and consider the paper-based forms and logbooks as our closest "competition"; and (3) design the application to support vertical and horizontal health information exchange, and incorporate report-generation features to make sure community health workers can make use of the health data that they generate at their level.

To develop and implement CHITS, these methods were applied to two health centers (Lagrosa and Malibay), each with an average coverage of 10,000 families and located in a progressive local government unit with which our university had established a memorandum of understanding for student deployments in community health centers. Figure 1 shows the map of the local government unit of Pasay City where the two health centers are located.

3. Results

We describe the project outcome below according to the objectives previously enumerated.

To design and develop a generic, reusable, open-source framework for primary care level health information systems. We had earlier developed a modular information system architecture called the Generic Architecture for a Modular Enterprise (GAME) Engine [12] that can serve as an applications development platform for other software development projects. This software engine runs on Linux, Apache Web Server, MySQL database and the PHP Scripting Language. GAME makes extensive use of previously published open-source code libraries like JPGRAPH for object-oriented graph display and FPDF, a PDF-generation engine for creating the summary reports. Using this platform, software development was carried out, resulting in the development of 44 software components together with lookup data libraries, including ICD10 Diagnosis Coding. Among these modules is a Clinical Reminders module that enables health center staff to send mobile phone Short Messaging System (SMS) messages, which are generated from system templates, and sent to patients to remind them of follow-up visits and encourage compliance with medication intake, particularly for tuberculosis treatment. New software modules, software upgrades and data dictionaries are uploaded as compressed files and automatically incorporated into the system. The CHITS application currently runs in an intranet environment with a Pentium 4 class server and 3 scaled down Pentium 4 workstations costing about $1,900 at 2003 hardware prices. For the first time since CHITS became operational in one health center, submission of electronic reports has become part of the health ministry procedures for quality accreditation.

To determine the feasibility of integrating vertical programs at the end user level. To integrate the vertical program "information system islands," we used the incremental development approach [13] (Figure 2), developed a single interface for vertical program modules, and integrated report generation tools for the end-user. Figure 3 shows how modules are positioned in CHITS. We involved the health center staff in interface development, and successfully streamlined their workflow as far as vertical programs are concerned. Most importantly, we were able to eliminate "paper forms" by six months.

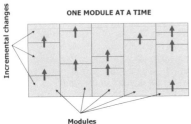

Modules

Figure 2 - Modular and incremental software development. Modules built incrementally and tested in a live environment over time, the red arrows indicating incremental buildup of each module (adapted from Heeks [13]).

To enable and empower health center staff to use this community based health information system through the development of a professionalized training course for community-based data managers. We studied health center culture and social organization using a scaled down ethnographic approach [14, 15] and worked with health center staff for six weeks. We were able to build relationships and an environment of mutual trust, enabling us to have smooth interactions with the health center staff. We incorporated capacity building to present a benevolent face to potential and obstinate change management areas, such as quality-adverse data habits. The end users became effective trainors themselves, proudly showing off not only their certificates but also their skills. This provided us with a possible solution to the problem of training staff from other health centers through "on-the-job" training. This also enables us to develop cohorts of technically-enabled end-users. Except for the health center physician module, community health workers operated most of the software modules from health center workstations.

To harness community resources for the sustainability of health information management activities. We were also able to create strategic alliances around CHITS. One example is the Tuberculosis (TB) registry vertical program which attracted the Philippine Coalition Against TB (PhilCAT), a well-funded implementing arm of the WHO Directly Observed Therapy for Short-Course Strategy chemotherapy (DOTS) for tuberculosis control. Between July and August 2004, two demonstration sessions were conducted for the city health offices of two neighboring local government units (the cities of Parañaque and Marikina). These LGUs have subsequently initiated CHITS deployment and secured their own internal and external funding. In the hardware area, the Advanced Science and Technology Institute (ASTI, http://asti.dost.gov.ph/) of the Department of Science and

Technology (ASTI, a government agency) developed a plug-in PC card that incorporates a GSM modem which enables CHITS to send clinical reminders and receive data by SMS. To support and complement CHITS implementation, we proposed two other projects to the national government: the National Telehealth Project, called BuddyWorks, and the Philippine National Health Information Infrastructure Project, to link health information stakeholders and enable information exchange. Both projects were subsequently funded through the e-government program of the national government and actually form part of the initial activities of the emerging Department of Information and Communications Technology. These projects provide a primary care and public health informatics environment where CHITS becomes an integral component.

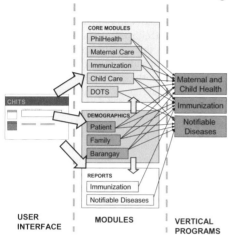

Figure 3 - Flow of information from user interface, processing within modules and reorganization of information to health ministry vertical programs in CHITS. Only selected modules and vertical programs are shown here.

4. Discussion

Designing community-based health information systems is a challenging task that involves simultaneous work along technical, social, political, and financial fronts. Chandrasekhar enumerates systemic constraints related to a developing country's economic status that are breeding grounds for skepticism towards the potential of information and communications technologies (ICTs) to have a positive impact on health services delivery. First, an overwhelming majority is likely not to have access to technology. Second, inadequate education would ensure people do not have adequate levels of competence or confidence to take part in transformational activities [16]. By using the rich library of open-source tools available online, by integrating capacity building, and harnessing external, national and local government political and funding support, we hope to have addressed these systemic constraints.

In this project, we have developed a generic, reusable, open-source framework and a community-based health information system that integrated vertical programs at the community level. There are three lessons we learned from this project: First, by paying close attention to health center culture and immersing ourselves in the end-user's social context, we captured an accurate model of their organizational and personal realities, and were able to gain insight into their needs and requirements. We then applied these insights, together with the health center information and data model, into software code – in a process called evolutionary software development using a modular approach with incremental introduction of change [13]. These insights were also applied to the design of a certificate data management course for community health workers that brought out their potential to be able to manage the change brought about by technology and allowed us to "indoctrinate" them about the importance of data quality and the bigger information ecosystem where health center data and information belong. Second, open-source software, aside from enabling us to decrease implementation costs, provided an environment for software code transparency for peer-review purposes and fostered shared learning. Traditional proprietary software development otherwise hides internal processes as it happens in a software "blackbox." Third, we discovered that it is important to have a heightened awareness of the "ecosystem" in which the health information system will function. Included in this ecosystem are the people who will make it work (community health workers), the people who make things possible, logistically and politically, and the enabling environment to use the system and derive benefits from it.

In the end, implementing this system became a battle for "hearts and minds" as we created and managed change in implementing a community-based health information system, first, by looking at how the people involved viewed things from their perspective, and then by giving them the software and knowledge tools to manage the change.

5. Acknowledgements

The authors wish to thank the local government unit of Pasay, the physicians and staff of the Lagrosa and Malibay Health Centers, and the faculty and staff of the Department of Family and Community Medicine for their support in implementing the project. The authors also wish to thank PANASIA-ICT, IDRC (International Development and Research Centre of Canada) and UNDP (United Nations Development Programme) for funding support to implement this project. Herman thanks Michael McNeill of the Centers for Disease Control and Prevention for providing insight into the menagerie of words that can be used to express the collaborative nature of the project.

6. References

[1]	Department of Health, Philippine Government. Philippine Health Sector Reform Agenda (HSRA). URL: http://www.doh.gov.ph/.
[2]	Jayasuria R. Health informatics from theory to practice: lessons from a case study in a developing country. MEDINFO95 Proceedings. Greenes et.al. (editors). IMIA 1995; pp 1603-1607.
[3]	Anonymous. An integrated approach to communicable disease surveillance. WHO Weekly Epidemiological Record (WER), Jan 7 2000, 75:1, page 1.
[4]	Kanshana S, Simonds RJ. National program for preventing mother-child HIV transmission in Thailand: successful implementation and lessons learned. AIDS. 2002 May 3;16(7):953-9. Review.
[5]	Kilmarx PH, Supawitkul S, Wankrairoj M, Uthaivoravit W, Limpakarnjanarat K, Saisorn S, Mastro TD. Explosive spread and effective control of human immunodeficiency virus in northernmost Thailand: the epidemic in Chiang Rai province, 1988-99. AIDS. 2000 Dec 1;14(17):2731-40.
[6]	Henderson DA. Victory over smallpox: interview with Donald A. Henderson. Popul Rep L. 1986 Mar-Apr(5):L172-3.
[7]	Fleck F. Should I stay or should I go [News]. Bulletin of the World Health Organization. August 2004; 82(8):634.
[8]	Jaymalin M. DOLE chief sees silver lining in exodus of doctors, nurses abroad. URL: http://www.newsflash.org/2004/02/hl/hl101202.htm. Last accessed: 3/14/2005.
[9]	Bach S. Migration patterns of physicians and nurses: still the same story? Bulletin of the World Health Organization. August 2004; 82(8): 624-625.
[10]	PANASIA-ICT web site. URL: http://web.idrc.ca/en/ev-51764-201-1-DO_TOPIC.html. See also URL: http://web.idrc.ca/en/ev-51764-201-1-DO_TOPIC.html.
[11]	Lorenzi N. The cornerstones of medical informatics. Journal of the American Medical Informatics Association. 2000; 7:204-205.
[12]	GAME Engine Sourceforge Web Site http://www.sourceforge.org/game-engine/.
[13]	Heeks R. Failure, Success and Improvisation of Information Systems Projects in Developing Countries. Institute for Development Policy and Management. Document last viewed at URL: http://www.man.ac.uk/idpm/idpm_dp.htm#devinf_wp. January 2002.
[14]	Friedman C. Subjectivist approaches to evaluation. In Evaluation Methods in Medical Informatics. Springer, New York. 1997; 205-221.
[15]	Myers M. Investigating information systems with ethnographic research. Communications of the Association for Information Systems. December 1999; 2(23).
[16]	Chandrasekhar CP, Gosh J. Information and communications technologies and health in low income countries: the potential and constraints. Bulletin of the World Health Organization. 2001; 79(9): 850-855.
[17]	Clements P [editor]. Constructing Superior Software, Software Quality Institute Series. MacMillan Publishing, USA, 2000. Page 59.

Address for Correspondence:

Herman D. Tolentino, MD, Medical Informatics Unit, University of the Philippines, College of Medicine, 547 Pedro Gil Street, Manila, Philippines 1000, Email: herman.tolentino@gmail.com

Connecting Medical Informatics and Bio-Informatics
R. Engelbrecht et al. (Eds.)
IOS Press, 2005

An eConsent-based System Architecture Supporting Cooperation in Integrated Healthcare Networks

Joachim Bergmann, Oliver J Bott, Ina Hoffmann, Dietrich P Pretschner

Technical University of Braunschweig, Braunschweig, Germany

Abstract

Objectives: The economical need for efficient healthcare leads to cooperative shared care networks. A virtual electronic health record is required, which integrates patient related information but reflects the distributed infrastructure and restricts access only to those health professionals involved into the care process. Our work aims on specification and development of a system architecture fulfilling these requirements to be used in concrete regional pilot studies.
Methods: Methodical analysis and specification have been performed in a healthcare network using the formal method and modelling tool MOSAIK-M. The complexity of the application field was reduced by focusing on the scenario of thyroid disease care, which still includes various interdisciplinary cooperation.
Results: Result is an architecture for a secure distributed electronic health record for integrated care networks, specified in terms of a MOSAIK-M-based system model. The architecture proposes business processes, application services, and a sophisticated security concept, providing a platform for distributed document-based, patient-centred, and secure cooperation. A corresponding system prototype has been developed for pilot studies, using advanced application server technologies. The architecture combines a consolidated patient-centred document management with a decentralized system structure without needs for replication management. An eConsent-based approach assures, that access to the distributed health record remains under control of the patient.
Conclusion: The proposed architecture replaces message-based communication approaches, because it implements a virtual health record providing complete and current information. Acceptance of the new communication services depends on compatibility with the clinical routine. Unique and cross-institutional identification of a patient is also a challenge, but will loose significance with establishing common patient cards.

Keywords:
Integrated Health Care Systems; Interdisciplinary Communication; Medical Record Linkage; Computerized Medical Record; Patient Data Privacy

1. Introduction

Economical needs for efficient healthcare in line with quality goals lead to a progressive diversification and specialization of health professions and processes, requiring enhanced communication, coordination, and documentation. Significant problems are well known in various clinical settings (see for instance [1], [2], [3]): the lack of current, complete and timely information, and shortcomings in control and coordination of care processes.

Instantiation of the shared care paradigm in regional healthcare networks is one approach to overcome these problems.

A common approach for building up an efficient communication system for integrated healthcare networks is the replacement of traditional paper-based messaging processes with their electronic equivalents. Pure messaging results in faster communications and may be appropriate for many tasks, but does not lead to an integrated lifelong medical record, because most parts of the record are fragmented and spread over various care providers like in paper-based systems. Advanced information system architectures supporting shared care should provide a patient-centred integrated health record as described in several approaches, e.g. Synapses [4], PICNIC [5], or government initiatives like e-toile [6], the Australian Health*Connect* and Canada Health Infoway. These architectures, enabling the authorized health professional to acquire current and complete information nearly whenever needed, require sophisticated security and administration concepts, because many distributed entities are going to provide and request information under different access conditions [7], using various data formats and patient ID schemes. Generally it has to be guaranteed, that access to a patient's medical information is restricted only to health professionals involved into the care process within the required scope [8].

This paper presents an architecture for secure information sharing in integrated healthcare networks addressing the requirements mentioned above.

2. Materials and methods

A methodical analysis has been performed in a healthcare network using MOSAIK-M [9], a framework and tool environment which supports modelling, simulation, and animation of information and communication systems in medicine. A generic process scheme guides projects in producing system models of high quality in terms of correctness, completeness and validity. A meta model defines the modelling language for these models. A UML-based modelling tool allows modelling of organizational structures, applications, and information structures, while processes are expressed with Petri nets. For a better participation of medical staff during modelling and specification phases, the model allows simulation and animation of communication and data processing activities.

The complexity of the analysis was reduced by focusing on the exemplary scenario of thyroid disease care. Thus it was possible to limit the number of communication processes and documents to a manageable amount, while the application field is comprehensive enough to show cooperation between various specialists.

Analysis of the problem domain resulted in an *"As is"-model* of the current situation of thyroid disease care. Subsequently, the model was transformed into a *"To be"-model*, which was validated and improved in a workshop with representative participants of the healthcare network. Based on this architecture model, an advanced prototype system was built, which is currently being evaluated in the European funded project INCA (INtelligent Control Assistant for diabetes, www.ist-inca.org) addressing telemedical issues in diabetes care, and in a project supporting the communication between general practitioners and a hospital in a regional setting.

3. Results

Result of analysis and specification is an architecture for distributed information processing in integrated healthcare networks, specified with means of a formal MOSAIK-M model and implemented as an advanced system prototype.

From analysis phase and recent publications, two basic requirements for a system architecture supporting efficient shared care are derived. First, the architecture should support migration from provider-based and isolated information management to consolidated patient-centred documentation [10]. Second, the architecture should reflect the decentralized infrastructure in integrated healthcare networks [6,8]. The proposed concept is intended to merge these apparently oppositional requirements of a consolidated but decentralized information management. It focuses on the virtual integration of distributed documents in order to share information between participating healthcare parties, allowing a health professional's information system to become part of the *Distributed Electronic Health Record* (DEHR).

Patient-oriented clinical document

Key elements are the *patient-oriented clinical documents* provided by healthcare institutions with respect to the following policy:

- The patient as subject of information recorded in the care process holds the *exploitation rights* to related documents. He is able to monitor, authorize and constrain document usage.

- A health professional providing care for the patient is a *trusted manager* of those documents he creates referring to the patient (stewardship).

- The patient *authorizes* a health professional, who is involved into the care process, to access the shared distributed health record. This authorization includes the right to forward granted privileges, e.g. in case of consultations or laboratory requests.

A clinical document is always assigned to an overall identified patient. This requires a common ID-service like a patient card or a master patient index.

Contribution, retrieval and messaging in a Distributed Electronic Health Record

The fundamental concept of a DEHR is, that each clinical document resides where it is originated without copying it to a central server or sending it to a receiver. Fig. 1 shows a simplified configuration of a healthcare network.

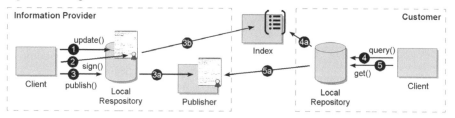

Fig. 1 – Simplified configuration of a shared healthcare network

Contribution. The document is processed locally (1) within the *Local Repository*, until the author or an executive declares it finished and to be of interest for the virtual record. The author signs the current version (2) and subsequently initiates the "publication" process (3), which stores the signed document onto the *Publisher* (3a) and forwards a characterizing reference to this document (so-called *Document Descriptor*) onto the patient's *Index* (3b).

Retrieval. Whenever access to a document is required, the client queries its Local Repository (4), which at first processes the query locally and subsequently adds the results from requesting the patient's index (4a). From this list of Document Descriptors, the health professional decides about relevant documents and subsequently requests them from the related Publisher (5, 5a). The resulting documents can either be exported from the DEHR or viewed with a DEHR viewer, provided from a *Catalogue* service (not depicted).

Messaging of information about a patient between two care providers, e.g. posting the order for an expert consultation or subsequently sending back the result, can also be seen as access to a document being part of DEHR. Additionally, a message referring to the document has to be transferred, indicating that it has become available.

In order to avoid multiple documentation in DEHR and in the locally used information systems, the Publisher concept allows integrating these legacy information systems (LIS) into DEHR by encapsulating them with a *Mounter* (see fig. 2).

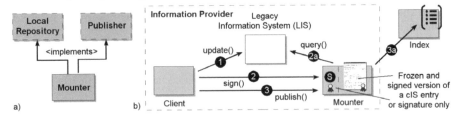

Fig. 2 – UML model (a) and functionality of a Mounter (b)

Information is processed within the LIS (1), until the health professional "freezes" a specific artefact of the legacy system with a digital signature onto the mounter (2, 2a) and publishes it like a generic document (3, 3a) under a common ID. For retrieval from outside, the mounter checks the authorisation of a query, maps the common ID-space into the LIS domain and forwards the resulting request to the LIS (not depicted). If the LIS allows to lock a document or a well-defined information unit as finished and invariant, the mounter only has to store a signature (S) instead of a whole document, with which integrity and authorship of the information unit are ensured.

Electronic consent

Since accessing medical documents in a DEHR is not limited to the health professional's own repository, the architecture has to ensure, that a query to the virtual record is permitted by the patient. Thus an eConsent-concept [11] is introduced, which electronically reproduces the contract between patient and health professional. The patient creates a digital certificate, referring to a health professional and including access privileges and a validity period:

$$eConsent^{p, h} := (p, h, v, R)$$ given patient p, health professional h, validity period v, and set of privileges R.

This certificate is always sent with a request and authorizes its owner to attend the distributed health record according to granted access privileges. To cover the case of consultation, a health professional is granted a non-transferable privilege to forward the eConsent to a further expert. This new eConsent represents a contract between the primary health professional and the expert to be consulted. It includes the original consent of the patient to prove the health professional's legitimation concerning patient p:

$$eConsent^{h, h'} :=$$
$$(h, h', eConsent^{p, h}, v', R')$$
given health professionals h and h', validity period v' covered by v, and privileges $R' \subseteq R$.

This concept implies a public key infrastructure (PKI) including equipment for creating qualified digital signatures.

Health professional authorization

Whenever a health professional requests a document, he has to authenticate to the remote service with an end-to-end-security challenge/response process, based on health professional cards [12]. The remote service checks the identity of the user and of the following transferred credentials:

- an eConsent object representing the patient's consent, and
- an attribute certificate, which is stored on the health professional card and represents the user's roles within the healthcare system. This certificate is supposed to be issued by the German association of CHI physicians in the near future.

After verification of the credentials against a Trusted Third Party, the service processes the request. Due to end-to-end authentication and the attribute certificates, there is no need for a common authentication service or a central repository of users and roles.

Proof of concept: trial system V-Net Med

The trial system V-Net Med (Virtual Medical Network) was developed to prove the architecture in pilot studies. Apache Web Services with SOAP messages are used, allowing flexible deployment and implementation-independent client systems. Clinical information is recorded in HL7 CDA Release 1 documents [13] and wrapped with a digital signature following the PKCS#7 Cryptographic Message Syntax Standard. "Black-box" documents containing any kind of information (e.g. PDF) are supported.

Although Apache's SSL connectivity with client authentication is used exclusively, the system operates through a VPN to enhance security. For digital signature, a commercially available qualified signature card (T-Systems PKS SigG card) is used.

4. Discussion and Conclusion

The requirement of a *consolidated patient-centred documentation* can be achieved by virtual integration of documents, where the unique and cross-institutional identification of a patient is done with the help of a patient card. The requirement of *distributed management of information* is achieved with publication services, providing documents directly from the source system (or from an outsourced storage node, if continuous availability cannot be guaranteed due to network configuration). This respects an author's properties of the information he has recorded, whereas a sophisticated security concept grants access only to the health professionals involved into the care process. The patient is always able to control and restrict the access to the shared record. Granting privileges derived from the original contract between patient and health professional allows a health professional to consult an expert and thus forward a constrained authorisation. The architecture provides a vision similar to a *Health Bank* [10, 14], with the patient deciding about the locations of his document collections (the indexes) and probably many institutions competing for his trust.

On the other side, some challenges currently constrain deployment of the proposed architecture. First, publication services have to guarantee high availability to provide a reliable shared record, which requires an advanced and probably expensive infrastructure within the healthcare network. Second, a common identification infrastructure has to be established. This could be achieved either by a patient card or a person identification service, which maps several ID domains together. Third, acceptance of the new communication services depends on a transparent fitting into clinical routine without disarranging well-working processes.

New architectures supporting cross-institutional cooperation are more and more requested from the increasing number of healthcare networks. A trend towards national platforms providing common services for integration of distributed information can be found in several countries. The report of the CEN/ISSS e-Health Standardization Focus Group [15] determines the necessity of coordinating these approaches and recommends a Europe-wide eHealth interoperability platform. There is a growing market for a new type of software connecting healthcare systems together. But concerning interoperability between legacy systems, not even the problem of interoperability on a functional level is currently solved. For instance, OMG's healthcare interoperability specifications are not widely used and the OASIS standards from the eBusiness field are recently being explored by medical informatics. The HL7 Clinical Document Architecture provides a helpful common syntax for information exchange in the presented project. But semantic interoperability remains a major issue. CDA Release 2 with its templates and Reference Information Model is an important step in this direction, as well as the two model approach (archetype and reference model) recently introduced into the CEN EN 13606 revision.

5. References

[1] Kvamme OJ, Olesen F, Samuelson M. Improving the interface between primary and secondary care: a statement from the European Working Party on Quality in Family Practice (EQuiP). *Qual Health Care.* 2001; 10:33-9.

[2] Wilson S, Ruscoe W, Chapman M, Miller R. General practitioner-hospital communications: a review of discharge summaries. *J Qual Clin Pract.* 2001; 21:104-8.

[3] Stiell A, Forster AJ, Stiell IG, van Walraven C. Prevalence of information gaps in the emergency department and the effect on patient outcomes. *CMAJ.* 2003; 169:1023-8.

[4] Grimson J, Stephens G, Jung B, Grimson W, Berry D, Pardon S. Sharing Health-Care Records over the Internet. *IEEE Internet Computing.* 2001; 5:49-58.

[5] Bruun-Rasmussen M, Bernstein K, Chronaki C. Collaboration--a new IT-service in the next generation of regional health care networks. *Int J Med Inform.* 2003; 70:205-14.

[6] Geissbuhler A, Spahni S, Assimacopoulos A, Raetzo M, Gobet G. Design of a Patient-centered, Multi-institutional Healthcare Information Network Using Peer-to-peer Communication in a Highly Distributed Architecture. *Medinfo.* 2004; 2004:1048-52.

[7] Scott RE, Jennett P, Yeo M. Access and authorisation in a Glocal e-Health Policy context. *Int J Med Inform.* 2004; 73:259-266.

[8] Van der Haak M, Wolff A, Brandner R, Drings P, Wannenmacher M, Wetter T. Data security and protection in cross-institutional electronic patient records. *Int J Med Inform.* 2003; 70:117-30.

[9] Bott OJ, Bergmann J, Hoffmann I, Vering T, Gomez EJ, Hernando ME, Pretschner DP. The INCA-Project: Specifying a Telemedical System for Closed-Loop Therapy of Diabetes using MOSAIK-M. Accepted for Proceedings of MIE 2005.

[10] Shabo A, Vortman P, Robson B. Who's Afraid of Lifetime Electronic Health Records. *Proceedings of 1st Annual Conference on Mobile and Wireless Healthcare Applications 11 - 14 November 2001, Café Royal, London.* 2001.

[11] O'Keefe C, Greenfield P, Goodchild A. A Decentralised Approach to Electronic Consent and Health Information Access Control. *J Res Prac Inf Tech.* 2004; 37:137-154.

[12] Wenzlaff P. The German electronic doctor's license: the introduction of a health professional card. *Stud Health Technol Inform.* 2003; 96:218-23.

[13] Dolin RH, Alschuler L, Beebe C et al. The HL7 Clinical Document Architecture. *J Am Med Inform Assoc.* 2001; 8:552-69.

[14] Ramsaroop P, Ball MJ. The 'Bank of Health' - A Model for More Useful Patient Health Records. *MD Computing.* 2000; 17:45-8.

[15] Report from the CEN/ISS e-Health Standardization Focus Group - Current and future standardization issues in the e-Health domain: Achieving interoperability. 2005.

Address for correspondence

Dipl.-Inform. Joachim Bergmann, Technical University of Braunschweig, Institute for Medical Informatics Muehlenpfordtstr. 23, D-38106 Braunschweig, Germany, J.Bergmann@mi.tu-bs.de
www.mi.tu-bs.de

Connecting Medical Informatics and Bio-Informatics
R. Engelbrecht et al. (Eds.)
IOS Press, 2005

The ISO/IEC 9126-1 as a Supporting Means for the System Development Process of a Patient Information Web Service

Alexander Hörbst[a], Kerstin Fink[a], Georg Goebel[b]

[a]Leopold-Franzens University Innsbruck, Innsbruck, Austria
[b]Medical University Innsbruck, Innsbruck, Austria

Abstract:

The development of patient information systems faces the mayor problems of increasing and more complex content as well as the introduction of new techniques of system implementation. An integrated development demands for a method to deal with both aspects. The ISO/IEC 9126-1 offers a framework where both views can be integrated to a general view of the system and can be used as a basis for further development. This article wants to introduce the ISO/IEC 9126-1 as a supporting means for the development of patient information systems considering the example of a web service for a patient information system.

Keywords:
Patient information system; ISO/IEC 9126; System development; Functional design; Technical design, Web service

1. Introduction

Patient information systems are becoming more and more important as the amount of information available on the health sector increases steadily [5]. But not only the availability and increasing amount of information determine the importance of patient information systems. Also the increasing need for organising and structuring the available information centres the development of patient information systems.

Apart from content concerns new techniques and concepts like Web Services or the Semantic Web technology offer a whole new range of applications to patient information systems [4,6]. Therefore also implicate increased demands on the development of patient information systems.

This states that the development of patient information systems faces two mayor challenges [6]:

- The process of system development must comply with the increasing complexity and amount of available content.
- The development has to integrate new available techniques in the implementation process of the system.

This implies that the cooperation of persons from different fields like computer science or medicine as well as the integration of their interests is a crucial factor for the success in developing such systems [3,7]. The need for cooperation and integration leads to the problem of organising those teams from different fields in a system development process.

2. The ISO/IEC 9126

The ISO/IEC 9126 is a considerable norm for the evaluation of software products and was issued by the International Standardization Organisation in cooperation with the International Electrotechnical Commission in the year 2001. The norm divides into 4 parts:

- Part 1: Quality model
- Part 2: External metrics
- Part 3: Internal metrics
- Part 4: Quality in use metrics

The first part of the norm, the quality model, primarily deals with the establishment of a system of characteristics and subcharacteristics for the definition of software quality.

The second, third and fourth part of the norm deal with the development of criteria for the actual measurement of the characteristics defined in part one.

In this context only the first part of the ISO/IEC 9126 is to be considered important for the support in the development of patient information systems. This can be traced back to the fact that the first part provides consistent terminology through the definition of characteristics and subcharacteristics for software product quality. These characteristics also provide a framework for specifying quality requirements for software, and making trade-offs between software product capabilities.[1]

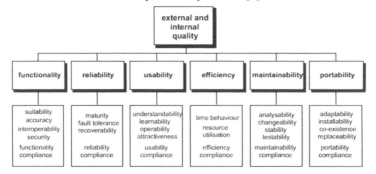

Figure 1 – External and internal quality characteristics [1]

The first part of the ISO 9126 is furthermore divided in 2 parts where the first part deals with external and internal quality and the second part covers quality in use. Quality in use offers characteristics how the quality of the system can be described from the user's point of view in a specific context or environment. Whereas internal and external quality requirements specify the level of required quality from the internal/external view of the product.[1] Figure one shows all the characteristics and subcharacteristics defined by the ISO 9126 for internal and external quality.

3. A Web Service for a patient information system

Figure 2 and figure 3 show the actual implementation of the ISO 9126-1 in the development of a Web Service for a patient information system.

The figures show the characteristics und subcharacteristics of the ISO 9126 as well as an extract from the developed requirements for this Web Service going from the root to the branches of the mind map. This list of requirements is not exhaustive. It should exemplify how the ISO 9126 can be used in an actual system development process. The concept of this Web Service was developed in [2] and aimed for the development of a Web Service to assist a patient during the process of a breast cancer treatment. The idea for the Web Service is based on a scenario which was developed together with physicians from the University Hospital in Innsbruck [8].

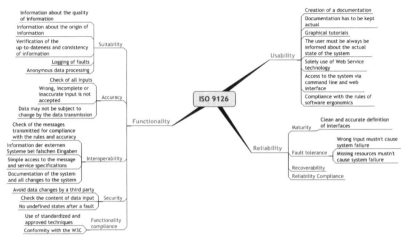

Figure 2 – Part 1: Actual implementation of the ISO 9126 in a Web Service for a patient information system

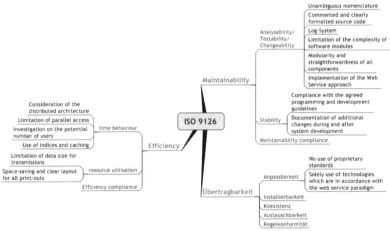

Figure 3 – Part 2: Actual implementation of the ISO 9126 in a Web Service for a patient information system

The figures show that the ISO 9126-1 with its terminology renders a structured approach for the developing team possible.

4. Discussion

The use of the ISO 9126 has a great impact on the system development process and helps to solve and assist respectively in solving several problems during the development process:

- The ISO 9126-1 provides the developing team with a consistent terminology and structure and offers a proofed framework.
- The norm helps with the definition of clear objectives for the further steps of the development process of the system.
- It can be used as a basis for a system specification.
- The ISO 9126 addresses functional as well as technical aspects in its framework.
- The integration of external and internal quality characteristics gives a complete overview of the system.
- The Framework can be used in different levels of development cause of the general terminology. This means that the ISO can be used as an accompanying throughout the whole development process.

However the ISO 9126 itself isn't sufficient to be solely used to describe all requirements of a patient information system in detail. The ISO 9126 can only be used as an initial means, to provide the further methods of system development with a structured basis of information.

5. Outlook

As mentioned in paragraph four, the ISO 9126 assists in the system development process but can not be used solely for the system description. The next step should be to define a complete system development process based on the use of the ISO 9126 as well as to further elaborate the characteristics and subcharacteristics given by the norm to better match the specific needs of the system development process in patient information system and health information systems respectively.

6. References

[1] International Organization for Standardization: ISO/IEC 9126 Software engineering – Product quality – Part1: Quality model. 15/06/2001.

[2] Hoerbst, A.: The use of Web Services with health information systems. 06/09/2004

[3] Balzert, Lehrbuch der Software-Technik, Spektrum akademischer Verlag, Heidelberg 1998

[4] Chaudhary, A.S.; Saleem, M.A.; Bukhari, H.Z.: Web Services in Distributed Applications Advantages and Problems. 2002. URL: http://citeseer.ist.psu.edu/548303.html [01/10/2004].

[5] Goebel, G.: A Datamodel for an Austrian Comsumer Health Information System. Dissertation Innsbruck University. 04/2002.

[6] Miksch, S.; Cheng, K.; Hayes-Roth, B.: An Intelligent Assistant for Patient Health Care. 1996. URL: http://citeseer.ist.psu.edu/miksch96intelligent.html [01/10/2004].

[7] National Library of Medicine: Medical Subject Headings. 15/04/2004; URL: http://www.nlm.nih.gov/mesh/meshhome.html [01/10/2004].

[8] Szolovits, P.; Doyle, J.; Long, W.J.: Guardian Angel: Patient Centered Health Information Systems. 1994. URL: http://citeseer.ist.psu.edu/szolovits94guardian.html [01/10/2004].

Address for correspondence:

Dr. Georg Goebel, Dept of Medical Statistics, Informatics and Health Economics, Medical University of Innsbruck, Schoepfstrasse 41, A-6020 Innsbruck, Austria, Email: Georg.Goebel@uibk.ac.at

Connecting Medical Informatics and Bio-Informatics
R. Engelbrecht et al. (Eds.)
IOS Press, 2005

Can *open*EHR Archetypes Empower Multi-Centre Clinical Research?

Sebastian Garde[a], Petra Knaup[b], Thilo Schuler[a,c], Evelyn Hovenga[a]

[a] *Health Informatics Research Group, Central Queensland University, Rockhampton, Australia*

[b] *University of Heidelberg, Department of Medical Informatics, Heidelberg, Germany*

[c] *University of Freiburg, Department of Medical Informatics, Freiburg, Germany*

Abstract

*The Electronic Health Record is of utmost importance to enable the provision of high-quality collaborative care; one prominent development is open*EHR*. On the other hand, a systematic approach to support the use of routine data for multi-centre clinical research is becoming increasingly important. One example of this is the extensible architecture for using routine data for additional purposes (**eardap**) which features comprehensive terminological support. However, as experiences in various medical fields have shown, the terminology-based approach is limited to specialized fields and it is argued that a comprehensive terminology is simply too complex and too difficult to maintain. As the open*EHR *archetype approach does not rely heavily on big standardized terminologies, it offers more flexibility during standardisation of clinical concepts and overcome the shortcomings of terminology-focused approaches. It is unknown, however, how far the more generic open*EHR *approach can also enable re-use of routinely collected data for clinical research purposes – the use case for which **eardap** was designed. We therefore explored the feasibility of using the open*EHR *approach to support multi-centre research in comparison to **eardap***. Generally speaking, our results show that both **eardap** and open*EHR *are suitable to enable the use of routine data for multi-centre clinical research. As the open*EHR *approach also ensures open, future-proof Electronic Health Records, we conclude that it is highly desirable that multi-centre clinical trials adopt open*EHR*.*

Keywords:
Electronic Health Record, Terminology, *open*EHR, Medical Informatics, Clinical Trials

1. Introduction

The Electronic Health Record (EHR) is of utmost importance to provide high-quality collaborative care. EHRs have the potential to offer simultaneous remote access to patient data, increased legibility of the documents, flexible data layout and analysis, integration of information resources, and tailored paper output [1]. In real life, however, a considerable amount of information stored in the records is obsolete, redundant, duplicated, or indecipherable or even contradictory to the extent that it does not benefit the patient at the point of care. To solve this problem, several approaches are currently being explored. Two prominent examples are the Clinical Document Architecture (CDA) [2] which is primarily focussed on documents and document exchange, and the *open*EHR approach ([3], http://www.openEHR.org) which focuses on the semantic interoperability of complete EHRs or EHR extracts and is the basis for the new European standard [4].

On the other hand, a systematic approach to support the use of routine data for clinical research is becoming more important. To support clinical trials in medical fields where the treatment is complex, the severity of the illness high or the incident rates low, collaborative research efforts are vital and information technology support is essential. Such multi-centre clinical trials may even cross national borders. There are powerful data collection, management and Remote Data Entry (RDE) systems for clinical trials ([5], [6]) and even multi-centre clinical trials ([7]). Some of them provide solutions for single terminological aspects like the translation of Case Report Forms (CRFs), for the administration of measurement units and conversion factors. However, there are very few offering a comprehensive terminological support which is useful for conventional trials, desirable in multi-centre trials and absolutely necessary in cooperative groups of multi-centre clinical trials [8]. One example that supports comprehensive terminological support is **eardap** [9].

Still, the terminology-based approach is limited to specialized fields as research in various medical fields has shown [10], [11] and it is argued that a comprehensive terminology is simply too complex and too difficult to maintain [12]. As the *open*EHR archetype approach does not rely on big standardized terminologies but micro-vocabularies [13], it would offer more flexibility during standardisation of clinical concepts and overcome the shortcomings of terminology-focused approaches. Further, *open*EHR provides the basis for future-proof, medico-legally sound EHR systems. While this is not in the focus of **eardap** it might still be valuable for ongoing multi-centre research.

It is unknown, however, how far the more generic *open*EHR approach for Electronic Health Records can also enable the use of routine data for multi-centre research purposes – the use case **eardap** was designed for. We therefore explored the feasibility of the *open*EHR approach to support this and compared its characteristics in detail with **eardap**.

The overall aim of this paper is to answer the research question - to what extent is *open*EHR suitable for multi-centre research environments. We will

- outline essential criteria for collaborative research environments,
- show to what extent these criteria are fulfilled by **eardap** and *open*EHR, and
- highlight differences, advantages and disadvantages between **eardap** and *open*EHR.

2. Material and methods

2.1.   *openEHR and archetypes*

The aim of *open*EHR is to enable the development of open specifications and software for EHR systems. *open*EHR is based on the results of the GEHR-Project of the European Union. GEHR is an acronym for Good European Health Record respectively later Good Electronic Health Record. Following GEHR several projects extended and refined its results (e.g. the Synapses and SynEx projects). All these projects influenced the *open*EHR architecture. *open*EHR has pioneered a two level modelling approach for EHRs ([3]). An overview of this approach is given in Figure 1. The first level is the reference information model which is pared down to the minimum to support the medico-legal requirements and record management functions. This ensures that clinicians can always send information to another provider and receive information which they can read – thus ensuring data interoperability. The second level involves the *open*EHR archetype methodology – a way of sharing evolving clinical information so that it can be processed by the receiving provider – thus ensuring semantic interoperability. A blood pressure archetype for example represents a description of all the information a clinician might want or has to report about a blood pressure measurement. Basically, one archetype therefore represents one clinical concept.

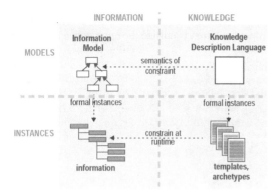

Figure 1: Overview of the openEHR two level modelling approach for EHRs ([3]).

Through the use of freely available archetype tools, e.g. the Archetype Editor, clinical groups are empowered to control the way that EHRs are built up, using designed structures to express the required clinical data and assuring that all necessary constraints on the values of record components are observed. This ensures that all data in an EHR system is valid at two levels, because it conforms both to an information model, and to domain-designed concept definitions. Design principles of *open*EHR are described in more detail in [14], but the key innovation of the *open*EHR architecture is that it separates record keeping concerns from clinical data collection using archetypes [15] and thus enabling **patient-centred, longitudinal, comprehensive** and **prospective** EHRs.

2.2.   eardap

eardap as an extensible architecture for using routine data for additional purposes was developed to suit the needs of multi-centre clinical research in a multi-hospital environment [9]. It focuses less on generic characteristics which Electronic Health Records must feature. **eardap** can be characterized as terminology-based and component-based architecture. **eardap** consists of 3 main components: core system, terminology management system (TMS) and module generator (*Figure 2*). Main advantage of **eardap** is the comfortable extensibility of any implemented architecture by new items and new research questions. Like *open*EHR **eardap** is concept-oriented. In contrast, however, its architecture is based on object-relational modelling supported by the TMS. The module generator is used each time a new module has to be generated or an existing one has to be adapted. If the underlying terminology has to be changed, the TMS is used: further modules will then be built upon the changed terminology. Once the definition of a terminological system for a trial in the TMS is finished, a consistent, corresponding relational database can be created within short time and without any informatics skills. The process of building forms takes place under strict terminological control. Generated research-specific modules can then be used by the **eardap** core system in the medical centres.

3.   Results

Based on our intensive requirements analyses with multi-centre trial environments (e.g. [8], [16]), we developed criteria that are desirable for a multi-centre research environment. These criteria are in harmony with other research (e.g. [5], [6], [17]) and are in the following applied to both **eardap** and *open*EHR. For each criterion a description of how well it is supported by either approach as well as an overall assessment is given (Table 1). Assessments are given using the following scale: ++, +, +–, –, ––. As a baseline, +– is given if the specification of the respective approach allows the criteria to be fulfilled but is either not yet implemented or the scope of the implementation is outside the approach.

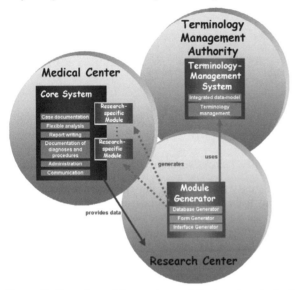

Figure 2: Overview of the eardap architecture in a typical eardap environment.

4. Discussion

Generally speaking, our results show that both **eardap** and *open*EHR are suitable to enable the use of routine data for multi-centre medical research. **eardap** excels in providing highly integrated tools for convenient analysis and report writing – exclusively based on the terminology provided and therefore usable for all scenarios. Further, mechanisms for high data quality are supported by **eardap** through its warning and error integrity constraints. *open*EHR excels in enabling a more flexible standardisation process and making internationalisation and localisation feasible through concept-oriented multi-language support and specialisation of archetypes. Further *open*EHR enables data and semantic interoperability via its generic information model, archetypes and EHR extracts.

Our experiences in paediatric oncology in Germany have shown the applicability of the **eardap** architecture for national research [9]. The functions of our core system – including additionally chemotherapy decision support based on the system – were in routine use in several hospitals all over Germany [16]. With **eardap** special emphasis has to be laid on interfaces to local hospital information systems and data security.

The *open*EHR approach is currently being trialed in Australia in the framework of Health*Connect* (http://www.healthconnect.gov.au), the Australian initiative for a national health information network and used in further projects [18]. First results are promising.

In this paper we have considered **eardap** and *open*EHR solely in the context of how well they support clinical research based on routine clinical data; the primary purpose of *open*EHR – laying the foundation for sound Electronic Health Records - of course is slightly different. Our criteria do not intend to generally assess approaches to Electronic Health Records.

Independent of the approach used, the degree of reuse of routine data for multi-centre research is highly dependant on the quality of the terminology used. Our experiences confirm that terminology harmonization, maintenance and general governance are key factors for success in this area and a challenging task in a multi-centre project. The greater flexibility during standardization processes offered by the *open*EHR archetyping is of great value here.

Table 1: Overview of all criteria and how well they are supported by eardap and openEHR.

Criteria	eardap		openEHR	
Usable for basic data set documentation	Yes.	++	Yes.	++
Data validation/integrity constraints	Sophisticated model for warning and error integrity constraints, intra- and inter-contextual.	++	Error integrity constraints can easily be applied in one archetype (one context). Warning constraints or inter-contextual constraints are indirectly supported by templates and invariants.	+
Support for multiple trial terminologies[1]	Yes, inbuilt.	++	Not inherently supported by *open*EHR. Achievable through specialized archetypes and external control which archetypes are to be applied.	–
Support for evolving terminologies	Yes, possible via new or adapted research-specific module based on terminology server and created by **eardap** module generator.	++	Yes, as *open*EHR features a standard information model. For incompatible changes a new version of the archetype and adequate update routines are needed.	++
Automatic form generation	Yes, via Form Building Component.	++	In the future, via templates, GUI-Generator.	+–
Specialisation of concepts allowed	Indirectly via specialized data in research-specific module.	+	Yes (basic feature of archetypes).	++
Supports rapid cross-patient analysis	Integrated (standard and flexible analysis based on terminology).	++	Possible to implement even retrospectively based on archetypes, but not integrated.	+–
Supports report writing	Integrated (based on terminology and templates).	++	Possible to implement, but not integrated.	+–
Provides data basis for decision support modules	Yes, but have to know database schema.	+	Yes, based on archetypes.	++
Export/Import of Data	Possible via HL7 or own protocols. Context has to be established.	+	Possible via *open*EHR EHR Extracts based on archetypes. Context is guaranteed.	++
Degree of standardization needed	Flexible through common terminology (e.g. basic data set) that is extendable by research-specific terminologies.	+	Even more flexible through specialisation and because only commonly used archetypes have to be standardized.	++
Degree of governance needed	Only essential to agree on basic data set by all parties. Further items can be standardised.	+	Only essential to agree on standardized archetypes that are used by all parties, more flexible.	++
Possibility for internationalisation (international trials)	Not easily achievable.	—	Yes, possible via context-based translation of archetypes.	++

While HL7 primarily defines messages between applications and HL7 CDA is a generic model for the communication of clinical documents, and in this is similar to openEHR Transactions, openEHR's focus is the EHR as a whole. The Clinical Data Interchange Standards Consortium Operational Data Model (CDISC ODM) as a format for clinical trial

---

[1] Various trial terminologies extending the basic terminology and are applied based on patient characteristics like diagnosis.

data exchange could support data exchange between openEHR and non-openEHR clinical trial systems.

5. Conclusion

It can be concluded that *open*EHR can support multi-centre research based on routine clinical data about as well as **eardap**. As, in addition, *open*EHR inherently offers valuable features of Electronic Health Records, we recommend that multi-centre clinical trials adopt the *open*EHR approach for their research activities. For higher efficiency and data quality, some of the features **eardap** excels in could be applied in addition to the *open*EHR methodology.

6. Acknowledgements

The authors wish to thank all those who have contributed with commitment and enthusiasm to the *open*EHR and **eardap** projects.

7. References

[1] Powsner SM, Wyatt JC, and Wright P. Opportunities for and challenges of computerisation. *Lancet* 1998; 352(9140):1617-22.
[2] Dolin RH, Alschuler L, Beebe C, Biron PV, Boyer SL, Essin D, Kimber E, Lincoln T, and Mattison JE. The HL7 Clinical Document Architecture. *J Am Med Inform Assoc* 2001; 8(6):552-69.
[3] Beale T. Archetypes: Constraint-based Domain Models for Future-proof Information Systems OOPSLA 2002 workshop on behavioural semantics., 2002.
[4] CEN/TC 251. EHRCOM prEN 13606-1. Health informatics — Electronic health record communication — Part 1: Reference model. 2004.
[5] Duftschmid G, Gall W, Eigenbauer E, and Dorda W. Management of data from clinical trials using the ArchiMed system. *Med Inform Internet Med* 2002; 27(2):85-98.
[6] Kuchinke W, Eich HP, and Ohmann C. Software for Remote Data Entry and Clinical Trials: Review of Commercial Solutions and Trends 46. annual meeting of Deutsche Gesellschaft für Medizinische Informatik, Biometrie und Epidemiologie (gmds), Urban & Fischer, Cologne, 2001. 205-6.
[7] Abdellatif M and Reda DJ. A Paradox-based data collection and management system for multi-center randomized clinical trials. *Comput Methods Programs Biomed* 2004; 73(2):145-64.
[8] Merzweiler A, Weber R, Garde S, Haux R, and Knaup-Gregori P. TERMTrial - Terminology-based documentation systems for cooperative clinical trials. *Comput Methods Programs Biomed* 2005; to appear
[9] Knaup P, Garde S, Merzweiler A, Graf N, Weber R, and Haux R. Towards shared patient records: An Architecture for Using Routine Data for Nationwide Research. *EuroMISE 2004: EFMI Symposium on Electronic Health Record, Health Registers and Telemedicine. Prague, 12.-15.4.2004.* 2004;
[10] Brown PJ. Coming to terms with datasets for diabetes care. *Diabetes Nutr Metab* 2000; 13(4):215-9.
[11] Cimino JJ. Terminology tools: state of the art and practical lessons. *Methods Inf Med* 2001; 40(4):298-306.
[12] Rector AL. Terminology and concept representation languages: where are we? *Artif Intell Med* 1999; 15(1):1-4.
[13] Health Level 7. HL7 EHR System Functional Model: A Major Development Towards Consensus on Electronic Health Record System Functionality - A White Paper. 2004.
[14] Beale T, Goodchild A, and Heard S. EHR Design Principles. *open*EHR Foundation; 2001.
[15] Goodchild A, Gibson K, Anderson L, and Bird L. The Brisbane Southside HealthConnect Trial: Preliminary Results Health Informatics Conference (HIC), Brisbane, 2004.
[16] Garde S, Baumgarten B, Basu O, Graf N, Haux R, Herold R, Kutscha U, Schilling F, Selle B, Spiess C, Wetter T, and Knaup P. A meta-model of chemotherapy planning in the multi-hospital/multi-trial-center-environment of pediatric oncology. *Methods Inf Med* 2004; 43(2):171-83.
[17] Silva JS, Ball MJ, Chute CG, Douglas JV, Langlotz CP, C. NJ, and Scherlis WL. *Cancer Informatics - Essential Technologies for Clinical Trials.* New York: Springer, 2002.
[18] Bird L, Goodchild A, and Tun Z. Experiences with a Two-Level Modelling Approach to Electronic Health Records. *Journal of Research and Practice in Information Technology* 2003; 35(2)

Address for correspondence

Dr. Sebastian Garde, Health Informatics Research Group, Faculty of Informatics and Communication, Central Queensland University, Rockhampton Qld 4702, Australia , s.garde@cqu.edu.au, Ph +61 (0)7 4930 6542, Fax +61 (0)7 4930 9729, http://infocom.cqu.edu.au/hi

Connecting Medical Informatics and Bio-Informatics
R. Engelbrecht et al. (Eds.)
IOS Press, 2005

Brazilian National Standard for Electronic Form Interchange among Private Health Plan and Healthcare Providers

Jussara Macedo Pinho Rötzsch, Rigoleta Dutra Mediano Dias, Marcia Franke Piovesan, Maria Angela Scatena, José Leôncio de Andrade Feitosa, José Ricardo Fragoso Peret Antunes, Ceres Albuquerque

National Supplementary Health Agency (NSHA), Rio de Janeiro, Brazil

Abstract

Since 1988 the Federal Constitution of Brazil declared health care as a public right to be provided as a duty of the state[1]. Thus the Unique Public System ("Sistema Único de Saúde-SUS"), Ministry of Health, a comprehensive health care system with full coverage, was created since then. But the private sector has nevertheless also been operating since 1960s but without any government regulation at all. It serves approximately twenty-five per cent of the Brazilian population (estimated at 180 million of people).
The National Supplementary Health Agency – NSHA ("Agência Nacional de Saúde Suplementar- ANS") was created in 2000 and is in charge of regulating and assisting the private health plan organizations. The public sector has been structuring its information systems for almost 15 years, defining standard schemes, such as the National Health Card Project, in order to institute a national unique identifier health care and to construct a national repository of health records.
The lack of widely common information standards in the private sector, however, and the difficulties involved in the complex information interchange among private health plan organizations and health providers have caused NSHA to work out a proposal for a national standard for electronic form interchange proposal, based on XML technology, known as the supplementary health information interchange (TISS – "Troca de Informação em Saúde Suplementar"). The TISS project aims integrating healthcare information nationwide; therefore it was developed in accordance with the National Health Card Project, using the same unique identifiers and others standard sets proposed by the Ministry of Health, such as unique identifiers of providers.
NSHA has presented the TISS project successfully to all stakeholders and is going to introduce legislation to enforce the standards. There are more than two thousands private health plan organizations in the whole country and more than ten thousands hospitals and clinics. Private health practioners, including dentists, will also have to adopt the standard. As a matter of fact, the TISS project not only focuses on the patient billing but also on epidemiological information. And the TISS project is not only for health provider claims, but also to all kinds of events such as consultation and exams.

Keywords:
Medical Informatics; Information Technology, Electronic Data Interchange, Health Information Systems, Health Plan Management, Health administration;

1. Introduction

The National Supplementary Health Agency (NSHA) was instituted in 2000 to regulate private health plan organizations and also to evaluate health care services [2]. This private sector has been operating since 1960s, even a little before, without any government regulation at all. There are different kinds of organizations such as physicians' and dentists' groups, insurance companies, employer sponsored, professional associations, philanthropic and odontological care organizations. All these kinds of organizations differ mainly in their forms of management. Some of them aim no profit, some share their profit within the group, and some do not provide a medical network but only free choices. Information asymmetry has led NSHA to acquire economic, demographic and epidemiological information from all the organizations.

Due to the complex relationship between private health plan organizations and health providers the reliability of the information collected about patient assistance has been extremely poor. With the Interamerican Development Bank (IDB) sponsor, which had defined only eleven months for the project development, the TISS project has been built and has established the electronic standards for information interchange related to such assistance. The beginning of the project was on August 2003 and ending on July 2004. NSHA adopted the strategy of researching some standards established in Brazil and also from abroad [3, 4, 5, 6, 7, 8, 9, 10], for instance, ISO/TC 215 [11], CEN/TC 251 [13]' Health Level Seven [14] and OpenEHR [15]. The unique keys to identifying beneficiaries, health plan organizations, health plan characteristics (types of coverage and regions code), providers and so on were a priority in the project. Afterwards the standards were presented to stakeholders who have found the project very important for defining strategic actions throughout the private health sector and even minimizing administrative costs.

The TISS project defined seven types of standard billing forms, covering consultation, exams and hospitalization data. The electronic technology chosen for the interchange was XML (Extensible Markup Language) because it is a simple and very flexible text format derived from SGML (ISO 8879) [16]. Originally designed to meet the challenges of large-scale electronic publishing XML is also playing an increasingly important role in the interchange of a wide variety of data on the Web and elsewhere. The DTD (Data Type Definition), which is a formal description in XML Declaration Syntax of a particular type of form, was defined with a list of elements for all seven types of billing forms. In addiction to the billing forms, a standard form as a return (called return-form) from the private health plan organizations to the providers was also designed. Nowadays few providers receive any describing what is going to be paid, or not, by the private health plan organization. The return-form also has a DTD to describe all the data covered.

2. Material and methods

More than fifty forms that are interchanged among private health plan organizations and providers were analyzed by NSHA. A matrix was designed containing all information in order to ascertain which are common ones. Several visits were also made to hospitals, clinics and private health plan organizations to permit identifying how the information interchange works. Many stakeholders were interviewed as well.

Some public health information systems were also analyzed to identify the national unique keys already in use in Brazil [17] such as:

- National Health Card [18], in order to adopt the same national unique beneficiaries identifier;

- national providers database [19], in order to adopt same national unique identifier for the providers. This database includes all types of medical and odontological providers: physicians, dentists, clinics, hospitals and so on.

Some private health information systems were also analyzed (these systems are developed by NSHA for information collection from the private health plan organizations) to identify the unique keys already in use in the private market such as:

- private health plan organizations database, in order to adopt one same national unique identifier for the health plan organization;
- health plan registration database, in order to adopt one same national unique identifier for the health plan.

Chart 1 shows private health information flow among private healthcare providers, health plan organizations, NSHA and SUS (Unique Public System).

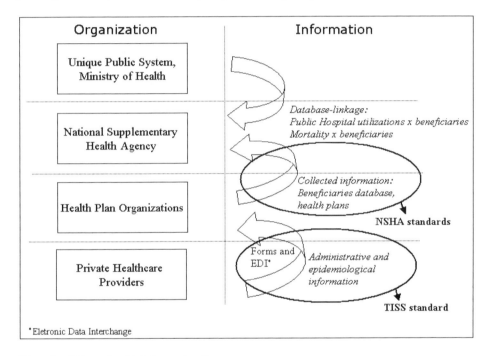

Chart 1 – Private health information flow

The TISS project also includes the development of downloadable and free software to permit those organizations to adopt the electronic standard interchange and have any difficulty in developing an information system. The TISS software is available for both private healthcare organizations and health care providers. The software is divided in two different kits:

- kit one: specifically for the private health plan organizations;
- kit two: specifically for all types of medical and odontological providers.

The kit one permits XML export for the return-form and import of the standard billing forms. The kit two permits just the opposite: XML export for the standard billing forms and import of the return-form. Web-based technology has not been chosen considering that this kind of technology would be difficult for some organizations because it would be necessary to maintain a great security structure. Delphi Borland compiler with Interbase database was the selected technology.

As eleven months were a short period for the project development it was necessary to choose an appropriate methodology. The use case methodology, associated with the relational database model, was then selected to define the requirements of the system, to act as a springboard for the software design, to validate the software design, for software test and quality assurance and also as an initial framework for the on-line help and user manual. Each kit contains around a hundred use cases. This methodology has been considered extremely relevant for the success of the software development, considering the short period of time for assembling it.

3. Results

The TISS project was then presented to stakeholders as a first approach to create a national standard for the claim forms and electronic interchange in the private market. Four seminars have held in different regions in Brazil since August 2004: Northeast region (State of Ceará), South region (State of Paraná), Southeast (States of Rio de Janeiro and São Paulo). NSHA has published claim forms and DTDs in its Web site. The software is still being tested in some organizations.

Several electronic mails have been received by NSHA with respect to the project, considered one of the most important projects for strategic purpose in the private health plan market. Nowadays few organizations interchange billing information electronically, even being aware of the gains in terms of administrative costs or as a factor for rationalization and for clarification of transactions among players. Some organizations have already changed their billing forms to adapt them to those ones proposed by NSHA.

Even the software, which at the beginning was considered not relevant to the standard, is now being requested by the organizations. Not only to use it, by also to analyze how the functions were defined and how the data model was built up to implement all the standards keys. Organizations consider that, in future, performance indicators will be much more easily established and even comparability among health plans for quality assurance[19].

The TISS standards will probably change the format of the information systems in the health organizations. So far NSHA has spent about 300,000 US Dollars in the project. It is still difficult to estimate the total cost so that all players become TISS standards-compliant because they can either adopt the TISS software or another low-cost software or, on the other extreme, pay much money to update their information system. NSHA is now actively working to determine what the savings will be and expects them to be substantial since the adoption of the standardization will improve the efficiency and quality of health care.

A permanent committee on health standards will be set up so that experts should discuss all possible changes in depth. The permanent committee will have to face some challenge in the coming years, for instance: adequate safeguards for the security and privacy of the information, the acquisition of indicators to measure performance, the information dissemination to society and so on. The permanent committee shall include representatives of private health plan organizations, providers, consumers, purchasers and policy- makers.

4. Discussion

NSHA is not itself a standard producer organization. Its intention is to stimulate the adoption of national information and terminology standards and unique keys identifiers in order to permit interoperability between different information systems throughout the public health system and the private sector in the country, minimize variability and data interpretation. This incentive will certainly support the national health information network. It is relevant to mention that NSHA already uses database-linkage methodology to identify beneficiaries of private health plan in the National Vital Statistics on Mortality [21] and in the SUS Database of Hospital Utilization [22].

Standardization is recognized as an essential discipline for all players within the economy, and Electronic Data Interchange (EDI) is increasing more and more. The expansion of EDI has occurred due to the expansion of techniques and technology. EDI has been adopted in many activities such as banks or information routes. In Brazil banks have already adopted a standard information interchange for compulsory use.

It is not different in health activities. Effective and efficient information interchange in health can certainly improve quality of healthcare. In the Unique Public System (SUS) all hospital claims are interchanged in electronic way. However in private health sector, EDI is far less common. The TISS project has started a nationwide discussion about this matter. Oftentimes all players have tried to implement a national standard information interchange, but with no success. It is now expected that NSHA will not only intermediate this discussion, but also enforce the adoption of national mandated standards, based on the premise that voluntary conformity leads to hybrid, with dilutes the proposal of standards 23. The proposed version of the TISS project standards was submitted to a two-month stakeholders comment on February 2005.

5. Conclusion

A standard electronic data interchange (EDI) on private health sector will enforce preparation for health organizations. It will probably demand some time before it is adopted, but it is strongly recommended in this sector. The TISS project has defined electronic standard for information interchange, but another standards will be necessary in the future: terminology, private classification of interventions and so on. Next steps should be related to the security information interchange concerning mainly the international code of diseases, which will also be interchanged.

NHSA considers that this project will be very relevant for the sector even with all the difficulties of implementing it. The process of managing a national standard for information interchange among private health plan and healthcare providers will be constantly evolving and broadly participative.

6. Acknowledgments

NHSA would like to thank all in-house staff involved with the TISS project and all outside groups for their contributions from many Brazilian States (Rio Grande do Sul, São Paulo, Rio de Janeiro), especially our consultant, Beatriz de Faria Leão [24], who kindly helped us to launch his project.

7. References

[1]   Ministério da Saúde. MS - Agência Nacional de Saúde Suplementar – http://www.ans.gov.br
[2]   International approaches to the electronic health record. Volume 3. Part one. Commonwealth of Australia, 2003 – ISBN: 0642823316
[3]   Object Management Group – http://www.omg.org
[4]   Digital Imaging and Communications in Medicine. DICOM - http://medical.nema.org

[5]   Association for Electronic Health Care Transactions. AFEHCT- http://www.afehct.org
[6]   National Uniform Billing Committee. NUBC - http://www.nubc.org
[7]   Australian Department of Health and Ageing - http://www.health.gov.au/healthonline
[8]   Canadá Health Infoway– http://www.infoway.ca
[9]   German Institute of Medical Documentation and Information -http://www.dimdi.de/de/ehealth/karte/index.htm
[10]   Health Insurance Portability Accountability Act. HIPAA – http://www.hipaa.org
[11]   International Standards Worldwide. ASTM – http://www.astm.org
[12]   International Organization for Standardization. ISO/TC 215
[13]   European Standardization of Health Informatics. CEN/TC 251 - http://www.tc251wgiv.nhs.uk/pages/default.asp
[14]   Health Level Seven. HL7-ANSI - http://www.hl7.org
[15]   Open Electronic Health Records. OpenEHR – http://www.openehr.org
[16]   World Wide Web Consortium. W3 - www.w3.org/XML/
[17]   Ministério da Saúde. MS – http://www.saude.gov.br
[18]   Ministério da Saúde. MS - Sistema Cartão Nacional de Saúde. SCNS - http://dtr2001.saude.gov.br/cartao/
[19]   Ministério da Saúde. MS - Cadastro Nacional de Estabelecimentos de Saúde - http://cnes.datasus.gov.br
[20]   National Committee for Quality Assurance. NCQA – http://ncqa.org
[21]   Ministério da Saúde. MS – http://tabnet.datasus.gov.br/tabnet/tabnet.htm#EstatVitais
[22]   Ministério da Saúde. MS – http://www.datasus.gov.br/
[23]   CIOS: Mandate Clinical Standards - http://www.healthmanagement.com/htlm/portalstory.cfm?type=gov%DID=12296
[24]   Leão BF. Padrões para representar informações em saúde. In: I Seminário Nacional de Informação e Saúde: O setor saúde no contexto da sociedade da informação. Série Fiocruz: eventos científicos, 3. Rio de Janeiro: Fundação Oswaldo Cruz, 2000; pp. 21

14. Address for correspondence

Avenida Augusto Severo– 84 – 10 andar –20021.040- Rio de Janeiro – Brazil
Phones: 55-21-2105-0157 /55 –21–2105-0356
email: tiss@ans.gov.br

Connecting Medical Informatics and Bio-Informatics
R. Engelbrecht et al. (Eds.)
IOS Press, 2005
983

Distributed and Mobile Collaboration for Real Time Epidemiological Surveillance during Forces Deployments

Hervé Chaudet[a,d], Jean-Baptiste Meynard[b], Gaëtan Texier[a], Olivier Tournebize[c], Liliane Pellegrin[d], Benjamin Queyriaux[a], Jean-Paul Boutin[a]

[a] Département d'Epidémiologie et de Santé Publique, IMTSSA, Marseille Armées, France

[b] Département d'Epidémiologie et de Santé Publique, EASSA, Paris Armées, France

[c] MEDES, Centre National d'Etudes Spatiales, Toulouse, France

[d] Laboratoire d'Informatique Fondamentale, UMR CNRS 6166, Faculté de Médecine, Marseille, France

Abstract

This paper presents a pilot project of a real time syndromic surveillance system in French armed forces for early warning of biological attack by mass destruction weapons. For simulating the situation of a theatre of operations and its organisation, an electronic syndromic surveillance system covering all branches of service in French Guiana (about 3,000 persons) has been deployed and connected to a surveillance centre in France. This system has been design taking in account a collaborative view of epidemiological surveillance and the mobility of forces in extreme conditions. Several kinds of hardware, from rugged personal digital assistant to desktop computer, and several telecommunication links, from PSTN to satellite data links, are used. This system allows a quick report of cases, which are georeferenced. In the first results, some problems associated with the human and the technical aspects have been reported, in association with some immediate advantages.

Keywords:
Public health informatics; Epidemiology; Syndromic surveillance; Tele-epidemiology; Real time surveillance; Biological warfare

1. Introduction

At their November 2002 meeting in Prague, NATO Heads of State and Government have decided to endorse the implementation of 5 defence initiatives against weapons of mass destruction, including the development of an interoperable disease surveillance system for early warnings [1]. Within this framework, and facing the increasing threat of mass destruction weapons during forces deployments, the French armed forces have decided to acquire the capacity of detecting biological attacks by the mean of a real time epidemiological surveillance system.

The objective of 2SEFAG project ("Surveillance Spatiale des Epidémies au sein des Forces Armées en Guyane") is precisely to build a pilot project of a real time surveillance system taking in account the medical, environmental, technical and organizational specificities of armed forces in deployment, in order to evaluate the feasibility and advantages of such a system before its generalisation.

Disease early warning system in this context has the special feature of being distributive and mobile. Distributive because keeping under surveillance the apparition of early clinical and biological symptoms in the forces requires a coordinated contribution from a large number of people representing several professional specialities (from medical aid to epidemiologist) that are distributed amongst the 4 branches of service (army, air and naval forces, gendarmerie) and the common services (e.g. military health service system), and localized in different distant places. Mobile because the population under surveillance and the observers shall operate in distant and difficult situations, as in deserts or equatorial forests, where communication links are sparse and uncertain, and where geolocation of epidemiological information is especially valuable. Despite these constraints the surveillance system must keep its real time and early warning capabilities.

The aim of this paper is to focus on the way the architecture of our pilot system of tele-epidemiology has taken in account the distributed and mobile aspects of surveillance activity and the first lessons learned.

2. Context and related works

From the military side, early warning capability has been a main concern for a long time. A recent review of these systems has been published in [2]. Near all these syndromic surveillance systems collect medical structure activities, as J95/EpiNATO, which has been used in the NATO forces in Balkans since 1996, or as EWORS and LEADERS systems from US Navy and US Air Force. Special mention must be made for the British PRISM system, which is based on a hand-held data input device connected to a portable phone. It allows sending a georeferenced set of signs and symptoms concerning a soldier to an analysis centre located in Great Britain. Although technically promising, the military physicians use only 10% of the PDAs currently deployed in the Gulf Area.

While biological attacks by mass destruction weapons concern armies, bioterrorist threat is a civilian matter, even if the same agents may be encountered in both situations. This is why the civilian world has also developed syndromic surveillance systems, essentially since the events of Fall 2001. However, civilian surveillance involves many different systems, concerns a large general population with a mass of medical structures and health indicators, and is less influenced by mobility problems [3,4]. The need to extend the diversity of "epidemiological sensors" to individual care providers, emergency calls, clinics, hospitals and laboratories, with their own information systems, raises the requisite for standard formats (e.g. HL7) and secure information technology infrastructure based on Internet connectivity integrated with existent infrastructure for public health surveillance [5]. But the risks of erroneously using data not initially intended for surveillance purpose and the barriers to electronically communicating information outside a healthcare structure in a context of wide syndromic surveillance have been emphasized [6]. Face to this diversity, which is a characteristic of civilian surveillance that is also met in joint task forces, the adoption of functional surveillance standards to facilitate data integration for proper threat assessment and response support has been advocated [7]. The closer civilian experience to our problem, from a technological point of view, is a training exercise for terrorism and disaster response using telehealth technologies [8].

3. Material and method

Design constraints

The design constraints of this project were to (a) enforce the circulation organisation of epidemiological information on operation theatre (Figure 1), which is a fundamental organisational requisite based on the circulation of general health information and command decisions; (b) be syndromic oriented to allow attack early warning; (c) georeference declared cases for allowing risk mapping; (d) be connected to the composition of the exposed population to identify secondary cases and epidemic potentials; (d) be used in extreme conditions; (e) cover and coordinate all branches of service existing in French forces; (f) simultaneously watch several high epidemic capacity diseases; (g) experience several modes of electronic transmission; (h) determine the constraints and limits of use of various hardware.

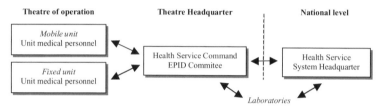

Figure 1: Circulation of epidemiological information on operation theatre

Face to these constraints, we have chosen to deploy our pilot project in French Guiana because its geographical characteristics and the military presence realistically mimic an operation theatre with extreme conditions (forest, humidity). All military personnel present in French Guiana were concerned by the surveillance system. For this pilot experiment, the medical personnel were required to electronically report the presence of about 40 clinical signs and symptoms for each case of fever, with a special orientation toward the detection of hemorrhagic signs due to the presence of arboviruses in this country.

Collaborative functional architecture of the surveillance system

The operational organisation of the human network associated with the surveillance system has been precisely drawn up. The result is summarised in Figure 2. The system architecture has been specifically designed according to this organisation. This leads us toward a secure collaborative system allowing (a) the building of a population database with the identity, appointment, and address of each member of the military personnel; (b) the building of a minimal electronic patient record that links identities with missions' compositions and GPS daily trackpoints, syndromic declarations, biological results and patient following; (c) the electronic circulation and exchange of information by email, including epidemiological information feedback; (d) access to all system functionalities wherever the user may be located and whatever the hardware.

Identity database updating is made in Unit Medical Centres and must especially reflect personnel transfers (about 1,500) that occur every 4 months. Before each mission departure, its composition is entered in the system. This allows identifying risk exposure and the history of exposure for each personnel member. Every member of medical personnel can enter epidemiological and medical data, depending on his access to patient's information. During a mission, syndromic information is georeferenced with the GPS positioning of the mission at declaration time. Otherwise, the declaration reference is given by the medical centre geolocation or may be the patient's address. During a mission, information (at least the daily mission track point) is sent every evening.

Epidemiologists directly made data validation and quality controls using electronic support, and information feedback possibilities.

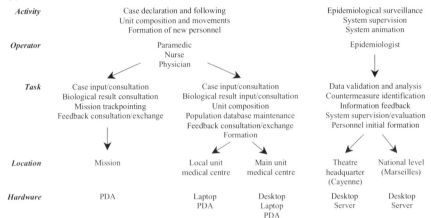

Activity	Case declaration and following Unit composition and movements Formation of new personnel		Epidemiological surveillance System supervision System animation	
Operator	Paramedic Nurse Physician		Epidemiologist	
Task	Case input/consultation Biological result consultation Mission trackpointing Feedback consultation/exchange	Case input/consultation Biological result input/consultation Unit composition Population database maintenance Feedback consultation/exchange Formation	Data validation and analysis Countermeasure identification Information feedback System supervision/evaluation Personnel initial formation	
Location	Mission	Local unit medical centre	Main unit medical centre	Theatre headquarter (Cayenne)	National level (Marseilles)
Hardware	PDA	Laptop PDA	Desktop Laptop PDA	Desktop Server	Desktop Server

Figure 2: Functional organisation of 2SEFAG, showing the tasks belonging to each network member depending on their specialisation, location and decisional level

Technical solutions

This project was the opportunity to demonstrate and test several telecommunication systems and kinds of computers depending on work location (Figure 3).

Missions were equipped with a 'PDA-pack' made up of a rugged (IEC529 – MIL STD810F) Personal Digital Assistants (GoBook Q100 Itronix®) with an internal GPRS card, a waterproof (IEC529 IPX7) Magellan GPS, and a CAPSAT® TT-3060A Mini-M Inmarsat station. A second battery pack was added for each electronic material.

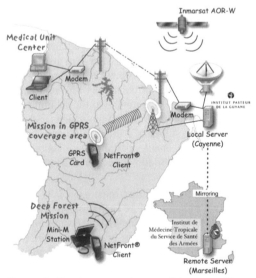

Figure 3: Deployment schema of the surveillance system in French Guyana, showing the technical solutions that have been adopted.

Each Unit Medical Centre is equipped with a 'Wintel' desktop or laptop computers (Windows® 2000/XP, line power protection, 56K V92 modem). The servers were Pentium based computers with Windows 2003, 56K V92 external modems, external ISDN 128K adaptors, internal Ethernet 100Mb cards and power protections.

The software development was based on Lotus Domino® / Notes®, Java enabled Internet Clients (NetFront®), and was conceived to reduce the bandwidth use. Due to the risk of retransmitting a same declaration, the system regularly verifies the presence of doubles. All communications are secured. The most complete securing is active between Medical Unit Centres and the servers, and is based on dedicated clients, point-to-point connection over PSTN using X.509 client certification authentication and using Secure Socket Layer (SSL) with 128 bits encryption. Because of technical constraints imposed by GPRS and satellite communication characteristics (restriction of communication to some usual ports), only SSL 128 bits encryption is used for these two channels, which use the Internet infrastructure between the reception antenna and the servers. The servers communicate directly by point-to-point connection over PSTN or ISDN using X.509 client certification and SSL encryption. The servers' Internet connections are protected by firewalls. Every computer involved in the surveillance network is dedicated to this activity and disconnected from other computers. The local server, in communication with each network client in French Guiana, was located in Cayenne's Pasteur Institute, and was used as production server. The database is mirrored every hour on the remote server in Marseilles. In case of difficulty, the remote server had the possibility of replacing the local server.

Deployment of the network to on board of patrol boats (P-400) via non-rugged PDA and satellite communications was planned but not currently implemented.

4. First results and lessons learned

Deploying the surveillance system required 5 weeks of 3-persons missions in French Guiana besides organisational and administrative works in the research team. These missions were used for informing the local commands, training the medical personnel and the future training officers about surveillance instructions, hardware and software (each training session was 2 days long), installing and testing the hardware, the communication links, and the software in each Unit Medical Centre and in Pasteur Institute.

A total of 8 medical centres have been equipped with the configurations described above and with 10 PDA-packs for the missions under their responsibilities, and their medical personnel have been trained. The surveillance network covers a susceptible population of about 3,000 people all over French Guiana. Since the beginning of the surveillance in October 2004, between 10 and 15 cases a month have been electronically declared, and no outbreak has been reported. The emailed exchanges were essentially made between unit doctors and epidemiologists.

During this period, 3 kinds of problems have been identified:

1. From a human point of view, the main problem is identity database updating. The amount of work associated to this task has required the development of specific software for importing the main part of this information from other military databases. Some other problems were associated with administrative relations with local telecommunication providers as this project aimed to use non-military telecommunication links. Another important human problem is the acceptability of the excess load of the PDA-pack in a mission backpack (about 3.5 Kg).

2. The instability of the electric power supply in remote medical centres that are at power line ends and some problem of reliability with PSTN links. The weak satellite bandwidth (2.4 kbps at best with Inmarsat data link) is also a concern.

3. The hardware was the origin of some connection instabilities and plug correspondence problems between the PDAs, the GPS and the Mini-M, and between the desktops and the external modems. Depending on the mission duration, the power autonomy of the PDA-pack may also be a concern, as solar chargers are unusable (missions stop only at evening when the sun is down and they represent another excess load).

We have however observed some immediate advantages concerning (a) the case declaration, which is processed within an hour (in comparison to a week for the usual declaration periodicity in the army); (b) the immediate identification of every potential contact subject from the mission or the unit composition; (c) the use of the network electronic infrastructure for informing the medical personnel about the case declaration quality and for use precisions at the user's request; (d) the possibility of using this same infrastructure for a specific information about local diseases coming from epidemiological intelligence, increasing in this way the clinical and epidemiological awareness of local medical teams; (e) the potential use of mission trackpoints for the research of geographical risks related to cases of parasitic diseases (e.g. leishmaniasis).

In conclusion, some perspectives may be drawn from this pilot project before its final evaluation. As a biological attack is quite improbable in French Guiana, and in the absence of a natural outbreak despite the presence of several arboviruses, there is a place for one or more real scale outbreak simulation. In this paper we have presented the network architecture, leaving aside the surveillance work of the epidemiologists. The concept of an "epidemiological operational centre" with automatic assistance to surveillance is currently in development and will complete this project.

5. Acknowledgments

We wish to thank here the Cayenne's Pasteur Institute for his participation to this project, and all military medical personnel in French Guiana for their support.

6. References

[1] NATO. Prague summit declaration. Press Release 2002;127 21 nov. 2002. http://www.nato.int/docu/pr/2002/p02-127e.htm.
[2] Meynard J-B, Texier G, Sbai Idrissi K, Ollivier L, Michel R, Gaudry M, Rogier C, Migliani R, Spiegel A, Boutin J-P. La surveillance épidémiologique en temps réel pour les armées. Médecine et armées 2004;32(4):360-65
[3] Lober WB, Karras BT, Wagner MM, Overhage JM, Davidson AJ, Fraser H, Trigg LJ, Mandl KD, Espino JU, Tsui F. Roundtable on bioterrorism detection: information system-based surveillance. J Am Med Inform Assoc 2002;9:105-15.
[4] Teich, JM, Wagner MM, Mackenzie CF, Schafer KO. The informatics response in disaster, terrorism, and war. J Am Med Inform Assoc 2002;9:97-104.
[5] Brennan PF. AMIA recommendations for national health threat surveillance and response. J Am Med Inform Assoc 2002;9:204-6.
[6] Buehler JW, Berkelman RL, Hartley DM, Peters CJ. Syndromic surveillance and bioterrorism-related epidemics. Emerg Infect Dis 2003;9(10):1197-204.
[7] Forslund DW, Joyce EL, Burr T, Picard R, Wokoun D, Umland E, Brillman JC, Froman P, Koster R. Setting standards for improved syndromic surveillance. IEEE Engin Med Biol Magazine 2004; 23(1): 65-70.
[8] Simmons SC, Murphy TA, Blanarovich A, Workman FT, Rosenthal DA, Carbone M. Telehealth technologies and applications for terrorism response: a report of the 2002 coastal North Carolina domestic preparedness training exercice. J Am Med Inform Assoc 2003;10:166-176.

Address for correspondence

Hervé Chaudet, Unité de Recherche Epidémiologique - Département d'Epidémiologie et de Santé Publique, Institut de Médecine Tropicale du Service de Santé des Armées – Le Pharo, 13998 Marseille Armées - France
Email : herve.chaudet@medecine.univ-mrs.fr

Connecting Medical Informatics and Bio-Informatics
R. Engelbrecht et al. (Eds.)
IOS Press, 2005

989

Metasurv: Web-Platform Generator for the Monitoring of Health Indicators and Interactive Geographical Information System.

Laurent Toubiana[a,b], *Stéphane Moreau*[a], *Gaétan Bonnard*[a]

[a]*INSERM U707 "Epidemiologie Systèmes d'Information et Modélisation ", Faculté de Médecine Saint Antoine-UPMC*
[b]*WHO collaborating center for electronic disease surveillance*

Abstract

The control of the transmissible epidemics of diseases requires fast and effective tools for data acquisition, analysis, and information feedback to the actors of health like to general public. We present a tool for the fast creation of platforms of monitoring on Internet allowing the collection and the analysis in real time of the epidemic data of any origin with the dynamic and interactive cartographic representation. A Web-based Geographic Information System (Web-GIS) has been designed for communicable diseases monitoring. The Web-GIS was coupled to a data warehouse and embedded in an n-tier architecture designed as the Multi-Source Information System. It allows to access views of communicable diseases. Thus it is a useful tool for supporting health care decision-making for communicable diseases. This tool is based on the 20 years experiment of the Network Sentinels, with the daily participation of the general practitioners.

Keywords:
Multi-Source Information System; Public Health Informatics, communicable diseases, Population Surveillance, Data warehouse, Internet, Geographic Information Systems, Web-GIS, Decision Support Systems, Management, Environmental Health, Environmental Monitoring/instrumentation/methods.

1. Introduction

During one recent past, several striking events in term of public health emerged with a rare impact. The epidemic of SRAS during the winter 2002-2003 has impressed people [1]. The introduction of New Communication and Information Technologies for help the decision-making in health allowed in many cases, and should still allow better in the future, detecting, locating and circumscribing quickly an unusual situation in term of public health [2,3,4].

The information and communication technologies highlighted their extraordinary capacity as early warning system in the field of the public health.

Since 1984, INSERM (the National Institute of Health and Medical Research in France) in collaboration with the Ministry for health developed an electronic monitoring system for contagious diseases [5,6,7]. On a voluntary basis, a sample accounting for approximately 1% of the French general practitioners, electronically transmits descriptions of the cases of 8 defined pathologies diagnosed during their exercise. This continuous monitoring system made it possible to collect in twenty years, one of the largest data bases of described cases. The demand in term of that kind of systems, allowing the electronic monitoring of the diseases, increases very quikly [8]. Early detection and monitoring systems for other international contagious diseases such as dengue, malaria, brucellosis, and cholera, are being studied. The demand of tools for the installation of systems allowing the remote data acquisition, real-time analysis and the redistribution of information is done increasingly speedily. These systems could show their effectiveness in case of disasters, wars or crises [9,10].

Within this framework, we present a technologic research program entitled MetaSurv. It aims to diffuse among health professionals, the means for the installation of complete monitoring "Sentinel" systems in record time. This device is equipped with graphic and cartographic interactive restitutions of the observed data and accessible on line.

2. Material and Methods

New information system based on n-tier architecture allowed fast and remote access of data sources. SentiWeb, the site of the Sentinels Network [11,12,13], is a typical example of this approach. By means of Internet, morbidity or mortality indicators became available in real time as well as health professionals and public at large. The main idea of the MetaSurv project is to take advantage of the twenty years experience of the sentinel network and the electronic monitoring principle. MetaSurv proposes a strong and highly configurable application in order to adapt to any type of monitoring needs. MetaSurv is very simple to deploy since it is entirely automated, and guides the user step by step. From the creation of a network to data visualization under various representations, the Web interface assists the user to data processing at all steps.

This on line system makes it possible to create very quickly a monitoring network without any special informatics skills. The system regularly profits of the updates without any intervention of users. All operations are supported by a web based interface at: www.scepid.org. Moreover, the fact that it is based on Web technologies, it is accessible everywhere in the world and by means of a simple connection to Internet.

MetaSurv is presented as a Community platform. It should be noted that it makes it possible for lots of users to collaborate within the same unit: the surveillance network. MetaSurv gives the possibility of generating its own surveillance network hosted on a dedicated server. Once the network is created, it is possible for the new administrator, to create as many monitoring modules as he wishes. It is particularly easy to create forms: number of supervised criteria is infinite and numerous types of data are available (Text, all types of number, drop-down list, check box, date). An assistance is available using "Tooltips" in order to precisely inform the sentinel general practitioner. With each creation of surveillance, a model is created that can be modified to be adapted for another new surveillances in order to accelerate the creation of surveillance procedure.

MetaSurv gives to the initiator of a monitoring project, tools making it possible to create and manage a network. We consider that the initiator of the project is likely to motivate sufficient number of medical practitioners to carry out his monitoring. The inscription procedure of practitioners by themselves on the site is the mean to establish and initiate the network. From this time, when the forms and the associated data base tables are generated, the monitoring can be started if there is a valid network in term of representativeness. Consequently, the system proposes to the administrator to forward a pre-written email announcing the setting up of new on line monitoring. The administrator only has to enter the name of the address book of the contacts he wants to participate in the monitoring network.

Once the system is installed and configured and health care professionals are registered to take part in the monitoring project, medical data can be collected via a protected Web interface and be stored in the data base. The use of the "sentinels" system does not require any particular knowledge in data processing. The recruitment of doctor Sentinels wanting to take part in a monitoring is probably one of the major points in the installation of a monitoring. This aspect largely exceeds the limits of this article; however it is important to be aware of the coherence of the sentinel network and the assiduity of these members for the participation in a monitoring. The management of such a network is a heavy task. The MetaSurv project has a large amont of functions facilitating the interactions with the system's users: news, forum, interactive repertory of personal cards, possibility of sharing documents, as well contextual help, automatic mailing generator are available to help the administrator to keeping the network coherent and giving information feedback.

MetaSurv offers several tools enabling access to a synthetic representation of information stored in the data base, as well as tools of early epidemiologic alert [13]. This site is in particular equipped with a geographical information system allowing the diffusion of maps.

This functionality allows the cartographic visualization of the space distribution of the cases reported during one period. These representations allow studying the epidemics spreading dynamics.

Any user can obtain epidemiologic information starting from a query interface common to all types of visualization. Data resulting from this query is presented as tables, graphs (curves and histograms) or charts (representations in space) and interactive maps in "choroplethe", or isocontours. It gives thus either more precise information or another mode of representation according to the context. It is possible to download the monitoring data into files compatible with all spreadsheet software. In the other way, there is an importation procedure to integrate data in MetaSurv.

It runs on a LAMP architecture (Linux, Apache, MySQL, PHP). The geographical maps, charts, and all representations are produced by using Macromedia Flash technology which is used as a technological basis for interactive graphs generation.

3. Results

Most of the functionalities validated in this project were used for the establishment of the SARS site of WHO http://oms.u444.jussieu.fr/ .

The interactive map generation system was selected because of its friendly interactive interface, its flexibility, its fast execution, and its reduced cost as well.

This system is currently used to generate the maps of the "Sentinel Network" http://www.sentiweb.org/ and to manage the sentinel general practitioners address list using the module "PaGeom" of geographical accesses system to the data.

Other sites use these functionalities as MapoFlash http://www.scepid.org/mapoflash/ and GripSite http://www.scepid.org/gripsite/ site of Influenza like Illness experimental epidemiology

4. Discussion

The INSERM Research Unit, U707 "Epidemiology, Information systems and Modeling" proposes through the MetaSurv project, a tool which allows the installation and application of epidemiologic monitoring in any part of the world. It is easy to use and allows dynamic and interactive cartographic representations. This approach not only makes it possible to create, manage and maintain monitoring (collection of information to the redistribution on a large scale of analyses on this information) but it also has several functions for the installation and animation of the networks participating in the process of monitoring. Our twenty years experiment in "Sentinel Surveillance" exhibits that this point is a crucial aspect of the monitoring system because an active participation of Sentinels general practitioners is an indispensable condition for this process. The permanent observation of the evolution in time and space of certain pathologies incidence such as influenza for example, also makes it possible to evaluate the adopted preventive policy (for example closing schools, mass vaccination, or use of antivirals). This tool meets a need for development and improvement of monitoring systems. Computers clearly modified the approach for the monitoring of environment and health. The use of the Internet is probably (currently) an optimal solution. "Sentinels" Systems must be reinforced in the near future, since they proved to be effective tools for the detection of epidemics, and the monitoring to the contagious diseases. As well, they can be employed for epidemiologic goals, but also for the entomological monitoring or to monitor any environmental indicator. This product is on line. It is operational immediately and requires a few minutes to set up any professional's network. Accessible at the address: http://www.scepid.org/metasurv

5. Acknowledgments

This research was funded by a grant from STIC-Santé-Inserm 2002, n°A02126ds, and by Paris 6 University. We thank students of Compiègne University of technology (UTC) and Troyes University of technology (UTT).

6. References

[1]	Teo, P., B.S. Yeoh, and S.N. Ong, SARS in Singapore: surveillance strategies in a globalising city. Health Policy, 2005. 72(3): p. 279-91.

[2]	Ritz, B., I. Tager, and J. Balmes, Can lessons from public health disease surveillance be applied to environmental public health tracking? Environ Health Perspect, 2005. 113(3): p. 243-9.

[3]	Foldy, S.L., et al., SARS Surveillance Project--Internet-enabled multiregion surveillance for rapidly emerging disease. MMWR Morb Mortal Wkly Rep, 2004. 53 Suppl: p. 215-20.

[4]	Toubiana, L. and A. Flahault, A space time criterion for early detection of epidemics of influenza like illness. Eur J Epidemiol, 1998. 14(5): p. 465 470

[5]	Valleron AJ, Bouvet E, Garnerin PH., Menares J, Heard I, Letrait S, Lefaucheux J. A computer network for the surveillance of communicable diseases: the French experiment. Am J Public Health 1986; 76:1289-1292.

[6]	Fourquet F, Drucker J.Communicable disease surveillance: the Sentinel network. Lancet, 1997; 349:794-795.

[7]	Toubiana L, Vibert JF, Garnerin P, Valleron AJ "SITIE: A health care workstation integration architecture for epidemiologists" Comput Biomed Res 1995; 28:100 115

[8]	Halperin W, Baker EL, Monson RR. Public health surveillance. Van Nostrand Reinhold, 1992 (238 pages).

[9]	Morse SS, Rosenberg BH, Woodall J, et coll. ProMED global monitoring of emerging diseases: design for a demonstration program. Health Policy, 1996; 135-153.

[10]	Garshnek V, Burkle FM. Application of telemedicine and telecommunications to disaster medicine. Historical and future perspectives. JAMIA 1999; 6:26-37.

[11]	Flahault A, Dias Ferrao V, Chabety P, Esteves K, Valleron AJ, Lavanchy D. FluNet as a tool for global monitoring of influenza on the Web. JAMA 1998 ; 280:1330-2.

[12] Toubiana L, Viboud C. Flahault A. Valleron AjV Geography and Health. Edition INSERM 1-228, Paris 2003 Boussard, E., Flahault, A., Vibert, J.F., Valleron, A.J., Sentiweb: French communicable disease surveillance on the
[13] World Wide Web. BMJ, 1996. 313: p. 1381-2.

Adress of correspondance

Laurent Toubiana, Inserm U707, Faculté de médecine Saint-Antoine UPCM , 27 rue Chaligny, F-75 571 Paris cedex 12, FRANCE.
Ph: +33 1 44 73 84 52; Fax:+33 1 44 73 84 54;
url : http://www.scepid.org
Email: laurent.toubiana@u444.jussieu.fr

994
Connecting Medical Informatics and Bio-Informatics
R. Engelbrecht et al. (Eds.)
IOS Press, 2005
© 2005 EFMI – European Federation for Medical Informatics. All rights reserved.

A Multi-Source Information System via the Internet for End-Stage Renal Disease: Scalability and Data Quality

Mohamed Ben Saïd[a], Loic Le Mignot[a], Claude Mugnier[a], Jean Baptiste Richard[a], Christine Le Bihan-Benjamin[a], Jean-Philippe Jais[a], Didier Guillon[b], Ana Simonet[b], Michel Simonet[b], Paul Landais[a]

[a]*Université Paris-Descartes ; Faculté de Médecine ; Assistance Publique-Hôpitaux de Paris ; EA222 ; Service de Biostatistique et d'Informatique Médicale, Hôpital Necker,149 rue de Sèvres 75743 Cedex 15 Paris - France*
[b]*Université J. Fourier, TIMC-IMAG, Grenoble, France*

Abstract

A Multi-Source Information System (MSIS), has been designed for the Renal Epidemiology and Information Network (REIN) dedicated to End-Stage Renal Disease (ESRD). MSIS aims at providing reliable follow-up data for ESRD patients. It is based on an n-tier architecture, made out of a universal client, a dynamic Web server connected to a production database and to a data warehouse. MSIS is operational since 2002 and progressively deployed in 9 regions in France. It includes 11,500 patients. MSIS facilitates documenting medical events which occur during the course of ESRD patient' health care and provides means to control the quality of each patient's record and reconstruct the patient trajectory of care. Consolidated data are made available to a data warehouse and to a geographic information system for analysis and data representation in support of public-health decision making.

Keywords:
Scalability; Data quality; Dynamic Web server; n-tier architecture; Multi-Source Information System; Internet; End-Stage Renal Disease.

1. Introduction

The lack of coordinated information about patients suffering from end-stage renal disease (ESRD) led a large panel of health care providers, decision makers, researchers and institution representatives to initiate the Renal Epidemiology and Information Network (REIN) [1]. REIN is organized, at national and regional levels, around a network of professionals involved in ESRD health care. A Multi-Source Information System (MSIS) [2] dedicated to collect continuous and exhaustive records of all ESRD cases and their clinical follow-up, was developed by Necker Hospital at University Paris-Descartes. MSIS collates in a standardized representation a minimal patient record elaborated by health professionals [3]. Progressive deployment in the regions since year 2002 allowed testing the MSIS performance, acceptance among users, workload impact and maintenance cost effectiveness. MSIS is operational via the Internet, in eight regions plus one virtual region devoted to follow paediatric cases.

Scalability remains a major issue in the design of the information system, especially during implementation and deployment phases. It remains a major issue as the system grows [4]. In a general definition, scalability is an overlap between structural scalability and load scalability [5]: "Structural scalability is the ability of a system to expand to a chosen dimension without major modifications to its architecture". A system is thought of "as being structurally scalable if its implementation or standards do not impede the growth of the number of objects it encompasses, or at least will not do so within a chosen time frame". "Load scalability is the ability of a system to perform gracefully as the offered traffic increases". A system is said to have "load scalability if it has the ability to function gracefully, without undue delay and without unproductive resource consumption or resource contention at light, moderate, heavy loads while making good use of available resources" [5].

In a previous paper [3], seek of scalability was one of the MSIS' aims. It influenced MSIS design, architecture and implementation. In the present paper we will focus on the efficiency of the technological choices made to support the organizational network of professionals at the regional level to build a reliable and methodological longitudinal resource of information for a nationwide cohort of ESRD patients.

2. Material and Methods

Organizational support

REIN national committee for guidance and follow-up involves several organizations: Société de Néphrologie, Société francophone de dialyse, INSERM, Paris Descartes University and Grenoble J. Fourier University, Agence de la Biomédecine, Caisse Nationale d'Assurance Maladie des Travailleurs Salariés (CNAMTS), Direction de l'Hospitalisation et de l'Organisation des Soins (DHOS), Institut de Veille Sanitaire (InVS) and representatives of patients' associations. Regional committees involve nephrologists, decision makers, public health insurers, epidemiologists and patients' associations. Each region elects a nephrologist as program coordinator. In each region, a public health and epidemiology department supports the professionals and decision makers by providing resources and expertise for methodology and epidemiology studies. A clinical research assistant performs the quality control at least once every year for every patient record.

Architecture and technical support

Architecture

MSIS is based on an n-tier architecture interfaced with a light-weighted universal client. MSIS uses a secure connection via the Internet. The client connects to the middle tier that is in relation with several databases: an identification database, a production database, a data warehouse and a geographical information system (Figure 1).

Security

Authorized users validate a certificate issued by MSIS system to exchange SSL encrypted messages. Client messages are analyzed by the firewall [6], which proceeds at the networking level. The firewall translates public IP addresses into local ones in order to filter IP addresses and TCP port accesses. Allowed messages are sent to the proxy [7]: a software component that rewrites public URL addresses and controls their validity and access-authorization. The proxy makes access-control decisions, to and from the production zone. It communicates with the production zone through the firewall. Outgoing messages to the client follow a reverse path (Figure 2).

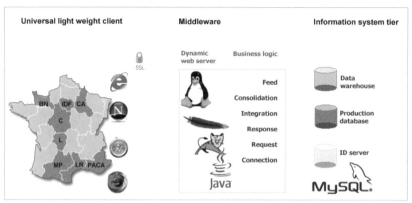

Figure 1: MSIS n-tier architecture. Universal light weighted clients connect from 8 administrative regions plus a "pediatrics virtual" region: Limousin (L), Languedoc-Roussillon (LR), Champagne-Ardenne (CA), Provence-Alpes-Côte d'Azur (PACA), Centre (C), Ile-de-France (IDF), Basse-Normandie (BN), Midi-Pyrénées (MP). The middleware uses free software (Linux™, Apache, Tomcat JSP/Servlet™ container, and Java™ programming language). It is organized into a dynamic web server tier, interfaced with the web client tier and into a business logic tier, interacting with the databases in the information system tier.

An intrusion detection system audits all the devices and analyzes connections according to an updated list of threats.

Deployment

At the client side, MSIS relies on existing local Internet networking facilities and on a widely spread computer configuration in medical settings: Pentium III processor computer or equivalent, 128 Megabytes of random access memory (RAM), 1024x768 pixels screen resolution, Acrobat Reader™ 4, a web browser allowing 128 character SSL encryption (Internet Explorer 6.0, Netscape 7.0, Safari 2.0, Mozilla FireFox 1.0). Maintenance and evolutions are made centrally which reduce deployment costs and delays.

Use of the system in the regions

The patient record is organized into three parts:

- a medical history, aetiology of ESRD and comorbidity at start of replacement therapy,
- a recent medical observation with information about access to the care facilities and to the national kidney-graft waiting list,
- an update of the actual renal dialysis method and context of treatment.

Admission, discharge and transfer event information are documented and updated annually on the anniversary of first ESRD treatment. A decease record file, including standard medical codification of the decease is documented when necessary. The coordinating nephrologists and the clinical research assistant relay local trainings and are the main interlocutors in daily use of the system. They also provide an exhaustive representation of dialysis units and request authorizations and profiles for the nephrologists in the region. MSIS access codes are delivered individually to the users.

Exhaustiveness control

Monitoring tools in MSIS provide means to control exhaustiveness on a monthly basis and on an annual basis for patients' follow-up update. The demand of care requires information about patients living in a neighbouring region and treated in the region of interest.

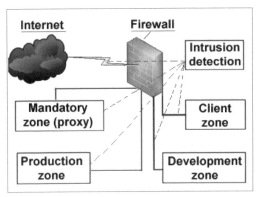

Figure 2: MSIS security system organization. Incoming and outgoing traffic passes through the firewall. Controls are made at the networking level. The proxy rewrites URL addresses and controls URL access-authorizations to and from the production zone. An intrusion detection listener audits the traffic.

Nephrologists of the neighbouring region are given an access MSIS in order to complete the missing information.

Quality control

More than ten mandatory information items are requested to create a patient record in the MSIS production database. Randomized study focused on the quality of information stored using MSIS in comparison with the information in the patient's hospital record. Appropriate correlation coefficients or kappa coefficients are calculated for quantitative and qualitative variables, respectively. The clinical research assistant with the support of the epidemiological department realizes this work.

MSIS functionalities

MSIS provides tools permitting users at the dialysis unit level, to access to reporting lists of descriptive statistics. At the region level, specific quality control functions are available to the coordinating nephrologists and to the clinical research assistant: they consist of recapitulative regional information and reminders for annual follow-up as well as a data extraction module. This latter is organized to facilitate answering questions in relation with the project: better knowledge of the demand of ESRD care and matching the offer of care to the demand. The demand of care is derived from the set of data of patients living in the region, whether or not treated in the region. The offer of ESRD care concerns the patients treated in the region during a period of time, whether or not residing in the region.

Identification server

A patient identification server is implemented to provide unique identifier for every patient in the system and to prevent from creating duplicates by detecting existing close spelling patient names. The patient unique identifier allows the link between the two kinds of information. The identification server algorithm focused on strings comparison between the user entry information and the information stored in MSIS database. The method is derived from Needleman and Wunsch (N&W) algorithm [8] searching for similarities in strings. A value of an "acceptable distance" between two strings is assigned. If the minimal computed distance is equal or lower than an acceptable distance, the information entered is considered as having a match in the system.

The identification server complies with the French law about privacy. Necessary agreements of the Commission Nationale Informatique et Libertés (CNIL) were obtained.

CNIL recommends separate transit over the network of explicit nominative data and of medical data.

MSIS' interface was adapted consequently: two separate requests-response processes connect to the identification server and to the production database. The results are displayed "simultaneously" on the same screen, the patient full name and identification information in one frame and the medical information in another frame. Since the identification server implementation in April 2004, workload generated by the management of duplicates, dropped significantly and the data quality of the system improved consequently.

Data consolidation and periodic feed of the data warehouse

The quality control process performed by the clinical research assistant provides consolidated information, which are then exported to the data warehouse. A geographical information system uses this information to generate dynamically graphical representations of the demand and offer of care. It is an aid for public health decision-making.

3. Results

As of May 24th 2005, 11424 patient records, 898 transplantations and 2295 ESRD patient decease cases are documented in the production database. The active file includes 8227 patients who undergo dialysis (detailed information are presented in table 1). According to the national survey of prevalent ESRD dialyzed patients in June 2003 [9], MSIS active file includes 26 % of the nation wide ESRD dialyzed patients.

MSIS and the organizational support

MSIS access codes were provided to more than 300 nephrologists and 50 codes to their collaborators. Ten clinical research assistants and nine physicians perform the quality control at the regional level. Eight university departments of medical informatics, and/or of epidemiology and/or of public health insure the patient data quality control using MSIS.

Table 1: MSIS deployment in the regions

Region	Date of inclusion	Population	Number of cases in the active file
Limousin	Jan 22nd 2002	711 000	382
Languedoc-Roussillon	Jun 2nd 2002	2 296 000	1,405
Champagne-Ardenne	Jan 1st 2003	1 342 000	682
Centre	Jan 1st 2004	2 440 000	1,306
Provence-Alpes-Côte-d'Azur	Jan 1st 2004	4 506 000	3,060
Ile-de-France	Nov 1st 2004	10 952 000	615
Midi-Pyrénées	Feb 1st 2005	2 552 000	285
Basse Normandie	Feb 1st 2005	1 422 000	378
Pediatrics virtual region	Jan 1st 2004	N/A	114

As longitudinal data accumulate, annual follow-up of the ESRD cohort are progressively and systematically taking place in the regions.

4. Discussion: scalability issues

Adding components fits within the n-tier architecture either as a database server, business logic or technologies such as XML data processing. Only few environmental changes occurred during last 3 years: migration to Java 1.4, to Tomcat 5.0 and to MySQL 4.0.

A reinforcement of the system security was an addition to MSIS rather than a rebuilt. Few changes of the data structure were necessary. This was the case when transactions were introduced into the system or when responding to the nephrologists' demand of adding new items in the patient record. The data conceptual model remained unaffected. The implementation of the identification server fitted within an n-tier modular architecture. Additional feed-back functionalities, focused on information retrieval and quality control. Scalability issues evolve with the system use. While MSIS online use for three years and progressive deployment in the regions confirmed choices made at the design and implementation phases, new workload is identified and needs to be addressed. It points to the need of further resources to support the efforts of the clinical research assistants in guaranteeing quality of the patient information entered in the system. MSIS showed a major stability and good performance in extending its use to new regions.

5. Conclusion

MSIS proved its usability and support to nephrologists and health care decision makers to follow a cohort of ESRD patients and to provide reliable longitudinal information for epidemiology and public health decision-making in the context of ESRD.

6. Acknowledgments

This research was funded by a grant from STIC-Santé-Inserm 2002, n°A02126ds, by Paris-Descartes University and by Assistance Publique-Hôpitaux de Paris. This work was also supported by grants provided by the Caisse Nationale d'Assurance Maladie des Travailleurs Salariés, the Institut de Veille Sanitaire and the Agence de la Biomédecine. The nephrologists in charge of the ESRD units of Limousin, Languedoc-Roussillon, Champagne Ardenne, Provence-Alpes-Côte-d'Azur, Centre, Ile-de-France, Basse-Normandie, Midi-Pyrénées and the pediatricians are especially acknowledged for their fruitful cooperation and comments. JP Necker and X Ferreira are acknowledged for their skilful help.

7. References

[1]   Landais P. L'insuffisance rénale terminale en France : offre de soins et prévention. *Presse Med*.2002; 31:176-85.

[2]   Landais P, Simonet A, Guillon D, Jacquelinet C, Ben Saïd M, Mugnier C, Simonet M. SIMS@REIN:Un Système d'Information Multi-Sources pour l'Insuffisance Rénale Terminale. CR Biol 2002;325:515-528.

[3]   Ben Said M, Simonet A, Guillon D, Jacquelinet C, Gaspoz F, Dufour E, Mugnier C, Jais JP, Simonet M, Landais P. A dynamic Web application within an n-tier architecture: a Multi-Source Information System for end-stage renal disease. Stud Health Technol Inform. 2003;95:95-100.

[4]   Arlitt M, Krishnamurthy D, Rolia J. Characterizing the Scalability of a Large Web-based Shopping System. ACM Transactions on Internet Technology, Vol. 1, No. 1, August 2001, Pages 44–69

[5]   Bondi AB Characteristics of Scalability and Their Impact On Performance. Proceedings of the second international workshop on Software and performance. WOSP 2000, Ontario, Canada - ACM 2000 1-58113-195-X/00/09.

[6]   Al-Tawil K, Al-Katham IA. Evaluation and Testing of Internet Firewalls. Int. J. Network Mgmt. 1999; 9:135-149

[7]   Burnside M, Clarke D, Mills T, Maywah A, Devadas S, Rivest R. Proxy-Based Security in Networked Mobile Devices. Proceedings of the 2002 ACM symposium on Applied computing - Madrid, Spain - 2002: 265 – 272

[8]   Le Mignot L, Mugnier C, Ben Saïd M, Jais JP, Le Bihan C, Richard JB, Taupin P, Landais P. Avoiding Doubles in Distributed Nominative Medical Databases: Optimization of the Needleman and Wunsch Algorithm. MIE 2005 (in press)

[9]   http://www.ameli.fr/174/DOC/1182/dp.html (document published on January 8th 2004 and observed on May 23rd 2005) or http://www.fehap.fr/sanitaire/dialyse/PrevalenceIRC09012004.pdf (document published on January 15th 2004 and observed on May 23rd 2005)

Address for correspondence

Pr Paul Landais, Service de Biostatistique et d'Informatique Médicale, Hôpital Necker-Enfants Malades, 149, rue de Sèvres, 75743 Paris cedex 15 - France. E-mail : landais@necker.fr

1000

Connecting Medical Informatics and Bio-Informatics
R. Engelbrecht et al. (Eds.)
IOS Press, 2005

The Necessity of an Electronic SOP Retrieval System

Katja Krockenberger,[a] Petra Knaup,[b] Kornelia Bez,[a] Christoph H Gleiter[a]

[a]KKS-UKT gGmbH, Tübingen, Germany
[b]University of Heidelberg, Institute of Medical Biometry and Informatics; Department of Medical Informatics, Heidelberg, Germany

Abstract

Objectives: Standard Operating Procedures (SOP) are part of the quality management system when carrying out clinical trials. It is therefore important for all those envolved to know about them and act accordingly. This survey should help to detect problems concerning the handling of SOP during clinical trials. Method: Anonymous survey of all employees of the Koordinierungszentren Klinische Studien (KKS) in Germany by means of standardised questionnaires (238 employees in August 2004 according to the KKS homepages). Result: 58,8% of all evaluation sheets were sent back proving that paper-based as well as electronic SOP systems are not sufficiently integrated into everyday work procedures. Conclusion: Steps will have to be taken in order to increase the use of SOP. We propose a computer-based retrieval tool (SOP Information Retrieval System)

Keywords:
Clinical Research, Clinical Trials, Standard Operating Procedures, SOP, Information Retrieval, Medical Informatics

1. Introduction

Due to new EU directives the quality standards required for clinical trials are higher than before[1][2]. These directives date back to May 1, 2004, providing that the new standards are binding for tests initiated by investigators [3] as well as for regular trials. Therefore, the creation of instruments assuring and improving quality (or making procedures easier) is an important goal.

The amendment no 12 to the law relating to the manufacture and distribution of medicines integrates the EU directive 2001/20/EG into German law [4]. It defines the requirements concerning clinical trials involving medicines and their control during GCP audits as well as official inspections. There is no longer any differentiation between regular trials and trials initiated by investigators (IIT). This amendment came to effect on August 6, 2004 [5].

In order to further improve quality standards centres for the coordination of clinical trials (Koordinierungszentren Klinische Studien, KKS) were founded all over Germany with the financial support of the Federal Ministry of Education and Research (Bundesministerium für Bildung und Forschung, BMBF) [6][7]. Today there are 12 of these centres located at university hospitals. Their goal is to support clinical trials (including IIT) concerning preparation, implementation, and evaluation in order to improve and maintain quality standards [8].

Part of this quality management are standardised procedures defined by the ISO/DIN-Norm (International Standard Organisation / Deutsche Industrienorm) [9]. These directives concerning SOP are obligatory for clinical research performed by GCP as well [10].

In order to guarantee utmost safety for the patient on the one hand and data quality on the other, it is imperative that the staff members are familiar with all relevant procedures. This can only be obtained by means of SOP [11].

These standardised procedures are manifold as well as complicated due to the involvement of different experts and legal requirements. As a result the SOP are likewise various and complex.

This variety of SOP leads to the assumption that their proper application can be a true challenge to staff members. Their tasks can probably only be performed with sufficient technical support. The first step to the creation of an electronic feature for SOP users was a survey in order to document the handling of SOP during clinical trials. Since the application of SOP should be documented in IIT as well as regular trials, the participation of employees connected with the KKS were of particular importance because of their assistance in regular trials as well as in IIT.

2. Objectives

According to ICH-GCP the sponsor of a clinical study is responsible for the observance of legal specifications and internal restrictions; the data has to be retrieved, documented and presented in accordance with those specifications [12]. In order to guarantee the observance of necessary limitations, the sponsor has to use SOP in the form of detailed written directives, for example [13]. If clinical trials are not carried out in accordance with those specifications recorded by the SOP, the validity of the entire clinical study can be called into question.

The sponsor has to guarantee furthermore that his staff members are familiar with SOP and that the access to the latest version of those procedures is ensured. This means that the sponsor has to carry out the following coordinational tasks: create, actualise, manage, examine, and replace obsolete SOP. Older versions of SOP have to be archived and supervised [14].

Due to the variety and complexity of SOP, the step-by-step retrievability of information is difficult. Staff members are therefore asked to keep the appropriate directives always at hand.

Searching for SOP demands a lot of time, especially when paper-based. A great effort is necessary to provide and record SOP for all persons involved because of their enormous impact on the quality and duration of a clinical study. This additional amount of time has to be refunded. Since especially the IIT lack money when completing a clinical study the reduction of cost-intensive factors such as working hours has to be kept in mind. It is therefore important that staff members work in accordance with SOP in order to be more effective.

This background shapes the following survey in order to determine possible improvements concerning the handling of SOP.

The following questions have to be answered:

Q1: How detailed is the staff's knowledge of the relevant SOP (existence)?

Q2: Do all persons involved have a SOP and is it available (availability)?

Q3: Is the latest version of the SOP available to each staff member (actuality)?

Q4: How do staff members work with SOP when attempting to retrieve information (efficiency)?

3. Method

To answer these questions a survey was conducted among employees of the 12 "Koordinierungszentren Klinischer Studien" in Germany by means of a standardised evaluation sheet.

In order to identify possible improvements concerning the handling of SOP, the focus of attention was the accessability as well as the feasibility of SOP. Furthermore, it is of great importance that all participants take notice of all existing and relevant SOP.

After evaluating all members of one centre final evaluation forms were sent to the chief managers of the KKS. They were asked to pass on those forms to their employees. According to the homepage of the KKS, 238 people were employed there at that time.

The survey started in August 2004. All forms sent back until October 4, 2004, were included. To guarantee anonymity a neutral person collected them. Standardised answers were analysed by means of descriptive statistics; textual answers were summarised by the first author of this article.

4. Result

140 forms were sent back until October 4, 2004, or 58,8% respectively.

After a first, rough analysis the following conclusions can be made. The participants stated

- a low access rate of SOP during every-day work procedures
- accessing SOP and searching for relevant information is regarded as being an effort. This applies to paper-based versions as well as electronic versions
- rather than consulting SOP the participants ask their colleagues for help
- informing each staff member about SOP is difficult

The final results are to be presented at the conference.

5. Discussion

The participation rate of more than 50 % suggests that the handling of SOP during everyday work procedures is important to staff members in order to maintain or even improve quality standards. It is therefore absolutely necessary to find out if all the persons involved in conducting clinical trials are sufficiently informed about those procedures. By means of this survey it will be possible to determine whether the access to and availability of SOP are guaranteed for paper-based as well as electronic SOP or not. Another important result of this survey concerns the relevance of SOP and the way each staff member gets relevant information. The participants of this study were further asked to define how data could be found more effectively in paper-based as well as electronic SOP in order to improve the retrieval of relevant information. This evaluation is therefore the starting-point for improving the usage and integration of SOP during clinical trials in accordance with internal restrictions, directives, and laws. Further plans involve the implementation of a computer-based retrieval tool (SOP Information Retrieval System) especially designed for clinical trials. This tool will be put to the test by further practical use. Another focus of attention is the improvement of SOP by means of a retrieval system whose design will also be based on the results of this survey.

6. Conclusion

After introducing the EU directive 2001/20/EG and the amendment no 12 to the law relating to the manufacture and distribution of medicines, certain quality standards concerning clinical trials have to be observed. A computer-based system may improve the usage and accessability of SOP in order to save money and improve the quality of clinical trials.

7.Acknowledgments

The authors would like to thank all employees of the KKS-UKT gGmbH in Tübingen for their assistance. Furthermore, we would like to thank all participating employees of the KKS in Germany for their valuable comments. We would also like to thank Edith Belz and Andrea Schröter of the KKS-UKT gGmbH for their assistance in conducting this survey.

The KKS-UKT gGmbH is sponsored by the Federal Ministry of Education and Research (BMBF, grant: 01GH0101)

8. References

[1] Kori-Lindner C. The 12th AMG amending law (part 1): consequences for clinical trials. *DGPharMed News* 2004: 4 piii: 9-27 (in German).

[2] O'Doherty E, Clumeck N. The EU-Directive: Practical Implications for Clinical Research Teams. *APPLIED CLINICAL TRIALS* 2004: May.

[3] Hoffman J. Investigator-Initiated Studies. *E-Liver Online* 2004 (http://www.eliveronline.com/2004_06/2004_06_ART1.htm, last access: 05-01-13).

[4] Directive 2001/20/EG of the European Parliament and of the European Council from April 4th, 2001 (http://www.kori-lindner.de/daten/eugcprichtlinie2001deutsch.pdf, last access: 05-01-14) (in German).

[5] 12th law changing AMG from July 30th, 2004. *Bundesgesetzblatt 2004: 41 piii: 2031-2053 (in German).*

[6] Ohmann C, Albrecht J. Coordination centers for clinical studies-structure and integration of non-university hospitals. *Kongressbd Dtsch Ges Chir Kongr 2001: 118 pii 804-808 (in German).*

[7] Ohmann C. Responsibilities of coordination centers for clinical studies and their status in general practice. *Internist (Berl)* 2002: 43(4) pii: 498-505 (in German).

[8] Mertens S. Clinical Trials: Less would be more. *Deutsches Ärzteblatt 2001: 48 pii: A-3174/B-2688/C-2495 (in German).*

[9] Leonhard KW, Naumann P. *Management Systems – Terms (DGQ-Band ; 11-04).* 7th ed. Berlin, Wien, Zürich: Beuth, 2002 (in German).

[10] Stapff M. Clinical Trials for drugs. 3nd ed. München, Bern, Wien New York: W. Zuckschwerdt Verlag, 2004 (in German).

[11] Ginsberg D. *The Investigator's Guide to Clinical Research.* 3nd ed. Boston: THOMSON – CenterWatch, 2002.

[12] ICH Harmonised Tripartite Guideline for Good Clinical Practice. (http://www.ich.org/MediaServer.jser?@_ID=482&@_MODE=GLB, last access: 05-01-14).

[13] Korteweg M. Quality assurance in Clinical Trials. In:Witte PU, Schenk J, Schwarz JA, Kori-Lindner C, eds. Methodical clinical trial – Good Clinical Practice. 5th ed. Habrich E., Verlag, 2000 (in German).

[14] Schwarz JA. *Clinical trials of drugs and medical devices.* 2nd ed. Aulendorf: ECV - EDITIO-CANTOR-VERLAG, 2000 (in German).

Address for Correspondence

Dipl.-Inform. Med. Katja Krockenberger, KKS-UKT gGmbH, Otfried-Müller-Str. 45, D-72076 Tübingen, Katja.Krockenberger@kks-ukt.de, http://www.kks-ukt.de

Connecting Medical Informatics and Bio-Informatics
R. Engelbrecht et al. (Eds.)
IOS Press, 2005

Investigating the Effect of Differences in Entry Criteria on Trial Populations: A Method with an Application in Severe Sepsis

Linda Peelen[a,c], **Niels Peek**[a], **Nicolette de Keizer**[a,c], **Evert de Jonge**[b,c]

[a]*Department of Medical Informatics* [b]*Department of Intensive Care*
[b]*Academic Medical Center – Universiteit van Amsterdam*
[c]*National Intensive Care Evaluation (NICE) foundation*

Abstract

Multiple clinical trials that investigate the same intervention often use different entry criteria to enroll patients into the trials. This variation in entry criteria might lead to the selection of patients with different characteristics. If these characteristics are related to the effect measure (e.g. baseline mortality in a trial investigating mortality reduction) the results of the trials cannot be compared straightforwardly. Therefore it is important to investigate whether the use of different entry criteria leads to the selection of patients with different characteristics.

To study differences in the characteristics of the study populations, one could use the data from the control groups of the trials. However, differences in characteristics of these study populations can be caused by differences in entry criteria as well as by clinical diversity. Based on the data from the trials these two causes cannot be distinguished. We propose a method to investigate the influence of differences in entry criteria on the characteristics of study populations. The method corrects for the effects of clinical diversity by simulating the patient selection process on an independent registry database. The method has been successfully applied in the area of severe sepsis.

Keywords:
Entry criteria; Heterogeneity; Registry; Meta analysis; Severe sepsis

1. Introduction

Clinical trials are conducted to investigate the effect of an intervention in a specific patient group. When multiple trials have studied the same intervention on the same type of patients, it is appealing to combine the results of the trials. Combination of the results may lead to a more precise estimate of the effect and a pooled effect may be found whereas the singular trials were too small to detect a significant effect. Often the effect of the intervention varies among the trials, which may hinder the combination of trial results. This heterogeneity with respect to the effect has to be investigated before calculating a pooled effect [1]. In the area of meta-analysis several methods exist to assess this *effect heterogeneity*.

Trials do not only differ in the effect of the intervention, but also with respect to the criteria that are used to enroll patients into the trial. These criteria can be divided into two types: *inclusion criteria* to select those patients that might benefit from the intervention and in whom a measurable effect is expected; and *exclusion criteria* to exclude patients for whom the treatment might be harmful (e.g. pregnant women), in whom the outcome might be distorted by competing risks (e.g. moribund patients in a trial with 28-day mortality as outcome), who are not able to give informed consent or who are likely not to adhere to the intervention protocol [2]. In this paper we use the term *entry criteria* for the combination of inclusion and exclusion criteria.

The variation in entry criteria among trials within a given domain can have several reasons. If different adverse effects are expected different exclusion criteria are required. Another reason for variation is the lack of consensus about the definition of the disease. Differences in entry criteria might lead to the selection of patients with different characteristics. We use the term *entry heterogeneity* to refer to differences in characteristics of the study population due to differences in entry criteria. If these characteristics are related to the effect measure (e.g. baseline mortality in a trial that investigates mortality reduction) this might be an underlying cause of the effect heterogeneity. Therefore it is important to investigate whether the use of different entry criteria leads to the selection of patients with different characteristics.

A straightforward way to assess entry-heterogeneity would be to compare the characteristics of the patients in the control groups of the clinical trials. In a randomized clinical trial this group of patients can be considered to be representative for the total study population of the trial. As these patients do not undergo the intervention, the effect of the intervention does not disturb the characteristic of interest (e.g. the mortality in the control group of the trial is considered the baseline mortality risk for all patients enrolled into the trial). However, often the sizes of the control groups of those trials are relatively small, which makes it difficult to detect possible entry-heterogeneity. Furthermore, the differences we observe in the characteristics of the control groups can be due to differences in entry criteria, but also to other factors such as participating countries and care organization, which is often summarized as 'clinical diversity'.

This paper presents a method (the *projection* method) to investigate entry-heterogeneity that overcomes the disadvantages of comparing control groups of the trials by making use of one large, uniform registry database for all trials. In Section 2 the method is explained. A case-study using the method in the field of severe sepsis is presented in Section 3. In Section 4 we discuss the possibilities and drawbacks of the method. For now, we restrict ourselves to dichotomous outcomes, using mortality as an example.

2. Methods

In a clinical trial entry criteria are developed in the design phase of the study and after that patients are enrolled into the study prospectively. The basis of the method we present here is that we mimic this patient selection process. However, the patient selection is performed retrospectively on a database containing prospectively collected patient information. Thereby we assume that all patients that could possibly be eligible for one of the trials are indeed registered within the database.

The projection method consists of three steps which are depicted in Figure 1. In Step 1 the entry criteria of the trials are expressed in terms of the variables that are collected in the database. Therefore the criteria have to be as specific as possible, preferably at the same level of detail as used in the registry. If necessary the investigators of the trials have to be contacted for further specification of the entry criteria. This step results in one database query per trial. In Step 2 we mimic the selection process of patients for the trial by applying each of the queries associated with a trial onto the registry database. This results in one dataset per trial, containing the patients from the registry database that would have been eligible for that trial. In most cases these datasets are overlapping, i.e. there exist patients that fulfill the criteria of more than one trial and therefore are included in more than one dataset. In clinical practice, patients are not enrolled into more than one trial at the same time (often 'already enrolled into other trial' is in fact one of the exclusion criteria). However, they can be eligible for more than one trial. In Step 3 the characteristics of the patients in the datasets of the trials are compared.

The datasets are compared in a pair-wise manner. Let the trials to be compared be denoted by I and II respectively. We define the mortality rate in the registry database subsets

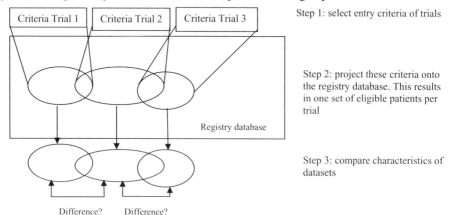

Figure 1 The projection method to compare the characteristics of patients selected by different entry criteria.

associated with these trials as p_I and p_{II}. The difference in these mortality rates, Δ, can be calculated as $p_I - p_{II}$. If the datasets were not overlapping a χ^2 test would have been appropriate to test whether Δ differs significantly from zero. However, as the datasets are overlapping, the uncertainty in Δ cannot be determined straightforwardly, because the variances of p_I and p_{II} are not independent. Using bootstrap sampling [3, 4], we estimate the uncertainty in the estimate of the difference in mortality, without making assumptions on the variance of the two mortality rates.

The following procedure is applied: we generate 10000 samples by drawing with replacement from the entire registry database. For each sample we apply the queries of the two trials from step 1 onto the sample and calculate $\Delta_i = p_{i,I} - p_{i,II}$, where $p_{i,I}$ is the mortality in the group of patients in sample i ($i = 1,..,10000$) that are selected by the entry criteria of trial I. The collection of $\Delta_I, ..., \Delta_{10000}$ yields an empirical distribution of the difference in mortality between patients selected by the entry criteria of trial I and trial II. Based on percentiles of this distribution a confidence interval for the difference in mortality is constructed. If multiple trials are to be compared using this pair-wise comparison method, the risks of multiple testing can be reduced by increasing the width of the confidence interval.

3. Application in the field of severe sepsis

Sepsis is a quite common condition which can be easily cured provided it is timely detected. However, if the disease progresses to severe sepsis, it can be life-threatening, as organ systems start to fail. In this stage of the disease treatment at the Intensive Care Unit is necessary to stabilize the function of the organ systems. Mortality among patients with such a severe form of sepsis is high, reported to be 20-50% [5]. A curative treatment is hardly available and very expensive. This is one of the reasons why many clinical trials are performed in this area. However, a patient with severe sepsis is difficult to characterize, which results in remarkable differences in entry criteria that are used in clinical trials. If differences in entry criteria lead to differences in the severity of illness in the study populations (which can be expressed by the baseline mortality) study results cannot be compared in a straightforward manner, as severity of illness influences the effect of the intervention. Using the method presented in this paper, we studied whether differences in entry criteria led to the selection of patients with a significantly different ICU mortality.

Based on a MEDLINE search, we selected all randomized controlled trials performed in the field of severe sepsis reported between 1999 and 2003, which included over 30 patients and

Table 1 Number of patients and mortality in the datasets

Trial Code	Number of patients (% of entire database)	ICU mortality (% ± SD)
A[7]	1650 (2.3)	34.2 ± 1.2
B [8]	3460 (4.8)	25.0 ± 0.7
C [9]	3920 (5.4)	27.4 ± 0.7
D [6]	2721 (3.8)	27.2 ± 0.8
E [10]	1103 (1.5)	31.6 ± 1.4
F [11]	4334 (6.0)	27.3 ± 0.6
G [12]	3912 (5.4)	26.9 ± 0.7
H [13]	1472 (2.0)	43.1 ± 1.2
I [14]	3561 (5.0)	28.9 ± 0.7

reported 28-day mortality [6-14]. From the resulting nine trials we analyzed the entry criteria used to enroll patients. For one trial [6] the main conductor of the trial was contacted to clarify some details with respect to the criteria. This resulted in nine sets of entry criteria, one set per trial.

We projected these sets of entry criteria on the database of the Dutch National Intensive Care Evaluation (NICE) registry [15]. This registry contains information on admissions at 29 Dutch Intensive Care Units (ICUs). The records in this database describe the general ICU population and contain 108 variables per admission, describing the physiological condition of the patient and the outcome. Stringent measures such as data checks and training of participants are taken to assure the quality of the data [16].

The nine sets of entry criteria have been applied onto all 71,929 records from the NICE database collected between December 1996 and February 2003. Not all items of the entry criteria were matched exactly to the NICE database. Together with expert intensivists some of the criteria were slightly adapted in order to match with the variables in the NICE database. The application of the nine sets of entry criteria onto the NICE database resulted in nine datasets, one per trial. Using bootstrapping as described in Section 2.2, we tested whether the ICU mortality rates differed significantly between these datasets. As 36 comparisons were made (each trial was compared to all other trials in a pair-wise manner), we have calculated 99.9% confidence intervals to reduce the effects of multiple testing.

Table 1 gives the number of patients and the ICU mortality for each dataset. The number of patients selected by these sets of criteria ranges from 1103 to 4334 (1.5% to 6.0% of the registry database respectively). The ICU mortality ranges from 25.0% to 43.1%. From the third column we already detect differences in ICU mortality: dataset B has a low mortality, whereas the ICU mortality in datasets A, E and H is remarkably higher. The results from the bootstrapping procedure show whether significant differences in ICU mortality are found when comparing these trials.

Table 2 presents the 99.9% confidence intervals for the difference in ICU mortality with the other datasets. We note that datasets C, D, F and G do not have a significantly different ICU mortality, as all pairwise comparisons among these datasets contain the value of zero within the 99.9% confidence interval. For trial B only the difference with trial G is non-significant and for trial E only the difference with trial I is non-significant. Furthermore we observe that the ICU mortality in datasets A and H differs significantly from all other datasets. We conclude that in 28 out of the 36 comparisons a difference in baseline ICU mortality was found. When comparing the effects of the intervention from the trials with a difference in baseline ICU mortality, these differences have to be taken into account, as baseline ICU mortality might have influenced the effect of the intervention that was found in the trials.

Table 2 - Results from the pair-wise comparison of the datasets associated with the entry criteria of the trials. Results represent the 99.9% confidence interval for the difference in ICU mortality between the datasets. Results marked with a * indicate non-significant results.

Trial Code	Confidence interval (99.9 %) for the difference in ICU mortality between datasets							
	A	B	C	D	E	F	G	H
A[8]	--	--	--	--	--	--	--	--
B [9]	-6.3, -12.0	--	--	--	--	--	--	--
C [10]	-3.7, -9.9	1.0, 4.0	--	--	--	--	--	--
D [7]	-4.0, -10.2	0.5, 5.9	-1.7, 1.2 *	--	--	--	--	--
E [11]	-6.7, -14.9	3.0, 10.2	0.4, 7.8	0.7, 8.2	--	--	--	--
F [12]	-3.9, -10.0	0.8, 3.9	-1.0, 0.8 *	-1.6, 1.8 *	-8.0, -0.4	--	--	--
G [13]	-4.5, -0.3	0.0, 3.6 *	-1.7, 0.6 *	-2.3, 1.4 *	-8.3, -1.0	-1.6, 0.6 *	--	--
H [14]	4.8, 13.0	14.7, 21.6	12.4, 18.9	12.3, 19.3	6.8, 16.2	12.6, 19.0	13.1, 19.5	--
I [15]	-2.2, -8.4	2.2, 5.6	0.5, 2.4	0.1, 3.3	-6.2, 1.1 *	0.5, 2.7	0.6, 3.4	-17.3, -11.0

4. Discussion and Conclusion

This paper presents a method to investigate whether differences in entry criteria lead to differences in the characteristics of the patients that are selected by these entry criteria. By mimicking the selection process of patients as performed in clinical trials, making use of a patient data stored in a large registry database, datasets of patients fulfilling the entry criteria of the trials can be obtained. Characteristics of the patients in these datasets can then be compared.

Although it is computationally more intensive than merely comparing the characteristics of the control groups of the original trials, our method has several advantages. First, because all entry criteria are applied onto the same database, other factors causing differences in population characteristics do not disturb the findings. Second, because the entry criteria are applied onto a large database, the size of the patient groups that are selected is larger than the sizes of the control groups in the trial, thereby providing a more precise estimate of the differences in characteristics. We realize that such a large, general database is not available for all diseases. However, more and more specialties set up registries for quality control and accountability.

The use of a large dataset can rather quickly lead to significant results just because of the number of patients. A statistically significant difference does not automatically imply a clinically relevant difference. However, the confidence intervals resulting from the bootstrapping procedure can also be used to assess clinically relevant differences.

The method presented in this paper makes use of a database from an existing registry. There are a few requirements to the database: it has to be large, describing a rather general patient population and the data has to be uniformly collected with a consistent quality. The fact that the registry describes a general population has the disadvantage that some of the criteria that are used to select the patients may not be collected in the registry or at least not in a desirable level of detail (e.g. the entry criteria use 'HIV positive with a CD4 count of less than 50' whereas the registry stores whether a patient is HIV positive). Then variables are to be matched as closely as possible. If the criteria that cannot be matched exactly are important criteria to distinguish one trial from the others, our method will underestimate the difference in ICU mortality because the associated registry database subsets are more similar than they should have been. In our case-study in severe sepsis, it turned out that most of the criteria that did not match with variables in the NICE database were present in all trials (such as contra-indications for treatment, pregnancy etc), so we do not expect that this strongly influenced the differences in ICU mortality that were found.

The methods that are used in the area of meta-analysis to investigate effect-heterogeneity often yield one single value indicating a 'degree of heterogeneity'. The pair-wise comparison of trials in our method enables the possibility to investigate which particular trials use entry criteria that lead to different patient characteristics. In the example of severe sepsis this enabled us to find four trials that all selected patients with a baseline ICU mortality that was not significantly different, although the entry criteria used in these four trials did show differences.

5. Acknowledgements

NICE / Linda Peelen received an educational grant of Eli Lilly. Niels Peek received a grant from the Netherlands Organisation for Scientific Research (NWO) under number 634.000.020.

6. References

[1] Thompson SG: Why sources of heterogeneity in meta-analysis should be investigated, *Br Med J 1994;* 309:1351-1355.

[2] Friedman LM, Furberg CD and DeMets, DL. *Fundamentals of clinical trials.* New York: Springer, 1998.

[3] Efron B: *The Jackknife, the Bootstrap and Other Resampling Plans.* CBMS-NSF Regional Conference Series in Applied Mathematics. Society for Industrial and Applied Mathematics, 1982.

[4] Davison AC, Hinkley DV: *Bootstrap methods and their applications.* Cambridge Series in Statistical and Probabilistic Mathematics. 2nd Edition, Cambridge University Press, 1997.

[5] Wheeler AP, Bernard GR: Treating patients with severe sepsis. *N Eng J Med* 1999;340:207-214

[6] Abraham E, Reinhart K, Opal S, et al: Efficacy and safety of Tifacogin (recombinant tissue factor pathway inhibitor) in severe sepsis: a randomized controlled trial. *JAMA* 2003; 290(2): 238-247

[7] Abraham E, Laterre PF, Garbino J, et al: Lenercept (p55 tumor necrosis factor receptor fusion protein) in severe sepsis and early septic shock: A randomized double-blind, placebo-controlled, multicenter phase III trial with 1,342 patients. *Crit Care Med* 2001; 29(3): 503-510

[8] Bernard GR, Vincent JL, Laterre PF, et al: Efficacy and safety of recombinant human activated protein C for severe sepsis. *N Engl J Med* 2001; 344(10): 699-709

[9] Abraham E, Naum C, Bandi V, et al: Efficacy and safety of LY315920Na/S-5920, a selective inhibitor of 14-kDa group IIA secretory phospholipase A_2, in patients with suspected sepsis and organ failure. *Crit Care Med* 2003; 31(3): 718-728

[10] Warren BL, Eid A, Singer P, et al: Caring for the critically ill patient: High-dose Antithrombin III in severe sepsis: A randomized controlled trial. *JAMA* 2001; 286(15): 1869-78

[11] Angus DC, Birmingham MC, Balk RA, et al: Caring for the critically ill patient: E5 murine monoclonal antiendotoxin antibody in gram-negative sepsis: A randomized controlled trial. *JAMA* 2000; 283(13):1723-1730

[12] Schuster DP, Metzler M, Opal S, et al: Recombinant platelet-activating factor acetylhydrolase to prevent acute respiratory distress syndrome and mortality in severe sepsis: Phase IIb, multicenter, randomized, placebo-controlled, clinical trial. *Crit Care Med* 2003; 31(6): 1612-1619

[13] Suputtamongkol Y, Intaranongpai S, Schmidt MD, et al: A double-blind placebo-controlled study of an infusion of Lexipafant (Platelet-activating factor receptor antagonist) in patients with severe sepsis. *Antimicrobial Agents & Chemotherapy* 2000; 44(3): 693-696

[14] Nemoto H, Nakamoto H, Okada H, et al: Newly developed immobilized Polymyxin B fibers improve the survival of patients with sepsis. *Blood Purif* 2001;19(4): 361-369

[15] National Intensive Care Evaluation (NICE) Foundation: http://www.stichting-nice.nl (also in English).

[16] Arts DGT, De Keizer NF, Scheffer GJ: Defining and Improving Data Quality in Medical Registries: A Literature Review, Case Study, and Generic Framework. *J Am Med Inform Assoc* 2002; 9(6): 600-611.

Address for Correspondence

Linda Peelen , Academic Medical Center -- Universiteit van Amsterdam, Department of Medical Informatics PO Box 22700, 1100 DE Amsterdam, The Netherlands, Email: l.m.peelen@amc.uva.nl

1010

Connecting Medical Informatics and Bio-Informatics
R. Engelbrecht et al. (Eds.)
IOS Press, 2005
© 2005 EFMI – European Federation for Medical Informatics. All rights reserved.

Ensuring the Quality of Aggregated General Practice Data: Lessons from the Primary Care Data Quality Programme (PCDQ)

Jeremy van Vlymen, Simon de Lusignan, Nigel Hague, Tom Chan, Billy Dzregah

St. George's - University of London, UK

Abstract

Background: There are large numbers of schemes that collect and aggregate data from primary care computer systems into large databases. These data are then used for market and academic research. How the data is aggregated, cleaned and processed is usually opaque. Making the method transparent allows researchers to compare methods, and users of the output to better understand the strengths and weaknesses of the data.
Objectives To define the stages of the process of aggregating, processing and cleaning clinical data from multiple data sources.
Methods: Identify errors in design, collection, staging, integration and analysis.
Results: An eight step process defined: (1) Design (2) Data: entry, (3) Extraction, (4) Migration, (5) Integration, (6) Cleaning, (7) Processing, and (8) Analysis.
Conclusions: This eight step method provides a taxonomy to enable researchers to compare their methods of data process and aggregation.

Keywords:
Medical Informatics, Databases, Primary Medical Care, Computers, Data collection, Computers, Vocabulary controlled

1. Introduction

Computer data routinely collected as part of primary medical care are widely used for research; and the volume of activity in England can be gained from the DocDat website (Directory of Clinical Databases) [1]. There are two methods used to access clinical data for audit, research or other purposes. Either all the data from the general practice computer system is downloaded and analysis conducted on a copy of the whole database or, individual practice systems are interrogated at a point of time using a query that extracts the data needed to answer a particular question. There are three well established databases in operation in the UK which extract the whole database (table 1). Two of these extract data from Torex-Isoft [2,3] computer systems; and one is from "In-Practice Systems" IPS [4]. There are also two new data repositories: one extracts data from IPS [5] the other from EMIS [6]. The collection of data from practices using one manufacturer's computer system avoids some of the inconsistency problems associated with aggregating data from different systems; and, studies have shown little difference is found when systems are compared [7,8]. These large databases aim to provide a national sample. Other investigators collect data on a more *ad hoc* basis; extracting the data needed for a particular audit or study. They collect data from across the range of different general practice computer systems; usually collecting a specific data set across one or more localities. The commonest tool used for data extraction is a UK Department of Health sponsored tool called MIQUEST (Morbidity Information Query and Export Syntax) [9].

Table 1: Large databases aggregating primary care data in England and Wales

Database	Reference providing information about the database:	Computer system	URL http://www
DIN Doctors Independent Network	Carey IM, Cook DG, De Wilde S, et al. Developing a large electronic primary care database (Doctors' Independent Network) for research. Int J Med Inform. 2004;73(5):443-53.	**Torex /** **iSoft**	isoftplc.com
IMS Mediplus (Intercontinental Medical Statistics)	de Lusignan S, Stephens PN, et al.,. Does feedback improve the quality of computerized medical records..J Am Med Inform Assoc. 2002;9(4):395-401.	**Torex /** **iSoft**	isoftplc.com
GPRD General Practice Research Network	Hollowell J. The General Practice Research Database: quality of morbidity data. Popul Trends. 1997;(87):36-40.	**IPS** In Practice Systems	inps.co.uk
Qresearch	Hippisley-Cox J, Stables D, Pringle M. QRESEARCH: a new general practice database for research. Inform Prim Care. 2004;12(1):49-50.	**EMIS**	emis-online.com
THIN The Health Improvement Network	Bourke A, Dattani H, Robinson M. Feasibility study and methodology to create a quality-evaluated database… Inform Prim Care. 2004;12(3):171-7.	**IPS** In Practice Systems	inps.co.uk

As the UK uses a single terminology to record structured data, the Read "codes"; in theory the extraction and aggregation of data should be straightforward. In reality things are far more complex. The range of clinical computer systems offer different user interfaces and will inevitably bias what data is collected and the nature of input errors. The terminology used to code the structured data within the computer system is undergoing constant modification. The early systems contributing to the General Practice Research Database (GPRD) used Oxford Medical Information Systems Codes (OXMIS), the EMIS [10] computer system has many of its own codes [11]. Practitioners using the Read Code system have migrated from version 1, to a 4-character version of version 2, to a 5-character version [12]; and some have now moved on to Version 3: Clinical Terms (CT v3) [13]. To these challenges have to be added the inherent problems associated with data warehousing and quality assurance [14]. Finally, there can be problems associated with the analysis such as sample attrition. Currently, little is written about the process of aggregating, processing and cleaning computer data within the medical literature; and the lessons learnt from this data may have relevance internationally to those involved in processing primary care data drawn from different sources. This paper describes the method used within the primary care data quality project (PCDQ) with the aim of promoting transparency and improving the quality of this process.

2. Method

We reviewed our process and errors that had occurred over the last eight years using eight categories: design, data entry, extraction, migration, integration, cleaning, processing and analysis. This taxonomy is adapted from an error classification published by Berndt et al. [14] who developed this in the context of quality assurance of the healthcare data warehouse. Successful or good quality output is defined using the definition of data quality used in total data quality management (TQDM) as data fit for purpose by its consumers [15]: i.e. in our case, data useable as an educational intervention to improve chronic disease management, to improve the health of populations and for research.

Design: The design process is driven by the purpose of the study or audit we are involved in.
Step 1:   Defining the research question or audit criteria for the study.
Step 2:   We identify the data set that needs to be extracted to answer the question defined in
Step 1. This step of the process includes identifying system specific (e.g. the EMIS computer
system has additional codes over and above the national set) or locality specific codes used to
record data. We also have to ensure we are collecting sufficient demographic data to define
the denominator and characterise individuals. We define labels for all variables, as well as
any associated dates and numerical values. These labels will be used in all the successive
phases of the process. We use a controlled vocabulary to define these precisely.
Step 3:   Identify the information governance issues that might relate to the study. These
will include: privacy, confidentiality, and data protection. Ethical committee or other
approval may be needed. Generally we extract de-identified data, and take steps to see it is
fully anonymised prior to analysis; however all data can be de-identified in its originating
practice.
Step 4:   Pilot the data extraction and processing. Important lessons may be learnt from this
that need to be fed back into the design process. Only once these changes have been
incorporated, is the design stage complete.

Data entry issues: Clinicians and clerical staff enter data into their operational computer
systems using the codes that their system presents. We set out to identify errors that might
occur around data entry. This includes the process of identification of how patients with a
clinical condition are represented within the coding system (e.g. what codes are used to
identify patients with raised blood pressure). The social context of data entry also has to be
considered. For example, a patient the clinician thinks is depressed may wish their problem
title to be "headache."

Extraction: We mainly use MIQUEST queries[9] to extract the data held within the
computer system; though we have also experimented with XML (extensible mark-up
language) and proprietary extraction tools. We looked to see what form of queries had been
most effective in extracting data, and their influence on the down stream processes of
migration, integration and analysis. Generally we find that extraction of data into a one line
per patient data table is the most flexible arrangement for later analysis. However, we also
develop queries that count the size of any dataset or subset. These are run at the same time as
an internal validity check – to verify that the correct number of lines of patient data have been
returned.

Migration: Migration of data from the general practice system to the data repository requires
the transmission of that data. We usually do this using a physical storage device (floppy disk
or flash memory card.)   The data then has to be migrated into a format whereby it can be
integrated into the data repository. We have to have a unique identifier in place throughout
the process, so that the data has referential integrity and all the data can, where necessary, be
linked to a single patient, practice and locality.

Integration: Different data tables, data about subsets of patients with one disease, serial data
collections all have to be linked; so that the project outputs can be delivered. We do this for
small projects in a customised Microsoft Access database or for larger projects in My-SQL.
De-duplication is performed at this stage.

Cleaning: The cleaning of the data takes place at this final stage. Here the issue of out of
range values, inconsistencies such as data entry in more than one type of unit (e.g. heights in
centimetres and metres), and other problems with the data are addressed. We usually
produce histograms of numerical variables so that we can see if they are normally distributed
or if mixed units account for a binomial or other distribution; and the extent to which any

outliers or strange values (e.g. one UK computer systems allocates a zero when a test request is made) are present.

Processing: Processing involves the conversion of extracted code into the plain English text assigned to that code by the coding system; e.g. the code H3z into "chronic obstructive pulmonary disease." It involves grouping these into categories relevant to the intended analysis; something usually done at the design phase; e.g. sorting anti-psychotic medications into new drugs recommended by national guidelines and older ones. Sometimes more that one variable will contribute information to generate a new derived variable; e.g. patients treated with thyroxine as well as patients with a diagnosis of hypothyroidism might be included in a diagnosis of myxeodema.

Analysis: The output from the processing stage is usually a "flat file". This will have one line per patient and variables in columns. The flat files always include the original un-cleaned data. Ensuring the accuracy of the denominator, and standardising prevalence's so that comparisons can be made between populations are critical parts of this process.

The first stage is assess the quality of the data (completeness, accuracy, consistency, currency) and where appropriate to calculate the sensitivity and positive predictive value of diagnostic and prescribing data.

Automated reports are generated from this data for feedback to practices or localities; or flat-file data tables for research which are migrated into a standard statistical package.

3. Results

Examples are provided of where we have used our method to produce scientific research.

Design: We conducted a study of the stroke risk of patients with atrial fibrillation for a primary care organisation. The research question was whether stroke was sub-optimally managed and what the scope was to improve management, especially the use of anti-coagulants. These clear audit criteria enabled us to develop and pilot a dataset to meet their needs [16].

Data entry: Data entry issues are often overlooked. Very different picking lists are offered by the different computer systems. The way that the same patients are represented in different computer systems is illustrated in our study of osteoporosis; where we found 100 fold differences in recorded prevalence and that the major UK computing system could not accept results of the gold-standard test for osteoporosis, because the scan result is often a negative number [17]. Coding of bronchitis (H3z if chronic; H06 if acute) is also fraught with difficulty because not only is the difference between chronic and acute easy to confuse when coding but asthma (H33) is a child code of obstructive airways disease (H3) [18].

Extraction: There are many practical issues associated with data extraction. The largest query set we have extracted is a study to identify patients with undiagnosed kidney disease. As there are so many possible causes of kidney disease the dataset is very large and has to be broken down into sections for extraction [19].

Migration: Migration of data involves coping with all the quirks of computer systems prior to integration. Although there is a national specification, data may be in different formats. We try to hold data as triplets of "date-code-numerical value (if present)" (i. e. Date the code was recorded, the code (e.g. 44p = cholesterol), and the value (e.g. 5 mmol/l.) However, the different clinical systems may export data in varying orders, which then adds to the burden of customising the migration process for particular data sources. Similarly systems may have different variants of the same coding system – e.g. the different versions of the Read "codes", and proprietary system codes [17].

Integration: We generate and use our own unique identifier (UPID) to make each patient's line of data unique. Most computer systems generate a unique ID for that system – but there is a chance it might be replicated elsewhere. We therefore compound this UPID with a unique reference for that practice, the research or audit they are participating in, and the local computer unique ID. This is converted into an ASCII format so that it can be used in non-case sensitive relational database joins. The final product, which we call "UPID ASCII" provides the data base with full referential integrity.

Cleaning: We could cite many examples of customised data cleaning. One of the best was discovering that one computer system missed out the decimal point in its haemoglobin estimations. It appears that the users of this system have mentally inserted the decimal – as there have been no complaints about it. However, it meant that we found a bimodal distribution of haemoglobin [19].

Processing: This step involves the writing of syntax to recode data into names with meaning, usually categorical variables. We have evolved a set protocol for doing this. We define ranges for numerical variables by consensus with the lead clinicians and remove outliers. We adjust for incorrect units. In an audit looking at the prevalence of obesity we wished to maximise the proportion of patients with a body mass index (BMI) recorded. To do this we extensively cleaned a lot of height and weight data (e.g. if we find "5f10" in a height field we will reinterpret as 5 feet 10 inches and convert to its metric equivalent [20].)

Analysis: This involves the use of a statistical package. Increasingly we are stratifying patient risk outside the computerised medical record e.g. Calculating kidney function and stage of chronic kidney disease [19], stratifying the risk of stroke [16], and so on.

4. Discussion

This paper describes an eight step process for processing primary care data. The process planning is tightly aligned with its purpose: answering a research question or conducting an audit. We would stress the importance of using a controlled vocabulary for variable naming and the importance of developing an understanding of any data entry issues. We believe that are potentially serious weaknesses in analysing data when the researcher does not understand the picking list or other data entry choices that are presented to the person making the data entry; or the social context in which that data entry is made. It is widely recognised that medical diagnostic labels carry stigma and that coding in the consultation is not a neutral process [21]. The volume of publications generated [16-20] from routinely collected data suggests that this represents a reliable process.

Other groups working with routinely collected data should look to put their processes in the public domain so that the generalisable principles can become part of the core theory of primary care informatics [22]. The principals of error classification applied to data warehousing and total data quality management [14,15] need to be more widely adopted by the health informatics community; but adapted to meet our needs. Health informaticians need to carefully evaluate whether other techniques within computer science would enable more effective data warehouse design. There have been very few critical evaluation or comparison of current clinical databases [8] and further research is needed to compare methods of processing data.

5. Conclusions

This eight-step method provides a taxonomy, as well as a guide to the steps involved in processing routinely collected data. We would recommend that all those involved in processing primary care data define and publish their process of analysis and that all study teams working with primary care data include at least one person familiar with using the clinical systems.

6. Acknowledgments

MSD is the principal sponsors of PCDQ through a series of unconditional educational grants.

7. References

[1]   London School of Hygiene and Tropical Medicine. Directory of Clinical Databases (DocDat). URL: http://www.lshtm.ac.uk/docdat

[2]   IMS Health, Mediplus database. URL: http://www.ims-global.com/index.html

[3]   DIN (Doctors Independent Network.) URL: http://www.dinweb.org/dinweb

[4]   GPRD General Practice Research Database. http://www.gprd.com/

[5]   QResearch. URL: http://www.qresearch.org

[6]   THIN The Health Improvement Network. URL: http://www. epic-uk.org/

[7]   Farmer RD, Lawrenson RA, Todd JC, Williams TJ, MacRae K. Oral contraceptives and venous thromboembolic disease. Analyses of the UK General Practice Research Database and the UK Mediplus database. *Hum Reprod Update*. 1999;5(6):688-706.

[8]   Carey IM, Cook DG, De Wilde S, Bremner SA, Richards N, Caine S, Strachan DP, Hilton SR. Implications of the problem orientated medical record (POMR) for research using electronic GP databases: a comparison of the Doctors Independent Network Database (DIN) and the General Practice Research Database (GPRD). *BMC Fam Pract*. 2003;4(1):14.

[9]   Clinical Information Consultancy. MIQUEST and Health Query Language. URL: http://www.clininfo.co.uk/main/miquest.htm

[10] Egton Medical Information Systems (EMS). URL: http://www.emis-online.com

[11] Tyrer F, Hambleton I, Lawrenson R, Pierce M. Building a research database from computerised general practice records *Journal of Informatics in Primary Care* 1996;(September):8-13. URL: http://www.primis.nottingham.ac.uk/informatics/sep96/sep3.htm

[12] Robinson D. Wanger K, Price C. The clinical terms and ICPC: Identifying equivalence and enabling compatibility for "Non-medical" terms. *British Computer Society, Primary Care Specialist Group Annual Conference 1998*. URL: http://phcsg.ncl.ac.uk/conferences/cambridge1998/robinson.htm

[13] O'Neil M, Payne C, Read JD. Read codes version 3—a user led terminology. *Methods Inf Med* 1995;34: 187-92.

[14] Berndt DJ, Fisher JW, Hevner AR, Studinicki J. Healthcare data warehousing and quality assurance. *IEEE Computer* 2001;34(12): 56-65.

[15] Wang, R.Y. and Strong, D.M. Beyond accuracy: what data quality means to data consumers. *Journal of Management Information Systems* 1996;12(4):5--34.

[16] de Lusignan S, Van Vlymen J, Hague N, Thana L, Chan T, Dzregah B. Preventing stroke in people with atrial fibrillation: a cross-sectional study. *Accepted for publication J Public Health (Oxf)*. 2004 Dec 8; [Epub ahead of print]

[17] de Lusignan S, Valentin T, Chan T, Hague N, Wood O, van Vlymen J, Dhoul N. Problems with primary care data quality: osteoporosis as an exemplar. *Inform Prim Care*. 2004;13(3):147-56.

[18] Falconer E, de Lusignan S. An eight step method for assessing diagnostic data quality in practice: Chronic obstructive pulmonary disease (COPD) as an exemplar. *Accepted for publication Informatics in Primary Care*.

[19] de Lusignan S, Chan T, Stevens P, O'Donoghue D, Hague N, Dzregah B, van Vlymen J, Walker M, Hilton S. Identifying patients with undiagnosed kidney disease from general practitioner computer records. *Accepted for publication Family Practice*.

[20] de Lusignan S, Dzregah B, Hague N, van Vlymen J, Thana L, Dhoul A, Chan T. A cross-sectional study of the prevalence and cardiovascular risk in overweight and obese people in England. *Submitted for publication EJGP*

[21] de Lusignan S, Wells SE, Hague NJ, Thiru K. Managers see the problems associated with coding clinical data as a technical issue whilst clinicians also see cultural barriers. *Methods Inf Med*. 2003;42(4):416-22.

[22] de Lusignan S. What is primary care informatics? J Am Med Inform Assoc. 2003 Jul-Aug;10(4):304-9.

Corresponding author

Jeremy van Vlymen, Primary Care Informatics, Division of Community Health Sciences, St. George's, University of London, SW17 0RE., jvanvlym@sgul.ac.uk

Connecting Medical Informatics and Bio-Informatics
R. Engelbrecht et al. (Eds.)
IOS Press, 2005

Central IT-Structures for Integrated Medical Research and Health Care of Viral Hepatitis - Hep-Net

Thomas H Müller

Institute for Medical Informatics, Biometry and Epidemiology,University of Munich, Munich, Germany

Abstract

Hep-Net is a German medical research and health care network dedicated to viral hepatitis. Its many activities include basic and clinical research, training and public awareness, and rely on modern information technology and the Internet. One major component is a central registry for medical data, serum and tissue samples. In order to build this registry, important legal and technological issues needed to be addressed. Specifically, commercially available electronic data capture systems for clinical trials are generally ill suited for this purpose. The framework of the solution described here may be the basis for similar networks dedicated to specific disease entities or other phenomena.

Keywords:
Telematics, Web technologies, Patient privacy

1. Introduction

Viral hepatitis is one the most common infectious diseases, worldwide. In Germany alone, nearly one million patients suffer from chronic viral hepatitis, an affliction that can lead to serious complications such as cirrhosis and cancer. In order to integrate and improve medical research and health care in the field of viral hepatitis, a network ("Kompetenznetz Hepatitis" or "Hep-Net") connecting medical research groups with physicians in hospitals and practices, was founded in the beginning of 2002 with the help of start-up funding provided by the German Ministry for Education and Research [1]. Its major goal is to enhance communication, both, between specialised research groups and across the tiers of the health care system. It serves the dual purpose of gaining new knowledge about the disease and its treatment, and of accelerating the transfer of new knowledge into the health care process. This is achieved through a wide range of activities carried out by Hep-Net, spanning from public-awareness activities, telephone hot-lines and web-based information resources for physicians and patients to clinical trials, long-term patient registries, and bio-material banks [2].

Many of Hep-Net's activities rely on modern information technology (IT) and, specifically, on the versatility and ubiquity of the Internet. The aim of the efforts described in this paper is to develop central IT structures needed to support the goals of Hep-Net and to sustain its activities. In addition to considerations of feasibility and practicability, special emphasis is placed on issues related to the protection of patients' privacy. The results may be useful for similar research and health care networks focused on other disease entities.

2. Methods

Patient privacy

With few exceptions, the capture, storage, and use of patient-related data in research-oriented settings is subject to regulation at the national and European levels. The common principles laid out in these documents (e.g., the Directive 95/46/EC of the European Parliament and of the Council) specify a number of requirements that must be observed wherever personal data is concerned. Among those that are of particular importance for medical information systems of the kind discussed here are:

1) the requirement for unambiguous consent (by the patient),

2) the requirement for an explicit, specific, and legitimate purpose,

3) the requirement for adequacy and relevance of the collected data items.

Unfortunately (from the viewpoint of a medical research and health care network), the latter two requirements are somewhat in conflict with the goals of long-term patient registries and bio-material banks. The very purpose of such long-term repositories – as opposed to databases for clinical trials – is to collect information and tissue or blood from a sample population at a time when the scientific issue addressed has not yet been precisely defined and the procedures that will be carried out have not yet been fully specified. Hence, when the patient is asked to consent at the time of sampling, the associated risks cannot be assessed. Following a very strict interpretation of the legal situation, this would entirely preclude even the possibility of giving consent. On the other hand, many scientific questions, including, for example, epidemiological issues, cannot be addressed in a practical manner without recourse to available samples collected over a long period of time. In order to resolve this dilemma, a consensus was sought between government officers responsible for privacy issues in public institutions (Beauftragte für den Datenschutz der Länder und des Bundes) and the Telematics Platform for Medical Research Networks (Telematikplattform für Medizinische Forschungsnetze; TMF) representing several research networks in Germany. The result of these consultations is a generic conceptual template for the design and operation of long-term repositories containing patient-related information [3].

Technical requirements

The central IT-systems and organisational structures developed for Hep-Net are based on this template. Out of the many specific issues covered by the generic template, the following bear considerable impact on IT-systems' design. First, registries may not be maintained as strictly anonymous case-repositories – at least when comprehensive datasets are collected – even if one could circumvent the problem of integrating follow-up data. This seemingly paradoxical requirement stems from the fact that the specific use made of the material is not known at the time of the donor's consent and, hence, the donor may not be deprived of the right to have his/her data and samples removed from the registry at any time. In addition, the organisation maintaining the registry must control access to the material for scientific use and must establish appropriate procedures to ensure that the material is used only in compliance with the registry's statement of purpose and to protect the donor from any harmful side-effects of the planned use.

The second major technical requirement is intended to minimise the risk of misuse of the material contained in the registry and states that medical data and patient identification data must be kept at separate locations and under the auspices of mutually independent persons. It should be noted that simply replacing the patient name by some openly used patient identifier in the medical database and keeping the patient list, i.e. the relation between patient name and identifier, in another place isn't considered an adequate technique. The circulation of such identifiers within the network must be avoided in order to prevent re-identification during the long period that the registry is maintained. Instead, the common key maintained in the patient list and the medical database must be kept secret. A temporary key is generated for entering or retrieving medical data. In this respect, registries differ markedly from data capture systems used for clinical trials.

At present, these requirements aren't met by commercially available software for electronic data capture in clinical trials. Furthermore, due to the integrating nature of Hep-Net, appropriate systems must rely on existing installations of workstations, local- and wide-area networks, and must accommodate local security policies such as those enforced by Internet firewalls. The implementation of the systems for Hep-Net is based on versatile and stable open source software packages (e.g., Linux, Apache) and a commercial database management system (Oracle). As an aside, it may be noted that open source database management software has made significant advances in recent years and might be considered a suitable replacement in future revisions of this registry implementation.

3. Results

The IT requirements of Hep-Net can be divided into three major areas: 1) the Internet presence and web-site, 2) the central Hep-Net patient registry described in more detail below, and 3) systems supporting clinical trials conducted by Hep-Net, such as a web-based central patient randomisation facility [4] and electronic data capture systems.

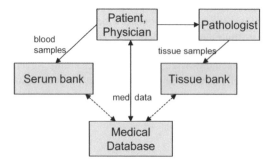

The central Hep-Net patient registry consists of three parts: a medical database, a serum bank and a tissue sample bank. Fig. 1 illustrates the flow of information and blood/tissue samples. Each of these is operated independently.

The treating and recruiting physician communicates information about the participating patient's medical history, social and economic situation, present condition, examination results, laboratory tests, etc. to the medical database, ideally upon every visit. Participating patients receive a Hep-Net identification card which they are asked to present when visiting any physician, including their general practitioner and specialists. This card improves the reliability of patient identification and is intended to allow on-line access to patient data entered by other participating physicians.

Patients are asked to provide a limited number of blood samples specifically for the Hep-Net registry. These samples are collected by the recruiting physician and forwarded to the central serum bank. Upon processing at the serum bank, the sample is registered on-line with the medical database and relabelled with a randomly generated key, linking it to the clinical data. No further identification is maintained at the serum bank. Tissue samples are handled in a similar manner, except that samples are explanted only if and when required for diagnostic purposes and are first processed by the co-operating pathologist. The pathologist is requested to forward any remaining material to the central tissue bank where it is registered in the medical database and re-labelled to remove any non-encrypted identification.

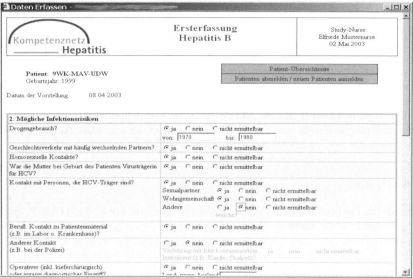

Fig. 2 - Screen shot of medical database

Hep-Net currently supports web-based on-line data entry (see Fig. 2) as well as paper-based data capture. The information submitted on paper forms is subsequently entered into the database at one of several regional offices maintained by Hep-Net.

During the first year after the initial launch in October 2003, 53 hospitals and 91 practices have registered as active participants in Hep-Net. One hundred of those have recruited at least one patient. These participants have recruited a total of 1178 patients, including at least one follow-up in 575 cases.

4. Discussion and conclusions

Medical research and health care networks such as Hep-Net must rely on powerful central IT-structures in order to achieve their goal of integrating the two areas, research and care. One major component of these structures is a central patient registry containing medical data, serum and tissue samples. For this, modern information technology – in particular the Internet – provide a powerful basis. On the other hand, both the Internet technology and the general principles upon which patient registries are constructed incur risks for participating patients that needed to be considered.

Commercial electronic data capture software for use in clinical trials is widely available. Although there are many similarities between registries and clinical trials, building a registry with this type of software proves more difficult than one might expect. Major requirements such as the separation of medical and identifying data are not supported. Furthermore, clinical trial data is more rigidly structured and is recorded uniformly at prescribed time points. By contrast, registry data generally calls for much greater flexibility.

Until significant developments occur in clinical trial software, its use for registries will be limited.

The Hep-Net registry for patients with viral hepatitis is one of several similar registries that are currently being installed in Germany and that are dedicated to specific disease entities. Current projects aim to create similar structures at the European level. For example, the European Network of Excellence "ViRgil" (for vigilance against viral resistance) is the first European surveillance network capable of addressing current and emerging antiviral drugs resistance developments. Perhaps, a common trait of these recent network registry projects as opposed to the well established cancer registries lies in focussing on a more specific disease while simultaneously entertaining many concurrent activities such as supporting basic and clinical research, promoting the development of guidelines, providing information for physicians and patients, and increasing public awareness. Until now, the efforts within Hep-Net regarding patient registry have been directed toward building the registries, addressing many legal and practical issues. Current and future projects analysing the compiled data will reveal the effectiveness of the approach.

4. Acknowledgment

Supported by the German Bundesministerium für Bildung und Forschung (BMBF; grant number 01 KI 0403; Kompetenznetz Hepatitis).

5. References

[1]   Manns MP, Meyer S, Wedemeyer S. The German Network of Excellence for Viral Hepatitis (Hep-Net) Hepatology 2003; 38:543-544

[2]   Wedemeyer H, Meyer S, Manns MP. Kompetenznetz Hepatitis (Hep-Net) Internist 2004; 45:415-421

[3]   Reng CM, Debold P, Adelhard K, Pommerening K. Akzeptiertes Datenschutzkonzept Dtsch. Ärztebl. 2003; 100:A2134-2137

[4]   Müller TH, Adelhard K. A web-based randomisation service for clinical studies. Studies in Health Technology and Informatics 2002; 90:587-590

6. Address for correspondence

Thomas H. Müller
IBE - Institut für Medizinische Informationsverarbeitung, Biometrie und Epidemiologie
Universität München
Marchioninistr. 15
81377 München, Germany
E-Mail: mueller@ibe.med.uni-muenchen.de

Connecting Medical Informatics and Bio-Informatics
R. Engelbrecht et al. (Eds.)
IOS Press, 2005

Real Association of Factors with Inappropriate Hospital Days

Bernard Huet[a,b], Maxime Cauterman[a]

[a]*Hôpital Avicenne (Assistance Publique – Hôpitaux de Paris), Université Paris XIII,*
Biostatistiques et Santé Publique, Informatique Médicale, Bobigny, France
[b]*Laboratoire d'Informatique de Paris 6 (lip6) CNRS UMR 7606, Université P. et M. Curie,*
Paris, France

Abstract

Several studies of inappropriate (in the sense of the AEP) hospital days highlighted associations between two factors (rate of inappropriateness and reasons for inappropriateness, rate of inappropriateness and appropriate setting of care,...). The aim of this communication is to present a study on real associations, at constant factor, between five factors associated with hospital inappropriate days: medical management process, reason for inappropriateness, scheduled admission, rate of inappropriateness, length of stay. We used the European version of Appropriateness Evaluation Protocol for evaluation of inappropriate days and the French protocol ;for analysis of inappropriate days. The study set in three Parisian hospitals, four clinical departments, three specialities. 523 patients were included in the study, 5663 days were evaluated on a wide variety of pathologies: 27 Medical Management Processes. Results show that there are real associations (elimination of transitive associations) between five factors : medical management process and discharge processes, reason for inappropriateness, scheduled admission, rate of inappropriate days, length of stay. Multiple Correspondence Analysis on all "groups of contiguous days related with the same reason for inappropriateness" shows five profiles of queues integrating various medical management processes.

Keywords:
Hospital; Iinappropriateness; Factors

1. Introduction

Reduction in hospital inappropriateness in the sense of the Appropriateness Evaluation Protocol (EU-AEP) [1] is a general objective for health care managers [2] as well as quality experts because this inappropriateness has heavy consequences: lower quality of care, lower quality of life for patients, lower performances,... Understanding the basic mechanism of the elaboration process of hospital inappropriateness is crucial for reduction of inappropriateness.

In this sense, our research differ from other studies which have looked for associations between two variables: rate of inappropriateness and reasons for inappropriateness [3] rate of inappropriateness and appropriate setting of care [4], rate of inappropriateness and position of inappropriate days in the stay [5], importance of admission and discharge processes [6] , importance of patient's age, availability of home care, medical speciality [7] . All these studies give associations without eliminating transitivity between factors.

The aim of this communication is to present a study on real associations, *at constant factor*, between five factors associated with hospital inappropriate days (medical management process, reason for inappropriateness, scheduled admission, rate of inappropriateness, length of stay).

We proceed as follows. In the next section we present tools used for evaluation and analysis, the setting of data collection, data analysis strategy (targeted on queue analysis & medical-management-process analysis. In the third section we present results with statistical tests and multivariate analysis. In the fourth section we discuss two supplementary computed variables for aid to decision and quality improvement projects.

2. Materials and Methods

Tools

Two tools were used for evaluation and analysis: first, EU-AEP [8] (24 clinical criteria) (for the purpose of the study, the EU-AEP was validated [9] for acute geriatrics), second, French Inappropriateness Analysis Protocol [10] (two parts: part one relates to reasons for inappropriateness (13 criteria in four subsets), part two relates to appropriate setting of care (8 criteria in two subsets).

Data Collection

All patients aged 18 or older and not under the care of a psychiatrist. were eligible for inclusion in the study provided they were admitted to gastro-enterology or to orthopaedic surgery (hôpital Avicenne), between may 11th 2000 and July 14th 2000 (and between September 4th and October 12th 2000 for orthopaedic surgery only), to acute geriatrics between November 21st 2001 and January 30th 2002 ("Hôpital Européen Georges Pompidou" and "Hôpital ND Bon Secours"). A trained physician (not part of the medical team) collected high quality and exhaustive data (1 per thousand missing data). Daily evaluation of appropriateness and analysis of inappropriateness was executed from to for each patient.

For each included patient, each day (from admission to discharge, except admission day - not evaluated, because criteria are different - and discharge day - not evaluated because it is not a full day-) appropriateness was evaluated from EU-AEP[8,] with no use of the override option; if inappropriate then analysis of inappropriateness was evaluated from the French Inappropriateness Analysis Protocol[10].

Demographic data were extracted from the hospital's computerized data: name, surname, sex, age, zip code, date of admission, date of discharge, mode of admission, mode of discharge. Clinician's discharge summary gave Medical Management Process and its associated discharge process. Social data (household status), administrative data (scheduled / not scheduled admission), medical data (reason for admission) were measured. Some variables by Medical Management Process were computed: total inappropriate days by reason for inappropriateness, total inappropriate days, total number of queues (with mean delay and sd), rate of inappropriateness (total inappropriate days / total evaluated days), length of stay, rate of scheduled admissions, distribution of appropriate settings of care.

Data analysis strategy

523 patients were included in the study, 5663 days were evaluated on a wide variety of pathologies: 27 Medical Management Processes (MMPs) in orthopaedic surgery, 14 MMPs in gastro-enterology, 12 MMPs in acute geriatrics. Grouping MMPs led to 4 MMPs in orthopaedic surgery, 3 MMPs in gastro-enterology, 3 MMPs in geriatrics. 46 patients were

excluded for grouping and for statistical tests (too small size groups). 477 patients were processed.

Data analysis aimed at two targets: queue analysis & medical management process analysis. For each target we developed a two-step analysis. First, a global analysis to highlight groups of queues and groups of Medical Management Processes (MMPs) that totalize big amounts of inappropriate days. Second, a detailed analysis to identify and to characterize precise queues and precise characteristics of inappropriateness by MMP.

The data were analysed using SAS (V8.2 / PC), 5% level of significance for statistical tests. Moreover, multiple correspondence analysis (MCA) was applied (SAS V8.2 / PC) to identify associations among sets of categorical variables for queues and for medical management processes; MCA was chosen for several reasons: our goal was an exploratory approach; no underlying distribution has to be assumed, no model has to be hypothesized. MCA analysis highlighted a compound variable of inappropriateness by queue and a compound weight of inappropriateness by medical management process.

3. Results

Global analysis

477 patients were analysed (114 in gastro-enterology, 174 in orthopaedic surgery, 189 in geriatrics) : 235 (49%) male, 242 (51%) female, 200 (42%) living alone, 277 (58%) not living alone, mean age 64.2 (SD 23.7). 218 patients (46%) had a fully appropriate stay while 259 (54%) were included in one (at least) queue, 153 (32%) had a scheduled admission, 172 (36%) were admitted in emergency.

Detailed analysis

In table 1, it is presented some details about the main reasons for inappropriate days.

Table 1 – main reasons for inappropriate days

cause of inappropriate episodes / medical management process	Total Inappropriate episodes/ mmp	Cause of inappropriate episodes			
		Internal cause to the ward	Internal cause to the hospit and external to the ward	External cause to the hospital	Cause linked with patient
Cutaneo-mucous Wound	1	1(100%)	0	0	0
Alcoholic detoxication	6	1 (16.7%)	1(16.7%)	1(16.7%)	3(50%)
Ablat oper equipment, short stay surgery	8	2 (25%)	1 (12.5%)	5 (62.5%)	0
Gastro-enterology	48	8 (16.7%)	23 (47.9%)	15 (31.2%)	2 (4.1%)
Simple fracture	19	5 (26.3%)	3 (15.8%)	11 (57.9%)	0
Int medicine (not ger)	21	3 (14.3%)	11 (52.4%)	7 (33.3%)	0
Complex fracture, long stay surgery	27	4 (14.8%)	3 (11.1%)	20 (74.1%)	0
Dem+ neuro-psy troubles	71	1 (1.4%)	18 (25.3%)	41 (57.7%)	11 (15.5%)
Dem + int med	132	9 (6.8%)	13 (9.8%)	84 (63.6%)	26 (19.7%)
Int medicine (ger)	91	1 (1.1%)	10 (11%)	56 (61.5%)	24 (26.4%)

In table 2, four essential factors related with inappropriate days are presented.

Table 2 – four factors related with inappropriate days

MMP	Nr pati ents	Length of stay ok	Mean inappropriate days per MMP	Rate Inapdays/ total days	Rate sched uled admission
cutaneo-mucous Wound	21	2.95 (SD 1.8)	0.10 (SD 0.43)	0.06 (SD0.2)	0%
Alcoholic detoxication	32	7.9 (SD 3.4)	0.31 (SD0.86)	0.08 (SD 0.2)	84%
Ablat oper equipment, short stay surgery	68	4.00 (SD3)	0.41 (SD 1.5)	0.06 (SD 0.2)	99%
Gastro-enterology	59	8.5 (SD 6.5)	2 (SD 3.1)	0.22 (SD 0.3)	41%
Simple fracture	43	6.4 (SD 4.2)	1.7 (SD 2.2)	0.24 (SD 0.3)	26%
Int medicine (not ger)	23	8.7 (SD 5.2)	2.8 (SD 3.3)	0.4 (SD 0.4)	9%
Complex fracture, long stay surgery	42	13 (SD 7.9)	3.9 (SD 5.5)	0.26 (SD 0.3)	21%
Dem+ neuro-psy troubles	47	18 (SD 10)	12.8 (SD 9.1)	0.66 (SD 0.3)	5%
Dem + int med	86	16.9 (SD 13.7)	7.7 (SD 7)	0.46 (SD 0.3)	5%
Int medicine (ger)	56	16 (SD 14)	8.1 (SD 12.4)	0.42 (SD 0.3)	13%

Results of associations between factors at constant factor are shown in table 3

Table 3 – Associations at constant factor

Association between	test at constant factor - result
Medical Management Process & reason for inappropriateness	Inappropriate days p<0.0001
Medical Management Process & rate of scheduled admissions	Inappropriate days p<0.0001
Medical Management Process & rate of scheduled admissions	Length of stay p<0.0001
Medical Management Process & length of stay	Inappropriate days p<0.0001
Medical Management Process & inappropriate days	Ratio Inappropriate days /Total days p=0.0063
Medical Management Process & ratio Inappropriate days /Total days	rate of scheduled admissions p<0.0001
Medical Management Process & rate of scheduled admissions	Inappropriate days p<0.0001
Medical Management Process & rate of scheduled admissions	Length of stay p<0.0001
Medical Management Process & Inappropriate days	Reason for inappropriateness p=0.05
Reason for inappropriateness & rate of scheduled admissions	Medical Management Process p=0.002
Reason for inappropriateness & Inappropriate days	Medical Management Process p<0.0001
Inappropriate days & rate of scheduled admissions	Length of stay p<0.0001
Inappropriate days & ratio Inappropriate days /Total days	Length of stay p<0.0001

The processing of all (424) "groups of contiguous days related with the same reason for inappropriateness" by Multiple Correspondence Analysis (SAS V8.2 / PC) shows that 81% of the variance can be modeled in two axes. The first axis (63%) depends essentially on the appropriate setting of care (60%), rate of scheduled admission (21%), cause of inappropriateness (19%) while the second axis (19%) is essentially composed of the appropriate setting of care (53%), cause of inappropriateness (26%), rate of scheduled admission (21%).

Five P profiles of queues (Fig.1) were found:

P1 : very low rate of scheduled admissions, appropriate setting of care is at home with no help, cause of inappropriateness is internal to the ward (cutaneo-mucous wound),

P2 : high rate of scheduled admissions, appropriate setting of care is at home with no help, cause of inappropriateness is external to the hospital (alcoholic detoxication and ablation of operative equipment),

P3 : low rate of scheduled admissions, very high rate of inappropriateness, appropriate setting of care is non acute medical ward, cause of inappropriateness is external to the hospital (dementia and neuro-psychic troubles, dementia and internal medicine, internal medicine in acute geriatrics).

P4 : low rate of scheduled admissions, appropriate structure is at home with help, internal cause to the hospital and external to the ward (gastro-enterology, internal medicine),

P5 : low rate of scheduled admissions, appropriate structure is at home with medical and paramedical help, external cause to the hospital (simple fracture or short stay surgery, complex fracture or long stay surgery).

4. Discussion

Computed factors for decision-makers.

We computed two supplementary factors for aid to decision.

"Relative weight of inappropriate days by reason for inappropriateness by functional unit" (total inappropriate days for this reason in this functional unit / total inappropriate days for all reasons in this functional unit). This relative weight gives a classification of reasons for inappropriate days from the "heavier reason" (reason that cumulates the biggest number of inappropriate days) to the « lighter one » (the smaller number).

"Relative weight of inappropriate days by Medical Management Process" by functional unit (total inappropriate days for this MMP in this functional unit / total inappropriate days for all MMPs in this functional unit). This relative weight gives a classification of medical management processes from the "heavier one" (medical management process that cumulates the biggest number of inappropriate days) to the "lighter one" (the smaller number).

A strategy for reducing inappropriate days

First, we recommend to collect information for evaluation of appropriate days and analysis of inappropriate days on the following factors: medical management and discharge processes, scheduled admission, reason for inappropriateness, rate of inappropriate days, length of stay, number of queues per patient.

Second to classify queues and medical management processes by "relative weight of inappropriate days".

Third, to launch "quality improvement projects" e.g. based on the Demming wheel to reduce inappropriate hospital days.

5. Conclusion

In this study, we showed that there are real associations (elimination of transitive associations) between five factors : medical management process and discharge processes, reason for inappropriateness, scheduled admission, rate of inappropriate days, length of stay.

6. References

[1] Gertman P.M., Restuccia D. The Appropriateness Evaluation Protocol : a technique for assessing unnecessary days of hospital care. *Med. Care* 1981;**19**: 855 – 871

[2] Payne M.C., Restuccia J.D., Ash A. *et al.* Using utilization review to improve hospital efficiency. *Hosp.Health Serv. Admin.* 1991; **36** : 473 – 490

[3] Ingold B.B., Yersin B., Wietlisbach V., Burckhardt P., Burnand B., Bula C.J. Characteristics associated with inappropriate hospital use in elderly patients admitted to a general internal medicine service. *Aging Clin. Exp. Res.* 2000; **12**: 430-438,

[4] Menu-Branthomme A., Benamouzig R., Bejou B., Coste T., Rautureau J., Huet B., Etude de la pertinence des journées d'hospitalisation dans un service de gastro-entérologie et médecine interne et analyse des causes de non-pertinence. Gastroentérol. Clin. Biol 2002 ; **26**: 29-37

[5] Houghton A., Bowling A., Jones I. Appropriateness of admission and the last 24 hours of hospital care in medical wards in an east London teaching group hospital. *Int. J. Qual. Health Care* 1996; **8**: 543 – 553

[6] Chopard P., Perneger T., Gaspoz JM., *et al.* Predictors of inappropriate hospital days in a department of internal medicine. *Int. J. Epid.* 1998; 27: 513 –519

[7] Panis L., Gooskens M., Verheggen F., *et al.* Predictors of inappropriate hospital stay: a clinical case study. *Int. J. Qual. Health Care* 2003; **15**: 57 – 65

[8] Lang T., Liberati A., Fellin G. *et al.*A European version of the Appropriateness Evaluation Protocol. *Int. J. Tech. Assessment Health Care* 1999; **15**:1, 185 – 197

[9] Somme D., Cauterman M., Durand-Gasselin B., Saint Jean O., Huet B. Une première approche de la pertinence technique de l'hospitalisation en gériatrie aigüe *Rev Med Bruxelles* 2002; **23**-S1:A129

[10] Lombard I., Lahmek P., Diène E., Monnet E., Logerot H., Levy Soussan M., Huet B., Six P., Yeu C., Lang T., Cause of inappropriate hospital stays : interobserver concordance using the French version of the Appropriateness Evaluation Protocol (2nd part). *Rev. Epidém. et Santé Publ.* 2001, **49**, 367 – 375 (in French – abstract in english)

Address for Correspondence:

bernard.huet@lip6.fr
Pr. Huet Bernard, Hôpital Avicenne / Université PARIS XIII, Unité de Biostatistiques et Santé Publique, Informatique Médicale, 125 Av de Stalingrad, 93000 BOBIGNY, FRANCE

Author Index